COMPREHENSIVE

Medical Terminology

Second Edition

Betty Davis Jones, RN, MA, CMA
Chairperson, Medical Assisting Department
Gaston College, Dallas, North Carolina

THOMSON
DELMAR LEARNING
Australia Canada Mexico Singapore Spain United Kingdom United States

THOMSON
DELMAR LEARNING

Comprehensive Medical Terminology, Second Edition
by Betty Davis Jones

Executive Director, Health Care Business Unit:
William Brottmiller

Executive Editor:
Cathy L. Esperti

Acquisitions Editor:
Sherry Gomoll

Developmental Editor:
Deb Flis

Executive Marketing Manager:
Dawn F. Gerrain

Channel Manager:
Jennifer McAvey

Editorial Assistant:
Jennifer Conklin

Executive Production Manager:
Karen Leet

Art/Design Coordinator:
Connie Lundberg-Watkins

Project Editor:
Shelley Esposito

Printed in Canada
7 8 XXX 07 06

For more information, contact Delmar Learning, 5 Maxwell Drive, Clifton Park, NY 12065

Or find us on the World Wide Web at http://www.delmarlearning.com

Library of Congress Cataloging-in-Publication Data
Jones, Betty Davis.
Comprehensive medical terminology/ Betty Davis Jones.—2nd ed.
p. cm.
Previous ed. published under the title: Delmar s comprehensive medical terminology.
Includes index.
ISBN-13: 978-1-4018-1004-7
ISBN-10: 1-4018-1004-7
1. Medicine N omenclature Examinations, questions, etc. 2. Medicine T erminology Examinations, questions, etc. I. Jones, Betty Davis. Delmar s comprehensive medical terminology. II. Title.

R123 .J685 2002
610'.1'4 dc21 2002023155

Notice to the Reader

Publisher does not warrant or guarantee any of the products described herein or perform any independent analysis in connection with any of the product information contained herein. Publisher does not assume, and expressly disclaims, any obligation to obtain and include information other than that provided to it by the manufacturer.

The reader is expressly warned to consider and adopt all safety precautions that might be indicated by the activities described herein and to avoid all potential hazards. By following the instructions contained herein, the reader willingly assumes all risks in connection with such instructions.

The publisher makes no representations or warranties of any kind, including but not limited to, the warranties of fitness for particular purpose or merchantability, nor are any such representations implied with respect to the material set forth herein, and the publisher takes no responsibility with respect to such material. The publisher shall not be liable for any special, consequential, or exemplary damages resulting, in whole or part, from the reader s use of, or reliance upon, this material.

Contents

Chapter 5

Chapter 6

Chapter 7

Chapter 8

Chapter 9

The Blood and Lymphatic Systems / 282

Chapter 10

The Cardiovascular System / 334

Chapter 11

The Respiratory System / 382

Chapter 12

The Digestive System / 420

Chapter 13

The Endocrine System / 472

Chapter 14

The Special Senses / 517

Chapter 15

The Urinary System / 571

Chapter 16

The Male Reproductive System / 617

Chapter 17

The Female Reproductive System / 653

Chapter 18

Obstetrics / 702

Chapter 19

Child Health / 748

Chapter 20

Radiology and Diagnostic Imaging / 787

Chapter 21

Oncology (Cancer Medicine) / 825

Chapter 22

Pharmacology / 861

Chapter 23

Mental Health / 895

Chapter 24

Gerontology / 940

Glossary/Index / 997

Dedication

This textbook is dedicated to Marjean D. Hughes, my sister, my friend.

Preface

Medical terminology is the key to unlocking a whole new world of knowledge. This knowledge will empower you to communicate on a highly technical level about medical disorders, disease processes, surgical procedures, and treatments. You will learn terms that will allow you to read and interpret medical terms in reports, charts, and other health care environments.

This text has been developed to provide you the lear ner w ith the skills you need to become an effective communicator in the highly technical world of medicine. Once you learn that medical terms have many interchangeable parts, you will realize that learning medical terms is not as difficult as you might have thought. Couple this with the appropriate word building rules and you re on your way to expanding your vocabulary by hundreds of new medical words!

Textbook Organization

First, you should familiarize yourself with the organization of this textbook and any supplementary materials that may be available to you such as the Activity CD-ROM and Audio CDs. Some of the key points regarding the organization are as follows:

The textbook begins with Chapter 1, Word Building Rules. It is important that you understand how word elements (parts) are put together to make up the many different medical terms. This knowledge will enable you to build words that you have never seen before, simply by knowing the meaning of the word elements and the appropriate way to put the elements together to form a medical term. Always remember that if you get confused on word building skills, you can return to Chapter 1 for guidance.

Chapters 2 through 4 concentrate on the basics of medical terminology: prefixes, suffixes, and whole body terminology. Chapters 5 through 24 concentrate on body systems and specialty areas of practice. The body systems are arranged in basically the same order as most anatomy and physiology textbooks. This seems to be the most logical approach to keeping the thought processes moving in an orderly pattern, by working from the outside of the body inward.

Chapter Organization

The basic organization for all applicable body systems and specialty chapters includes the following elements: chapter content, key competencies, anatomy and physiology, vocabulary, word elements, pathological conditions, diagnostic techniques and procedures, common abbreviations, written and audio terminology review, chapter review exercises, and answers to chapter review exercises.

Chapter content and key competencies present learners with a basis for what they are about to learn. They are then grounded with basic information about the specific body system in the anatomy and physiology sections and proceed to the vocabulary and word elements sections to specifically learn the medical terms and word parts appropriate to that chapter. The pathological conditions and diagnostic techniques and procedures sections reinforce and elaborate through basic and more extensive definitions many of the terms that have already been introduced in the vocabulary and word part sections. The abbreviation section presents the most common abbreviations appropriate to that chapter. The written and audio terminology review allows students to write out the definitions and study the pronunciations for the major terms; the chapter review exercises test and assess the information to which the learner has been exposed. Additional information on some of these elements is included in the Pedagogical Features section below and in the About the Book section.

Pedagogical Features

Key Competencies

Each chapter opens with a list of key competencies that introduce main areas to target for mastery within the chapter. Competencies have been developed to include standards for learners to attain competency specifically in medical terminology. The review exercises are tied directly to these competencies to help learners assess themselves and determine if they have mastered them.

Word Elements

Each chapter contains a word element review activity after the vocabulary list. The word elements are accompanied by a phonetic pronunciation. You are encouraged to pronounce these words twice to reinforce your pronunciation skills, and indicate that you have achieved success by entering a check mark in the box provided. Each word element has an example word that includes the word element, followed by a space for you to enter the definition of the word. The definitions for the example words are not included in the text. This was done intentionally, because everyone who studies medical terminology needs to know how to use a medical dictionary! These definitions should be looked up in your medical dictionary and recorded in the space provided in your textbook. This is an extra challenge designed to expand your knowledge base. Be careful though, a medical dictionary is a contagious thing!

Color Photos and Illustrations

The body systems and specialty chapters contain over 300 color photographs and drawings that have been selected to reinforce the specific topic of discussion. Most of the photographs appear beside the discussion or immediately following the discussion, for immediate reinforcement of your comprehension of the topic. The old saying, A picture is worth a thousand words is very true in this case. The quality of the photographs and the detail of the artist s illustrations in this textbook will allow you to form a clear mental image of the structure, disease process, or technique being discussed. This will prove particularly helpful when you are reading about a disease or treatment with which you are not familiar.

Written and Audio Terminology Review

At the end of each chapter you will find an alphabetized list of key terms that were introduced in the chapter. You will write the definition of each term and check it in the glossary/index. A phonetic pronunciation is included for each term as well as a check box to indicate mastery of the pronunciation.

The review list can be used in a variety of ways:

- If you have the Audio CDs available, listen to each term, pronounce it, and check the box next to the term in your textbook once you are comfortable saying the word.
- Listen to the terms pronounced in the Listening Activity on the Activity CD-ROM in the back of the text. Pronounce the words during each pause and check the box next to the term in the textbook.
- Test your accuracy in transcription of medical terms. Listen to the pronunciation of terms on the Audio CDs and key them into the computer. When the list is complete, check your accuracy against the written list in your textbook.
- Use the list to review the key terms, their definitions, and pronunciations.

Chapter Review Exercises

Each chapter has numerous review exercises designed to check your comprehension of the chapter material. You will note that each review activity provides a space for recording your score at the end of the exercise. Each exercise question is valued at either 5 or 10 points, with the maximum number of points possible being 100. Your goal will be to earn a minimum 80% on each activity. You will be able to gain instant feedback on your level of success, by computing your score. Scores lower than 80% indicate a need to go back and review that particular area.

Glossary/Index

A comprehensive glossary/index has been developed to allow you to check one place for the page number as well as the definition of major terms in the text. Terms with glossary definitions are in color.

Special Features

Simple to Complex Definitions

The presentation of medical terms and conditions in this textbook present the opportunity to learn a simple basic definition of words, along with its component parts or to learn the basic definition along with a more comprehensive discussion of the disease process, diagnostic techniques and procedures, signs and symptoms, routes of drug administration, and mental disorders. You will note that the medical term and **the basic**

definition are in bold type. The more comprehensive discussion of the condition follows in regular type. An example follows:

carcinoma, basal cell
(car-sih-**NOH**-mah, **BAY**-sal sell)
carcin/o = cancer
-oma = tumor

The most common malignant tumor of the epithelial tissue, occurring most often on areas of the skin that are exposed to the sun. See **Figure 5-18.**

Basal cell carcinoma presents as a slightly elevated nodule with a depression or ulceration in the center that becomes more obvious as the tumor grows.

If not treated, the basal cell carcinomas will invade surrounding tissue, which can lead to destruction of body parts (such as a nose). Treatment includes surgical excision, curettage and electrodesiccation, cryosurgery, or radiation therapy (see the section on diagnostic tests and procedures for description of these).

Basal cell carcinomas rarely metastasize, but they tend to recur, especially those that are larger than 2 cm in diameter.

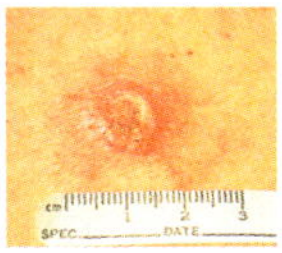

Figure 5-18 Basal cell carcinoma (Courtesy of Robert A. Silverman, M.D., Pediatric Dermatology, Georgetown University)

carcinoma, squamous cell
(car-sih-**NOH**-ma, **SKWAY**-mus sell)
carcin/o = cancer
-oma = tumor

A malignancy of the squamous, or scalelike, cells of the epithelial tissue, which is a much faster growing cancer than basal cell carcinoma and which has a greater potential for metastasis if not treated. See **Figure 5-19.**

These squamous cell lesions are seen most frequently on sun-exposed areas such as the:

1. top of the nose,
2. forehead,
3. margin of the external ear,
4. back of the hands, and
5. lower lip.

The squamous cell lesion begins as a firm, flesh-colored or red papule, sometimes with a crusted appearance. As the lesion grows it may bleed or ulcerate and become painful. When squamous cell carcinoma recurs, it can be quite invasive and create an increased risk of metastasis.

Treatment is surgical excision with the goal of removing the tumor completely, along with a margin of healthy surrounding tissue. Cryosurgery for low-risk squamous cell carcinomas is also common.

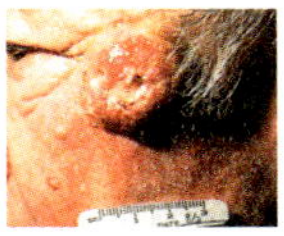

Figure 5-19 Squamous cell carcinoma (Courtesy of Robert A. Silverman, M.D., Pediatric Dermatology, Georgetown University)

dermatitis
(der-mah-**TYE**-tis)
dermat/o = skin
-itis = inflammation

Inflammation of the skin, seen in several forms. Dermatitis **may be acute or chronic, contact or seborrheic.**

Contact dermatitis occurs as the skin responds to an irritant or allergen with redness, pruritus (itching), and various skin lesions. Two forms of contact dermatitis are allergic contact dermatitis and irritant contact dermatitis.

Allergic contact dermatitis develops by sensitization. When coming in contact with a substance for the first time, no immediate inflammation occurs,

- ◆ Basic definition in bold
- ◆ More comprehensive discussion

Word Elements are Reinforced Throughout the Text

The study of word elements is integrated throughout the book. You will note that word elements are repeated in the chapters, to reinforce their meaning again and again, as you expand your studies from basic medical terms to signs and symptoms, disease conditions, and procedures. Note that the medical term will appear in the left-hand column usually with a phonetic pronunciation immediately beneath the word. The component parts of the medical term (word elements) will be listed directly beneath the phonetic pronunciation. This format will also allow you to see the word in context (as it relates to the particular disease process) while continuing to reinforce the word elements.

- ◆ Pronunciation
- ◆ Word elements and definition

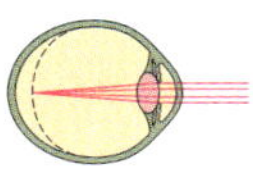

Myopia (nearsightedness)
Light rays focus in front of the retina

verified through an ophthalmoscopic examination and corrected through the use of contact lenses or eyeglasses. Treatment includes a surgical procedure called a radial keratotomy, which involves creating microscopic incisions in the outside segment of the cornea, making it flatten in specific areas. This procedure has been successful, but it is not without potential complications.

Figure 14-9 Myopia (nearsightedness)

nyctalopia
(night blindness)
(nik-tah-**LOH**-pee-ah)
nyct/o = night
-opia = visual condition

Inadequate vision at night or in faint lighting following reduction in the synthesis of rhodopsin, a compound in the rods of the retina that enables the eye to adjust to low-density light.

Retinal deterioration, vitamin A deficiency, or a congenital defect may cause nyctalopia.

nystagmus
(niss-**TAG**-mus)

Vertical, horizontal, rotary, or mixed rhythmic involuntary movements of the eye(s) caused by use of alcohol or certain drugs, lesions on the brain or inner ear, congenital abnormalities, nerve injury at birth, or abnormal retinal development. Nystagmus **may not be apparent to the patient.**

Nystagmus can be acquired when a lesion is produced in the brain or inner ear due to another disease process. With congenital nystagmus, the child often has poor vision that also arises from the congenital abnormalities.

Diagnosis of nystagmus is made from the visualization of the involuntary eye movements. Treatment is aimed at managing the underlying condition, if indicated. Congenital nystagmus often cannot be successfully treated and therefore remains with the individual for life.

ophthalmia neonatorum
(off-**THAL**-mee-ah nee-oh-nay-**TOR**-um)
ophthalm/o = eye
-ia = condition
ne/o = new
nat/i = pertaining to birth

A purulent **(contains pus) inflammation of the conjunctiva and/or cornea in the newborn.**

The cause of the keratitis and conjunctivitis results from the newborn's exposure to viral, bacterial, chemical, or chlamydial agents.

One category of ophthalmia neonatorum is Neisseria gonorrheal conjunctivitis, which is spread to the neonate while passing through the birth canal. This type is rare in the United States due to the preventive antibiotic ointment applied to the newborn's eyes after birth. Another category of ophthalmia neonatorum is chlamydial conjunctivitis, also transmitted to the newborn while passing through the birth canal.

presbyopia
(prez-bee-**OH**-pee-ah)
presby/o = old, elderly
-opia = visual condition

A refractive error occurring after the age of 40, when the lens of the eye(s) cannot focus on an image accurately due to its decreasing loss of elasticity resulting in a firmer and more opaque lens.

This results in decreased color vision and a decline in refraction and accommodation for close vision. Presbyopia is also called farsightedness due to better clarity of distant objects.

"Do This" and "Say It" Segments

Where appropriate, we have incorporated Do This instructions to actively involve you in the learning process. For example, in the chapter on muscles, the Do This instructions are designed to help you learn muscle actions such as extension, flexion, and abduction by having you respond to the directions by actually performing the action. This should reinforce your knowledge of the actions of the various muscles of the body. The Say It segments are designed to have you repeat words and/or word elements when studying them. Pronouncing the words aloud should help you remember how the word sounds, which can also help you spell correctly when you hear the words pronounced by your instructor or by a physician on a transcription tape. Many times students misspell words they have not heard before and/or have not taken the time to familiarize themselves with the sound of the word.

Activity CD-ROM

A free Activity CD-ROM is packaged with each textbook. The software is designed to offer the students additional practice with terminology by providing: diagram exercises; review exercises in choice of completion, matching, multiple choice, true and false questions; as well as several games and practice tests. It also includes the pronunciation of over 1,200 terms, feedback, for the right and wrong answers, plus a scoring feature. See the How to Use the Activity CD-ROM section.

Changes to the Second Edition

- A new chapter on gerontology presents information on the aging process for each system and pathological conditions that pertain to the elderly.
- Definitions of word elements are more consistent throughout the textbook. The more complete definition is listed each time the word element appears.
- Additional exercises were added to the end of each chapter. Beginning with Chapter 4, each chapter has at least 10 review exercises.
- The Glossary/Index was thoroughly updated: Terms omitted in the first edition were added and additional cross-references for terms were included.
- Pronunciations for all terms in the Written and Audio Terminology Review are included on the Activity CD-ROM.
- Word Building Guidelines for Pronunciation were added to Chapter 1.
- The number of color prefixes was increased in Chapter 2 to include those prefixes that are actually combining forms used as prefixes, such as *erythr/o*, which means red.
- A discussion on fistula and electrodesiccation was added to Chapter 5.
- A discussion on Homan s sign was added to Chapter 10.
- A discussion on LASIK procedure was added to Chapter 14.
- A discussion of residual urine specimen was added to Chapter 15.
- A discussion on the Lunelle injection as a newer method of birth control was added to Chapter 17.
- A discussion on bimanual examination as part of the female annual examination was added to Chapter 17.
- Discussion of cephalocaudal and proximodistal development principles and general-to-specific development was expanded in Chapter 19.
- A discussion of umbilical hernia was added to Chapter 19.
- The 2002 Immunization Schedule for Infants and Children was added to Chapter 19.
- A new drug classification, Antidiuretics, was added to Chapter 22.

Complete Teaching/Learning Package

Audio CD ISBN: 1-4018-10101

The Audio CDs accompanying this text have been developed to allow students to listen to each term and repeat it aloud for pronunciation practice. Students may also use the CDs to listen to the terms while they follow along with the Written and Audio Terminology Review section of the chapters.

Also Available: **Text/Audio CDs Value Package ISBN: 1-4018-2241-X**

Computerized Test Bank ISBN: 1-4018-1005-5

The computerized test bank includes over 1,000 questions with answers and is available in Windows format (CD-ROM) to easily create a variety of testing materials with your personal computer. You can even add your own questions to the test bank.

Instructor's Manual ISBN: 1-4018-1006-3

The instructor s manual includes a sample course syllabus, crossover guide, suggested classroom activities, transcription word list exercises, chapter review sheets, and sample tests for all chapters.

Online Companion

An online companion is available to accompany the text that includes term to definition and definition to term quick access tables for prefixes, suffixes, combining forms, and abbreviations that appear in the textbook. The tables can be used as a quick reference when learners forget the meaning of a word element or when they remember the meaning but forget the particular word element. To access the companion, go to http://www.delmarhealthcare.com. Click on the online companion link.

WebTUTOR™ Advantage

Designed to compliment the text, WebTUTOR“ is a c ontent rich, web-based teaching and learning aid that reinforces and clarifies complex concepts. Animations enhance learning and retention of material. The WebCT“ and Blackboar d“ platfor ms also provide rich communication tools to instructors and students, including a course calendar, chat, e-mail, and threaded discussions.

WebTUTOR“ Advantage on WebCT“ (ISBN 1-4018-1007-1)

Text Bundled with WebTUTOR“ Advantage on WebCT“ (1-4018-3682-8)

Text Bundled with WebTUTOR“ Advantage on WebCT“ and Audio CDs (1-4018-6557-7)

WebTUTOR“ Advantage on Blackboard“ (1-4018-1008-X)

Text Bundled with WebTUTOR“ Advantage on Blackboard“ (1-4018-4316-6)

Text Bundled with WebTUTOR“ Advantage on Blackboard“ and Audio CDs (1-4018-7752-4)

Delmar Learning's Medical Terminology Image Library, 2E, ISBN: 1-4018-1009-8

This CD-ROM includes over 600 graphic files. These files can be incorporated into a PowerPoint, Microsoft® Word, or WordPerfect® presentation, used directly off the CD-ROM in a classroom presentation, or used to make color transparencies. The Image Library is organized around body systems and medical specialties. The library will include various anatomy, physiology, and pathology graphics of different levels of complexity. Instructors will be able to search and select the graphics that best apply to their teaching situation. This is an ideal resource to enhance your teaching presentation of medical terminology or anatomy and physiology.

Delmar's Medical Terminology CD-ROM Institutional Version ISBN: 0-7668-0979-X

This is an exciting interactive reference, practice, and assessment tool designed to compliment any medical terminology program. Features include the extensive use of multimedia animations, video, graphics, and activities to present terms and word building features. Difficult functions, processes, and procedures are included, so learners can more effectively learn from a textbook.

Delmar's Medical Terminology Video Series

This series of 14 medical terminology videotapes is designed for allied health and nursing students who are enrolled in medical terminology courses. The videos may be used in class to supplement a lecture or in a resource lab by users who want additional reinforcement. The series can also be used in distance learning programs as a telecourse. The videos simulate a typical medical terminology class, and are organized by body system. The on-camera instructor leads students through the various concepts, interspersing lectures with graphics, video clips, and illustrations to emphasize points. This comprehensive series is invaluable to students trying to master the complex world of medical terminology.

Complete set of videos ISBN 0-7668-0976-5 (Videos can also be purchased individually.)

Delmar's Medical Terminology Flash!: Computerized Flashcards ISBN 0-7668-4320-3

Learn and review over 1,500 medical terms using this unique electronic flashcard program. Flash! is a computerized flashcard-type question and answer association program designed to help users learn correct spellings, definitions, and pronunciations. The use of graphics and audio clips makes it a fun and easy way for users to learn and test their knowledge of medical terminology.

This vast new world of medical terminology is just a turn of the key away from your fingertips. Open the door (your textbook) and enter a new and exciting world of medical terminology. Enjoy your trip!

Betty Davis Jones

About the Author

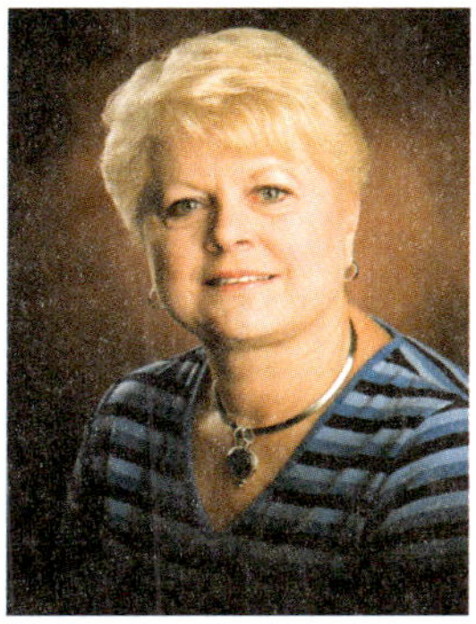

Betty Davis Jones, RN, MA, CMA, is the department chairperson for medical assisting at Gaston College, Dallas, North Carolina. She earned her Bachelor of Science Degree in Nursing from the University of South Carolina, and her Master of Arts Degree in Management form Central Michigan University.

Jones, who has taught at Gaston College for over 20 years, has been instrumental in the development of the medical assisting, phlebotomy, and veterinary medical technology programs at Gaston. She is a member of the American Association of Medical Assistants, the North Carolina Society of Medical Assistants, the Gaston County Chapter of Medical Assistants, and the North Carolina Association of Medical Assisting Educators. Jones has previous credits as a contributing author for several medical assisting textbooks.

Contributor

Dianne Spearman George, RN, BSN, MSN, is presently in nursing education at the associate degree level at Gaston College, Dallas, North Carolina, where she has taught for over 18 years. George is a registered nurse with 26 years of nursing practice focused on leadership and the needs of the family. Her experience in practicing and teaching health care has been diversified among medical assisting, child health, adult health, mental health, and hospice. As former director of nursing at a local hospice, George was instrumental in the opening of a new hospice inpatient and residential facility.

Acknowledgments

A textbook is never written solely by one individual. There may be one name on the cover, but there is input from many who support and challenge the author to achieve his or her goal. To the following individuals, I owe a special thanks!

To Deb Flis, Developmental Editor, a very big thank you. Thank you for guiding me and for offering your support throughout this second edition.

Also, my thanks to the staff at Delmar who have worked enthusiastically to see this project through to completion. I never realized just how many individuals were involved in the revision of a textbook!

Acquisitions Editor: Sherry Gomoll

Developmental Editor: Deb Flis

Editorial Assistant: Jennifer Conklin

Project Editor: Shelley Esposito

Art and Design Coordinator: Connie Lundberg-Watkins

Production Coordinator: Nina Lontrato

Thanks to my husband, Dean, for believing in my abilities and for continuing to support my writing projects. You have taken on added responsibilities in order to help me achieve my goal and have cheered me on all the way!

To my son, Mark, who has grown up with this textbook. You have been supportive and have willingly shared the computer with me e ven when you really wanted to use it! It s yours once again.

To my daughter, Marla, who is now a registered nurse, a special thanks for all the creative ideas that you have offered for reinforcing medical terminology terms and for helping me to see things from the student s perspective. Many of your suggestions are reflected in this textbook.

To Lynn King, B.S., CMA, medical assisting instructor at Gaston College: a special thanks for serving as a mentor throughout this project. You offered many helpful suggestions that have been incorporated into this textbook. Your support and enthusiasm for my success in this project are greatly appreciated. You are a wonderful friend and colleague.

Thank you to the members of the nursing department at Gaston College who offered their support by sharing their reference books with me and answering my many questions. A special thanks to Ann Sprinkle, RN, MSN who read and critiqued the textbook chapter on Gerontology.

Thanks to Ms. Jackie Ramseur, Manager of Library Services at Gaston Memorial Hospital, for helping me locate those difficult resources, and to Kandy Penley, our department secretary, for listening to my ideas and for staying after work and assisting me in proofing material.

A special thanks to my brother-in-law, Dr. E.M. Hughes of Newberry, SC, for assisting me with improvements in the Radiology and Diagnostic Imaging chapter.

And finally to the Gastonia area pharmacists, physicians, medical office managers and staff, who so willingly answered my questions and shared valuable literature with me: Thank you!

Reviewers

I am particularly grateful to the reviewers who have been an invaluable resource in guiding this book as it has evolved. Their insights, comments, suggestions, and attention to detail were extremely important in developing this textbook.

Paul David Bell, MS, RHIA, CTR
East Carolina University
School of Allied Health Sciences
Health Information Management Program
Greenville, North Carolina

Jeffrey L. Beinke, BS, REMT-P
Division Chair
Allied Health Technology
Montgomery Community College
Troy, North Carolina

Janice A. Edelstein, RN-CS, EdD
Associate Professor of Nursing
Mariann College of Fond du Lac
Fond du Lac, Wisconsin

Rebecca Hageman, RHIA, CCS
Instructor, Health Information
Technology Program
Hutchinson Community College
Hutchinson, Kansas

Barbara Hogg, MLT, RN, BSN
Former Instructor, Medical Terminology

Maria Moran, RN
Staff Development Coordinator
SunBridge Rehabilitation and
Alzheimer s Unit
Fort Collins, Colorado

Sharon Newton, PhD, RN, CDMS
Home Health Consultant
Healthcare ConsultLink, Inc.
Azle, Texas

Karen Somer, PT
Faculty, Houston Community College
Clinician, Memorial Hermann Hospital
Houston, Texas

Terri D. Wyman, CMA
Director of Medical Billing and Coding
Program
Ultrasound Diagnostic School
Springfield, Massachusetts

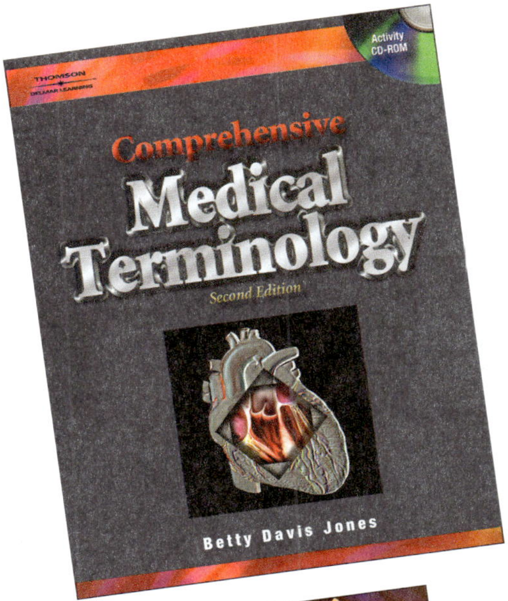

About the Book and Components

Review these two pages to understand how each chapter has been designed to help you learn medical terminology in the context of human body systems and medical specialties. A typical body system chapter includes anatomy (structure of the body), physiology (how the system works), pathology (conditions and diseases), and diagnostic techniques and procedures (examinations, tests, and treatments).

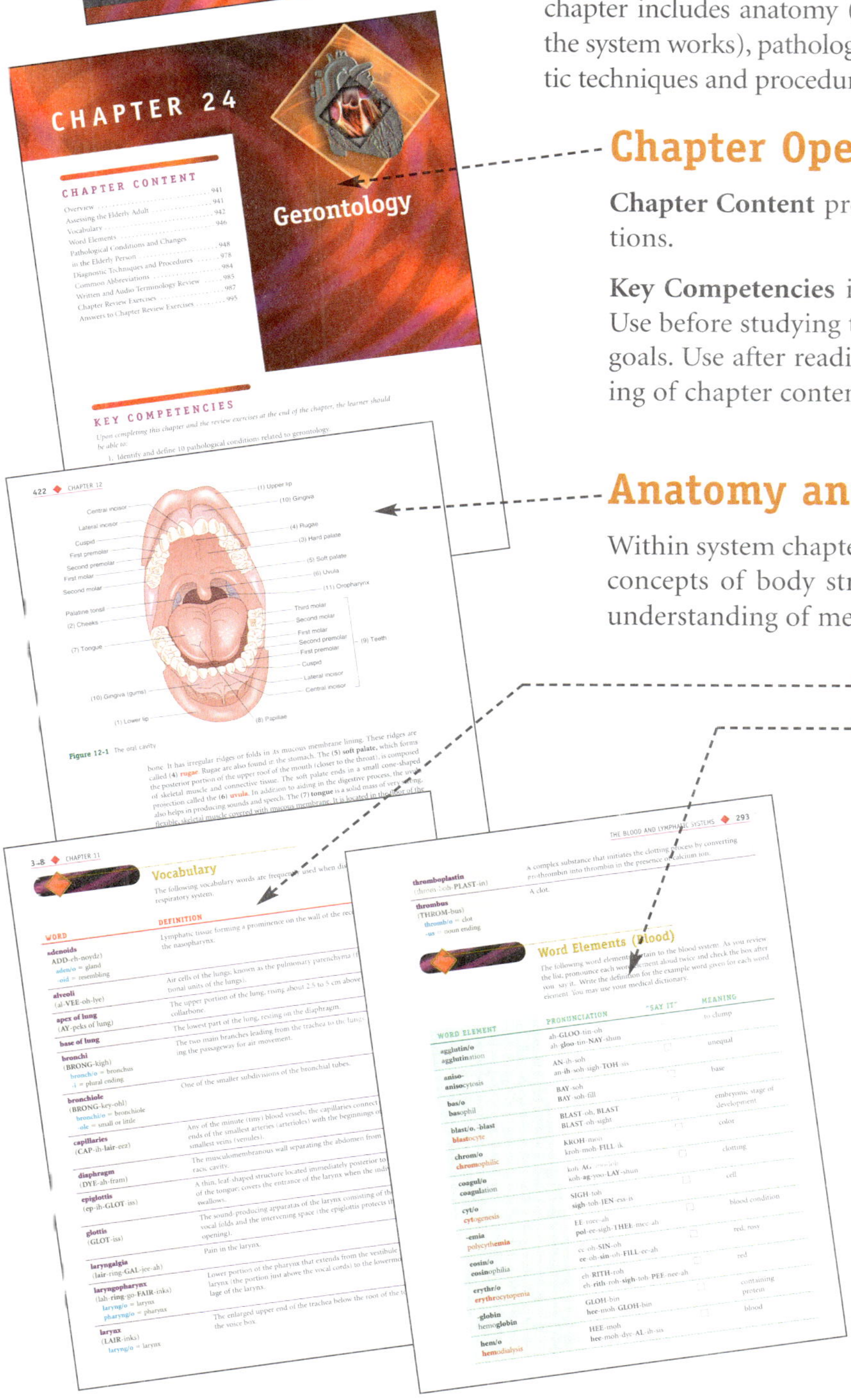

Chapter Opener

Chapter Content provides an outline of major chapter sections.

Key Competencies identify the key objectives for learning. Use before studying the chapter to understand your learning goals. Use after reading the chapter to test your understanding of chapter content.

Anatomy and Physiology

Within system chapters, these sections introduce you to basic concepts of body structure and function to provide better understanding of medical terms.

Vocabulary and Word Elements

Here is your first practice with medical terms and word parts.

- Study the **Vocabulary** section to learn term definitions plus word part breakdowns and definitions.
- Study and work through the **Word Elements** section to learn more about prefixes, combining forms, and suffixes. It s important to notice how pronunciations differ when the same word part is used in a complete term.

Pathological Conditions

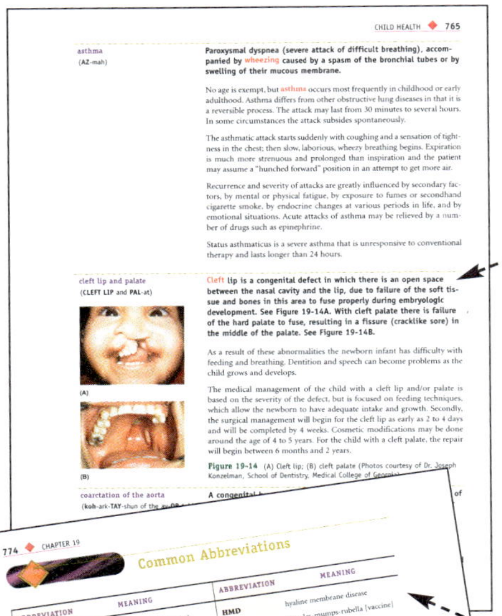

Diagnostic Techniques and Procedures

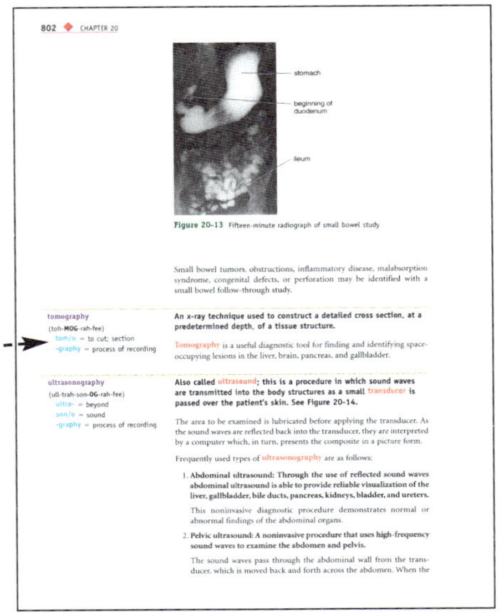

This book includes comprehensive coverage of major diseases, conditions, treatments, and techniques.

- Basic definitions are in **bold** type.
- Terms are broken into word parts to reinforce learning.

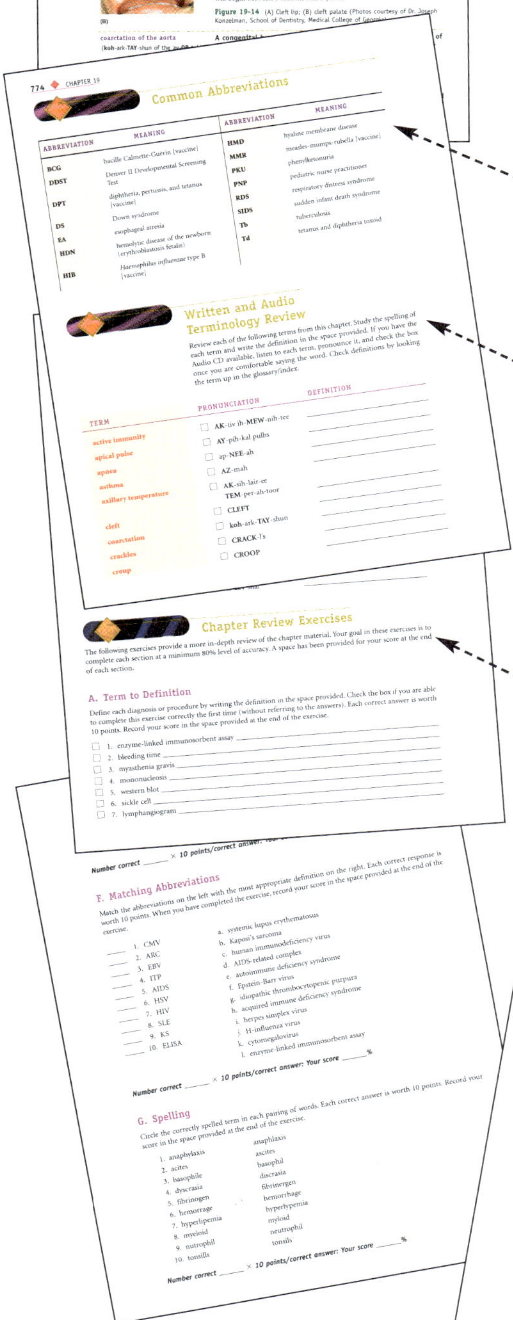

Common Abbreviations

This section presents the most common abbreviations used in today's health care environment.

Written and Audio Terminology Review

This review includes an alphabetical list of medical terms presented in each chapter.

- Use for review of written definitions—check your definition to those listed in the glossary/index.
- Use this section to review the pronunciations on the Audio CDs.

Chapter Review Exercises

Extensive exercises at the end of each chapter help reinforce what you have learned. All exercises include self-assessment scoring to help you immediately determine your competency. Answers are provided at the end of each chapter. Additionally, 1,200 review exercises and over 1,200 pronunciations are on the free Activity CD-ROM that accompanies this textbook.

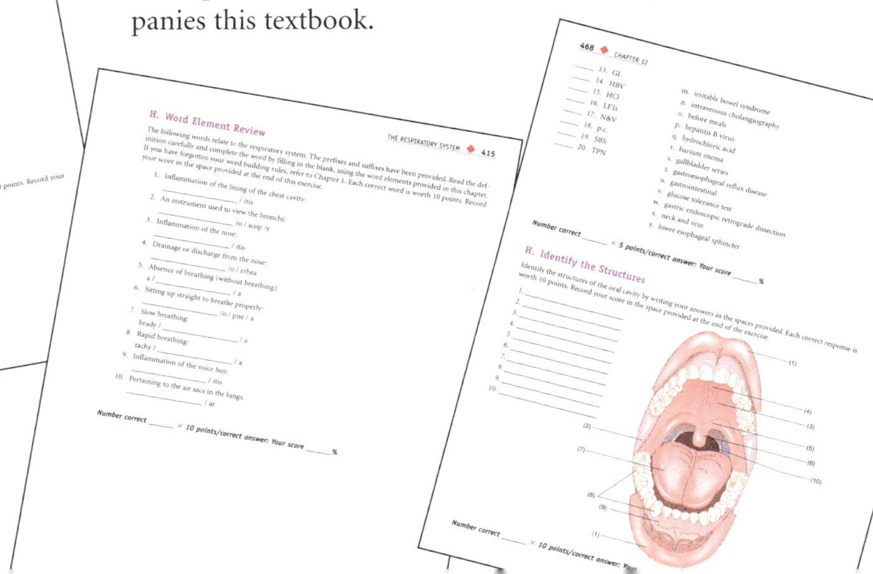

How to Use the Activity CD-ROM

The Activity CD-ROM has been designed to accompany *Comprehensive Medical Terminology,* second edition, so you can learn even the toughest medical terms plus anatomy, physiology, pathology, and diagnostic techniques and procedures. By using these exercises and games, you ll challenge yourself to make your study of medical terms more effective, and have fun!

Getting Started

Getting started is easy. Follow these simple steps to install the program on your computer:

1. Double click on my Computer.
2. Double click the Control Panel icon.
3. Double click Add/Remove Programs.
4. Click the Install button and follow the on-screen prompts from there.

Now you can take advantage of the following features.

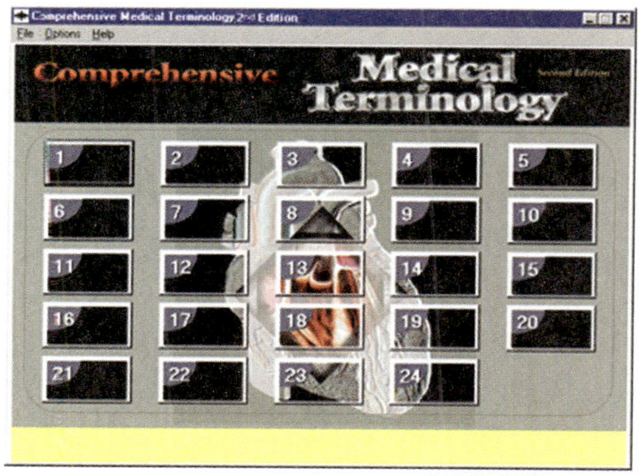

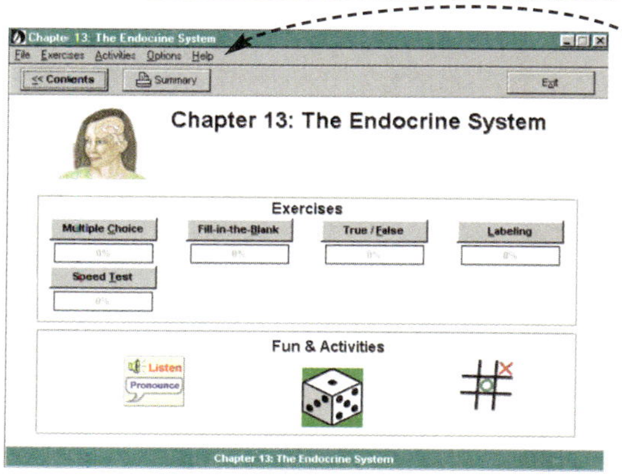

Main Menu

The main menu follows the chapter organization of the text exactly w hich makes it easy for you to find your way around. Just click on the button for the chapter opener screen to select the exercises and games for that chapter.

As you navigate through the software, check the toolbar for other exercises, games, and resetting and printing features. The button bar allows you to retrace your steps, while the Exit button lets you end your practice session quickly and easily.

Online Help

If you get stuck, just press F1 or click Help on the toolbar for assistance. The online help includes instructions for all parts of the practice software.

Basic System Requirements

- Microsoft¤ Windows¤ 95 or better

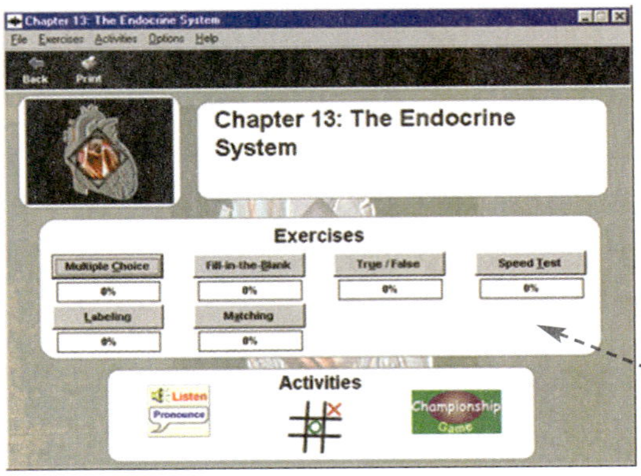

- Pentium or faster processor
- 24 MB or more of RAM
- Double-spin CD-ROM drive
- 10 MB or more free hard drive space

Chapter Screen

The program lets you choose how you want to learn the material. Select one of the exercises for practice, review, or self-testing. Or click on an activity to practice chapter terms in a fun format.

Exercises

The software acts as your own private tutor. For each exercise, it chooses from a bank of over 1,200 questions covering all 24 chapters. To start, simply choose an exercise from those displayed, such as **multiple choice, fill-in, matching,** or **labeling,** whichever appeals to you. Highlighted terms throughout the exercises are directly hyperlinked to the audio pronunciation of that term. Simply click the term to hear it pronounced.

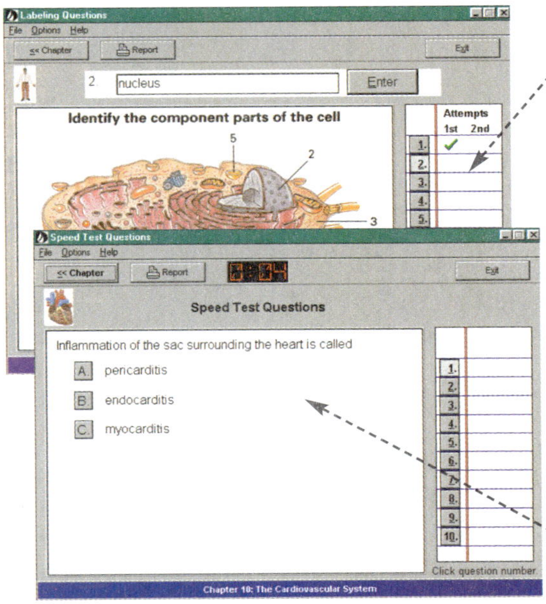

- Each exercise offers you a series of 10 questions randomly selected from that chapter s bank of questions. Each question gives you two chances to answer correctly.
- Instant **feedback** tells you whether you are right or wrong. **Rationales** explain why an answer was correct and **critical thinking hints** are provided when your first-choice answer is incorrect.
- The percentage of correct answers displays on the chapter screen. An on-screen score sheet (which you can print) lets you track correct and incorrect answers.
- Review of previous questions and answers for an exercise provides more in-depth understanding. Or start an exercise over with a new, random set of questions.
- When you re ready for an additional challenge, try the timed **Speed Test.** Once you ve finished, it displays your score and the time you took to complete the test, so you can see how much you ve learned.

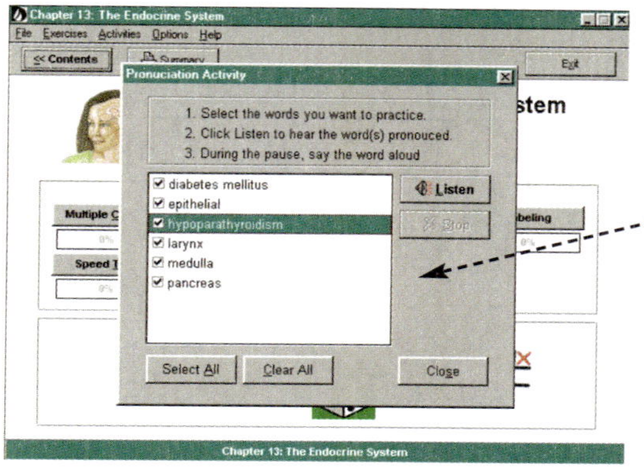

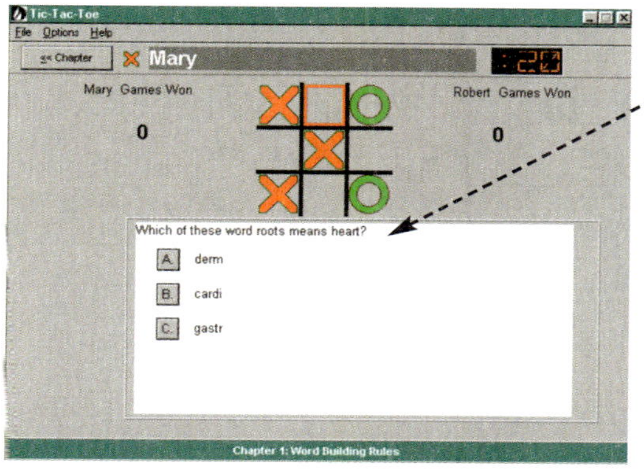

Activities

To further reinforce your skill and knowledge, here are three more activities that you can enjoy alone, with a partner, or on teams.

- **Listen and Pronounce:** In this powerful feature, you select words you want to hear and practice speaking. The program automatically plays term after term from those you selected. Practice all the terms in each chapter, or just the ones that give you trouble.
- **Board Game:** Challenge your classmates and increase your knowledge by playing this question-and-answer game.
- **Tic-Tac-Toe:** You or your team must correctly answer a medical question before placing an **X** or an **O.**

CHAPTER 1

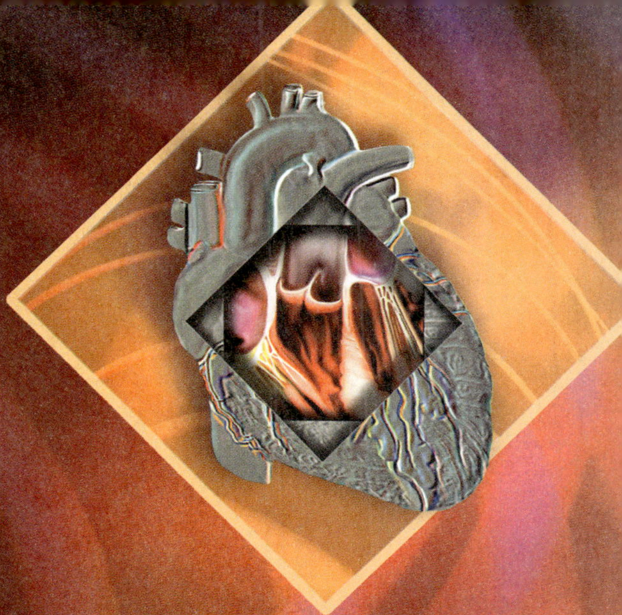

Word Building Rules

CHAPTER CONTENT

KEY COMPETENCIES

Upon completing this chapter and the review exercises at the end of the chapter, the learner should be able to:

1. List the three basic component parts of a word.
2. Correctly state the rule for joining prefixes to a word root.
3. Accurately define the terms *word root, suffix, prefix, combining vowel,* and *combining form.*
4. Correctly state the rule for attaching a suffix to a word root.
5. Correctly state the rule for using multiple word roots in a compound word.
6. Demonstrate the ability to apply the word building rules by accurately completing the review exercises located at the end of this chapter.

OVERVIEW

Studying the language of medicine—that is, medical terminology—is very similar to learning a foreign language. There are rules that must be applied to make the "language" understandable. As a health care professional, you have chosen to learn the language, to master it, and to use it appropriately in the field of medicine. In order to do this, you must learn the word building rules necessary to expand your knowledge and understanding of medical terminology. Once you have accomplished this, you will possess the power to define words you never thought possible. Sounds exciting, doesn't it? It is! Let's get started.

Word Parts, Combining Forms, and Word Building Rules

Before you begin, remember: **It will be critical for you to learn the word parts, and the rules for combining word parts to create words, in order to be successful with medical terminology.** It is impossible to memorize thousands of words over the course of one or two quarters or semesters. It *is* possible, however, to memorize the word parts and the rules that will enable you to build the thousands of words you will need to function effectively as a health care professional. As you study this chapter on word building rules, understand that you will probably not master all of the rules in the beginning. This chapter will serve as a reference as you progress through the textbook. When you find that you have difficulty understanding how the words are put together, or how to pronounce certain words, return to this chapter and review the word building rules and pronunciation guidelines.

Medical words, like English words, consist of three basic component parts: word roots, prefixes, and suffixes. How you combine the component parts, or word elements, determines the meaning of the word. For example, if one part is changed, the meaning of the word also changes. Review the English word *port* and see the different words you can create by adding to it different prefixes and suffixes. Prefixes appear at the beginning of the word root, whereas suffixes appear at the end of the word root. Notice that the prefixes and the suffixes are bold to emphasize how these word elements can change the meaning of the word root *port.*

port

report

import

support

export

transport

port**er**

port**able**

Let's now examine the word parts that we will be using and identifying throughout this text.

1. **Word root: A word root is the basic foundation of a word, to which component parts are added.** By adding other word elements to the root, the meaning of the word changes. A word root is also called the stem of a word or the base of a word, and usually has a Greek or Latin origin. All medical words have at least one word root; some have multiple roots that are joined by a vowel called a combining vowel.

Example: In the word *cardiologist,* the word root is *cardi,* which means "heart." When you see *cardi* (or *card*) as part of a word, you know that the meaning will have something to do with the heart. Another example can be found in *dermatology;* the root is *dermat,* which means "skin." Anytime you see *dermat* (or *derm*) as part of a word, the meaning will have something to do with the skin.

Word roots keep their same meaning throughout; adding prefixes and suffixes to the roots, however, changes the meaning of the word. Look at the following words, which contain either the root *cardi, card, dermat,* or *derm,* and see how the meaning changes by adding word parts. In each word, the root is in color.

WORD	MEANING
cardiologist (car-dee-**ALL**-oh-jist)	**One who specializes in the study of diseases and disorders of the heart;** *-logist* (one who specializes) is a suffix; *o* is the combining vowel.
cardiology (car-dee-**ALL**-oh-gee)	**The study of the heart;** *-logy* (the study of) is a suffix; *o* is the combining vowel.
carditis (car-**DYE**-tis)	**Inflammation of the heart;** *-itis* (inflammation) is a suffix.
cardiac (**CAR**-dee-ak)	**Pertaining to the heart;** *-ac* (pertaining to) is a suffix.
dermatologist (der-mah-**TALL**-oh-jist)	**One who specializes in the study of diseases and disorders of the skin;** *-logist* (one who specializes) is a suffix; *o* is the combining vowel.
dermatology (der-mah-**TALL**-oh-gee)	**The study of the skin;** *-logy* (the study of) is a suffix; *o* is the combining vowel.
dermatitis (der-mah-**TYE**-tis)	**Inflammation of the skin;** *-itis* (inflammation) is a suffix.
dermatosis (der-mah-**TOH**-sis)	**Any condition of the skin;** *-osis* (condition) is a suffix.
acro**dermat**itis (ack-roh-der-mah-**TYE**-tis)	**Inflammation of the skin of the extremities;** *-itis* (inflammation) is a suffix; *dermat* is a word root; *acr* (extremities) is a word root; *o* is the combining vowel.
hypo**derm**ic (high-poh-**DER**-mik)	**Pertaining to under the skin;** *-ic* (pertaining to) is a suffix; *hypo-* (under) is a prefix.

2. **Combining form: A combining form is created when a word root is combined with a vowel.** This vowel, known as a combining vowel, is usually an *o,* but occasionally it is an *i.* The combining vowel is used to join the word parts appropriately when creating words; it also helps in pronunciation by allowing the word to flow as opposed to being choppy without the aid of the vowel.

Rule: ***Generally, when using more than one word root, as in a compound word, a combining vowel is needed to separate the different word roots, regardless if the second or third word root begins with a vowel. (There are exceptions to the rule!)***

Example 1: In the word ***cardi*o*my*o*pathy***, which means "any disease that affects the structure and function of the heart (i.e., the heart muscle)," there are two word roots: *cardi* meaning "heart" and *my* meaning "muscle," followed by the suffix *-pathy* which means "disease." The best way to determine the number of word roots in a compound word is to look for the combining vowels and divide, or separate, the word into elements. Let's divide the word *cardiomyopathy* to illustrate.

cardi	/	*o*	/	*my*	/	*o*	/	*-pathy*
↑		↑		↑		↑		↑
root	+	vowel	+	root	+	vowel	+	suffix

Example 2: In the word ***my*o*electric***, which means "pertaining to the electrical properties of the muscle," there are two word roots; *my* meaning "muscle" and *electr* meaning "electric," followed by the suffix *-ic* which means "pertaining to." The combining vowel is still used even though the word root *electric* begins with a vowel.

my	/	*o*	/	*electr*	/	*-ic*
↑		↑		↑		↑
root	+	vowel	+	root	+	suffix

Example 3: Now comes an exception to the rule. In the word ***lymphaden*o*pathy,*** which literally means "any disease of the lymph nodes" (but refers to enlargement of the lymph nodes, by dictionary definition), there are two roots; *lymph* meaning "lymph" and *aden* meaning "gland," followed by the suffix *-pathy* which means "disease." The combining vowel is not used in this word to separate the two roots, as it is in the others. There is not always a clear-cut explanation as to why the vowel is used in combining some roots and not in others, but the rule of using the vowel to separate the word roots in compound words applies more often than not. One might speculate that it is easier to pronounce *lymphadenopathy* without using the *o* than it would be if using the *o* to separate the two roots in this compound word.

lymph	/	*aden*	/	*o*	/	*-pathy*
↑		↑		↑		↑
root	+	root	+	vowel	+	suffix

Rule: ***A word cannot end in a combining form (word root + vowel); the combining vowel must be dropped and a suffix added, making the word a noun or an adjective.***

Example: One word that means "enlargement of the heart" is ***megal*o*card*ia** (megal/o/card/ia).

megal	/	*o*	/	*card*	/	*-ia*
↑		↑		↑		↑
root	+	vowel	+	root	+	suffix

(root + vowel) combining form = *megal/o*

Note that the word root *megal* (enlargement or enlarged) becomes a combining form by adding the vowel *o*; the word root *card* cannot be used as a combining form to end the word because this would create *megalocardo*, which is not a word. These words must use a suffix as an ending. Therefore, the *o* is not used after *card*, and the suffix *-ia* is added to make the word a noun.

3. **Suffix: A suffix is a word element that is attached at the end of the word root.** Adding a suffix to a word changes the meaning of the word, just as adding different prefixes changes the meaning of the word. Are you beginning to see a pattern here? Just think, a change at the beginning, a change at the end, and you have increased your word building power significantly! All medical words have an ending, or suffix, unless the root is a word itself.

Example: In the word **cardiomegaly,** the suffix is *-megaly* (enlargement or enlarged). When you see the suffix *-megaly* as part of a word, it is referring to something being enlarged.

Note: *-megaly* and *megal/o* are both acceptable word elements; *-megaly* is a suffix and *megal/o* is a combining form. As you continue learning medical terms, you will find other word elements that work as either a suffix or a combining form. Each suffix carries its same meaning regardless of the root to which it is attached.

As you look at the following words using the word root *cardi,* notice how the different suffixes allow you to make several words, all with different meanings, but all referring to the heart. The suffix is in color in each word.

WORD	MEANING
cardi**algia** (car-dee-**AL**-jee-ah)	**Pain in the heart, heart pain;** *-algia* (pain) is a suffix. Note that a combining vowel was not used with this word because the suffix begins with a vowel.
cardio**centesis** (car-dee-oh-sen-**TEE**-sis)	**Surgical puncture of the heart;** *-centesis* (surgical puncture) is a suffix. The combining vowel was needed with this word because the suffix begins with a consonant.
cardiomegaly (car-dee-oh-**MEG**-ah-lee)	**Enlargement of the heart;** *o* is the combining vowel, which is needed because the suffix begins with a consonant; *-megaly* (enlargement) is a suffix.

Now that we have explored how changing the suffix also changes the meaning of the word, let's see how a particular suffix dictates whether or not you use a combining vowel.

Rule: ***If the suffix begins with a vowel, the root will attach directly to it. If, however, the suffix begins with a consonant (anything other than a, e, i, o, u, y), the root will need a combining vowel before attaching to the suffix.***

Example: In the word *cardiogram* (cardi/o/gram), which means "a record of the heart's activity," the word root *cardi* (heart) is joined to the suffix *-gram* (record) by the combining vowel *o* because the suffix begins with a consonant.

Now you try the next one! Look at the word **cardialgia**. Identify the word root and the suffix. Was a combining form necessary? Why or why not?

Check your answers in the box immediately following the exercise.

Word root: ______

Suffix: ______

Combining vowel used? ______

If yes, why? ______

If no, why? ______

Answers

Word root: cardi

Suffix: -algia

Combining vowel used? No

If yes, why? ______

If no, why? The suffix -algia begins with a vowel, so the combining vowel is not needed.

How about another one for good measure! Look at the word **carditis**. Identify the word root and the suffix. Was a combining form necessary? Why or why not?

Word root: ______

Suffix: ______

Combining vowel used? ______

If yes, why? ______

If no, why? ______

Answers

Word root: card

Suffix: -itis

Combining vowel used? No

If yes, why? ______

If no, why? The suffix -itis begins with a vowel, so the combining vowel is not needed.

Before we continue with word building rules pertaining to prefixes, it is important to note that Chapters 2 and 3 are devoted to the discussion of prefixes and suffixes, respectively. Word roots, however, are addressed in each "system" chapter throughout the text. Each word, when possible, is separated into its word elements followed by a definition of the element. This appears in the left column next to the medical term.

4. **Prefix: A prefix is a word element that is added at the beginning of the word.** When a prefix is used with a root, it changes, or alters, the meaning of the word. Prefixes are not a part of all medical words.

Rule: ***Prefixes are attached directly to the beginning of the word.***

Example: In the word *endocardium*, the prefix is *endo-*, which means "within or inner." You will always be discussing the inner part, or within, when using the prefix *endo-*. Prefixes keep the same meaning whenever they are attached to a word. What does this mean? If the root doesn't change, and the prefix doesn't change, how does the word change? The same root can change its meaning in a word each time a new prefix is added to it, as we have already seen in the previous example with the word root *port*.

Look at the following words that contain the root *cardi* or *card* and see how using different prefixes makes several words, all with different meanings, but all referring to the heart. In each word the prefix is in color.

WORD	MEANING
endocardium (en-doh-**CAR**-dee-um)	**Within the heart, the inner lining of the heart;** *endo-* (within) is a prefix; *-um* (structure, tissue, or thing) is a noun suffix.
intracardiac (in-trah-**CAR**-dee-ak)	**Pertaining to within the heart (i.e., pertaining to the interior of the heart chambers);** *intra-* (within) is a prefix; *-ac* (pertaining to) is an adjective suffix.
pericardial (pair-ih-**CAR**-dee-ul)	**Pertaining to around the heart (i.e., pertaining to the pericardium, which is the sac that surrounds the heart);** *peri-* (around) is a prefix; *-al* is an adjective suffix. When you first begin to build medical terms, it is important to define each word part (e.g., pertaining to around the heart). Once you become more comfortable you may give a briefer definition with some of the word endings being understood without actually saying them (e.g., around the heart).

Now, look at the following words containing the root *ur*, which means "urine," to see how the different prefixes in these words change the meaning while continuing to refer to urine. Again, the prefix is in color in each word.

anuria (an-**YOU**-ree-ah)	**Absence of urine;** *an-* (without or absence of) is a prefix; *-ia* (condition) is a noun suffix.
dysuria (dis-**YOU**-ree-ah)	**Painful or difficult urination;** *dys-* (difficult or painful) is a prefix; *-ia* (condition) is a noun suffix.
polyuria (pol-ee-**YOU**-ree-ah)	**Excessive amount of urine;** *poly-* (excessive or more than normal) is a prefix; *-ia* (condition) is a noun suffix.

Word Structure

Now that we have identified the word elements (word roots, combining forms, prefixes, and suffixes), let's see how they fit together to build medical words. There is a logical order to building medical words:

Rule: ***A prefix is placed at the beginning of the word. (Applies: always)***

Rule: ***A suffix is placed at the end of the word root. (Applies: always)***

Rule: ***The use of more than one word root in a word creates the need for combining vowels to connect the roots. This, in turn, creates combining forms that are used in compound words. (Applies: words that have several components)***

Rule: ***Compound words are usually composed in the following order: combining form + word root + suffix.***

Example: *leuk/o* + *cyt* + *-osis* = leukocytosis

leuk = word root; o = vowel; leuk/o = combining form; cyt = word root; -osis = suffix

When several combining forms are used, the order is as follows: combining form + combining form + word root + suffix.

Example: *dermat/o* + *fibr/o* + *sarc* + *-oma* = dermatofibrosarcoma

leuk/o + *erythr/o* + *blast* + *-ic* = leukoerythroblastic

When defining a medical word, there is also a logical approach.

Rule: ***The definition of a medical word usually begins with defining the suffix (the word ending) first and continuing to "read" backwards through the word as you define it.***

Example: For the word *carditis,* the definition is inflammation (*-itis*) of the heart (*card*).

For the word *cardiomegaly,* the definition is enlargement (*-megal*) of the heart (*cardi*). The *y* is a noun ending and the *o* is a combining vowel for the two word roots.

For the word *cyanosis,* the definition is condition (*-osis*) of blueness (*cyan*)

Rule: ***When a medical word has a prefix, the definition of the word usually begins with defining the suffix first, the prefix second, and the root(s) last.***

Example: For the word *intracardiac*, the definition is pertaining to (*-ac*) within (*intra-*) the heart (*cardi*).

For the word *pericardial*, the definition is pertaining to (*-al*) around (*peri-*) the heart (*cardi*).

For the word *hypoglycemia,* the definition is blood condition (*-emia*) of low or less than normal (*hypo-*) sugar (*glyc*).

For the word *hyperhidrosis,* the definition is condition (*-osis*) of excessive (*hyper-*) sweating (*hidr*).

Rule: ***When a medical word identifies body systems or parts, the definition of the word usually begins with defining the suffix first, then defining the organs in the order in which they are studied in the particular body system.***

Example: In the word *cardiopulmonary,* the definition is pertaining to (*-ary*) the heart (*cardi*) and lungs (*pulmon*). The *o* is a combining vowel for the two word roots.

In the word *cardioarterial,* the definition is pertaining to (*-al*) the heart (*cardi*) and the arteries (*arteri*). The *o* is a combining vowel for the two word roots.

In the word *hysterosalpingectomy,* the definition is removal of (*-ectomy*) the uterus (*hyster*) and fallopian tubes (*salping*). The *o* is a combining vowel for the two word roots.

In the word *nasopharyngitis,* the definition is inflammation (*-itis*) of the nose (*nas*) and throat (*pharyng*). The *o* is a combining vowel for the two word roots.

Guidelines for Pronunciation

As you continue your study of medical terminology and the word building rules, you must also incorporate a few pronunciation rules or guidelines to help you pronounce the words correctly. Sometimes a medical word is spelled exactly like it sounds; other times it is spelled with a letter, or letters, that produces the same phonetic sound. Let's look at some example words and guidelines for looking up the words in a dictionary.

Note: In the pronunciation of the example words, the part of the word that receives the strongest accent is written in bold, uppercase letters. For your convenience, the rules have been simplified in Tables 1-1 and 1-2. These tables can be used as references when a particular word stumps you.

***Guidelines for words beginning with the "f" sound: Notice if the word begins with* f *or with* ph.**

1. If the word begins with *f,* it will have the "f" sound, as in the word *febrile,* which is pronounced "**FEE**-brill."
2. If the word begins with *ph,* it will also have the "f" sound, as in the word *physiology,* which is pronounced "fizz-ee-**ALL**-oh-gee."

***Guidelines for words beginning with the "j" sound: Notice if the word begins with* j *or with* g.**

1. If the word begins with *j,* it will have the "j" sound, as in the word *jejunum,* which is pronounced "jee-**JOO**-num."
2. If the word begins with *g* and is followed by the letter *e, i,* or *y,* it will have a "j" sound:
   - If the *g* is followed by *e* as in the word *genesis,* which is pronounced "**JEN**-ee-sis."
   - If the *g* is followed by *i* as in the word *gingivitis,* which is pronounced "jin-jih-**VYE**-tis."
   - If the *g* is followed by the *y* as in the word *gyrus,* which is pronounced "**JYE**-russ."

***Guidelines for words beginning with the "k" sound: Notice if the word begins with* k, c, ch, *or* qu.**

1. If the word begins with *k,* it may have the "k" sound, as in the word *kyphosis,* which is pronounced "ki-**FOH**-sis"; however, some words that begin with the letter *k,* as in *knee,* do not have the "k" sound. This variation will be discussed in another pronunciation guideline.
2. Some words that begin with the letter *c* will have the "k" sound, as in the word *cornea,* which is pronounced "**COR**-nee-ah."
3. Some words that begin with the letters *ch* will have the "k" sound, as in the word *chorion,* which is pronounced "**KOR**-ree-on."
4. Words that begin with the letters *qu* will have the "k" sound, as in the word *quadruplet,* which is pronounced "kwah-**DROOP**-let."

***Guidelines for words having the "n" sound: Notice if the word begins with* n, pn, *or* kn.**

1. If the word begins with *n* it will have the "n" sound, as in the word *neonatal,* which is pronounced "nee-oh-**NAY**-tl."

Table 1-1 Pronunciation Guideline Chart

"SOUNDS LIKE"	OBSERVATION	EXAMPLE WORD	PRONUNCIATION
Words beginning with the "f" sound	Notice if the word begins with *f*.	febrile	"**FEE**-brill"
	Notice if the word begins with *ph*.	physiology	"fizz-ee-**ALL**-oh-gee"
Words beginning with the "j" sound	Notice if the word begins with *j*.	jejunum	"jee-**JOO**-num"
	Notice if the word begins with *g* and is followed by an *e*.	genesis	"**JEN**-ee-sis"
	Notice if the word begins with *g* and is followed by an *i*.	gingivitis	"jin-jih-**VYE**-tis"
	Notice if the word begins with *g* and is followed by a *y*.	gyrus	"**JYE**-russ"
Words beginning with the "k" sound	Notice if the word begins with *k*.	kyphosis	"ki-**FOH**-sis"
	Notice if the word begins with *c*.	cornea	"**KOR**-nee-ah"
	Notice if the word begins with *ch*.	chorion	"**KOR**-ree-on"
	Notice if the word begins with *qu*.	quadruplet	"kwah-**DROOP**-let"
Words beginning with the "n" sound	Notice if the word begins with *n*.	neonatal	"nee-oh-**NAY**-tl"
	Notice if the word begins with *pn*.	pneumonia	"new-**MOH**-nee-ah"
	Notice if the word begins with *kn*.	knee	"**NEE**"
Words beginning with the "s" sound	Notice if the word begins with *s*.	sarcoma	"sar-**KOM**-ah"
	Notice if the word begins with *c*.	cervix	"**SIR**-viks"
	Notice if the word begins with *ps*.	psychology	"sigh-**KALL**-oh-jee"
Words beginning with the "sk" sound	Notice if the word begins with *sk*.	skeleton	"**SKELL**-eh-ton"
	Notice if the word begins with *sc*.	sclera	"**SKLAIR**-ah"
	Notice if the word begins with *sch*.	schizophrenia	"skiz-oh-**FREN**-ee-ah"
Words beginning with the "z" sound	Notice if the word begins with *z*.	zygomatic	"zeye-go-**MAT**-ik"
	Notice if the word begins with *x*.	xanthoma	"zan-**THOH**-mah"

2. Some words that have the "n" sound begin with *pn,* as in the word *pneumonia,* which is pronounced "new-**MOH**-nee- ah."

3. Some words that have the "n" sound begin with *kn,* as in the word *knee,* which is pronounced "**NEE**."

***Guidelines for words beginning with the "s" sound: Notice if the word begins with* s, c, *or* ps.**

1. If the word begins with *s,* it will have the "s" sound, as in the word *sarcoma,* which is pronounced "sar-**KOM**-ah."

2. Some words that begin with *c* will have the "s" sound, as in the word *cervix,* which is pronounced "**SIR**-viks."

3. Words that begin with *ps* will have the "s" sound because the *p* will be silent, as in the word *psychology,* which is pronounced "sigh-**KALL**-oh-jee."

Table 1-2 Additional Rules for Variations in Pronunciations

BEGINNING/ENDING	RULE	PRONUNCIATION	EXAMPLE WORD
Word begins with ***c***	If the *c* is followed by *e*	Pronounced as a soft "c" and has a "s" sound	cervix ("**SIR**-viks")
	If the *c* is followed by *i*	Pronounced as a soft "c" and has a "s" sound	"circumduction" ("sir-kum-**DUCK**-shun")
	If the *c* is followed by *y*	Pronounced as a soft "c" and has a "s" sound	cyst ("**SIST**")
	If the *c* is followed by *a*	Pronounced as a hard "c" and has a "k" sound	cancer ("**KAN**-ser")
	If the *c* is followed by *o*	Pronounced as a hard "c" and has a "k" sound	collagen ("**KOL**-ah-jen")
	If the *c* is followed by *u*	Pronounced as a hard "c" and has a "k" sound	cuticle ("**KEW**-tikl")
	If the *c* is followed by a consonant	Pronounced as a hard "c" and has a "k" sound	cheiloplasty ("**KYE**-loh-plas-tee")
Word root ends with ***g***	If the *g* is followed by *e*	Pronounced as a soft "g" and has a "j" sound	laryngectomy ("lah-rin-**JEK**-toh-me")
	If the *g* is followed by *i*	Pronounced as a soft "g" and has a "j" sound	pharyngitis ("fair-rin-**JYE**-tiss")
	If the *g* is followed by *a*	Pronounced as a hard "g" and has a "guh" sound	laryngalgia ("lah-rin-**GAL**-jee-ah")
	If the *g* is followed by *o*	Pronounced as a hard "g" and has a "guh" sound	meningocele ("men-**IN**-goh-seel")
	If the *g* is followed by a consonant	Pronounced as a hard "g" and has a "guh" sound	glossal ("**GLOSS**-al")

***Guidelines for words beginning with the "sk" sound: Notice if the word begins with* sk, sc, *or* sch.**

1. Words that begin with *sk* will have the "sk" sound, as in the word *skeleton,* which is pronounced "**SKELL**-eh-ton."
2. Some words that begin with *sc* will have the "sk" sound, as in the word, *sclera,* which is pronounced "**SKLAIR**-ah."
3. Some words that begin with *sch* will have the "sk" sound, as in the word *schizophrenia,* which is pronounced "skiz-oh-**FREN**-ee-ah."

***Guidelines for words having the "z" sound: Notice if the word begins with* z *or* x.**

1. If the word begins with *z* it will have the "z" sound, as in the word *zygomatic,* which is pronounced "zeye-go-**MAT**-ik."

2. Some words that begin with *x* will have the "z" sound, as in the word *xanthoma*, which is pronounced "zan-**THOH**-mah."

Let's take a look at some additional words and explore the rules for variations in pronunciations.

Rule: ***When a word begins with the letter* c, *the rule is as follows: If the* c *is followed by* e, i, *or* y, *then the* c *is pronounced as a soft "c" and has an "s" sound.***

Example: In the word *cervix,* the *c* is followed by *e* and the *c* is pronounced as a soft "c." The word is pronounced "**SIR**-viks."

In the word *circumduction,* the *c* is followed by *i* and the *c* is pronounced as a soft "c." The word is pronounced "sir-kum-**DUCK**-shun."

In the word *cyst,* the *c* is followed by *y* and the *c* is pronounced as a soft "c." The word is pronounced "**SIST**."

Rule: ***When a word begins with the letter* c, *the rule is as follows: If the* c *is followed by* a, o, u, *or a consonant, then the* c *is pronounced as a hard "c" and has a "k" sound.***

Example: In the word *cancer,* the *c* is followed by *a,* and the *c* is pronounced as a hard "c." The word is pronounced "**KAN**-ser."

In the word *collagen,* the *c* is followed by *o,* and the *c* is pronounced as a hard "c." The word is pronounced "**KOL**-ah-jen."

In the word *cuticle,* the *c* is followed by *u,* and the *c* is pronounced as a hard "c." The word is pronounced "**KEW**-tikl."

In the word *cheiloplasty,* the *c* is followed by a consonant, and the *c* is pronounced as a hard "c." The word is pronounced "**KYE**-loh-plas-tee."

Rule: ***When building words with word elements that end in g, such as* laryng *and* pharyng, *the rule is as follows: If the* g *is followed by* e *or* i, *then the* g *is pronounced as a soft "g" and has a "j" sound.***

Example: In the word *laryngectomy,* the *g* is followed by *e,* and the *g* is pronounced as a soft "g." The word is pronounced "lah-rin-**JEK**-toh-me."

In the word *pharyngitis,* the *g* is followed by *i,* and the *g* is pronounced as a soft "g." The word is pronounced "fair-rin-**JYE**-tiss."

Rule: ***When building words with word elements that end in g, such as* laryng, pharyng, *and* mening, *the rule is as follows: If the* g *is followed by* a *or* o, *then the* g *is pronounced as a hard "g" and has a "guh" sound.***

Example: In the word *laryngalgia,* the *g* is followed by *a,* and the *g* is pronounced as a hard "g." The word is pronounced "lah-rin-**GAL**-jee-ah."

In the word *meningocele,* the *g* is followed by *o,* and the *g* is pronounced as a hard "g." The word is pronounced "men-**IN**-goh-seel."

Rule: ***When building words with word elements that end in g, the rule is as follows: If the* g *is followed by a consonant, then the* g *is pronounced as a hard "g" and has a "guh" sound.***

Example: In the word *glossal,* the *g* is followed by a consonant, and the *g* is pronounced as a hard "g." The word is pronounced "**GLOSS**-al."

Written and Audio Terminology Review

Review each of the following terms from this chapter. Study the spelling of each term and write the definition in the space provided. If you have the Audio CD available, listen to each term, pronounce it, and check the box once you are comfortable saying the word. Check definitions by looking the term up in the glossary/index.

TERM	PRONUNCIATION	DEFINITION
acrodermatitis	☐ ack-roh-der-mah-**TYE**-tis	______
anuria	☐ an-**YOU**-ree-ah	______
cardiac	☐ **CAR**-dee-ak	______
cardialgia	☐ **car**-dee-**AL**-jee-ah	______
cardiocentesis	☐ car-dee-oh-sen-**TEE**-sis	______
cardiologist	☐ car-dee-**ALL**-oh-jist	______
cardiology	☐ car-dee-**ALL**-oh-gee	______
cardiomegaly	☐ **car**-dee-oh-**MEG**-ah-lee	______
carditis	☐ car-**DYE**-tis	______
dermatitis	☐ der-mah-**TYE**-tis	______
dermatologist	☐ der-mah-**TALL**-oh-jist	______
dermatology	☐ der-mah-**TALL**-oh-gee	______
dermatosis	☐ der-mah-**TOH**-sis	______
dysuria	☐ dis-**YOU**-ree-ah	______
endocardium	☐ en-doh-**CAR**-dee-um	______
hypodermic	☐ high-poh-**DER**-mik	______
intracardiac	☐ in-trah-**CAR**-dee-ak	______
pericardial	☐ pair-ih-**CAR**-dee-ul	______
polyuria	☐ pol-ee-**YOU**-ree-ah	______

Chapter Review Exercises

The following exercises provide a general review of the chapter material. Your goal in these exercises is to complete each section at a minimum 80% level of accuracy. A space has been provided for your score at the end of each section.

A. Matching

Match the term or definition on the left with the correct definition or term on the right. Each correct answer is worth 10 points. Record your score in the space provided at the end of the exercise.

_____	1. word root	a. prefix
_____	2. prefix	b. word ending
_____	3. suffix	c. word root + suffix
_____	4. combining vowel	d. combining form
_____	5. combining form	e. usually an *o*, sometimes an *i*
_____	6. compound word	f. attached directly to the beginning of a word
_____	7. does not need a vowel for attachment to root	g. basic foundation of a word h. word root + vowel
_____	8. requires a combining vowel for attachment when it begins with a consonant	i. combining form + word root + suffix j. suffix k. word roots, prefixes, suffixes, and combining vowels l. *dermatitis*
_____	9. a word cannot end with this word element	m. prefix + vowel
_____	10. component parts of words	

Number correct _______ × 10 points/correct answer: Your score _______%

B. Identify the Word Roots

Identify the word root(s) in each word by separating them with slash marks (/). Remember the word building rules concerning the attachment of suffixes to word roots. **The suffix, when used, appears in bold print in the first four (4) words. After that, you will have to identify the word root without the help of a bold suffix.** All answers appear within this chapter. Each correct answer is worth 10 points. Record your score in the space provided at the end of the exercise.

1. Definition: Enlargement of the heart.
   Root: cardi (the *o* is needed because the suffix *-megaly* begins with a consonant)
   Word: c a r d i o **m e g a l y**
2. Definition: Condition in which there is a decrease in the number of white blood cells.
   Root: cyt (the *o* is needed because the suffix *-penia* begins with a consonant)
   Word: l e u k o c y t o **p e n i a**

3. Definition: Inflammation of the skin of the extremities.
   Root: dermat (the *o* is not needed because the suffix *-itis* begins with a vowel)
   Word: a c r o d e r m a **t i t i s**
4. Definition: One who specializes in the study of diseases and disorders of the heart.
   Root: cardi (the *o* is needed because the suffix *-logist* begins with a consonant) (This one may appear to be wrong because *cardi* ends with a vowel, but remember, it is the beginning of the suffix that determines whether to use the vowel.)
   Word: c a r d i o **l o g i s t**
5. Definition: Any condition of the skin.
   Root: ____________________
   Word: d e r m a t o s i s
6. Definition: Painful urination.
   Root: ____________________
   Word: d y s u r i a
7. Definition: Pain in the heart.
   Root: ____________________
   Word: c a r d i a l g i a
8. Definition: One who specializes in the study of diseases and disorders of the skin.
   Root: ____________________
   Word: d e r m a t o l o g i s t
9. Definition: Condition of blueness.
   Root: ____________________
   Word: c y a n o s i s
10. Definition: Inflammation of the heart.
    Root: ____________________
    Word: c a r d i t i s

Number correct _______ × 10 points/correct answer: Your score _______%

C. What Is Wrong with This Word?

Each of the following words have been created incorrectly according to the word building rules. Review each word carefully and circle the mistake. Rewrite the word correctly in the space provided, and state your rationale for the change. You may need to refer to the word building rules in the chapter for help. Each correct answer is worth 10 points. Record your score in the space provided at the end of the exercise.

Example:

Wrong: a n u r o i a
Correct: *a n u r i a*
Rationale: *The suffix begins with a vowel; therefore, the combining vowel is not needed.*

1. Wrong: m e g a l y c a r d i o
   Correct: ____________________
   Rationale: ____________________
   ____

2. Wrong: p e n i a l e u k o c y t o
   Correct: ______
   Rationale: ______

3. Wrong: d e r m a t o i t i s a c r o
   Correct: ______
   Rationale: ______

4. Wrong: m e g a l y g a s t r o
   Correct: ______
   Rationale: ______

5. Wrong: o s i s d e r m a t o
   Correct: ______
   Rationale: ______

6. Wrong: d y s u r o i a
   Correct: ______
   Rationale: ______

7. Wrong: c a r d i o a l g i a
   Correct: ______
   Rationale: ______

8. Wrong: l o g i s t d e r m a t o
   Correct: ______
   Rationale: ______

9. Wrong: o s i s c y a n o
   Correct: ______
   Rationale: ______

10. Wrong: i t i s c a r d o
    Correct: ______
    Rationale: ______

Number correct ______ × 10 points/correct answer: Your score ______%

D. Completion

Read the following statements about word elements and complete the statement with the correct answer. The spaces provided indicate the number of words in the answer. Each correct answer is worth 10 points. Record your score in the space provided at the end of the exercise.

1. When building a medical word, remember that a word cannot end with a ______________ ______________; you must drop the vowel and add a ______________.
2. The basic foundation of a word is known as the ______________ ______________.
3. Word roots, prefixes, suffixes, and combining vowels are known as ______________ ______________ ______________.
4. The word element that is attached directly to the beginning of a word is known as a ______________.
5. The word element that requires a combining vowel for attachment when it begins with a consonant is known as a ______________.
6. The component part of a word that is usually an *o* or sometimes an *i* is called the ______________ ______________.
7. The word ending is called a ______________.
8. A word root + a vowel is known as a ______________ ______________.
9. The word element that attaches to the beginning of a word and does not need a vowel for attachment to the root is a ______________.
10. A medical word that is made up of a combining form + a word root + a suffix is known as a ______________.

Number correct _______ × 10 points/correct answer: Your score _______%

E. Review the Rules

Read each statement carefully and select the correct answer from the options listed. Each correct answer is worth 10 points. Record your score in the space provided at the end of the exercise.

1. When using more than one word root, as in a compound word, a ______________ is needed to separate the different word roots. This is done regardless if the second or third word root begins with a vowel.
   a. prefix
   b. suffix
   c. combining vowel
   d. hyphen
2. If a suffix begins with a vowel, the ______________ will attach directly to it.
   a. word root
   b. prefix
   c. combining form
   d. hyphen
3. If a suffix begins with a consonant (anything other than *a, e, i, o, u, y*), the root will need a(n) ______________ before attaching to the suffix.
   a. prefix
   b. hyphen
   c. combining vowel
   d. extra word root

4. A word element that is added at the beginning of the word is a:
    a. prefix
    b. suffix
    c. combining vowel
    d. hyphen
5. Compound words are usually composed in the following order:
    a. combining form + word root + suffix
    b. combining form + suffix
    c. word root + suffix
    d. prefix + word root
6. The definition of a medical word usually begins with defining the ______________ first and continuing to "read" backwards through the word as you define it.
    a. prefix
    b. combining form
    c. word root
    d. suffix
7. When a medical word has a prefix, the definition of the word usually begins with defining the suffix first, the prefix ______________, and the root(s) last.
    a. third
    b. second
    c. fourth
    d. after the root
8. When a medical word identifies body systems or parts, the definition of the word usually begins with defining the suffix first, then defining the organs ______________ in the particular body system.
    a. in the order in which they are studied
    b. in alphabetical order
    c. in reverse order
    d. in any order desired
9. In the medical word *cardiocentesis* (cardi + o + centesis), the word element *-centesis* is a suffix. The combining vowel *o* is used in building this word because:
    a. the suffix always has to have a combining vowel.
    b. the suffix begins with a consonant.
    c. the root *cardi* ends in a vowel.
    d. the vowel is not needed, this word is misspelled.
10. In the medical word *cardialgia* (cardi + algia), the word element *-algia* is a suffix. The combining vowel *o* is not used in building this word because:
    a. the suffix *-algia* begins with a vowel and a combining vowel is not necessary.
    b. the vowel is needed, this word is misspelled.
    c. the root *cardi* ends in a vowel.
    d. a suffix never needs a combining vowel.

Number correct _______ × 10 points/correct answer: Your score _______%

Answers to Chapter Review Exercises

A. Matching

1. g
2. f
3. b
4. e
5. h
6. i
7. a
8. j
9. d
10. k

B. Identify the Word Roots

1. cardi
2. cyt
3. dermat
4. cardi
5. dermat
6. ur
7. cardi
8. dermat
9. cyan
10. card

C. What Is Wrong with This Word?

1. **Correct:** cardiomegaly
   Rationale: A word cannot end with a combining form. The suffix *-megaly* should go at the end of the word.
2. **Correct:** leukocytopenia
   Rationale: The suffix *-penia* should go at the end of the word. The combining vowel *o* should remain with the root *cyt* because the suffix begins with a consonant.
3. **Correct:** acrodermatitis
   Rationale: A word cannot end with a combining form; therefore, the vowel *o* should be dropped and the suffix *-itis* should be added at the end of the word. The combining vowel is not needed because the suffix begins with a vowel.
4. **Correct:** gastromegaly
   Rationale: The suffix *-megaly* should go at the end of the word. The combining vowel *o* should remain with the root because the suffix begins with a consonant.
5. **Correct:** dermatosis
   Rationale: A word cannot end with a combining form; therefore, the vowel *o* should be dropped and the suffix *-osis* should be added at the end of the word. The combining vowel is not needed because the suffix begins with a vowel.
6. **Correct:** dysuria
   Rationale: The vowel *o* should be dropped from the root *ur* and the suffix *-ia* should be added at the end of the word. The combining vowel is not needed because the suffix begins with a vowel.
7. **Correct:** cardialgia
   Rationale: The vowel *o* should be dropped from the root *cardi* and the suffix *-algia* should be added at the end of the word. The combining vowel is not needed because the suffix begins with a vowel.
8. **Correct:** dermatologist
   Rationale: The suffix *-logist* should go at the end of the word. The combining vowel *o* should remain with the root because the suffix begins with a consonant.
9. **Correct:** cyanosis
   Rationale: The suffix *-osis* should go at the end of the word. The combining vowel *o* should be dropped from the root *cyan* because the suffix begins with a vowel.
10. **Correct:** carditis
    Rationale: A word cannot end with a combining form; therefore, the vowel *o* should be dropped and the suffix *-itis* should be added at the end of the word. The combining vowel is not needed because the suffix begins with a vowel.

D. Completion

1. combining form; suffix
2. word root
3. component parts of words
4. prefix
5. suffix
6. combining vowel
7. suffix
8. combining form
9. prefix
10. compound word

E. Review the Rules

1. c
2. a
3. c
4. a
5. a
6. d
7. b
8. a
9. b
10. a

CHAPTER 2

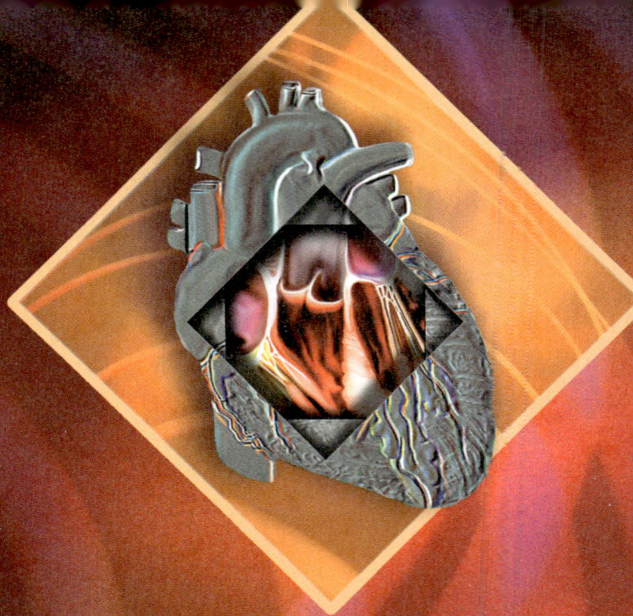

Prefixes

CHAPTER CONTENT

KEY COMPETENCIES

Upon completing this chapter and the review exercises at the end of the chapter, the learner should be able to:

1. Define a prefix and state the rule for using prefixes in words.
2. Correctly identify at least 20 prefixes that deal with numbers, color, measurements, and negatives.
3. Correctly identify at least 10 prefixes that deal with position and direction.
4. Correctly identify at least 30 prefixes.
5. Demonstrate the ability to create at least 10 new words using prefixes by completing the appropriate exercises at the end of the chapter.

OVERVIEW

Have you ever drawn a **dia**gram? Have you ever taken a **pre**test? Have you ever taken **anti**biotics? Have you ever received a blood **trans**fusion? Have you ever thought about the many prefixes we use on a daily basis?

While studying this chapter, you will discover many new prefixes. You will also find that some of the prefixes that are part of your regular vocabulary are also used in medical terminology.

Every medical word has a root. Every medical word has an ending, which is either a suffix or a root that is itself a word. Not every medical word, however, has a prefix, but when prefixes are used, they are attached directly to the beginning of the word.

The meaning of a prefix will not change from word to word. For example, *hyper-* always means "excessive or more than normal." Any word that has *hyper-* as its prefix will mean "in an excessive or more than normal state." Words with the same root, however, will have different meanings depending on the prefix attached. Look at the following example. Although each word has the same root *pne,* meaning "breathing," the addition of different prefixes gives each word a different definition.

WORD	PREFIX	+	ROOT	+	ENDING		DEFINITION
dyspnea	**dys**		pne		a	=	**difficult** breathing
apnea	**a**		pne		a	=	**absence of** breathing
bradypnea	**brady**		pne		a	=	**slow** breathing

Prefixes are attached to words to express numbers, measurements, position, direction, negatives, and color. This chapter concentrates on various categories of prefixes and their meanings.

Numbers

Prefixes that express numbers indicate, for example, whether there is one, two, or three; whether it is single, double, or half. Look at some of the more commonly used prefixes and see how they relate to numbers.

PREFIX	MEANING	EXAMPLE
bi-	two, double	**bi**cuspid (having two cusps or points)
hemi-	half	**hemi**plegia (paralysis of one side [half] of the body)
milli-	one-thousandth	**milli**liter (one-thousandth of a liter)
mono-	one, single	**mono**cyte (a white cell with a singular nucleus)
nulli-	none	**nulli**para (a woman who has borne no children)
primi-	first	**primi**gravida (first pregnancy)

quadri-	four	**quadri**plegia (paralysis of all four extremities)
semi-	half	**semi**conscious (half conscious)
tetra-	four	**tetra**plegia (paralysis of both arms and both legs; also known as quadriplegia)
tri-	three	**tri**ceps ("a muscle" having three heads)
uni-	one	**uni**nuclear ("a cell" having one nucleus)

Measurement

Prefixes that express measurement indicate quantity such as much, many, or excessive. They often refer to multiples without specifically referring to a number; they also refer to excessive (above normal) conditions. The following prefixes relate to measurements.

PREFIX	MEANING	EXAMPLE
hyper-	excessive	**hyper**lipemia (an excessive or above normal level of blood fats)
hyp-	under, below, beneath, less than normal	**hyp**oxemia (less than normal blood oxygen level)
hypo-	under, below, beneath, less than normal	**hypo**glycemia (less than normal blood sugar)
multi-	many	**multi**para (to bear many "children")
poly-	many, much	**poly**arthritis (inflammation of many joints) **poly**uria (the excretion of large amounts of [much] urine)

Position and/or Direction

Prefixes that express position and/or direction are used to describe a location. The location may be in the middle of, between, under, before, or after a particular body structure, or it may be around, upon, near, or outside an area or structure. The prefixes listed are examples.

PREFIX	MEANING	EXAMPLE
ab-	from, away from	**ab**duct (to move away from the midline of the body)
ad-	toward, increase	**ad**duct (movement toward the midline of the body)
ambi-	both, both sides	**ambi**dextrous (able to use both hands well)
ante-	before, in front	**ante**cubital ("the space" in front of the elbow)
circum-	around	**circum**oral (around the mouth)

de-	down, from	**de**scend (to come down from)
dia-	through	**dia**gnosis (knowledge through testing)
ecto-	outside	**ecto**pic (outside of its normal location)
endo-	within	**endo**cervical (pertaining to the inner lining of the cervix)
epi-	upon, over	**epi**gastric (upon the stomach)
ex-	out, away from, outside	**ex**tract (to remove a tooth from [away from] the oral cavity)
extra-	outside, beyond	**extra**hepatic (outside of the liver)
hypo-	under, below, beneath, less than normal	**hypo**glossal (under the tongue)
in-	in, inside, within, not	**in**tubate (to insert a tube inside [into] an organ or body cavity)
infra-	beneath, below, under	**infra**patellar (below the knee)
inter-	between	**inter**costal (between the ribs)
intra-	within	**intra**venous (within a vein)
juxta-	near, beside	**juxta**articular (pertaining to a location near a joint)
meso-	middle	**meso**derm (the middle of the three layers of the skin)
para-	near, beside, beyond, two like parts	**para**cervical (near, or beside, the cervix)
peri-	around	**peri**anal (around the anus)
pre-	before, in front	**pre**cordial (the region "of the chest wall" in front of the heart)
pro-	in front, before	**pro**gravid (preceding pregnancy)
retro-	backward, behind	**retro**flexion (an abnormal position of an organ in which the organ is tilted backward)
sub-	under, below	**sub**lingual (under the tongue)
supra-	above, over	**supra**pubic (above, or over, the pubic area)
trans-	across, through	**trans**urethral (across, or through, the urethra)

Color

Prefixes that express color can, for example, indicate color in reactions, the color of growths or rashes, and the color of body fluids. Some of the following word elements are pure prefixes; others are combining forms used as prefixes. Most dictionaries identify these forms relating to color as "combining forms" not prefixes, but their constant placement at the beginning of the word identifies them more as a prefix than as a combining form, thus the reason for their insertion in this section. The list contains examples

Table 2-1 Prefixes and Combining Forms for Color

COLOR	PREFIX/COMBINING FORM
black	melan/o
blue	cyan/o
gray, silver	glauc/o
	poli/o
green	chlor/o
purple	purpur/o
red	erythr/o
	eosin/o
	rube-
white	alb-
	albin/o
	leuk/o
yellow	cirrh/o
	jaund/o
	xanth/o

of prefixes, and combining forms used as prefixes, that express color. The list is summarized in Table 2-1 for easy reference, listing only the color and the appropriate prefix/combining form.

PREFIX	MEANING	EXAMPLE
alb-	white	**alb**ino (person who has a marked deficiency of pigment in the eyes, hair, and skin; has abnormally white skin)
albin/o	white	**albin**ism (condition of abnormally white skin; characterized by absence of pigment in the skin, hair, and eyes)
chlor/o	green	**chlor**ophyll (green pigment in plants that accomplishes photosynthesis)
cirrh/o	yellow, tawny	**cirrh**osis (chronic degenerative disease of the liver with resultant yellowness of the liver and of the skin)
cyan/o	blue	**cyan**oderma (slightly bluish, grayish, slatelike, or dark discoloration of the skin)
eosin/o	red, rosy	**eosin**ophil (bilobed leukocyte that stains a red, rosy color with an acid dye)
erythr/o	red	**erythr**ocyte (mature red blood cell)
glauc/o	gray, silver	**glauc**oma (disorder of the eye due to an increase in intraocular pressure; creates a dull gray gleam of the affected eye)
jaund/o	yellow	**jaund**ice (yellow discoloration of the skin)

leuk/o	white	**leuk**oplakia (white, hard, thickened patches firmly attached to the mucous membrane in areas such as the mouth, vulva, or penis)
melan/o	black	**melan**oma (darkly pigmented cancerous tumor)
poli/o	gray	**poli**omyelitis (inflammation of the gray matter of the spinal cord)
purpur/o	purple	**purpur**a (collection of blood beneath the skin in the form of pinpoint hemorrhages appearing as red/purple skin discolorations)
rube-	red	**rube**lla (contagious viral disease characterized by fever, coldlike symptoms, and a diffuse, fine, red rash)
xanth/o	yellow	**xanth**oderma (yellow coloration of the skin)

Negatives

Prefixes that express negatives indicate such things as not, without, lack of, and against.

PREFIX	MEANING	EXAMPLE
a-	without, not, no	apnea (without breathing) **Note:** When *a* is used as a prefix it means "without, not, no"; *a* can also be used as a suffix.
an-	without, not	**an**esthesia (without feeling)
ana-	not, without	**ana**plasia (without formation or development)
anti-	against	**anti**dote (a drug or other substance that opposes [works against] the action of a poison)
contra-	against	**contra**ceptive (any device or technique that prevents [works against] conception)
dis-	free of, to undo	**dis**charge (to release a substance or object [to free it from its location])
im-	not	**im**potence (an adult male's inability [not able] to achieve penile erection)
in-	in, inside, within, not	**in**competent (not capable)
non-	not	**non**invasive (pertaining to a diagnostic or therapeutic technique that does not require the skin to be broken [not invaded] or a cavity or organ to be entered)

Common Prefixes

An alphabetical listing of prefixes commonly used in medical terminology is included here for easy reference. As you read the list, note that the prefixes just discussed in the "categories" sections are repeated. Additionally, some of the prefixes appear throughout the text as they relate to discussions of specific body systems.

Note: The combining forms used as prefixes to express color have also been included in this list.

PREFIX	MEANING	EXAMPLE
a-	without, not	**a**pnea (without breathing)
ab-	from, away from	**ab**errant (wandering away from)
ad-	toward, increase	**ad**duct (movement toward the midline of the body)
alb-	white	**alb**ino (person who has a marked deficiency of pigment in the eyes, hair, and skin; has abnormally white skin)
albin/o	white	**albin**ism (condition of abnormally white skin; characterized by absence of pigment in the skin, hair, and eyes)
ambi-	both, both sides	**ambi**dextrous (able to use both hands well)
an-	without, not	**an**esthesia (without feeling)
ante-	before, in front	**ante**cubital ("the space" in front of the elbow)
anti-	against	**anti**dote (a drug or other substance that opposes [works against] the action of a poison)
auto-	self	**auto**graft (a graft transferred from one part of a patient's body to another)
bi-	two, double	**bi**cuspid (having two cusps or points)
bio-	life	**bio**logy (the study of life)
brady-	slow	**brady**cardia (slow heartbeat)
chlor/o	green	**chloro**phyll (green pigment in plants that accomplishes photosynthesis)
circum-	around	**circum**duction (movement around in a circle)
cirrh/o	yellow, tawny	**cirrh**osis (chronic degenerative liver disease with resultant yellowness of the liver and skin)
con-	together, with	**con**genital (born with)
contra-	against	**contra**indication (against what is indicated)
cyan/o	blue	**cyano**derma (slightly bluish, grayish, slatelike, or dark discoloration of the skin)
de-	down, from	**de**scend (to come down from)
dia-	through	**dia**gnosis (knowledge through testing)
dis-	free of, to undo	**dis**location (the displacement [undoing] of any part of the body from its normal position)
dys-	bad, difficult, painful, disordered	**dys**pnea (difficult breathing)
ecto-	outside	**ecto**pic (outside of its normal location, as in an ectopic pregnancy, which occurs in the fallopian tubes instead of the uterus)

endo-	within, inner	**endo**scope (instrument used to look inside the body)
eosin/o	red, rosy	**eosin**ophil (bilobed leukocyte that stains a red, rosy color with an acid dye)
epi-	upon, over	**epi**gastric (pertaining to the region over the stomach)
erythr/o	red	**erythr**ocyte (mature red blood cell)
eu-	well, easily, good, normal	**eu**pnea (normal breathing)
ex-	out, away from, outside	**ex**hale (to breathe out)
extra-	outside, beyond	**extra**hepatic (outside of the liver)
glauc/o	gray, silver	**glauc**oma (disorder of the eye due to increased intraocular pressure; creates a dull gray gleam of the affected eye)
hemi-	half	**hemi**plegia (paralysis of one side [half] of the body)
hetero-	different	**hetero**geneous (composed of different or unlike substances)
homeo-	likeness, same	**homeo**stasis (a relative constancy [likeness] in the internal environment of the body)
homo-	same	**homo**genesis (having the same origins)
hydro-	water	**hydro**cephalus (an abnormal accumulation of fluid [water] within the head)
hyp-	under, below, beneath, less than normal	**hyp**oxemia (less than normal blood oxygen level)
hyper-	excessive	**hyper**emesis (excessive vomiting)
hypo-	under, below, beneath, less than normal	**hypo**glycemia (less than normal blood sugar; low blood sugar level)
idio-	individual	**idio**syncrasy (an individual sensitivity to effects of a drug caused by inherited or other bodily constitution factors)
im-	not	**im**potence (an adult male's inability [not able] to achieve penile erection)
in-	in, inside, within, not	**in**competent (not capable) **in**born (acquired during intrauterine life)
infra-	beneath, below, under	**infra**orbital (beneath the bony cavity in which the eyeball is located)
inter-	between	**inter**costal (between the ribs)
intra-	within	**intra**venous (within a vein)
jaund/o	yellow	**jaund**ice (yellow discoloration of the skin)
juxta-	near, beside	**juxta**articular (pertaining to a location near a joint)
leuk/o	white	**leuk**oplakia (white, hard, thickened patches firmly attached to the mucous membrane in areas such as the mouth, vulva, or penis)

melan/o	black	**melan**oma (a darkly pigmented cancerous tumor)
meso-	middle	**meso**derm (the middle of the three layers of the skin)
meta-	beyond, after	**meta**carpals (pertaining to the bones after the carpal [wrist] bones, i.e., the hand bones)
milli-	one-thousandth	**milli**liter (one-thousandth of a liter)
mono-	one	**mono**cyte (a white cell with a singular nucleus)
multi-	many	**multi**para (to bear many "children")
non-	not	**non**invasive (pertaining to a diagnostic or therapeutic technique that does not require the skin to be broken [not invaded] or a cavity or organ to be entered)
pan-	all	**pan**carditis (inflammation of the entire heart [all])
para-	near, beside, beyond, two like parts	**para**cervical (near, or beside, the cervix)
per-	through	**per**cussion (striking through)
peri-	around	**peri**anal (around the anus)
poli/o	gray	**poli**omyelitis (inflammation of the gray matter of the spinal cord)
poly-	many, much, excessive	**poly**arthritis (inflammation of many joints) **poly**uria (the excretion of large amounts of [much] urine)
post-	after, behind	**post**cibal (after meals)
pre-	before, in front	**pre**cordial (the region "of the chest wall" in front of the heart)
primi-	first	**primi**gravida (first pregnancy)
pseudo-	false	**pseudo**anorexia ("false anorexia"; a condition in which an individual eats secretly while claiming a lack of appetite and inability to eat)
purpur/o	purple	**purpur**a (collection of blood beneath the skin in the form of pinpoint hemorrhages appearing as red/purple skin discolorations)
quadri-	four	**quadri**plegia (paralysis of all four extremities)
retro-	backward, behind	**retro**cecal (pertaining to the region behind the cecum)
rube-	red	**rub**ella (a contagious viral disease characterized by fever, coldlike symptoms, and a diffuse, fine red rash [also German measles])
semi-	half	**semi**conscious (half conscious)
sub-	under, below	**sub**cutaneous (under the skin)
supra-	above, over	**supra**pubic (above, or over, the pubic area)
sym-	joined, together	**sym**pathetic (displaying compassion for another's grief; literally, "joined in disease")

syn-	joined, together	**syn**drome (a group of symptoms joined by a common cause; "running together")
tachy-	rapid	**tachy**cardia (rapid heartbeat)
trans-	across, through	**trans**urethral (across, or through, the urethra)
tri-	three	**tri**ceps ("a muscle" having three heads)
ultra-	beyond, excess	**ultra**sound (sound waves at the very high frequency of over 20,000 vibrations per second)
uni-	one	**uni**nuclear ("a cell" having one nucleus)
xanth/o	yellow	**xanth**oderma (any yellow coloration of the skin)

Chapter Review Exercises

The following exercises provide a more in-depth review of the chapter material. Prefixes and combining forms that are used as prefixes are treated the same and are called prefixes in the exercises. Your goal is to complete each section at a minimum 80% level of accuracy. A space has been provided for your score at the end of each section.

A. Matching

Match the prefixes on the left with the appropriate definition on the right. Each correct answer is worth 5 points. Record your score in the space provided at the end of the exercise.

______ 1. bi-	______ 13. non-	a. bad, difficult	m. first
______ 2. hemi-	______ 14. dys-	b. from, away from	n. between
______ 3. mono-	______ 15. ambi-	c. before, in front of	o. all
______ 4. primi-	______ 16. inter-	d. outside	p. both, both sides
______ 5. tri-	______ 17. pseudo-	e. two	q. after, behind
______ 6. ab-	______ 18. pan-	f. half	r. not
______ 7. ante-	______ 19. post-	g. one	s. near
______ 8. circum-	______ 20. endo-	h. within	t. across
______ 9. ecto-		i. three	u. many, much
______ 10. trans-		j. around	v. without
______ 11. a-		k. one-thousandth	w. against
______ 12. anti-		l. false	

Number correct ______ × 5 points/correct answer: Your score ______%

B. Create a Word

Using the prefixes listed, create a word that best completes each statement dealing with position and direction. If you need assistance, refer to your list of prefixes within the chapter. After you have determined the correct prefix, write the word, without the divisions, in the space provided. Each correct answer is worth 10 points. Record your score in the space provided at the end of the exercise.

inter-	intra-	ambi-	peri-
epi-	dia-	hypo-	supra-
trans-	ab-		

Create a word that means:

1. To move away from the midline of the body

	+	duct	=	
(prefix)	+	(root)	=	(complete word)

2. Able to use both hands well

	+	dextr	+	ous	=	
(prefix)	+	(root)	+	(suffix)	=	(complete word)

3. Around the mouth

	+	or	+	al	=	
(prefix)	+	(root)	+	(suffix)	=	(complete word)

4. Knowledge through testing

	+	gnos	+	is	=	
(prefix)	+	(root)	+	(suffix)	=	(complete word)

5. Under the tongue

	+	gloss	+	al	=	
(prefix)	+	(root)	+	(suffix)	=	(complete word)

6. Within a vein

	+	ven	+	ous	=	
(prefix)	+	(root)	+	(suffix)	=	(complete word)

7. Above the pubis

	+	pub	+	ic	=	
(prefix)	+	(root)	+	(suffix)	=	(complete word)

8. Across, or through, the urethra

	+	urethr	+	al	=	
(prefix)	+	(root)	+	(suffix)	=	(complete word)

9. Pertaining to the region upon the stomach

	+	gastr	+	ic	=	
(prefix)	+	(root)	+	(suffix)	=	(complete word)

10. Between the ribs

______	+	cost	+	al	=	______
(prefix)	+	(root)	+	(suffix)	=	(complete word)

Number correct* ______ × *10 points/correct answer: Your score* ______ *%

C. Crossword Puzzle

Complete the crossword puzzle by entering the appropriate prefix for each definition in the spaces provided. Each crossword answer is worth 5 points. When you have completed the puzzle, total your points and enter your score in the space provided.

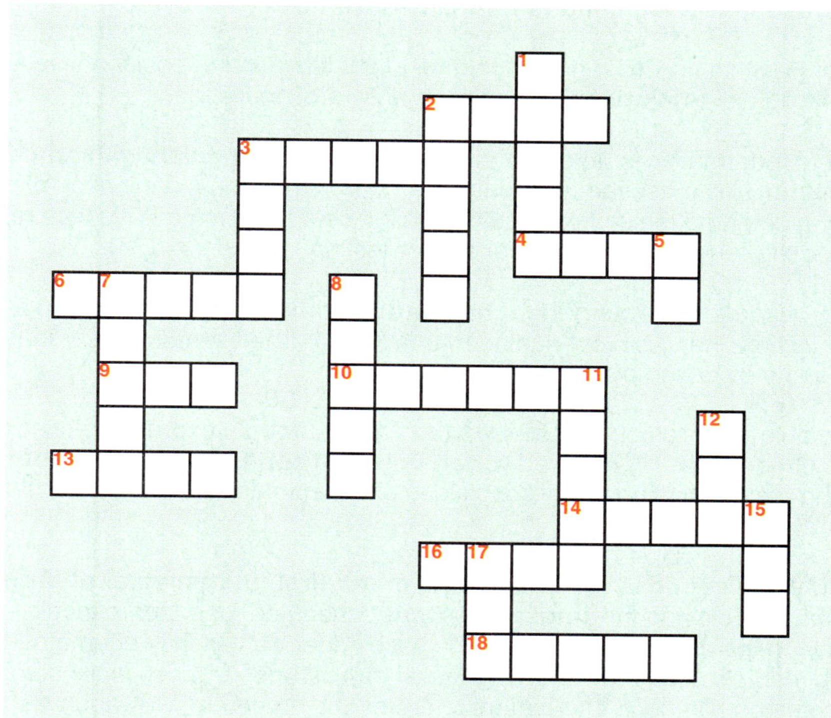

ACROSS

2 One
3 First
4 Against
6 Slow
9 Three
10 Around
13 Same
14 Across, through
16 Half
18 Between

DOWN

1 Within
2 One-thousandth
3 Many, much
5 In, within, not
7 Backward, behind
8 Rapid
11 Many
12 Together, with
15 Joined, together
17 Upon, over

Number correct* ______ × *5 points/correct answer: Your score* ______ *%

D. Proofreading Skills

Read the following consultation report and identify 10 misspelled prefixes by circling them in the script. Lines that have errors are numbered and are printed in bold. After you have identified the errors, write each prefix correctly and define it in the space provided. Each correct answer is worth 10 points. Record your score in the space provided at the end of the exercise.

PATIENT: Ms. Kelli Greene

IDENTIFICATION NUMBER: 620378

DATE: February 25, 2003

SUMMARY: Ms. Kelli Greene is a 26-year-old female who was seen by Dr. George White numerous times for repeated complaints **(1) of epygastric pain and was referred to me after** the last episode. She states that the pain radiates to her shoulder and back, and is so severe at times that she experiences diplopia.

(2) Physical examination shows no trachycardia, no cyanosis of nail beds. Blood pressure is 120/78 mmHg; pulse 82; respiration 14. Visual acuity examination reveals that patient **(3) has ambeopia. Microscopic examination of urine reveals no erythrocytes.**

Leukocyte count is within normal range except for slight elevation of eosinophil level. This appears to be negligible. **(4) Patient has no complaints of pollyuria.**

A slight case of acrodermatitis is noted on the left side in **(5) particular, with some hiperplasia of skin and scaling.** Will prescribe cortisone cream for this. Close examination of the right arm reveals a darkly pigmented mole which could possibly be a melanoma. This was removed in my office and sent to the regional laboratory for further testing.

(6) Past history reveals that this patient had endacarditis at age 14 following a streptococcal infection. Her recovery has been uneventful. She expressed fear that this may be resurfacing. I see no evidence of this, however.

Palpation of the epigastric region was met with resistance and an expression of considerable discomfort. Ms. Greene was **(7) referred for an upper GI series and an ultersound of the gallbladder.** The results confirmed my suspicions of inflammation of the gallbladder with presence of gallstones.

(8) The fact that Ms. Greene is a primagravida in her first (9) trymester of pregnancy, did not create a need for delaying the surgery. She was scheduled for a laparoscopic cholecystectomy on the 28th of this month. The gallbladder was slightly edematous but was removed without complications under **(10) general annesthesia. There were several stones blocking the** common bile duct. The patient tolerated the procedure well and was discharged three days later.

Two-week, follow-up visit revealed no complications. Patient is progressing well. Pathology report of mole on right forearm was negative. No further visits are deemed necessary and patient was instructed to return to family physician and personal obstetrician as needed.

DIAGNOSIS:
1. Acute cholecystitis with cholelithiasis
2. Possible melanoma of right forearm

TREATMENT:
1. Laparoscopic cholecystectomy
2. Excisional biopsy of mole on right forearm, negative

FOLLOW-UP
1. Return to family physician as needed
2. Copy of consultation report mailed to Dr. George White on 4-30-03.

Cole Black, M.D.

1. Correct spelling of the prefix: ______________________________
   Definition of the prefix: ______________________________
   ____
2. Correct spelling of the prefix: ______________________________
   Definition of the prefix: ______________________________
   ____
3. Correct spelling of the prefix: ______________________________
   Definition of the prefix: ______________________________
   ____
4. Correct spelling of the prefix: ______________________________
   Definition of the prefix: ______________________________
   ____
5. Correct spelling of the prefix: ______________________________
   Definition of the prefix: ______________________________
   ____
6. Correct spelling of the prefix: ______________________________
   Definition of the prefix: ______________________________
   ____
7. Correct spelling of the prefix: ______________________________
   Definition of the prefix: ______________________________
   ____
8. Correct spelling of the prefix: ______________________________
   Definition of the prefix: ______________________________
   ____
9. Correct spelling of the prefix: ______________________________
   Definition of the prefix: ______________________________
   ____
10. Correct spelling of the prefix: ______________________________
    Definition of the prefix: ______________________________
    ____

Number correct _______ × 10 points/correct answer: Your score _______%

E. Completion

Complete each statement with the most appropriate prefix. **Note:** Because you are just beginning your study of medical terminology, the meaning of the prefix has been italicized for you. Each correct answer is worth 10 points. Record your score in the space provided at the end of the exercise.

1. A tooth having *two* cusps or points is known as a _________cuspid tooth.
2. A person who is paralyzed on *one half* (one side) of the body is known to have _________plegia.
3. A woman who is pregnant for the *first* time is termed a _________gravida.
4. The excretion of large amounts of urine (*much* urine) is known as _________uria.
5. The medical term that means "being *without* pain," or refers to an agent that is given to relieve pain, is _________algesic.

6. A person who is able to use *both* hands well is said to be _________dextrous.
7. A medication that is placed *under* the tongue is a _________lingual medication.
8. An _________venous medication is one that is administered *within* a vein.
9. The term _________charge means "release of a substance or object in order (*to free it from* its location."
10. A diagnostic or therapeutic technique that does not require the skin to be broken (*not* invaded) or a cavity or organ to be entered is said to be a _________invasive procedure.

Number correct _______ × 10 points/correct answer: Your score _______%

Answers to Chapter Review Exercises

A. Matching

1. e
2. f
3. g
4. m
5. i
6. b
7. c
8. j
9. d
10. t
11. v
12. w
13. r
14. a
15. p
16. n
17. l
18. o
19. q
20. h

B. Create a Word

1. ab- (abduct)
2. ambi- (ambidextrous)
3. peri- (perioral)
4. dia- (diagnosis)
5. hypo- (hypoglossal)
6. intra- (intravenous)
7. supra- (suprapubic)
8. trans- (transurethral)
9. epi- (epigastric)
10. inter- (intercostal)

C. Crossword Puzzle

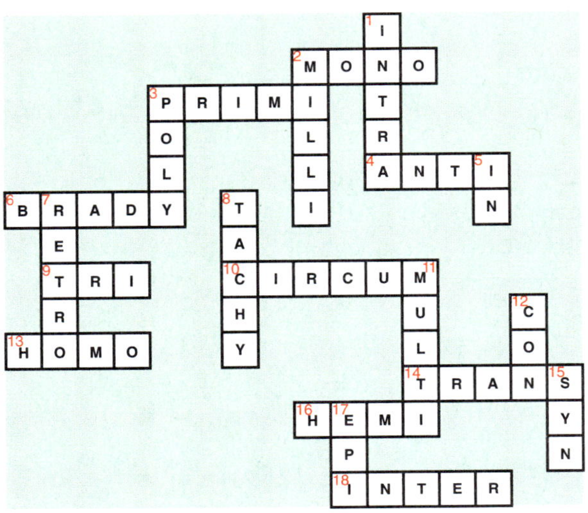

Note: #15 down can also be "sym"
Note: #16 down can also be "semi"

D. Proofreading Skills

1. epi- (upon, over)
2. tachy- (rapid)
3. ambi- (both, both sides)
4. poly- (many, much)
5. hyper- (excessive)
6. endo- (within)
7. ultra- (beyond, excess)
8. primi- (first)
9. tri- (three)
10. an- (without, not)

E. Completion

1. bi-
2. hemi-
3. primi-
4. poly-
5. an-
6. ambi-
7. sub-
8. intra-
9. dis-
10. non-

CHAPTER 3

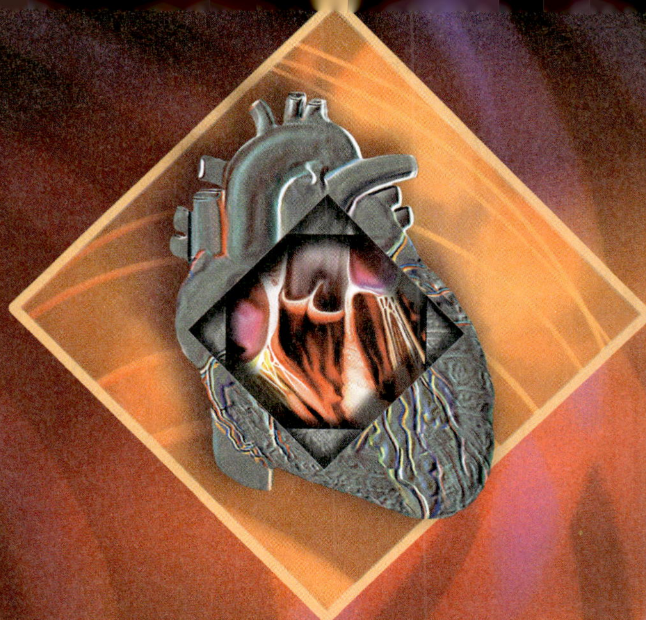

Suffixes

CHAPTER CONTENT

KEY COMPETENCIES

Upon completing this chapter and the review exercises at the end of the chapter, the learner should be able to:

1. Define a suffix and state the rule for using suffixes in words.
2. Correctly identify at least 10 suffixes that make a word a noun.
3. Correctly identify at least 10 suffixes that make a word an adjective.
4. Correctly identify at least 10 suffixes that deal with instruments, and diagnostic and surgical procedures.
5. Identify and define at least 8 suffixes that deal with specialties and specialists.

OVERVIEW

A suffix is the ending of a word. The root to which a suffix is attached may or may not need a combining vowel, depending on whether the suffix begins with a consonant or a vowel.

Example: Combining Vowel Needed: *cephal + o + dynia* = **cephalodynia**
Cephal is a word root meaning "head;" *-dynia* is a suffix meaning "pain." Because *-dynia* begins with a consonant (*d*), it is necessary to use the combining vowel *o* to make the word *cephalodynia,* which means "pain in the head."

Rule: ***When a suffix begins with a consonant, a combining vowel is used with the word root that attaches to the suffix.***

Example: Combining Vowel *Not* Needed: *cephal + algia* = **cephalalgia**
Cephal is a word root meaning "head;" *-algia* is a suffix meaning "pain." Because *-algia* begins with a vowel (*a*), it is not necessary to use a combining vowel to make the word *cephalalgia,* which means "pain in the head."

Rule: ***When a suffix begins with a vowel, the word root attaches directly to the suffix without the aid of a combining vowel.***

A suffix makes a word either a noun or an adjective. When the noun ending *-um* is attached to the word root *duoden,* the newly created word *duodenum* is a noun. When the adjective ending *-al* is attached to the same word root, the new word becomes the adjective *duodenal.* In this chapter we classify the suffixes as either noun endings or adjective endings. Seeing the suffixes in a grouping such as this should help you as you continue to create medical words.

As mentioned in Chapter 2 on prefixes, the meaning of a particular suffix does not change from word to word; thus, *-itis* always means "inflammation." Any word that has *-itis* as its suffix denotes inflammation. A word with the same root does change its meaning, however, each time a new suffix is attached. For example, use the word root *gastr,* meaning "stomach," and look at the various definitions that result with the addition of different suffixes. Notice that in each word the suffix is bold, as is the definition of the suffix.

WORD	WORD ROOT	+ SUFFIX		DEFINITION
gastr**algia**	gastr	**-algia**	=	**pain** in the stomach
gastr**itis**	gastr	**-itis**	=	**inflammation** of the stomach
gastr**ic**	gastr	**-ic**	=	**pertaining to** the stomach
gastr**ostomy**	gastr	**-ostomy**	=	**creating a new opening into** the stomach

Suffixes indicate, among other things, surgical procedures, types of surgeries, specialties, specialists, and conditions. Defining medical terms usually begins with the meaning of the suffix. For example, the definition of *gastr**itis*** begins with defining the suffix first, followed by defining the word root. Therefore, the definition of *gastritis* is "**inflammation of** the stomach."

Rule: ***When defining a medical term, begin the definition by defining the suffix first, the prefix second, and the root(s) last.***

The remainder of this chapter concentrates on the various categories of suffixes and their meanings. The review exercises at the end of the chapter will reinforce your understanding of suffixes and how to use them appropriately in medical terms.

Noun Suffixes

Most of the suffixes in this chapter make a word a noun. They can be categorized by their relationship to specialties, surgeries, specialists, conditions, and so on. Some of the basic noun suffixes addressed in this section are used in all categories when building words that have noun endings.

SUFFIX	MEANING	EXAMPLE
-a	(*a* is a noun ending)	cyanoderm**a** (skin with a bluish discoloration) **Note:** When *a* is used as a suffix, it is a noun ending; *a* can also be used as a prefix.
-ate	something that . . .	hemolys**ate** (something that results from hemolysis)
-e	(*e* is a noun ending)	dermatom**e** (instrument used to cut the skin; e.g., thin slices of skin for grafting)
-emia	blood condition	hypergly**cemia** (blood condition in which a greater than normal level of glucose is present in the blood; high blood sugar)
-er	one who	radiograph**er** (one who takes and processes x-rays)
-esis	condition of	enur**esis** (condition of urinary incontinence; bed-wetting)
-ia	condition (*ia* is a noun ending)	parapleg**ia** (condition of paralysis of the lower half of the body)
-iatry	medical treatment, medical profession	pod**iatry** (treatment of diseases and disorders of the foot)
-ion	action, process	conduct**ion** (process in which heat is transferred from one substance to another)
-ism	condition	hirsut**ism** (condition of excessive body hair in a male distribution pattern)
-ist	practitioner	pharmac**ist** (practitioner who prepares/dispenses drugs/medications)
-ole	small or little	arteri**ole** (smallest branch of the arterial circulation; small artery)
-osis	condition	cyan**osis** (condition of blueness)

-tion	process of	relaxa**tion** (the process of reducing tension, as in a muscle when it relaxes after contraction)
-ula	small, little	mac**ula** (small, pigmented spot that appears separate from the surrounding tissue)
-ule	"small one"	ven**ule** (smallest vein that collects blood from a capillary)
-um	a suffix that identifies singular nouns	duoden**um** (first part of the small intestine)
-us	a suffix that identifies singular nouns	cocc**us** (singular bacterium)
-y	(*y* is a noun ending)	myopath**y** (abnormal condition of the muscle)

Plural Words

When a word changes from singular to plural form, the ending of the word also changes. For example, you may have only one cris**is** (singular) or you may have many cris**es** (plural). Use the following rules when changing from singular to plural forms of words.

Rule: ***When the singular form of a word ends in -a, change the a to ae to form the plural.***

Example: The singular form *pleur**a*** becomes *pleur**ae*** in the plural form.

Rule: ***When the singular form of a word ends in -ax, change the ax to aces to form the plural.***

Example: The singular form *thor**ax*** becomes *thor**aces*** in the plural form.

Rule: ***When the singular form of a word ends in -is, change the is to es to form the plural.***

Example: The singular form *cris**is*** becomes *cris**es*** in the plural form.

Rule: ***When the singular form of a word ends in -ix, -ex, or -yx change the ix, ex, or yx to ices to form the plural.***

Example: The singular form *append**ix*** becomes *append**ices*** in the plural form. The singular form *ap**ex*** becomes *ap**ices*** in the plural form.

Rule: ***When the singular form of a word ends in -on, change the on to a to form the plural.***

Example: The singular form *gangli**on*** becomes *gangli**a*** in the plural form.

Rule: ***When the singular form of a word ends in -um, change the um to a to form the plural.***

Example: The singular form *bacteri**um*** becomes *bacteri**a*** in the plural form.

Rule: ***When the singular form of a word ends in -us, change the us to i to form the plural.***

Example: The singular form *thromb**us*** becomes *thromb**i*** in the plural form.

Rule: ***When the singular form of a word ends in -ma, change the ma to mata to form the plural.***

Example: The singular form *fibro**ma*** becomes *fibro**mata*** in the plural form.

The rules for changing singular form to plural are recapped in the examples in Table 3-1.

Table 3-1 Singular to Plural Suffix Changes

SINGULAR FORM		PLURAL FORM
pleur**a**	becomes	pleur**ae**
thor**ax**	becomes	thor**aces**
cris**is**	becomes	cris**es**
append**ix**	becomes	append**ices**
ap**ex**	becomes	ap**ices**
ganglion	becomes	gangli**a**
bacter**ium**	becomes	bacteri**a**
thromb**us**	becomes	thromb**i**
fibro**ma**	becomes	fibro**mata**

Adjective Suffixes

Adjective suffixes are normally used to describe the root word to which they are attached. They usually mean "pertaining to," "relating to," "characterized by," or "resembling." There are no specific rules governing which adjective endings go with which words; sometimes more than one ending will work with the same word root. Understanding the definition and use of a word will help in selecting the most appropriate adjective suffix. The following is a list of some frequently used adjective suffixes.

SUFFIX	MEANING	EXAMPLE
-ac	pertaining to	cardi**ac** (pertaining to the heart)
-al	pertaining to	duoden**al** (pertaining to the duodenum)
-ar	pertaining to	ventricul**ar** (pertaining to the ventricle)
-ary	pertaining to; relating to	pulmon**ary** (pertaining to the lungs)
-eal	pertaining to	esophag**eal** (pertaining to the esophagus)
-ic	pertaining to	thorac**ic** (pertaining to the thorax)
-ical	pertaining to (*-ical* is the combination of *ic* + *al*)	neurolog**ical** (pertaining to the study of nerves)
-ile	pertaining to; capable	febr**ile** (pertaining to fever)
-oid	resembling	muc**oid** (resembling mucus)
-ory	pertaining to; characterized by	audit**ory** (pertaining to hearing)
-ous	pertaining to	ven**ous** (pertaining to veins)
-tic	pertaining to	cyano**tic** (pertaining to blueness)

Specialties and Specialists

Suffixes that indicate specialties and/or specialists are presented throughout the study of medical terminology, particularly as you learn more about specialties, subspecialties, and the physicians who choose to pursue these specialties as lifelong careers. By the time a physician has earned the title of Board Certified or Diplomate in a particular field of study, this person may have invested as much as 3 to 7 years studying beyond the basic medical degree.

The following list identifies the most frequently used suffixes that denote specialties and/or specialists.

SUFFIX	MEANING	EXAMPLE
-ician	specialist in a field of study	obstetr**ician** (specialist in the field of study of pregnancy and childbirth)
-iatrics	relating to medicine, physicians, or medical treatment	ped**iatrics** (field of medicine that deals with children)
-iatry	medical treatment, medical profession	psych**iatry** (field of medicine that deals with the diagnosis, treatment, and prevention of mental illness)
-iatrist	one who treats; a physician	psych**iatrist** (specialist in the study, treatment, and prevention of mental illness)
-ian	specialist in a field of study	geriatric**ian** (specialist in the field of study of the aging)
-ist	practitioner	pharmac**ist** (one who is licensed to prepare and dispense medications)
-logist	one who specializes in the study of	bio**logist** (one who specializes in the study of living things)
-logy	the study of	bio**logy** (the study of living things)

Instruments, Surgical and Diagnostic Procedures

The following suffixes indicate some type of instrument or a surgical or diagnostic procedure. The procedures vary from those that are performed in a medical office or outpatient setting to those performed in hospital surgery settings. The instruments are used primarily for diagnostic purposes.

SUFFIX	MEANING	EXAMPLE
-centesis	surgical puncture	amnio**centesis** (surgical puncture of the amniotic sac to remove fluid for laboratory analysis; an obstetrical procedure)

-clasis	crushing or breaking up	osteo**clasis** (intentional surgical fracture of a bone to correct a deformity)
-desis	binding or surgical fusion	arthro**desis** (fixation of a joint by a procedure designed to accomplish fusion of the joint surfaces)
-ectomy	surgical removal	append**ectomy** (surgical removal of the appendix)
-gram	record or picture	electrocardio**gram** (record of the electrical activity of the heart)
-graph	an instrument used to record	electrocardio**graph** (instrument used to record the electrical activity of the heart)
-graphy	process of recording	electrocardio**graphy** (the process of recording the electrical activity of the heart)
-ize	to make; to treat or combine with	anesthet**ize** (to induce a state of anesthesia; to make one "feelingless")
-lysis	destruction or detachment	dia**lysis** (the removal or detachment of certain elements from the blood or lymph by passing them through a semipermeable membrane)
-meter	an instrument used to measure	pelvi**meter** (instrument used to measure the diameter and capacity of the pelvis)
-metry	the process of measuring	pelvi**metry** (process of measuring the dimensions of the pelvis)
-pexy	surgical fixation	colpo**pexy** (surgical fixation of a relaxed vaginal wall)
-plasty	surgical repair	rhino**plasty** (surgical repair of the nose in which the structure of the nose is changed)
-rrhaphy	suturing	nephro**rrhaphy** (the operation of suturing the kidney)
-scope	an instrument used to view	ophthalmo**scope** (instrument used to view the interior of the eye)
-scopy	the process of viewing with a scope	ophthalmo**scopy** (the process of using an ophthalmoscope to view the interior of the eye)
-stomy	the surgical creation of a new opening	colo**stomy** (surgical creation of a new opening between the colon and the surface of the body)
-tomy	incision into	phlebo**tomy** (incision into a vein)
-tripsy	intentional crushing	litho**tripsy** (crushing of a stone in the bladder; may be accomplished by ultrasound or by laser)

Common Suffixes

An alphabetical listing of suffixes commonly used in medical terminology is included here for easy reference. As you read the list, note that the suffixes just discussed in the "categories" section are repeated in this list. Some of the suffixes also appear throughout the text as they relate to discussions of the body.

SUFFIX	MEANING	EXAMPLE
-a	(*a* is a noun ending)	cyanoderm**a** (skin with a bluish discoloration) **Note:** When *a* is used as a suffix, it is a noun ending; *a* can also be used as a prefix.
-ac	pertaining to	cardi**ac** (pertaining to the heart)
-ad	toward, increase	caud**ad** (toward the tail or end of the body)
-al	pertaining to	duoden**al** (pertaining to the duodenum)
-algesia	sensitivity to pain	an**algesia** (without sensitivity to pain)
-algia	pain	cephal**algia** (pain in the head; a headache)
-ar	pertaining to	ventricul**ar** (pertaining to the ventricle)
-ary	pertaining to; relating to	pulmon**ary** (pertaining to the lungs)
-ate	something that . . .	hemolys**ate** (something that results from hemolysis)
-blast	embryonic stage of development	leuko**blast** (immature white blood cell)
-cele	swelling or herniation	cysto**cele** (herniation or protrusion of the urinary bladder through the wall of the vagina)
-centesis	surgical puncture	amnio**centesis** (surgical puncture of the amniotic sac to remove fluid for laboratory analysis; an obstetrical procedure)
-cide	to kill; to destroy	spermi**cide** (chemical substance that kills spermatozoa)
-clasis	crushing or breaking up	osteo**clasis** (the intentional surgical fracture of a bone to correct a deformity)
-cyte	cell	leuko**cyte** (white blood cell)
-desis	binding or surgical fusion	arthro**desis** (fixation of a joint by a procedure designed to accomplish fusion of the joint surfaces)
-dynia	pain	cephalo**dynia** (pain in the head; a headache)
-e	(*e* is a noun ending)	dermatom**e** (instrument used to cut the skin; i.e., thin slices of skin for grafting)
-eal	pertaining to	esophag**eal** (pertaining to the esophagus)
-ectasia	stretching or dilatation	gastr**ectasia** (stretching or dilatation of the stomach)
-ectomy	surgical removal	append**ectomy** (surgical removal of the appendix)
-emia	blood condition	hyperglyc**emia** (blood condition in which there is a higher than normal level of glucose in the blood; high blood sugar)
-er	one who	radiograph**er** (one who takes and processes x-rays)
-esis	condition of	enur**esis** (condition of urinary incontinence)
-gen	that which generates	glyco**gen** ("that which generates sugar")
-genesis	generating; formation	litho**genesis** (the formation of stones)

-genic	pertaining to, formation, producing	litho**genic** (pertaining to the formation of stones)
-gram	record or picture	electrocardio**gram** (record of the electrical activity of the heart)
-graph	an instrument used to record	electrocardio**graph** (instrument used to record the electrical activity of the heart)
-graphy	process of recording	electrocardio**graphy** (the process of recording the electrical activity of the heart)
-gravida	pregnancy	multi**gravida** (a woman who has been pregnant more than once; "many pregnancies")
-ia	condition (*ia* is a noun ending)	parapleg**ia** (condition of paralysis of the lower half of the body)
-ian	specialist in a field of study	geriatric**ian** (specialist in the field of study of the aging)
-iasis	presence of an abnormal condition	cholelith**iasis** (abnormal presence of gallstones in the gallbladder)
-iatric(s)	relating to medicine, physicians, or medical treatment	ped**iatrics** (field of medicine that deals with children)
-iatrician	one who treats; a physician	ped**iatrician** (physician who treats children)
-iatrist	one who treats; a physician	psych**iatrist** (specialist in the study, treatment, and prevention of mental illness)
-iatry	medical treatment, medical profession	psych**iatry** (field of medicine that deals with the diagnosis, treatment, and prevention of mental illness)
-ic	pertaining to	thorac**ic** (pertaining to the thorax)
-ical	pertaining to (*-ical* is the combination of *ic* + *al*)	neurolog**ical** (pertaining to the study of nerves)
-ician	specialist in a field of study	obstet**rician** (specialist in the field of study of pregnancy and childbirth)
-ile	pertaining to; capable	febr**ile** (pertaining to fever)
-ion	action; process	conduct**ion** (process in which heat is transferred from one substance to another)
-ism	condition	hirsut**ism** (condition of excessive body hair in a masculine distribution pattern)
-ist	practitioner	pharmac**ist** (practitioner who is licensed to prepare and dispense medications)
-itis	inflammation	appendic**itis** (inflammation of the appendix)
-ize	to make; to treat or combine with	anesthet**ize** (to induce a state of anesthesia; to make one "feelingless")
-lepsy	seizure, attack	narco**lepsy** (seizure or sudden attack of sleep)
-lith	stone	rhino**lith** (stone or calculus in the nose)

-lithiasis	presence or formation of stones	chole**lithiasis** (presence of gallstones)
-logy	the study of	bio**logy** (the study of living things)
-logist	one who specializes in the study of	bio**logist** (one who specializes in the study of living things)
-lysis	destruction or detachment	dia**lysis** (removal or detachment of certain elements from the blood or lymph by passing them through a semipermeable membrane)
-lytic	destruction	kerato**lytic** (agent used to destroy hardened skin)
-mania	a mental disorder; a "madness"	megalo**mania** (mental disorder characterized by delusions of grandeur: the patient believes he or she is someone of great importance)
-megaly	enlargement	cardio**megaly** (enlargement of the heart)
-meter	an instrument used to measure	pelvi**meter** (instrument used to measure the diameter and capacity of the pelvis)
-metry	the process of measuring	pelvi**metry** (the process of measuring the dimensions of the pelvis)
-oid	resembling	muc**oid** (resembling mucus)
-ole	small or little	arteri**ole** (smallest branch of the arterial circulation; a "small" artery)
-oma	tumor	lip**oma** (fatty tumor)
-opia	visual condition	my**opia** (a condition of nearsightedness)
-opsia	visual condition	heman**opsia** (blindness in one half of the visual field)
-ory	pertaining to; characterized by	audit**ory** (pertaining to hearing)
-osis	condition	cyan**osis** (condition of blueness)
-ous	pertaining to	ven**ous** (pertaining to veins)
-pathy	disease	adeno**pathy** (disease of a gland)
-penia	decrease in; deficiency	leukocyto**penia** (decrease in the number of white blood cells)
-pexy	surgical fixation	colpo**pexy** (surgical fixation of a relaxed vaginal wall)
-philia	attracted to	necro**philia** (abnormal attraction to dead bodies)
-phobia	abnormal fear	necro**phobia** (abnormal fear of death and dead bodies)
-plasia	formation or development	hyper**plasia** (excessive formation or development)
-plasty	surgical repair	rhino**plasty** (surgical repair of the nose in which the structure of the nose is changed)
-plegia	paralysis	hemi**plegia** (paralysis of half of the body, of one side of the body)
-pnea	breathing	dys**pnea** (difficult breathing)

-ptosis	drooping or prolapse	colpo**ptosis** (prolapse of the vagina)
-rrhagia	excessive flow, discharge	gastro**rrhagia** (bursting forth of blood from the stomach)
-rrhaphy	suturing	nephro**rrhaphy** (operation of suturing the kidney)
-rrhea	discharge; flow	rhino**rrhea** (flow or drainage from the nose)
-rrhexis	rupture	arterio**rrhexis** (rupture of an artery)
-scope	an instrument used to view	ophthalmo**scope** (instrument used to view the interior of the eye)
-scopy	the process of viewing with a scope	ophthalmo**scopy** (the process of using an ophthalmoscope to view the interior of the eye)
-stasis	stopping or controlling	hemo**stasis** (stopping or controlling the flow of blood) veno**stasis** (the trapping or "standing still" of blood in an extremity)
-stomy	the surgical creation of a new opening	colo**stomy** (surgical creation of a new opening between the colon and the surface of the body)
-tic	pertaining to	cyano**tic** (pertaining to blueness)
-tion	process of	relaxa**tion** (the process of reducing tension, as when a muscle relaxes after contraction)
-tomy	incision into	phlebo**tomy** (incision into a vein)
-tripsy	intentional crushing	litho**tripsy** (the crushing of a stone in the bladder; may be accomplished by ultrasound or by laser)
-ula	small, little	mac**ula** (small pigmented spot that appears separate from the surrounding tissue)
-ule	"small one"	ven**ule** (smallest vein that collects blood from a capillary)
-um	a suffix that identifies singular nouns	duoden**um** (first part of the small intestines)
-uria	a characteristic of the urine	hemat**uria** (presence of blood in the urine)
-us	a suffix that identifies singular nouns	cocc**us** (singular bacterium)
-y	(*y* is a noun ending)	myopath**y** (abnormal condition of the muscles)

Chapter Review Exercises

The following exercises provide a more in-depth review of the chapter material. Your goal in these exercises is to complete each section at a minimum 80% level of accuracy. A space has been provided for your score at the end of each section.

A. Replacing

Read each sentence carefully and replace the terms in bold with the appropriate noun ending. Each correct answer is worth 10 points. Record your score in the space provided at the end of the exercise.

-algia -emia -iatry -um

-cele -er -itis

-dynia -genesis -ole

1. **One who** takes and processes x-rays is known as a radiograph_________.
2. A **blood condition** in which there is a higher than normal level of glucose in the blood is known as hyperglyc_________.
3. The **treatment** of diseases and disorders of the foot is known as pod_________.
4. The **smallest** branch of the arterial circulation is the arteri_________.
5. To change the word **duodenal** from its adjective form, you would drop the *-al* and add _________ to make the word a noun.
6. **Pain** in the head, or headache, is known as cephal_________.
7. **Herniation** of the bladder through the wall of the vagina is known as a cysto_________.
8. **Pain** in the head can also be called cephalo_________.
9. The **formation of** stones is known as litho_________.
10. **Inflammation** of the appendix is termed appendic_________.

Number correct _______ × 10 points/correct answer: Your score _______%

B. Crossword Puzzle

In this puzzle, you will be working with suffixes that indicate instruments and diagnostic or surgical procedures. Each crossword answer is worth 10 points. When you have completed the crossword puzzle, total your points and enter your score in the space provided.

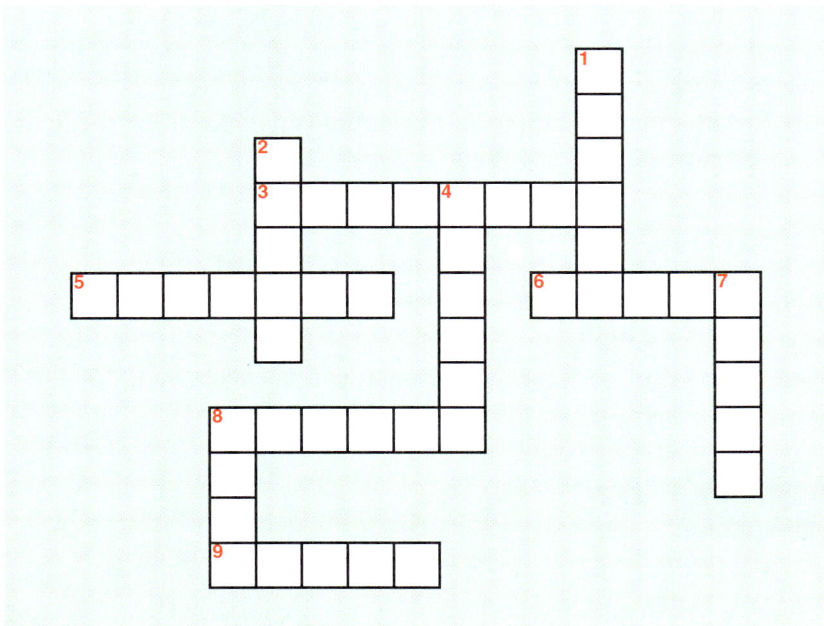

ACROSS

3 Surgical puncture
5 Suturing
6 Destruction
8 Process of recording
9 Instrument used to measure

DOWN

1 Surgical repair
2 Process of viewing
4 Surgical removal
7 Creation of a new opening
8 Record or picture

Number correct _______ × 10 points/correct answer: Your score _______%

C. Create a Word

Using the suffixes listed, create a word that best completes each statement dealing with specialties, specialists, and specialty instruments. If you need assistance, refer to your list of suffixes within the chapter. After you have determined the correct suffix, write the word, without the divisions, in the space provided. Each correct answer is worth 10 points. Record your score in the space provided at the end of the exercise.

-logist	-scope	-iatrics	-ician
-ist	-logy	-mania	
-iatrist	-iatry	-ian	

Create a word that means:

1. A specialist in the field of study of the aging

   geriatric + ______ = ______

   (word root) + (suffix) = (complete word)

2. The study of living things

   bio + ______ = ______

   (word root) + (suffix) = (complete word)

3. A specialist in the field of study of pregnancy and childbirth

   obstetr + ______ = ______

   (word root) + (suffix) = (complete word)

4. A pediatrician would use this instrument for viewing the interior of the eye

   ophthalm + o + ______ = ______

   (root) + (vowel) + (suffix) = (complete word)

5. A specialist in the study, treatment, and prevention of mental illness

   psych + ______ = ______

   (word root) + (suffix) = (complete word)

6. The field of medicine that deals with children

   ped + ______ = ______

   (word root) + (suffix) = (complete word)

7. One who is licensed to prepare and dispense medications

   pharmac + ______ = ______

   (word root) + (suffix) = (complete word)

8. A psychiatrist might treat this mental disorder, which is characterized by delusions of grandeur (the patient believes he or she is someone of great importance)

   megal + o + ______ = ______

   (root) + (vowel) + (suffix) = (complete word)

9. The field of medicine that deals with the diagnosis, treatment, and prevention of mental illness

   psych + ______ = ______

   (word root) + (suffix) = (complete word)

10. One who specializes in the study of living things

bi	+	o	+		=	
(root)	+	(vowel)	+	(suffix)	=	(complete word)

Number correct ______ × 10 points/correct answer: Your score ______%

D. Word Search

Using the definitions listed, identify the appropriate adjective word and then find and circle it in the puzzle. The words may be read up, down, diagonally, across, or backward. Each correct answer is worth 10 points. Record your score in the space provided at the end of the exercise.

Example: pertaining to veins *venous*

1. pertaining to the heart ______
2. pertaining to the duodenum ______
3. pertaining to the ventricle ______
4. pertaining to the lungs ______
5. pertaining to the thorax ______
6. pertaining to the nerves ______
7. pertaining to fever ______
8. resembling mucus ______
9. pertaining to hearing ______
10. pertaining to blueness ______

C	A	R	V	E	N	O	U	S	D	I	A	C	B
A	C	R	F	E	B	R	I	L	E	T	Y	O	R
L	U	E	O	Y	N	T	I	C	H	A	P	Y	I
M	U	C	O	I	D	T	A	O	N	E	B	R	L
N	E	A	U	R	O	L	R	O	T	H	O	O	E
M	U	R	S	C	O	A	T	I	I	D	R	T	F
P	U	D	L	M	C	I	O	N	C	U	A	I	R
F	E	I	B	I	C	R	I	L	E	U	V	D	E
N	O	A	C	U	Y	R	A	N	O	M	L	U	P
S	A	C	U	D	I	D	U	O	D	E	N	A	L
L	A	C	I	G	O	L	O	R	U	E	N	T	R

Number correct ______ × 10 points/correct answer: Your score ______%

E. Matching

Match the suffixes on the left with the correct definition on the right. Each correct answer is worth 10 points. Record your score in the space provided at the end of the exercise.

_____	1. -oid	a. discharge; flow
_____	2. -clasis	b. rupture
_____	3. -ectomy	c. instrument used to record
_____	4. -gram	d. surgical fixation
_____	5. -graph	e. surgical removal
_____	6. -pexy	f. record or picture
_____	7. -plasty	g. suturing
_____	8. -rrhaphy	h. surgical repair
_____	9. -rrhea	i. resembling
_____	10. -rrhexis	j. crushing or breaking up

Number correct _______ × 10 points/correct answer: Your score _______%

F. Singular to Plural

Look at the singular form of the words below and change each word ending to the plural form, following the rules presented in this chapter. (HINT: You do not have to change the spelling of the complete word, just the ending to make it a plural form.) The singular ending is printed in bold. Each correct answer is worth 10 points. Record your score in the space provided at the end of the exercise.

SINGULAR FORM	PLURAL FORM
Example: cocc**us**	Example: cocc**i**
1. pleur**a**	1. ____________________
2. thor**ax**	2. ____________________
3. cris**is**	3. ____________________
4. append**ix**	4. ____________________
5. ap**ex**	5. ____________________
6. gangli**on**	6. ____________________
7. bacteri**um**	7. ____________________
8. thromb**us**	8. ____________________
9. fibro**ma**	9. ____________________
10. diagnos**is**	10. ____________________

Number correct _______ × 10 points/correct answer: Your score _______%

Answers to Chapter Review Exercises

A. Replacing

1. -er
2. -emia
3. -iatry
4. -ole
5. -um
6. -algia
7. -cele
8. -dynia
9. -genesis
10. -itis

B. Crossword Puzzle

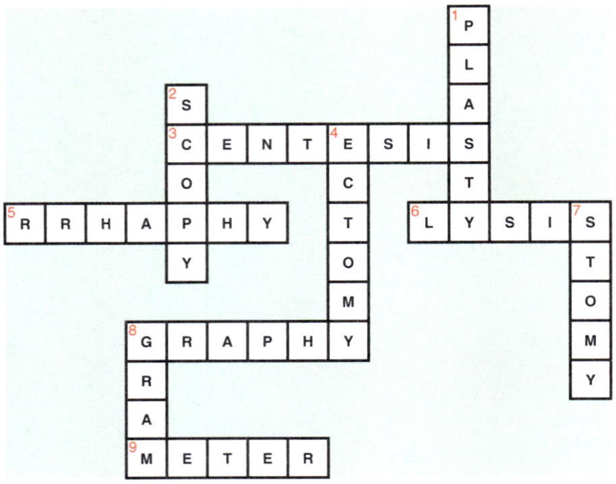

C. Create a Word

1. -ian (geriatrician)
2. -logy (biology)
3. -ician (obstetrician)
4. -scope (ophthalmoscope)
5. -iatrist (psychiatrist)
6. -iatrics (pediatrics)
7. -ist (pharmacist)
8. -mania (megalomania)
9. -iatry (psychiatry)
10. -logist (biologist)

D. Word Search

1. cardiac
2. duodenal
3. ventricular
4. pulmonary
5. thoracic
6. neurological
7. febrile
8. mucoid
9. auditory
10. cyanotic

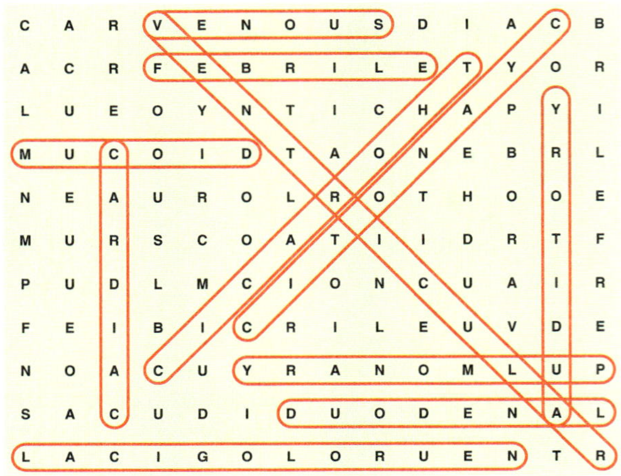

E. Matching

1. i
2. j
3. e
4. f
5. c
6. d
7. h
8. g
9. a
10. b

F. Singular to Plural

1. pleur**ae**
2. thora**ces**
3. cris**es**
4. append**ices**
5. ap**ices**
6. gangl**ia**
7. bacter**ia**
8. thromb**i**
9. fibrom**ata**
10. diagnos**es**

CHAPTER 4

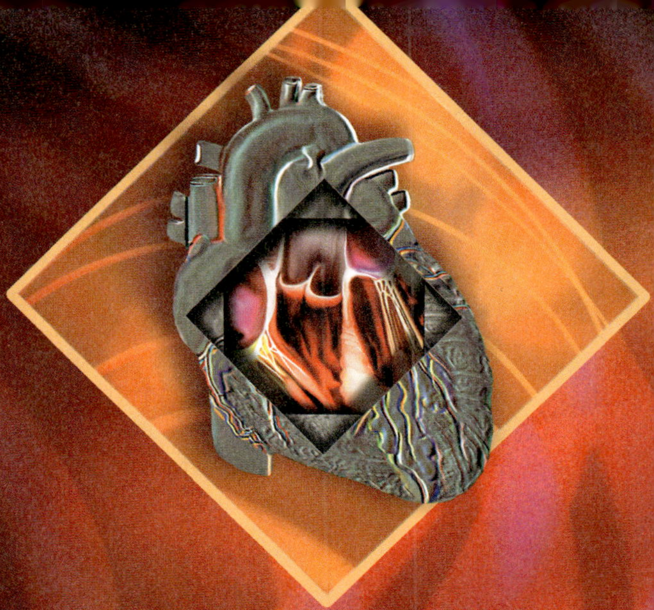

Whole Body Terminology

CHAPTER CONTENT

KEY COMPETENCIES

Upon completing this chapter and the review exercises at the end of the chapter, the learner should be able to:

1. List the five body cavities identified in this chapter.
2. List the organs contained within the five body cavities as identified in the chapter reading.
3. Define at least 10 general terms relating to the body as a whole.
4. Correctly spell and pronounce each new term introduced in this chapter using the Activity CD-ROM and Audio CD, if available.
5. Identify the nine body regions studied in this chapter.
6. Identify at least eight terms relating to structural organization of the body.
7. Identify at least 10 directional terms relating to the body as a whole.
8. Create at least 10 medical terms relating to the body as a whole.

OVERVIEW

So far we have discussed prefixes that are placed at the beginning of a word, suffixes that are placed at the end of a word, and word roots that are the foundation of a word. We have also reviewed the word building rules used to construct medical terms, using any combination of prefixes, word roots, and suffixes.

In addition to the ability to build medical terms that relate to the various body systems and particular disease, disorders, and treatments, it is important to know terms that relate to the body as a whole. Whole body terms are an important part of medical terminology because they help define the makeup of the various body systems.

Medical terms are used to describe the structural organization of the body, from the cellular level to the systemic level. They are used to describe body cavities; divisions of the spinal column; and regions, quadrants, and planes of the body. In addition, whole body terms provide information about position, direction, and location of organs in relation to each other within the body. Knowledge of whole body terminology provides the necessary foundation for a better understanding of the body systems that follow.

Structural Organization

Although the organization of the body begins at the chemical level, our discussion of terms begins at the cellular level and builds from that point. Cells that are grouped together to perform specialized functions are known as **tissue**. Tissues that are arranged together to perform a special function are known as **organs**. Organs that work together to perform the many functions of the body as a whole are called **systems**.

Cells

The **cell** is the smallest and most numerous structural unit of living matter. Refer to **Figure 4-1.** All cells are surrounded by a **(1) cell membrane**, which is the cell's outer covering. The cell membrane is a semipermeable barrier that allows certain substances to pass through while blocking others. The cell membrane is also known as the plasma membrane. The central controlling body within a living cell is the **(2) nucleus**, which is enclosed within the cell membrane. The nucleus is made up of threadlike structures, called **chromosomes** (molecules of deoxyribonucleic acid, or DNA), that control the functions of growth, repair, and reproduction for the body. The chromosomes contain segments or regions called **genes** that transmit hereditary characteristics. Each body cell, with the exception of the female ovum and the male spermatozoa, contains 23 pairs of chromosomes that determine its genetic makeup. The female ovum (egg) and the male spermatozoa (sperm) each contain only 23 chromosomes. When the female ovum and the male sperm unite, resulting in fertilization of the ovum, the newly formed embryo contains 23 pairs of chromosomes (half coming from the ovum and half coming from the sperm).

Surrounding the nucleus of the cell is the **(3) cytoplasm**. The cytoplasm is a gel-like substance containing cell organs, called organelles, that carry out the essential functions of the cell. A few examples of organelles are **(4) mitochondria**, which provide the energy needed by the cell to carry on its essential functions, and **(5) lysosomes**, which contain various kinds of enzymes capable of breaking down all the main components of cells. When bac-

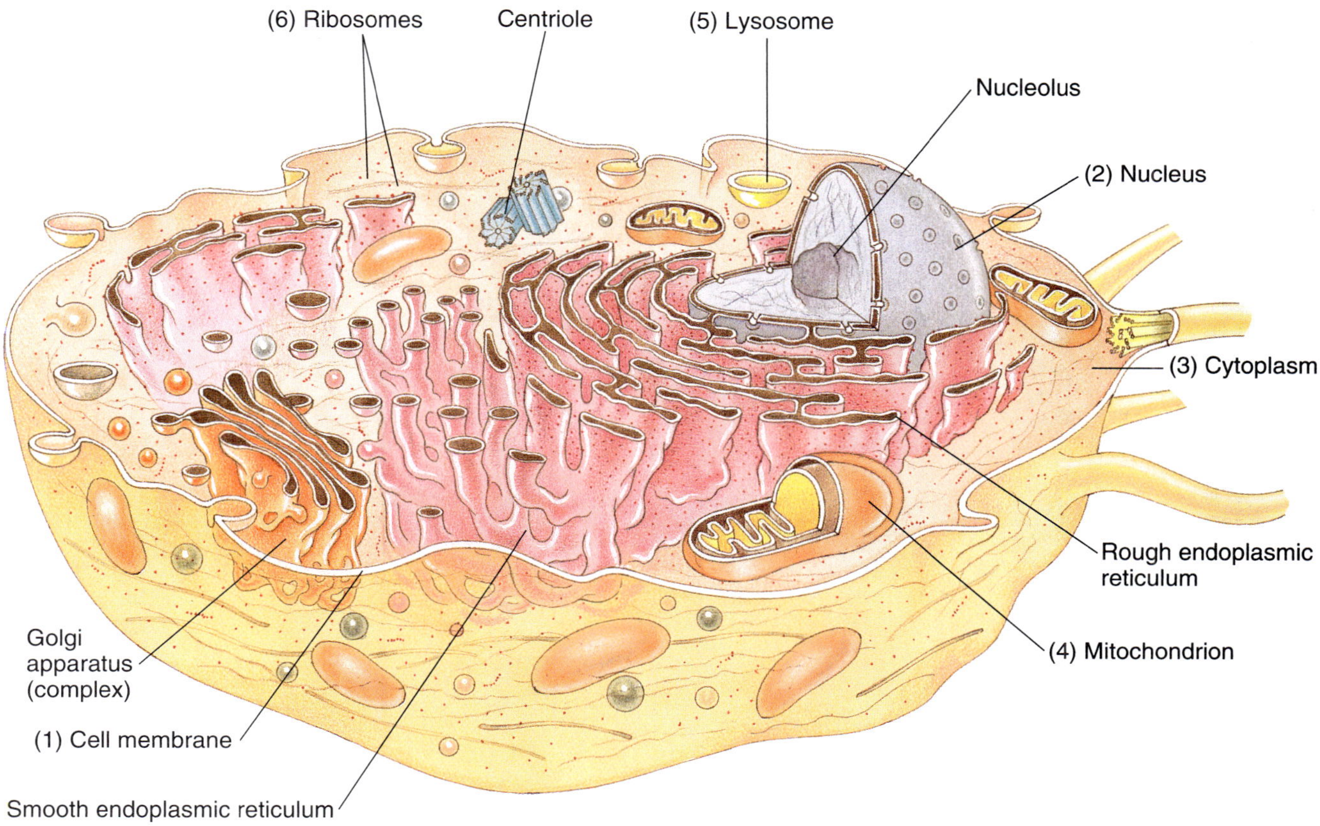

Figure 4-1 Component parts of a cell

teria enter the cells, the lysosome enzymes destroy the bacteria by digesting them. The **(6) ribosomes**, which synthesize proteins, are often called the cell's "protein factories."

The following terms relate to cellular growth.

WORD	MEANING
anaplasia (an-ah-**PLAY**-zee-ah) **ana-** = not, without **-plasia** = formation, growth	A change in the structure and orientation of cells, characterized by a loss of differentiation and reversion to a more primitive form.
aplasia (ah-**PLAY**-zee-ah) **a-** = without, not **-plasia** = formation, growth	A developmental failure resulting in the absence of any organ or tissue.
dysplasia (dis-**PLAY**-zee-ah) **dys-** = bad, difficult, painful, disordered **-plasia** = formation, growth	Any abnormal development of tissues or organs ("disordered formation").

hyperplasia (**high**-per-**PLAY**-zee-ah) **hyper-** = excessive **-plasia** = formation, growth	An increase in the number of cells of a body part ("excessive formation").
hypoplasia (**high**-poh-**PLAY**-zee-ah) **hypo-** = under, below, beneath, less than normal **-plasia** = formation, growth	Incomplete or underdeveloped organ or tissue, usually the result of a decrease in the number of cells.
neoplasia (**nee**-oh-**PLAY**-zee-ah) **ne/o** = new **-plasia** = formation, growth	The new and abnormal development of cells that may be benign or malignant.

Tissues

Tissue is composed of groups of similar cells that perform specialized or common functions. The four main types of tissue are connective, epithelial, muscle, and nervous.

1. **Connective tissue** supports and binds other body tissue and parts. Connective tissue may be liquid (as in blood), fatty (as in protective padding), fibrous (as in tendons and ligaments), cartilage (as in the rings of the trachea), or solid (as in bone).
2. **Epithelial tissue** covers the internal and external organs of the body. It also lines the vessels, body cavities, glands, and body organs.
3. **Muscle tissue** is capable of producing movement of the parts and organs of the body through the contraction and relaxation of its fibers. The three types of muscle tissue in the body are (a) **skeletal muscle**, which is attached to bone and is responsible for the movement of the skeleton, (b) **smooth muscle** (also known as **visceral muscle**), which is found in the walls of the hollow internal organs of the body, such as the stomach and intestines, and (c) **cardiac muscle**, which makes up the muscular wall of the heart.
4. **Nervous tissue** transmits impulses throughout the body, thereby activating, coordinating, and controlling the many functions of the body.

The term **membrane** describes a thin layer of tissue that covers a surface, lines a cavity, or divides a space, such as the **abdominal** membrane that lines the abdominal wall. A specific membrane, the **peritoneum**, is an extensive serous membrane that covers the entire abdominal wall of the body and is reflected over the contained viscera.

A medical specialist in the study of tissues is known as a **histologist**. The study of cells is known as **cytology**.

Organs

Organs are made up of tissues arranged together to perform a particular function. Examples of various organs are the liver, spleen, stomach, and ovaries. The term **visceral** refers to the internal organs. In the remaining chapters of this textbook, the various organs of the body will be discussed in their specific system chapter.

Systems

The organization of different organs so they can perform the many functions of the body as a whole is known as a system. Most of the remaining chapters in this textbook focus on the primary body systems including:

integumentary	cardiovascular
skeletal	respiratory
muscles and joints	digestive
nervous	urinary
special senses	male reproductive
endocrine	female reproductive
blood and lymphatic	

Body Planes

To identify the position of various parts of the body in the study of anatomy, the body can be visually divided into areas called **planes**. These imaginary slices, or cuts, are made as if a dividing sheet were passed through the body at a particular angle and in a particular direction. For example, if you were physically able to divide the body straight down the middle into equal halves, you would create the midsagittal plane. If you separated those two halves of the body, laying them open like a book, you could view the inner structures of the body, on the left side and on the right side. The **midsagittal plane** divides the body or structure into equal right and left portions. See **Figure 4-2.**

The "line" created when the body is divided into equal right and left halves is referred to as the **midline** of the body. When we discuss directional terms, notice that many of the terms are described in relation to the midline of the body and the imaginary lines created by the various planes of the body.

The following is a list of the planes of the body.

frontal plane — Any of the vertical planes passing through the body from the head to the feet, perpendicular to the sagittal planes and dividing the body into front and back portions. Also known as the coronal plane. See Figure 4-3.

transverse plane — Any of the planes cutting across the body, perpendicular to the sagittal and the frontal planes and dividing the body into superior (upper) and inferior (lower) portions. See Figure 4-4.

Although we can visualize the cuts through the body that create the various planes, based on our sense of direction and our knowledge of anatomy,

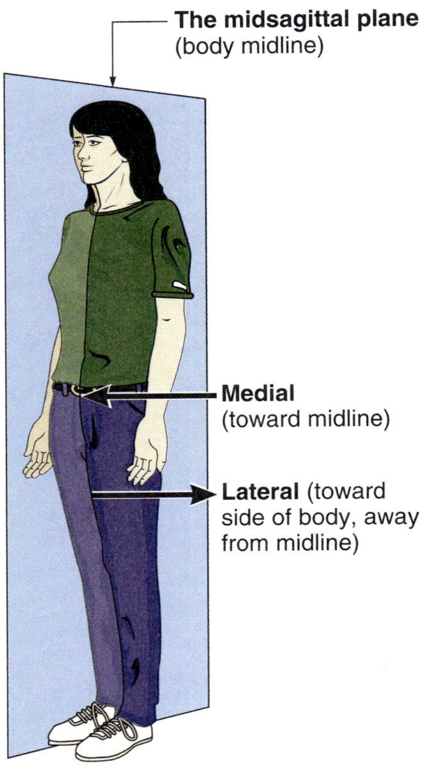

Figure 4-2 Midsagittal plane

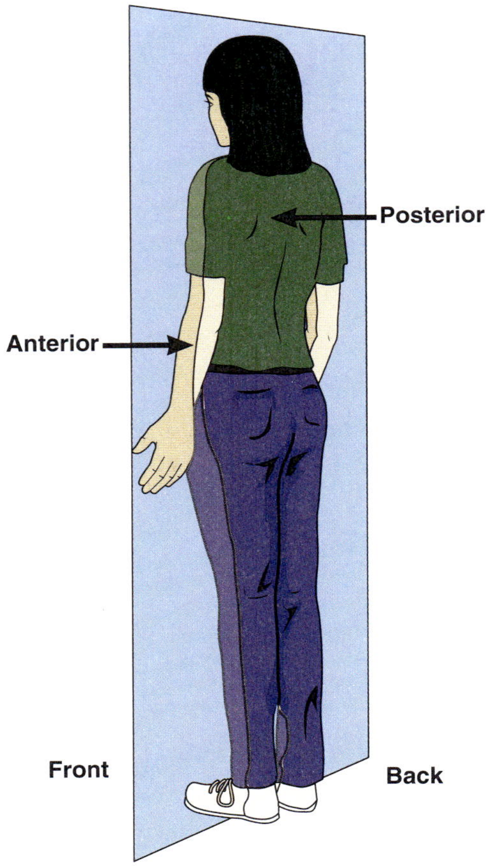

Figure 4-3 Frontal (coronal) plane

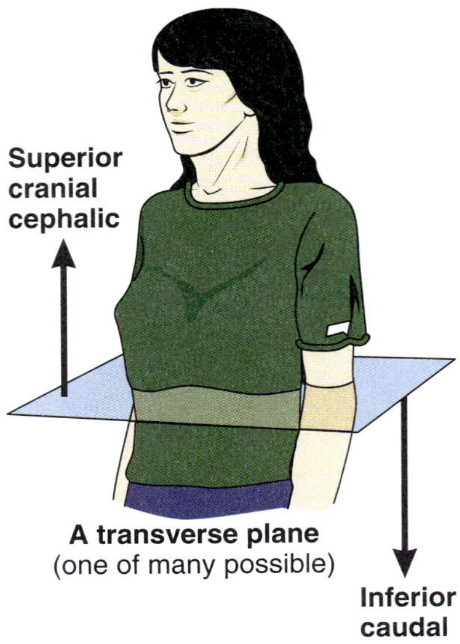

Figure 4-4 Transverse plane

medical technology has advanced to the point where computers can produce a cross-sectional image of the body. This image, produced by computerized axial tomography, or CAT scan, represents a detailed cross section of the tissue structure being examined. (CAT scans are discussed in later chapters.)

Body Regions and Quadrants

In addition to planes, areas of the body can be further divided into regions and quadrants. Anatomists have divided the abdomen into nine imaginary sections, called regions, that are helpful in identifying the location of particular abdominal organs. Moreover, regions are useful for describing the location of pain.

Figure 4-5 shows the nine abdominal regions, which are identified from the left to the right, moving from top to bottom one row at a time. The most superficial organs in these regions are also identified.

region 1

Right hypochondriac region Located in the upper-right section of the abdomen, beneath the cartilage of the lower ribs, the superficial organs visible in the right hypochondriac region include the right lobe of the liver and the gallbladder.

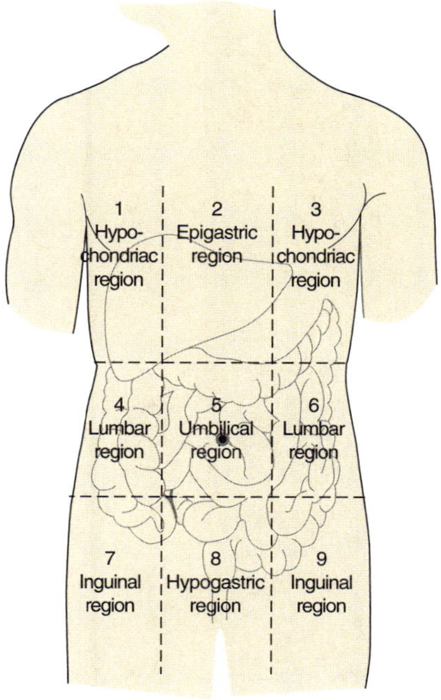

Figure 4-5 Abdominal regions

region 2	Epigastric region Located between the right and left hypochondriac regions in the upper section of the abdomen, beneath the cartilage of the lower ribs; the superficial organs visible in the epigastric region include parts of the right and left lobes of the liver and a major portion of the stomach.
region 3	Left hypochondriac region Located in the upper-left section of the abdomen, beneath the cartilage of the lower ribs; the superficial organs visible in the left hypochondriac region include a small portion of the stomach and a portion of the large intestine.
region 4	Right lumbar region Located in the middle-right section of the abdomen, beneath the right hypochondriac region; the superficial organs visible in the right lumbar region include portions of the large and small intestines.
region 5	Umbilical region Located in the middle section of the abdomen, between the right and left lumbar regions and directly beneath the epigastric region; the superficial organs visible in the umbilical region include a portion of the transverse colon and portions of the small intestine.
region 6	Left lumbar region Located in the middle-left section of the abdomen, beneath the left hypochondriac region; the superficial organs visible in the left lumbar region include portions of the small intestine and part of the colon.
region 7	Right inguinal (iliac) region Located in the lower-right section of the abdomen, beneath the right lumbar region; the superficial organs visible in the right inguinal region include portions of the small intestine and the cecum.

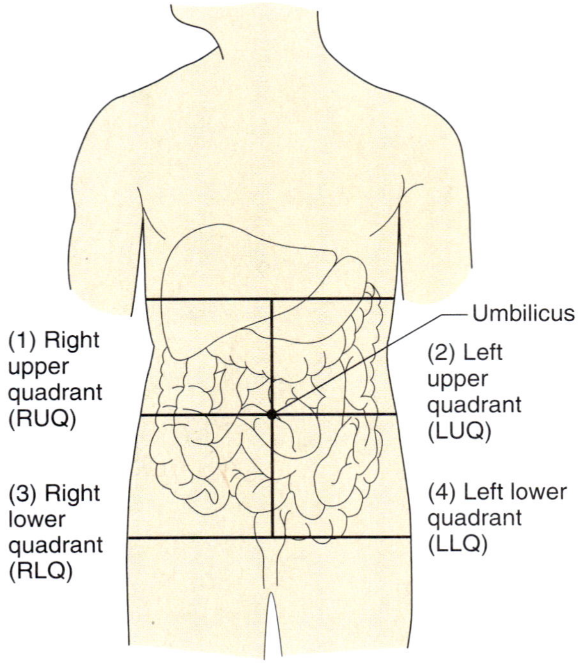

Figure 4-6 Abdominal quadrants

region 8 Hypogastric region Located in the lower-middle section of the abdomen, beneath the umbilical region; the superficial organs visible in the hypogastric region include the urinary bladder, portions of the small intestine, and the appendix.

region 9 Left inguinal (iliac) region Located in the lower-left section of the abdomen, beneath the left lumbar region; the superficial organs visible in the left inguinal region include portions of the colon and the small intestine.

Anatomists have also divided the abdomen into quadrants. These four imaginary divisions provide reference points for physicians and health professionals when describing the location of abdominopelvic pain or when locating areas of involvement in certain diseases or conditions. The landmark on the external abdominal wall for dividing the abdomen into quadrants is the **umbilicus**, or **navel** (sometimes referred to as the belly button). To divide the abdomen into quadrants, an imaginary line is drawn vertically and horizontally through the umbilicus, creating the four abdominal quadrants: **(1) right upper quadrant (RUQ), (2) left upper quadrant (LUQ), (3) right lower quadrant (RLQ),** and **(4) left lower quadrant (LLQ). Figure 4-6** shows the four abdominal quadrants.

Two additional reference points on the abdomen that use the umbilicus as a landmark are Munro's point and McBurney's point. **Munro's point** is located on the left side of the abdomen, halfway between the umbilicus and the anterior bony prominence of the hip. Surgeons often use this as a point of entry for abdominal puncture when performing laparoscopic ("viewing the abdomen") surgery. **McBurney's point** is located on the right side of the abdomen, about two-thirds of the distance between the umbilicus and the anterior bony prominence of the hip. When tenderness

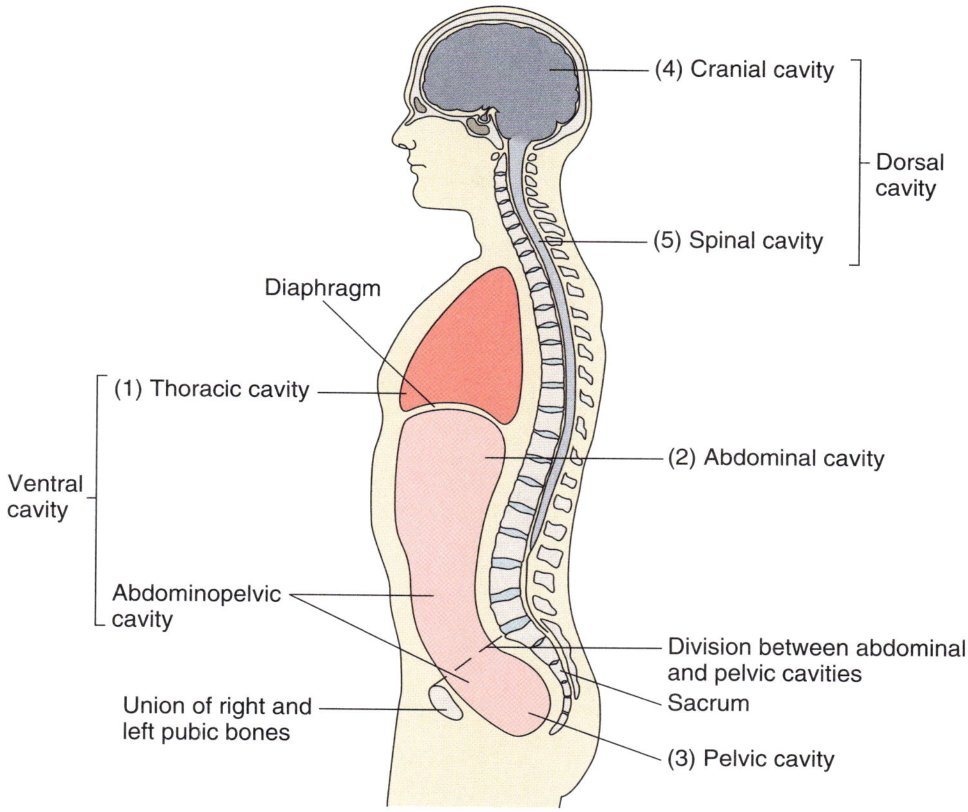

Figure 4-7 Major body cavities and subdivisions

exists upon McBurney's point, a physician might suspect appendicitis (inflammation of the appendix).

Body Cavities

The body has two major cavities, or hollow spaces, which contain orderly arrangements of internal body organs. These main body cavities are the **ventral** cavity and the **dorsal** cavity. Each of these is further divided into smaller cavities containing specific organs. **Figure 4-7** provides a visual reference for the major body cavities and their subdivisions.

Ventral Cavity Subdivisions

The ventral cavity, which contains the organs on the front, or "belly side," of the body, is subdivided into the thoracic cavity (chest cavity), the abdominal cavity, and the pelvic cavity.

(1) thoracic cavity
thorac/o = chest
-ic = pertaining to

The thoracic cavity contains the lungs, heart, aorta, esophagus, and trachea.

(2) abdominal cavity
abdomin/o = abdomen
-al = pertaining to

The **abdominal cavity** is separated from the thoracic cavity by the diaphragm (the muscle that aids in the process of breathing). The abdominal cavity contains the liver, gallbladder, spleen, stomach, pancreas, intestines, and kidneys.

(3) pelvic cavity
pelv/i = pelvis
-ic = pertaining to

The **pelvic cavity** contains the urinary bladder and reproductive organs. The pelvic cavity and the abdominal cavity are often addressed collectively as the **abdominopelvic cavity**, which refers to the space between the diaphragm and the groin.

Dorsal Cavity Subdivisions

The dorsal cavity, which contains the organs of the back side of the body, is subdivided into the cranial cavity and the spinal cavity.

(4) cranial cavity
crani/o = skull
-al = pertaining to

The cranial cavity contains the brain.

(5) spinal cavity
spin/o = spine
-al = pertaining to

The spinal cavity contains the nerves of the spinal cord.

Divisions of the Back

The back is subdivided into five sections that relate to the proximity (nearness) of each section to the vertebrae of the spinal column. The sections are named for the vertebrae located in that particular area of the back, as shown in **Figure 4-8.**

(1) cervical vertebrae
cervic/o = neck
-al = pertaining to

The cervical vertebrae, consisting of the first seven segments of the spinal column, make up the bones of the neck (cervic/o 5 neck). The abbreviations for the cervical vertebrae range from C1 to C7; these abbreviations are used to pinpoint the exact area of involvement with the cervical vertebrae.

(2) thoracic vertebrae
thorac/o = chest
-ic = pertaining to

The thoracic vertebrae, consisting of the next 12 segments, or vertebrae of the spinal column, make up the vertebral bones of the chest (thorac/o 5 chest or thorax). The abbreviations for the thoracic vertebrae range from T1 to T12; these abbreviations are also used to pinpoint the exact area of or involvement with the thoracic vertebrae.

(3) lumbar vertebrae
lumb/o = loins, lower back
-ar = pertaining to

The lumbar vertebrae consist of five large segments of the movable part of the spinal column. Identified as L1 through L5, the lumbar vertebrae are the largest and strongest of the vertebrae of the spinal column.

(4) sacrum
sacr/o = sacrum
-um = noun ending

The sacrum, located below the lumbar vertebrae, is the fourth segment of the spinal column. This single, triangular-shaped bone is a result of the fusion of the five individual sacral bones in the child.

(5) coccyx
(COCK-siks)

The fifth segment of the vertebral column is the coccyx. It is located at the very end of the vertebral column and is also called the tailbone.

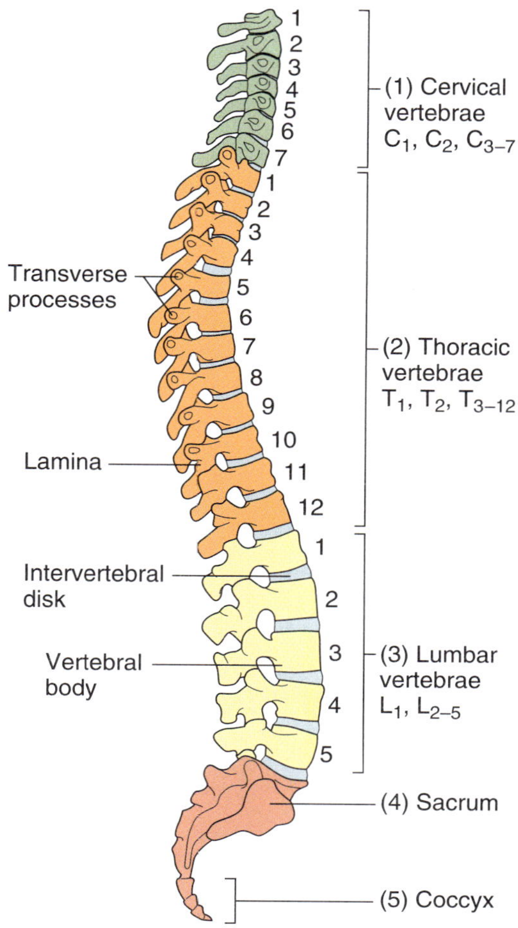

Figure 4-8 Divisions of the back

The adult coccyx is a single bone that is the result of the fusion of the four individual coccygeal bones in the child.

Direction

Directional terms are used by health professionals to define the specific location of a structure, to increase understanding when stating the relationship between body areas, and to indicate the position of the body for particular procedures. The standard reference position for the body as a whole, which gives meaning to these directional terms, is known as **anatomical position.** Anatomical position means that the person is standing with the arms at the sides and the palms turned forward. The individual's head and feet are also pointing forward. Directional terms often use the anatomical position and the midline of the body as reference points. **Figure 4-9** is a visual reference for the anatomical position and the directional terms.

The following is a list of the most commonly used directional terms (and definitions) that use the anatomical position and/or the midline of the body as reference points. Terms marked with an asterisk (*) are immediately followed by a term with the opposite meaning.

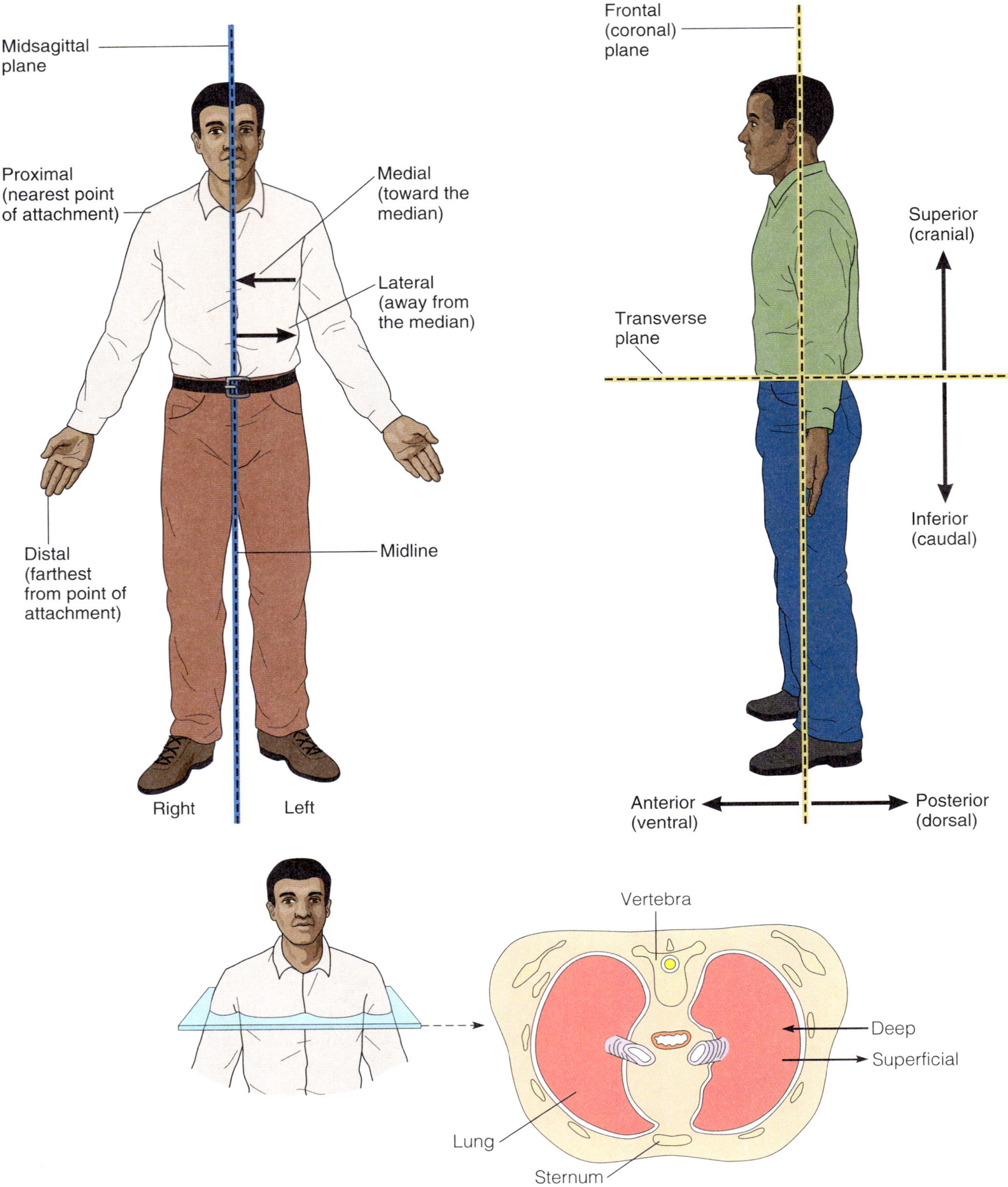

Figure 4-9 Anatomical position

WORD	MEANING
superficial*	Pertaining to the surface of the body, or near the surface.
deep	Away from the surface.
anterior* (an-**TEE**-ree-or)	Pertaining to the front of the body, or toward the belly of the body.
posterior (poss-**TEE**-ree-or)	Pertaining to the back of the body.
ventral* (**VEN**-tral) **ventr/o** = belly, front side **-al** = pertaining to	Of or pertaining to a position toward the belly of the body; frontward; **anterior**.
dorsal (**DOR**-sal) **dors/o** = back **-al** = pertaining to	Pertaining to the back or **posterior**.
medial* (**MEE**-dee-al) **medi/o** = middle **-al** = pertaining to	Toward the midline of the body.
lateral (**LAT**-er-al) **later/o** = side **-al** = pertaining to	Toward the side of the body, away from the midline of the body.
superior* (soo-**PEE**-ree-or)	Above or upward toward the head.
inferior (in-**FEE**-ree-or)	Below or downward toward the tail or feet.
cranial* (**KRAY**-nee-al) **crani/o** = skull **-al** = pertaining to	Pertaining to the head.
caudal (**KAWD**-al)	Pertaining to the tail.
distal* (**DISS**-tal)	Away from or farthest from the trunk of the body, or farthest from the point of origin of a body part.
proximal (**PROK**-sim-al) **proxim/o** = near **-al** = pertaining to	Toward or nearest to the trunk of the body, or nearest to the point of origin of a body part.

The following terms do not use the midline of the body as a reference point.

supine* (soo-**PINE**) 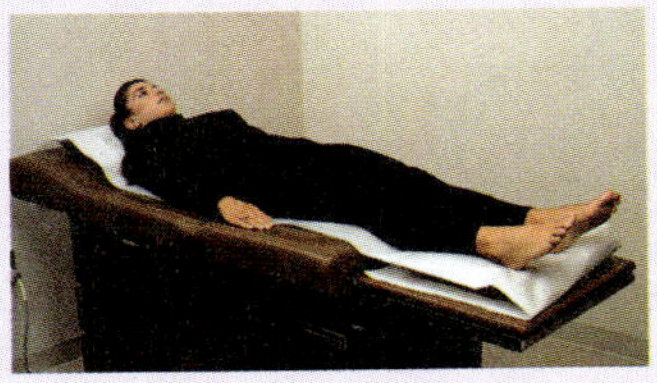	Lying horizontally on the back, faceup (see **Figure 4-10A**). **Figure 4-10A** Supine position
prone (**PROHN**) 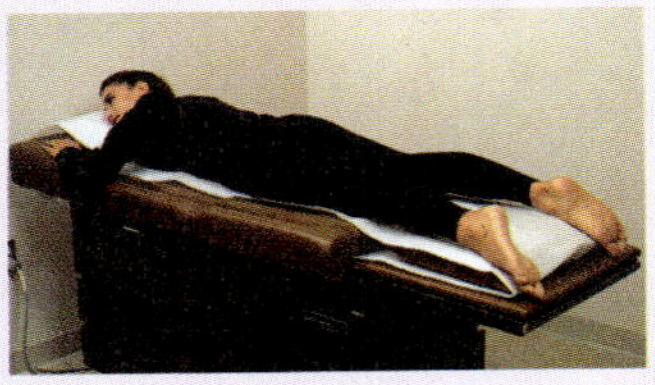	Lying facedown on the abdomen (see **Figure 4-10B**). **Figure 4-10B** Prone position
supination* (**soo**-pin-**AY**-shun)	A movement that allows the palms of the hands to turn upward or forward.
pronation (proh-**NAY**-shun)	A movement that allows the palms of the hands to turn downward and backward.
plantar* (**PLANT**-ar)	Pertaining to the sole or bottom of the foot.
dorsum (**DOR**-sum)	The back or posterior surface of a part; in the foot, the top of the foot.

Vocabulary

The following vocabulary words are frequently used when discussing the human body.

WORD	DEFINITION
abdominal cavity abdomin/o = abdomen -al = pertaining to	The cavity beneath the thoracic cavity that is separated from the thoracic cavity by the diaphragm; contains the liver, gallbladder, spleen, stomach, pancreas, intestines, and kidneys.
abdominopelvic cavity abdomin/o = abdomen pelv/i = pelvis -ic = pertaining to	A term that describes the abdominal and pelvic cavity collectively; refers to the space between the diaphragm and the groin.
anaplasia (an-ah-**PLAY**-zee-ah) ana- = not, without -plasia = formation, growth	A change in the structure and orientation of cells, characterized by a loss of differentiation and reversion to a more primitive form.

anatomical position	The standard reference position for the body as a whole: The person is standing with arms at the sides and palms turned forward; the individual's head and feet are also pointing forward.
anterior	Pertaining to the front of the body or toward the belly of the body.
aplasia (ah-**PLAY**-zee-ah) a- = without, not -plasia = formation, growth	A developmental failure resulting in the absence of any organ or tissue.
cardiac muscle cardi/o = heart -ac = pertaining to	The muscle that makes up the muscular wall of the heart.
caudal (**KAWD**-al)	Pertaining to the tail.
cell	The smallest and most numerous structural unit of living matter.
cell membrane	The semipermeable barrier that is the outer covering of a cell.
cervical vertebrae (**SER**-vic-al **VER**-teh-bray) cervic/o = neck -al = pertaining to	The first seven segments of the spinal column; identified as C1–C7.
chromosomes (**KROH**-moh-sohm)	The threadlike structures within the nucleus that control the functions of growth, repair, and reproduction for the body.
coccyx (**COCK**-siks)	The tailbone. Located at the end of the vertebral column, the coccyx results from the fusion of four individual coccygeal bones in the child.
connective tissue	Tissue that supports and binds other body tissue and parts.
cranial (**KRAY**-nee-al) crani/o = skull -al = pertaining to	Pertaining to the skull or cranium.
cranial cavity crani/o = skull -al = pertaining to	The cavity that contains the brain.
cytology (sigh-**TALL**-oh-jee) cyt/o = cell -logy = the study of	The study of cells.
cytoplasm (**SIGH**-toh-plazm) cyt/o = cell -plasm = living substance	A gel-like substance that surrounds the nucleus of a cell. The cytoplasm contains cell organs, called organelles, which carry out the essential functions of the cell.
deep	Away from the surface.
distal	Away from or farthest from the trunk of the body, or farthest from the point of origin of a body part.

dorsal dors/o = back -al = pertaining to	Pertaining to the back.
dorsum dors/o = back -um = noun ending	The back or posterior surface of a part; in the foot, the top of the foot.
dysplasia (dis-**PLAY**-zee-ah) dys- = bad, difficult, painful, disordered -plasia = formation, growth	Any abnormal development of tissues or organs.
epigastric region (**ep**-ih-**GAS**-trik **REE**-jun) epi- = upon, over gastr/o = stomach -ic = pertaining to	The region of the abdomen located between the right and left hypochondriac regions in the upper section of the abdomen, beneath the cartilage of the ribs.
epithelial tissue (**ep**-ih-**THEE**-lee-al **TISH**-oo)	The tissue that covers the internal and external organs of the body; it also lines the vessels, body cavities, glands, and body organs.
frontal plane	Any of the vertical planes passing through the body from the head to the feet, perpendicular to the sagittal planes and dividing the body into front and back portions.
genes	Segments of chromosomes that transmit hereditary characteristics.
histologist (hiss-**TALL**-oh-jist) hist/o = tissue -logist = one who specializes	A medical scientist who specializes in the study of tissues.
hyperplasia (**high**-per-**PLAY**-zee-ah) hyper- = excessive -plasia = formation, growth	An increase in the number of cells of a body part.
hypochondriac region (**high**-poh-**KON**-dree-ak **REE**-jun) hypo- = under, below, beneath, less than normal chondr/i = cartilage -ac = pertaining to	The right and left regions of the upper abdomen, beneath the cartilage of the lower ribs; located on either side of the epigastric region.
hypogastric region (**high**-poh-**GAS**-trik **REE**-jun) hypo- = under, below, beneath, less than normal gastr/o = stomach -ic = pertaining to	The middle section of the lower abdomen, beneath the umbilical region.

hypoplasia (**high**-poh-**PLAY**-zee-ah) hypo- = under, below, beneath, less than normal -plasia = formation, growth	Incomplete or underdeveloped organ or tissue, usually the result of a decrease in the number of cells.
inferior	Below or downward toward the tail or feet.
inguinal region (**ING**-gwih-nal) inguin/o = groin -al = pertaining to	The right and left regions of the lower section of the abdomen; also called the iliac region.
lateral later/o = side -al = pertaining to	Toward the side of the body, away from the midline of the body.
lumbar region lumb/o = loins -ar = pertaining to	The right and left regions of the middle section of the abdomen.
lumbar vertebrae lumb/o = loins, lower back -ar = pertaining to	The largest and strongest of the vertebrae of the spinal column, located in the lower back. The lumbar vertebrae consist of five large segments of the movable part of the spinal column; identified as L1–L5.
lysosomes (**LIGH**-soh-sohmz)	Cell organs, or organelles, that contain various kinds of enzymes capable of breaking down all of the main components of cells; lysosomes destroy bacteria by digesting them.
McBurney's point	A point on the right side of the abdomen, about two-thirds of the distance between the umbilicus and the anterior bony prominence of the hip.
medial (**MEE**-dee-al) medi/o = middle -al = pertaining to	Toward the midline of the body.
mediolateral (**MEE**-dee-oh-**LAT**-er-al) medi/o = middle later/o = side -al = pertaining to	Pertaining to the middle and side of a structure.
membrane	A thin layer of tissue that covers a surface, lines a cavity, or divides a space, such as the abdominal membrane that lines the abdominal wall.
midline of the body	The imaginary "line" that is created when the body is divided into equal right and left halves.
midsagittal plane (mid-**SAJ**-ih-tal)	The plane that divides the body or a structure into right and left equal portions.
mitochondria (my-toh-**KON**-dree-ah)	Cell organs, or organelles, which provide the energy needed by the cell to carry on its essential functions.

Munro's point (mun-**ROHZ**)	A point on the left side of the abdomen, about halfway between the umbilicus and the anterior bony prominence of the hip.
muscle tissue	The tissue that is capable of producing movement of the parts and organs of the body by contracting and relaxing its fibers.
navel (**NAY**-vel)	The umbilicus; the belly button.
neoplasia (**nee**-oh-**PLAY**-zee-ah) ne/o = new -plasia = formation, growth	The new and abnormal development of cells that may be benign or malignant.
nervous tissue	Tissue that transmits impulses throughout the body, thereby activating, coordinating, and controlling the many functions of the body.
nucleus (**NOO**-klee-us) nucle/o = nucleus -us = noun ending	The central controlling body within a living cell that is enclosed within the cell membrane.
organ	Tissues that are arranged together to perform a special function.
pelvic cavity pelv/i = pelvis -ic = pertaining to	The lower front cavity of the body, located beneath the abdominal cavity; contains the urinary bladder and reproductive organs.
peritoneum (pair-ih-toh-**NEE**-um) peritone/o = peritoneum -um = noun ending	A specific, serous membrane that covers the entire abdominal wall of the body and is reflected over the contained viscera.
plane	Imaginary slices, or cuts, made through the body as if a dividing sheet were passed through the body at a particular angle and in a particular direction, permitting a view from a different angle.
plantar (**PLANT**-ar)	Pertaining to the sole or bottom of the foot.
posterior (poss-**TEE**-ree-or)	Pertaining to the back of the body.
pronation (proh-**NAY**-shun)	A movement that allows the palms of the hands to turn downward and backward.
prone (**PROHN**)	Lying facedown on the abdomen.
proximal (**PROK**-sim-al) proxim/o = near -al = pertaining to	Toward or nearest to the trunk of the body, or nearest to the point of origin of a body part.
ribosomes (**RYE**-boh-sohmz)	Cell organs, or organelles, that synthesize proteins; often called the cell's "protein factories."

sacrum (**SAY**-krum) sacr/o = sacrum -um = noun ending	The singular, triangular-shaped bone that results from the fusion of the five individual sacral bones of the child.
skeletal muscle (**SKELL**-eh-tal) skelet/o = skeleton -al = pertaining to	Muscle that is attached to bone and is responsible for the movement of the skeleton.
smooth muscle	Muscle that is found in the walls of the hollow internal organs of the body such as the stomach and intestines.
spinal cavity spin/o = spine -al = pertaining to	The cavity that contains the nerves of the spinal cord; also known as the spinal canal.
superficial	Pertaining to the surface of the body, or near the surface.
superior	Above or upward toward the head.
supination (**soo**-pin-**AY**-shun)	A movement that allows the palms of the hands to turn upward or forward.
supine (soo-**PINE**)	Lying horizontally on the back, faceup.
system	Organs that work together to perform the many functions of the body as a whole.
thoracic cavity (tho-**RASS**-ik) thorac/o = chest -ic = pertaining to	The chest cavity, which contains the lungs, heart, aorta, esophagus, and trachea.
thoracic vertebrae (tho-**RASS**-ik) thorac/o = chest -ic = pertaining to	The second segment of 12 vertebrae that make up the vertebral bones of the chest; identified as T1–T12.
tissue	A group of cells that perform specialized functions.
transverse plane (trans-**VERS**)	Any of the planes cutting across the body perpendicular to the sagittal and the frontal planes, dividing the body into superior (upper) and inferior (lower) portions.
umbilical region umbilic/o = navel -al = pertaining to	The region of the abdomen located in the middle section of the abdomen, between the right and left lumbar regions and directly beneath the epigastric region.
umbilicus umbilic/o = navel -us = noun ending	The navel; also called the belly button.
ventral ventr/o = belly, front side -al = pertaining to	Pertaining to the front; belly side.

visceral
viscer/o = internal organs
-al = pertaining to

Pertaining to the internal organs.

visceral muscle
viscer/o = internal organs
-al = pertaining to

See *smooth muscle*.

Word Elements

The following word elements pertain to the body as a whole. As you review the list, pronounce each word element aloud twice and check the box after you "say it." Write the definition for the example word given for each word element. You may use your medical dictionary.

WORD ELEMENT	PRONUNCIATION	"SAY IT"	MEANING
abdomin/o **abdominal**	ab-**DOM**-ih-no ab-**DOM**-ih-nal	☐	abdomen
ana- **ana**plasia	an-ah **an**-ah-**PLAY**-zee-ah	☐	not, without
anter/o **anter**ior	an-**TEE**-ree-oh an-**TEE**-ree-or	☐	front
cervic/o **cervic**al	**SER**-vih-ko **SER**-vih-kal	☐	neck; cervix
coccyg/o **coccyg**eal vertebrae	**COCK**-si-goh cock-**SIJ**-ee-al **VER**-teh-bray	☐	coccyx
crani/o **crani**al	**KRAY**-nee-oh **KRAY**-nee-al	☐	skull, cranium
cyt/o **cyt**ology	**SIGH**-toh sigh-**TALL**-oh-jee	☐	cell
dors/o **dors**um	**DOR**-so **DOR**-sum	☐	back
dys- **dys**plasia	**DIS** dis-**PLAY**-zee-ah	☐	bad, difficult, painful, disordered
epi- **epi**gastric	**EP**-ih **ep**-ih-**GAS**-trik	☐	upon, over
hist/o **hist**ologist	**HISS**-toh hiss-**TALL**-oh-jist	☐	tissue

hypo- **hypo**chondriac region	**HIGH**-poh **high**-poh-**KON**-dree-ak	☐	under, below, beneath, less than normal
-iac card**iac** muscle	**EE**-ak **CAR**-dee-ak	☐	pertaining to
ili/o **ili**ac	**ILL**-ee-oh **ILL**-ee-ak	☐	ilium
inguin/o **inguin**al region	**ING**-gwih-no **ING**-gwih-nal	☐	groin
inter- **inter**vertebral	**IN**-ter in-ter-**VER**-teh-bral	☐	between
-ion supinat**ion**	**SHUN** **soo**-pin-**AY**-shun	☐	action, process
later/o **later**al	**LAT**-er-oh **LAT**-er-al	☐	side
lumb/o **lumb**ar vertebrae	**LUM**-boh **LUM**-bar	☐	loins, lower back
medi/o **medi**olateral	**MEE**-dee-oh **MEE**-dee-oh-**LAT**-er-al	☐	middle
nucle/o **nucle**ic acid	**NOO**-klee-oh **NOO**-klee-ic	☐	nucleus
pelv/i **pelv**ic cavity	**PELL**-vih **PELL**-vik	☐	pelvis
-plasm neo**plasm**	**PLAZM** **NEE**-oh-plazm	☐	living substance
poster/o **poster**ior	**POSS**-tee-roh poss-**TEE**-ree-or	☐	back
proxim/o **proxim**al	**PROK**-sim-oh **PROK**-sim-al	☐	near
sacr/o **sacr**um	**SAY**-kroh **SAY**-krum	☐	sacrum
-some chromo**some**	**SOHM** **KROH**-moh-sohm	☐	"a body" of a specified sort
spin/o **spin**al canal	**SPY**-noh **SPY**-nal	☐	spine

thorac/o **thoracic** vertebrae	**THO**-rah-koh tho-**RASS**-ik **VER**-teh-bray	☐	chest
umbilic/o **umbilical** region	um-**BILL**-ih-koh um-**BILL**-ih-kal	☐	navel
ventr/o **ventral**	**VEN**-troh **VEN**-tral	☐	belly, front side
vertebr/o **vertebral** column	**VER**-teh-broh **VER**-teh-bral	☐	vertebra
viscer/o **visceral** cavity	**VISS**-er-oh **VISS**-er-al	☐	internal organs

Common Abbreviations

ABBREVIATIONS	MEANING
RUQ	right upper quadrant
LUQ	left upper quadrant
RLQ	right lower quadrant
LLQ	left lower quadrant

Written and Audio Terminology Review

Review each of the following terms from the chapter. Study the spelling of each term and write the definition in the space provided. If you have the Audio CD available, listen to each term, pronounce it, and check the box once you are comfortable saying the word. Check definitions by looking the term up in the glossary/index.

TERM	PRONUNCIATION	DEFINITION
abdominal	☐ ab-**DOM**-ih-nal	________________
abdominal cavity	☐ ab-**DOM**-ih-nal **CAV**-ih-tee	________________
anaplasia	☐ **an**-ah-**PLAY**-zee-ah	________________
anterior	☐ an-**TEE**-ree-or	________________
aplasia	☐ ah-**PLAY**-zee-ah	________________

Term	Pronunciation	Definition
cardiac muscle	☐ **CAR**-dee-ak **MUS**-cle	______
caudal	☐ **KAWD**-al	______
cell membrane	☐ **SELL MEM**-brayn	______
cervical	☐ **SER**-vih-kal	______
cervical vertebrae	☐ **SER**-vih-kal **VER**-teh-bray	______
chromosomes	☐ **KROH**-moh-sohmz	______
coccygeal	☐ cock-**SIJ**-ee-al	______
coccyx	☐ **COCK**-siks	______
connective tissue	☐ kon-**NEK**-tiv **TISH**-yoo	______
cranial	☐ **KRAY**-nee-al	______
cranial cavity	☐ **KRAY**-nee-al **CAV**-ih-tee	______
cytology	☐ sigh-**TALL**-oh-jee	______
cytoplasm	☐ **SIGH**-toh-plazm	______
distal	☐ **DISS**-tal	______
dorsal	☐ **DOR**-sal	______
dorsum	☐ **DOR**-sum	______
dysplasia	☐ dis-**PLAY**-zee-ah	______
epigastric	☐ ep-ih-**GAS**-trik	______
epithelial	☐ **ep**-ih-**THEE**-lee-al	______
frontal	☐ **FRONT**-al	______
genes	☐ **JEENS**	______
histologist	☐ hiss-**TALL**-oh-jist	______
hyperplasia	☐ **high**-per-**PLAY**-zee-ah	______
hypochondriac	☐ **high**-poh-**KON**-dree-ak	______
hypogastric	☐ **high**-poh-**GAS**-trik	______
hypoplasia	☐ **high**-poh-**PLAY**-zee-ah	______
iliac	☐ **ILL**-ee-ak	______
inferior	☐ in-**FEE**-ree-or	______
inguinal	☐ **ING**-gwih-nal	______
intervertebral	☐ **in**-ter-**VER**-teh-bral	______
lateral	☐ **LAT**-er-al	______

Term	Pronunciation	
lumbar	☐ **LUM**-bar	______
lumbar vertebrae	☐ **LUM**-bar **VER**-teh-bray	______
lysosomes	☐ **LIGH**-soh-sohmz	______
McBurney's point	☐ Mc-**BURN**-eez **POINT**	______
medial	☐ **MEE**-dee-al	______
mediolateral	☐ **mee**-dee-oh-**LAT**-er-al	______
membrane	☐ **MEM**-brayn	______
midline	☐ **MID**-line	______
midsagittal	☐ **mid**-**SAJ**-ih-tal	______
mitochondria	☐ **my**-toh-**KON**-dree-ah	______
Munro's point	☐ mun-**ROHZ POINT**	______
muscle	☐ **MUS**-cle	______
navel	☐ **NAY**-vel	______
neoplasia	☐ **nee**-oh-**PLAY**-zee-ah	______
neoplasm	☐ **NEE**-oh-plazm	______
nervous	☐ **NER**-vus	______
nucleic acid	☐ **NOO**-klee-ic **ASS**-id	______
nucleus	☐ **NOO**-klee-us	______
organ	☐ **OR**-gan	______
pelvic cavity	☐ **PELL**-vik **CAV**-ih-tee	______
peritoneum	☐ **pair**-ih-toh-**NEE**-um	______
plane	☐ **PLANE**	______
plantar	☐ **PLANT**-ar	______
posterior	☐ poss-**TEE**-ree-or	______
pronation	☐ proh-**NAY**-shun	______
prone	☐ **PROHN**	______
proximal	☐ **PROK**-sim-al	______
ribosomes	☐ **RYE**-boh-sohmz	______
sacrum	☐ **SAY**-krum	______
skeletal muscle	☐ **SKELL**-eh-tal **MUS**-cle	______
smooth muscle	☐ **SMOOTH MUS**-cle	______

spinal canal	☐ **SPY**-nal kah-**NAL**	______
spinal cavity	☐ **SPY**-nal **CAV**-ih-tee	______
superficial	☐ **soo**-per-**FISH**-al	______
superior	☐ soo-**PEE**-ree-or	______
supination	☐ **soo**-pin-**AY**-shun	______
supine	☐ soo-**PINE**	______
system	☐ **SIS**-tem	______
thoracic	☐ tho-**RASS**-ik	______
thoracic cavity	☐ tho-**RASS**-ik **CAV**-ih-tee	______
tissue	☐ **TISH**-yoo	______
transverse	☐ trans-**VERS**	______
umbilical	☐ um-**BILL**-ih-kal	______
umbilicus	☐ um-**BILL**-ih-kus	______
ventral	☐ **VEN**-tral	______
vertebral column	☐ **VER**-teh-bral **CALL**-um	______
visceral	☐ **VISS**-er-al	______
visceral cavity	☐ **VISS**-er-al **CAV**-ih-tee	______
visceral muscle	☐ **VISS**-er-al **MUS**-cle	______

Chapter Review Exercises

The following exercises provide a more in-depth review of the chapter material. Your goal in these exercises is to complete each section at a minimum 80% level of accuracy. A space has been provided for your score at the end of each section.

A. Term to Definition

Define each term by writing the definition in the space provided. Check the box if you are able to complete this exercise correctly the first time (without referring to the answers). Each correct answer is worth 10 points. Record your score in the space provided at the end of the exercise.

☐ 1. prone ______

☐ 2. cervical vertebrae ______

☐ 3. cytology ______

☐ 4. dorsum ______

☐ 5. epigastric ______

☐ 6. supination ____________________

☐ 7. pronation ____________________

☐ 8. lateral ____________________

☐ 9. mediolateral ____________________

☐ 10. supine ____________________

Number correct _______ × 10 points/correct answer: Your score _______%

B. Labeling

Label the nine regions of the body. Each correct response is worth 10 points. If you get all nine regions correct, without referring to your textbook, give yourself a bonus of 10 points for a total of 100 points. Record your score in the space provided at the end of the exercise.

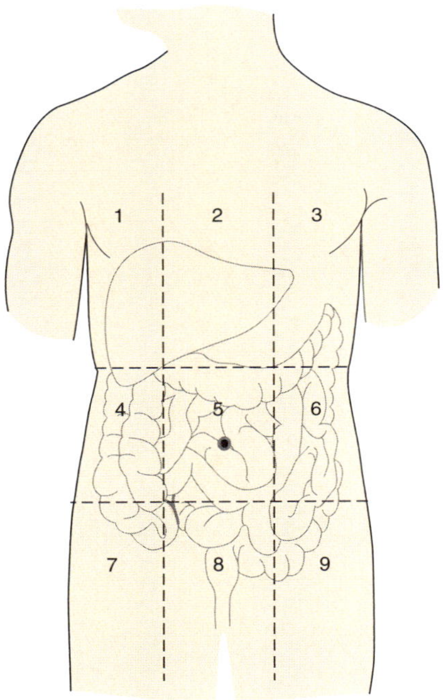

1. ____________________
2. ____________________
3. ____________________
4. ____________________
5. ____________________
6. ____________________
7. ____________________
8. ____________________
9. ____________________

Number correct _______ × 10 points/correct answer: Subtotal _______

10-point bonus for getting all answers correct + _______

Total number of points earned _______

C. Crossword Puzzle

Each crossword answer is worth 10 points. When you have completed the crossword puzzle, total your points and enter your score in the space provided.

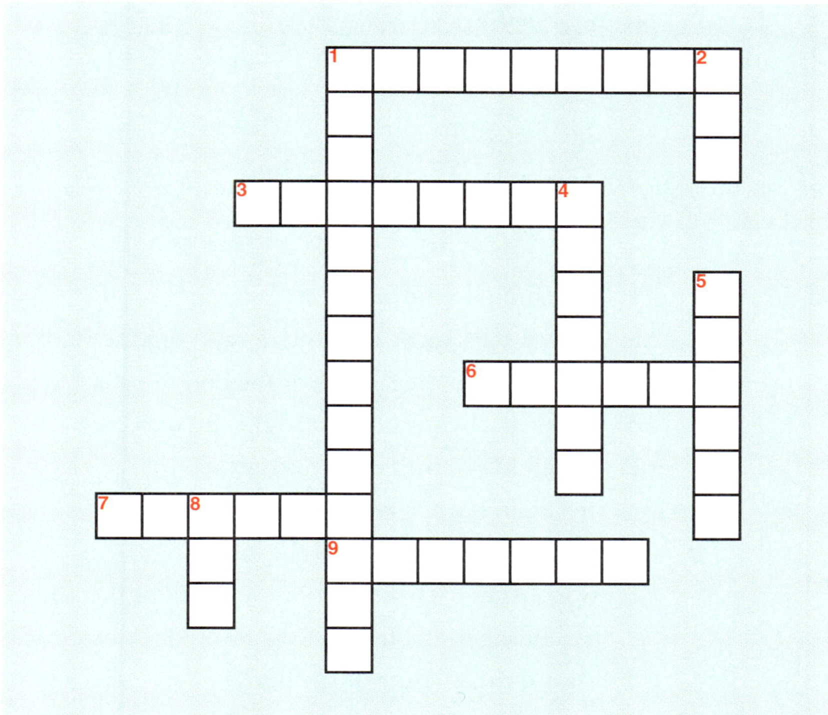

ACROSS

1 Pertaining to the abdomen
3 Cavity that contains the lungs
6 Cavity that contains spinal cord nerves
7 Pertains to the back side of body
9 "Belly side" of the body

DOWN

1 Cavity between diaphragm and groin
2 Left upper quadrant (abbreviation)
4 Cavity that contains the brain
5 Cavity that contains reproductive organs
8 Right lower quadrant (abbreviation)

***Number correct* _______ × *10 points/correct answer: Your score* _______%**

D. Completion

Complete each sentence with the most appropriate answer. Each correct answer is worth 10 points. Record your score in the space provided at the end of the exercise.

1. The fourth segment of the spinal column is a fused, triangular-shaped bone that once consisted in the child as five individual bones; it is called the ______________________________.
2. The tailbone is known as the ______________________________.
3. The smallest and most numerous unit of living matter is the ______________________________.
4. The semipermeable barrier that surrounds the cell is known as the ______________________________.
5. The central controlling body within a living cell is known as the ______________________________.
6. The gel-like substance that surrounds the nucleus of the cell is the ______________________________.
7. The term that describes any abnormal development of tissues or organs is ______________________________.
8. The term that describes new and abnormal development of cells that may be benign or malignant is ______________________________.

9. The term that refers to a developmental failure resulting in the absence of any organ or tissue is ______________________________.

10. The term that refers to an increase in the number of cells of a body part is ______________.

Number correct ______ × 10 points/correct answer: Your score ______%

E. Matching the Directional Terms

Match the descriptions on the right with the appropriate directional term on the left. Each correct answer is worth 10 points. Record your answers in the space provided at the end of the exercise.

______	1. superficial	a. pertaining to the head
______	2. anterior	b. toward the side of the body, away from the midline of the body
______	3. dorsal	c. pertaining to the surface of the body, or near the surface
______	4. medial	d. below or downward toward the tail or feet
______	5. lateral	e. pertaining to the back or posterior
______	6. superior	f. pertaining to the tail
______	7. inferior	g. above or upward toward the head
______	8. cranial	h. away from or farthest from the trunk of the body
______	9. caudal	i. pertaining to the front of the body, or toward the belly of the body
______	10. distal	j. toward the midline of the body

Number correct ______ × 10 points/correct answer: Your score ______%

F. Spelling

Circle the correctly spelled term in each pairing of words. Each correct answer is worth 10 points. Record your score in the space provided at the end of the exercise.

1. coccyx	coccyxx
2. midsaggital	midsagittal
3. MacBurney's	McBurney's
4. mediolateral	medialateral
5. peritoneum	peritoneim
6. ribosomes	ribysomes
7. viseral	visceral
8. umbilicus	umbillicus
9. navul	navel
10. dysplasia	dysplacia

Number correct ______ × 10 points/correct answer: Your score ______%

G. Definition of Term

Identify and provide the medical term to match the definition provided. Each correct answer is worth 10 points. Record your score in the space provided at the end of the exercise.

1. Pertaining to the abdomen.

   ____

2. The study of cells.

   ____

3. Without development.

   ____

4. One who specializes in the study of tissues.

   ____

5. New and abnormal development of cells that may be benign or malignant.

   ____

6. Pertaining to the sole or bottom of the foot.

   ____

7. The threadlike structures within the nucleus of the cell that control the functions of growth, repair, and reproduction for the body.

   ____

8. Pertaining to the skull or cranium.

   ____

9. The umbilicus; the belly button.

   ____

10. Tissues that are arranged together to perform a special function.

   ____

Number correct _______ × 10 points/correct answer: Your score _______%

H. Multiple Choice

Read each statement carefully and select the correct answer from the options listed. Each correct answer is worth 10 points. Record your score in the space provided at the end of the exercise.

1. A change in the structure and orientation of cells, characterized by a loss of differentiation to a more primitive form ("without formation"), is known as:
   a. neoplasia
   b. anaplasia
   c. dysplasia
   d. hypoplasia
2. The new and abnormal development of cells that may be benign or malignant ("new formation") is known as:
   a. neoplasia
   b. anaplasia
   c. dysplasia
   d. hypoplasia

3. A developmental failure resulting in the absence of any organ or tissue ("without formation") is known as:
    a. hyperplasia
    b. hypoplasia
    c. aplasia
    d. neoplasia
4. Any abnormal development of tissues ("disordered formation") is known as:
    a. neoplasia
    b. aplasia
    c. dysplasia
    d. anaplasia
5. An increase in the number of cells of a body part ("excessive formation") is known as:
    a. hyperplasia
    b. hypoplasia
    c. aplasia
    d. neoplasia
6. Incomplete or underdeveloped organ or tissue, usually the result of a decrease in the number of cells ("less than, under formation"), is known as:
    a. hyperplasia
    b. hypoplasia
    c. aplasia
    d. neoplasia
7. When a person is standing with the arms at the sides and the palms turned forward, with the head and feet pointing forward, the individual is said to be in what position?
    a. supine
    b. anatomical
    c. prone
    d. lateral
8. The medical term that means "pertaining to the tail" is:
    a. caudal
    b. cranial
    c. dorsal
    d. ventral
9. The imaginary "line" created when the body is divided into equal right and left halves is called the:
    a. transverse plane
    b. midline of the body
    c. frontal plane
    d. coronal plane
10. The navel, or belly button, is also known as the:
    a. umbilicus
    b. nucleus
    c. Monroe's point
    d. McBurney's point

Number correct _______ × 10 points/correct answer: Your score _______%

I. Word Element Review

The following words relate to the chapter on whole body terms. The prefixes, suffixes, and combining vowels have been provided. Read the definition carefully and complete the word by filling in the space, using the word elements provided in the chapter. Each correct answer is worth 10 points. Record your score in the space provided at the end of the exercise.

1. Pertaining to the abdomen
   ______________/ al
2. Pertaining to the neck
   ______________/ al
3. The study of cells
   ______________/o/ logy
4. Pertaining to the side
   ______________/ al
5. Pertaining to the belly or front side
   ______________/ al
6. A new growth ("cell or tissue substance")
   neo/ ______________
7. Without formation or growth
   ______________/ plasia
8. Pertaining to the skull
   ______________/ al
9. Pertaining to between the vertebrae
   ______________/ vertebral
10. Pertaining to internal organs
    ______________/ al

Number correct _______ × 10 points/correct answer: Your score _______%

J. Labeling

The figures below illustrate directional terms and various planes of the body. Study the figures carefully and label the numbered items appropriately. Each correct response is worth 10 points. Record your score in the space provided at the end of the exercise.

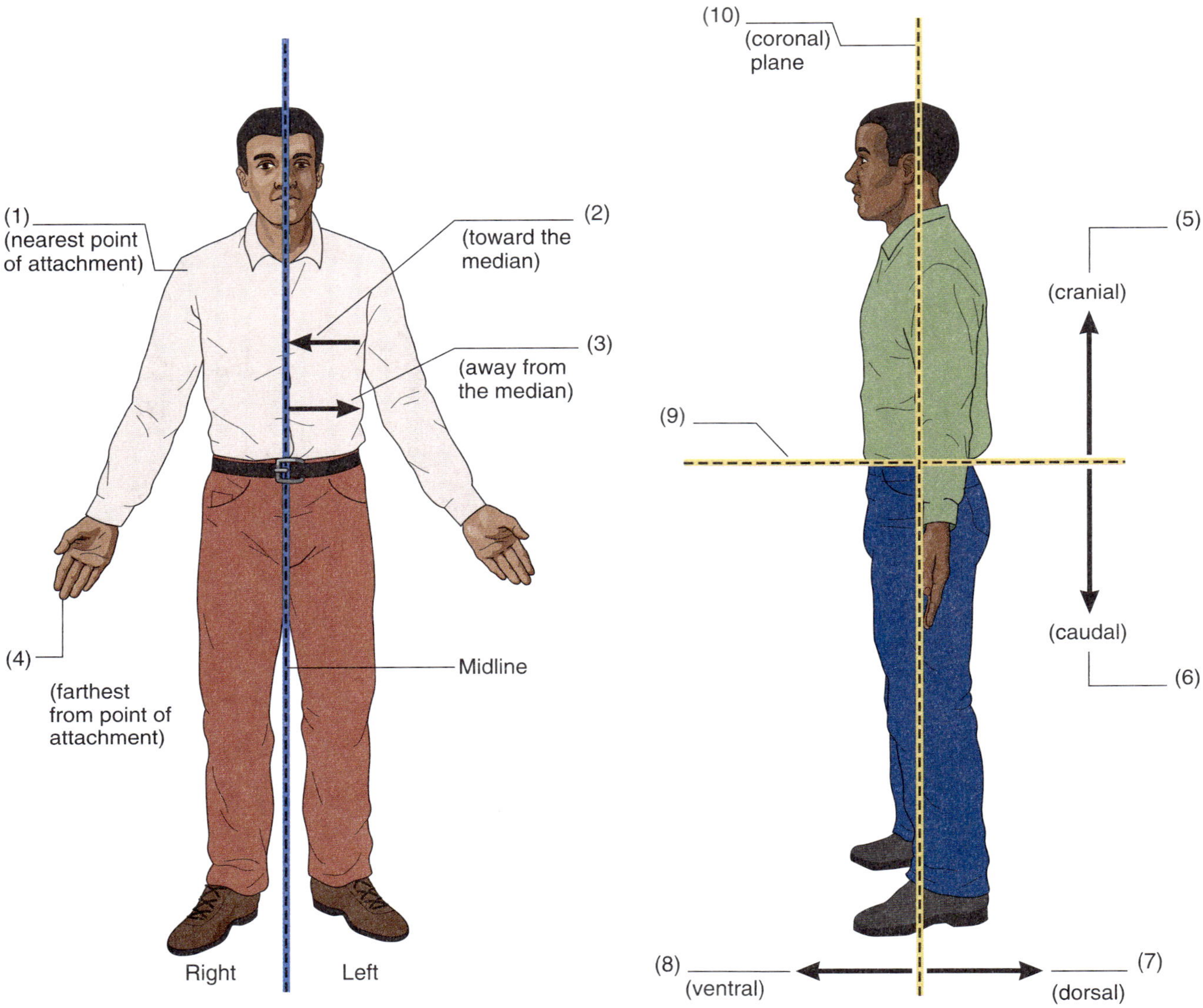

1. ______________________________
2. ______________________________
3. ______________________________
4. ______________________________
5. ______________________________
6. ______________________________
7. ______________________________
8. ______________________________
9. ______________________________
10. ______________________________

Number correct _______ × 10 points/correct answer: Your score _______%

Answers to Chapter Review Exercises

A. Term to Definition

1. Lying facedown on the abdomen.
2. The first seven segments of the spinal column.
3. The study of cells.
4. The back or posterior surface of a part; in the foot, the top of the foot.
5. The region of the abdomen located between the right and left hypochondriac regions, in the upper section of the abdomen, beneath the cartilage of the ribs.
6. A movement that allows the palms of the hands to turn upward or forward.
7. A movement that allows the palms of the hands to turn downward and backward.
8. Toward the side of the body, away from the midline.
9. Pertaining to the middle and side of a structure.
10. Lying horizontally on the back, faceup.

B. Labeling

1. Right hypochondriac region
2. Epigastric region
3. Left hypochondriac region
4. Right lumbar region
5. Umbilical region
6. Left lumbar region
7. Right inguinal region
8. Hypogastric region
9. Left inguinal region

C. Crossword Puzzle

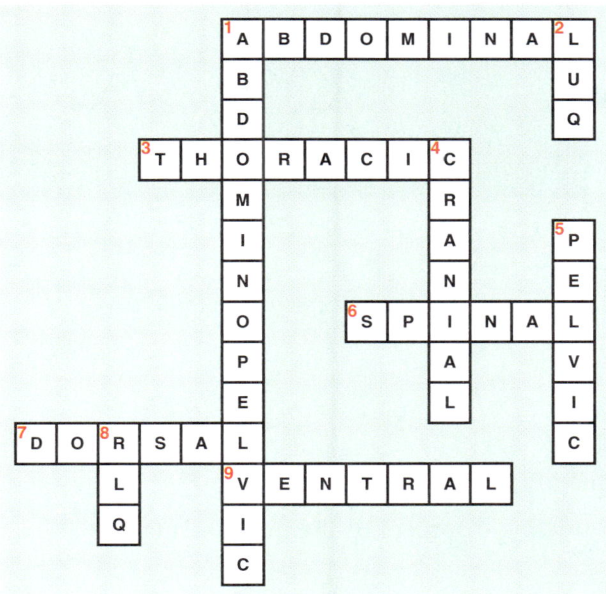

D. Completion

1. sacrum
2. coccyx
3. cell
4. cell membrane
5. nucleus
6. cytoplasm
7. dysplasia
8. neoplasm
9. aplasia
10. hyperplasia

E. Matching the Directional Terms

1. c
2. i
3. e
4. j
5. b
6. g
7. d
8. a
9. f
10. h

F. Spelling

1. coccyx
2. midsagittal
3. McBurney's
4. mediolateral
5. peritoneum
6. ribosomes
7. visceral
8. umbilicus
9. navel
10. dysplasia

G. Definition of Term

1. abdominal
2. cytology
3. aplasia
4. histologist
5. neoplasm
6. plantar
7. chromosomes
8. cranial
9. navel
10. organs

H. Multiple Choice

1. b
2. a
3. c
4. c
5. a
6. b
7. b
8. a
9. b
10. a

I. Word Element Review

1. abdomin
2. cervic
3. cyt
4. later
5. ventr
6. plasm
7. ana
8. crani
9. inter
10. viscer

J. Labeling

1. proximal
2. medial
3. lateral
4. distal
5. superior
6. inferior
7. posterior
8. anterior
9. transverse plane
10. frontal plane

CHAPTER 5

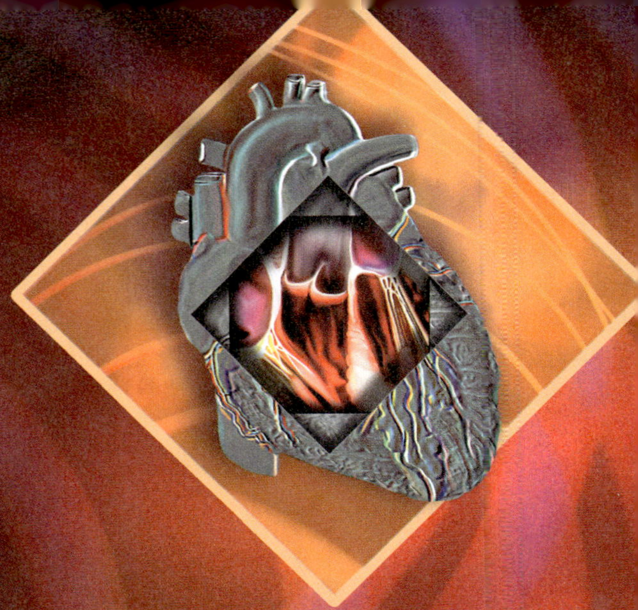

The Integumentary System

CHAPTER CONTENT

KEY COMPETENCIES

Upon completing this chapter and the review exercises at the end of the chapter, the learner should be able to:

1. Identify the major structures of the skin.
2. List five functions of the skin.
3. Identify and define 20 pathological conditions of the integumentary system.
4. Identify at least 10 diagnostic techniques used in treating disorders of the integumentary system.
5. Correctly spell and pronounce each new term introduced in this chapter using the Activity CD-ROM and Audio CD, if available.
6. Identify at least 10 skin lesions, based on their descriptions.
7. Create at least 10 medical terms related to the integumentary system and identify the appropriate combining form(s) for each term.
8. Identify at least 20 abbreviations common to the integumentary system.

OVERVIEW

One of the body's most important organs is the skin. This protective covering is part of the **integumentary system,** which consists of the skin, hair, nails, sweat glands, and oil glands. Also known as the **integument** or the **cutaneous membrane,** the skin has five basic functions:

1. The skin protects the body against invasion by microorganisms and protects underlying body structures and delicate tissues from injury. The pigment melanin, which provides color to the skin, further protects the skin from the harmful effects of the ultraviolet rays of the sun.
2. The skin regulates body temperature by protecting the body from excessive loss of heat and fluids from underlying tissues. **Sweat glands,** which are located under the skin, secrete a watery fluid that cools the body as it evaporates from the surface of the skin.
3. The skin serves as a sensory receptor for sensations such as touch, pressure, pain, and temperature; these sensations are detected by the nerve endings within the skin and then are relayed to the brain. The appearance of the skin, in the form of facial expressions (e.g., grimaces, shivering, frowns, or smiles), is sometimes visible evidence of the sensations felt by the skin.
4. The skin provides for elimination of body wastes in the form of perspiration. Substances such as water, salts, and some fatty substances are excreted through the **pores** (openings) of the skin.
5. The skin is responsible for the first step in the synthesis of vitamin D, which is essential for bone growth and development. When exposed to the ultraviolet rays of the sun, molecules within the skin are converted to a chemical which is transported in the blood to the liver and kidneys, where it is converted into vitamin D.

The study of the skin is known as **dermatology**. The physician who specializes in the treatment of diseases and disorders of the skin is known as a **dermatologist.**

Anatomy and Physiology

The main structures of the skin include the epidermis, dermis, and subcutaneous layers. As we discuss these structures, refer to **Figure 5-1** for a visual reference.

Epidermis

The (**1**) **epidermis,** the outer layer of the skin, contains no blood or nerve supply. It consists of squamous epithelial cells, which are flat, scalelike, and arranged in layers (strata). The epidermis actually has about five different layers of stratified epithelium cells, each carrying on specific functions. The two layers of the epidermis that will be mentioned here are the stratum basale and the stratum corneum. The base layer (**stratum basale**) is where new cells are continually being reproduced, pushing older cells toward the outermost surface of the skin. The basal layer also contains **melanocytes,** which provide color to the skin and some protection from the harmful effects of the ultraviolet rays of

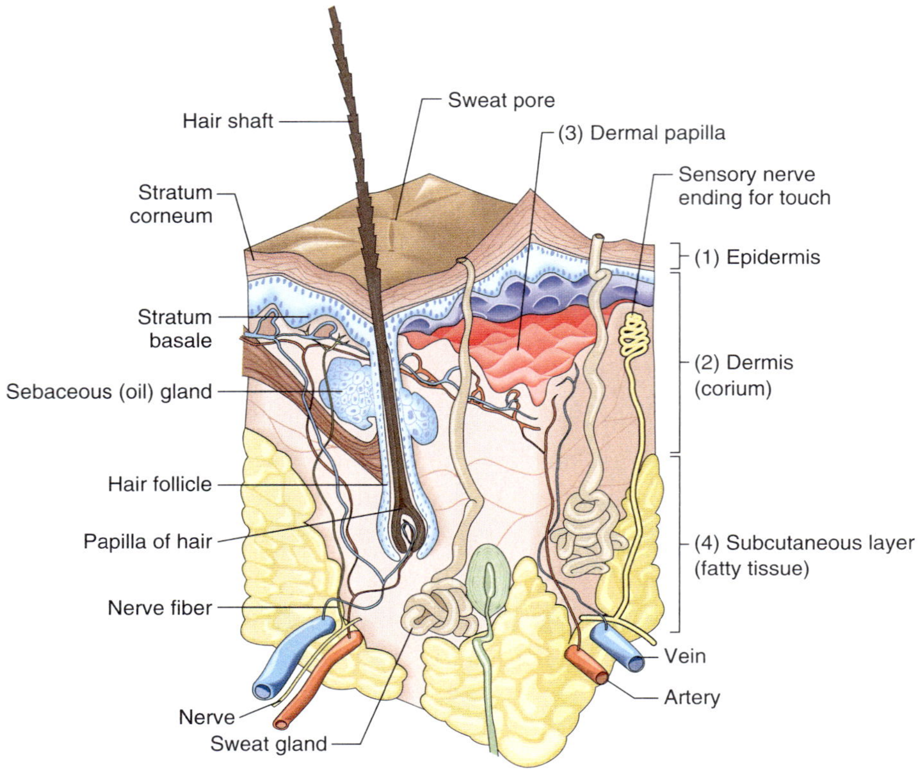

Figure 5-1 Layers and structures of the skin

the sun. The outermost layer of the epidermis is the **stratum corneum,** where the dead skin cells are constantly being shed and replaced. When the cells reach the outermost layer of the epidermis and die, they become filled with a hard, water-repellant protein called **keratin.** This characteristic of keratin (waterproofing the body) creates a barrier, or a first line of defense for the body, by not allowing water to penetrate the skin or to be lost from the body, and by not allowing microorganisms to penetrate the unbroken skin. If the skin is injured and the barrier layer is damaged, microorganisms and other contaminants can easily pass through the epidermis to the lower layers of the skin, and fluids can escape the body (as occurs with burns).

Dermis

The (2) **dermis** is the inner, thicker layer of skin lying directly beneath the epidermis; it is also known as the **corium.** It protects the body against mechanical injury and compression and serves as a reservoir (storage area) for water and electrolytes. Composed of living tissue, the dermis contains capillaries, lymphatic channels, and nerve endings. The hair follicles, sweat glands, and **sebaceous** (oil) glands are also embedded in the dermis. The dermis contains both connective tissue and elastic fibers to give it strength and elasticity. If the elastic fibers of the dermis are overstretched as a result of rapid increase in size of the abdomen, for example, due to obesity or during pregnancy, the fibers will weaken and tear. These linear tears in the dermis are known as **stretch marks** or **stria.** They begin as pinkish-blue streaks with jagged edges and may be accompanied by itching. As they heal and lose their color, the stria remain as silvery-white scar lines.

The thickness of the dermis varies from the very thin, delicate layers of the eyelids to the thicker layers of the palms of the hands and soles of the feet. Look at your hands and

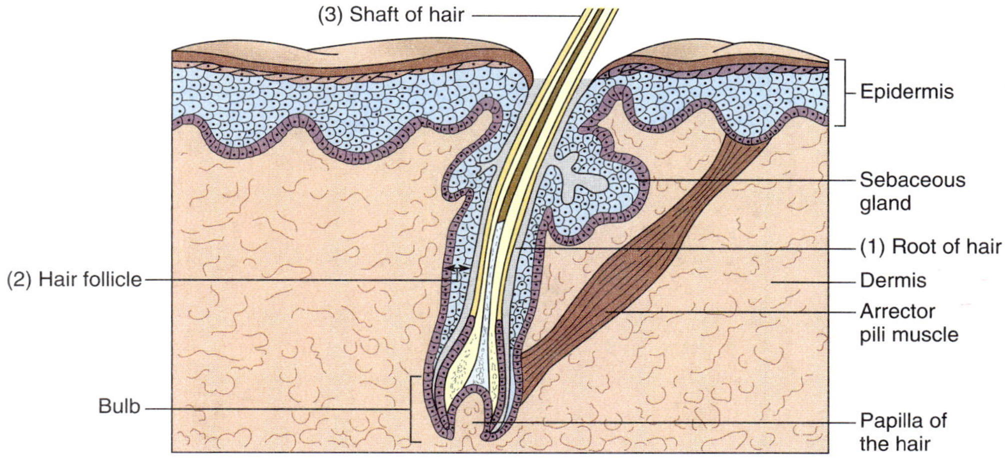

Figure 5-2 Structure of the hair

notice the distinct pattern of ridges on your fingertips. These ridges provide friction for grasping objects and are a result of the papillae (projections) of the superficial layer of the dermis that extend into the epidermis. The thin layer of the epidermis conforms to the ridges of the **(3)** dermal papillae, forming the characteristic ridges that you are observing on your fingertips. In each of us, these ridges form a unique pattern that is genetically determined. These patterns are the basis of fingerprints and footprints.

Subcutaneous Layer

The **(4)** **subcutaneous tissue,** which lies just beneath the dermis, consists largely of loose connective tissue and adipose (fatty) tissue that connects the skin to the surface muscles. It is sometimes called the superficial fascia or subcutaneous fascia. The subcutaneous, or fatty, tissue serves as insulation for the body and protects the deeper tissues. It is rich in nerves and nerve endings, including those that supply the dermis and epidermis. The major blood vessels that supply the skin pass through the subcutaneous layer, and sweat glands and hair roots extend from the dermis down into the subcutaneous layer. The thickness of the subcutaneous layer varies, from the thinnest layer over the eyelids to the thickest layer over the abdomen.

Accessory Structures

The accessory structures of the skin consist of the hair, nails, and glands.

Hair

A strand of hair, **Figure 5-2,** is a long slender filament of keratin that consists of a (1) hair **root,** which is embedded in the (2) hair **follicle,** and a (3) hair **shaft,** which is the visible part of the hair. Each hair develops within the hair follicle, with any new hair forming from the keratin cells located at the bottom of the follicles.

Hair covers most of the human body, with the exception of the palms of the hands, the soles of the feet, the lips, nipples, and some areas of the genitalia. Toward the end of the second trimester of pregnancy (around the fifth month), the developing fetus is almost completely covered with a soft, downy (very fine) hair known as **lanugo.** This hairy

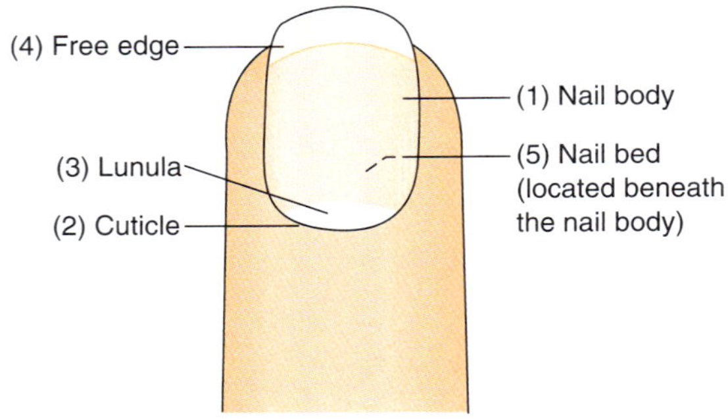

Figure 5-3 Structure of the nail

coating is almost completely gone by birth, with any remaining lanugo disappearing shortly after birth. When present at birth, lanugo appears as a very fine, velvety coating of hair over the baby's skin.

Hair gets its color from the melanocytes (darkly pigmented cells) that surround the core of the hair shaft. These cells produce **melanin**, which gives hair a black or brown color, depending on the amount produced. A unique type of melanin containing iron is responsible for red hair. When hair turns grey or white, usually due to the aging process, the amount of melanin has decreased significantly in the hair.

Nails

The fingernails and toenails are protective coverings for the tips of the fingers and toes. These hard, keratinized nail beds cover the dorsal surface of the last bone of each finger or toe. See **Figure 5-3.**

The visible part of the nail is called the **(1) nail body.** The fold of skin at the base of the nail body is known as the **(2) cuticle.** Beneath the cuticle is the extension of the nail body known as the root of the nail; it lies in a groove hidden by the cuticle. At the base of the nail body nearest the root is a crescent-shaped white area known as the **(3) lunula.** The **(4) free edge** of the nail extends beyond the tip of the finger tip or toe. Nails grow approximately 0.5 mm per week. The nail body is nourished by the **(5) nail bed,** which is an epithelial layer located directly beneath it. The rich supply of blood vessels contained in the nail bed generate the pink color you can see through the translucent nail bodies.

Glands

The glands of the skin complete the accessory structures of the skin. Refer to **Figure 5-4.**

The **(1) sweat,** or **sudoriferous, gland** is a small structure that originates deep within the dermis and ends at the surface of the skin with a tiny opening called a **(2) pore.** The sweat glands are found on almost all body surfaces, particularly the palms of the hands, soles of the feet, forehead, and armpits (axillae). Two main functions of the sweat glands are to cool the body by evaporation and to eliminate waste products through their pores.

The sweat glands produce a clear watery fluid known as **sweat** or **perspiration,** which travels from the gland to the surface of the skin where it is excreted through the pores.

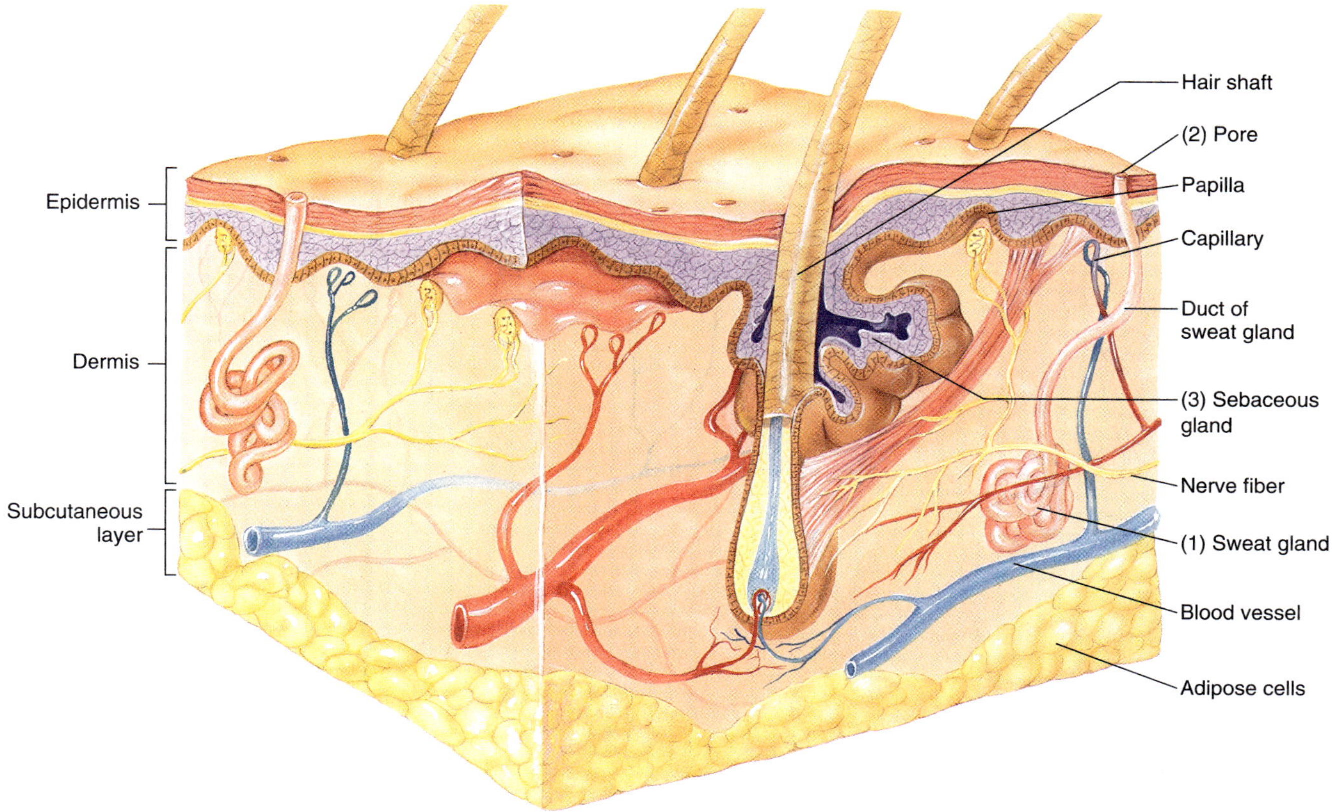

Figure 5-4 Glands of the skin

As the sweat evaporates from the surface of the skin into the air, it creates a cooling effect on the body.

In addition to being clear or colorless, sweat is odorless. It is made up of mostly water containing a small amount of dissolved substances such as salts, ammonia, uric acid, urea, and other waste products. These waste products are eliminated from the body through the pores of the sweat glands. As the sweat comes in contact with the bacteria present on the surface of the skin, it becomes contaminated and decomposes. This interaction of the sweat with the bacteria found on the surface of the skin creates the odor we often associate with sweating.

The (**3**) **sebaceous gland,** also known as the **oil gland,** secretes a substance necessary for lubricating the hair and keeping the skin soft and waterproof. This substance, known as **sebum,** is secreted along the shaft of the hair follicles and directly onto the skin through ducts that open directly onto the epidermis.

Secretion of sebum is influenced by the sex hormones and increases during adolescence. As a result of this increased secretion of sebum, the sebaceous gland ducts often become blocked and a **pimple** or **blackhead** may develop. The sebaceous glands, present throughout most of the body, are more numerous on the scalp, forehead, face, and chin; they are absent on the palms of the hands and the soles of the feet.

The **ceruminous gland** is actually classified as a modified sweat gland. Opening onto the free surface of the external ear canal, the ceruminous glands lubricate the skin of the ear canal with a yellowish-brown waxy substance, called **cerumen,** also known as ear wax.

Vocabulary

The following vocabulary words are frequently used when discussing the integumentary system.

WORD	DEFINITION
abrasion (ah-**BRAY**-zhun)	A scraping or rubbing away of skin or mucous membrane as a result of friction to the area.
abscess (**AB**-sess)	A localized collection of pus in any part of the body.
albino (al-**BYE**-noh)	An individual with a marked deficiency of pigment in the eyes, hair, and skin.
alopecia (al-oh-**PEE**-she-ah) 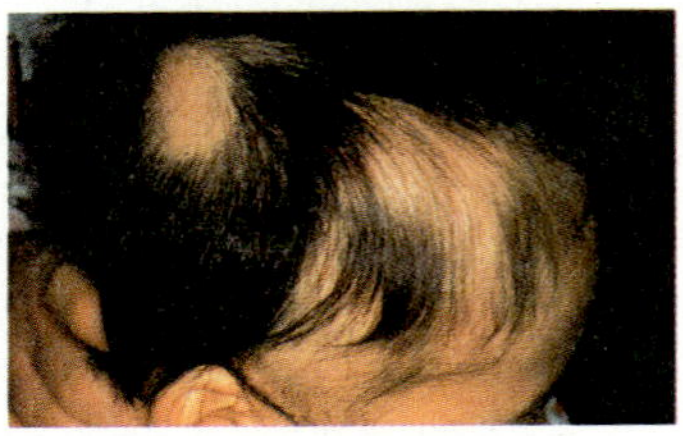	Partial or complete loss of hair. **Alopecia** may result from normal aging, a reaction to a medication such as anticancer medications, an endocrine disorder, or some skin disease. See **Figure 5-5.** **Figure 5-5** Alopecia (Courtesy of Robert A. Silverman, M.D., Clinical Associate Professor, Department of Pediatrics, Georgetown University)
amputation (am-pew-**TAY**-shun)	The surgical removal of a part of the body or a limb or a part of a limb; performed to treat recurrent infections or gangrene of a limb.
basal layer (**BAY**-sal layer)	The deepest of the five layers of the skin.
bedsore 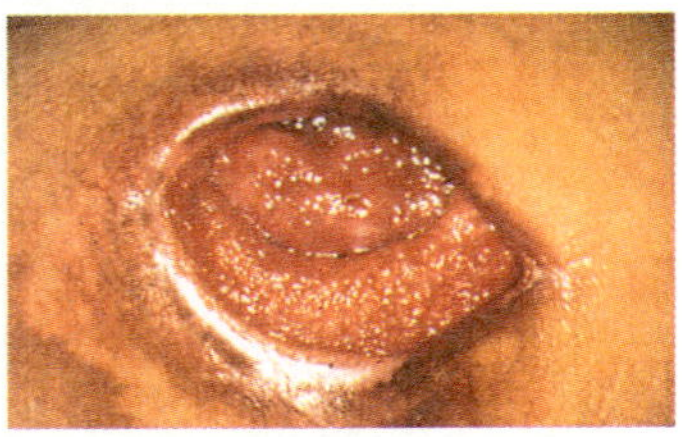	An inflammation, sore, or **ulcer** in the skin over a bony prominence of the body, resulting from loss of blood supply and oxygen to the area due to prolonged pressure on the body part; also known as a pressure ulcer. See **Figure 5-6.** **Figure 5-6** Stage IV pressure sore (Permission to reproduce this copyrighted material has been granted by the owner, Hollister Incorporated.)
blackhead	An open **comedo,** caused by accumulation of keratin and sebum within the opening of a hair follicle.
blister	A small, thin-walled, skin lesion containing clear fluid; a **vesicle.**
boil	A localized pus-producing infection originating deep in a hair follicle; a **furuncle.**
bruise	A bluish-black discoloration of an area of the skin or mucous membrane caused by an escape of blood into the tissues as a result of an injury to the area; see *ecchymosis*.
bulla (**BOO**-lah)	A large blister.

carbuncle (**CAR**-bung-kl)	A circumscribed inflammation of the skin and deeper tissues that contains pus, which eventually discharges to the skin surface.
cellulitis (sell-you-**LYE**-tis)	A diffuse, acute infection of the skin and subcutaneous tissue, characterized by localized heat, deep redness, pain, and swelling.
cerumen (seh-**ROO**-men)	Ear wax.
ceruminous gland (seh-**ROO**-mih-nus gland)	A modified sweat gland that lubricates the skin of the ear canal with a yellowish-brown waxy substance called cerumen or ear wax.
cicatrix (**SIK**-ah-trix *or* sik-**AY**-trix)	A scar; the pale, firm tissue that forms in the healing of a wound.
collagen (**KOL**-ah-jen)	The protein substance that forms the glistening inelastic fibers of connective tissue such as tendons, ligaments, and fascia.
comedo (**KOM**-ee-doh)	The typical lesion of acne vulgaris, caused by accumulation of keratin and sebum within the opening of a hair follicle (closed comedo = whitehead; open comedo = blackhead).
contusion (kon-**TOO**-zhun)	An injury to a part of the body without a break in the skin.
corium (**KOH**-ree-um)	The dermis; the layer of the skin just under the epidermis.
cryosurgery (cry-oh-**SER**-jer-ee) cry/o = cold	A noninvasive treatment that uses subfreezing temperature to freeze and destroy the tissue. Coolants such as liquid nitrogen are used in the metal probe.
curettage (koo-**REH**-tazh)	The process of scraping material from the wall of a cavity or other surface for the purpose of removing abnormal tissue or unwanted material.
cutaneous membrane (kew-**TAY**-nee-us) cutane/o = skin -ous = pertaining to	The skin. See *integument.*
cuticle (**KEW**-tikl)	A fold of skin that covers the root of the fingernail or toenail.
cyanosis (sigh-ah-**NOH**-sis) cyan/o = blue -osis = condition	A condition of a bluish discoloration of the skin.
cyst (**SIST**)	A closed sac or pouch in or within the skin that contains fluid, semi-fluid, or solid material.
debridement (day-breed-**MON**)	Removal of debris, foreign objects, and damaged or necrotic tissue from a wound in order to prevent infection and to promote healing.

dermatitis
(der-mah-**TYE**-tis)
dermat/o = skin
-itis = inflammation

Inflammation of the skin. See **Figure 5-7.**

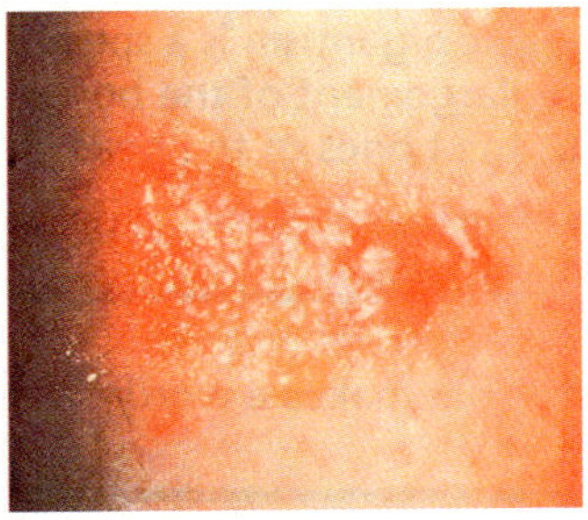

Figure 5-7 Dermatitis (Courtesy of Timothy Berger, M.D., Clinical Professor, Department of Dermatology, University of California, San Francisco)

dermatologist
(der-mah-**TALL**-oh-jist)
dermat/o = skin
-logist = specialist in the study of

A physician who specializes in the treatment of diseases and disorders of the skin.

dermatology
(der-mah-**TALL**-oh-jee)
dermat/o = skin
-logy = the study of

The study of the skin.

dermis
(**DER**-mis)
derm/o = skin
-is = noun ending

The layer of skin immediately beneath the epidermis; the corium.

diaphoresis
(**dye**-ah-foh-**REE**-sis)

The secretion of sweat.

ecchymosis
(ek-ih-**MOH**-sis)

A bluish-black discoloration of an area of the skin or mucous membrane caused by an escape of blood into the tissues as a result of injury to the area; also known as a bruise or a black-and-blue mark. See **Figure 5-8.**

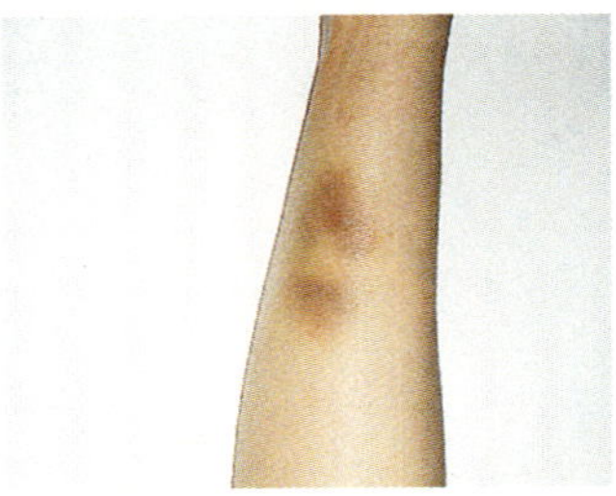

Figure 5-8 Ecchymosis

electrodesiccation
(ee-lek-troh-**des**-ih-**KAY**-shun)

A technique that uses an electrical spark to burn and destroy tissue; used primarily for the removal of surface lesions.

epidermis
(ep-ih-**DER**-mis)
epi- = upon, over
derm/o = skin
-is = noun ending

The outermost layer of the skin.

epidermoid cyst (ep-ih-**DER**-moid) **epi-** = upon, over **derm/o** = skin **-oid** = resembling	A cyst filled with a cheesy material composed of sebum and epithelial debris that has formed in the duct of a sebaceous gland; also known as a sebaceous cyst.
epithelium (ep-ih-**THEE**-lee-um)	The tissue that covers the internal and external surfaces of the body.
erythema (er-ih-**THEE**-mah)	Redness of the skin due to capillary dilatation. An example of **erythema** is nervous blushing or a mild sunburn.
erythremia (**er**-ih-**THREE**-mee-ah) **erythr/o** = red **-emia** = blood condition	An abnormal increase in the number of red blood cells; polycythemia vera.
erythroderma (eh-**rith**-roh-**DER**-mah) **erythr/o** = red **derm/o** = skin **-a** = noun ending	See *erythema.*
excoriation (eks-koh-ree-**AY**-shun)	An injury to the surface of the skin caused by trauma, such as scratching or abrasions.
exfoliation (eks-foh-lee-**AY**-shun)	Peeling or sloughing off of tissue cells, as in peeling of the skin after a severe sunburn.
fissure (**FISH**-er)	A cracklike sore or groove in the skin or mucous membrane.
fistula (**FISS**-tyoo-lah)	An abnormal passageway between two tubular organs (e.g., rectum and vagina) or from an organ to the body surface.
furuncle (**FOO**-rung-kl)	A localized pus-producing infection originating deep in a hair follicle; a boil. See **Figure 5-9.**

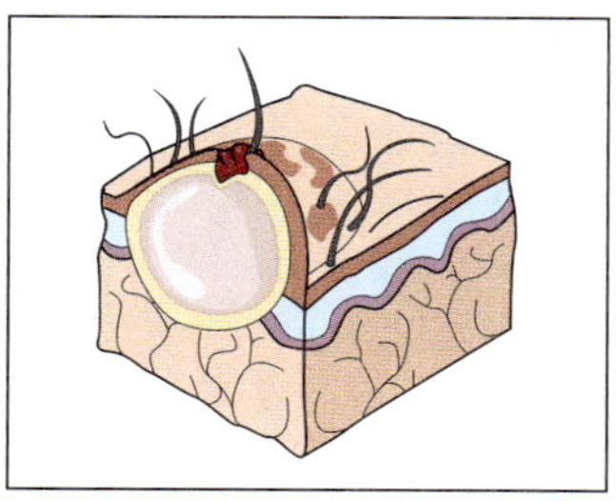

Figure 5-9 Furuncle

gangrene (**GANG**-green)	Death of tissue, most often involving the extremities. **Gangrene** is usually the result of ischemia (loss of blood supply to an area), bacterial invasion, and subsequent putrefaction (decaying) of the tissue.
hair follicle (**FALL**-ikl)	The tiny tube within the dermis that contains the root of a hair shaft.
hair root	The portion of a strand of hair that is embedded in the hair follicle.
hair shaft	The visible part of the hair.

hemangioma
(hee-**man**-jee-**OH**-mah)
hem/o = blood
angi/o = vessel
-oma = tumor

A benign (nonmalignant) tumor that consists of a mass of blood vessels and has a reddish-purple color. See **Figure 5-10.**

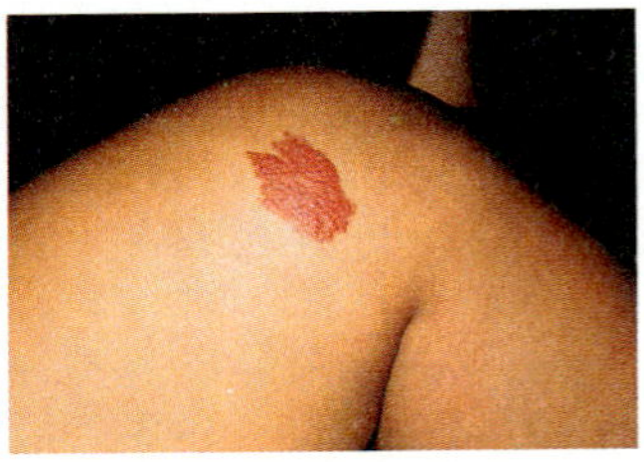

Figure 5-10 Hemangioma

heparin
(**HEP**-er-in)

A natural anticoagulant substance produced by the body tissues; **heparin** is also produced in laboratories for therapeutic use as heparin sodium.

hirsutism
(**HUR**-soot-izm)

Excessive body hair in an adult male distribution pattern, occurring in women.

histamine
(**HISS**-tah-min or
(**HISS**-tah-meen)

A substance, found in all cells, that is released in allergic, inflammatory reactions.

histiocyte
(**HISS**-tee-oh-sight)
histi/o = tissue
cyt/o = cell
-e = noun ending

Macrophage; a large phagocytic cell (cell that ingests microorganisms, other cells, and foreign particles) occurring in the walls of blood vessels and loose connective tissue.

hives

A circumscribed, slightly elevated lesion of the skin that is paler in the center than its surrounding edges; see *wheal.*

hydrocele
(**HIGH**-droh-seel)
hydr/o = water
-cele = swelling or herniation

A collection of fluid located in the area of the scrotal sac in the male.

ichthyosis
(**ik**-thee-**OH**-sis)
ichthy/o = fishlike, scaly
-osis = condition

An inherited dermatological condition in which the skin is dry, hyperkeratotic (hardened), and fissured, resembling fish scales.

integument
(in-**TEG**-you-ment)

The skin. See *cutaneous membrane.*

integumentary system
(in-teg-you-**MEN**-tah-ree)

The body system composed of the skin, hair, nails, sweat glands, and sebaceous glands.

keratin
(**KAIR**-ah-tin)

A hard, fibrous protein that is found in the epidermis, hair, nails, enamel of the teeth, and horns of animals.

keratolytic
(**KAIR**-ah-toh-**LIT**-ic)
kerat/o = hard, horny; also refers to cornea of the eye
-lytic = destruction

An agent used to break down or loosen the horny (hardened) layer of the skin.

laceration (**lass**-er-**AY**-shun)	A tear in the skin.
lanugo (lan-**NOO**-go)	Soft, very fine hair that covers the body of the developing fetus; this hairy coating is almost completely gone by birth.
lesion (**LEE**-zhun)	Any visible damage to the tissues of the skin, such as a wound, sore, rash, or boil.
lipocyte (**LIP**-oh-sight) lip/o = fat cyt/o = cell -e = noun ending	A fat cell.
lunula (**LOO**-noo-lah)	The crescent-shaped pale area at the base of the fingernail or toenail.
macrophage (**MACK**-roh-fayj) macr/o = large phag/o = to eat -e = noun ending	A large phagocytic cell (cell that ingests microorganisms, other cells, and foreign particles) occurring in the walls of blood vessels and loose connective tissue; see *histiocyte*.
macule (**MACK**-yool)	A small, flat discoloration of the skin that is neither raised or depressed.
mast cell	A cell, found within the connective tissue, that contains heparin and **histamine**; these substances are released from the mast cell in response to injury and infection.
melanin (**MEL**-an-in) melan/o = black	A black or dark pigment, produced by melanocytes within the epidermis, that contributes color to the skin and helps to filter ultraviolet light.
melanocytes (**MEL**-an-oh-sights *or* mel-**AN**-oh-sights) melan/o = black cyt/o = cell -es = noun ending	Cells responsible for producing melanin.
nail body	The visible part of the nail.
nodule (**NOD**-yool)	A small, circumscribed swelling protruding above the skin.
oil gland	One of the many small glands located in the dermis; its secretions provide oil to the hair and surrounding skin; see *sebaceous gland*.
onycholysis (**on**-ih-**CALL**-ih-sis) onych/o = nail -lysis = destruction or detachment	Separation of a fingernail from its bed, beginning at the free margin. This condition is associated with dermatitis of the hand, psoriasis, and fungal infections.

onychomycosis (**on**-ih-koh-my-**KOH**-sis) onych/o = nail; myc/o = fungus; -osis = condition	Any fungal infection of the nails.
onychophagia (**on**-ih-koh-**FAY**-jee-ah) onych/o = nail; phag/o = to eat; -ia = noun ending	The habit of biting the nails.
pachyderma (pak-ee-**DER**-mah) pachy = thick; derm/o = skin; -a = noun ending	Abnormal thickening of the skin.
papule (**PAP**-yool)	A small, solid, circumscribed elevation on the skin.
paronychia (par-oh-**NIK**-ee-ah) par/o = beside, beyond, near; onych/o = nail; -ia = condition	Inflammation of the fold of skin surrounding the fingernail; also called run-around. See **Figure 5-11.**

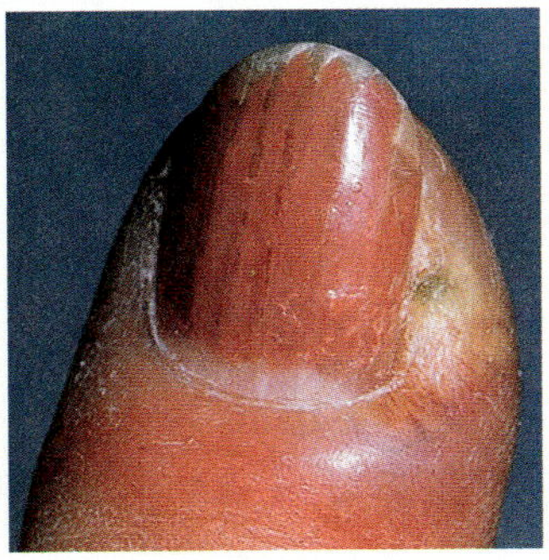

Figure 5-11 Paronychia

pediculosis (pee-dik-you-**LOH**-sis)	Infestation with lice.
perspiration	The clear, watery fluid produced by the sweat glands; see *sweat.*
petechia (pee-**TEE**-kee-ee)	Small, pinpoint hemorrhages of the skin.
pimple	A papule or pustule of the skin.
polyp (**PAL**-ip)	A small, stalklike growth that protrudes upward or outward from a mucous membrane surface, resembling a mushroom stalk.
pores	Openings of the skin through which substances such as water, salts, and some fatty substances are excreted.
pruritus (proo-**RYE**-tus)	Itching.

purpura (**PER**-pew-ah)	A group of bleeding disorders characterized by bleeding into the skin and mucous membranes; small, pinpoint hemorrhages are known as **petechia** and larger hemorrhagic areas are known as **ecchymoses** or bruises.
pustule (**PUS**-tool)	A small elevation of the skin filled with pus; a small **abscess**.
scales	Thin flakes of hardened **epithelium** that are shed from the epidermis.
sebaceous cyst (see-**BAY**-shus)	A cyst filled with a cheesy material composed of sebum and epithelial debris that has formed in the duct of a sebaceous gland; also known as an **epidermoid** cyst.
sebaceous gland (see-**BAY**-shus)	An oil gland located in the dermis; its secretions provide oil to the hair and surrounding skin.
seborrhea (seb-or-**EE**-ah) seb/o = sebum -rrhea = flow, drainage	Excessive secretion of sebum, resulting in excessive oiliness or dry scales.
sebum (**SEE**-bum) seb/o = sebum -um = noun ending	The oily secretions of the sebaceous glands.
skin tags	A small brownish or flesh-colored outgrowth of skin occurring frequently on the neck; also known as a cutaneous papilloma.
squamous epithelial cells (**SKWAY**-mus ep-ih-**THEE**-lee-ul)	Flat scalelike cells that are arranged in layers (strata).
squamous epithelium (**SKWAY**-mus ep-ih-**THEE**-lee-um)	The single layer of flattened platelike cells that cover internal and external body surfaces.
stratified (**STRAT**-ih-fyd)	Layered; arranged in layers.
stratum (**STRAT**-um)	A uniformly thick sheet or layer of cells.
stratum basale (**STRAT**-um **BAY**-sil)	The layer of skin where new cells are continually being reproduced, pushing older cells toward the outermost surface of the skin.
stratum corneum (**STRAT**-um **COR**-nee-um)	The outermost layer of skin (composed of dead cells that have converted to keratin), which continually sluffs off or flakes away; known as the keratinized or "horny" cell layer (kerat/o = horn).
stretch marks	Linear tears in the dermis which result from overstretching from rapid growth. They begin as pinkish-blue streaks with jagged edges and may be accompanied by itching. As they heal and lose their color, the stria remain as silvery-white scar lines.

subcutaneous tissue (**sub**-kew-**TAY**-nee-us) sub- = beneath, under, below cutane/o = skin -ous = pertaining to	The fatty layer of tissue located beneath the dermis.
subungual hematoma (sub-**UNG**-gwall) sub = beneath, under, below ungu/o = nail hemat/o = blood -oma = tumor	A collection of blood beneath a nail bed, usually the result of trauma (injury).
sudoriferous gland (soo-door-**IF**-er-us)	A sweat gland.
sweat	The clear, watery fluid produced by the sweat glands; also known as perspiration.
sweat gland	One of the tiny structures within the dermis that produces sweat, which carries waste products to the surface of the skin for excretion; also known as a sudoriferous gland.
ulcer (**ULL**-ser)	A circumscribed, open sore or lesion of the skin that is accompanied by inflammation.
urticaria (er-tih-**KAY**-ree-ah) 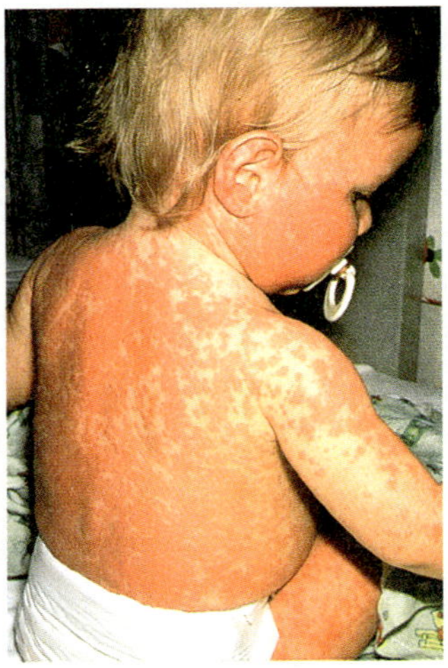	A reaction of the skin in which there is an appearance of smooth, slightly elevated patches (**wheals**) that are redder or paler than the surrounding skin and often accompanied by severe itching (**pruritus**). See **Figure 5-12.** **Figure 5-12** Urticaria (Courtesy of Robert A. Silverman, M.D., Pediatric Dermatology, Georgetown University)
vesicle (**VESS**-ikl)	A small, thin-walled, skin lesion containing clear fluid; a blister.
vitiligo (vit-ill-**EYE**-go)	A skin disorder characterized by nonpigmented white patches of skin of varying sizes that are surrounded by skin with normal pigmentation.
wheal (**WEEL**)	A circumscribed, slightly elevated lesion of the skin that is paler in the center than its surrounding edges; hives.

whitehead	A closed comedo, caused by accumulation of keratin and sebum within the opening of a hair follicle; the contents within are not easily expressed.
xanthoderma (**zan**-thoh-**DER**-mah) xanth/o = yellow derm/o = skin -a = noun ending	Any yellow coloration of the skin.
xeroderma (zee-roh-**DER**-mah) xer/o = dry derm/o = skin -a = noun ending	A chronic skin condition characterized by roughness and dryness.

Word Elements

The following word elements pertain to the integumentary system. As you review the list, pronounce each word element aloud twice and check the box after you "say it." Write the definition for the example word given for each word element. You may use your medical dictionary.

WORD ELEMENT	PRONUNCIATION	"SAY IT"	MEANING
adip/o **adip**ofibroma	**ADD**-ih-poh add-ih-poh-fih-**BROH**-mah	☐	fat
albin/o **albin**ism	al-**BYE**-noh **AL**-bin-izm	☐	white
caut/o **caut**ery	**KAW**-toh **KAW**-ter-ee	☐	burn
cutane/o sub**cutane**ous	kew-**TAY**-nee-oh sub-kew-**TAY**-nee-us	☐	skin
derm/o **derm**abrasion	**DERM**-oh **DERM**-ah-bray-shun	☐	skin
dermat/o **dermat**itis	der-**MAT**-oh der-mah-**TYE**-tis	☐	skin
erythr/o **erythr**algia	air-**IH**-thro air-ih-**THRAL**-jee-ah	☐	red
hidr/o **hidr**osis	**HIGH**-droh high-**DROH**-sis	☐	sweat
hist/o **hist**ology	**HISS**-toh hiss-**TALL**-oh-jee	☐	tissue

ichthy/o **ichthy**osis	**IK**-thee-oh ik-thee-**OH**-sis	☐	fish
kerat/o **kerat**osis	kair-**AH**-toh kair-ah-**TOH**-sis	☐	hard, horny; also refers to cornea of the eye
leuk/o **leuk**oderma	**LOO**-koh loo-koh-**DER**-mah	☐	white
lip/o **lip**ohypertrophy	**LIP**-oh lip-oh-high-**PER**-troh-fee	☐	fat
melan/o **melan**oma	mell-**AH**-noh mell-ah-**NOH**-mah	☐	black
myc/o **myc**osis	**MY**-koh my-**KOH**-sis	☐	fungus
onych/o **onych**ogryposis	**ON**-ih-koh on-ih-koh-grih-**POH**-sis	☐	nails
pil/o **pil**onidal	**PYE**-loh pye-loh-**NYE**-dal	☐	hair
scler/o **scler**oderma	**SKLAIR**-oh sklair-ah-**DER**-mah	☐	hard; also refers to sclera of the eye
squam/o **squam**ous epithelium	**SKWAY**-moh **SKWAY**-mus ep-ih-**THEE**-lee-um	☐	scales
trich/o **trich**iasis	**TRIK**-oh trik-**EYE**-ah-sis	☐	hair
xanth/o **xanth**osis	**ZAN**-thoh zan-**THOH**-sis	☐	yellow
xer/o **xer**oderma	**ZEE**-roh zee-roh-**DER**-mah	☐	dryness

Skin Lesions

A skin **lesion** is any circumscribed area of injury to the skin or a wound to the skin. The following are the most commonly known skin lesions.

abrasion
(ah-**BRAY**-zhun)

A scraping or rubbing away of skin or mucous membrane as a result of friction to the area.

An example of an **abrasion** is "carpet burn," which can occur in children who run and slide across the carpet on their knees.

abscess
(**AB**-sess)

A localized collection of pus in any body part that results from invasion of pus-forming bacteria.

The area is surrounded by inflamed tissue; a small abscess on the skin is also known as a **pustule.**

bedsore

An inflammation, sore, or ulcer in the skin over a bony prominence of the body, resulting from loss of blood supply and oxygen to the area due to prolonged pressure on the body part; also known as a pressure ulcer. Refer back to Figure 5-6.

blister

A small, thin-walled, skin lesion containing clear fluid; a vesicle.

bulla
(**BOO**-lah)

A large blister.

carbuncle
(**CAR**-bung-kl)

A circumscribed inflammation of the skin and deeper tissues that contains pus, which eventually discharges to the skin surface.

The lesion begins as a painful node covered by tight, reddened skin. The skin later thins out and perforates, discharging pus through several small openings. Treatment may include administration of antibiotics and use of warm compresses.

comedo
(**KOM**-ee-doh)

The typical lesion of acne vulgaris, caused by the accumulation of keratin and sebum within the opening of a hair follicle.

When a comedo is closed, it is called a **whitehead,** and the contents within are not easily expressed. When a comedo is open, it is called a **blackhead,** and the oily contents are easily expressed. Both forms of comedos are usually located on the face but may also appear on the back and chest.

cyst
(**SIST**)

A closed sac or pouch in or within the skin that contains fluid, semifluid, or solid material.

A common example of a fluid-filled cyst is a **hydrocele,** which is a collection of fluid located in the area of the scrotal sac in the male. A common example of a solid-filled cyst is a **sebaceous cyst,** which is a cyst filled with a cheesy material composed of sebum and epithelial debris that has formed in the duct of a sebaceous gland; also known as an epidermoid cyst. Sebaceous cysts frequently form on the scalp and may grow quite large.

fissure
(**FISH**-er)

A cracklike sore or groove in the skin or mucous membrane.

An example of a **fissure** is the cracklike sore in the skin that occurs with athlete's foot or the groovelike sore, known as an anal fissure, that occurs in the mucous membrane near the anus. For an example of a fissure in the mucous membrane, see **Figure 5-13.**

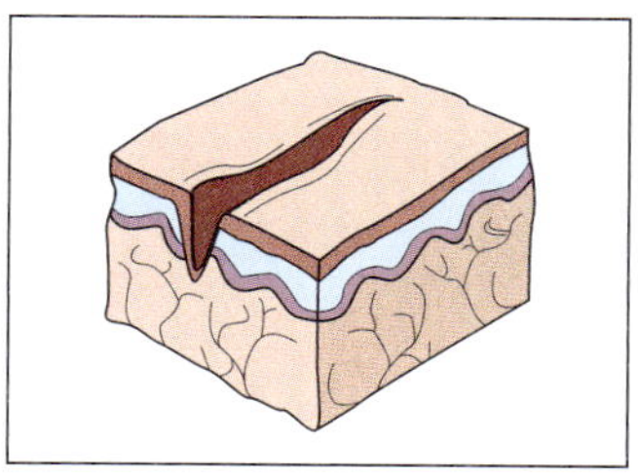

Figure 5-13 Fissure

fistula
(**FISS**-tyoo-lah)

An abnormal passageway between two tubular organs (such as the rectum and vagina, etc.); or from an organ to the body surface.

Some fistulas are created surgically for therapeutic purposes and others may be the result of congenital defects, infection, or injury to the body. An example of a surgically created fistula is an arteriovenous fistula created for the purpose of hemodialysis. (Refer to the discussion of hemodialysis in Chapter 15.) A rectovaginal fistula results from an abnormal passageway between the rectum and vagina. This opening allows feces from the rectum or anal canal to escape into the vaginal canal. The rectovaginal fistula can result from trauma during childbirth.

furuncle
(**FOO**-rung-kl)

A localized pus-producing (pyogenic) infection originating deep in a hair follicle, characterized by pain, redness, and swelling; also known as a boil. Refer back to Figure 5-9.

Because a furuncle is caused by a staphylococcal infection, it is important to avoid squeezing or irritating the lesion in order to prevent the possible spread of the infection to surrounding tissue.

hives

Circumscribed, slightly elevated lesion of the skin that is paler in the center than its surrounding edges; see *wheal.*

laceration
(**lass**-er-**AY**-shun)

A tear in the skin; a torn, jagged wound.

macule
(**MACK**-yool)

A small, flat discoloration of the skin that is neither raised nor depressed. Some common examples of **macules** are bruises, freckles, and the rashes of measles and roseola. See **Figure 5-14.**

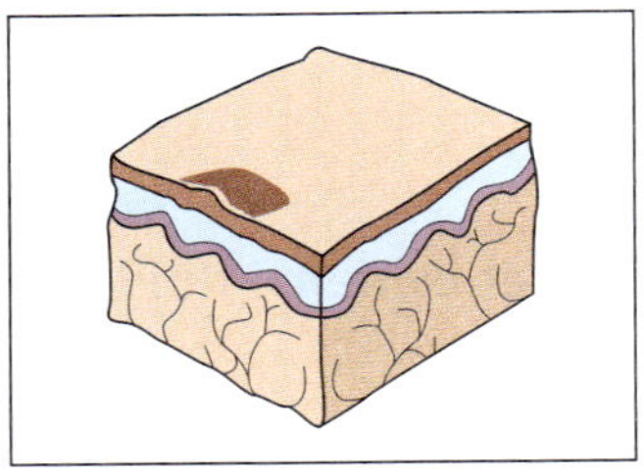

Figure 5-14 Macule

nodule
(**NOD**-yool)

A small, circumscribed swelling protruding above the skin; a small node.

papule
(**PAP**-yool)

A small, solid, circumscribed elevation on the skin.

Examples of a **papule** include a pimple, a wart, and an elevated nevus (mole). See **Figure 5-15.**

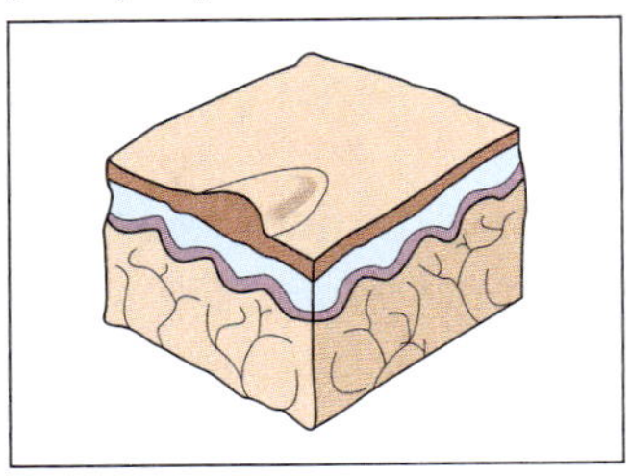

Figure 5-15 Papule

polyp
(**PALL**-ip)

A small, stalklike growth that protrudes upward or outward from a mucous membrane surface, resembling a mushroom stalk.

An example of a **polyp** is a nasal polyp.

pustule
(**PUS**-tool)

A small elevation of the skin filled with pus; a small abscess on the skin.

scales

Thin flakes of hardened epithelium that are shed from the epidermis.

ulcer
(**ULL**-ser)

A circumscribed, open sore or lesion of the skin that is accompanied by inflammation.

A decubitus ulcer, also known as a bedsore, is the breakdown of skin and underlying tissues resulting from constant pressure to bony prominences of the skin and inadequate blood supply and oxygenation to the area.

vesicle
(**VESS**-ikl)

A small, thin-walled, skin lesion containing clear fluid; a blister.

The small, fluid-filled blisters that occur with poison ivy are vesicles. See **Figure 5-16.**

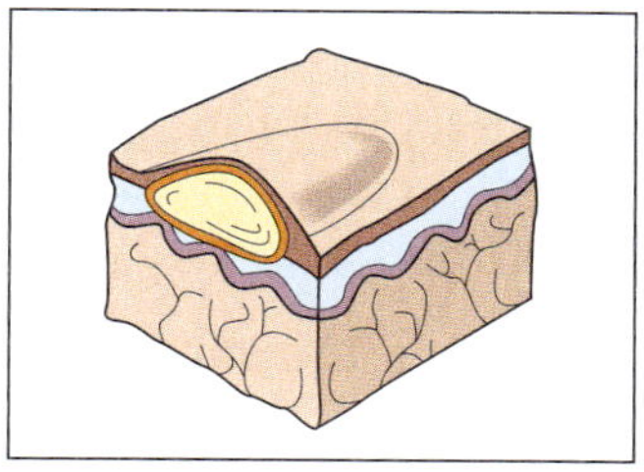

Figure 5-16 Vesicle

wheal
(**WEEL**)

A circumscribed, slightly elevated lesion of the skin that is paler in the center than its surrounding edges; hives.

A wheal is usually accompanied by intense itching and is of short duration. A mosquito bite is an example of a wheal. An allergic reaction to something may result in numerous wheals of varying sizes and intense itching, which is known as **urticaria.**

Pathological Conditions

As you study the pathological conditions of the integumentary system, note that the **basic definition** is in bold print, followed by a detailed description in regular print. The phonetic pronunciation is directly beneath each term, and a breakdown of the component parts of the term when appropriate.

acne vulgaris
(**ACK**-nee vul-**GAY**-ris)

A common inflammatory disorder seen on the face, chest, back, and neck, and which appears as papules, pustules, and comedos; commonly known as acne.

Acne vulgaris typically begins during adolescence due to the influence of sex hormones, largely androgens. Because it is a major cosmetic concern for the teenage population, acne should never be dismissed as trivial.

This condition is characterized by:

1. the formation of comedos, papules, and pustules on the face, chest, back, and neck,

2. the increased secretion of sebum as evidenced by greasy skin, and
3. **hyperkeratosis** at the opening of the hair follicle, which blocks the discharge of sebum and promotes the colonization of anaerobic bacteria.

The formation of blackheads (open comedos) and whiteheads (closed comedos) occurs as a result of the growth of anaerobic bacteria, which can live without air. The degree of involvement varies from the small comedos to obstruction of the entire follicle when large pustules or abscesses form. Picking, scratching, or pressing of these lesions can lead to secondary infections and scarring.

Although there is no cure for acne, treatment is directed at the following:

1. keeping the skin free of excess oil and bacteria through frequent cleansing,
2. avoiding heavy makeup and creams that can clog up the pores,
3. controlling infection with local antibiotics, and
4. decreasing the keratinization (hardening) of follicles by using **keratolytic** agents or *retinoic acid.*

---

albinism
(**AL**-bin-izm)
albin/o = white
-ism = condition

A condition characterized by absence of pigment in the skin, hair, and eyes.

Individuals with **albinism** lack the inherited ability to produce a brown skin coloring pigment, melanin. Persons with this inherited disorder:

1. are hypersensitive to light (photophobia),
2. are susceptible to skin cancer,
3. are prone to visual disturbances such as nearsightedness,
4. have pink or very pale blue eyes,
5. must avoid the sun in order to protect their eyes and skin from burning.

The widespread incidence of albinism is 1 in 20,000 births, equally male and female. The prevalence of albinism is higher in African Americans than Caucasians.

---

burns

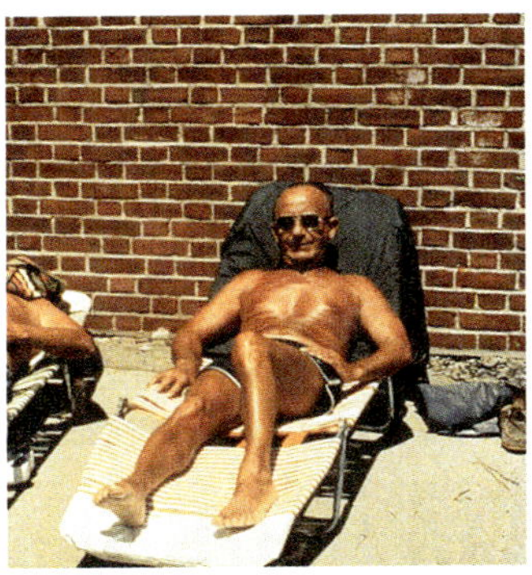

Figure 5-17A
First-degree burn

Tissue injury produced by flame, heat, chemicals, radiation, electricity, or gases. The extent of the damage to the underlying tissue is determined by the mode and duration of exposure, the thermal intensity or temperature, and the anatomic site of the burn. Burn degree is classified according to the depth of injury. See **Figures 5-17A through C.**

First-degree or superficial burns:

1. produce redness and swelling of the epidermis,
2. are painful, and
3. heal spontaneously with peeling in about 3 to 6 days and produce no scar.

An example of a first-degree or superficial burn is sunburn. See Figure 5-17A.

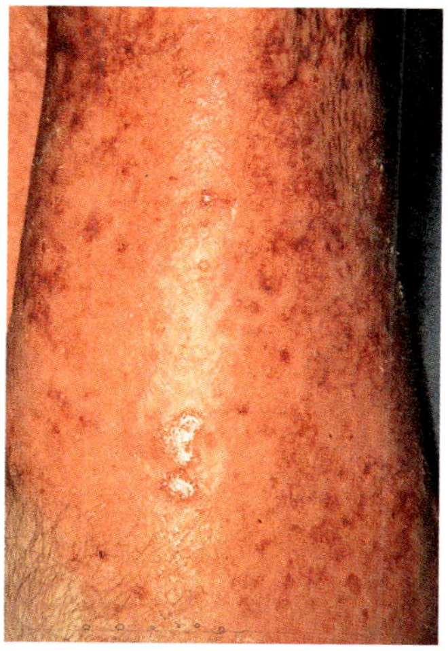

Figure 5-17B Second-degree burn

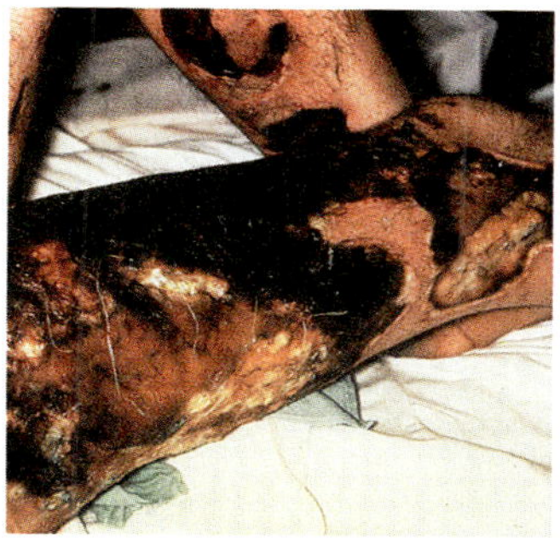

Figure 5-17C Third-degree burn (A, B, and C courtesy of The Phoenix Society for Burn Survivors, Inc.)

Second-degree or partial-thickness burns:

1. exhibit a blistering pink to red color and some swelling,
2. involve the epidermis and upper layer of the dermis,
3. are very sensitive and painful, and
4. heal in approximately 2 weeks without a scar if no wound infection or trauma occurs during the healing process.

An example of a second-degree or partial-thickness burn is flash contact with hot objects, such as boiling water. See Figure 5-17B.

Third-degree or full-thickness burns:

1. cause tissue damage according to the duration and temperature of the heat source,
2. involve massive necrosis of the epidermis and entire dermis, and may include part of the subcutaneous tissue or muscle,
3. appear brown, black, tan, white, or deep cherry red (will not blanch) and are wet or dry, sunken, with eschar (dry crust) and coagulated capillaries,
4. produce pain according to the amount of nerve tissue involved (where nerve endings are destroyed pain will be absent), and
5. will take a long time to heal and will likely require debridement(s) and grafting. See Figure 5-17C.

The classification of burns as first, second, or third degree helps to evaluate the severity of the burn; however, other factors influence the severity, such as:

1. the age of person burned,
2. the percentage of body surface burned,
3. the location of burn on the body, and
4. concurrent injuries.

---

callus
(**CAL**-us)

A common, usually painless thickening of the epidermis at sites of external pressure or friction, such as the weight-bearing areas of the feet and on the palmar surface of the hands. This localized hyperplastic area of up to 1 inch in size is also known as a callosity.

A callus may be caused by pressure or friction from ill-fitting shoes, deformities of the foot, or improper weight bearing; it may also be the result of repeated trauma to the skin such as that which occurs with manual labor or strumming a string instrument (guitar, banjo, etc.).

Treatment for calluses involves relieving the pressure or friction points on the skin. Metatarsal pads may also provide relief. The best treatment is prevention (i.e., by wearing shoes that fit well and avoiding unnecessary trauma to the hands and feet).

carcinoma, basal cell
(car-sih-**NOH**-mah, **BAY**-sal sell)
carcin/o = cancer
-oma = tumor

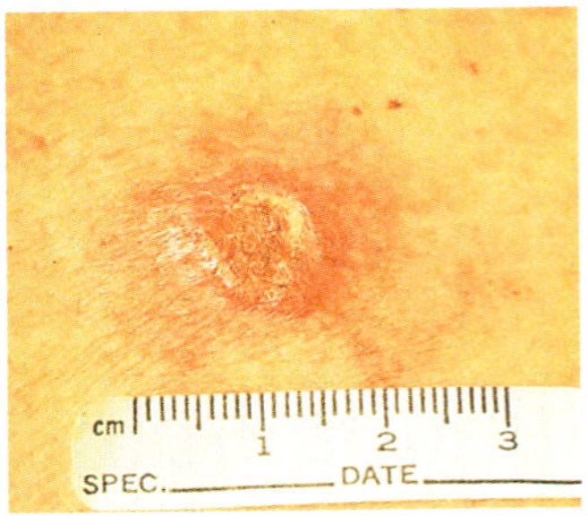

Figure 5-18 Basal cell carcinoma (Courtesy of Robert A. Silverman, M.D., Pediatric Dermatology, Georgetown University)

The most common malignant tumor of the epithelial tissue, occurring most often on areas of the skin that are exposed to the sun. See **Figure 5-18.**

Basal cell carcinoma presents as a slightly elevated nodule with a depression or ulceration in the center that becomes more obvious as the tumor grows.

If not treated, the basal cell carcinomas will invade surrounding tissue, which can lead to destruction of body parts (such as a nose). Treatment includes surgical excision, curettage and electrodesiccation, cryosurgery, or radiation therapy (see the section on diagnostic tests and procedures for description of these).

Basal cell carcinomas rarely metastasize, but they tend to recur, especially those that are larger than 2 cm in diameter.

carcinoma, squamous cell
(car-sih-**NOH**-ma, **SKWAY**-mus sell)
carcin/o = cancer
-oma = tumor

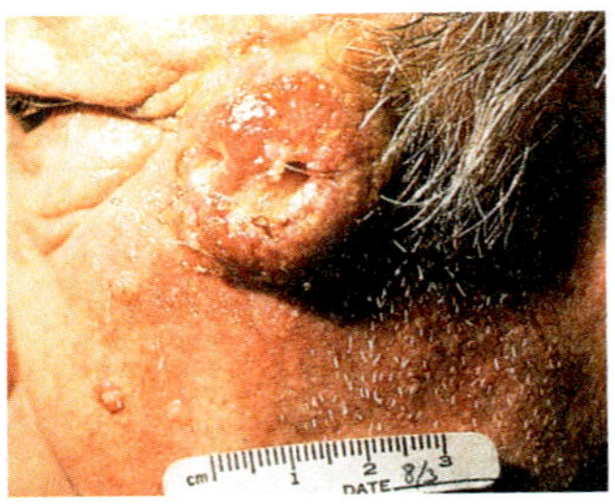

Figure 5-19 Squamous cell carcinoma (Courtesy of Robert A. Silverman, M.D., Pediatric Dermatology, Georgetown University)

A malignancy of the squamous, or scalelike, cells of the epithelial tissue, which is a much faster growing cancer than basal cell carcinoma and which has a greater potential for metastasis if not treated. See **Figure 5-19.**

These squamous cell lesions are seen most frequently on sun-exposed areas such as the:

1. top of the nose,
2. forehead,
3. margin of the external ear,
4. back of the hands, and
5. lower lip.

The squamous cell lesion begins as a firm, flesh-colored or red papule, sometimes with a crusted appearance. As the lesion grows it may bleed or ulcerate and become painful. When squamous cell carcinoma recurs, it can be quite invasive and create an increased risk of metastasis.

Treatment is surgical excision with the goal of removing the tumor completely, along with a margin of healthy surrounding tissue. Cryosurgery for low-risk squamous cell carcinomas is also common.

dermatitis
(der-mah-**TYE**-tis)
dermat/o = skin
-itis = inflammation

Inflammation of the skin, seen in several forms. Dermatitis may be acute or chronic, contact or seborrheic.

Contact dermatitis occurs as the skin responds to an irritant or allergen with redness, pruritus (itching), and various skin lesions. Two forms of contact dermatitis are allergic contact dermatitis and irritant contact dermatitis.

Allergic contact dermatitis develops by sensitization. When coming in contact with a substance for the first time, no immediate inflammation occurs, but future exposure to this substance will result in severe acute inflammation with pruritic red vesicular oozing lesions at the area of contact.

Common causes of allergic contact dermatitis include plants such as poison oak (refer back to Figure 5-7) and poison ivy; drugs; some metals such as copper, silver, mercury, and jewelry; and many industrial cleaners.

Irritant contact dermatitis occurs following repeated exposure of a mild irritant or initial exposure of a strong irritant. This severe inflammatory reaction is characterized by a fine, itchy rash of clearly defined red papules and vesicles. The chronic features of irritant contact dermatitis are dryness and scaling with a dull reddened appearance.

Some of the common causes of irritant contact dermatitis are soaps, detergents, oven cleaners, and bleaches.

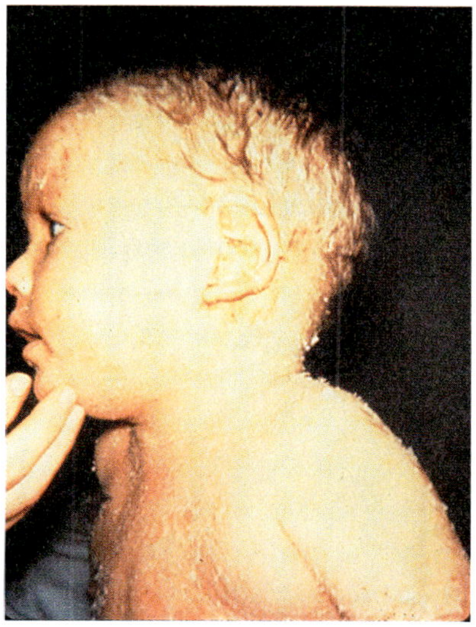

Figure 5-20 Seborrheic dermatitis (Courtesy of Robert A. Silverman, Clinical Associate Professor, Department of Pediatrics, Georgetown University)

Seborrheic (**seb**-oh-**REE**-ik) dermatitis is a very common inflammatory condition seen in areas where the oil glands are most prevalent, such as the:

1. scalp,
2. area behind the ears,
3. eyebrows,
4. sides of the nose,
5. eyelids, and
6. middle of the chest.

The skin affected by seborrheic dermatitis appears redden with a greasy, yellowish crusting or scales. If itching occurs it is usually mild. The most common form of seborrheic dermatitis is seen in infants from birth to 12 months of age and is called cradle cap (see **Figure 5-20**). It may also occur in adults, and statistics show it is higher in persons:

1. with disorders of the central nervous system, such as Parkinson's disease,
2. recovering from a stressful medical crisis, such as a heart attack,
3. confined for long periods of time in the hospital or a long-term care facility, and
4. with disorders of the immune system, such as AIDS.

---

eczema
(**EK**-zeh-mah)

An acute or chronic inflammatory skin condition characterized by erythema, papules, vesicles, pustules, scales, crusts, or scabs, and is accompanied by intense itching.

These lesions may occur alone or in any combination. They may be dry or they may produce a watery discharge with resultant itching.

Long-term effects of eczema may result in thickening and hardening of the skin, known as lichenification, which is due to irritation caused from repeated scratching of the itchy area. Redness and scaling of the skin may also accompany this. Severe itching predisposes the areas to secondary infections and possible invasion by viruses.

An estimated 9% to 12% of the population is affected by eczema, occurring most commonly during infancy and childhood. The incidence decreases in adolescence and adulthood. There is no exact cause known; however, statistics support a convincing genetic component in that children whose mother and father are affected have an 80% chance of developing eczema. This inflammatory response is believed to be initiated by histamine release with lesions usually occurring on the flexor surfaces of the arms and legs, the hands, the feet, and the upper trunk of the body.

Although there is no specific treatment to cure eczema, local and systemic medications may be prescribed to prevent itching. It is important to stress daily skin care and avoidance of known irritants. Chronic eczema is often frustrating to control and may recur throughout most of the individual's life.

---

exanthematous viral diseases
(eks-an-**THEM**-ah-tus)

A skin eruption or rash accompanied by inflammation, having specific diagnostic features of an infectious viral disease.

There are over 50 known viral agents that cause exanthems (eruptions of the skin accompanied by inflammation). The most common viral agents cause childhood communicable infections such as:

1. rubella (German measles),
2. roseola infantum,
3. rubeola (measles), and
4. erythema infectiosum (fifth disease).

These childhood diseases will be discussed further in Chapter 19.

---

gangrene

Tissue death due to the loss of adequate blood supply, invasion of bacteria, and subsequent decay of enzymes, especially proteins, producing an offensive, foul odor.

Gangrene can occur in two forms:

1. **dry gangrene,** seen in an extremity that is dry, cold, and shriveled, and which has a blackening appearance (late complication of diabetes mellitus), and
2. **moist gangrene,** follows the cessation of blood flow to tissue after a crushing injury, embolism, tourniquet, or tight bandage; if untreated, it will progress quickly to death.

The necrotic tissue must be removed through **debridement** or **amputation** in order to restore healing. Treatment should be aimed at the prevention of gangrene.

---

herpes zoster (shingles)
(**HER**-peez **ZOS**-ter)

An acute viral infection characterized by painful, vesicular eruptions on the skin following along the nerve pathways of underlying spinal or cranial nerves.

Ten to 20% of the population are affected by **herpes zoster,** with the highest incidence in adults over 50. This acute eruption is caused by

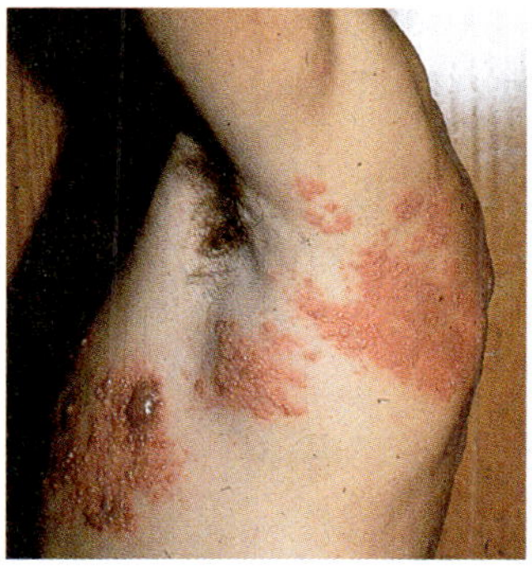

Figure 5-21 Herpes zoster (Courtesy of Robert A. Silverman, M.D., Clinical Associate Professor, Department of Pediatrics, Georgetown University)

reactivation of latent varicella virus (the same virus that causes chickenpox). See **Figure 5-21.**

Symptoms of herpes zoster include:

1. severe pain before and during eruption,
2. fever,
3. itching,
4. GI disturbances,
5. headache,
6. general tiredness, and
7. increased sensitivity of the skin around the area.

The lesions usually take 3 to 5 days to erupt, then progress to crusting and drying with recovery in approximately 3 weeks.

Treatment involves the use of antiviral medications, analgesics, and sometimes corticosteroids, which aid in decreasing the severity of symptoms.

---

hyperkeratosis
(**high**-per-**kair**-ah-**TOH**-sis)
hyper- = excessive
kerat/o = hard, horny; also refers to cornea of the eye
-osis = condition

An overgrowth of the horny layer of the epidermis.

This overgrowth occurs when the keratinocyte moves from the basal cell to the stratum corneum in 7 days instead of the normal 14 days, resulting in the formation of thick, flaky scales, along with excess growth of the cornified layer of epithelium. This process occurs in psoriasis and in the formation of calluses and corns.

---

impetigo
(im-peh-**TYE**-goh *or* im-peh-**TEE**-goh)

Contagious superficial skin infection characterized by serous vesicles and pustules filled with millions of staphylococcus or streptococcus bacteria, usually forming on the face.

Impetigo progresses to pruritic erosions and crusts with a honey-colored appearance. The discharge from the lesions allows the infection to be highly contagious. Treatment includes:

1. cleaning lesions with antibacterial soap and water using individual washcloths,
2. administration of oral and topical antibiotics,
3. Burrow's solution compresses, and
4. good handwashing

It is important to instruct the individual to complete the entire regime of systemic antibiotics in order to prevent the possibility of complications due to secondary infections, such as acute glomerulonephritis and/or rheumatic fever.

Kaposi's sarcoma
(**CAP**-oh-seez sar-**KOH**-ma)
sarc/o = flesh
-oma = tumor

Rare malignant lesions that begin as soft purple-brown nodules or plaques on the feet and gradually spread throughout the skin.

This systemic disease also involves the GI tract and lungs. **Kaposi's sarcoma** occurs most often in men, and there is an increased incidence in men infected with AIDS; it is also associated with diabetes and malignant lymphoma.

Radiotherapy and chemotherapy are usually recommended as methods of treatment. Kaposi's sarcoma may also be treated with cryosurgery or laser surgery.

keloid
(**KEE**-loyd)
kel/o = fibrous growth
-oid = pertaining to

An enlarged, irregularly shaped, and elevated scar that forms due to the presence of large amounts of collagen during the formation of the scar.

keratosis
(kair-ah-**TOH**-sis)
kerat/o = hard, horny; also refers to cornea of the eye
-osis = condition

Skin condition in which there is a thickening and overgrowth of the cornified epithelium.

seborrheic keratosis
(seb-oh-**REE**-ik kair-ah-**TOH**-sis)

Appears as brown or waxy yellow wartlike lesion(s), 5 to 20 mm in diameter, loosely attached to the skin surface.

Seborrheic keratosis is also known as senile warts.

actinic keratosis
(ak-**TIN**-ic kair-ah-**TOH**-sis)

A premalignant, gray or red-to-brown, hardened lesion caused by excessive exposure to sunlight. Also called solar keratosis.

leukoplakia
(loo-koh-**PLAY**-kee-ah)
leuk/o = white

White, hard, thickened patches firmly attached to the mucous membrane in areas such as the mouth, vulva, or penis.

Oral **leukoplakia** varies in size and occurs gradually over a period of several weeks. It begins without symptoms, but eventually develops sensitivity to hot or highly seasoned foods.

Causes of oral leukoplakia vary from irritating tobacco smoke to friction caused by a rough tooth or dentures. A biopsy should be performed when oral leukoplakia persists for more than 2 to 3 weeks because approximately 3% develop into cancerous lesions.

malignant melanoma
(mah-**LIG**-nant **mel**-ah-**NOH**-mah)
melan/o = black, dark
-oma = tumor

Malignant skin tumor originating from melanocytes in preexisting nevi, freckles, or skin with pigment; darkly pigmented cancerous tumor.

These tumors have irregular surfaces and borders, have variable colors, and are generally located on the trunk in men and on the legs in women. The diameter of most **malignant melanomas** measures more than 6 mm. Around the primary lesion, small satellite lesions 1 to 2 cm in diameter are often noted.

Persons at risk for malignant melanomas include those with a family history of melanoma and those with fair complexions. There is also an increased risk to develop particular forms of malignant melanomas with excessive sun exposure. Generally most melanomas are extremely invasive and spread first to the lymphatic system and then metastasize throughout the body to any organ, with fatal results.

All nevi and skin should be inspected and self-examined regularly, remembering the ABCDs of malignant melanoma:

> ***A**symmetry*—any pigmented lesion that has flat and elevated parts should be considered potentially malignant.
>
> ***B**orders*—any leakage across the borders of brown pigment or margins irregularly shaped are suspicious.
>
> ***C**olor*—variations whether red, black, dark brown, or pale are suspicious.
>
> ***D**iameter*—any lesions with the preceding characteristics measuring more than 6 mm in diameter should be removed.

Treatment is surgical removal, and for distant metastases chemotherapy and radiation therapy. The depth of surgical dissection and the prognosis depends on the staging classification of the tumor. The 5-year survival rate is approximately 60% for all forms of malignant melanomas.

---

nevus (mole)
(**NEV**-us)

A visual accumulation of melanocytes, creating a flat or raised rounded macule or papule with definite borders.

Nevi should be monitored for changes in size, color, thickness, itching, or bleeding. When any of these changes are noted, immediate professional assessment should be sought because of the potential for a malignant melanoma.

---

onychocryptosis
(**on**-ih-koh-krip-**TOH**-sis)
- **onych/o** = nail
- **crypt/o** = hidden
- **-osis** = condition

Ingrown nail. The nail pierces the lateral fold of skin and grows into the dermis, causing swelling and pain.

Ingrown nails most commonly involve the large toe.

---

onychomycosis
(**on**-ih-koh-my-**KOH**-sis)
- **onych/o** = nail
- **myc/o** = fungus
- **-osis** = condition

A fungal infection of the nails.

The nail becomes opaque, white, thickened, and friable (easily broken).

---

pediculosis
(pee-**dik**-you-**LOH**-sis)

A highly contagious parasitic infestation caused by blood-sucking lice.

Pediculosis may occur on any of the following parts of the body:

1. head (pediculosis capitis),
2. body (pediculosis corporis),
3. eyelashes and eyelids (pediculosis palpebrarum), and
4. pubic hair (pediculosis pubis)

With all types of pediculosis, a rash or wheals, intense pruritus, and the presence of louse eggs (nits) on the skin, hair shafts, or clothing are characteristic. When nits are present on the hair shaft, they appear as tiny, silvery-gray beads that cling to the hair strand. When thumping the hair strand, the nit will not fall off of the strand as would dandruff. Pediculosis can be spread directly through close physical contact or indirectly through articles of clothing, brushes, bed linens, and towels.

Treatment includes use of a special shampoo followed by removal of the nits with a fine-tooth comb; the treatment must be repeated weekly until nits are no longer present. Lice on the eyelid and lashes require a special ophthalmic ointment. Due to the intense itching, secondary infections can be a concern requiring antibiotic treatment.

---

pemphigus
(**PEM**-fih-gus)

A rare, incurable disorder manifested by blisters in the mouth and on the skin and spreading to involve large areas of the body, including the chest, face, umbilicus, back, and groin.

These painful blisters ooze, form crusts, and put off a musty odor. The serious risk is the secondary infection with the large areas of skin involved. Treatment involves administration of drugs, prevention of excessive fluid loss, and prevention of infection.

---

pilonidal cyst
(**pye**-loh-**NYE**-dal)

A closed sac located in the sacrococcygeal area of the back sometimes noted at birth as a dimple.

The cyst is of no bother unless it becomes acutely infected. When the **pilonidal cyst** is infected, an incision and drainage are indicated, followed by removal of the cyst or sac.

---

psoriasis
(soh-**RYE**-ah-sis)

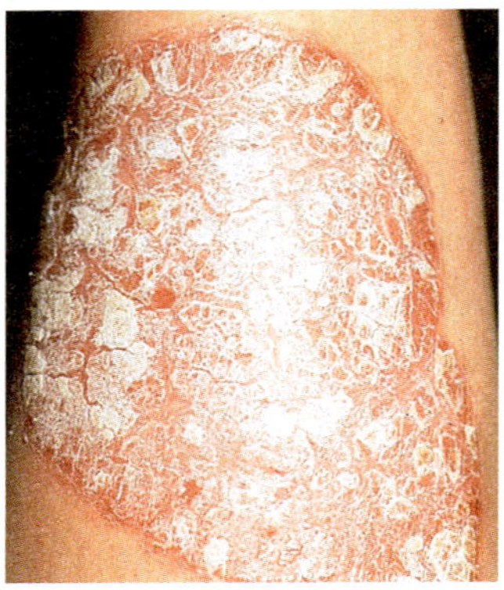

A common, noninfectious, chronic disorder of the skin manifested by silvery-white scales over round, raised, reddened plaques producing itching (pruritus).

The process of hyperkeratosis produces various-sized lesions occurring mainly on the scalp, ears, extensor surfaces of the extremities, bony prominences, perianal and genital areas. See **Figure 5-22** for a visual reference.

Treatment for **psoriasis** includes topical application of various medications, phototherapy, and ultraviolet light therapy in an attempt to slow the hyperkeratosis.

Figure 5-22 Psoriasis (Courtesy of Robert A. Silverman, M.D., Pediatric Dermatology, Georgetown University)

---

scabies
(**SKAY**-beez)

A highly contagious parasitic infestation caused by the "human itch mite," resulting in a rash, pruritus, and a feeling in the skin of "something crawling."

Scabies are seen most frequently on the genital area, armpits, waistline, hands, and breasts. Scabies can be spread directly through close physical contact or indirectly through articles of clothing, brushes, bed linens, and towels.

Treatment includes the use of special sulfur preparations, shampoos, and topical ointments. Due to the intense itching, secondary infections can be a concern requiring antibiotic treatment.

scleroderma
(**sklair**-ah-**DER**-mah)
scler/o = hard; also refers to sclera of the eye
derm/o = skin
-a = noun ending

A gradual thickening of the dermis and swelling of the hands and feet to a state in which the skin is anchored to the underlying tissue.

The severity of this disease varies from a mild localized form only affecting the skin (seen in persons in the 30-to-50-year age group), to a generalized form known as progressive systemic scleroderma (PSS) with progressive systemic involvement (persons die from pulmonary, cardiac, GI, renal, or pulmonary involvement).

No cure is available for scleroderma; therefore, the treatment is aimed at decreasing symptoms and treating the involved system with medications appropriate to the dysfunction. Physiotherapy may be recommended for some patients to restore and maintain musculoskeletal function as much as possible.

systemic lupus erythematosus
(sis-**TEM**-ic **LOO**-pus air-ih-them-ah-**TOH**-sis)

A chronic, multisystem, inflammatory disease characterized by lesions of the nervous system and skin, renal problems, and vasculitis. A red rash known as the "butterfly rash" is often seen on the nose and face.

Skin lesions may also spread to the mucous membranes or other tissues. Pain and swelling of the joints, along with weakness, weight loss, and fatigue, are symptoms of the disease process.

Treatment consists of the use of the systemic steroids, topical steroids on skin lesions, salicylates to relieve joint pain and swelling, and protection from sunlight.

tinea
(**TIN**-ee-ah)

More commonly known as ringworm, a chronic fungal infection of the skin that is characterized by scaling, itching, and sometimes painful lesions. The lesions are named according to the body part affected. See Figures 5-23A through C.

tinea capitis
(**TIN**-ee-ah **CAP**-ih-tis)
capit/o = head
-is = noun ending

Ringworm of the scalp is more common in children.

The infection may lead to hair loss. Symptoms of tinea capitis include severe itching and scaling of the scalp. Treatment with topical antifungal agents is sufficient for clearing the condition. See Figure 5-23A.

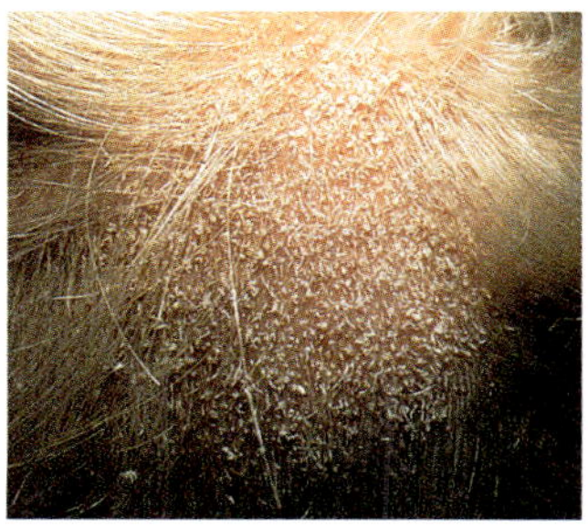

Figure 5-23A Tinea capitis (Courtesy of Robert A. Silverman, M.D., Clinical Associate Professor, Department of Pediatrics, Georgetown University)

tinea corporis
(**TIN**-ee-ah **COR**-poh-ris)
corpor/o = body
-is = noun ending

Ringworm of the body is characterized by round patches with elevated red borders of pustules, papules, or vesicles that affect the nonhairy skin of the body. The lesion actually looks like a circle and is raised. See Figure 5-23B.

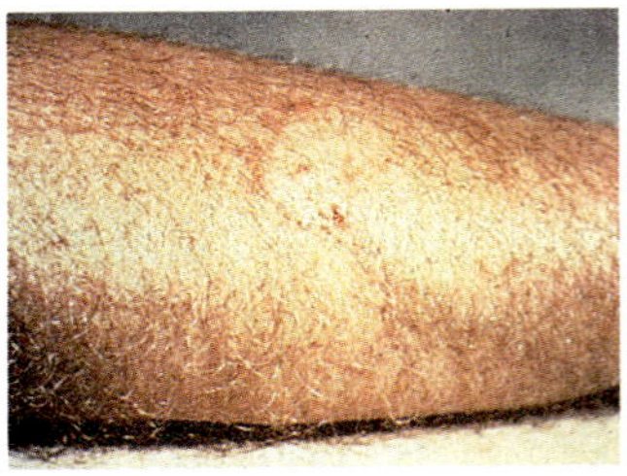

Ringworm of the body is most common in hot, humid climates and in rural areas. Tinea corporis can be spread through skin contact with an infected person or skin contact with an infected domestic animal, especially cats.

Figure 5-23B Tinea corporis (Courtesy of the Centers for Disease Control and Prevention [CDC])

tinea cruris
(**TIN**-ee-ah **KROO**-ris)
crur/o = leg or thigh
-is = noun ending

Ringworm of the groin is also known as jock itch.

This type of ringworm occurs more commonly in adult males. It is characterized by red, raised, vesicular patches in the groin area that are accompanied by pruritus.

Tinea cruris is more likely to occur during the hot, humid summer months and is aggravated by heat, physical activity, tight-fitting clothes, and perspiration. Topical antifungal agents are recommended for treatment.

tinea pedis
(**TIN**-ee-ah **PED**-is)
ped/o = foot
-is = noun ending

Ringworm of the foot is also known as athlete's foot.

It affects the space between the toes and the soles of the feet, with lesions varying from dry and peeling to draining, painful fissures with a foul odor and pruritus. Adults are most susceptible to tinea pedis. See Figure 5-23C.

Drying the feet well after bathing and applying powder between the toes will keep the moisture from building up and help to prevent the recurrence of the fungal infection. Treatment with topical antifungal agents is helpful in clearing the condition, although recurrence is common.

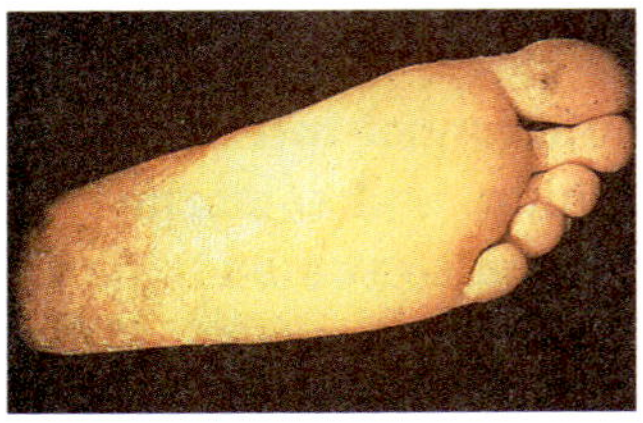

Treatment for all types of tinea that are severe or resistant to the topical antifungal agents includes the administration of oral antifungal medications that act systemically. If this becomes necessary, the drug of choice is griseofulvin.

Figure 5-23C Tinea pedis (Courtesy of the Centers for Disease Control and Prevention [CDC])

wart (verruca)
(ver-**ROO**-kah)

A benign, circumscribed, elevated skin lesion that results from hypertrophy of the epidermis; caused by the human papilloma virus.

The virus can be spread by touch or contact with the skin shed from a wart. They may occur alone or in clusters.

The **common wart** (verruca vulgaris) occurs on the face, elbow, fingers, or hands. These are seen largely in children and young adults.

Plantar warts occur either singly or in clusters on the sole of the foot. These warts can be painful, causing individuals to feel as if they have a stone in their shoe. Plantar warts occur primarily at points of pressure, such as over the metatarsal heads and the heel of the foot.

Condyloma acuminata or **venereal warts** are transmitted via sexual contact and are found on the female genitalia, the penis, or the rectum. These warts develop near the mucous membrane/skin junctures on the prepuce of the penis or on the female vulva. The growths appear as small, soft, moist, pinkish or purplish projections and may appear singly or in clusters.

Seborrheic warts or **seborrheic keratoses** are seen in the elderly population. These are benign, circumscribed, slightly raised lesions that occur on the face, neck, chest, or upper back and are often accompanied by itching. The lesions range from yellowish-tan to dark brown and are covered with either a greasy scale or a rough, dry scale depending on the location. Treatment for seborrheic warts includes curettage, cryotherapy, or electrodesiccation in conjunction with a local anesthetic. These methods of treatment will be discussed later in the chapter.

Diagnostic Techniques and Procedures

allergy testing

Various procedures used to identify specific allergens in an individual by exposing the person to a very small quantity of the allergen.

The intradermal, patch, and scratch test are among the most common allergy tests used.

cautery
(**KAW**-ter-ee)

Heat or caustic substances that burn and scar the skin (coagulation of tissue).

cryosurgery
(**cry**-oh-**SER**-jer-ee)
cry/o = cold

A noninvasive treatment that uses subfreezing temperature to freeze and destroy the tissue.

A local anesthetic is applied to the surface of the lesion, followed by the application of liquid nitrogen, which freezes and destroys tumor tissue.

Cryosurgery is used for low-risk squamous cell malignancies and primary basal cell carcinomas. This procedure causes very little pain and has good cosmetic results. It may also be used to remove warts.

Cryosurgery requires a prolonged healing time during which the wound tends to be painful and swollen with some inflammation and blistering.

curettage and electrodesiccation
(koo-**REH**-tahz and ee-**lek**-troh-**des**-ih-**KAY**-shun)

A combination procedure of curettage, which involves scraping away abnormal tissue, and electrodesiccation, which involves destroying the tumor base with a low-voltage electrode.

This treatment is used for basal cell cancers that are superficial, recur due to poor margin control, or are less than 2 cm in diameter. It is also used to treat primary squamous cell carcinomas with distinct edges when the diameter is less than 1 cm.

Good cosmetic results and preservation of normal tissue have been noted as advantages of **curettage and electrodesiccation.** Disadvantages are that healing time is longer and it is very difficult to confirm that all tumor margins have been excised.

debridement
(day-breed-**MON**)

Removal of debris, foreign objects, and damaged or necrotic tissue from a wound in order to prevent infection and to promote healing.

This may be a surgical or medical procedure. When debriding a burn, it may be done along with hydrotherapy.

---

dermabrasion
(**DERM**-ah-**bray**-shun)

Removal of the epidermis and a portion of the dermis with sandpaper or brushes in order to eliminate superficial scars or unwanted tatoos.

A chemical is used to cause light freezing of the skin prior to the use of the brushes and sandpaper.

---

dermatoplasty
(**DER**-mah-toh-**plas**-tee)
dermat/o = skin
-plasty = surgical repair

Skin transplantation to a body surface damaged by injury or disease.

---

electrodesiccation
(ee-lek-troh-**des**-ih-**KAY**-shun)

A technique using an electrical spark to burn and destroy tissue; used primarily for the removal of surface lesions.

Electrodesiccation involves the destruction of tissue by burning it with an electrical spark upon contact—the spark desiccates (dries) the tissue by dehydration. Although it is used primarily for removing small surface lesions, it may also be used to eliminate abnormal tissue deeper in the skin using a local anesthetic.

---

electrosurgery
(ee-**lek**-troh-**SER**-jer-ee)

The removal or destruction of tissue with an electrical current.

The variety of electrosurgeries include:

1. electrodesiccation, which is destruction of superficial tissue,
2. electrocoagulation, which is destruction of deeper tissue, and
3. electrosection, which is cutting through skin and tissue.

---

escharotomy
(es-kar-**OT**-oh-mee)

An incision made into the necrotic tissue resulting from a severe burn.

This scab, or dry crust, which forms after a severe full-thickness burn, is known as an eschar. Removal of this necrotic tissue is necessary to prevent a wound infection of the burn site.

The eschar is incised with a scalpel or by electrocautery for relief of tightness in the affected area. This sterile surgical incision allows for expansion of tissue created by the edema and also aides in promoting blood flow to the area and preventing gangrene.

---

fulguration
(ful-goo-**RAY**-shun)

See *electrodesiccation*.

liposuction
(**LIP**-oh-suck-shun)
lip/o = fat

Aspiration of fat through a suction cannula or curette to alter the body contours.

Liposuction is usually done on younger persons because of the elasticity of their skin. A pressure dressing is applied after the procedure to aide the skin in adapting to the new tissue size.

skin biopsy
(**BYE**-op-see)

The removal of a small piece of tissue from skin lesions for the purpose of examining it under a microscope to confirm or establish a diagnosis.

Types of skin biopsies are:

1. **excisional biopsy,** which is removal of the complete tumor or lesion for analysis,
2. **incisional biopsy,** in which a portion of the lesion is removed with a scalpel,
3. **punch biopsy,** which is removal of a small specimen of tissue in the "cookie cutter" fashion, and
4. **shave biopsy,** which uses the scalpel or a razor blade to shave lesions that are elevated above the skin.

skin graft

A process of placing tissue on a recipient site, taken from a donor site, in order to provide the protective mechanisms of skin to an area unable to regenerate skin, as in third-degree burns.

Skin grafting is successful when the base of the wound aides the donor tissue in developing a new blood supply and is found to be effective in wounds:

1. that are free of infection,
2. that have a good blood supply, and
3. in which bleeding can be controlled.

Full-thickness (both epidermis and dermis) or split-thickness (epidermis with a segment of dermis) grafts may be used. Types of grafting include:

1. **autografting,** in which the donor tissue comes from the person receiving the graft; transplanting tissue from one part of the body to another location in the same individual,
2. **homografting** or **allografting,** in which the donor tissue is harvested from a cadaver, and
3. **heterograft** or **xenograft,** in which the donor tissue is obtained from an animal.

Wood's lamp

An ultraviolet light that is used to examine the scalp and skin for the purpose of observing fungal spores.

The light causes hairs infected with a fungus, such as ringworm of the scalp (tinea capitis), to appear as a bright fluorescent blue-green color; also called Wood's light, black light, or Wood's rays.

The procedure is performed in a darkened room and the light beam is focused on the affected area. If the fungal spores are present, they will appear brilliantly fluorescent, as described.

Common Abbreviations

ABBREVIATION	MEANING	ABBREVIATION	MEANING
Bx, bx	biopsy	**PPD**	purified protein derivative
decub.	decubitus (ulcer); bedsore	**PSS**	progressive systemic scleroderma
derm.	dermatology	**SC**	subcutaneous
DLE	discoid lupus erythematosus	**SLE**	systemic lupus erythematosus
EAHF	eczema, asthma, and hay fever	**TENS**	transcutaneous electrical nerve stimulation
FANA	fluorescent antinuclear antibody	**ung.**	ointment
FS	frozen section	**UV**	ultraviolet (light)
ID	intradermal	**XP, XDP**	xeroderma pigmentosum
I&D	incision and drainage		
LE	(systemic) lupus erythematosus		

Written and Audio Terminology Review

Review each of the following terms from this chapter. Study the spelling of each term and write the definition in the space provided. If you have the Audio CD available, listen to each term, pronounce it, and check the box once you are comfortable saying the word. Check definitions by looking the term up in the glossary/index.

TERM	PRONUNCIATION	DEFINITION
abrasion	☐ ah-**BRAY**-zhun	______
abscess	☐ **AB**-sess	______
acne vulgaris	☐ **ACK**-nee vul-**GAY**-ris	______
actinic keratosis	☐ ak-**TIN**-ic kair-ah-**TOH**-sis	______
adipofibroma	☐ add-ih-poh-fib-**BROH**-mah	______
albinism	☐ **AL**-bin-izm	______
albino	☐ al-**BYE**-noh	______
alopecia	☐ **al**-oh-**PEE**-she-ah	______

Term	Pronunciation	Definition
amputation	☐ **am**-pew-**TAY**-shun	________
basal cell carcinoma	☐ **BAY**-sal sell **car**-sih-**NOH**-mah	________
basal layer	☐ **BAY**-sal layer	________
bulla	☐ **BOO**-lah	________
callus	☐ **CAL**-us	________
carbuncle	☐ **CAR**-**bung**-kl	________
carcinoma	☐ **car**-sih-**NOH**-mah	________
cautery	☐ **KAW**-ter-ee	________
cellulitis	☐ sell-you-**LYE**-tis	________
cerumen	☐ seh-**ROO**-men	________
ceruminous gland	☐ seh-**ROO**-mih-nus gland	________
cicatrix	☐ sik-**AY**-trix	________
collagen	☐ **KOL**-ah-jen	________
comedo	☐ **KOM**-ee-doh	________
condyloma acuminata	☐ con-dih-**LOH**-mah ah-**kew**-min-**AH**-tah	________
contusion	☐ kon-**TOO**-zhun	________
corium	☐ **KOH**-ree-um	________
cryosurgery	☐ **cry**-oh-**SER**-jer-ee	________
curettage	☐ **koo**-**REH**-tazh	________
curettage and electrodesiccation	☐ **koo**-**REH**-tazh and ee-**lek**-troh-**des**-ih-**KAY**-shun	________
cyanosis	☐ sigh-ah-**NOH**-sis	________
cyst	☐ **SIST**	________
debridement	☐ day-breed-**MON**	________
dermabrasion	☐ **DERM**-ah-**bray**-shun	________
dermatitis	☐ der-mah-**TYE**-tis	________
dermatology	☐ der-mah-**TALL**-oh-jee	________
dermatoplasty	☐ **DER**-mah-toh-plas-tee	________
dermis	☐ **DER**-mis	________
diaphoresis	☐ **dye**-ah-foh-**REE**-sis	________
ecchymosis	☐ ek-ih-**MOH**-sis	________

Term		Pronunciation	
eczema	☐	**EK**-zeh-mah	
electrodesiccation	☐	ee-**lek**-troh-**des**-ih-**KAY**-shun	
electrosurgery	☐	ee-**lek**-troh-**SIR**-jeh-ree	
epidermis	☐	**ep**-ih-**DER**-mis	
epidermoid	☐	ep-ih-**DER**-moid	
epithelium	☐	ep-ih-**THEE**-lee-um	
erythema	☐	**er**-ih-**THEE**-mah	
erythralgia	☐	air-ih-**THRAL**-jee-ah	
erythremia	☐	**er**-ih-**THREE**-mee-ah	
erythroderma	☐	eh-**rith**-roh-**DER**-mah	
escharotomy	☐	es-**kar**-**OT**-oh-mee	
exanthematous	☐	**eks**-an-**THEM**-ah-tus	
excoriation	☐	eks-**koh**-ree-**AY**-shun	
exfoliation	☐	**eks**-foh-lee-**AY**-shun	
fissure	☐	**FISH**-er	
fistula	☐	**FISS**-tyoo-lah	
follicle	☐	**FALL**-ikl	
fulguration	☐	ful-goo-**RAY**-shun	
furuncle	☐	**FOO**-rung-kl	
gangrene	☐	**GANG**-green	
hemangioma	☐	hee-**man**-jee-**OH**-mah	
heparin	☐	**HEP**-er-in	
herpes zoster	☐	**HER**-peez **ZOS**-ter	
hidrosis	☐	high-**DROH**-sis	
hirsutism	☐	**HUR**-soot-izm	
histamine	☐	**HISS**-tah-min *or* **HISS**-tah-meen	
histiocyte	☐	**HISS**-tee-oh-sight	
histology	☐	hiss-**TALL**-oh-jee	
hydrocele	☐	**HIGH**-droh-seel	
hyperkeratosis	☐	**high**-per-**kair**-ah-**TOH**-sis	
ichthyosis	☐	ik-thee-**OH**-sis	

Term	Pronunciation	
impetigo	☐ im-peh-**TYE**-goh *or* im-peh-**TEE**-goh	______
integument	☐ in-**TEG**-you-ment	______
integumentary	☐ in-**TEG**-you-**MEN**-tah-ree	______
Kaposi's sarcoma	☐ **CAP**-oh-seez sar-**KOH**-mah	______
keloid	☐ **KEE**-loyd	______
keratin	☐ **KAIR**-ah-tin	______
keratolytic	☐ **kair**-ah-toh-**LIT**-ic	______
keratosis	☐ kair-ah-**TOH**-sis	______
laceration	☐ lass-er-**AY**-shun	______
lanugo	☐ lan-**NOO**-go	______
lesion	☐ **LEE**-zhun	______
leukoderma	☐ loo-koh-**DER**-mah	______
leukoplakia	☐ **loo**-koh-**PLAY**-kee-ah	______
lipocyte	☐ **LIP**-oh-sight	______
lipohypertrophy	☐ lip-oh-high-**PER**-troh-fee	______
liposuction	☐ **LIP**-oh-suck-shun	______
lunula	☐ **LOO**-noo-lah	______
macule	☐ **MACK**-yool	______
malignant melanoma	☐ mah-**LIG**-nant **mel**-ah-**NOH**-mah	______
melanin	☐ **MEL**-an-in	______
melanocyte	☐ mel-**AN**-oh-sight *or* **MEL**-an-oh-sight	______
melanoma	☐ **mel**-ah-**NOH**-mah	______
mycosis	☐ my-**KOH**-sis	______
nevus	☐ **NEV**-us	______
nodule	☐ **NOD**-yool	______
onychocryptosis	☐ **on**-ih-koh-krip-**TOH**-sis	______
onychogryposis	☐ **on**-ih-koh-grih-**POH**-sis	______
onycholysis	☐ **on**-ih-**CALL**-ih-sis	______
onychomycosis	☐ **on**-ih-koh-my-**KOH**-sis	______

Term		Pronunciation	
onychophagia	☐	**on**-ih-koh-**FAY**-jee-ah	______
pachyderma	☐	pak-ee-**DER**-mah	______
papule	☐	**PAP**-yool	______
pediculosis	☐	pee-**dik**-you-**LOH**-sis	______
pemphigus	☐	**PEM**-fih-gus	______
petechia	☐	pee-**TEE**-kee-ee	______
pilonidal cyst	☐	**pye**-loh-**NYE**-dal cyst	______
plantar warts	☐	**PLAN**-tar warts	______
polyp	☐	**PALL**-ip	______
pruritus	☐	proo-**RYE**-tus	______
psoriasis	☐	soh-**RYE**-ah-sis	______
purpura	☐	**PER**-pew-rah	______
pustule	☐	**PUS**-tool	______
scabies	☐	**SKAY**-beez	______
scleroderma	☐	**sklair**-ah-**DER**-mah	______
sebaceous	☐	see-**BAY**-shus	______
sebaceous cyst	☐	see-**BAY**-shus cyst	______
seborrhea	☐	seb-or-**EE**-ah	______
seborrheic dermatitis	☐	**seb**-oh-**REE**-ik der-mah-**TYE**-tis	______
seborrheic keratoses	☐	seb-oh-**REE**-ik **kair**-ah-**TOH**-seez	______
seborrheic keratosis	☐	**seb**-oh-**REE**-ik **kair**-ah-**TOH**-sis	______
seborrheic warts	☐	**seb**-oh-**REE**-ik warts	______
sebum	☐	**SEE**-bum	______
skin biopsy	☐	skin **BYE**-op-see	______
squamous cell carcinoma	☐	**SKWAY**-mus sell **car**-sih-**NOH**-mah	______
squamous epithelium	☐	**SKWAY**-mus ep-ih-**THEE**-lee-um	______
stratified	☐	**STRAT**-ih-feyed	______
stratum	☐	**STRAT**-um	______

Term		Pronunciation	
stratum basale	☐	**STRAT**-um **BAY**-sil	______
stratum corneum	☐	**STRAT**-um **COR**-nee-um	______
subcutaneous tissue	☐	**sub**-kew-**TAY**-nee-us tissue	______
subungual	☐	sub-**UNG**-gwall	______
sudoriferous	☐	soo-door-**IF**-er-us	______
systemic lupus erythematosus	☐	sis-**TEM**-ic **LOO**-pus air-ih-them-ah-**TOH**-sus	______
tinea	☐	**TIN**-ee-ah	______
tinea capitis	☐	**TIN**-ee-ah **CAP**-ih-tis	______
tinea corporis	☐	**TIN**-ee-ah **COR**-poh-ris	______
tinea cruris	☐	**TIN**-ee-ah **KROO**-ris	______
tinea pedis	☐	**TIN**-ee-ah **PED**-is	______
trichiasis	☐	trik-**EYE**-ah-sis	______
ulcer	☐	**ULL**-ser	______
urticaria	☐	er-tih-**KAY**-ree-ah	______
verruca	☐	ver-**ROO**-kah	______
verruca vulgaris	☐	ver-**ROO**-kah vul-**GAY**-ris	______
vesicle	☐	**VESS**-ikl	______
vitiligo	☐	vit-ill-**EYE**-go	______
wheal	☐	**WEEL**	______
xanthoderma	☐	**zan**-thoh-**DER**-mah	______
xanthosis	☐	zan-**THOS**-sis	______
xeroderma	☐	zee-roh-**DER**-mah	______

Chapter Review Exercises

The following exercises provide a more in-depth review of the chapter material. Your goal in these exercises is to complete each section at a minimum 80% level of accuracy. A space has been provided for your score at the end of each section.

A. Spelling

Circle the correctly spelled term in each pairing of words. Each correct answer is worth 10 points. Record your score in the space provided at the end of the exercise.

1. alopecia	alopeshea	6. petechii	petechia
2. eccymosis	ecchymosis	7. pruritus	pruritis
3. gangreen	gangrene	8. sudoriferous	sudoiferous
4. hirsutism	hirtsutism	9. xanthoderma	zanthoderma
5. icthyosis	ichthyosis	10. histocyte	histiocyte

***Number correct* _______ × *10 points/correct answer: Your score* _______%**

B. Term to Definition

Define each term by writing the definition in the space provided. Check the box if you are able to complete this exercise correctly the first time (without referring to the answers). Each correct answer is worth 10 points. Record your score in the space provided at the end of the exercise.

☐ 1. pruritus ______________________________

☐ 2. vitiligo ______________________________

☐ 3. sudoriferous gland ______________________________

☐ 4. onycholysis ______________________________

☐ 5. keratin ______________________________

☐ 6. hirsutism ______________________________

☐ 7. erythema ______________________________

☐ 8. exfoliation ______________________________

☐ 9. ecchymosis ______________________________

☐ 10. cellulitis ______________________________

***Number correct* _______ × *10 points/correct answer: Your score* _______%**

C. Matching Abbreviations

Match the abbreviations on the left with the appropriate definition on the right. Each correct response is worth 10 points. Record your score in the space provided at the end of the exercise.

_____ 1. Bx	a.	ointment
_____ 2. decub.	b.	dermatology
_____ 3. SC	c.	purified protein derivative
_____ 4. PPD	d.	fluorescent antinuclear antibody
_____ 5. FANA	e.	transcutaneous electrical nerve stimulation
_____ 6. FS	f.	frozen section
_____ 7. ID	g.	ultraviolet (light)
_____ 8. SLE	h.	decubitus ulcer; bedsore
_____ 9. PSS	i.	progressive systemic scleroderma
_____ 10. ung.	j.	biopsy
	k.	subcutaneous
	l.	systemic lupus erythematosus
	m.	intradermal

***Number correct* _______ × *10 points/correct answer: Your score* _______%**

D. Crossword Puzzle

Each crossword answer is worth 10 points. When you have completed the crossword puzzle, total your points and enter your score in the space provided.

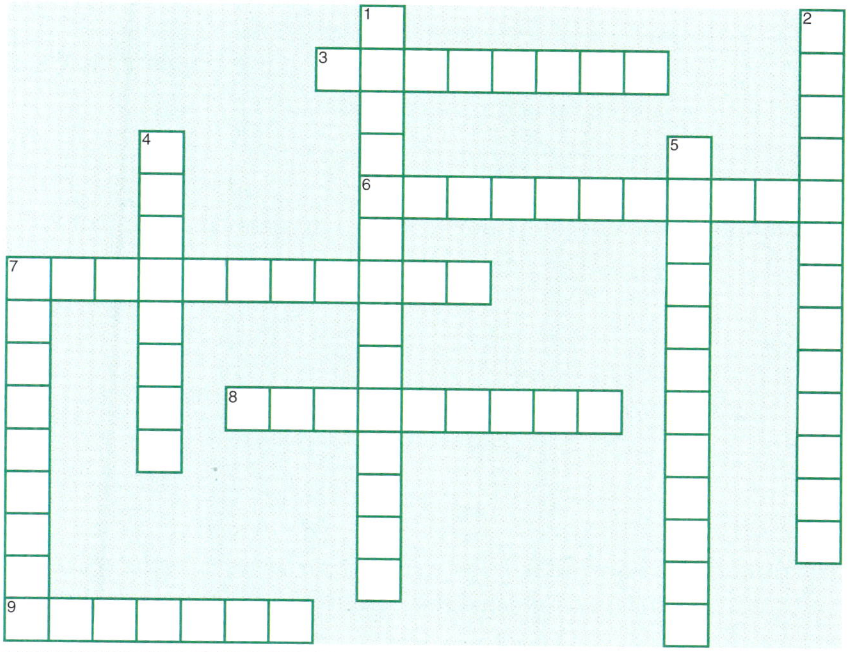

ACROSS

3 Death of tissue/no blood supply
6 Hardening of the skin
7 Infestation with lice
8 Hyperkeratosis of the skin cells
9 Infestation with the itch mite

DOWN

1 Malignment lesion, associated with AIDS
2 Ringworm of the body
4 Absence of melanin in skin
5 Painful vesicles (shingles)
7 Painful blisters with musty odor

Number correct _______ × 10 points/correct answer: Your score _______ %

E. Definition to Term

Identify and provide the medical word to match the following definitions. Write the word in the first space and the appropriate combining form for the word in the second space. Each correct answer is worth 5 points. Record your score in the space provided at the end of the exercise.

1. Inflammation of the skin

   ______________________________ ______________________________

   (word) (combining form)

2. Condition of bluish discoloration

   ______________________________ ______________________________

   (word) (combining form)

3. Layer of skin immediately beneath the epidermis

   ______________________________ ______________________________

   (word) (combining form)

4. Abnormal increase in the number of red blood cells (hint: "blood condition")

   ______________________________ ______________________________

   (word) (combining form)

5. Benign tumor consisting of a mass of blood vessels

_______________ _______________

(word) (combining form) + (combining form)

6. Large cell that ingests (eats) microorganisms, other cells, and foreign particles in the blood vessels

_______________ _______________

(word) (combining form) + (combining form)

7. Condition of a hidden toenail (i.e., an ingrown toenail)

_______________ _______________

(word) (combining form) + (combining form)

8. Chronic skin condition characterized by roughness and dryness (i.e., skin that is dry)

_______________ _______________

(word) (combining form) + (combining form)

Number correct _______ × 5 points/correct answer: Your score _______%

F. Labeling

Label the following structures of the skin and nails by writing your answers in the spaces provided. Each correct answer is worth 10 points. When you have completed this exercise, record your score in the space provided at the end of the exercise.

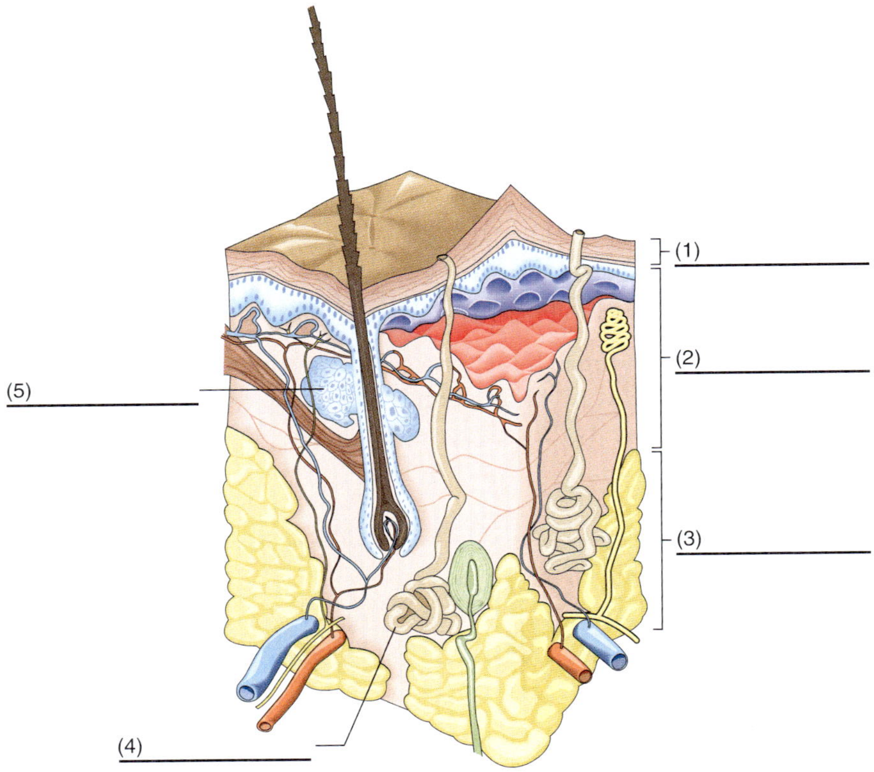

1. _______________
2. _______________
3. _______________
4. _______________
5. _______________

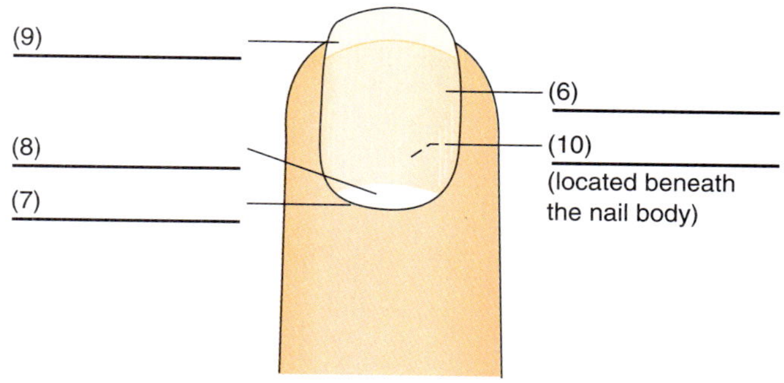

6. ______________________
7. ______________________
8. ______________________
9. ______________________
10. ______________________

***Number correct* _______ × *10 points/correct answer: Your score* _______%**

G. Identify and Define

Circle the correct spelling of each word, then write the definition for the correctly spelled word in the space provided. Refer to your text for assistance with definitions. Each correct answer is worth 5 points. Record your answer in the space provided at the end of the exercise.

1. psoriasis poriasis
____
2. infantigo impetigo
____
3. cryiosurgery cryosurgery
____
4. hyperkeratosis hyperkarotosis
____
5. albinism albinoism
____
6. gangreen gangrene
____
7. exzema eczema
____
8. pediculosis peddiculosis
____
9. leukaplakia leukoplakia
____
10. melonama (malignant) melanoma (malignant)
____

***Number correct* _______ × *5 points/correct answer: Your score* _______%**

H. Matching Procedures

Match the following procedures on the left with their descriptions on the right. Each correct answer is worth 10 points. When you have completed the exercise, record your score in the space provided at the end of the exercise.

_____ 1. debridement
_____ 2. dermabrasion
_____ 3. escharotomy
_____ 4. cautery
_____ 5. allergy testing
_____ 6. curettage
_____ 7. cryosurgery
_____ 8. electrodesiccation
_____ 9. skin biopsy
_____ 10. skin graft

a. An incision made into the eschar with a scalpel or by electrocautery for relief of tightness in a person with a burn
b. Removal of small pieces of tissue from skin lesions for diagnosis
c. Destruction of a tumor base with a low-voltage electrode
d. Removal of foreign objects and damaged or necrotic tissue from a wound in order to prevent infection and promote healing
e. A process of placing tissue on a recipient site taken from a donor site
f. Scraping away abnormal tissue
g. Heat or caustic substances that burn and scar the skin
h. Removal of the epidermis and a portion of the dermis with sandpaper or brushes
i. Procedures used to identify specific allergens in an individual by exposing the person to a very small quantity of the allergen
j. A noninvasive treatment for nonmelanoma skin cancer using liquid nitrogen

Number correct _______ × 10 points/correct answer: Your score _______%

I. Completion

The following statements describe various pathological conditions of the integumentary system. Complete each sentence with the most appropriate pathological condition. Each correct answer is worth 10 points. Record your score in the space provided at the end of the exercise.

1. The most common malignant tumor of the epithelial tissue is:

   ____

2. An inflammatory skin reaction characterized by intense itching, predisposing the person to secondary infections and long-term chronic lichenification, is known as:

   ____

3. Rash or wheals, intense pruritus, and the presence of louse eggs (nits) on the skin, hair shafts, or clothing is known as:

   ____

4. An inflammatory disorder seen on the face, chest, back, and neck, which appears as papules, pustules, and comedos, is known as:

   ____

5. Skin tumors with irregular surfaces, uneven borders, and variable colors, originating from melanocytes, are known as:

   ____

6. Blisters form with some swelling, involving the epidermis and upper layer of the dermis, and are very sensitive and painful when this condition occurs:

   ____

7. The noninfectious, chronic disorder of the skin that is manifested by silvery-white scales over round, raised, reddened plaques producing pruritus is:

____

8. A contagious skin infection characterized by serous vesicles and pustules filled with millions of staphylococci or streptococcal bacteria is known as:

____

9. A skin cancer with scalelike cells that has a potential for metastasis if not treated is:

____

10. A condition that involves massive necrosis of the epidermis and entire dermis, and may include part of the subcutaneous tissue, is known as:

____

Number correct _______ × 10 points/correct answer: Your score _______%

J. Matching Skin Lesions

Match the skin lesions on the left with the appropriate description on the right. Each correct answer is worth 10 points. Record your score in the space provided at the end of the exercise.

_____	1. abrasion	a. a circumscribed, open sore or lesion of the skin that is accompanied by inflammation
_____	2. bulla	b. a small elevation of the skin filled with pus
_____	3. fissure	c. a small stalklike growth that protrudes upward or outward from a mucous membrane surface
_____	4. furuncle	d. a blister
_____	5. macule	e. thin flakes of hardened epithelium that are shed from the epidermis
_____	6. polyp	f. a cracklike sore or groove in the skin or mucous membrane
_____	7. pustule	g. a large blister
_____	8. scales	h. a small flat discoloration of the skin that is neither raised nor depressed
_____	9. vesicle	i. a boil
_____	10. ulcer	j. a scraping or rubbing away of skin or mucous membrane as a result of friction to the area

Number correct _______ × 10 points/correct answer: Your score _______%

Answers to Chapter Review Exercises

A. Spelling

1. alopecia
2. ecchymosis
3. gangrene
4. hirsutism
5. ichthyosis
6. petechia
7. pruritus
8. sudoriferous
9. xanthoderma
10. histiocyte

B. Term to Definition

1. itching
2. a skin disorder characterized by nonpigmented white patches of skin of varying sizes that are surrounded by skin with normal pigmentation
3. a sweat gland

4. separation of a fingernail from its bed, beginning at the free margin
5. a hard, fibrous protein that is found in the epidermis, hair, nails, enamel of the teeth, and the horns of animals
6. excessive body hair in an adult male distribution pattern, occurring in women
7. redness of the skin due to capillary dilatation
8. peeling or sloughing off of tissue cells
9. a bruise or a black-and-blue mark
10. a diffuse, acute infection of the skin and subcutaneous tissue; characterized by localized heat, deep redness, pain, and swelling

C. Matching Abbreviations

1. j	6. f
2. h	7. m
3. k	8. l
4. c	9. i
5. d	10. a

D. Crossword Puzzle

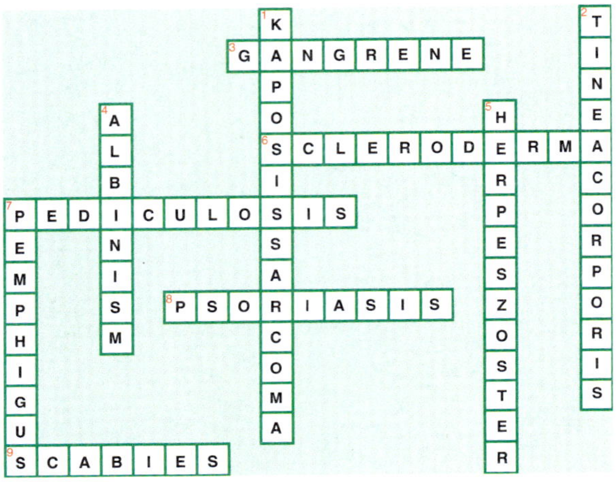

E. Definition to Term

1. dermatitis	dermat/o	
2. cyanosis	cyan/o	
3. dermis, or corium	derm/o, or cori/o	
4. erythremia	erythr/o	
5. hemangioma	hem/o	angi/o
6. macrophage	macr/o	phag/o
7. onychocryptosis	onych/o	crypt/o
8. xeroderma	xer/o	derm/o

F. Labeling

1. epidermis	6. nail body
2. dermis	7. cuticle
3. subcutaneous layer	8. lunula
4. sweat gland	9. free edge
5. oil gland	10. nail bed

G. Identify and Define

1. psoriasis: a common noninfectious chronic disorder of the skin manifested by silvery-white scales over round raised reddened plaques producing pruritus
2. impetigo: contagious superficial skin infection characterized by serous vesicles and pustules filled with millions of staphylococcus or streptococcus bacteria, usually forming on the face
3. cryosurgery: a noninvasive treatment for nonmelanoma skin cancer using liquid nitrogen, which freezes the tissue
4. hyperkeratosis: an overgrowth of the horny layer of the epidermis
5. albinism: a condition characterized by absence of pigment in the skin, hair, and eyes
6. gangrene: tissue death due to the loss of adequate blood supply, invasion of bacteria, and subsequent decay of enzymes, especially proteins, producing an offensive, foul odor
7. eczema: an acute or chronic inflammatory skin condition characterized by erythema, papules, vesicles, pustules, scales, crusts, or scabs
8. pediculosis: a highly contagious parasitic infestation caused by blood-sucking lice
9. leukoplakia: white, hard, thickened patches firmly attached to the mucous membrane in areas such as the mouth, vulva, or penis
10. melanoma (malignant): darkly pigmented cancerous tumor

H. Matching Procedures

1. d	6. f
2. h	7. j
3. a	8. c
4. g	9. b
5. i	10. e

I. Completion

1. basal cell carcinoma
2. eczema
3. pediculosis
4. acne vulgaris
5. malignant melanoma
6. second-degree burn
7. psoriasis
8. impetigo
9. squamous cell carcinoma
10. third-degree burn

J. Matching Skin Lesions

1. j	6. c
2. g	7. b
3. f	8. e
4. i	9. d
5. h	10. a

CHAPTER 6

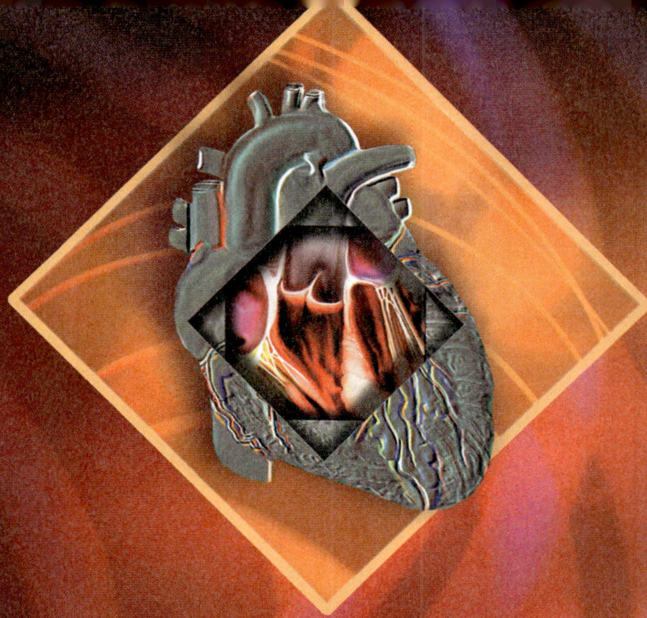

The Skeletal System

CHAPTER CONTENT

KEY COMPETENCIES

Upon completing this chapter and the review exercises at the end of the chapter, the learner should be able to:

1. Identify five functions of the skeletal system.
2. Identify four classifications of bones.
3. Correctly identify 10 different bone markings.
4. Correctly identify at least 10 major bones of the body by labeling the skeletal diagram provided in the chapter review exercises.
5. Define at least 10 pathological conditions of the skeletal system.
6. Identify and define at least 10 different types of bone fractures.
7. Correctly spell and pronounce each new term introduced in this chapter using the Activity CD-ROM and Audio CD, if available.
8. Correctly construct words relating to the skeletal system.
9. Identify at least 10 abbreviations common to the skeletal system.
10. Proof and correct the chapter's transcription exercise relative to the skeletal system.

OVERVIEW

The thigh bone's connected to the knee bone, the knee bone's connected to the leg bone, the leg bone's connected to the ankle bone, and on, and on, and on. . . . If you've ever heard the words of the song about "them bones," you will often be reminded of it as you discuss the skeletal system. You will also discover that in the human skeleton, the thigh bone (femur) *is* connected to the knee bone (patella), and the knee bone *is* connected to the leg bone (fibula and the tibia), and on, and on, and on . . . !

The human skeleton, which consists of 206 bones, performs several important functions. First, the bones of the skeleton serve as the supporting framework of the body. They provide shape and alignment to the body and support to the soft tissues. Second, the hard bones of the skeleton protect the vital internal organs from injury. The brain, for example, is protected by the bones of the skull, and the spinal cord is protected by the bones of the vertebrae. Third, the skeleton plays an important role in movement by providing points of attachment for muscles, ligaments, and tendons. This connection of muscles to bones allows for movement of the jointed bones as the muscles contract or relax. Fourth, the bones of the skeleton serve as a reservoir for storing minerals. The principal minerals stored in the bone are calcium and phosphorus. Fifth, the red marrow of the bones is responsible for blood cell formation. This process of blood cell formation is known as **hematopoiesis.**

The bones of the skeleton are classified according to their shape as either long, short, flat, irregular, or sesamoid. **Long bones** are longer than they are wide, with distinctively shaped ends. Examples of long bones are the bones of the upper arm (humerus), lower arm (radius and ulna), thigh (femur), lower leg (tibia, fibula), and the fingers and toes (phalanges). **Short bones** are about as long as they are wide, with a somewhat box-shaped structure. Examples of short bones are the bones of the wrist (carpals) and the ankle (tarsals). **Flat bones** are broad and thin, having a flat, sometimes curved, surface. Examples of flat bones are the breastbone (sternum), ribs, shoulder blade (scapula), and pelvis. **Irregular bones** come in various sizes and shapes, and they are often clustered in groups. Examples of irregular bones are the bones of the spinal column (vertebrae) and the face. **Sesamoid bones** are unique, irregular bones that are embedded in the substance of tendons and are usually located around a joint. Only the few tendons that are subjected to compression or unusual exertion-type stress have these bones. The kneecap is a good example of a sesamoid bone. In addition to the kneecap, the most common locations for sesamoid bones are around the hand-to-finger joints (metacarpophalangeal joints) and the foot-to-toe joints (metatarsophalangeal joints).

Anatomy and Physiology

Bone Structure

As we discuss the structure of a long bone, look at **Figure 6-1** to identify each part.

The **(1)** **diaphysis** is the main shaftlike portion of a long bone. It has a hollow, cylindrical shape and is composed of thick compact bone. The **(2)** **epiphysis** is located at each

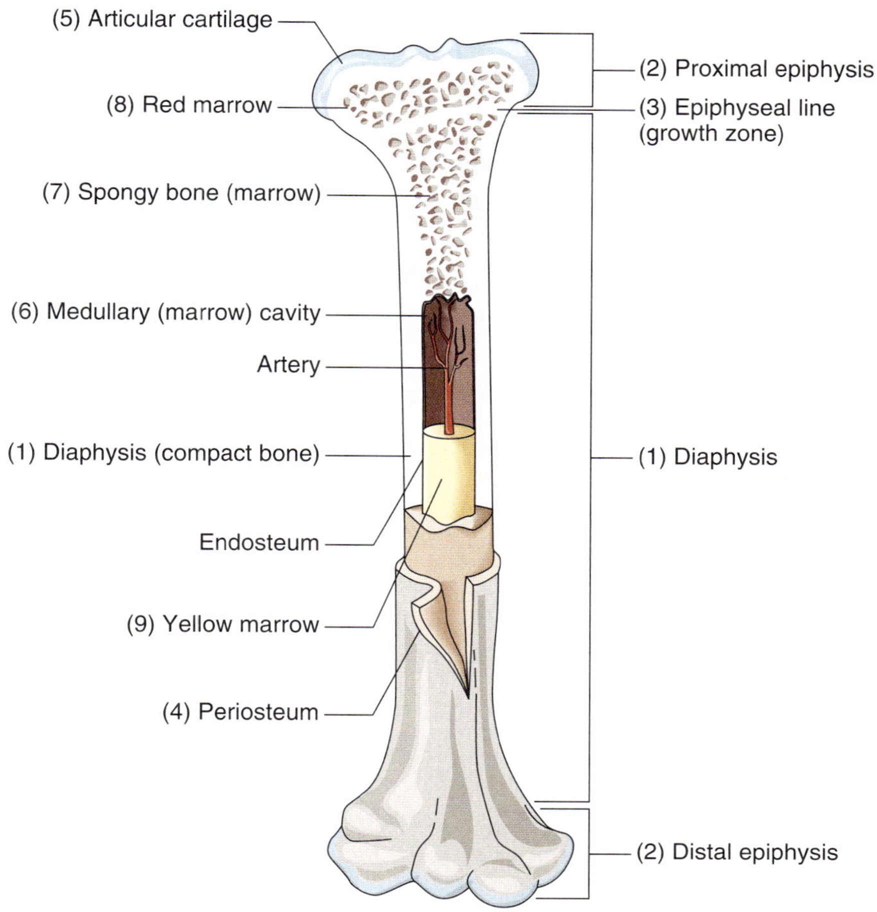

Figure 6-1 Structure of a long bone

end of a long bone. The epiphyses have a bulblike shape that provides ample space for muscle attachments. The epiphyseal plate/**(3) epiphyseal line** is a layer of cartilage that separates the diaphysis from the epiphysis of the bone. In children and young adults, the epiphyseal cartilage provides the means for the bone to increase in length. During periods of growth, the epiphyseal cartilage multiplies and thickens, generating new cartilage. When this occurs, the edges of the epiphyseal cartilage nearest the diaphysis are replaced by new bony tissue. Because the older cartilage is replaced with new bony tissue, the bone as a whole grows in length. When skeletal growth is complete, the epiphyseal cartilage will have been completely replaced by bone, causing the epiphyseal line to disappear on x-rays.

The **(4) periosteum** is the thick, white fibrous membrane that covers the surface of the long bone, except at joint surfaces (i.e., at the ends of the epiphyses). These joint surfaces are covered with **(5) articular cartilage.** The articular cartilage is a thin layer of cartilage that covers the ends of the long bones and the surface of the joints.

Bones differ not only in size and shape, but also in the types of bone tissue found in them. Look again at Figure 6-1, as we take a closer look at the structural components of bone.

Compact bone is the hard, outer shell of the bone. It lies just under the periosteum. The diaphysis, or shaft, of a long bone is composed of a hollow cylinder of compact bone. Within the center of this hollow area is the **(6) medullary (marrow) cavity,** which contains yellow marrow. Compact bone has a system of small canals, called the **haversian** canals, that extends lengthwise through the bone. The haversian canals contain blood vessels, lymphatic vessels, and nerves; the blood vessels transport nutrients and oxygen to the bone cells. Cancellous **bone,** also called (7) **spongy bone** or trabeculae **bone,** is not as dense as compact bone. The trabeculae are needlelike bony spicules that give the cancellous bone its spongy appearance; they are arranged along lines of stress, giving added strength to the bone.

The spaces between the trabeculae are filled with **(8) red bone marrow.** It is in the red marrow that blood cell production occurs throughout one's life. In an infant or child, almost all of the bones contain red marrow. In the adult, the bones that still contain red marrow include the ribs, the vertebrae, the epiphyses of the humerus (upper arm bone) and the femur (thigh bone), the sternum (breastbone), and the pelvis. The red marrow that was present in childhood is gradually replaced with yellow marrow as the individual grows into adulthood. The **(9) yellow marrow** stores fat and is not an active site for blood cell production in the adult.

Bone Formation

Now that we know how many bones we have and the structure of bones from the outside to the inner core, let's take it a step further. How are the bones formed?

The bones of the human skeleton begin their formation before birth. They begin as soft, flexible bones consisting of mostly cartilage and fibrous connective tissue. The cartilage and fibrous connective tissue are gradually replaced by stronger, calcified bone tissue as the skeleton continues to develop. Calcium salts are deposited into the gel-like matrix of the developing bones through the action of various enzymes, and **osteoblasts** (immature bone cells) actively produce the bony tissue that replaces the cartilage. The conversion of the fibrous connective tissue and cartilage into bone or a bony substance is known as **ossification.**

Bone is living tissue that is constantly being replaced and remodeled throughout life. This constant altering of bones occurs through growth in length and diameter. Earlier we discussed the bone's growth in length, occurring at the epiphyseal line. Bones also grow in diameter by the combined action of the osteoblasts and the **osteoclasts.** The osteoclasts are large cells that digest, or absorb, bony tissue. They help to hollow out the central portion of the bone by eating away at—or destroying the old bone tissue from—the inner walls of the medullary cavity, thus enlarging the diameter of the medullary cavity. This process of removing the old bone tissue, or destroying it so that its components can be absorbed into the circulation, is known as **resorption.** At the same time resorption is occurring through the action of the osteoclasts, the osteoblasts from the inner layer of the periosteum are depositing new bone around the outside of the bone. This concurrent process forms a larger bone structure from the smaller one. Osteoblasts become mature bone cells when the surrounding intercellular material hardens around them. They are then called **osteocytes** (mature bone cells). These osteocytes are living cells that continue to maintain the bone without producing new bone tissue.

Bone Markings

Now that we have discussed the structure and formation of bone, let us examine some of the specific features of individual bones, known as **bone markings.** These markings, which create characteristic features, include enlargements that extend out from the bone and openings or hollow regions within the bone. These areas may serve as points

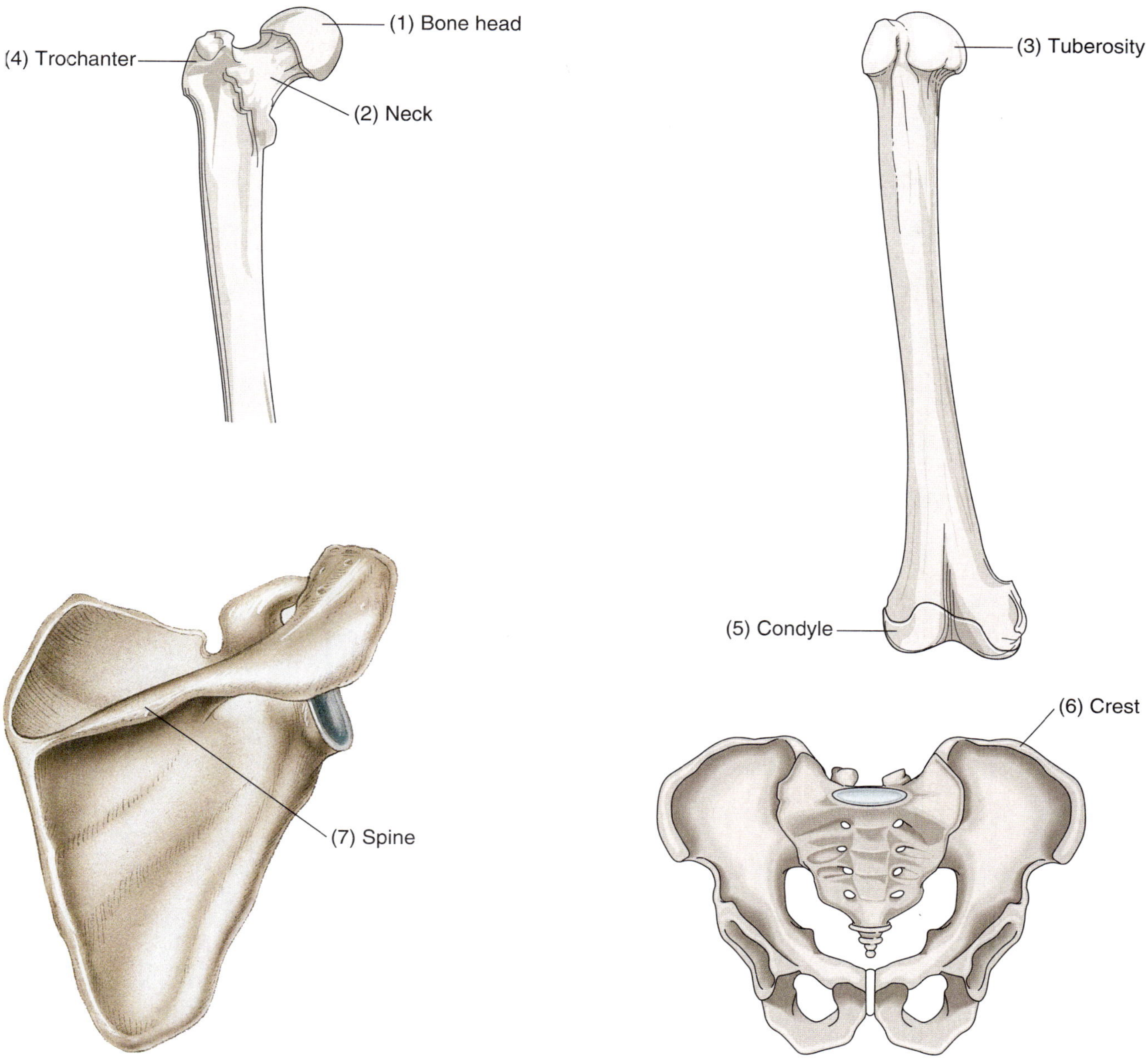

Figure 6-2 Bone processes

of attachment for muscles and tendons, join one bone to another, or provide cavities and passage for nerves and blood vessels.

Bone processes are projections or outgrowths of bone; they help to form joints or serve as points of attachment for muscles and tendons. Here are some of the more commonly known bone processes (see **Figure 6-2**).

(1) bone head	A rounded knoblike end of a long bone, separated from the shaft of the bone by a narrow portion (the neck of the bone).
(2) neck	A constricted or narrow section that connects with the head, as in the neck connecting to the head or the neck of the femur.

(3) tuberosity (too-ber-**OSS**-ih-tee)	An elevated, broad, rounded process of a bone, usually for attachment of muscles or tendons.
(4) trochanter (tro-**KAN**-ter)	Large bony process located below the neck of the femur, for attachment of muscles.
(5) condyle (**CON**-dill)	A knucklelike projection at the end of a bone; usually fits into a fossa of another bone to form a joint.
(6) crest	A distinct border or ridge; an upper, elevated edge as in the upper part of the hip bone (the iliac crest); generally a site for muscle attachment.
(7) spine	A sharp projection from the surface of a bone, similar to a crest; for example, the spine of the scapula (shoulder blade), used for muscle attachment.

Bone depressions are concave (indented) areas, or openings, in a bone. They help to form joints or serve as points of attachment for muscle.

sulcus (SULL-kus)	A groove or depression in a bone; a fissure.
sinus (**SIGH**-nus)	An opening or hollow space in a bone, as in the paranasal sinuses or the frontal sinus.
fissure (**FISH**-er)	Same as *sulcus*.
fossa (FOSS-ah)	A hollow or shallow concave depression in a bone.
foramen (for-**AY**-men)	A hole within a bone that allows blood vessels or nerves to pass through, as in the foramen magnum of the skull that allows the cranial nerves to pass through it.

Specific Skeletal Bones

Thus far, we have discussed the structure and formation of bones and their distinguishing markings. Let us now study specific bones of the skeletal system. These bones will be listed in order, from the head to the toe, and will include the majority of the bones of the skeleton. Throughout this section, refer to the figures for visual reinforcement of the bones being discussed.

Cranial Bones

The cranium is the bony skull that envelops the brain. It is composed of eight bones, which are immovable. The borders of the cranial bones meet to form **sutures**, or immovable joints. Refer to **Figure 6-3** as you study the bones of the cranium.

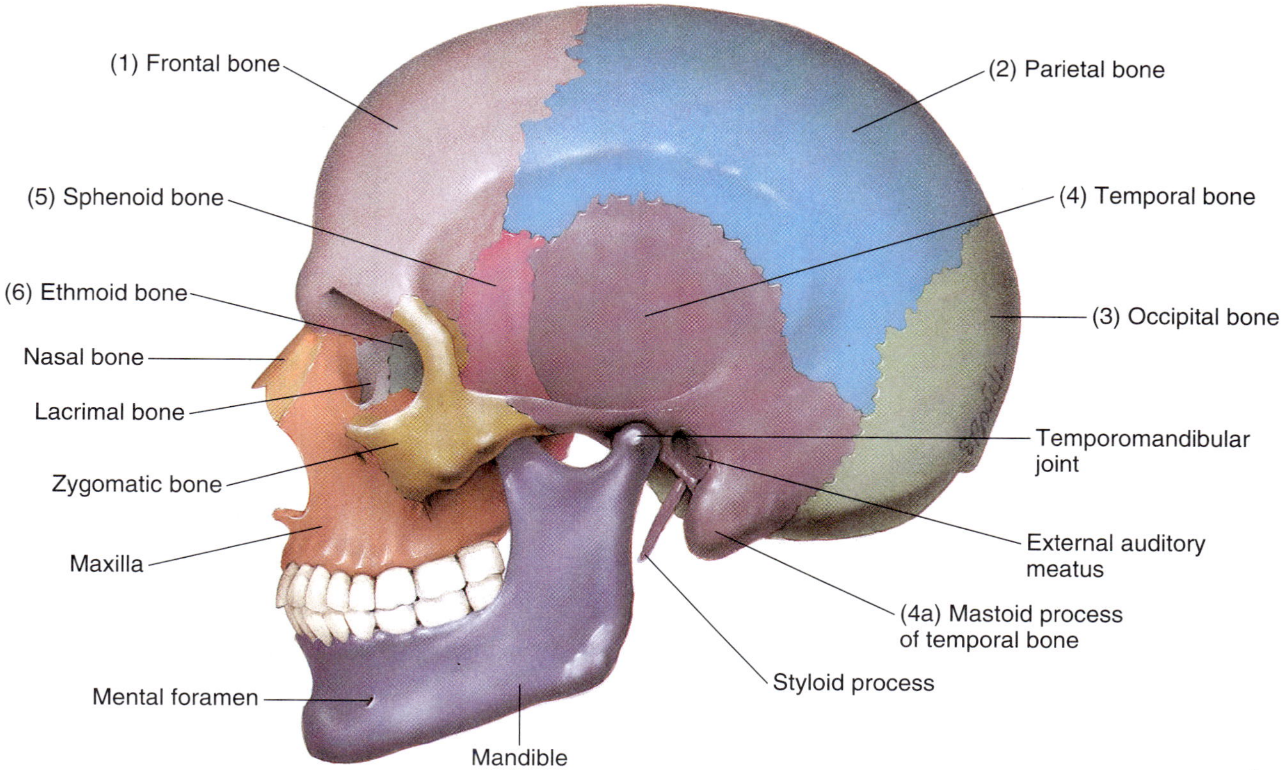

Figure 6-3 Cranial bones

(1) frontal bone	The frontal bone forms the forehead (front of the skull) and the upper part of the bony cavities that contain the eyeballs. The frontal sinuses are located in this bone, just above the area where the frontal bone joins the nasal bones.
(2) parietal bones (pah-REYE-eh-tall)	Moving toward the back of the head, just behind the frontal bones ("posterior to the frontal bones"), are the two **parietal** bones. They form most of the top and the upper sides of the cranium.
(3) occipital bone (ock-**SIP**-itle)	The single occipital bone forms the back of the head and the base of the skull (the back portion of the floor of the cranial cavity). The occipital bone contains the foramen magnum (a large opening in its base) through which the spinal cord passes.
(4) temporal bones (**TEM**-por-al)	The two temporal bones form the lower sides and part of the base of the skull (cranium). These bones contain the middle and inner ear structures. They also contain the mastoid sinuses. Immediately behind the external part of the ear is the **temporal** bone, which projects downward to form the **(4a) mastoid process,** which serves as a point of attachment for muscles.
(5) sphenoid bone (**SFEE**-noyd)	The **sphenoid** bone is a bat-shaped bone (resembling a bat with outstretched wings) that is located at the base of the skull in front of the temporal bones. It extends completely across the middle of the cranial floor, joining with and anchoring the frontal, parietal, occipital,

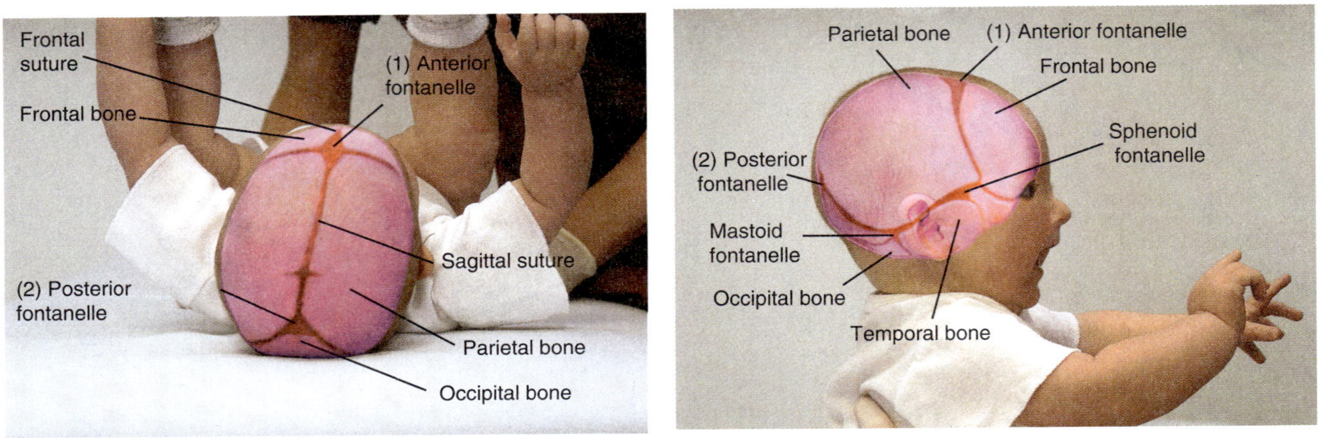

Figure 6-4 Fontanels in the newborn cranium

temporal, and ethmoid bones. The sphenoid bones form part of the base of the eye orbits.

---

(6) ethmoid bone
(**ETH**-moyd)

The **ethmoid** bone lies just behind the nasal bone, in front of the sphenoid bone. It also forms the front of the base of the skull, part of the eye orbits, and the nasal cavity. The ethmoid bone also contains the ethmoid sinuses.

As mentioned, the adult cranial bones are fused together by immovable joints known as sutures, permitting no movement of the cranial bones. This is different in the newborn. See **Figure 6-4.**

Within the cranial bones of a newborn are two points of union where a space is present between the bones. These spaces are called **fontanelles** ("soft spots"), also spelled **fontanel.** A fontanelle is a space between bones of an infant's cranium that is covered by a tough membrane. The (1) **anterior fontanelle,** also called the **frontal fontanelle,** is the diamond-shaped space between the frontal and the parietal bones. It normally closes between 18 and 24 months of age. The (2) **posterior fontanelle,** also called the **occipital fontanelle,** is the space between the occipital and parietal bones, and is much smaller than the anterior fontanelle. It normally closes within 2 months after birth.

The fontanelles in the newborn permit the bones of the roof of the skull to override one another during the birth process, narrowing the skull slightly as the head is exposed to the pressures within the birth canal. This may mold the newborn's head into an asymmetrical shape during the birthing process; the head generally assumes its normal shape in a week. The complete ossification of the cranial sutures (making them immovable joints) does not occur for some years after birth. The cranial bones are held together by fibrous connective tissue until ossification occurs, allowing some movement of the infant's skull bones. This feature permits additional growth of the skull to accommodate the normal development of the brain.

Facial Bones

The facial part of the skull is given its distinctive shape by two bones: the maxillae (upper jaw bones) and the mandible (lower jaw bone). These

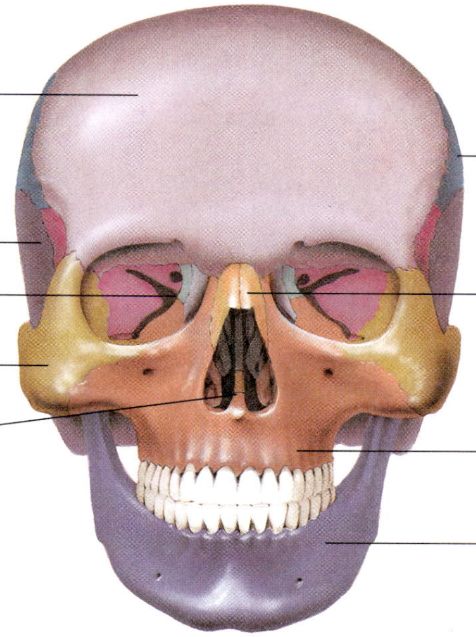

Figure 6-5 Facial bones

bones and 12 others make up the facial bones. All of the facial bones are connected by immovable joints (sutures), with the exception of the mandible (the only movable joint of the skull). Refer to **Figure 6-5** as you study the facial bones.

(1) mandibular bone (man-**DIB**-yoo-lar)	The **mandibular** bone, or mandible, is the lower jaw bone. It is the largest, strongest bone of the face and is the only movable bone of the skull. The mandibular bone meets the temporal bone in a movable joint called the **temporomandibular joint**, or **TMJ**. The mandible contains sockets for the teeth along its upper margin.
(2) maxillary bones (**MACK**-sih-**ler**-ee)	The two **maxillary** bones (maxillae) are the bones of the upper jaw. They are fused in the midline by a suture. These two bones form not only the upper jaw, but also the hard palate (front part of the roof of the mouth). The maxillary bones contain the maxillary sinuses, and the sockets for the teeth along the lower margin.
(3) zygomatic bones (zeye-go-**MAT**-ik)	The two **zygomatic** bones—one on each side of the face—form the high part of the cheek and the outer border of the eye orbits.
(4) nasal bones (**NAY**-zl)	The two slender nasal bones give shape to the nose by forming the upper part of the bridge. The lower part of the nose is formed by septal cartilage. The nasal bones meet at the midline of the face; they also join the frontal bone, the ethmoid bone, and the maxillae.
(5) lacrimal bones (**LACK**-rim-al)	The two small **lacrimal** bones are paper-thin and shaped somewhat like a fingernail. They are located at the inner corner of each eye, forming the sidewall of the nasal cavity and the middle wall of the eye orbit. The lacrimal bones join the cheek bones on each side to form the fossa, which houses the tear, or lacrimal, duct.

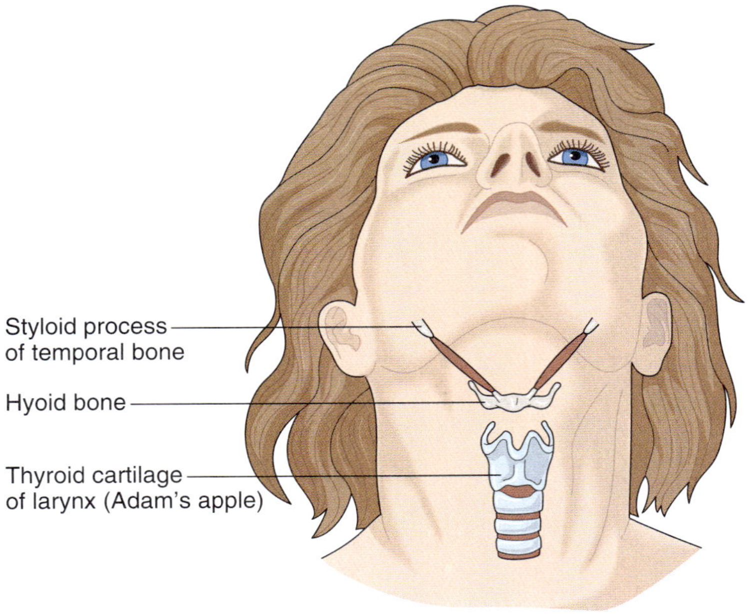

Figure 6-6 Hyoid bone

(6) vomer (**VOH**-mer)

The **vomer** is a thin, flat bone that forms the lower portion of the nasal septum. It joins with the sphenoid, palatine, ethmoid, and maxillary bones.

Other facial bones that are not shown in the illustration include the following:

palatine bones (**PAL**-ah-tine)

The two **palatine** bones are shaped like the letter L: They have a vertical and a horizontal portion. The vertical portion of the palatine bones forms the sidewall of the back of the nasal cavity. The horizontal portion of the palatine bones joins in the midline to form the back (posterior) part of the roof of the mouth, or hard palate. The palatine bones also join with the maxillae and sphenoid bone.

nasal conchae (**NAY**-zl **KONG**-kee)

The two inferior **nasal conchae** bones help to complete the nasal cavity by forming the side and lower wall. These bones connect with the maxilla, lacrimal, ethmoid, and palatine bones.

Hyoid Bone

The **hyoid** (**HIGH**-oyd) **bone** is located just above the larynx and below the mandible (see **Figure 6-6**). It does not connect with any other bone to form a joint, but it is suspended from the temporal bone by ligaments. The hyoid bone serves as points of attachment for muscles of the tongue and throat.

Vertebral Bones

The bones of the vertebral column form the long axis of the body. Also referred to as the spinal column or the "backbones," the vertebral column consists of 24 **vertebrae,** the sacrum, and the coccyx. It offers protection to the spinal cord as it passes through the central opening of each vertebra

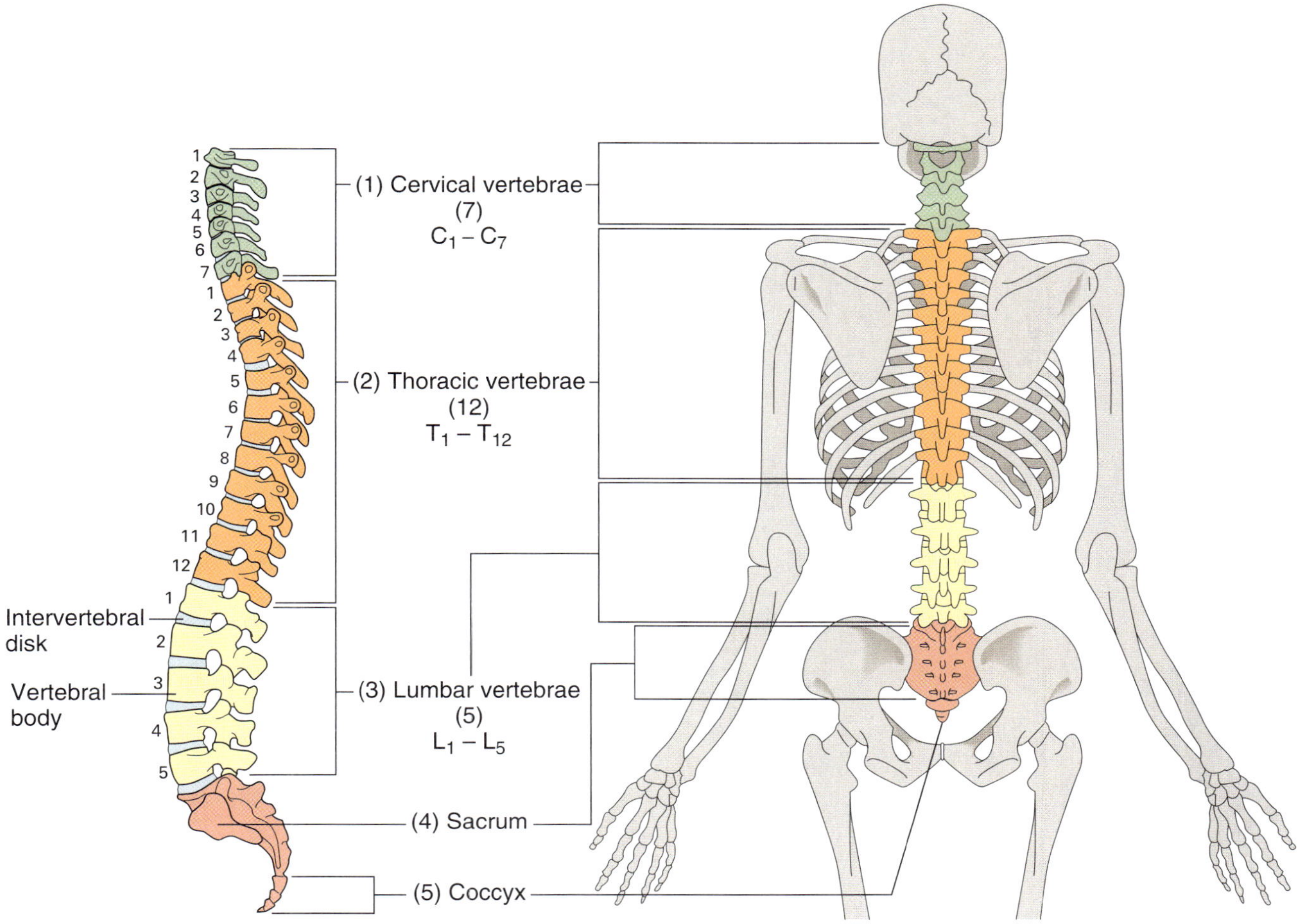

Figure 6-7 Divisions of a vertebral column

for the length of the column. The vertebral column, which connects with the skull, the ribs, and the pelvis, is divided into five segments, or divisions. The first three of these segments—the cervical, thoracic, and lumbar vertebrae—provide some flexibility in movement to the spinal column because each vertebra is separated by a cartilaginous disk. As you study the divisions of the vertebral column, refer to **Figure 6-7.**

(1) cervical vertebrae
(**SIR**-vih-kal **VER**-teh-bray)

The first segment of the vertebral column is the **cervical vertebrae,** which consists of the first seven bones of the vertebral column. These are neck bones that do not communicate with the ribs. The cervical vertebrae are identified specifically as C1–C7. The first cervical vertebra, which connects the spine with the occipital bone of the head, is also known as "atlas," after the Greek god Atlas, who supported the world on his shoulders. The second cervical vertebra is known as "axis," because atlas rotates about this bone, providing the rotating movements of the head.

(2) thoracic vertebrae
(tho-**RASS**-ik **VER**-teh-bray)

Progressing down the vertebral column, the second segment is the **thoracic** vertebrae, consisting of the next 12 vertebrae. These vertebrae connect with the 12 pairs of ribs and are identified specifically as T1–T12.

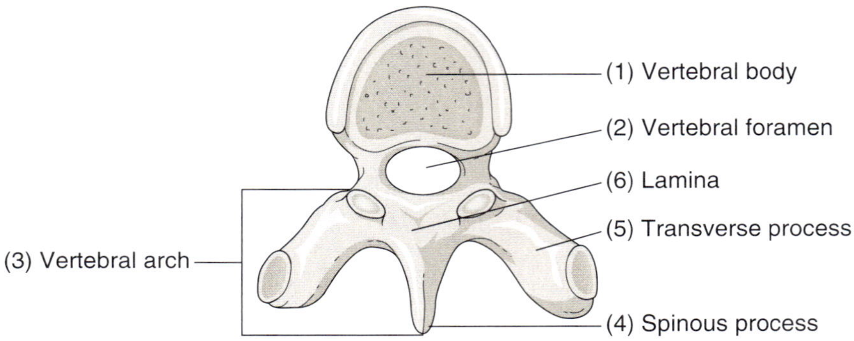

Figure 6-8 Structure of a vertebra

(3) lumbar vertebrae
(**LUM**-bar **VER**-teh-bray)

The third segment is the **lumbar vertebrae,** consisting of the next five vertebrae. The lumbar vertebrae are larger and heavier than the other vertebrae, and support the back and lower trunk of the body. These vertebrae do not communicate with the ribs. They are identified specifically as L1–L5.

(4) sacrum
(**SAY**-crum)

The fourth segment of the vertebral column—the **sacrum**—is located below the lumbar vertebrae. The adult sacrum is a single, triangular-shaped bone that resulted from the fusion of the five individual sacral bones of the child. The sacrum is wedged between the two hip bones and is attached to the pelvic girdle.

(5) coccyx
(**COCK**-six)

The fifth segment of the vertebral column is the **coccyx** (also called the "tailbone"), located at the very end of the vertebral column. The adult coccyx is a single bone that resulted from the fusion of four individual coccygeal bones in the child.

We shall now examine the vertebral column more closely by taking a look at the structure of a vertebra. Refer to **Figure 6–8** as you read.

Although the vertebrae within the spinal column vary considerably from segment to segment, they do have basic similarities. For example, each vertebra has a body called the **(1) vertebral body.** This thick, anterior portion of the vertebra is drum-shaped and serves as the weight-bearing part of the spinal column. Each of the vertebral bodies of the spinal column is separated by a disc of cartilage called the **intervertebral disk.** These cartilaginous discs are flat, circular, platelike structures that serve as shock absorbers, or cushions, between the vertebral bodies. The discs also provide some flexibility to the spinal column. With the exception of the sacrum and the coccyx, the center of each vertebra contains a large opening, called the **(2) vertebral foramen,** which serves as a passageway for the spinal cord. The vertebral column, as a unit, forms a bony spinal canal that protects the spinal cord. The posterior part of the vertebra is called the **(3) vertebral arch,** which consists of a **(4) spinous process** projecting from the midline of the back of the vertebral arch, a **(5) transverse process,** which extends laterally from the vertebral arch, and a space between the transverse process and the spinous process known as the **(6) lamina.** The spinous and transverse processes of the vertebrae serve as points of attachment for muscles and ligaments.

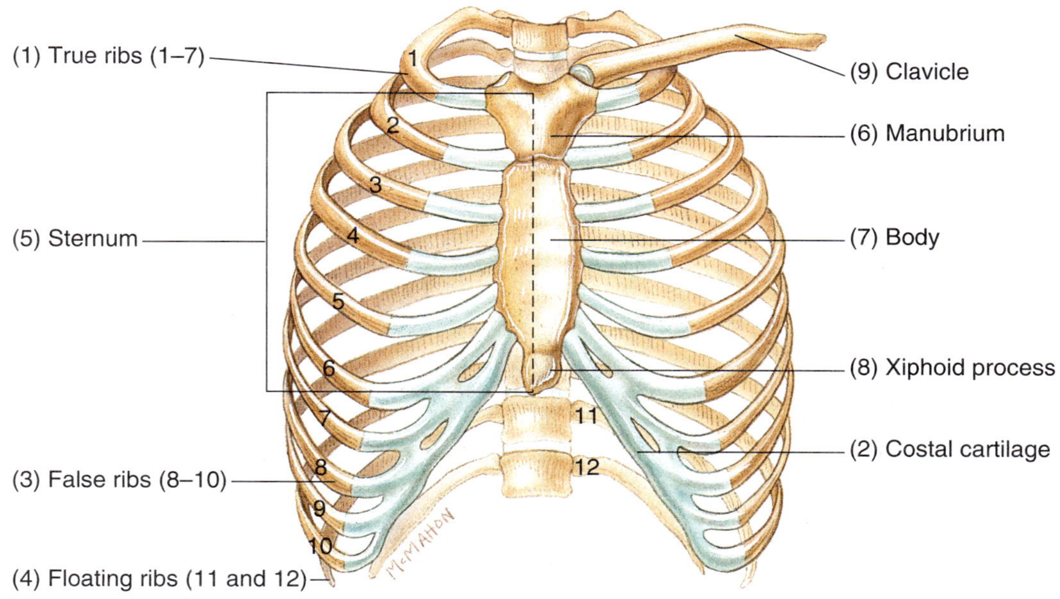

Figure 6-9 Bones of the thorax

Bones of the Thorax

The bones that create the shape of the thoracic cavity (chest cavity) are the ribs and the sternum, with the thoracic vertebrae forming the center back support. As you study these bones, refer to **Figure 6-9.**

The 12 pairs of ribs that shape the thorax are divided into three categories: true ribs, false ribs, and floating ribs. The **(1) true ribs** are the first 7 pairs of ribs (ribs 1–7). They are called true ribs because they attach to the sternum in the front and to the vertebrae in the back. The ribs attach to the sternum by means of **(2) costal cartilage,** which extends from each individual rib. The **(3) false ribs** consist of the next 3 pairs of ribs (ribs 8–10). They get the name false ribs because they connect in the back to the vertebrae but not with the sternum in the front. Instead they attach to the cartilage of the rib above (the seventh rib). The last 2 pairs of ribs (11 and 12) are called **(4) floating ribs.** Although these ribs attach to the vertebrae in the back, they are completely free of attachment in the front. The spaces between the ribs, called the intercostal spaces, contain the blood vessels, nerves, and muscles.

The **(5) sternum** is also called the breastbone. It is a flat, elongated bone (somewhat sword-shaped) that forms the midline portion of the front of the thorax. The broad, upper end of the sternum is called the **(6) manubrium;** it connects with each clavicle (collarbone) while the sides of the manubrium connect with the first pair of ribs. The elongated **(7) body** of the sternum connects on its sides with the second through seventh pair of ribs. The lower portion of the sternum is called the **(8) xiphoid process.** The **(9) clavicle,** also called the collarbone, is a slender bone with two shallow curves that helps to support the shoulder by connecting laterally to the scapula and anteriorly to the sternum.

The **scapula,** a large triangular-shaped bone, is also called the shoulder blade (see **Figure 6-10**). The portion of the scapula that can be felt in the

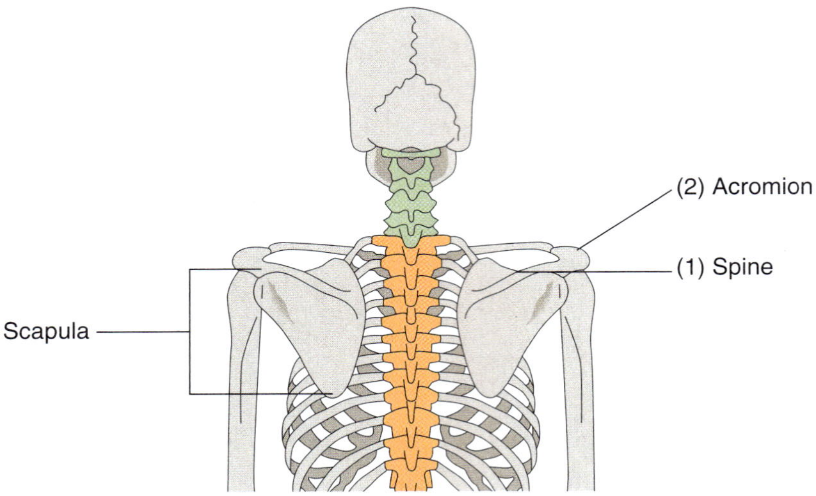

Figure 6-10 Scapula

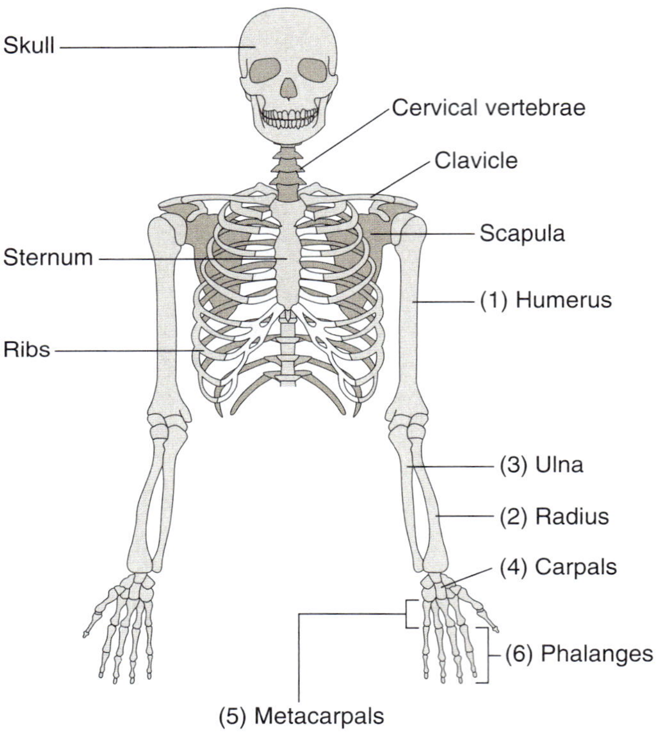

Figure 6-11 Bones of the upper extremities

back, behind the shoulder, is the raised ridge called the **(1) spine.** This area serves as points of attachment for muscles. The (2) **acromion** is the somewhat spoon-shaped projection of the scapula that connects with the clavicle to form the highest point of the shoulder.

Bones of the Upper Extremities

The bones of the upper extremities, shown in **Figure 6-11,** include the following.

(1) humerus (**HYOO**-mer-us)	The **humerus** is the upper arm bone. It joins the scapula above and the radius and ulna below.
(2) radius (**RAY**-dee-us)	The **radius** is one of the two lower arm bones that joins the humerus above and the wrist bones below; it is on the lateral, or thumb, side of the arm.
(3) ulna (**UHL**-nah)	The **ulna** is the second of the two lower arm bones that joins the humerus above and the wrist bones below; it is on the medial, or little finger, side of the arm. The ulna has a large projection at its end called the **olecranon** process. It is the olecranon that forms the point of the elbow.
(4) carpals (**CAR**-pals)	The bones of the wrist are known as the **carpals.** Each wrist has eight carpal bones (two rows of four bones each).
(5) metacarpals (met-ah-**CAR**-pals)	The bones of the hand are known as the **metacarpals**; they form the bones of the hand. The word *metacarpal* literally means "beyond the carpals." The metacarpals join with the carpals at their upper (proximal) end, and with the phalanges (fingers) at their lower (distal) end.
(6) phalanges (fah-**LAN**-jeez)	The bones of the fingers are known as the phalanges (as are the bones of the toes). Each finger has three phalangeal bones; the thumb has only two.

Pelvic Bones

The **pelvis,** shown in **Figure 6-12,** is the bony structure formed by the innominate (hip) bones (the ilium, ischium, and pubis), the sacrum, and the coccyx. The pelvis is the lower part of the trunk of the body and serves as a support for the vertebral column and as a connection with the lower extremities. The term **pelvic girdle** refers to the bony ring formed by the hip bones, the sacrum, and the coccyx—the bony ring that forms the walls of the pelvis.

If you place your hand just below your waist, on your hip, the bone your hand is resting on is the ilium. The **(1) ilium** is the largest of the three hip bones; it is the upper flared portion of the hip bones. The **(2) iliac crest** is

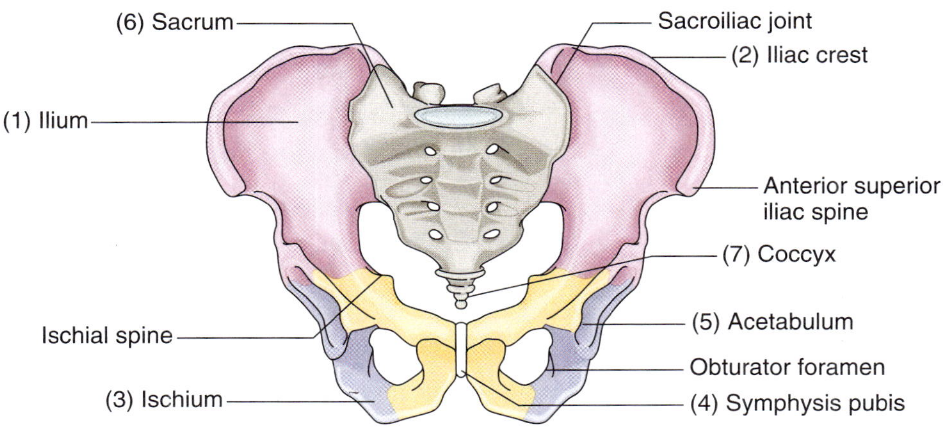

Figure 6-12 Bones of the pelvis

the upper curved edge of the ilium. The iliac crest has an anterior projection (toward the front of the body) called the anterior iliac crest, or the anterior iliac spine. It also has a posterior projection that is not as prominent. As you look at the illustration, notice the broad shape of the ilium. This flat bone is a good source for red bone marrow, as we studied earlier.

The **(3) ischium** is the lowest part of the hip bones and is the strongest of the pelvic bones. If you are sitting in a chair as you read this material, the bony part of your body that rests on the seat of the chair is your ischium (unless, of course, you are sitting on your feet!). The ischium has a projection on either side, at the back of the pelvic outlet, known as the **ischial** spine. The ischial spine takes on a great degree of importance in determining the adequacy of the diameter of the pelvic outlet for childbirth; it also serves as a point of reference in relation to how far a baby's head has progressed down the birth canal during labor.

The pubis is the anterior (front) part of the hip bones. The two bones of the pubis meet at the anterior midline of the pelvis and are connected by a cartilaginous joint. This point of connection of the two **pubic** bones is called the **(4) symphysis pubis.**

Segments of the ilium, ischium, and pubis form the **(5) acetabulum,** which is the socket that serves as the connecting point for the femur (thigh bone) and the hip. This is also known as the hip joint. The (6) sacrum and the (7) coccyx are actually part of the vertebral column and have been discussed earlier; they are, however, noted in Figure 6-12 to show their correlation with the pelvis.

Bones of the Lower Extremities

As you study the bones of the lower extremities, refer to **Figure 6-13** for a visual reference. The bones of the lower extremities include the following.

(1) femur (**FEE**-mer)	The **femur** is the thigh bone. It is the longest, heaviest, and strongest bone in the body. The proximal end of the femur (the end nearest the pelvis) has a large rounded head (somewhat ball-shaped) that fits into the acetabulum of the hip bones, forming the hip joint. The neck of the femur connects the head with the shaft of the bone. The greater **trochanter** is the large lateral projection at the point where the neck and the shaft meet. This projection, and the lesser trochanter, serves as a site for muscle attachment. The greater trochanter takes on significant importance as a landmark when selecting the site for the ventrogluteal intramuscular injection.
(2) patella (pah-**TELL**-ah)	The **patella** is the knee bone, or kneecap. It is the largest sesamoid bone in the body. Located in the tendon of the large anterior thigh muscle (quadriceps femoris), the patella covers and protects the knee joint, which is the point of connection between the thigh bone (femur) and one of the lower leg bones (tibia).
(3) tibia (**TIB**-ee-ah)	The **tibia** is the larger and stronger of the two lower leg bones. Also called the shin bone, the tibia is located on the great toe side of the

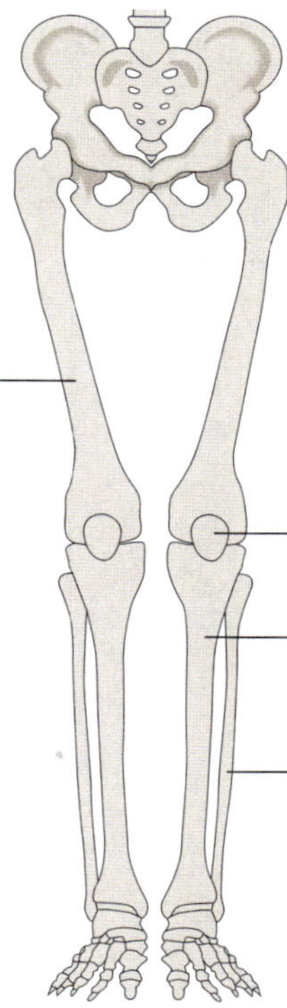

Figure 6-13 Bones of the lower extremities

lower leg. If you move your hand down the center front of your lower leg, you will feel the sharp anterior crest of the tibia.

The proximal end of the tibia connects with the femur to form the knee joint. The tibial **tuberosity** serves as an anchoring point for the tendons of the muscles from the thigh (those that enclose the patella). The distal end of the tibia connects with the tarsal bones; it has a downward projection called the medial malleolus, which is the bony prominence on the inner aspect of the ankle (place your hand on the inside of your ankle to feel this bony prominence).

(4) fibula
(**FIB**-yoo-lah)

The **fibula** is the more slender of the two lower leg bones and is lateral to the tibia. The proximal end of the fibula connects with the lateral condyle of the tibia. The distal end of the fibula projects downward to form the lateral malleolus, which is the bony prominence on the outer aspect of the ankle (place your hand on the outside of your ankle to feel this bony prominence). The fibula connects again with the tibia just above the lateral malleolus and, therefore, is not a weight-bearing bone.

The bones of the ankle (shown in **Figure 6-14A**) are known as the (1) **tarsals.** There are seven tarsal bones; the largest is the (2) **calcaneus.** The calcaneus, also known as the heel bone, serves as a point of attachment for several of the muscles of the calf. Just above the calcaneus is the (3) **talus** bone, which joins with the tibia and fibula to form the ankle joint. The impact of a person's entire body weight is received by the talus bone at this point of connection and is then distributed to the other tarsal bones.

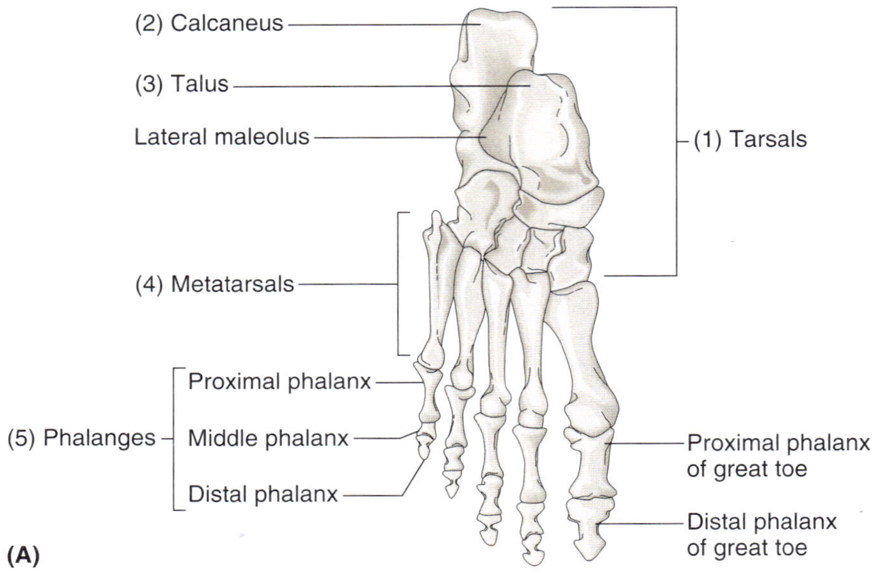

Figure 6-14A Bones of the ankle and foot

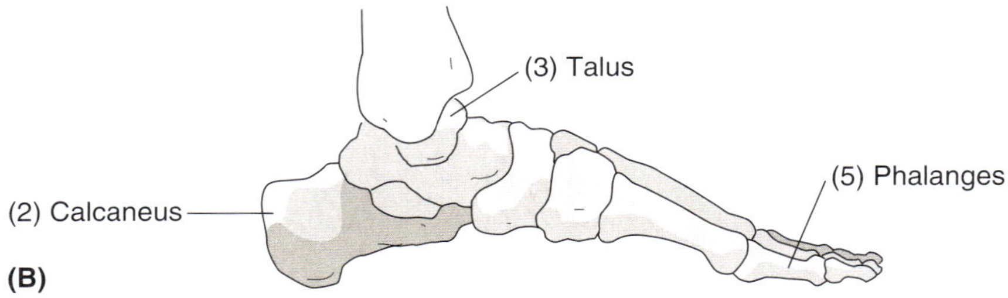

Figure 6-14B Bones of the ankle and foot

The bones of the foot (also shown in Figure 6-14A) are known as the **(4) metatarsals.** The heads of the metatarsal bones form the ball of the foot. The metatarsal bones, plus the tarsal bones, form the arch of the foot. The structural design of the arches of the foot, along with support from strong ligaments and tendons, makes the tarsal and metatarsal bones architecturally sound for weight bearing. The bones of the toes (shown in **Figure 6-14B**) are known as the **(5) phalanges** (as are the bones of the fingers). Each toe has three phalangeal bones, except for the great toe, which has only two.

Vocabulary

The following vocabulary words are frequently used when discussing the skeletal system.

WORD	DEFINITION
articular cartilage (ar-**TIK**-u-lar **CAR**-tih-lij)	Thin layer of cartilage that covers the ends of the long bones and the surfaces of the joints.
bone depressions	Concave, indented areas or openings in bones.

bone markings	Specific features of individual bones.
bone processes	Projections or outgrowths of bones.
cancellous bone (**CAN**-sell-us)	Spongy bone, not as dense as compact bone.
cervical vertebrae (**SIR**-vih-kal **VER**-teh-bray) cervic/o = neck -al = pertaining to	Vertebrae or bones of the neck, C1–C7.
compact bone	Hard outer shell of the bone.
condyle (**CON**-dill)	Knucklelike projection at the end of a bone.
crest	Distinct border or ridge, as in iliac crest.
diaphysis (**dye**-**AFF**-ih-sis)	Main shaftlike portion of a bone.
epiphyseal line (**ep**-ih-**FIZZ**-e-al)	A layer of cartilage that separates the diaphysis from the epiphysis of a bone; also known as the epiphyseal plate.
epiphysis (eh-**PIFF**-ih-sis)	The end of a bone.
false ribs	Rib pairs 8–10, which connect to the vertebrae in the back but not to the sternum in the front because they join the seventh rib in the front.
fissure (**FISH**-er)	A groove or depression in a bone; a sulcus.
flat bones	Bones that are broad and thin with flat or curved surfaces, such as the sternum.
floating ribs	Rib pairs 11–12, which connect to the vertebrae in the back but are free of any attachment in the front.
fontanelle or **fontanel** (**fon**-tah-**NELL**)	Space between the bones of an infant's cranium; "soft spot."
foramen (for-**AY**-men)	Hole in a bone through which blood vessels or nerves pass.
fossa (**FOSS**-ah)	Hollow or concave depression in a bone.
haversian canals (ha-**VER**-shan)	System of small canals within compact bone that contain blood vessels, lymphatic vessels, and nerves.
hematopoiesis (**hem**-ah-toh-poy-**EE**-sis) hemat/o = blood -poiesis = formation of	The normal formation and development of blood cells in the bone marrow.

intercostal spaces (in-ter-**COS**-tal) inter- = between cost/o = ribs -al = pertaining to	Spaces between the ribs.
intervertebral disc (in-ter-**VER**-teh-bral) inter- = between vertebr/o = vertebra -al = pertaining to	A flat, circular platelike structure of cartilage that serves as a cushion, or shock absorber, between the vertebrae.
long bones	Bones that are longer than they are wide and with distinctive shaped ends, such as the femur.
lumbar vertebrae (**LUM**-bar **VER**-teh-bray) lumb/o = loins, lower back -ar = pertaining to	The vertebrae of the lower back, L1–L5.
medullary cavity (**MED**-u-lair-ee)	The center portion of the shaft of a long bone containing the yellow marrow.
ossification (**oss**-sih-fih-**KAY**-shun)	The conversion of cartilage and fibrous connective tissue to bone; the formation of bone.
osteoblasts (**OSS**-tee-oh-blasts) oste/o = bone -blast = immature, embryonic	Immature bone cells that actively produce bony tissue.
osteoclasts (**OSS**-tee-oh-clasts) oste/o = bone -clast = something that breaks	Large cells that absorb or digest old bone tissue.
osteocytes (**OSS**-tee-oh-sites) oste/o = bone cyt/o = cell -e = noun ending	Mature bone cells.
periosteum (pair-ee-**AH**-stee-um) peri- = around oste/o =bone -um = noun ending	The thick, white, fibrous membrane that covers the surface of a long bone.
red bone marrow	The soft, semifluid substance located in the small spaces of cancellous bone that is the source of blood cell production.
resorption (ree-**SORP**-shun)	The process of removing or digesting old bone tissue.

sesamoid bones (**SES**-a-moyd)	Irregular bones imbedded in tendons near a joint, as in the kneecap.
short bones	Bones that are about as long as they are wide and somewhat box-shaped, such as the wrist bone.
sinus (**SIGH**-nuss)	An opening or hollow space in a bone; a cavity within a bone.
spine	A sharp projection from the surface of a bone, similar to a crest.
sulcus (**SULL**-kus)	A groove or depression in a bone; a fissure.
sutures (**SOO**-chers)	Immovable joints, such as those of the cranium.
thoracic vertebrae (tho-**RASS**-ik **VER**-teh-bray) thorac/o = chest -ic = pertaining to	The 12 vertebrae of the chest, T1–T12.
trabeculae (trah-**BEK**-u-lay)	Needlelike bony spicules within cancellous bone that contribute to the spongy appearance; their distribution along lines of stress add to the strength of the bone.
trochanter (tro-**CAN**-ter)	Large bony process located below the neck of the femur.
true ribs	The first seven pairs of ribs, which connect to the vertebrae in the back and to the sternum in the front.
tubercle (**TOO**-ber-kl)	A small rounded process of a bone.
tuberosity (too-ber-**OSS**-ih-tee)	An elevated, broad, rounded process of a bone.
vertebral foramen (**VER**-teh-bral for-**AY**-men)	A large opening in the center of each vertebra that serves as a passageway for the spinal cord.
yellow marrow	Located in the diaphysis of long bones, yellow marrow is composed of fatty tissue and is inactive in the formation of blood cells.

Word Elements

The following word elements pertain to the skeletal system. As you review the list, pronounce each word element aloud twice and check the box after you "say it." Write the definition for the example word given for each word element. You may use your medical dictionary.

WORD ELEMENT	PRONUNCIATION	"SAY IT"	MEANING
acetabul/o **acetabul**ar	ass-eh-**TAB**-yoo-loh ass-eh-**TAB**-yoo-lar	☐	acetabulum

Word Part / Example	Pronunciation		Definition
-blast, blast/o **osteo**blast	**BLAST**-oh **OSS**-stee-oh-blast	☐	embryonic stage of development
calc/o, calc/i hypo**calc**emia	**KALK**-oh, **KALK**-sigh **high**-poh-**kal**-**SEE**-mee-ah	☐	calcium
calcane/o **calcane**odynia	kal-**KAY**-nee-oh kal-**kay**-nee-oh-**DIN**-ee-ah	☐	heel bone
carp/o **carp**al	**CAR**-poh **CAR**-pal	☐	wrist
-clast, -clastic osteo**clast**	**CLAST, CLAST**-ic **OSS**-stee-oh-clast	☐	to break
clavicul/o supra**clavicul**ar	klah-**VIK**-yoo-loh **soo**-prah-klah-**VIK**-yoo-lar	☐	collarbone
coccyg/o **coccyg**eal	**COCK**-si-goh cock-**SIJ**-ee-al	☐	coccyx
cost/o **cost**ochondral	**KOSS**-toh **koss**-toh-**CON**-dral	☐	ribs
crani/o **crani**otomy	**KRAY**-nee-oh kray-nee-**OTT**-oh-mee	☐	skull, cranium
femor/o **femor**al	**FEM**-or-oh **FEM**-or-al	☐	femur
fibul/o **fibul**ar	**FIB**-yoo-loh **FIB**-yoo-lar	☐	fibula
gen/o osteo**gen**esis	**JEN**-oh oss-tee-oh-**JEN**-eh-sis	☐	to produce
humer/o **humer**al	**HYOO**-mor-oh **HYOO**-mor-al	☐	humerus
ili/o **ili**ac	**ILL**-ee-oh **ILL**-ee-ac	☐	ilium
ischi/o **ischi**al	**ISS**-kee-oh **ISS**-kee-al	☐	ischium
kyph/o **kyph**osis	**KI**-foh ki-**FOH**-sis	☐	humpback; pertaining to a hump
lamin/o **lamin**ectomy	**LAM**-ih-no **lam**-ih-**NEK**-toh-mee	☐	lamina
lord/o **lord**osis	**LOR**-doh lor-**DOH**-sis	☐	swayback; bent

lumb/o **lumb**ar	**LUM**-boh **LUM**-bar	☐	loins, lower back
-malacia osteo**malacia**	mah-**LAY**-she-ah **oss**-tee-oh-mah-**LAY**-she-**ah**	☐	softening
mandibul/o **mandibul**ar	man-**DIB**-yoo-loh man-**DIB**-yoo-lar	☐	mandible (lower jaw bone)
mastoid/o **mastoid**itis	mass-**TOYD**-oh mass-toyd-**EYE**-tis	☐	mastoid process
maxill/o **maxill**ary	**MACK**-sih-loh **MACK**-sih-**ler**-ee	☐	upper jaw
metacarp/o **metacarp**als	met-ah-**CAR**-poh met-ah-**CAR**-pals	☐	hand bones
metatars/o **metatars**algia	met-ah-**TAR**-soh met-ah-tar-**SAL**-jee-ah	☐	foot bones
myel/o osteo**myel**itis	**MY**-ell-oh **oss**-tee-oh-**my**-ell-**EYE**-tis	☐	spinal cord or bone marrow
olecran/o **olecran**on	oh-**LEK**-ran-oh oh-**LEK**-ran-on	☐	elbow
orth/o **orth**opedics	**OR**-thoh or-thoh-**PEE**-diks	☐	straight
oste/o **oste**oma	**OSS**-tee-oh oss-tee-**OH**-mah	☐	bone
patell/o, patell/a **patell**ar	pah-**TELL**-oh, pah-**TELL**-ah pah-**TELL**-ar	☐	kneecap
pelv/i **pelv**imetry	**PELL**-vigh pell-**VIM**-eh-tree	☐	pelvis
phalang/o **phalang**itis	fal-**AN**-goh **fal**-an-**JYE**-tis	☐	fingers, toes
-physis dia**physis**	**FIH**-sis dye-**AFF**-ih-sis	☐	growth, growing
-porosis osteo**porosis**	por-**ROW**-sis **oss**-tee-oh-por-**ROW**-sis	☐	passage or pore
pub/o **pub**ic	**PYOO**-boh **PYOO**-bik	☐	pubis
rach/i **rach**itis	**RAH**-kigh rah-**KIGH**-tis	☐	spinal column

radi/o **radi**al	**RAY**-dee-oh **RAY**-dee-al	☐	radiation; also refers to the radius
scapul/o **scapul**ar	**SKAP**-yoo-loh **SKAP**-yoo-lar	☐	shoulder blade
scoli/o **scoli**osis	**SKOH**-lee-oh skoh-lee-**OH**-sis	☐	crooked, bent
spondyl/o **spondyl**osis	**SPON**-dih-loh spon-dih-**LOH**-sis	☐	vertebra
stern/o sub**stern**al	**STER**-noh sub-**STER**-nal	☐	sternum
tars/o **tars**als	**TAR**-soh **TAR**-sals	☐	ankle bones
tempor/o **tempor**al	**TEM**-por-oh **TEM**-por-al	☐	temples of the head
vertebr/o inter**vertebr**al	ver-**TEE**-broh in-ter-ver-**TEE**-bral	☐	vertebra

Pathological Conditions

As you study the pathological conditions of the skeletal system, note that the **basic definition** is in bold print, followed by a detailed description in regular print. The phonetic pronunciation is directly beneath each term and a breakdown of the component parts of the term when appropriate.

osteoporosis
(oss-tee-oh-poh-**ROW**-sis)
- oste/o = bone
- por/o = cavity, passage
- -osis = condition

Osteoporosis literally means porous bones; that is, bones that were once strong become fragile due to loss of bone density.

The patient is more susceptible to fractures, especially in the wrist, hip, and vertebral column. Osteoporosis occurs most frequently in postmenopausal women, in sedentary or immobilized individuals, and in patients on long-term steroid treatment.

A major factor in osteoporosis is hormonal: Postmenopausal women are at a high risk for osteoporosis because estrogen production and bone calcium storage decrease with menopause. Hereditary risk factors include traits such as having blonde or red hair, fair skin, and freckles (characteristic of people of Scandinavian or northern European descent).

Classic characteristics of osteoporosis are fractures that occur in response to normal activity or minimal trauma, a loss of standing height of greater than 2 inches, and the development of the typical cervical kyphosis (dowager's hump). See **Figure 6-15.**

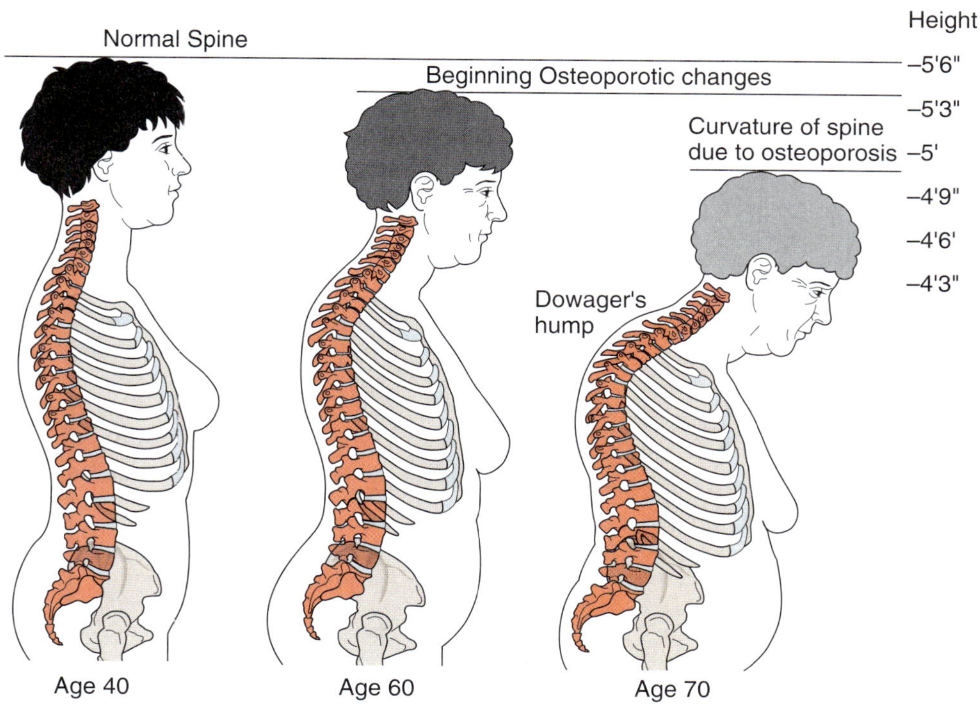

Figure 6-15 Structural changes due to osteoporosis

Treatment includes, but is not limited to, prescribing drug therapy such as estrogen replacement therapy and calcium supplements, promoting calcium intake, and promoting active weight-bearing exercises.

---

osteomalacia
(oss-tee-oh-mah-**LAY**-she-ah)
oste/o = bone
-malacia = softening

Osteomalacia is a disease in which the bones become abnormally soft due to a deficiency of calcium and phosphorus in the blood (which is necessary for bone mineralization). This disease results in fractures and noticeable deformities of the weight-bearing bones. When the disease occurs in children, it is called rickets.

The deficiency of these minerals is due to a lack of vitamin D, which is necessary for the absorption of calcium and phosphorus by the body. The vitamin D deficiency may be caused by a diet lacking in vitamin D, by a lack of exposure to sunlight, or by a metabolic disorder causing **malabsorption.**

Treatment includes daily administration of vitamin D and a diet sufficient in calcium and phosphorus, as well as protein; supplemental calcium may also be prescribed.

---

osteomyelitis
(oss-tee-oh-my-ell-**EYE**-tis)
oste/o = bone
myel/o = bone marrow
-itis = inflammation

Osteomyelitis is a local or generalized infection of the bone and bone marrow, resulting from a bacterial infection that has spread to the bone tissue through the blood.

Osteomyelitis is most frequently caused by a staphylococcal infection, but it may also be caused by a viral or fungal infection. The infection usually spreads from adjacent infected tissue to the bone marrow; it may also be introduced directly into the bone tissue as a result of injury or surgery.

Although symptoms vary with individuals, generalized symptoms of osteomyelitis include a sudden onset of fever (above 101°F), pain or tenderness, **erythema** (redness) and swelling over the affected bone, **anorexia** (loss of appetite), headaches, and general **malaise** (vague feeling of discomfort). There may be an open wound in the skin over the affected bone, with **purulent** (pus-containing) drainage.

Treatment for osteomyelitis includes bed rest and administration of intravenous or intramuscular antibiotics for 4 to 6 weeks. If the antibiotic therapy is not effective, surgical treatment may be necessary to drain the bone of pus and to remove any dead bone tissue.

Ewing's sarcoma
(**YOO**-wings sar-**KOH**-mah)
sarc/o = related to the flesh
-oma = tumor

Ewing's sarcoma is a malignant tumor of the bones common to young adults, particularly adolescent boys.

It usually develops in the long bones or the pelvis and is characterized by pain, swelling, fever, and **leukocytosis.**

Treatment includes **chemotherapy, radiation,** and surgery to remove the tumor. Patients who respond well to this therapy may not lose the extremity to amputation. The **prognosis** with the combination therapies is around 65% cure rate.

---

osteogenic sarcoma
(oss-tee-oh-**JEN**-ic sar-**KOH**-mah)
oste/o = bone
gen/o = to produce
-ic = pertaining to
sarc/o = related to the flesh
-oma = tumor

Osteogenic sarcoma is a malignant tumor arising from bone. Also known as osteosarcoma, it is the most common malignant bone tumor, with common sites being the distal femur (just above the knee), the proximal tibia (just below the knee), and the proximal humerus (just below the shoulder joint).

Early complaint of pain is often described as an intermittent and dull aching; night pain is common. As the disease rapidly progresses, the pain increases in intensity and duration. Other symptoms include weight loss, general malaise, and loss of appetite (anorexia).

Bone biopsy, x-ray films, **CAT scan,** and **MRI** are used to confirm the diagnosis and determine the location and size of the tumor.

Treatment includes radiation, chemotherapy, and surgery to remove the tumor. Patients who respond well to this combination therapy may not lose the extremity to amputation (which historically has been the treatment of choice). The prognosis for osteogenic sarcoma has improved with the combination therapies.

---

osteochondroma
(oss-tee-oh-kon-**DROH**-mah)
oste/o = bone
chondr/o = cartilage
-oma = tumor

An osteochondroma is the most common benign bone tumor. The femur and the tibia are most frequently involved.

Usually located within the bone marrow cavity, osteochondromas are covered by a cartilaginous cap. The onset of an osteochondroma is usually in childhood, but it may not be diagnosed until adulthood. Approximately 10% of all osteochondromas develop into malignant tumors (sarcomas).

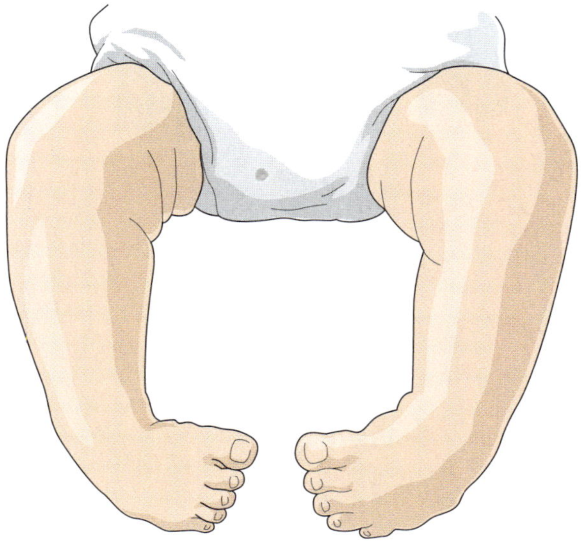

Figure 6-16 Talipes

talipes
(**TAL**-ih-peez)

Clubfoot; the complete name is talipes equinovarus (**eh**-kwine-oh-**VAIR**-us). See **Figure 6-16.**

The infant's foot is fixed in plantar flexion (turned downward) and deviates medially (turned inward), and the heel is in an elevated position; therefore, the infant's foot cannot remain in normal position with the sole of the foot firmly on the floor.

abnormal curvature of the spine

In this section we will define three abnormal curvatures of the spine. For a visual reference, refer to **Figure 6-17.**

(A) Kyphosis (ki-**FOH**-sis) **is an abnormal outward curvature of a portion of the spine, commonly known as humpback or hunchback.**

(B) Lordosis (lor-**DOH**-sis) **is an abnormal inward curvature of a portion of the spine, commonly known as swayback.**

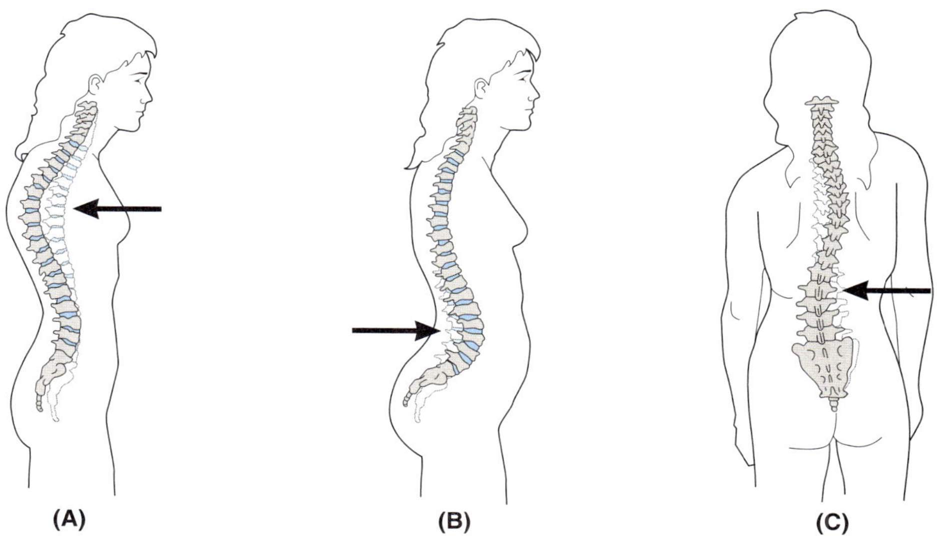

Figure 6-17 Abnormal curvatures of the spine

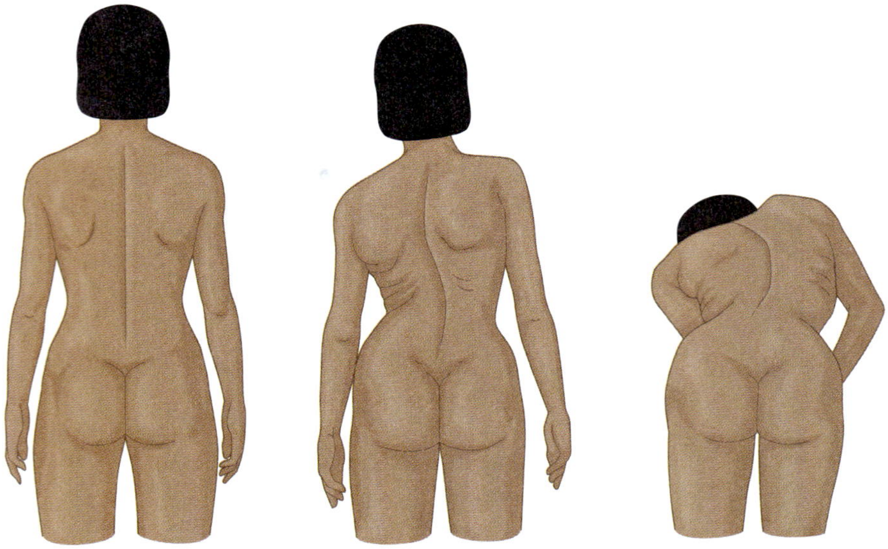

Figure 6-18 Scoliosis screening: (A) Normal spine; (B) patient with scoliosis standing erect (iliac crests are not symmetrical); (C) patient with scoliosis bending forward (shoulders are not symmetrical)

(C) Scoliosis (skoh-lee-**OH**-sis) **is an abnormal lateral (sideward) curvature of a portion of the spine;** the curvature may be to the left or to the right.

These abnormal curvatures of the spine may affect children or adults. The cause may be unknown (**idiopathic**), or it may be due to defects of the spine at birth (**congenital**) or some disease process (**pathological**).

Symptoms of any one of these abnormal curvatures of the spine may range from complaining of chronic fatigue and backache, to noticing that a skirt/dress hemline is longer on one side than the other, to noticing that shoulders are uneven. Scoliosis is sometimes picked up in a general health screening by performing a scoliosis screening. The individual should not be wearing shoes and should be disrobed, at least from the waist up. While the patient is standing erect, and then while the patient is bending forward, the health professional looks for symmetry of the shoulders, iliac crests, and normal alignment of the spinal column (see **Figure 6-18**).

If scoliosis is suspected, an x-ray will confirm or deny the suspicion. Treatment for abnormal curvature of the spine depends on the type and severity of the curvature. It may vary from physical therapy, exercises, or back braces, to surgical intervention for correcting the deformity.

---

fracture

A fracture is a broken bone; a sudden breaking of a bone.

As you read about the different types of fractures, refer to the various illustrations provided.

Classifications of fractures:

Fractures are classified according to the severity of the break. A **closed fracture** (**Figure 6-19A**) is also known as a simple fracture. There is a break in

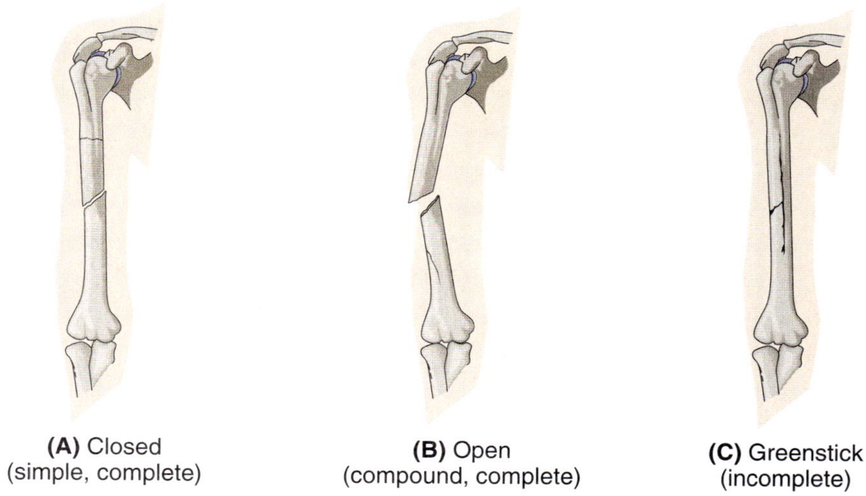

Figure 6-19 (A) Closed fracture (simple, complete); (B) open (compound, complete); (C) greenstick fracture (incomplete)

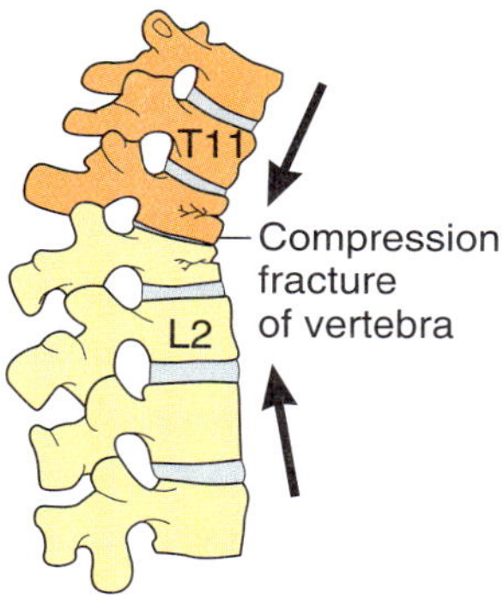

Figure 6-20 Compression fracture

a bone but no open wound in the skin. An **open fracture** (**Figure 6-19B**) is also known as a compound fracture. There is a break in a bone, as well as an open wound in the skin. A **complete fracture** is a break that extends through the entire thickness of the bone. An incomplete fracture is also known as a **greenstick fracture** (**Figure 6-19C**). It is a break that does not extend through the entire thickness of the bone; that is, one side of the bone is broken and one side of the bone is bent. An incomplete fracture gets the name greenstick fracture because its break is similar to trying to snap a "green stick or branch" from a tree; the break is incomplete, with one side breaking and the other side bending considerably but not breaking.

A **compression fracture** is caused by bone surfaces being forced against each other, as in the compression of one vertebra against another. Compression fractures are often associated with osteoporosis. See **Figure 6-20.**

An **impacted fracture** occurs when a direct force causes the bone to break, forcing the broken end of the smaller bone into the broken end of the larger bone. See **Figure 6-21.**

A **comminuted fracture** occurs when the force is so great that it splinters or crushes a segment of the bone. See **Figure 6-22.**

A **Colles' fracture** occurs at the lower end of the radius, within 1 inch of connecting with the wrist bones. See **Figure 6-23.**

A **hairline fracture** is also known as a **stress fracture.** It is a minor fracture in which the bone continues to be in perfect alignment; the fracture appears on an x-ray as a very thin "hair line" between the two segments; it does not extend through the entire surface of the bone. This type of fracture may occur in runners who run too much or too fast on hard surfaces, or who wear improper shoe support. The hairline fracture usually is not visible until 3 to 4 weeks after the onset of symptoms. A **pathological fracture** occurs when a bone, which is weakened by a preexisting disease, breaks in response to a force that would not cause a normal bone to break. Examples of some underlying causes of pathological fractures include, but are not limited to, rickets, osteomalacia, and osteoporosis.

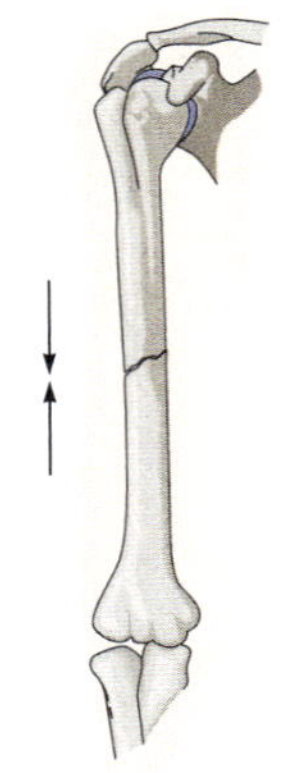

Figure 6-21
Impacted fracture

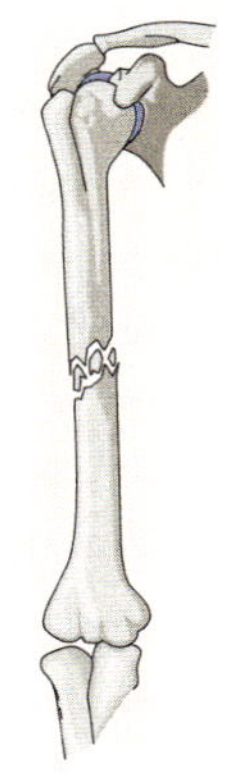

Figure 6-22
Comminuted fracture

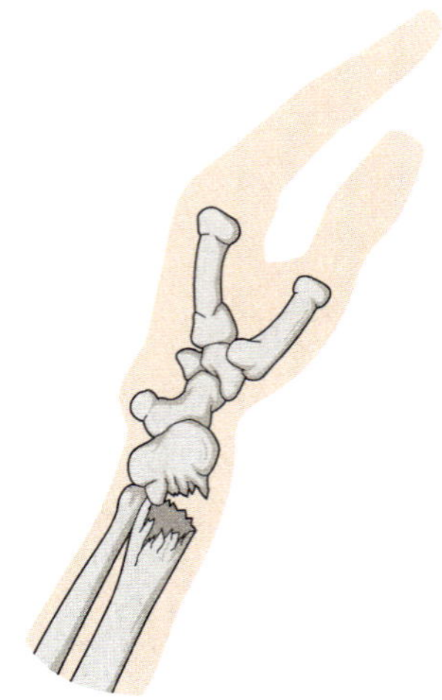

Figure 6-23
Colles' fracture

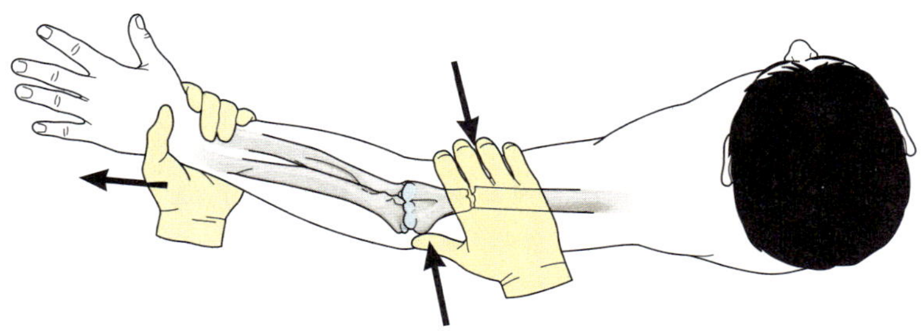

Figure 6-24 Closed reduction of a fracture

Treatment of Fractures

The specific method of treatment for fractures depends on the type of fracture sustained, its location, and any related injuries. An x-ray may be used to confirm and determine the severity of the fracture.

When a bone breaks, the normal anatomic alignment of the bone is displaced. To restore the bone to normal alignment, the fracture must be "reduced"; that is, the fragmented bone ends must be brought back together into a straight line, eliminating or "reducing" the fracture. The reduction of a fracture may be accomplished through closed reduction or open reduction.

Closed reduction of a fracture consists of aligning the bone fragments through manual manipulation or traction, without making an incision into the skin. See **Figure 6-24.**

Once the fracture is reduced, the bone is immobilized to maintain the position of the bone until healing occurs. Examples of devices used to stabilize the realigned bone are a cast, splint, or immobilizer. These devices protect the realigned bone and maintain support. See **Figure 6-25** for immobilization devices.

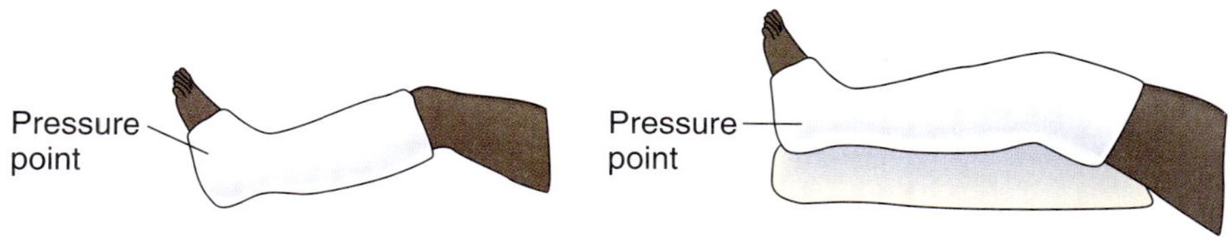

(A) Short leg cast

(B) Long leg cast

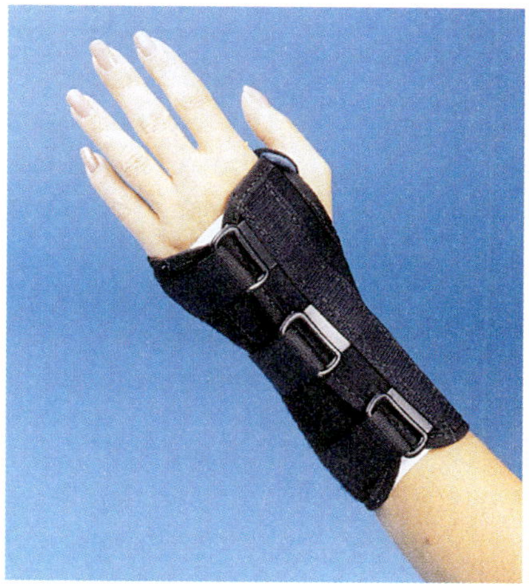

(C) Wrist Immobilizer

Figure 6-25 Devices used to stabilize fractures

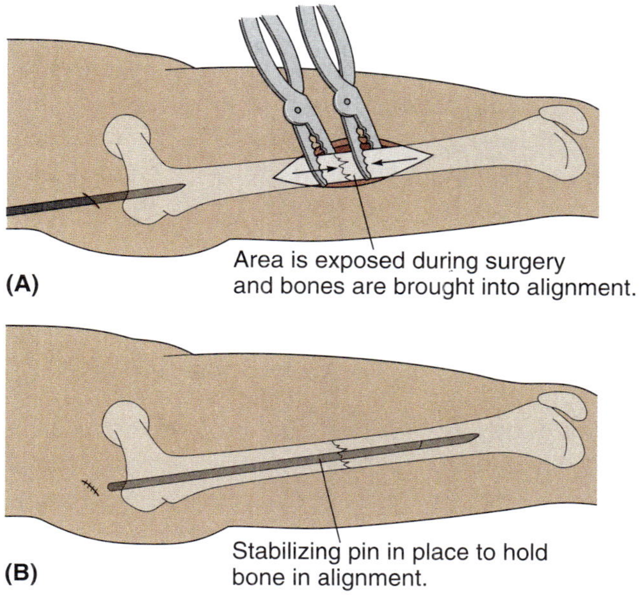

Figure 6-26 Open reduction of a fracture

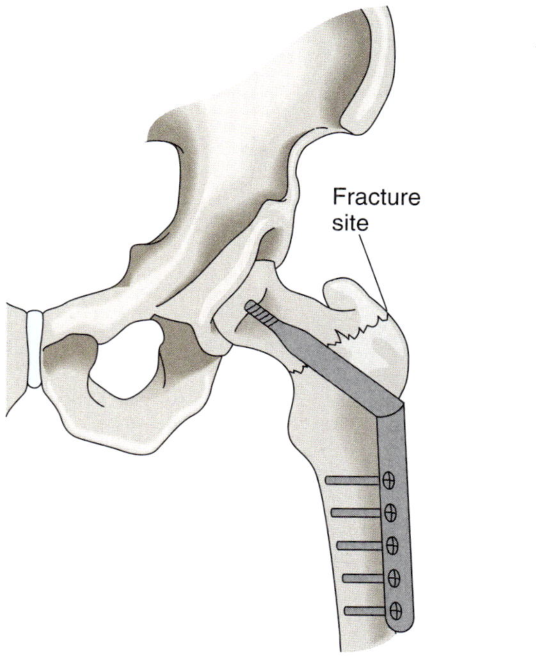

Figure 6-27 Internal fixation devices

Open reduction of a fracture consists of realigning the bone under direct observation during surgery. See **Figure 6-26.** Devices such as screws, pins, wires, and nails may be used to internally maintain the bone alignment while healing takes place. These devices, known as **internal fixation devices,** are more commonly used with fractures of the femur and fractures of joints. See **Figure 6-27.**

Diagnostic Techniques and Procedures

bone scan

A bone scan involves the intravenous injection of a radioisotope, which is absorbed by bone tissue. After approximately 3 hours, the skeleton is scanned with a gamma camera (scanner), moving from one end of the body to the other. The scanner detects the areas of radioactive concentration (areas where the bone absorbs the isotope) and converts the radioactive image to a screen where the concentrations show up as pinpoint dots cast in the image of a skeleton.

Areas of greater concentration of the radioisotope appear darker than other areas of distribution and are called "hot spots." Follow-up x-rays are then conducted to determine the cause of the hot spots.

A bone scan is primarily used to detect the spread of cancer to the bones (metastasis), osteomyelitis, and other destructive changes in the bone. It can be used to detect bone fractures when pathological fractures are suspected and multiple x-rays are not in the best interest of the patient: The "hot spots" on the scan will pinpoint the areas needing x-ray.

bone marrow aspiration

A bone marrow aspiration is the process of removing a small sample of bone marrow from a selected site with a needle for the purpose of examining the specimen under a microscope.

This common method of obtaining a bone marrow sample is used for patients with severe anemia, acute leukemia, neutropenia (decreased number of white blood cells, i.e., neutrophils), and thrombocytopenia (decreased number of platelets). The preferred sites for bone marrow aspiration are (1) the sternum, (2) the iliac crest, and (3) the broad end of the tibia. See **Figure 6-28.**

A bone marrow aspiration is performed using sterile technique in order to prevent osteomyelitis. After the skin has been **anesthetized** (numbed), the aspiration needle is inserted through the skin down to the periosteum.

The periosteum is then anesthetized to lessen the pain of the procedure. When the marrow cavity is entered, the marrow stylet (a long, closed cylinder that keeps the lumen of the aspiration needle closed during entry) is removed, and a sterile syringe is attached to the needle for aspiration of the marrow specimen.

The patient may experience a brief, sharp, burning-type pain as the marrow is aspirated. After the marrow is removed, a pressure dressing is applied to the site for a few minutes; bleeding should be minimal.

When a larger specimen of bone marrow is required, a bone marrow biopsy is performed using a larger lumen biopsy needle, which is designed to obtain a core of bone marrow. The procedure is basically the same as for a bone marrow aspiration.

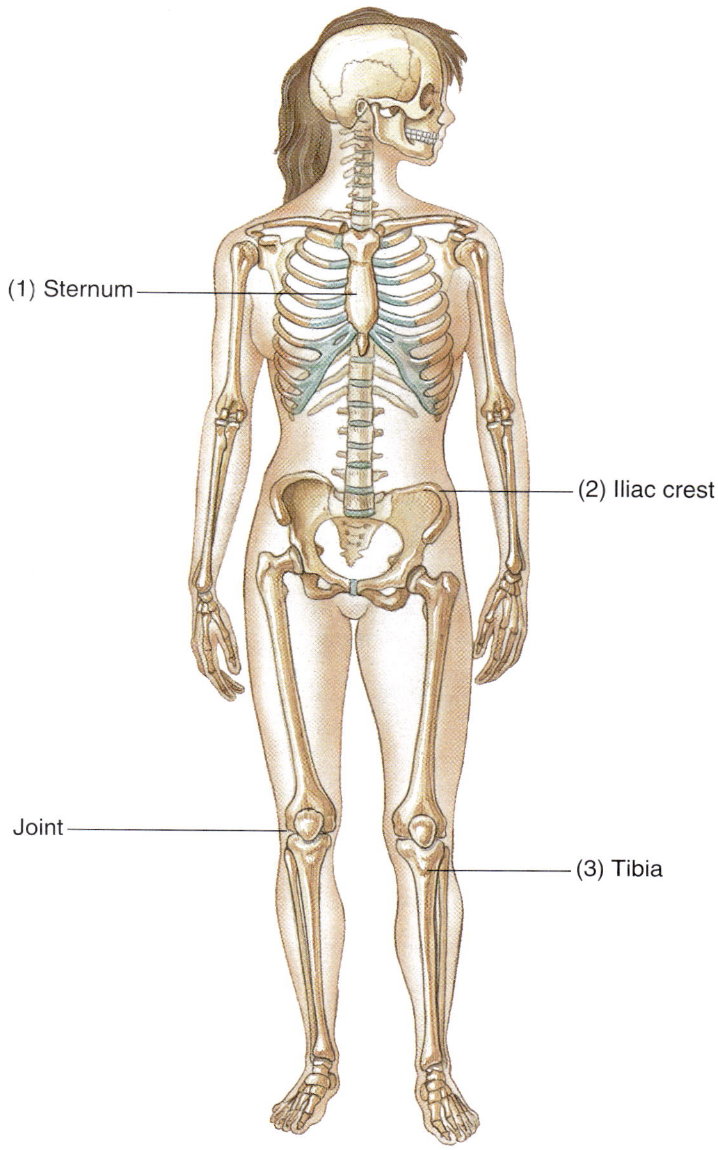

Figure 6-28 Sites for bone marrow aspiration

Bone Density Evaluation

The measurement of bone mineral density is important in providing helpful information regarding treatment and prevention of osteoporosis. The two methods of evaluating bone density discussed here are (1) dual photon absorptiometry and (2) dual energy x-ray absorptiometry (DEXA).

dual photon absorptiometry
(dual **FOH**-ton ab-sorp-she-**AHM**-eh-tree)

Dual photon absorptiometry is a noninvasive procedure that involves beaming a minimal amount of radiation (from a radioactive isotope) through the bones. A computer then evaluates the amount of radiation absorbed by the bones and summarizes the findings, which are then interpreted by the physician.

This procedure measures the bone density within 2% to 3% accuracy of the bone's actual density.

dual energy x-ray absorptiometry (DEXA)
(ab-sorp-she-**AHM**-eh-tree)

Dual energy x-ray absorptiometry (DEXA) is a noninvasive procedure that measures bone density. In the DEXA procedure, an x-ray machine generates the energy photons that pass through the bones. A computer then evaluates the amount of radiation absorbed by the bones, and the findings are interpreted by a physician.

This procedure measures the bone density more accurately than the dual photon absorptiometry, takes less time, and emits less radiation to the patient.

Common Abbreviations

ABBREVIATION	MEANING	ABBREVIATION	MEANING
C1, C2, C3, . . .	cervical vertebra 1, 2, 3, etc.	**S1**	sacrum (When transcribing, you may hear a medical report refer to the disc space between the last lumbar vertebra and the sacrum as L5–S1.)
DEXA	dual energy x-ray absorptiometry	**T1, T2, T3, . . .**	thoracic vertebra 1, 2, 3, etc.
DIP	distal interphalangeal (joint)	**THR**	total hip replacement
Fx	fracture	**TKR**	total knee replacement
L1, L2, L3, . . .	lumbar vertebra 1, 2, 3, etc.	**TMJ**	temporomandibular joint
MCP	metacarpophalangeal (joint)		
MTP	metatarsophalangeal (joint)		
PIP	posterior interphalangeal (joint)		

Written and Audio Terminology Review

Review each of the following terms from this chapter. Study the spelling of each term and write the definition in the space provided. If you have the Audio CD available, listen to each term, pronounce it, and check the box once you are comfortable saying the word. Check definitions by looking the term up in the glossary/index.

TERM	PRONUNCIATION	DEFINITION
acetabular	☐ ass-eh-**TAB**-yoo-lar	____________
articular cartilage	☐ ar-**TIK**-u-lar **CAR**-tih-laj	____________
calcaneodynia	☐ kal-**kay**-nee-oh-**DIN**-ee-ah	____________
cancellous	☐ **CAN**-sell-us	____________
carpals	☐ **CAR**-pals	____________

Term	Pronunciation	
cervical vertebrae	☐ **SIR**-vih-kal **VER**-teh-bray	________
coccygeal	☐ cock-**SIJ**-ee-al	________
coccyx	☐ **COCK**-six	________
condyle	☐ **CON**-dial	________
costochondral	☐ koss-toh-**CON**-dral	________
craniotomy	☐ kray-nee-**OTT**-oh-mee	________
diaphysis	☐ dye-**AFF**-ih-sis	________
dual energy x-ray absorptiometry	☐ dual energy x-**RAY** ab-sorp-she-**AHM**-eh-tree	________
dual photon absorptiometry	☐ dual **FOH**-ton ab-sorp-she-**AHM**-eh-tree	________
epiphyseal	☐ ep-ih-**FIZZ**-e-al	________
epiphysis	☐ eh-**PIFF**-ih-sis	________
equinovarus	☐ eh-kwine-oh-**VAIR**-us	________
ethmoid	☐ **ETH**-moyd	________
Ewing's sarcoma	☐ **YOO**-wings sar-**KOH**-mah	________
femoral	☐ **FEM**-or-al	________
femur	☐ **FEE**-mer	________
fibula	☐ **FIB**-yoo-lah	________
fibular	☐ **FIB**-yoo-lar	________
fissure	☐ **FISH**-er	________
fontanelle or fontanel	☐ fon-tah-**NELL**	________
foramen	☐ for-**AY**-men	________
fossa	☐ **FOSS**-ah	________
haversian	☐ ha-**VER**-shan	________
hematopoiesis	☐ **hem**-ah-toh-poy-**EE**-sis	________
humeral	☐ **HYOO**-mer-al	________
humerus	☐ **HYOO**-mer-us	________
hyoid	☐ **HIGH**-oyd	________
iliac	☐ **ILL**-ee-ac	________
intervertebral	☐ in-ter-**ver**-teh-bral	________
ischial	☐ **ISS**-kee-al	________

Term		Pronunciation	
kyphosis	☐	ki-**FOH**-sis	______
lacrimal	☐	**LACK**-rim-al	______
laminectomy	☐	lam-ih-**NEK**-toh-mee	______
lordosis	☐	lor-**DOH**-sis	______
lumbar	☐	**LUM**-bar	______
lumbar vertebrae	☐	**LUM**-bar **VER**-teh-bray	______
mandibular	☐	man-**DIB**-yoo-lar	______
mastoiditis	☐	mass-toyd-**EYE**-tis	______
maxillary	☐	**MACK**-sih-**ler**-ee	______
medullary	☐	**MED**-u-lair-ee	______
metacarpals	☐	met-ah-**CAR**-pals	______
metatarsalgia	☐	**met**-ah-tar-**SAL**-jee-ah	______
metatarsals	☐	met-ah-**TAR**-sals	______
nasal conchae	☐	**NAY**-zl **KONG**-kee	______
occipital	☐	ock-**SIP**-itle	______
olecranon	☐	oh-**LEK**-ran-on	______
orthopedics	☐	or-thoh-**PEE**-diks	______
ossification	☐	oss-sih-fih-**KAY**-shun	______
osteoblasts	☐	**OSS**-tee-oh-blasts	______
osteochondroma	☐	oss-tee-oh-kon-**DROH**-mah	______
osteoclasts	☐	**OSS**-tee-oh-clasts	______
osteocytes	☐	**OSS**-tee-oh-sites	______
osteogenic sarcoma	☐	oss-tee-oh-**JEN**-ic sar-**KOH**-mah	______
osteoma	☐	oss-tee-**OH**-mah	______
osteomalacia	☐	oss-tee-oh-mah-**LAY**-she-ah	______
osteomyelitis	☐	oss-tee-oh-my-ell-**EYE**-itis	______
osteoporosis	☐	oss-tee-oh-poh-**ROW**-sis	______
palatine	☐	**PAL**-ah-tine	______
parietal	☐	pah-**REYE**-eh-tall	______
patella	☐	pah-**TELL**-ah	______
patellar	☐	pah-**TELL**-ar	______

Term		Pronunciation	
pelvimetry	☐	pell-**VIM**-eh-tree	______
periosteum	☐	pair-ee-**AH**-stee-um	______
phalanges	☐	fah-**LAN**-jeez	______
phalangitis	☐	fal-an-**JYE**-tis	______
pubic	☐	**PYOO**-bik	______
rachitis	☐	rah-**KIGH**-tis	______
radial	☐	**RAY**-dee-al	______
radius	☐	**RAY**-dee-us	______
resorption	☐	re-**SORP**-shun	______
sacrum	☐	**SAY**-crum	______
scapular	☐	**SKAP**-yoo-lar	______
scoliosis	☐	skoh-lee-**OH**-sis	______
sesamoid	☐	**SES**-a-moyd	______
sinus	☐	**SIGH**-nuss	______
sphenoid	☐	**SFEE**-noyd	______
spondylosis	☐	spon-dih-**LOH**-sis	______
substernal	☐	sub-**STER**-nal	______
sulcus	☐	**SULL**-kuss	______
supraclavicular	☐	**soo**-prah-klah-**VIK**-yoo-lar	______
sutures	☐	**SOO**-chers	______
talipes	☐	**TAL**-ih-peez	______
tarsals	☐	**TAR**-sals	______
temporal	☐	**TEM**-por-al	______
thoracic	☐	tho-**RASS**-ik	______
tibia	☐	**TIB**-ee-ah	______
trabeculae	☐	trah-**BEK**-u-lay	______
trochanter	☐	tro-**KAN**-ter	______
tubercle	☐	**TOO**-ber-kl	______
tuberosity	☐	too-ber-**OSS**-ih-tee	______
ulna	☐	**UHL**-nah	______
vertebrae	☐	**VER**-teh-bray	______

vertebral foramen	☐ **VER**-teh-bral for-**AY**-men	______________
vomer	☐ **VOH**-mer	______________
zygomatic	☐ zeye-go-**MAT**-ik	______________

Chapter Review Exercises

The following exercises provide a more in-depth review of the chapter material. Your goal in these exercises is to complete each section at a minimum 80% level of accuracy. A space has been provided for your score at the end of each section.

A. Labeling

Write the names of the bones in the appropriate spaces. Each correct bone name is worth 10 points. When you have completed the exercise, total your points and record your score in the space provided at the end of the exercise.

Name of Bone

1. Femur
2. Patella
3. Tibia
4. Fibula
5. Sacrum
6. Radius
7. Sternum
8. Humerus
9. Ilium
10. Ulna

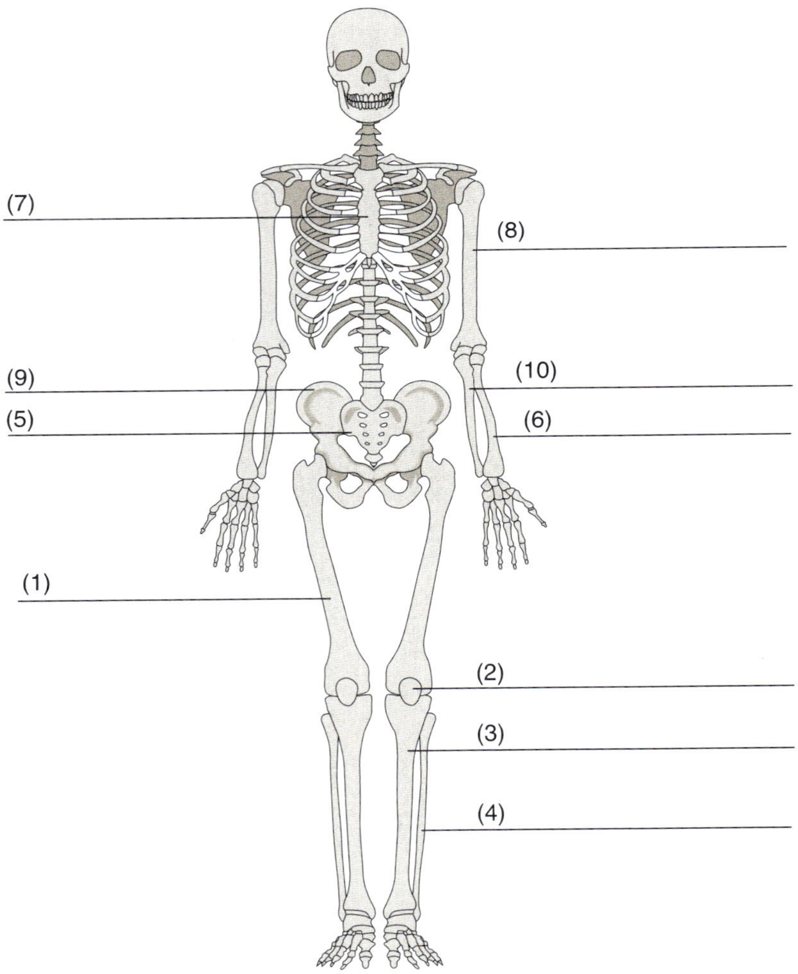

Number correct ______ × *10 points/correct answer: Your score* ______ %

B. Completion

The following is a discussion of the structure and formation of bone. Complete the sentences with the most appropriate word. Each correct answer is worth 10 points. Record your score in the space provided at the end of the exercise.

1. The main shaftlike portion of a bone is the diaphysis.
2. When skeletal growth is complete, the epiphyseal line will not show up on x-ray.
3. The periosteum is the thick, white fibrous membrane that covers the surface of the long bones.
4. Dense bone tissue that is the hard outer shell of the bone is known as compact bone.
5. Compact bone has a system of small canals which contain blood vessels, lymphatic vessels, and nerves. These canals are called the haversian canals.
6. osteoblasts are the immature bone cells that are actively producing bony tissue that replaces cartilage.
7. The conversion of fibrous connective tissue and cartilage into bone or a bony substance is known as ossification.
8. osteoclasts are large cells that digest (or absorb) bony tissue, helping to hollow out the central portion of the bone.
9. A mature bone cell is called an osteocytes.
10. Blood cell formation occurs in the bone marrow

Number correct ______ × 10 points/correct answer: Your score ______ %

C. Matching

Match the following bone markings in the left column with the most appropriate description on the right. Each correct answer is worth 10 points. Record your score in the space provided at the end of the exercise.

d 1. trochanter
f 2. crest
g 3. fissure
k 4. fossa
h 5. foramen
e 6. sinus
j 7. condyle
c 8. neck
a 9. tuberosity
i 10. spine

a. an elevated, broad, rounded process of a bone, usually for muscle or tendon attachment
b. a sharp projection from the surface of a bone
c. a constricted or narrow section that connects with the head
d. the large bony process located below the neck of the femur; for muscle attachment
e. an opening or hollow space in a bone
f. a distinct border or ridge; an upper, elevated edge
g. a groove or depression in a bone
h. a hole within a bone through which blood vessels or nerves pass
i. a sharp projection from the surface of a bone, similar to a crest; used for muscle attachment
j. a knucklelike projection at the end of a bone
k. a hollow or shallow concave depression in a bone

Number correct ______ × 10 points/correct answer: Your score ______ %

D. Spelling

Circle the correctly spelled term in each pairing of words. Each correct answer is worth 10 points. Record your score in the space provided at the end of the exercise.

1. sinus	sinous
2. temperal	temporal
3. mandibuler	mandibular
4. thoracic	thoraxic
5. xiphoid	zyphoid
6. acromian	acromion
7. meticarpals	metacarpals
8. acetabelum	acetabulum
9. maleolus	malleolus
10. condyle	condile

Number correct _______ × 10 points/correct answer: Your score _______%

E. Multiple Choice

Read each statement carefully and select the correct answer from the options listed. Each correct answer is worth 10 points. Record your score in the space provided at the end of the exercise.

1. A disease in which the bones become abnormally soft due to a deficiency of calcium and phosphorus in the blood is known as:
   a. osteoporosis
   b. osteomalacia
   c. osteomyelitis
   d. Ewing's sarcoma
2. Bones that are longer than they are wide and with distinctive-shaped ends, such as the femur, are known as:
   a. compact bones
   b. sesamoid bones
   c. short bones
   d. long bones
3. A flat, circular, platelike structure of cartilage that serves as a cushion, or shock absorber, between the vertebrae is known as:
   a. intercostal space
   b. intervertebral disc
   c. epiphyseal line
   d. bone process
4. A hollow or concave depression in a bone is called a:
   a. fossa
   b. foramen
   c. crest
   d. spine

5. The large bony process located below the neck of the femur is the:
   a. tuberosity
   b. trabeculae
   c. trochanter
   d. condyle
6. A disease that is characterized by bones that were once strong becoming fragile due to loss of bone density is called:
   a. osteomalacia
   b. osteoporosis
   c. osteomyelitis
   d. osteochondroma
7. The medical term for an abnormal outward curvature of a portion of the spine, commonly known as humpback or hunchback, is:
   a. scoliosis
   b. lordosis
   c. kyphosis
   d. osteochondroma
8. The medical term for an abnormal inward curvature of a portion of the spine, commonly known as swayback, is:
   a. osteochondroma
   b. kyphosis
   c. lordosis
   d. scoliosis
9. The medical term for an abnormal lateral (sideward) curvature of a portion of the spine to the left or to the right is:
   a. lordosis
   b. scoliosis
   c. kyphosis
   d. osteochondroma
10. A layer of cartilage that separates the diaphysis from the epiphysis of a bones is the:
    a. epiphyseal line
    b. intervertebral disk
    c. crest
    d. cancellous bone

Number correct _______ × 10 points/correct answer: Your score _______%

F. Proofreading Skills

Read the following report. For each bold term, provide a brief definition and indicate if the term is spelled correctly. If it is misspelled, provide the correct spelling. Each correct answer is worth 10 points. Record your score in the space provided at the end of the exercise.

HILLCREST Medical Center

NAME: Quinn, Mrs. Daisy **ROOM NO.** 678 **HOSPITAL NO:** 190278

EXAMINATION OF: Skull and nose **X-RAY NO:** 978

ATTENDING PHYSICIAN: Dr. Thoreau M. Abone **DATE:** 3-8-03

Anteroposterior, cerebellar, stereoscopic right lateral, and Water's view of the skull, and lateral and occlusal views of the nose show a stellate fracture of the left side of the frontal bone including the anterior and posterior walls of the left frontal **sinous**. The anterior wall of this sinus is comminuted, a few of the fragments being slightly elevated and at least one of the fragments being slightly depressed. No significant depression of the inner table is seen. This fracture extends into the left **orbital** plate, one fragment of which is slightly elevated and another slightly depressed. There is a suggestion that the fracture extends posteriorly to involve the left **sfenoid** ridge. The bones, **sutures**, and vascular markings of the **cranial** vault otherwise appear normal. The sella turcica is normal in size and contour, and there is no evidence of increased **intercranial** pressure. The pineal body cannot be seen with certainty. The petrous pyramids are intact, and the internal auditory **meatusis** appear normal. There is a deformity of the distal half of one of the **nasal** bones, which is tilted slightly downward. This could represent a recent fracture, and apparently involves the right nasal bone. Slight thickening of the lining membrane of the left **maxilary** sinus is noted.

IMPRESSION:

1. Stellate, **comminuted** fracture of the left side of the **frontel** bone involving the anterior and posterior walls of the left frontal sinus, a fragment of the anterior wall being very slightly depressed. This extends into the left orbital plate with slight elevation of one fragment and slight apparent depression of another.

2. Fracture of the right nasal bone with slight deformity.

Thoreau M. Abone

Example:

meatusis *openings*

Spelled correctly? ☐ Yes ☑ No *meatuses*

1. **sinous** yes

Spelled correctly? ☑ Yes ☐ No

2. **orbital**

Spelled correctly? ☑ Yes ☐ No

3. **sfenoid**

Spelled correctly? ☑ Yes ☐ No

4. **sutures**

Spelled correctly? ☑ Yes ☐ No

5. **cranial**

Spelled correctly? ☑ Yes ☐ No

6. **intercranial**

Spelled correctly? ☑ Yes ☐ No

7. **nasal**

Spelled correctly? ☑ Yes ☐ No

8. **maxilary**

Spelled correctly? ☑ Yes ☐ No

9. **comminuted**

Spelled correctly? ☑ Yes ☐ No

10. **frontel**

Spelled correctly? ☐ Yes ☐ No

Number correct _____ × 10 points/correct answer: Your score _____%

G. Crossword Puzzle

Each crossword answer is worth 10 points. When you have completed the crossword puzzle, total your points and enter your score in the space provided.

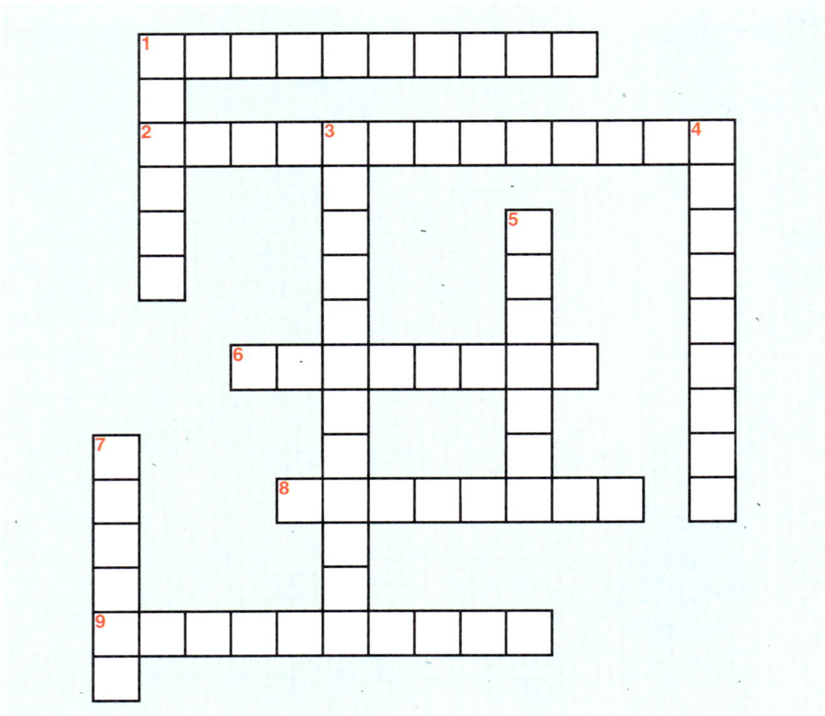

ACROSS

1 Splintered, crushed fracture
2 Inflammation of the bone and marrow
6 Humpback
8 Swayback
9 One side broken; other side bent

DOWN

1 Fracture with no open wound
3 Loss of bone density; brittle bones
4 Lateral curvature of spinal column
5 Clubfoot
7 Malignant bone tumor in young adult

Number correct _______ × 10 points/correct answer: Your score _______%

H. Word Element Review

The following words relate to the skeletal system. The prefixes and suffixes have been provided. Read the definition carefully and complete the word by filling in the space with the word elements provided in this chapter. If you have forgotten your word building rules, refer to Chapter 1. Each correct word is worth 10 points. Record your score in the space provided at the end of the exercise.

1. Pertaining to the acetabulum
   acetabul/ar
2. Low blood calcium level
   hypo/calc/emia
3. Pertaining to the cartilage and the ribs
   costo/chondr/al
4. Incision into the skull
   crani/otomy

5. Softening of bone tissue
   osteo/malacia
6. Pertaining to the jaw bone
   mandibul/ar
7. Inflammation of the spinal column
   rach/itis
8. Pertaining to below the sternum
   sub/stern/al
9. Pertaining to between the vertebrae
   inter/vertebr/al
10. A benign tumor of a bone
    oste/oma

Number correct _______ × 10 points/correct answer: Your score _______%

I. Matching Fractures

Can you name these fractures? Let's see! Match the names of the fracture types on the left with the appropriate description on the right. Each correct answer is worth 10 points. Record your answer in the space provided at the end of the exercise.

c 1. closed fracture
j 2. open fracture
i 3. complete fracture
h 4. greenstick fracture
d 5. compression fracture
g 6. impacted fracture
b 7. comminuted fracture
e 8. Colles' fracture
f 9. hairline fracture
a 10. pathological fracture

a. occurs when a bone is weakened by a preexisting disease
b. the force is so great that the bone is splintered or crushed
c. a break in the bone, but no open wound in the skin
d. caused by bone surfaces being forced against each other
e. occurs at the lower end of the radius, within 1 inch of the wrist
f. a minor fracture; the bone stays in perfect alignment; x-ray shows a small thin line at the site of the fracture (also called a stress fracture)
g. the force of the break causes the broken end of the smaller bone to be jammed into the broken end of the larger bone
h. one side of the bone is broken and the other side is bent; an incomplete fracture
i. a break that extends through the entire thickness of the bone
j. a break in the bone and an open wound in the skin

Number correct _______ × 10 points/correct answer: Your score _______%

J. Matching Abbreviations

Match the abbreviations on the left with the correct definition on the right. Each correct answer is worth 20 points. Record your score in the space provided at the end of the exercise.

f	1. Fx	a. temporomandibular joint
b	2. DEXA	b. dual energy x-ray absorptiometry
d	3. C1, C2, C3, . . .	c. total knee replacement
a	4. TMJ	d. cervical vertebra 1, 2, 3, etc.
h	5. THR	e. lumbar vertebra 1, 2, 3, etc.
		f. fracture
		h. total hip replacement

Number correct _______ × 20 points/correct answer: Your score _______%

K. Word Search

Using the definitions, write the appropriate answer in the space provided. After you have written each answer, find it in the word search puzzle and circle the word. The words may be read up, down, diagonally, across, or backward. Each correct answer is worth 10 points. Record your answer in the space provided at the end of the exercise.

Example: A hollow or concave depression in a bone.

fossa

1. The type of rib pairs 11–12 that connect to the vertebrae in the back but are free of any attachment in the front.

____

2. A knucklelike projection at the end of a bone.

____

3. The first seven pairs of ribs that connect to the vertebrae in the back and to the sternum in the front.

____

4. Immovable joints, such as those of the cranium.

____

5. Mature bone cells.

____

6. A hole in a bone through which blood vessels or nerves pass.

____

7. The end of a bone.

____

8. The large bony process located below the neck of the femur.

____

9. A sharp projection from the surface of a bone, similar to a crest.

____

10. The type of irregular bones imbedded in tendons near a joint, as in the kneecap.

____

F	L	O	A	T	I	N	G	I	O	L	E	M	I	C
A	C	Y	N	G	E	S	M	S	I	D	A	S	T	T
M	I	O	T	T	M	N	M	E	T	T	R	N	V	R
C	A	O	N	E	E	O	O	S	D	I	C	C	B	O
I	L	C	S	D	T	N	L	I	E	O	O	I	T	S
N	U	H	E	I	Y	T	T	O	T	E	L	N	L	T
C	R	O	P	H	L	L	B	I	U	A	E	C	O	E
O	U	S	T	N	P	N	E	M	A	R	O	F	E	O
N	U	R	R	P	O	I	P	I	A	T	E	O	E	C
T	U	V	O	D	A	I	I	N	D	E	Y	S	M	Y
E	A	L	C	G	R	S	P	I	N	E	C	S	E	T
N	I	E	H	A	R	C	H	I	S	I	S	A	I	E
E	S	P	A	D	R	U	Y	A	R	D	I	S	G	S
N	U	L	N	I	R	E	S	I	D	U	A	L	D	T
C	R	A	T	B	L	O	I	I	U	A	T	C	O	A
E	E	N	E	R	H	C	S	U	T	U	R	E	S	A
F	R	E	R	U	U	R	I	S	M	E	M	N	I	C
P	E	R	I	T	O	N	D	I	O	M	A	S	E	S

***Number correct* _______ × *10 points/correct answer: Your score* _______%**

Answers to Chapter Review Exercises

A. Labeling

1. femur
2. patella
3. tibia
4. fibula
5. sacrum
6. radius
7. sternum
8. humerus
9. ilium
10. ulna

B. Completion

1. diaphysis
2. epiphyseal line
3. periosteum
4. compact bone
5. haversian
6. osteoblasts
7. ossification
8. osteoclasts
9. osteocyte
10. bone marrow

C. Matching

1. d
2. f
3. g
4. k
5. h
6. e
7. j
8. c
9. a
10. i

D. Spelling

1. sinus
2. temporal
3. mandibular
4. thoracic
5. xiphoid
6. acromion
7. metacarpals
8. acetabulum
9. malleolus
10. condyle

E. Multiple Choice

1. b
2. d
3. b
4. a
5. c
6. b
7. c
8. c
9. b
10. a

F. Proofreading Skills

1. **sinus** opening or hollow space in a bone
   Spelled correctly? No
2. **orbital** bone in the skull that houses the eyeball
   Spelled correctly? Yes
3. **sphenoid** bat-shaped bone located at the base of the skull
   Spelled correctly? No
4. **sutures** immovable joints that fuse the cranial bones together, permitting no movement
   Spelled correctly? Yes
5. **cranial** bones that envelop the brain (eight bones that are immovable)
   Spelled correctly? Yes
6. **intracranial** within the cranium
   Spelled correctly? No
7. **nasal** nasal bones give shape to the nose by forming the upper part of the bridge of the nose
   Spelled correctly? Yes
8. **maxillary** bones of the upper jaw
   Spelled correctly? No
9. **comminuted** a fracture resulting in the splintering or crushing of a segment of a bone
   Spelled correctly? Yes
10. **frontal** the frontal bone forms the forehead (front of the skull) and the upper part of the bony cavities that contain the eyeballs
    Spelled correctly? No

G. Crossword Puzzle

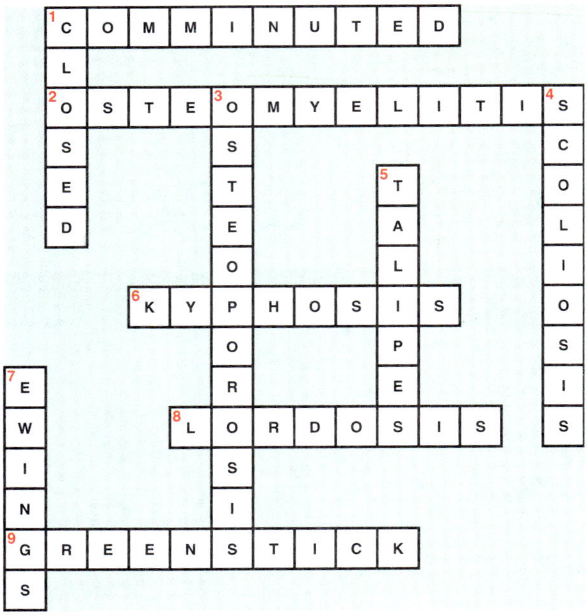

H. Word Element Review

1. **acetabul**/ar
2. hypo/**calc**/emia
3. **costo**/chondr/al
4. **crani**/otomy
5. **osteo**/**malac**/ia
6. **mandibul**/ar
7. **rach**/itis
8. sub/**stern**/al
9. inter/**vertebr**/al
10. **oste**/oma

I. Matching Fractures

1. c
2. j
3. i
4. h
5. d
6. g
7. b
8. e
9. f
10. a

J. Matching Abbreviations

1. f
2. b
3. d
4. a
5. h

K. Word Search

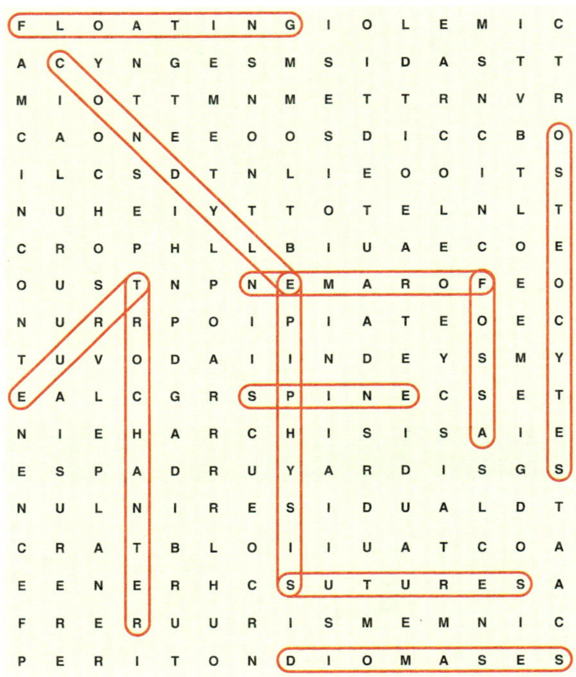

CHAPTER 7

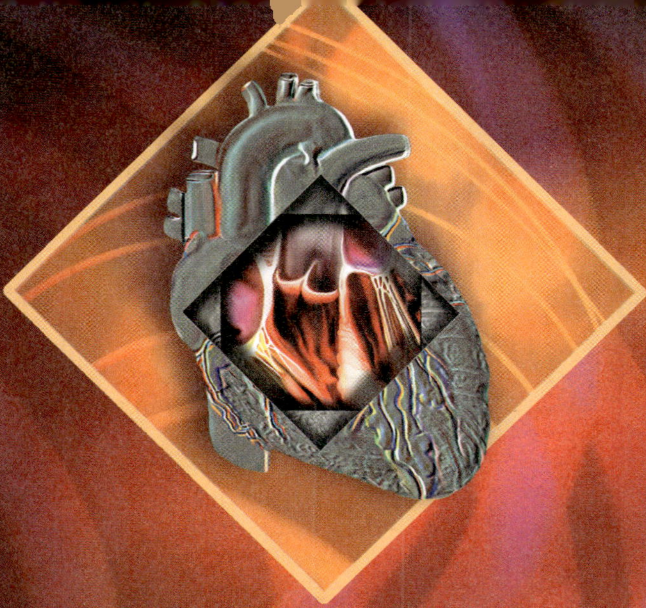

Muscles and Joints

CHAPTER CONTENT

KEY COMPETENCIES

Upon completing this chapter and the review exercises at the end of the chapter, the learner should be able to:

1. Identify three different types of muscles and indicate the control under which each type functions.
2. Correctly identify at least five major muscles of the body by labeling the muscle diagram provided in the chapter review exercises.
3. Define at least 10 pathological conditions of the muscles and joints.
4. Identify a minimum of 10 abbreviations common to the muscles and joints.
5. Demonstrate the ability to create at least 10 medical words pertaining to the muscles and joints.
6. Define 10 different range-of-motion movements of the skeletal muscles.
7. Identify at least five diagnostic techniques used in treating patients with disorders of the muscles or joints.
8. Proof and correct one transcription exercise relative to the muscles and joints.
9. Correctly spell and pronounce each new term introduced in this chapter using the Activity CD-ROM and Audio CD, if available.

OVERVIEW OF MUSCULAR SYSTEM

When you picked up this book, opened it, and turned the pages to this chapter on the muscles and joints, you used *many* of the more than 600 skeletal muscles of your body without much thought about muscle movement! If you were to close this book, put it down, and decide *not* to read this chapter on muscles and joints, you would still use many of the muscles you used when you picked it up . . . so, let's keep it open and continue reading!

The skeleton, as we have studied, provides points of attachment and support for the muscles. However, it cannot move itself; it must have help. The ability of the muscles to **contract** and extend produces body movement, allowing us to move about freely. In addition to movement of the body, the muscles have two other important functions.

Muscles support and maintain body posture through a low level of continual contraction; that is, a continual pull against gravity keeps the body in good alignment. Good body posture places the least amount of strain on the body's muscles, ligaments, and bones. Skeletal muscles also have a great effect on body temperature because they produce a substantial amount of heat when they contract. Think about the last time you were cold and you shivered; you used the energy generated by the contraction of your muscles to raise your body temperature. This response is controlled by your "built-in thermostat," the hypothalamus, which is an endocrine gland that we will discuss in Chapter 13.

In this chapter we concentrate on the major muscles of the body, leaving the detailed study of the muscular system to anatomy and physiology textbooks. We also study the **articulations** (joints) of the body and how they create the possibility for movement by the muscles.

Anatomy and Physiology (Muscles)

Types of Muscles

The body contains three types of muscles: skeletal muscle, smooth muscle, and cardiac muscle.

Skeletal muscles attach to the bones of the skeleton. They are also known as **voluntary muscles** because they operate under conscious control. All voluntary muscles, however, are not skeletal muscles: Some voluntary muscles are not attached to the skeleton; they are responsible for movement of the face, eyes, tongue, and pharynx. Skeletal muscles are also called **striated muscles** because they have a striped appearance when viewed under a microscope.

Many of the skeletal muscles work in pairs, creating coordinated movement through the opposing actions of **contraction** and relaxation. For example, when muscle A contracts (or shortens) to flex the arm, muscle B must relax; this action brings the arm closer to the body. Conversely, to extend the arm, muscle A must relax (returning to its normal resting length) while muscle B contracts; this action moves the arm away from the body.

Smooth muscles, also called **visceral muscles**, are found in the walls of hollow organs and tubes such as the stomach, intestines, respiratory passageways, and blood vessels. When viewed under a microscope, smooth muscles lack the striations (stripes) visible in striated muscles. Smooth muscles are *not* under the conscious control of the individual; accordingly, they are also known as **involuntary muscles.** The contraction of smooth, or involuntary, muscles is regulated by hormones and the autonomic nervous system. The autonomic nervous system regulates involuntary vital function, including the activity of the cardiac muscle, smooth muscles, and glands.

Cardiac muscle is a specialized type of muscle that forms the wall of the heart. It, too, is controlled by the autonomic nervous system and is an involuntary muscle. When viewed through a microscope, cardiac muscle is striated in appearance.

Attachment of Muscles

Each skeletal muscle is composed of individual muscle cells called **muscle fibers.** These fibers are held together by thin sheets of fibrous connective tissue called **fascia**, which penetrate and cover the entire muscle. The fascia and the partitions within the muscle extend to form a strong fibrous band of tissue called a **tendon**. The tendon attaches the muscle to the bone as it becomes continuous with the periosteum of the bone.

The attachments of muscles to bones are strategically placed so that muscles can cause movement of the bones when they contract or relax. Most of our muscles cross at least one joint, attaching to both of the bones forming the articulation. When movement occurs, one of the bones moves more freely than the other. The point of attachment of the muscle to the bone that is *less movable* is called the **origin** (the name of that particular bone will name the "point of origin" for the muscle). The point of attachment of the muscle to the bone that it *moves* is called the **insertion** (the name of that particular bone will name the point of insertion for the muscle). See **Figure 7-1.**

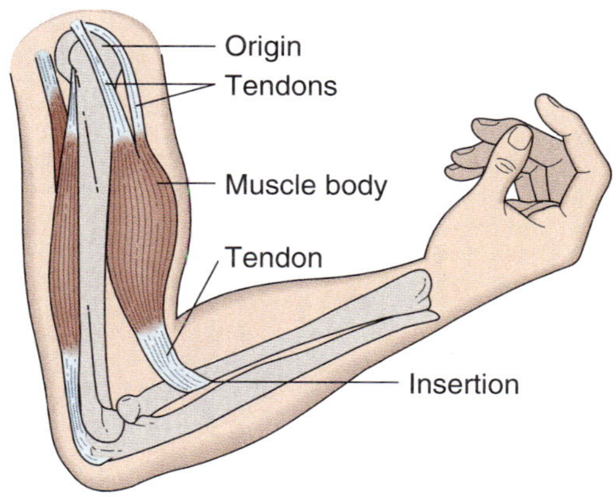

Figure 7-1 Origin and insertion points of a muscle

Groups of Muscles

This chapter concentrates on several of the major muscles near the body surface.

Note: This discussion does not cover all of the muscles of the body.

Many of the muscles discussed here will take on greater importance when you study administration of medications by injection, range-of-motion exercises, and other medical procedures. Although these muscles are generally described in the singular form, most of them are present on both sides of the body.

Each description, when possible, includes a "Do This" section that is designed to have you locate the muscle being discussed by participating in the exercise.

Muscles that Move the Head and Neck

For a visual reference as you study these muscles, refer to **Figure 7-2.**

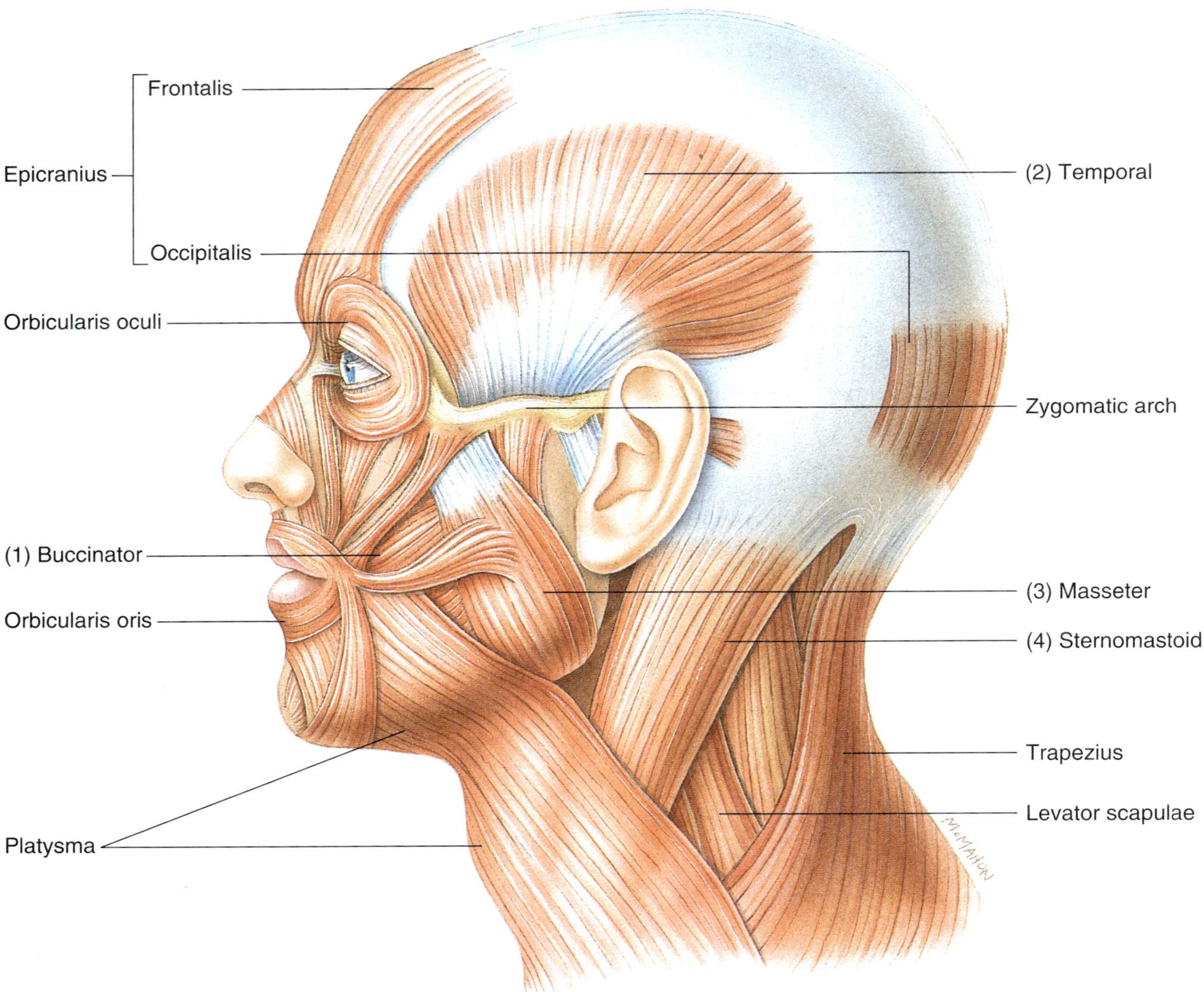

Figure 7-2 Muscles of the head and neck

(1) buccinator (**BUCK**-sin-ay-tor) bucc/o = cheek	The **buccinator** muscle is located in the fleshy part of the cheek. *(Do This: Suck in your cheeks; now release them. Blow as if you were blowing out a candle; now whistle. Smile! You have used your buccinator muscle to respond to each of these commands.)*
(2) temporal (**TEM**-po-ral) tempor/o = temporal	The **temporal** muscle is located above and near the ear. *(Do This: Open and close your jaws as if you were biting and chewing a piece of meat. To do this you have used your temporal muscle.)*
(3) masseter (mass-**SEE**-ter)	The **masseter** muscle, located at the angle of the jaw, also raises the mandible and closes the jaw. It is used when biting and chewing.
(4) sternomastoid (**stir**-no-**MASS**-toyd) stern/o = sternum mastoid/o = mastoid process	The **sternomastoid** muscle is sometimes called the sternocleidomastoid muscle. It extends from the sternum upward along the side of the neck to the mastoid process. *(Do This: Bend your neck, bringing your chin toward your chest; now raise your head back to normal position and turn your head from side to side. You are using your sternomastoid muscle.)*

Muscles that Move the Upper Extremities

For a visual reference as you study these muscles, refer to **Figure 7-3.**

(1) trapezius (trah-**PEE**-zee-us)	The **trapezius** muscle is a triangular-shape muscle that extends across the back of the shoulder, covers the back of the neck, and inserts on the clavicle and scapula. *(Do This: Raise your shoulders as if you were shrugging them; now pull them back. You have just used your trapezius muscles to accomplish this movement.)*
(2) latissimus dorsi (lah-**TIS**-ih-mus **DOR**-sigh) dors/o = back	The **latissimus dorsi** muscle originates from the vertebrae of the lower back, crosses the lower half of the thoracic region, and passes between the humerus and scapula to insert on the anterior surface of the humerus. It forms the posterior border of the axilla (armpit). *(Do This: Lean slightly forward; straighten or extend your arms over your head and begin moving your arms in a swimming motion. This extension of the arms and bringing them down forcibly is accomplished by using the latissimus dorsi muscle.)*
(3) pectoralis major (**peck**-toh-**RAY**-lis) pector/o = chest	The **pectoralis** major muscle is a large, fan-shape muscle that crosses the upper part of the front of the chest. It originates from the sternum and crosses over to the humerus. It forms the anterior border of the axilla (armpit). *(Do This: Cross your right arm over your chest and touch the back part of your left shoulder. To do this, your pectoralis major muscle flexed, causing the arm to adduct [come toward the body], pulling the arm across the shoulder.)*
(4) deltoid (**DELL**-toyd)	The **deltoid** muscle covers the shoulder joint. It originates from the clavicle and the scapula, and inserts on the lateral side of the humerus. The deltoid muscle is one of the muscles used for intramuscular injections. *(Do This: Hold your left arm straight down beside your body. Now raise your left arm out, away from your body, until it is in a horizontal*

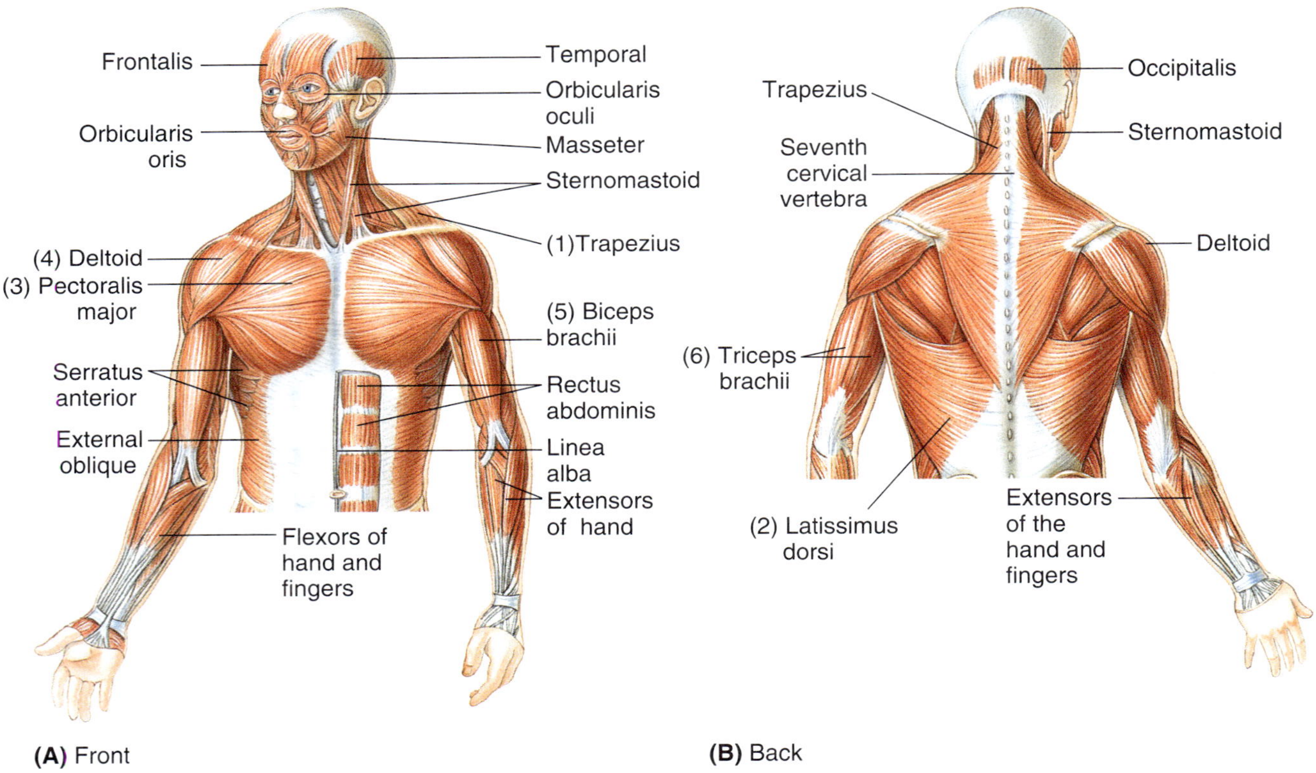

Figure 7-3 Muscles of the upper extremities

position. The contraction of the deltoid muscle is responsible for abducting the arm [moving it away from the body].)

(5) biceps brachii
(**BYE**-seps **BRAY**-kee-eye)

The **biceps brachii** muscle has two heads, both of which originate from the scapula and insert on the radius. *(Do This: Bend your right elbow to bring your lower arm up toward the right upper arm, holding the position tightly enough to flex your muscle. Now relax your right arm; extend it out in front of you and turn your palm up. Your biceps brachii muscle was responsible for flexing your lower arm and for supinating your palm, that is, turning the palm up.)*

(6) triceps brachii
(**TRY**-seps **BRAY**-kee-eye)

The **triceps brachii** muscle has three heads, which originate from the scapula and the humerus and insert onto the olecranon process of the ulna (at the elbow). *(Do This: Extend your right arm, straightening your elbow as if to throw a boxing blow—be sure no one is near enough to receive that blow! Your triceps brachii muscle is responsible for straightening the elbow.)*

Muscles of the Trunk of the Body

The **trunk** is the main part of the body, to which the head and the extremities are attached. It is also called the **torso**. The muscles of the trunk include the **diaphragm** and the muscles of the abdomen and perineum. A discussion of these muscles can be found in most anatomy textbooks.

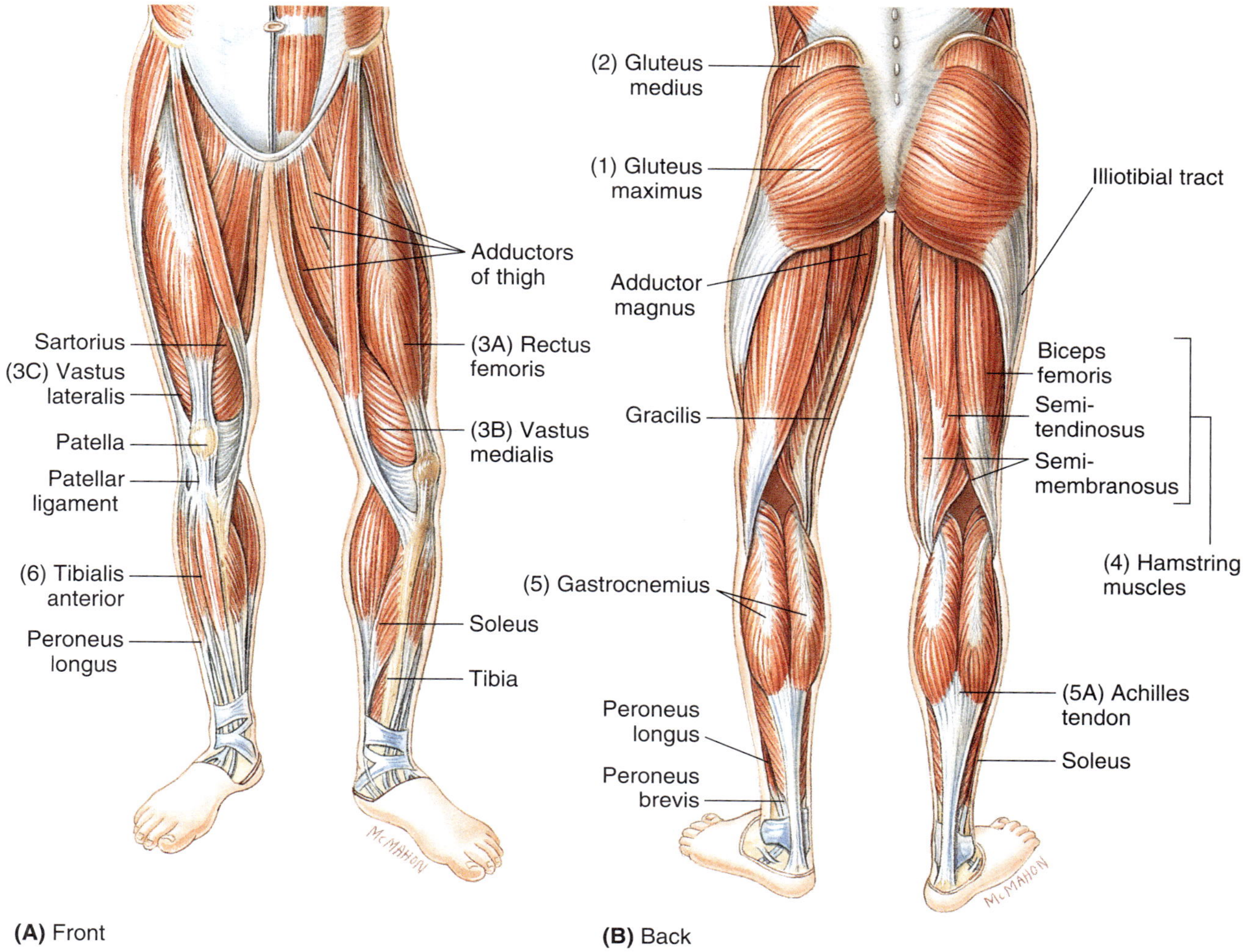

Figure 7-4 Muscles of the lower extremities

Muscles that Move the Lower Extremities

The muscles of the lower extremities, which are longer and stronger than those of the upper extremities, provide strength, stability, and movement to the lower extremities. For a visual reference as you study these muscles, refer to **Figure 7-4.**

(1) gluteus maximus (**GLOO**-tee-us **MACKS**-ih-mus)	The gluteus maximus muscle forms most of the fleshy part of the buttock. It is a large muscle that offers support when an individual is standing. This muscle originates from the ilium and inserts in the femur. It is responsible for causing the thigh to rotate, or turn, outward; that is, it extends the thigh. If you are sitting properly in a chair as you read this material, you are sitting on your gluteus maximus muscle.
(2) gluteus medius (**GLOO**-tee-us **MEE**-dee-us)	The gluteus medius muscle is a smaller muscle located above the upper outer quadrant of the gluteus maximus muscle. It originates from the posterior part of the ilium and inserts in the greater trochanter of the femur. The gluteus medius muscle also helps to abduct the thigh,

rotating it outward. The gluteus medius muscle is one of the muscles used for an intramuscular injection.

(3) quadriceps femoris
(**KWAHD**-rih-seps **FEM**-or-iss)

The anterior part of the thigh has five muscles that work together to extend the thigh, as in extending the leg to kick a ball. Four of these muscles are actually part of one large muscle (the **quadriceps femoris**) even though they are named individually. For study purposes, we will discuss them individually.

The **(3A) rectus femoris** muscle covers the center of the anterior part of the thigh. Originating from the ilium, it inserts on the patellar tendon. The rectus femoris muscle is used as an intramuscular injection site. The **(3B) vastus medialis** is located on the inner side of the femur. The **(3C) vastus lateralis** is located on the outer side of the femur; it is often used as a site for intramuscular injections. The fourth head of the quadriceps femoris muscle is the **vastus intermedius,** which is deeper in the center of the thigh. Each of these muscle heads, except the rectus femoris, originates from the femur and inserts on the patellar tendon.

(4) hamstring muscles
(**HAM**-string muscles)

Located in the posterior part of the thigh are the **hamstring muscles** (biceps femoris, semimembranosus, and the semitendinosus), which are responsible for flexing the leg on the thigh, as in kneeling. They also extend the thigh. These muscles originate from the ischium and insert on the fibula and the tibia. If you feel the area behind your knee, you can feel the hamstring muscle tendons.

(5) gastrocnemius
(**gas**-trok-**NEE**-mee-us)

The **gastrocnemius** muscle is the main muscle of the calf. It attaches to the calcaneus (heel bone) by way of the **(5A) Achilles tendon**. The gastrocnemius muscle is used in standing on tiptoe (plantar flexing the foot) and in flexing the toes. If you are a ballerina you will certainly exercise your gastrocnemius muscle!

(6) tibialis anterior
(tib-ee-**AY**-lis an-**TEER**-ee-or)

The **tibialis anterior** muscle is positioned on the front of the leg. It is responsible for turning the foot inward (inversion) and for dorsiflexing the foot (i.e., pulling the foot back up toward the leg). If you choose to walk on your heels, raising the ball of your foot and your toes up off the ground, you will be using your tibialis anterior muscle.

Vocabulary (Muscles)

The following vocabulary words are frequently used when discussing the muscular system.

WORD	DEFINITION
arthralgia (ar-**THRAL**-jee-ah) arthr/o = joint -algia = pain	Pain in the joints; symptom associated with polymyositis.

atrophy (**AT**-roh-fee) a = without troph/o = development -y = noun ending	Wasting away; literally "without development."
cardiac muscle (**CAR**-dee-ack muscle) cardi/o = heart -ac = pertaining to	Specialized type of muscle that forms the wall of the heart; cardiac muscle is a type of involuntary muscle.
contract/contraction (con-**TRACK**-shun)	A reduction in size, especially of muscle fibers.
contracture (con-**TRACK**-cher)	An abnormal, usually permanent bending of a joint into a fixed position; usually caused by atrophy and shortening of muscle fibers.
fascia (**FASH**-ee-ah)	Thin sheets of fibrous connective tissue that penetrate and cover the entire muscle, holding the fibers together.
insertion (in-**SIR**-shun)	The point of attachment of a muscle to a bone that it moves.
involuntary muscle	Muscles that act without conscious control; they are controlled by the autonomic nervous system and hormones.
muscle fiber	The name given to the individual muscle cell.
origin	The point of attachment of a muscle to a bone that is less movable (i.e., the more fixed end of attachment).
pelvic girdle weakness (**PELL**-vik **GER**-dl **WEAK**-ness)	Weakness of the muscles of the pelvic girdle (the muscles that extend the hip and the knee). In muscular dystrophy, the pelvic girdle weakness causes the child to use one or both hands to assist in rising from a sitting position by "walking" the hands up the lower extremities until he or she is in an upright position.
pseudohypertrophic muscular dystrophy (**soo**-doh-**hy**-per-**TROH**-fic **MUSS**-kew-lar **DIS**-troh-fee) pseud/o = false hyper- = excessive troph/o = development -ic = pertaining to	A form of muscular dystrophy that is characterized by progressive weakness and muscle fiber degeneration without evidence of nerve involvement or degeneration of nerve tissue; also known as Duchenne's muscular dystrophy.
skeletal muscle (**SKELL**-eh-tal muscle)	Muscles that attach to the bones of the skeleton; also known as striated muscle. Skeletal muscles act voluntarily.
smooth muscle	Muscles that are found in the walls of hollow organs and tubes such as the stomach, intestines, respiratory passageways, and blood vessels; also known as visceral muscles. Smooth muscles act involuntarily.
striated muscle (**STRY**-ay-ted muscle)	Muscles that have a striped appearance when viewed under a microscope; skeletal and cardiac muscles are examples.

tendon (**TEN**-dun)	A strong fibrous band of tissue that extends from a muscle, attaching it to the bone by becoming continuous with the periosteum of the bone.
torso (**TOR**-soh)	See *trunk*.
trunk	The main part of the body, to which the head and the extremities are attached; also called the torso.
visceral muscle (**VISS**-er-al muscle) viscer/o = pertaining to the internal organs of the body	Muscles of the internal organs. Refer to *smooth muscle*.
voluntary muscle (**VOL**-un-**ter**-ee muscle)	Muscles, such as skeletal muscles, that operate under conscious control. Those that are responsible for movement of the face, eyes, tongue, and pharynx are under voluntary control.

Word Elements (Muscles)

The following word elements pertain to the muscular system. As you review the list, pronounce each word element aloud twice and check the box after you "say it." Write the definition for the example word given for each word element. You may use your medical dictionary.

WORD ELEMENT	PRONUNCIATION	"SAY IT"	MEANING
bi- **bi**ceps	**BYE** **BYE**-seps	☐	two, double
bucc/o **bucc**al	**BUCK**-oh **BUCK**-al	☐	cheek
dors/o **dors**al	**DOR**-soh **DOR**-sal	☐	back
dys- **dys**tonia	**DIS** dis-**TOH**-nee-ah	☐	bad, difficult, painful, disordered
electr/o **electr**omyogram	ee-**LEK**-troh ee-**lek**-troh-**MY**-oh-gram	☐	electrical, electricity
fasci/o **fasci**otomy	**FASH**-ee-oh fash-ee-**OTT**-oh-mee	☐	band of fibrous tissue
fibr/o **fibr**oma	**FIH**-broh fih-**BROH**-mah	☐	fiber

-graphy electroneuromyo**graphy**	**GRAH**-fee ee-**lek**-troh-**noo**-roh-my-**OG**-rah-fee	☐	process of recording
-itis myos**itis**	**EYE**-tis my-oh-**SIGH**-tis	☐	inflammation
leiomy/o **leiomy**ofibroma	lye-oh-**MY**-oh **lye**-oh-**my**-oh-fih-**BROH**-mah	☐	smooth muscle
my/o **my**algia	**MY**-oh my-**AL**-jee-ah	☐	muscle
pector/o **pector**al	peck-**TOR**-oh **PECK**-toh-ral	☐	pertaining to the chest
rhabdomy/o **rhabdomy**osarcoma	rab-**DOH**-my-oh **rab**-doh-**my**-oh-sar-**KOH**-mah	☐	striated muscle; skeletal muscle
tri- **tri**ceps	**TRY** **TRY**-seps	☐	three
troph/o dys**troph**y	**TROH**-foh **DIS**-troh-fee	☐	development

Pathological Conditions (Muscles)

Diseases and disorders of the muscles may occur at any age. Some conditions are chronic and may require medications, treatments, and possibly surgery to correct the injury; others may be disease conditions with which the individual will live throughout his or her life. As you study the pathological conditions of the muscular system, note that the **basic definition** is in bold print, followed by a detailed description in regular print. The phonetic pronunciation is directly beneath each term, and a breakdown of the component parts of the term when appropriate.

muscular dystrophy
(**MUSS**-kew-lar **DIS**-troh-fee)
dys- = bad, difficult, painful, disordered
troph/o = development
-y = noun ending

Muscular dystrophy is a group of genetically transmitted disorders characterized by progressive weakness and muscle fiber degeneration without evidence of nerve involvement or degeneration of nerve tissue. The onset of muscular dystrophy is early in life.

Muscle weakness is characteristic of all types of muscular dystrophy. Diagnostic tests are performed to confirm the diagnosis of muscular dystrophy; these findings include elevated enzyme tests (CPK), abnormal **muscle biopsy** results, and an abnormal **electromyogram**.

There are numerous types of muscular dystrophy. One of the most common types is **Duchenne's muscular dystrophy,** with symptoms generally appearing by the age of 3. As the disease progresses, the muscles **atrophy** (waste away) and contractures form. Muscle tissue is replaced with fat as the muscle fibers degenerate. The muscle weakness may first appear as pelvic girdle weakness, then will progress to include weakness of the shoulder muscles, and will finally involve extreme weakness of all muscles, including those controlling respiration. Scoliosis is common in the late stages of muscular dystrophy.

Treatment includes exercise programs, possible corrective surgery for the scoliosis, braces to support the weakened muscles, and breathing exercises.

The progression of Duchenne's muscular dystrophy is rapid, with death resulting from respiratory complications occurring in late adolescence.

---

polymyositis
(**pol**-ee-my-oh-**SIGH**-tis)
poly- = many, much, excessive
my/o = muscle
-itis = inflammation

Polymyositis is a chronic, progressive disease affecting the skeletal (striated) muscles. It is characterized by muscle weakness and degeneration (atrophy).

The disease is termed dermatomyositis when the patient also has a rash on the face, neck, shoulders, chest, and upper extremities. This chronic disease is also characterized by periods of remission ("symptom free") and relapse (symptoms return).

The onset of polymyositis is gradual, with patients first experiencing weakness of the hips and shoulders. They may have difficulty getting out of a chair or the bath tub, difficulty climbing stairs, or difficulty reaching for things on the upper shelf of a cabinet or closet; they may experience arthralgia (painful joints) accompanied by edema. As the disease progresses, the neck muscles may become so weak that the patient may not be able to raise his or her head from the pillow.

The cause of polymyositis is unknown. It is thought to be caused by an autoimmune reaction. It occurs twice as often in women as in men and appears most commonly between the ages of 40 and 60.

Treatment includes high doses of corticosteroids and immunosuppressive drugs, along with reduction of the patient's activities until the inflammation subsides. Response to treatment has resulted in satisfactory, long periods of remission in some patients and recovery in others.

---

strains

A strain is an injury to the body of the muscle or attachment of the tendon, resulting from overstretching, overextension, or misuse (i.e., a "muscle pull"). Vigorous exercise may cause intense muscle strain when the individual is unaccustomed to this type of activity. Chronic muscle strain may result from repetitious muscle overuse.

Strains may vary from mild to severe. Patient symptoms may vary from the gradual onset of muscle spasms, some discomfort, decreased motion of the affected area, with no bruising, to severe muscle spasms, intense pain and tenderness, a sensation of a "sudden tearing" in the area, and swelling. An x-ray of the affected area may be ordered to rule out the possibility of a fracture.

Treatment includes rest, ice packs to the affected area for the first 24 to 48 hours to decrease the swelling, compression of the area with an elastic bandage to prevent swelling, and elevation of the affected part. Muscle relaxants may be prescribed if the muscle spasms continue after the injury.

The healing process for a muscle strain may take 4 to 6 weeks; activity should be limited during this time to avoid a recurrence of injury.

Diagnostic Techniques and Procedures (Muscles)

muscle biopsy
(muscle **BYE**-op-see)

Muscle biopsy is the extraction of a specimen of muscle tissue, through either a biopsy needle or an incisional biopsy, for the purpose of examining it under a microscope. Muscle biopsy may be performed for the purpose of diagnosing muscle atrophy, as in muscular dystrophy, or for diagnosing inflammation, as in polymyositis.

If an **incisional biopsy** of muscle tissue is needed, the procedure is carried out under local anesthesia. A surgical incision is made and the desired specimen is obtained. A pressure dressing is applied after the procedure. The affected extremity is immobilized for a period of 12 to 24 hours after the procedure. The biopsy is usually taken from the deltoid or quadriceps muscles.

If a **needle biopsy** of muscle tissue is needed, the procedure is carried out under local anesthesia. The biopsy needle is inserted, the inner trochar is removed, and the specimen is aspirated. Usually a Band-Aid over the biopsy site is the only dressing needed.

electromyography
(ee-**lek**-troh-my-**OG**-rah-fee)
electr/o = electrical, electricity
my/o = muscle
graph/o = record
-y = noun ending

Electromyography is the process of recording the strength of the contraction of a muscle when it is stimulated by an electric current.

The procedure is performed using either a surface electrode applied to the skin or a needle electrode inserted into the muscle. The muscle is electrically stimulated and the response is recorded with an oscilloscope (an instrument that displays a visual representation of electrical variations on a fluorescent screen).

Common Abbreviations (Muscles)

ABBREVIATION	MEANING
IM	intramuscular
MD	muscular dystrophy
DTR	deep tendon reflexes
EMG	electromyography

OVERVIEW OF JOINTS

We have discussed the skeletal system, our means of support and structure, and the muscular system, our means of movement. Now let's take a look at the system that determines our degree of movement: the joints of the body. A joint is a point at which two individual bones connect. It is also called an **articulation.** The type of joint present between the bones determines the range of motion for that body part. When we think of the joints of the body, we usually think of those that permit considerable movement, making it possible for us to perform the many activities of our day- to-day life. Some of the joints, however, allow no movement. **Sutures** are immovable joints; their purpose is to bind bones together. Other joints permit only limited motion. For example, the joints between the vertebrae of the spinal column provide strong support to the spinal column while allowing a narrow range of movement. Let's continue our study by discussing some of the different classifications of joints.

Classifications of Joints

Joints may be classified according to their structure or according to their function. The structural classification is based on the type of connective tissue that joins the bones together, or by the presence of a fluid-filled joint capsule. The functional classification is based upon the degree of movement allowed. Examples of the joint classifications follow.

Structural Classification

The following is a listing of joints according to the type of connective tissue that joins the bones together.

fibrous joint
(**FIH**-bruss *or* **FYE**-bruss)

In a **fibrous** joint, the surfaces of the bones fit closely together and are held together by fibrous connective tissue, as in a suture between the skull bones. This is an immovable joint. See Figure 7-5.

cartilaginous joint
(car-tih-**LAJ**-ih-nus)

In a **cartilaginous** joint, the bones are connected by cartilage as in the symphysis (joint between the pubic bones of the pelvis). This type of joint allows limited movement. See Figure 7-6.

synovial joint
(sin-**OH**-vee-al)

In a **synovial** joint (Figure 7-7), the bones have a space between them, called the **(1)** joint cavity. The joint cavity is lined with a **(2)** **synovial membrane**, which secretes a thick, lubricating fluid called the **synovial fluid**. The bones of the synovial joint are held together by **ligaments**. The surfaces of the connecting bones are protected by a thin layer of cartilage, called the **(3)** **articular cartilage**. A synovial joint allows free movement.

Located near some synovial joints are small sacs containing synovial fluid. Each sac, called a (4) **bursa**, lubricates the area around the joint where

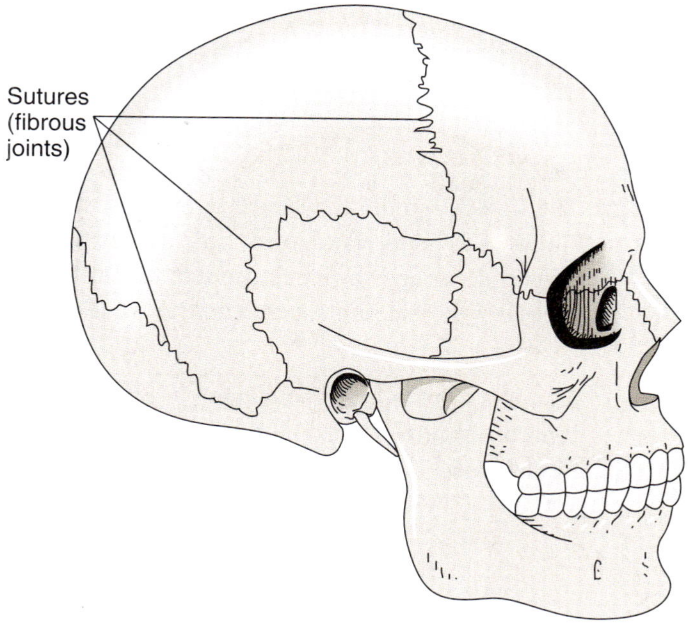

Figure 7-5 Fibrous joint

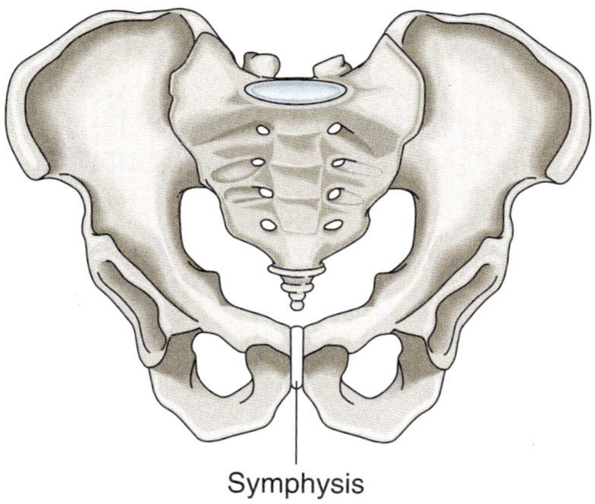

Figure 7-6 Cartilaginous joint

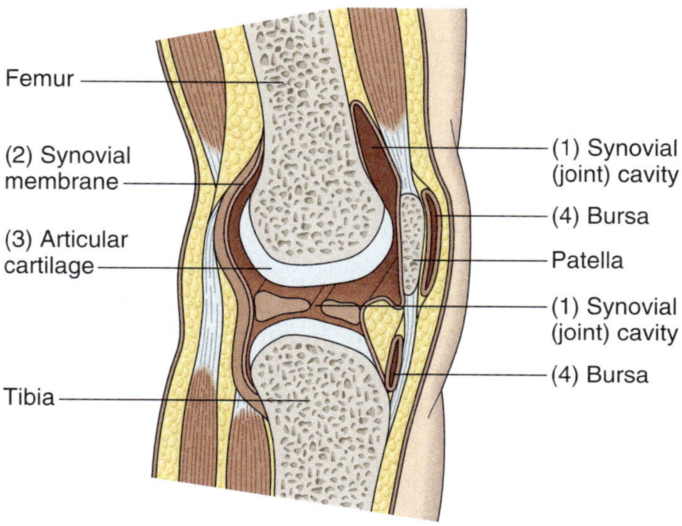

Figure 7-7 Synovial joint and bursa

friction is most likely to occur. A bursa tends to be associated with bony prominences, such as the elbow, knee, or shoulder.

Functional Classification

The synovial joints are the freely movable joints. The action of these joints allows us to bend, stand, turn, run, jump, walk—all necessary movements to carry out our day-to-day routines of life. The following is an example of two types of synovial joints, based on the amount of movement they permit.

hinge joint
(**HINJ** joint)

A **hinge joint** allows movement in one direction—a back and forth type of motion. An example of a hinge joint is the elbow. See **Figure 7-8**.

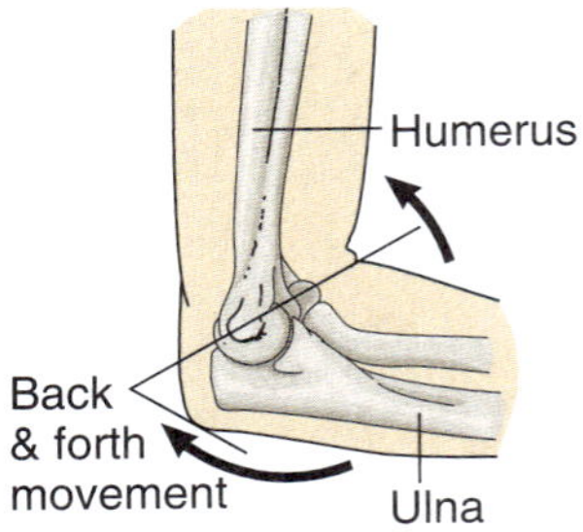

Figure 7-8 Hinge joint

ball-and-socket joint

A ball-and-socket joint allows movements in many directions around a central point. A ball-shaped head that fits into the concave depression of another bone allows the bone with the ball-shaped head to move in many directions. Examples of a ball-and-socket joint are the shoulder joint and the hip joint. See **Figure 7-9.**

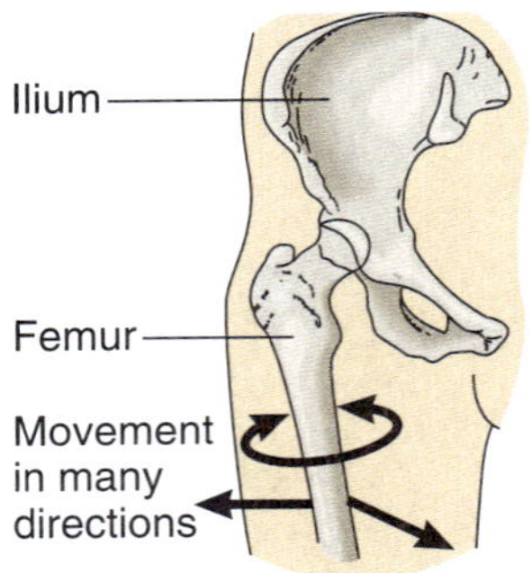

Figure 7-9 Ball-and-socket joint

Movements of Joints

The coordination of the muscular contractions and the range of motion of the joints allows for the many movements of the body. The joints allow the bending or extending of the elbow, the stooping to pick up an object from the floor, the fine finger grasp to pick up a small object, the turning of one's head, and so on. Let's take a look at some of the various movements of the synovial joints. Each description includes a "Do This" section that is designed to have the learner perform the range-of-motion exercise being discussed by participating in the exercise. For a visual reference as you study these movements, refer to **Figure 7-10A through F.**

flexion
(**FLEK**-shun)

Flexion is a bending motion. It decreases the angle between two bones. *(Do This: Bend your right elbow and touch the side of your neck with your fingertips. By bending the elbow, you decreased the angle*

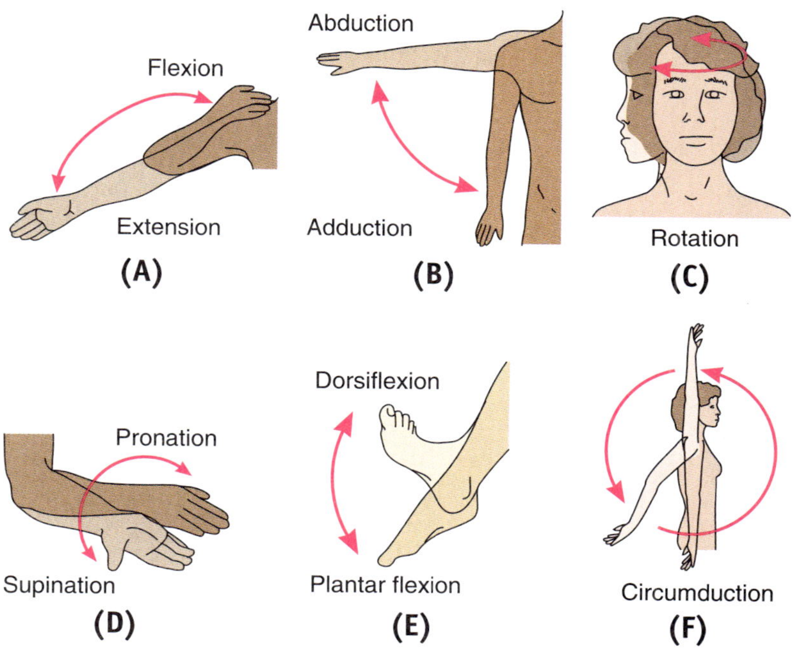

Figure 7-10 Movement of joints

between the lower arm bones and the upper arm bone by bringing them closer together. Keep your arm in this position as you read the next movement description.)

---

extension (eks-**TEN**-shun)

Extension is a straightening motion. It increases the angle between two bones. *(Do This: Remove your fingertips from the side of your neck and straighten your right arm, extending it as if you were going to shake someone's hand. You may now relax your arm. By completing this movement, you increased the angle between the lower arm bones and the upper arm bone by moving them farther apart.)*

---

abduction (ab-**DUCK**-shun)

Abduction is the movement of a bone away from the midline of the body. *(Do This: Raise your left arm out from your side until it is almost parallel with your left shoulder. You may now relax your arm. This action moved your arm away from the midline of your body, thus accomplishing the movement of abduction.)*

---

adduction (ad-**DUCK**-shun)

Adduction is the movement of a bone toward the midline of the body. *(Do This: First, place both of your hands on top of your head. Now remove your hands from the top of your head and return them to your side. This action moved your arms toward the midline of your body, thus accomplishing the movement of adduction.)*

---

rotation (roh-**TAY**-shun)

Rotation is the movement that involves the turning of a bone on its own axis. *(Do This: Turn your head from side to side as if to say "no." This twisting or turning of the head accomplishes the movement of rotation, that is, rotation of the neck.)*

---

supination (soo-pin-**NAY**-shun)

Supination is the act of turning the palm up or forward. *(Do This: Place your right hand out, as if to receive change from a cashier.*

	This upward turning of your palm is called supination. Next, place your hands by your side, arms relaxed; turn your palms so they face forward. This forward turning of your palms is also called supination.)
pronation (proh-**NAY**-shun)	**Pronation** is the act of turning the palm down or backward. *(Do This: Place your left hand out, as if to show a ring you are wearing. This downward turning of your palm is called pronation. Next, place your hands by your side, arms relaxed; turn your palms so they face backward. This backward turning of your palms is also called pronation.)*
dorsiflexion (dor-see-**FLEK**-shun)	**Dorsiflexion** of the foot narrows the angle between the leg and the top of the foot (i.e., the foot is bent backward, or upward, at the ankle).
plantar flexion (**PLAN**-tar **FLEK**-shun)	**Plantar flexion** of the foot increases the angle between the leg and the top of the foot (i.e., the foot is bent downward at the ankle with the toes pointing downward, as in toe dancing).
circumduction (sir-kum-**DUCK**-shun)	**Circumduction** is the movement of an extremity around in a circular motion. This motion can be performed with ball-and-socket joints, as in the shoulder and hip. *(Do This: Extend your right arm out beside your body and move your arm around in a circular motion. When you do this, you are performing a circumduction motion on your shoulder joint.)*

Vocabulary (Joints)

The following vocabulary words are frequently used when discussing the joints.

WORD	DEFINITION
abduction (ab-**DUCK**-shun) ab- = from, away from	Movement of a bone away from the midline of the body.
adduction (ad-**DUCK**-shun) ad- = toward, increase	Movement of a bone toward the midline of the body.
arthralgia (ar-**THRAL**-jee-ah) arthr/o = joint -algia = pain	Joint pain.
articular cartilage (ar-**TIK**-yoo-lar **CAR**-tih-laj)	Thin layer of cartilage protecting and covering the connecting surfaces of the bones.
articulation joint (ar-tik-yoo-**LAY**-shun)	The point at which two bones come together.

ball-and-socket joint	A joint that allows movements in many directions around a central point.
bunionectomy (bun-yun-**ECK**-toh-mee) -ectomy = surgical removal	Surgical removal of a bunion; removing the bony overgrowth and the bursa.
bursa (**BER**-sah) burs/o = bursa -a = noun ending	A small sac that contains synovial fluid; for lubricating the area around the joint where friction is most likely to occur.
closed manipulation	The manual forcing of a joint back into its original position without making an incision; also called closed reduction.
closed reduction	See *closed manipulation.*
crepitation (crep-ih-**TAY**-shun)	Clicking or crackling sounds heard upon joint movement.
dorsiflexion (dor-see-**FLEK**-shun) dors/i = back	Dorsiflexion of the foot is bending the foot backward, or upward, at the ankle.
extension (eks-**TEN**-shun)	A straightening motion that increases the angle between two bones.
flexion (**FLEK**-shun)	A bending motion that decreases the angle between two bones.
ganglionectomy (gang-lee-on-**ECK**-toh-mee) ganglion/o = ganglion -ectomy = surgical removal	Surgical removal of a ganglion.
hinge joint (**HINJ** joint)	A joint that allows movement in one direction; a back-and-forth motion.
joint cavity	The space between two connecting bones.
kyphosis (kye-**FOH**-sis) kyph/o = humpback; pertaining to a hump -osis = condition	Humpback.
ligaments (**LIG**-ah-ments)	Connective tissue bands that join bone to bone, offering support to the joint.
malaise (mah-**LAYZ**)	A vague feeling of weakness.
needle aspiration (needle ass-per-**AY**-shun)	The insertion of a needle into a cavity for the purpose of withdrawing fluid.
photosensitivity (**foh**-toh-**sen**-sih-**TIH**-vih-tee)	Increased reaction of the skin to exposure to sunlight.

plantar flexion (**PLAN**-tar **FLEK**-shun)	Plantar flexion of the foot is bending the foot downward, at the ankle, as in toe dancing.
pronation (proh-**NAY**-shun)	The act of turning the palm down or backward.
rotation (roh-**TAY**-shun)	The turning of a bone on its own axis.
sciatica (sigh-**AT**-ih-kah)	Inflammation of the sciatic nerve, marked by pain and tenderness along the path of the nerve through the thigh and leg.
subluxation (**sub**-luks-**AY**-shun)	An incomplete dislocation.
supination (soo-pin-**AY**-shun)	The act of turning the palm up or forward.
suture (**soo**-cher)	An immovable joint.
synovial fluid (sin-**OH**-vee-al)	A thick, lubricating fluid located in synovial joints.
synovial membrane (sin-**OH**-vee-al **MEM**-brayn)	The lining of a synovial joint cavity.
viscous (**VISS**-kus)	Sticky; gelatinous.

Word Elements (Joints)

The following word elements pertain to the joints. As you review the list, pronounce each word element aloud twice and check the box after you "say it." Write the definition for the example word given for each word element. You may use your medical dictionary.

WORD ELEMENT	PRONUNCIATION	"SAY IT"	MEANING
ankyl/o **ankyl**osis	**ANG**-kih-loh ang-kih-**LOH**-sis	☐	stiff
arthr/o **arthr**itis	**AR**-throh ar-**THRY**-tis	☐	joint
articul/o **articul**ar	ar-**TIK**-yoo-loh ar-**TIK**-yoo-lar	☐	joint
burs/o **burs**itis	**BER**-soh ber-**SIGH**-tis	☐	bursa
-centesis arthro**centesis**	sen-**TEE**-sis ar-throh-sen-**TEE**-sis	☐	surgical puncture

-desis arthro**desis**	**DEE**-sis ar-throh-**DEE**-sis	☐	binding or surgical fusion
-graphy arthro**graphy**	**GRAH**-fee ar-**THROG**-rah-fee	☐	process of recording
-itis tendin**itis**	**EYE**-tis ten-din-**EYE**-tis	☐	inflammation
ligament/o **ligament**al	lig-ah-**MEN**-toh lig-ah-**MEN**-tal	☐	ligament
oste/o **oste**oarthritis	**OSS**-tee-oh oss-tee-oh-ar-**THRY**-tis	☐	bone
-plasty arthro**plasty**	**PLAS**-tee **AR**-throh-**plas**-tee	☐	surgical repair
-scopy arthro**scopy**	**SKOH**-pee ar-**THROS**-koh-pee	☐	process of viewing with an endoscope
ten/o, tendin/o, tend/o **ten**osynovitis	**TEN**-oh, ten-**DIN**-oh, **TEN**-doh, **ten**-oh-**sin**-oh-**VY**-tis	☐	tendon

Pathological Conditions (Joints)

As you study the pathological conditions of the joints, note that the **basic definition** is in bold print, followed by a detailed description in regular print. The phonetic pronunciation is directly beneath each term, and a breakdown of the component parts of the term when appropriate.

arthritis
(ar-**THRY**-tis)
arthr/o = joint
-itis = inflammation

Arthritis is inflammation of joints.

The discussion of arthritis will be limited to four types: ankylosing spondylitis, gout, osteoarthritis, and rheumatoid arthritis (entries are listed alphabetically).

ankylosing spondylitis
(**ang**-kih-**LOH**-sing
spon-dil-**EYE**-tis)
ankyl/o = stiff
spondyl/o = spine; vertebra
-itis = inflammation

Ankylosing spondylitis is a type of arthritis that affects the vertebral column and causes deformities of the spine.

It is also known as Marie-Strumpell disease and as rheumatoid spondylitis.

Patient symptoms include other joint involvement, arthralgia (pain in the joints), weight loss, and generalized **malaise** (weakness). As the disease progresses, the spine becomes increasingly stiff, with fusion of the spine into a position of **kyphosis** (humpback).

Treatment includes anti-inflammatory medications to decrease the inflammation and relieve the pain, and physical therapy to keep the spine as straight as possible and promote mobility.

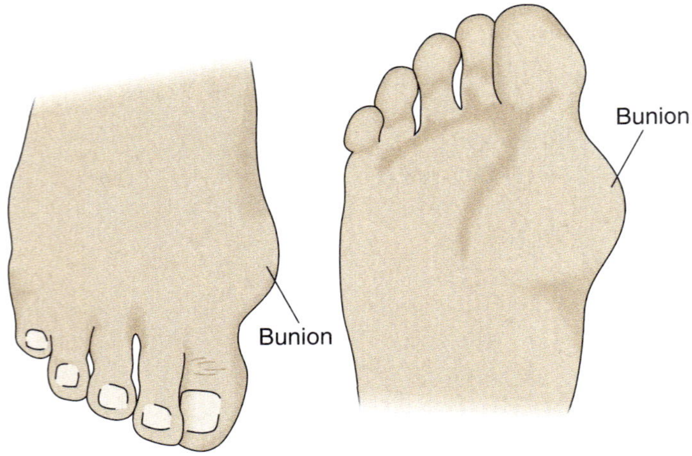

Figure 7-11 Bunion

bunion (hallux valgus)
(**BUN**-yun) (**HAL**-uks **VAL**-gus)

A bunion, or hallux valgus, is an abnormal enlargement of the joint at the base of the great toe. See Figure 7-11.

The great toe deviates laterally, causing it to either override or undercut the second toe. As the condition worsens, the bony prominence enlarges at the base of the great toe, causing pain and swelling of the joint.

A bunion often occurs as a result of arthritis or as a result of chronic irritation and pressure from wearing poorly fitting shoes, although it can be congenital. Treatment for a bunion may include application of padding between the toes or around the bunion to relieve pressure when wearing shoes, medications to relieve the pain and inflammation, or a bunionectomy, which involves removal of the bony overgrowth and the bursa.

dislocation
(diss-loh-**KAY**-shun)

A dislocation is the displacement of a bone from its normal location within a joint, causing loss of function of the joint.

If the dislocation is not complete (i.e., the bone is not completely out of its joint), it is termed a partial dislocation or subluxation. A dislocation can occur in any synovial joint, but it is more common in the shoulder, fingers, hip, and knee.

Dislocations are most often the result of an injury that exerts a force great enough to tear the joint ligaments (remember that the ligaments hold the bones in place at the joint). If this happens, the joint will be extremely painful, there will be rapid swelling at the site, the shape of the joint will be altered, and the patient will be unable to move the joint without severe pain.

Treatment involves the **closed manipulation,** or **reduction,** of the joint (forcing it back into its original position). This should be performed by a physician as soon after the dislocation as possible (within 30 minutes) because of the extensive swelling that occurs with a dislocation. Prior to the procedure, a sedative is administered intravenously to the patient. The procedure may be performed under local or general anesthesia. After the joint is returned to its normal position, it is immobilized with a cast, splint, or bandage until healing takes place.

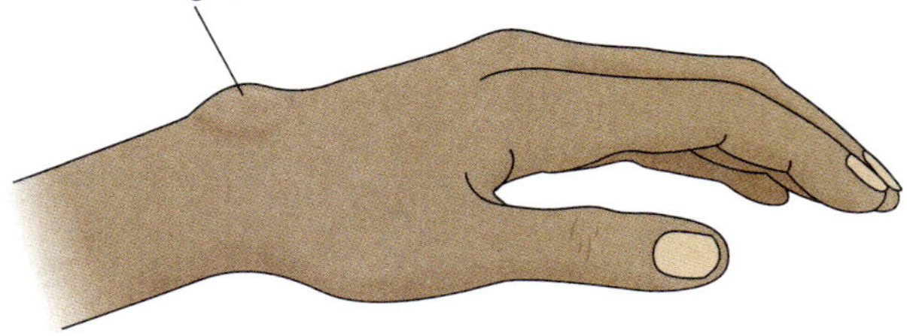

Figure 7-12 Ganglion

ganglion
(**GANG**-lee-on)

A ganglion is a cystic tumor developing on a tendon; sometimes occurs on the back of the wrist. See Figure 7-12.

The ganglion, which is filled with a jellylike substance, surfaces as a smooth lump just under the skin. It can be painless or somewhat bothersome to the wrist movements.

Treatment for a ganglion is unwarranted if the patient is not experiencing pain, disfigurement, or interference with wrist function. If, however, these symptoms are present and the patient is experiencing discomfort from the ganglion, a **ganglionectomy** (surgical removal of a ganglion) can be performed. The physician may favor a needle aspiration procedure to remove the fluid from within the cyst, followed by injection of cortisone.

gout
(**GOWT**)

Gout is a form of acute arthritis that is characterized by inflammation of the first metatarsal joint of the great toe.

It is an hereditary disease in which the patient does not metabolize uric acid properly. Large amounts of uric acid accumulate in the blood and in the synovial fluid of the joints. (The body produces uric acid from metabolism of ingested purines in the diet, especially from eating red meats). The uric acid crystals are responsible for the inflammatory reaction that develops in the joint, causing intense pain. The pain reaches a peak after several hours and then gradually declines; the attack may be accompanied by a slight fever and chills.

Treatment for gout may include bed rest, immobilizing the affected part, and application of a cold pack (if the area is not too painful to touch). Anti-inflammatory medications may be given to lessen the inflammation of the area; analgesics may be given to relieve the pain; and medications, such as allopurinol, may be prescribed to lower the uric acid level in the blood. The patient will be instructed to avoid eating foods high in purine (i.e., decrease the intake of red meat) and increase fluid intake.

herniated disk
(**HER**-nee-ay-ted disk)

A herniated disk is the rupture of the central portion, or nucleus, of the disk through the disk wall and into the spinal canal. A herniated disk is also called a ruptured disk or a slipped disk. See Figure 7-13.

Herniation may occur as a result of injury, an abrupt movement, or a degeneration of the vertebrae, or it may be the result of accumulated

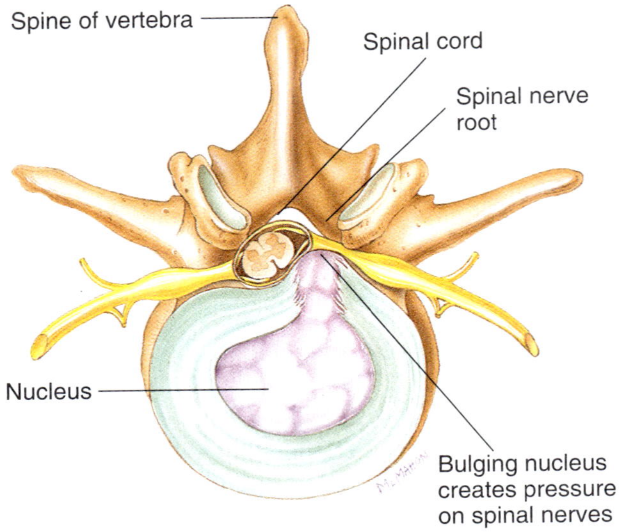

Figure 7-13 Herniated disk

trauma to the vertebrae. It occurs most often between the fourth and fifth lumbar vertebrae.

When a herniation occurs, the patient may experience a severe, burning, or knifelike pain that worsens on movement. This would indicate pressure on the spinal nerves. If the sciatic nerve is being pinched, the pain will radiate down the buttocks and back of the leg; this is known as **sciatica**.

Treatment consists of conservative measures such as bed rest, analgesics to relieve the pain, muscle relaxants, and physical therapy. If this approach is not successful, surgical intervention may become necessary to remove the herniated disk.

Lyme disease
(**LYME** dih-**ZEEZ**)

Lyme disease is an acute, recurrent inflammatory infection, transmitted through the bite of an infected deer tick.

It is characterized by a circular rash (a red, itchy rash with a circular center) and influenza-like symptoms: weakness, chills, fever, headaches, and muscle or joint pain. If these symptoms occur following a camping or hiking trip, the possibility of Lyme disease should be considered. The individual should inspect his or her skin for the presence of a tick, and remove it if one is found.

Treatment with antibiotics, such as tetracycline, is usually effective. Medications will also be given to relieve the fever, headaches, and muscle or joint pain.

---

osteoarthritis
(**oss**-tee-oh-ar-**THRY**-tis)
oste/o = bone
arthr/o = joint
-itis = inflammation

Osteoarthritis is also known as degenerative joint disease. It is the most common form of arthritis and results from wear and tear on the joints, especially weight-bearing joints such as the hips and knees.

As this chronic disease progresses, the repeated stress to the joints results in degeneration of the joint cartilage. The joint space becomes narrower, taking on a flattened appearance. See **Figure 7-14.**

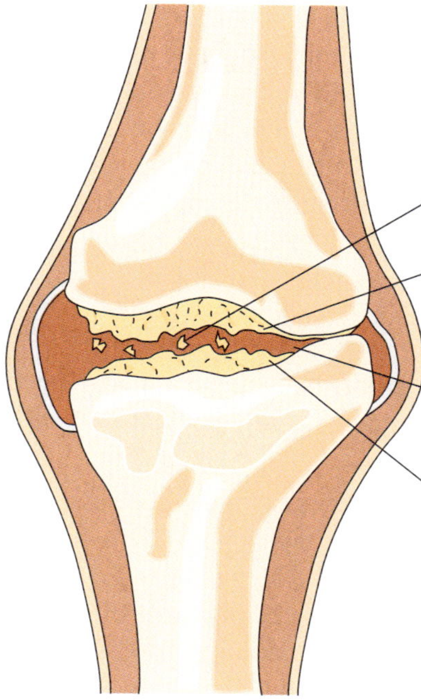

Figure 7-14 Osteoarthritis (knee joint)

Symptoms include joint soreness and pain; stiffness, especially in the mornings; and aching, particularly with changes in the weather. Joint movement may elicit clicking or crackling sounds, known as **crepitation**. The patient may also experience a decrease in the range of motion of a joint and increased pain with use of the joint.

The objectives of treatment for osteoarthritis are to reduce inflammation, lessen the pain, and maintain the function of the affected joints. Osteoarthritis cannot be cured. Medications may be prescribed to reduce the inflammation and to relieve the pain. Physical therapy may be prescribed to promote the function of the joint. If the condition becomes severe, joint replacement surgery may become necessary.

---

rheumatoid arthritis
(**ROO**-mah-toyd ar-**THRY**-tis)
arthr/o = joint
-itis = inflammation

Rheumatoid arthritis is a chronic, systemic, inflammatory disease that affects multiple joints of the body—mainly the small peripheral joints, such as in those of the hands and feet.

Larger peripheral joints such as the wrists, elbows, shoulders, ankles, knees, and hips may also be affected. This disease usually occurs in people between the ages of 20 and 40 and is characterized by periods of remission and relapse. Women are affected 2 to 3 times more often than men.

Rheumatoid arthritis is characterized by joint pain, stiffness, limitation of movement, and fatigue. The patient usually experiences pain upon arising in the morning and after periods of idleness. The joints of the hands and feet are usually swollen and painful. As the disease progresses, the severe inflammation may lead to deformity of the hands and feet. See **Figure 7-15.**

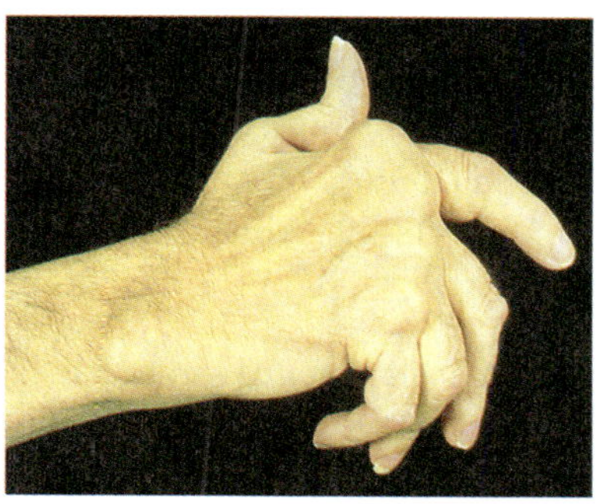

Figure 7-15 Rheumatoid hand deformity

The main objectives of treatment for rheumatoid arthritis are to reduce the inflammation and pain in the joints, to maintain the function of the joints, and to prevent joint deformity. Treatment includes salicylates, such as aspirin, to relieve the pain and inflammation (given in high doses), rest, and physical therapy. If aspirin is not tolerated well, nonsteroidal anti-inflammatory medications may be given to relieve the inflammation. Joint replacement surgery may become necessary for advanced cases of rheumatoid arthritis.

sprains

A sprain is an injury involving the ligaments that surround and support a joint, caused by a wrenching or twisting motion.

Movements, such as those associated with sports activities that overstress a joint or trying to break a fall, can be the cause of sprains to the upper extremities. Movements that twist the ankle, causing it to invert (turn inward), can be the cause of a sprained ankle. Movements such as whiplash (a sudden jerking or violent back-and-forth movement of the head and neck) can cause a cervical sprain.

A sprain can vary from mild (the ligament is not weakened because only a few fibers are torn), to severe (the ligament is completely torn, either away from its attachment or within itself, with resultant tissue bleeding).

If the sprain is severe, the patient may indicate a feeling that something has snapped or torn, and that the joint feels loose. The affected area will be tender to the touch. Other symptoms include swelling, decreased motion, severe pain, and discoloration. Increased tissue swelling following the injury will result in disability of the affected area.

Immediate treatment includes elevating the injured joint and applying ice to the area to prevent swelling. An x-ray of the affected area may be ordered to rule out the possibility of a fracture. The joint may be immobilized with either a splint or a cast. For a less severe sprain, taping the joint may be sufficient.

The healing process for a severe sprain may take 4 to 6 weeks; the joint may be immobilized for 3 to 4 weeks. Activity should be limited during this time to avoid recurrence of injury.

systemic lupus erythematosus
(sis-**TEM**-ic **LOO**-pus er-**ih**-them-ah-**TOH**-sis)

Systemic lupus erythematosus is a chronic, inflammatory connective-tissue disease affecting the skin, joints, nervous system, kidneys, lungs, and other organs. The most striking symptom of the disease is the "butterfly rash" that appears on the face. See Figure 7-16.

The disease may begin acutely with fever, arthritic joint pain, and weakness, or it may develop over the course of years with periodic fever and weakness. The butterfly rash covers both cheeks and connects by crossing the nose. The rash is aggravated by exposure to the sun (**photosensitivity**).

Mild cases of lupus may be treated with anti-inflammatory medicines, including aspirin, to control the joint pain and fever. More severe cases may be treated with corticosteroid medications.

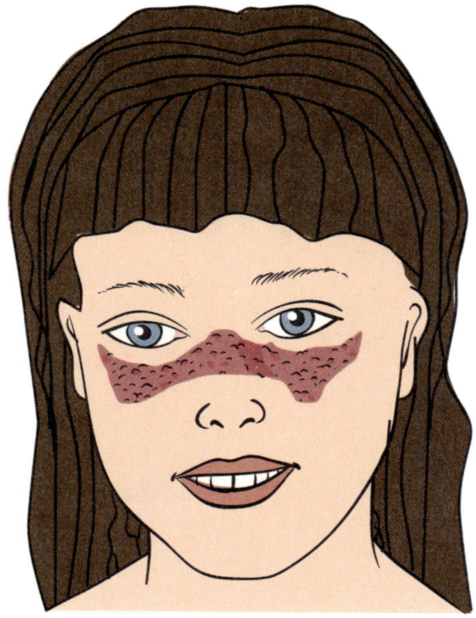

Figure 7-16 Butterfly rash often seen in SLE

Diagnostic Techniques and Procedures (Joints)

arthrocentesis
(ar-throh-sen-**TEE**-sis)
arthr/o = joint
-centesis = surgical puncture

An arthrocentesis is the surgical puncture of a joint with a needle for the purpose of withdrawing fluid for analysis.

A local anesthetic is used and the puncture needle is inserted using sterile technique. Normal synovial fluid is clear, straw colored, and slightly sticky; when mixed with glacial acetic acid, it will form a white, **viscous** (sticky) clot. When inflammation is present, as in rheumatoid arthritis, the synovial fluid will be watery and cloudy; the mixture of synovial fluid with the glacial acetic acid will result in a clumplike clot that is easily broken.

arthrography
(ar-**THROG**-rah-fee)
arthr/o = joint
-graphy = process of recording

Arthrography is the process of x-raying the inside of a joint, after a contrast medium (a substance that makes the inside of the joint visible) has been injected into the joint.

arthroplasty
(**AR**-throh-**plas**-tee)
arthr/o = joint
-plasty = surgical repair

Arthroplasty is the surgical repair of a joint.

It involves the surgical reconstruction or replacement of a painful, degenerated repair joint to restore mobility. It is used as a treatment method for osteoarthritis and rheumatoid arthritis, as well as to correct congenital deformities of the joint.

arthroscopy
(ar-**THROSS**-koh-pee)
arthr/o = joint
-scopy = process of viewing

Arthroscopy is the visualization of the interior of a joint using an endoscope.

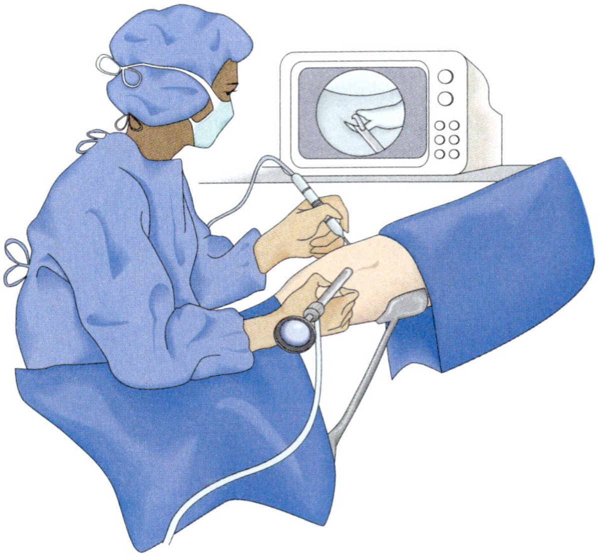

(A) Arthroscope in use

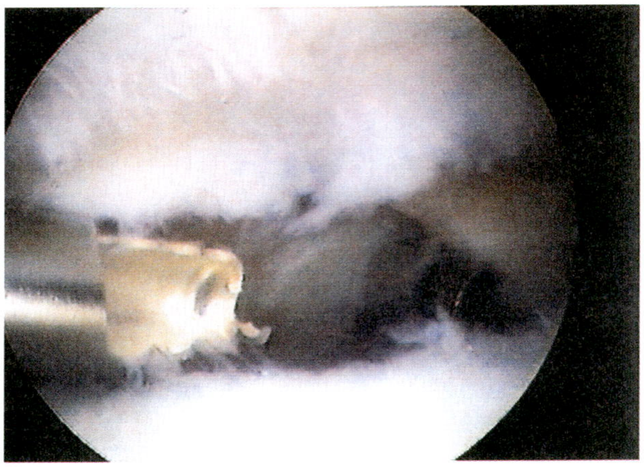

(B) Internal view of the knee during arthroscopy

Figure 7-17 Arthroscopy of the knee

A specially designed endoscope is inserted through a small incision into the joint. This procedure is used primarily with knee problems and is useful for obtaining a biopsy of cartilage or synovial membrane for analysis. See **Figure 7-17.**

rheumatoid factor
(**ROO**-mah-toyd factor)

The rheumatoid factor test is a blood test that measures the presence of unusual antibodies that develop in a number of connective tissue diseases, such as rheumatoid arthritis.

erythrocyte sed rate
(eh-**RITH**-roh-sight sed rate)
erythr/o = red
cyt/o = cell
-e = noun ending

The erythrocyte sedimentation (sed) rate is a blood test that measures the rate at which erythrocytes (red blood cells) settle to the bottom of a test tube filled with unclotted blood.

Elevated sed rates are associated with inflammatory conditions; the more elevated the sed rate, the more severe the inflammation. This test may be helpful in determining the degree of inflammation in rheumatoid arthritis.

Common Abbreviations (Joints)

ABBREVIATION	MEANING	ABBREVIATION	MEANING
DIP	distal interphalangeal	**RA**	rheumatoid arthritis
LLE	left lower extremity	**RF**	rheumatoid factor
LUE	left upper extremity	**RLE**	right lower extremity
MCP	metacarpophalangeal (joint)	**RUE**	right upper extremity
MTP	metatarsophalangeal (joint)	**sed rate**	sedimentation rate
PIP	proximal interphalangeal (joint)	**SLE**	systemic lupus erythematosus

Written and Audio Terminology Review

Review each of the following terms from this chapter. Study the spelling of each term and write the definition in the space provided. If you have the Audio CD available, listen to each term, pronounce it, and check the box once you are comfortable saying the word. Check definitions by looking the term up in the glossary/index.

TERM	PRONUNCIATION	DEFINITION
abduction	☐ ab-**DUCK**-shun	______________
adduction	☐ ad-**DUCK**-shun	______________
ankylosing spondylitis	☐ **ang**-kih-**LOH**-sing spon-dil-**EYE**-tis	______________
ankylosis	☐ **ang**-kih-**LOH**-sis	______________
arthralgia	☐ ar-**THRAL**-jee-ah	______________
arthritis	☐ ar-**THRY**-tis	______________
arthrocentesis	☐ ar-throh-sen-**TEE**-sis	______________
arthrodesis	☐ ar-throh-**DEE**-sis	______________
arthrography	☐ ar-**THROG**-rah-fee	______________
arthroplasty	☐ **AR**-throh-**plas**-tee	______________
arthroscopy	☐ ar-**THROSS**-koh-pee	______________
articular	☐ ar-**TIK**-yoo-lar	______________
articular cartilage	☐ ar-**TIK**-yoo-lar **CAR**-tih-laj	______________
articulation	☐ ar-tik-yoo-**LAY**-shun	______________
atrophy	☐ **AT**-troh-fee	______________
biceps	☐ **BYE**-seps	______________
biceps brachii	☐ **BYE**-seps **BRAY**-kee-eye	______________
buccal	☐ **BUCK**-al	______________
buccinator	☐ **BUCK**-sin-ay-tor	______________
bunion	☐ **BUN**-yun	______________
bunionectomy	☐ bun-yun-**ECK**-toh-mee	______________
bursa	☐ **BER**-suh	______________
bursitis	☐ ber-**SIGH**-tis	______________
cardiac muscle	☐ **CAR**-dee-ak muscle	______________

Term	Pronunciation	
cartilaginous	☐ **car**-tih-**LAJ**-ih-nus	______
circumduction	☐ sir-kum-**DUCK**-shun	______
contraction	☐ con-**TRACK**-shun	______
contracture	☐ con-**TRACK**-cher	______
crepitation	☐ crep-ih-**TAY**-shun	______
deltoid	☐ **DELL**-toyd	______
diaphragm	☐ **DYE**-ah-fram	______
dislocation	☐ diss-loh-**KAY**-shun	______
dorsal	☐ **DOR**-sal	______
dorsiflexion	☐ dor-see-**FLEK**-shun	______
dystonia	☐ dis-**TOH**-nee-ah	______
dystrophy	☐ **DIS**-troh-fee	______
electromyogram	☐ ee-**lek**-troh-**MY**-oh-gram	______
electromyography	☐ ee-**lek**-troh-my-**OG**-rah-fee	______
electroneuromyography	☐ ee-**lek**-troh-**noo**-roh-my-**OG**-rah-fee	______
erythrocyte sed rate	☐ eh-**RITH**-roh-sight sed rate	______
extension	☐ eks-**TEN**-shun	______
fascia	☐ **FASH**-ee-ah	______
fasciotomy	☐ fash-ee-**OTT**-oh-mee	______
fibroma	☐ fih-**BROH**-mah	______
fibrous	☐ **FIH**-bruss *or* **FYE**-bruss	______
flexion	☐ **FLEK**-shun	______
ganglion	☐ **GANG**-lee-on	______
gastrocnemius	☐ **gas**-trok-**NEE**-mee-us	______
gout	☐ **GOWT**	______
hallux valgus	☐ **HAL**-uks **VAL**-gus	______
hamstring muscles	☐ **HAM**-string muscles	______
herniated disk	☐ **HER**-nee-ay-ted disk	______
hinge joint	☐ **HINJ** joint	______
insertion	☐ in-**SIR**-shun	______
latissimus dorsi	☐ lah-**TIS**-ih-mus **DOR**-sigh	______

Term		Pronunciation	
leiomyofibroma	☐	**lye**-oh-**my**-oh-fih-**BROH**-mah	___
ligamental	☐	lig-ah-**MEN**-tal	___
ligaments	☐	**LIG**-ah-ments	___
Lyme disease	☐	**LYME** dih-**ZEEZ**	___
masseter	☐	mass-**SEE**-ter	___
muscle biopsy	☐	muscle **BYE**-op-see	___
muscular dystrophy	☐	**MUSS**-kew-lar **DIS**-troh-fee	___
myalgia	☐	my-**AL**-jee-ah	___
myositis	☐	my-oh-**SIGH**-tis	___
needle aspiration	☐	needle ass-per-**AY**-shun	___
osteoarthritis	☐	**oss**-tee-oh-ar-**THRY**-tis	___
pectoral	☐	**PECK**-toh-ral	___
pectoralis	☐	peck-toh-**RAY**-lis	___
pelvic girdle	☐	**PELL**-vik **GER**-dl	___
photosensitivity	☐	**foh**-toh-**sen**-sih-**TIH**-vih-tee	___
plantar flexion	☐	**PLAN**-tar **FLEK**-shun	___
polymyositis	☐	**pol**-ee-my-oh-**SIGH**-tis	___
pronation	☐	proh-**NAY**-shun	___
pseudohypertrophic muscular dystrophy	☐	**soo**-doh-**hy**-per-**TROH**-fic **MUSS**-kew-ler **DIS**-troh-fee	___
quadriceps femoris	☐	**KWAHD**-rih-seps **FEM**-or-iss	___
rhabdomyosarcoma	☐	**rab**-doh-**my**-oh-sar-**KOH**-mah	___
rheumatoid arthritis	☐	**ROO**-mah-toyd ar-**THRY**-tis	___
rheumatoid factor	☐	**ROO**-mah-toyd factor	___
rotation	☐	roh-**TAY**-shun	___
sciatica	☐	sigh-**AT**-ih-kah	___
skeletal muscle	☐	**SKELL**-eh-tal muscle	___
sternomastoid	☐	stir-no-**MASS**-toyd	___
striated muscle	☐	**STRY**-ay-ted muscle	___
subluxation	☐	sub-luks-**AY**-shun	___
supination	☐	soo-pin-**NAY**-shun	___

suture	☐ **SOO**-cher	______
synovial	☐ sin-**OH**-vee-al	______
synovial membrane	☐ sin-**OH**-vee-al **MEM**-brayn	______
systemic lupus erythrematosus	☐ sis-**TEM**-ic **LOO**-pus er-**ih**-them-ah-**TOH**-sis	______
temporal	☐ **TEM**-po-ral	______
tendinitis	☐ **ten**-din-**EYE**-tis	______
tendon	☐ **TEN**-dun	______
tenosynovitis	☐ **ten**-oh-**sin**-oh-**VY**-tis	______
tibialis anterior	☐ tib-ee-**AY**-lis an-**TEER**-ee-or	______
torso	☐ **TOR**-soh	______
trapezius	☐ trah-**PEE**-zee-us	______
triceps	☐ **TRY**-seps	______
triceps brachii	☐ **TRY**-seps **BRAY**-kee-eye	______
visceral muscle	☐ **VISS**-er-al muscle	______
viscous	☐ **VISS**-kus	______
voluntary muscle	☐ **VOL**-un-tair-ee muscle	______

Chapter Review Exercises

The following exercises provide a more in-depth review of the chapter material. Your goal in these exercises is to complete each section at a minimum 80% level of accuracy. A space has been provided for your score at the end of each section.

A. Matching Abbreviations

Match the abbreviations on the left with the correct definition on the right. Each correct answer is worth 20 points. Record your score in the space provided at the end of this exercise.

_____ 1. IM		a. rheumatoid arthritis
_____ 2. MD		b. intramuscular
_____ 3. EMG		c. systemic lupus erythematosus
_____ 4. RA		d. muscular dystrophy
_____ 5. SLE		e. electromyography
		f. rheumatoid factor
		g. sedimentation rate
		h. deep tendon reflex

Number correct ______ × 20 points/correct answer: Your score ______%

B. Matching Terms

Match the terms on the left with the most appropriate description on the right. Each correct answer is worth 10 points. Record your score in the space provided at the end of the exercise.

_____ 1. skeletal muscle
_____ 2. insertion
_____ 3. origin
_____ 4. striated muscle
_____ 5. visceral muscle
_____ 6. involuntary muscle
_____ 7. voluntary muscle
_____ 8. muscle fiber
_____ 9. fascia
_____ 10. tendon

a. thin sheets of fibrous connective tissue, covering a muscle
b. found in the walls of hollow organs and tubes such as the stomach, intestines, blood vessels, and respiratory passageways
c. attach to the bones of the skeleton; responsible for moving the bones of the skeleton
d. strong fibrous band of tissue that attaches muscle to bone
e. point of attachment of the muscle to the bone that it moves
f. acts under the control of the autonomic nervous system
g. has a striped appearance when viewed under the microscope
h. point of attachment of the muscle to the bone that is less movable
i. individual muscle cells
j. so named because it acts under conscious control

Number correct _______ × 10 points/correct answer: Your score _______%

C. Labeling

Label the following diagrams for the muscles by writing your answers in the spaces provided. Each correct response is worth 10 points. Record your score in the space provided at the end of the exercise.

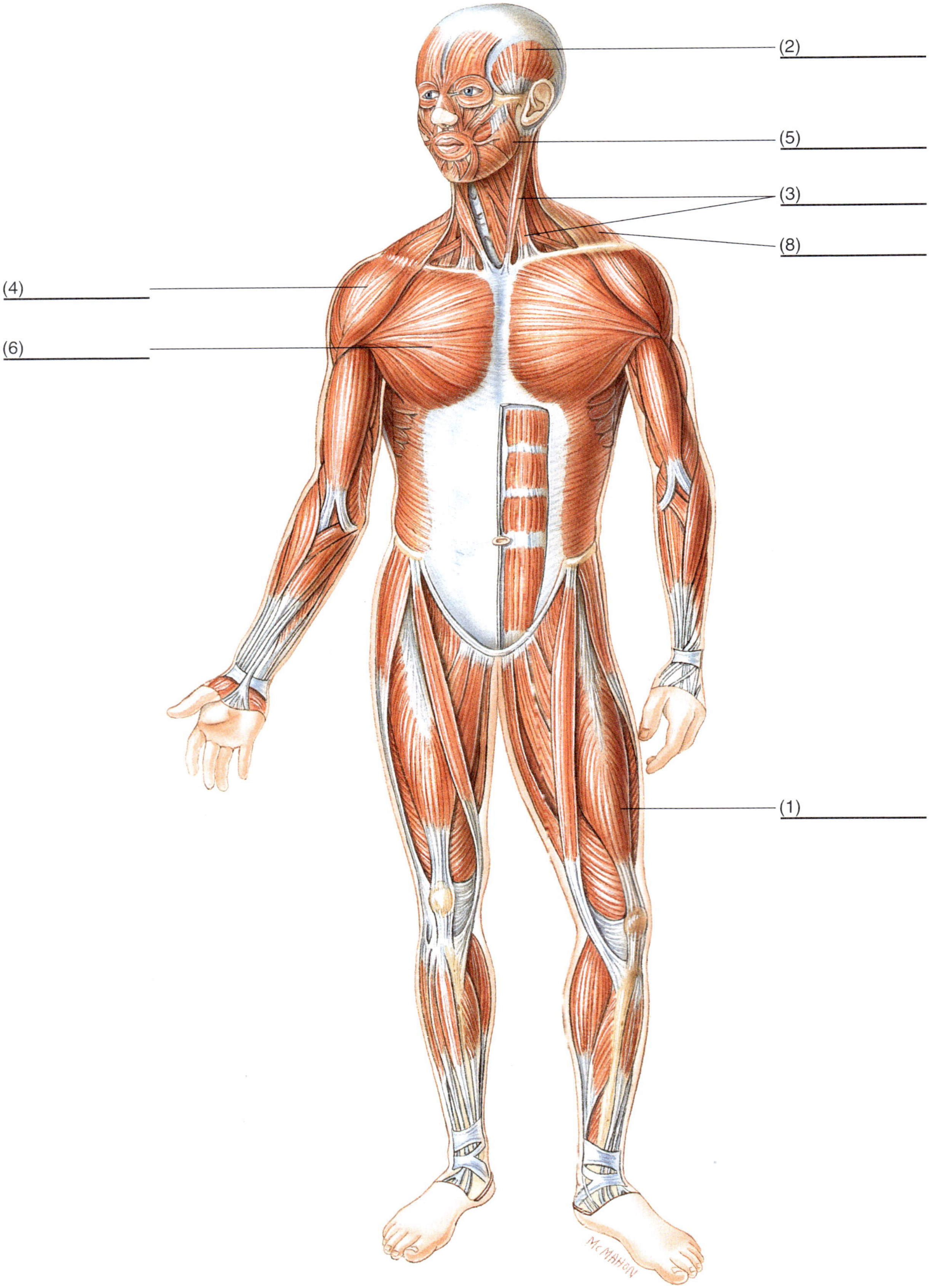

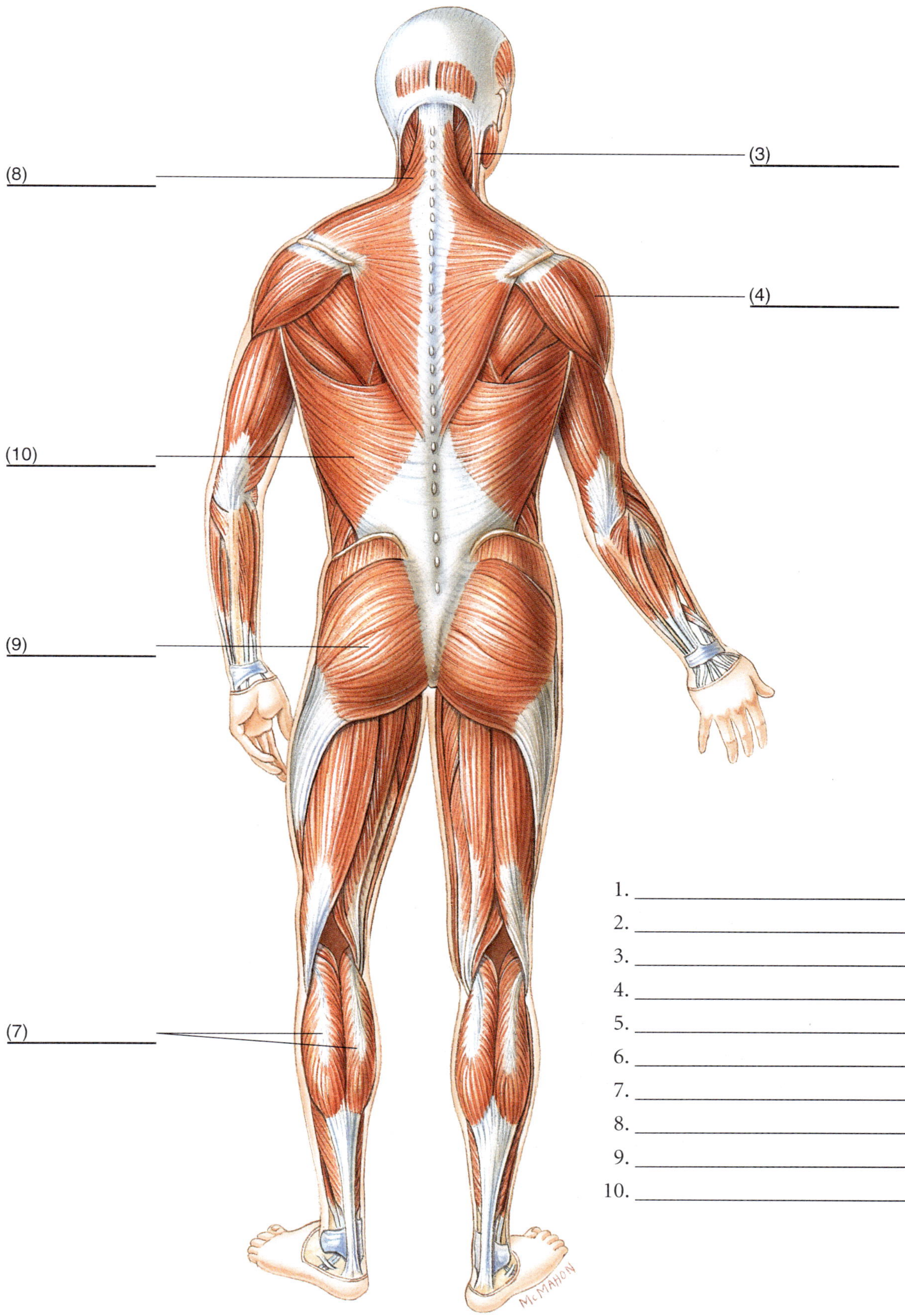

1. ______________________
2. ______________________
3. ______________________
4. ______________________
5. ______________________
6. ______________________
7. ______________________
8. ______________________
9. ______________________
10. ______________________

Number correct ______ × 10 points/correct answer: Your score ______%

D. Spelling

Circle the correctly spelled term in each pairing of words. Each correct answer is worth 10 points. Record your score in the space provided at the end of the exercise.

1.	brachi	brachii
2.	dystrophy	dystrophe
3.	polymyocytis	polymyositis
4.	arthritis	artheritis
5.	viscos	viscous
6.	visceral	viceral
7.	adduction	aduction
8.	soupination	supination
9.	rheumatoid	rumatoid
10.	siatica	sciatica

Number correct _______ × 10 points/correct answer: Your score _______%

E. Crossword Puzzle

The topic of this crossword puzzle is pathological conditions of the muscles and joints. Each crossword answer is worth 10 points. When you have completed the crossword puzzle, total your points and enter your score in the space provided.

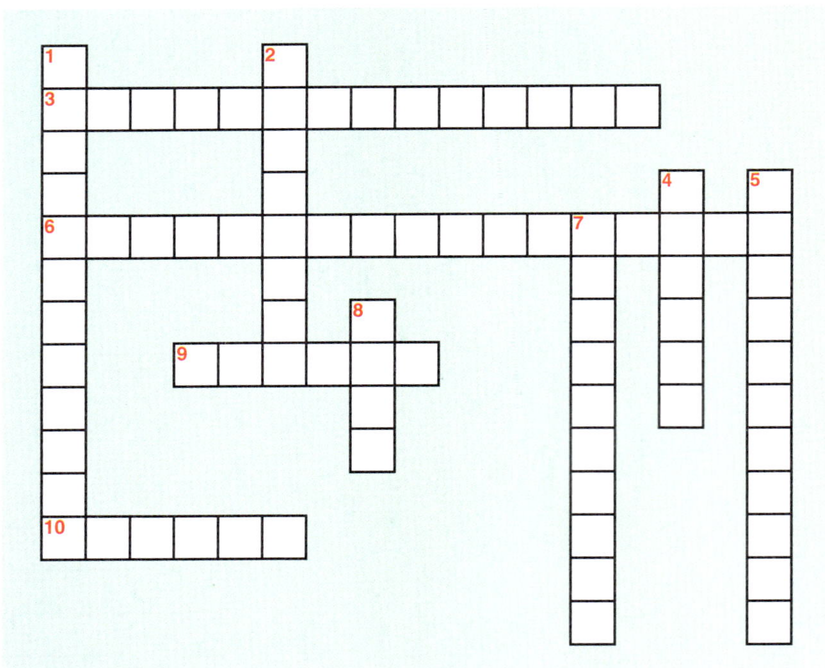

ACROSS
3 Degenerative joint disease
6 Disease: progressive muscle weakness
9 Enlargement of joint of great toe
10 Injury to the body of a muscle

DOWN
1 Inflammation of many muscles
2 Cystic tumor developing on a tendon
4 Injury involving twisted ligaments
5 Transmitted by infected deer tick
7 Arthritis affecting small joints
8 Due to accumulations of uric acid

Number correct _______ × 10 points/correct answer: Your score _______%

F. Completion

Complete each sentence with the most appropriate word. Each correct answer is worth 10 points. Record your score in the space provided at the end of the exercise.

1. Pain in the joints is termed ____________________.
2. The point of attachment of a muscle to the bone that it moves is called ____________________.
3. Another name for an individual muscle cell is a(n) ____________________.
4. The muscles that attach to the bones of the skeleton are known as the ____________________ muscles.
5. The main part of the body to which the head and the extremities are attached is the ____________________.
6. Another name for a joint is a(n) ____________________.
7. A clicking or crackling sound heard upon joint movement is known as ____________________.
8. A small sac, located near a joint, that contains synovial fluid for lubricating areas of increased friction is known as a(n) ____________________.
9. The proper term for an incomplete dislocation of a joint is ____________________.
10. An immovable joint is called a(n) ____________________.

Number correct ______ × 10 points/correct answer: Your score ______ %

G. Word Element Review

The following words relate to the muscles and joints. The prefixes and suffixes have been provided. Read the definition carefully and complete the word by filling in the space, using the word elements provided in the chapter. Each correct answer is worth 10 points. Record your score in the space provided at the end of this exercise.

1. Pertaining to the cheek
   ____________/al
2. A fibrous tumor
   ____________/oma
3. A painful muscle
   ____________/algia
4. Pertaining to the chest
   ____________/al
5. Bad, or poor, development
   dys/____________/y
6. Condition of stiffness, as in a stiff joint
   ____________/osis
7. Surgical puncture of a joint
   arthro/____________
8. Inflammation of a tendon
   ____________/itis
9. Surgical repair of a joint
   arthro/____________
10. The process of viewing the interior of a joint with a scope
    arthro/____________

Number correct ______ × 10 points/correct answer: Your score ______ %

H. Word Search

Using the definitions, write the appropriate range-of-motion word in the space provided, and then find and circle it in the puzzle. The words may be read up, down, diagonally, across, or backward. Each correct answer is worth 10 points. Record your score in the space provided at the end of this exercise.

Example: Another word for walking: *ambulation*

1. A bending motion that decreases the angle between two bones: ______
2. The act of turning the palm up or forward: ______
3. A straightening motion that increases the angle between two bones: ______
4. The movement of a bone toward the midline of the body: ______
5. A movement that involves turning a bone on its own axis: ______
6. The act of turning the palm down or backward: ______
7. The movement of a bone away from the midline of the body: ______
8. A foot movement that bends the foot downward as in toe dancing: ______
9. A foot movement that bends the foot upward toward the leg: ______
10. Movement of an extremity around in a circular motion: ______

C	A	D	O	R	S	I	F	L	E	X	I	O	N	A
B	I	S	N	O	I	T	A	N	O	R	P	C	D	M
A	O	R	U	E	T	L	I	M	B	R	I	C	E	B
D	N	E	C	P	F	L	E	X	I	O	N	A	R	U
D	A	X	N	U	I	N	O	I	T	A	T	O	R	L
U	T	T	O	I	M	N	E	X	T	E	N	S	I	A
C	I	E	I	R	C	D	A	R	O	T	A	T	I	T
T	O	N	T	A	L	Y	U	T	A	D	D	U	C	I
I	N	S	C	D	O	R	S	C	I	P	R	O	N	O
O	S	I	U	I	R	C	U	M	T	O	S	U	P	N
N	O	O	D	F	L	E	X	I	O	I	N	R	A	T
D	U	N	B	S	U	P	I	N	A	T	O	N	I	L
E	R	O	A	D	O	R	S	I	F	L	E	N	X	N
P	L	A	N	T	A	R	F	L	E	X	I	O	N	O

Number correct ______ × 10 points/correct answer: Your score ______%

I. Proofreading Skills

Read the following operation report. For each boldfaced term, provide a brief definition and indicate if the term is spelled correctly; if it is misspelled, provide the correct spelling. Each correct answer is worth 10 points. Record your score in the space provided at the end of the exercise.

NAME: John Smith **ROOM NO.:** 123 **HOSPITAL NO.:** 436725

SURGEON: Dr. M. Gude Asnew **DATE:** 3-25-03

PREOPERATIVE DIAGNOSIS:

1. Cerebral palsy, with spastic **hemiplegia**, right
2. Internal rotation and flexion deformity, right lower leg and knee

POSTOPERATIVE DIAGNOSIS:

1. Cerebral palsy, with spastic hemiplegia, right
2. Internal rotation and **flexion** deformity, right lower leg and knee
3. **Bunion,** first **metatarsophalangeal** joint of great toe, left foot

ANESTHESIA: General

OPERATION:

1. Transfer of gracilis and semitendinosus tendons to the lateral aspect of the femur
2. Lengthening of the posterior tibial **tendon** of the right lower leg
3. **Bunionectomy,** left great toe

INDICATIONS:

This cerebral palsy patient has marked spastic hemiplegia. When walking, he has a flexed knee and internal **rotation** gait on the right. He also has a **contracture** of the right knee joint. He also has a cavovarus deformity from over-pulling of the posterior tibial tendon. It is felt that transfer of the semitendinosus and gracilis tendons would weaken the deformity caused by the hamstring muscles and would improve the internal rotation forces on the right femur. Lengthening the posterior tibial tendon should relieve the disfiguring forces on the deformity of the foot. It is also noted that he has a rather large bunion formation on the first metatarsophalangeal joint of the great toe, left foot. Although this is accessory to the problems, it is deemed advisable to remove this during surgery.

PROCEDURE:

Under general anesthesia, the semitendinosus and gracilis tendons were identified on the medial aspect of the thigh by entering through a longitudinal incision over the distal end of these muscles. The muscles were resected from their distal **insertion** point and the **fascia** around the muscles was stripped to allow transfer to the right outer portion of the femur. An incision was made over the lateral aspect of the thigh, and by entering the thigh in the interval between the **vastus lateralis** and the hamstrings the femur was identified. Drill holes were made in the femur and the tendons were transferred and sutured in place with #2.0 chromic suture. The fascia was then closed with interrupted #2.0 chromic suture and the subcutaneous tissue, and both incisions were closed with #3.0 plain suture. The skin was closed with #4.0 nylon.

A bunionectomy was then performed on the left foot. The bony overgrowth and bursa were removed without difficulty. The subcutaneous tissue was closed with interrupted #3.0 plain suture, and the skin was closed with interrupted #4.0 nylon. A pressure dressing was applied to the area.

The posterior tibial tendon was exposed by making a longitudinal incision over the distal portion of the medial aspect of the right leg. By sharp dissection, this tendon was identified and was lengthened and was then resutured with a #2.0 chromic suture. The subcutaneous tissue was closed with interrupted #3.0 plain suture, and the skin was closed with interrupted #4.0 nylon. A short-leg plaster cast was then applied, holding the foot in neutral position.

The patient tolerated the procedure well and was taken to the recovery room in good condition. Bleeding was within normal expectations.

SPONGE COUNT: One missing; second count reported correct

DICTATED BY: Dr. M. Gude Asnew **DATE OF DICTATION**: 3-25-03

M. Gude Asnew M.D.
Signature of Surgeon

Example:

hemiplegia *paralysis of one side of the body*
Spelled correctly? ☑ Yes ☐ No

1. **flexion**
   Spelled correctly? ☐ Yes ☐ No
2. **bunion**
   Spelled correctly? ☐ Yes ☐ No
3. **metatarsophalangeal**
   Spelled correctly? ☐ Yes ☐ No
4. **tendon**
   Spelled correctly? ☐ Yes ☐ No
5. **bunionectomy**
   Spelled correctly? ☐ Yes ☐ No
6. **rotation**
   Spelled correctly? ☐ Yes ☐ No
7. **contracture**
   Spelled correctly? ☐ Yes ☐ No

8. **insertion** ______________________________

Spelled correctly? ☐ Yes ☐ No ______________________________

9. **fascia** ______________________________

Spelled correctly? ☐ Yes ☐ No ______________________________

10. **vastus lateralis** ______________________________

Spelled correctly? ☐ Yes ☐ No ______________________________

Number correct ______ × 10 points/correct answer: Your score ______%

J. Matching Diagnostics

Match the diagnostic techniques or tests on the left with the most appropriate definition on the right. Each correct response is worth 20 points. Record your score in the space provided at the end of this exercise.

______	1. muscle biopsy	a. measures the rate at which red blood cells settle to the bottom of a test tube filled with unclotted blood
______	2. electromyography	b. surgical puncture of a joint for the purpose of withdrawing fluid
______	3. arthrocentesis	c. extraction of a specimen of muscle tissue for the purpose of diagnosis
______	4. arthroscopy	d. the process of recording the strength of the contraction of a muscle when it is stimulated by an electric current
______	5. ESR	e. the process of viewing the interior of a joint using an endoscope

Number correct ______ × 20 points/correct answer: Your score ______%

Answers to Chapter Review Exercises

A. Matching Abbreviations

1. b
2. d
3. e
4. a
5. c

B. Matching Terms

1. c
2. e
3. h
4. g
5. b
6. f
7. j
8. i
9. a
10. d

C. Labeling

1. rectus femoris
2. temporal
3. sternomastoid
4. deltoid
5. masseter
6. pectoralis major
7. gastrocnemius
8. trapezius
9. gluteus maximus
10. latissimus dorsi

D. Spelling

1. brachii
2. dystrophy
3. polymyositis
4. arthritis
5. viscous
6. visceral
7. adduction
8. supination
9. rheumatoid
10. sciatica

E. Crossword Puzzle

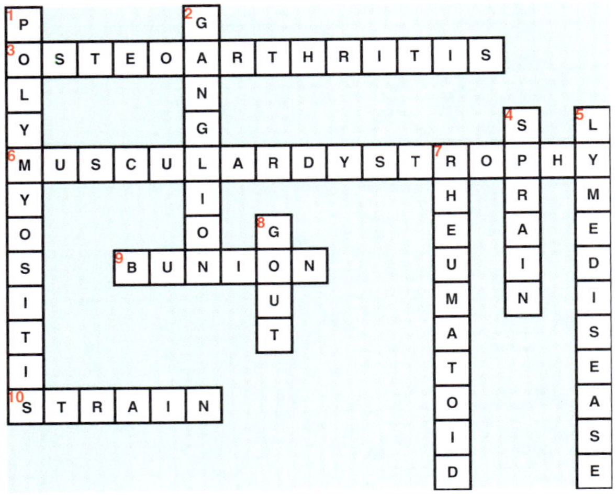

F. Completion

1. arthralgia
2. insertion
3. muscle fiber
4. skeletal
5. trunk
6. articulation
7. crepitation
8. bursa
9. subluxation
10. fibrous joint (*or* suture)

G. Word Element Review

1. **bucc**/al
2. **fibr**/oma
3. **my**/algia
4. **pector**/al
5. dys/**troph**/y
6. **ankyl**/osis
7. arthro/**centesis**
8. **tendin**/itis
9. arthro/**plasty**
10. arthro/**scopy**

H. Word Search

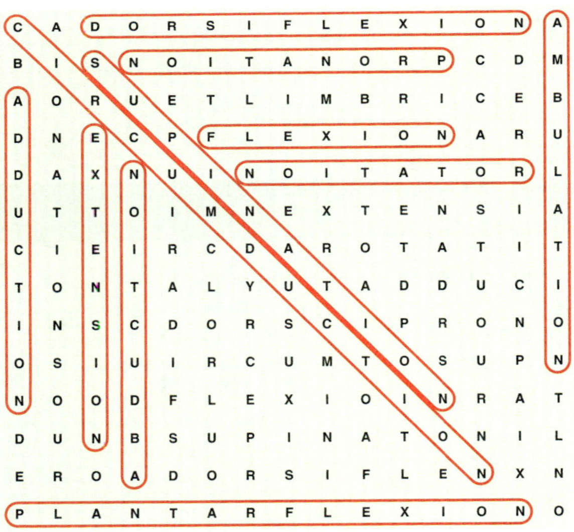

I. Proofreading Skills

1. **flexion:** bending motion decreasing the angle between two bones
   Spelled correctly? Yes
2. **bunion:** abnormal enlargement of the joint at the base of the great toe
   Spelled correctly? Yes
3. **metatarsophalangeal:** joint connecting the metatarsal of the foot with the phalange of the great toe
   Spelled correctly? Yes
4. **tendon:** strong fibrous band of tissue that attaches the muscle to the bone
   Spelled correctly? Yes
5. **bunionectomy:** removal of the bony overgrowth and the bursa at the base of the great toe
   Spelled correctly? Yes
6. **rotation:** the movement that involves the turning of a bone on its own axis
   Spelled correctly? Yes
7. **contracture:** an abnormal, usually permanent, bending of a joint into a fixed position
   Spelled correctly? Yes
8. **insertion:** point of attachment of a muscle to a bone that it moves
   Spelled correctly? Yes
9. **fascia:** thin sheets of fibrous connective tissue that penetrate as well as cover the entire muscle holding the fibers together
   Spelled correctly? Yes
10. **vastus lateralis:** a muscle located on the outer side of the femur, often used for intramuscular injections
    Spelled correctly? Yes
    (Note to learner: Were you surprised to find that all of the words in this exercise were spelled correctly?)

J. Matching Diagnostics

1. c
2. d
3. b
4. e
5. a

CHAPTER 8

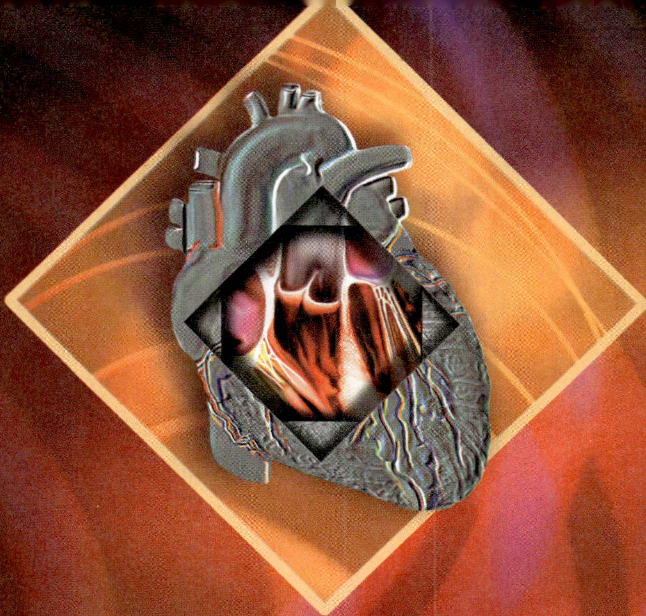

The Nervous System

CHAPTER CONTENT

KEY COMPETENCIES

Upon completing this chapter and the review exercises at the end of the chapter, the learner should be able to:

1. Correctly identify at least 10 anatomical terms relating to the nervous system.
2. Identify the structures common to the central nervous system.
3. Correctly spell and pronounce each new term introduced in this chapter using the CD-ROM Activity and Audio CD, if available.
4. Demonstrate the ability to create at least 10 medical words pertaining to the nervous system.
5. Identify the structures of the brain by labeling them on the diagrams provided in the chapter review exercises.
6. Identify at least 10 abbreviations common to the nervous system.
7. Identify at least 10 diagnostic procedures common to the nervous system.
8. Identify at least 30 pathological conditions common to the nervous system.
9. State the difference between afferent and efferent nerves.
10. List the structures of the central nervous system and the peripheral nervous system.
11. Correctly form the plurals of words ending in *-ion*, *-ite*, and *-us* by completing the appropriate chapter review exercise.

OVERVIEW

Think of the computer with all of its many wires throughout the system that enable it to perform its many functions. This massive system of wires and networks sends and receives messages. There are numerous wires that are twisted together into a braid, called the power cable, which connects the computer to the electricity that gives it the necessary power to operate.

Now think of the nervous system with all of its many nerves throughout the body that enable the body to carry on its many functions. This system of nerves sends and receives messages. There are many nerve fibers that are twisted together into bundles, called nerves, that connect the brain and the spinal cord with various parts of the body, relaying messages back and forth. Complicated? Yes!

The nervous system is perhaps the most intricate of all body systems. Consisting of the brain, spinal cord, and nerves, the nervous system functions to regulate and coordinate all body activities and to detect changes in the internal and external environment, evaluate the information, and respond to the stimuli by bringing about bodily responses. It is the center of all mental activity including thought, learning, and memory.

The study of the nervous system and its disorders is known as **neurology**. The physician who specializes in treating the diseases and disorders of the nervous system is known as a **neurologist**. Any surgery involving the brain, spinal cord, or peripheral nerves is known as **neurosurgery**, and the physician who specializes in surgery of the brain, spinal cord, or peripheral nerves is known as a **neurosurgeon**.

Anatomy and Physiology

The nervous system is divided into two subdivisions: the **central nervous system (CNS)**, consisting of the brain and spinal cord, and the **peripheral nervous system (PNS)**, consisting of 12 pairs of cranial nerves and 31 pairs of spinal nerves. The central nervous system is responsible for processing and storing sensory and motor information, and for controlling consciousness. The peripheral nervous system is responsible for transmitting sensory and motor impulses back and forth between the central nervous system and the rest of the body.

The Peripheral Nervous System

The peripheral nervous system is made up of nerves and ganglia. A **nerve** is a cordlike bundle of nerve fibers that transmits impulses to and from the brain and spinal cord to other parts of the body; a nerve is macroscopic (i.e., able to be seen without the aid of a microscope). A **ganglion** is a knotlike mass of nerve cell bodies located outside the central nervous system.

The peripheral nervous system contains **afferent (sensory) nerves** that carry impulses from the body to the central nervous system, and **efferent (motor) nerves** that carry impulses from the central nervous system to the muscles and glands, causing the target organs to do something in response to the commands received.

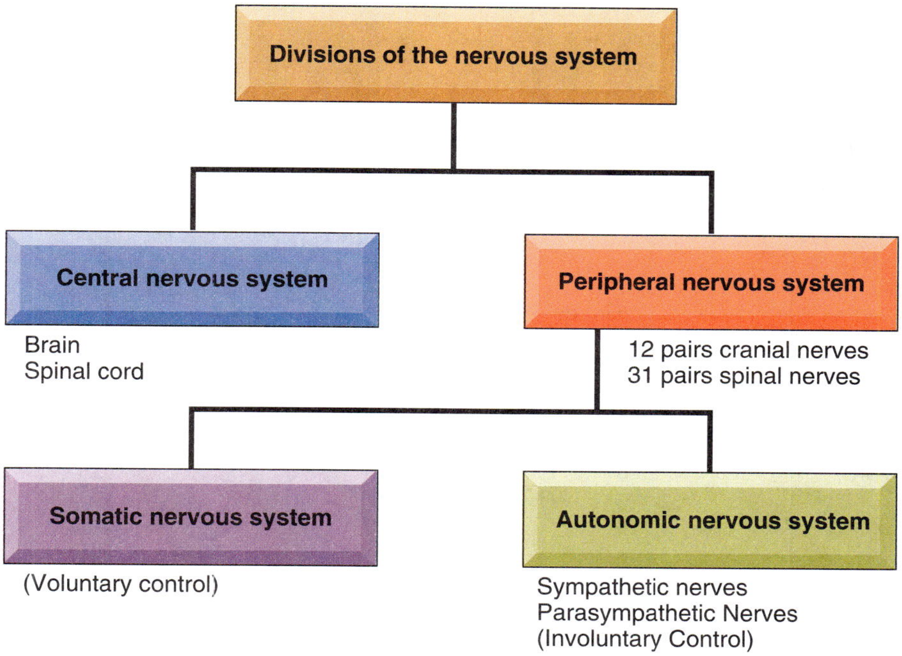

Figure 8-1 Divisions of the nervous system

The peripheral nervous system is further broken down into the somatic nervous system and the autonomic nervous system. The **somatic nervous system** (**SNS**) provides voluntary control over skeletal muscle contractions, and the **autonomic nervous system** (**ANS**) provides involuntary control over smooth muscle, cardiac muscle, and glandular activity and secretions in response to the commands of the central nervous system. The autonomic nervous system contains two types of nerves: sympathetic and parasympathetic. **Sympathetic nerves** regulate involuntary, essential body functions such as increasing the heart rate, constricting blood vessels, and raising the blood pressure; responding to the "fight-or-flight response," the body prepares to deal with immediate threats to the internal environment. The **parasympathetic nerves** regulate involuntary, essential body functions such as slowing the heart rate, increasing peristalsis of the intestines, increasing glandular secretions, and relaxing sphincters, thus serving as a complement to the sympathetic nervous system and returning the body to a more restful state. **Figure 8-1** illustrates the divisions of the nervous system.

Cells of the Nervous System

There are two main types of cells found in the nervous system tissue: neurons and neuroglia. The **neuron**, known as the functional unit, is the actual nerve cell; it transmits the impulses of the nervous system. A neuron consists of three basic parts: a cell body, one axon, and one or more dendrites. As you read about the structure of the neuron, refer to **Figure 8-2.**

The (1) **cell body** is the structure that contains the nucleus and cytoplasm, as do other cells. The (2) **axon** is a single, slender projection that extends from the cell body. Axons conduct impulses away from the cell body. Some axons are covered with a **myelin sheath,** which protects the axon and speeds the transmission of the impulses. Axons that are covered with this myelin sheath appear white, making up the **white matter** of the nervous system. Axons that are not covered with the myelin sheath appear gray, making up the **gray matter** of the nervous system. The (3) **dendrites** branch extensively from the cell body,

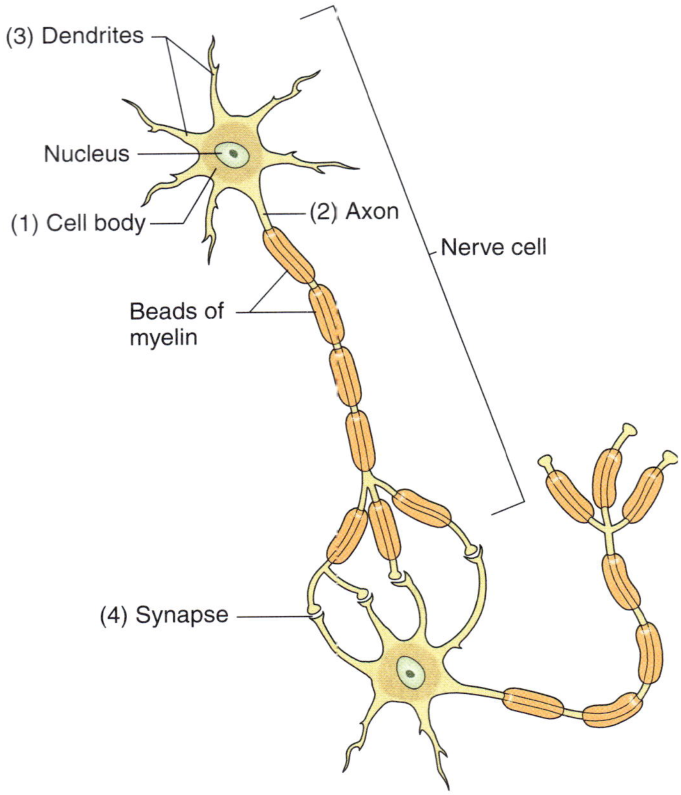

Figure 8-2 The neuron

somewhat like tiny trees. The dendrites conduct impulses toward the cell body. Neurons are not continuous with one another throughout the body; instead, a small space exists between the axon of one neuron and the dendrite of another neuron. This space between the two nerves over which the impulse must cross is known as a **(4) synapse**. Chemical substances are released into the synapse to activate or inhibit the transmission of nerve impulses across the synapses; these substances are known as **neurotransmitters**.

Nerves are classified according to the direction in which they transmit impulses. Afferent nerves transmit impulses toward the brain and spinal cord; they are also known as sensory nerves. Efferent nerves transmit impulses away from the brain and spinal cord; they are also known as motor nerves. The central nervous system also contains connecting neurons that conduct impulses from afferent nerves to (or toward) motor nerves; these are known as **interneurons**.

The **neuroglia**, a special type of connective tissue for the nervous system, provide a support system for the neurons. Neuroglia do not conduct impulses; they protect the nervous system through **phagocytosis** by engulfing and digesting any unwanted substances. There are three types of neuroglia cells: astrocytes, microglia, and oligodendrocytes (see **Figure 8-3**). **(1) Astrocytes** are star-shaped cells with numerous radiating processes for attachment. They are the largest and most numerous of the neuroglial cells and are found only in the central nervous system. The astrocytes wrap themselves around the brain's blood capillaries, forming a tight sheath. This sheath, plus the wall of the capillary, forms the **blood-brain barrier** that prevents the passage of harmful substances from the bloodstream into the brain tissue or cerebrospinal fluid.

(2) Microglia are small interstitial cells that have slender branched processes stemming from their bodies.

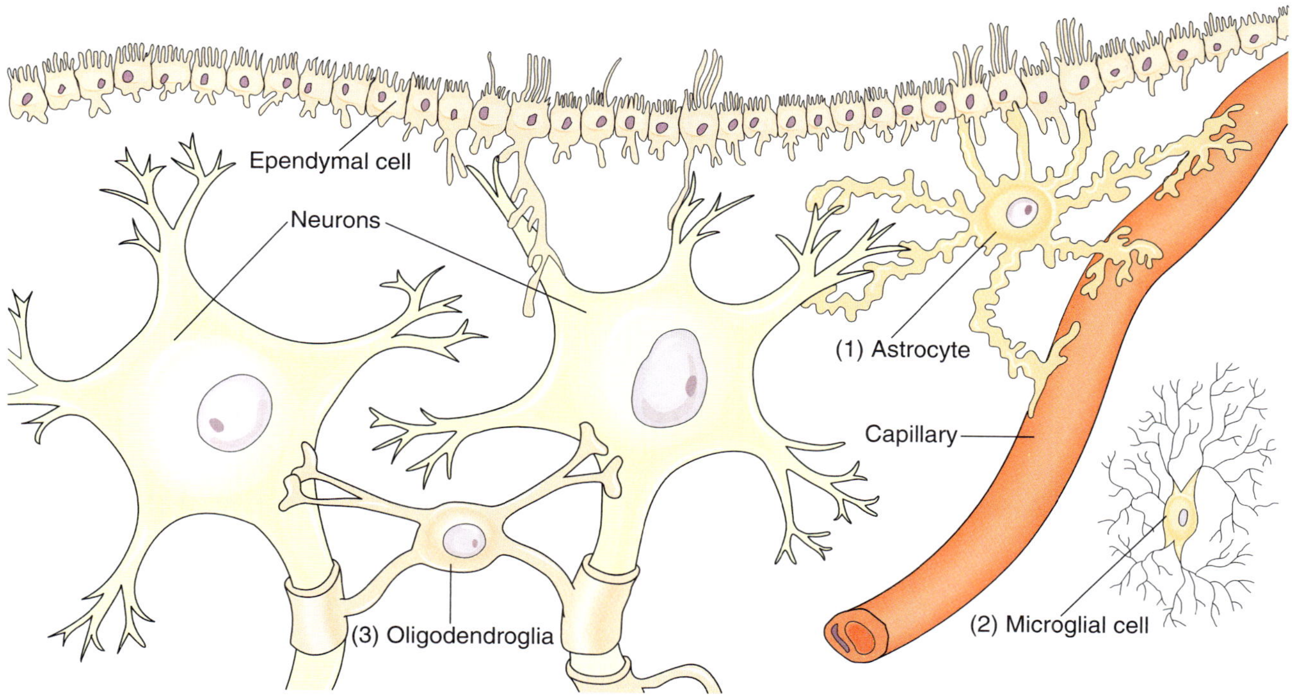

Figure 8-3 Neuroglia cells

Microglial cells are phagocytic in nature and engulf cellular debris, waste products, and pathogens within the nerve tissue. During times of injury or infection of the nerve tissue, the number of microglial cells dramatically increase, and these cells migrate to the damaged or infected area.

(3) **Oligodendrocytes** are found in the interstitial nervous tissue. They are smaller than astrocytes and have fewer processes. The processes of the oligodendrocytes fan out from the cell body and coil around the axons of many neurons to form the protective myelin sheath that covers the axons of many nerves in the body. The myelin sheath acts as an electrical insulator and helps to speed the conduction of nerve impulses.

The Central Nervous System

The central nervous system, consisting of the brain and the spinal cord, is highly complex in structure and function. We will first discuss the protective coverings of the brain and spinal cord and then will concentrate on the structures of the brain.

The spinal cord and the brain are surrounded by bone for protection: The brain is enclosed in the cranium (skull), and the spinal cord is protected by the vertebrae of the spinal column. In addition to the protection offered by the cranium and the vertebrae, the brain and spinal cord are surrounded by connective tissue membranes, called meninges, and by cerebrospinal fluid.

The **meninges** are three layers of protective membranes that surround the brain and spinal cord. See **Figure 8-4.** The outermost layer of the meninges is called the (1) **dura mater**, which is a tough, white connective tissue. Located beneath the dura mater is a cavity called the **subdural space,** which is filled with serous fluid. There is also a space immediately outside of the dura mater called the **epidural space.** This space contains a supporting cushion of fat and other connective tissues. The middle layer of the

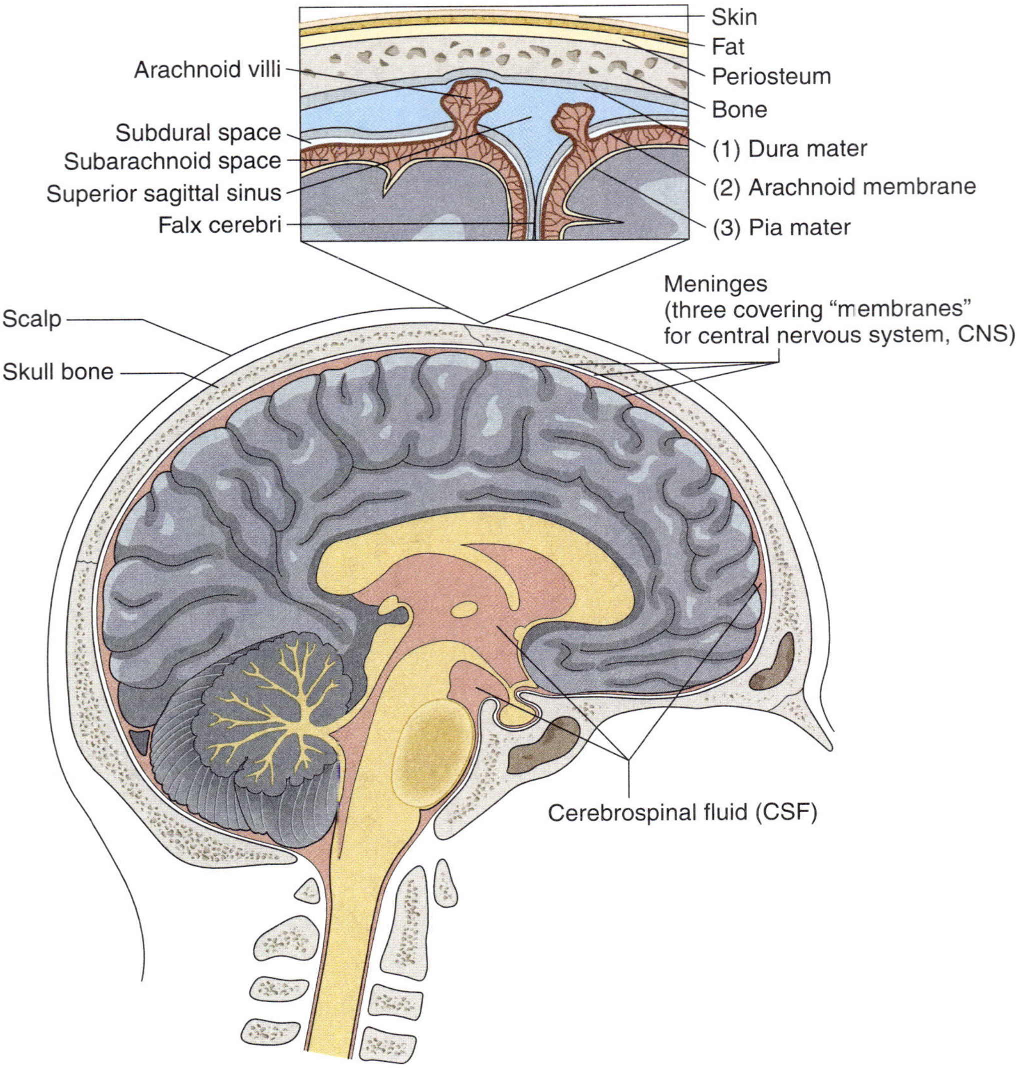

Figure 8-4 The meninges

meninges is called the **(2)** **arachnoid membrane**, which resembles a spider web in appearance. This thin layer has numerous threadlike strands that attach to the innermost layer of the meninges. The space immediately beneath the arachnoid membrane is the **subarachnoid space,** which contains **cerebrospinal fluid** **(CSF)**. This fluid provides additional protection for the brain and spinal cord by serving as a shock absorber. The innermost layer of the meninges is the **(3)** **pia mater**, which is tightly bound to the surface of the brain and spinal cord.

The cushion of cerebrospinal fluid flows in and around the organs of the central nervous system: from the blood, through the ventricles of the brain, the central canal of the spinal cord, the subarachnoid spaces around the brain and the spinal cord, and back into the blood. The cerebrospinal fluid contains proteins, glucose, urea, salts, and some white blood cells; it provides some nutritive substances to the central nervous system. A constant volume of CSF is maintained within the central nervous system because the fluid is absorbed as rapidly as it is formed. Any interference with the absorption of the CSF will result in an abnormal collection of fluid within the brain, which is termed hydrocephaly (or hydrocephalus). This condition will be discussed later in the pathological conditions section.

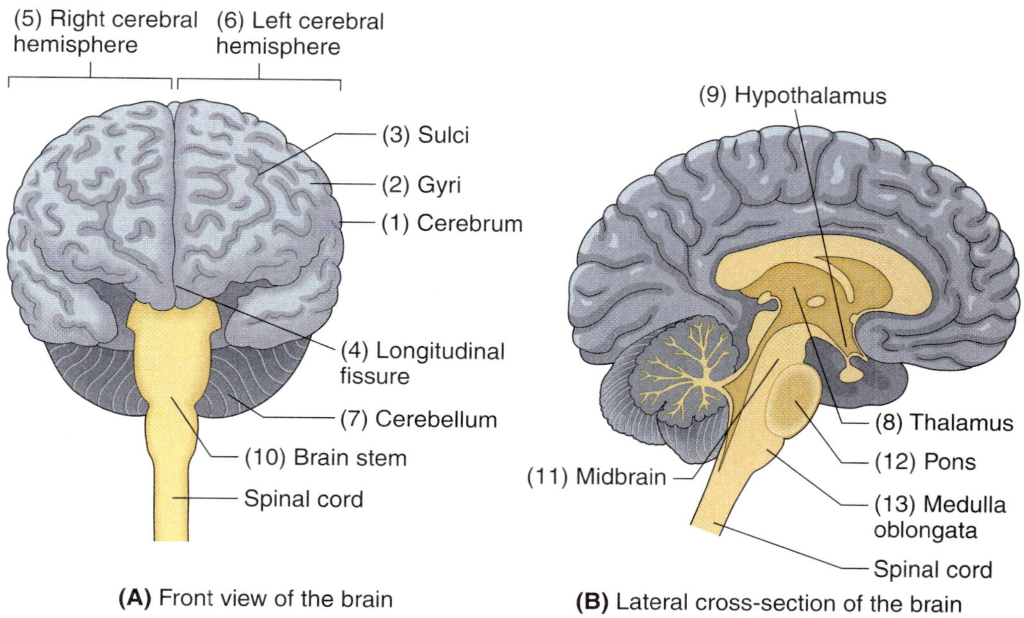

(A) Front view of the brain

(B) Lateral cross-section of the brain

Figure 8-5 Structures of the brain

Structures of the Brain

The brain is one of the largest organs in adults. It weighs approximately 3 pounds in most adults. The brain grows rapidly during the first 9 years or so of life, reaching full size by approximately 18 years of life. This very complex structure, which coordinates almost every physical and mental activity of the body, is divided into four major divisions for discussion: (1) the cerebrum, (2) the cerebellum, (3) the diencephalon, and (4) the brain stem. **Figures 8-5A** and **B** serve as a visual reference to our discussion of the brain.

The **(1)** **cerebrum** is the largest part and the uppermost portion of the brain. It controls consciousness, memory, sensations, emotions, and voluntary movements. The surface of the cerebrum is known as the **cerebral cortex**. The striking feature of the cerebral cortex is the presence of convolutions, or elevations, that are known as **(2) gyri** (singular: **gyrus**), which are separated by grooves known as **(3) sulci** (singular: **sulcus**). The gyri give the appearance of encased sausage folded upon itself many times. The cerebrum is divided by a deep **(4)** **longitudinal fissure** into the two hemispheres: the **(5) right cerebral hemisphere** and the **(6) left cerebral hemisphere.**

The **(7)** **cerebellum** is attached to the brain stem. It has an essential role in maintaining muscle tone and coordinating normal movement and balance.

The **diencephalon** is located between the cerebrum and the midbrain. It consists of several structures, with the main ones being the thalamus, hypothalamus, and the pineal gland. The **(8)** **thalamus** receives all sensory stimuli (except those of smell) and relays them to the cerebral cortex. The **(9)** **hypothalamus**, a small region located just below the thalamus, is responsible for activating, controlling, and integrating the peripheral autonomic nervous system, endocrine system processes, and many sensory functions such as body temperature, sleep, and appetite. The **pineal body** is a small, cone-shaped structure that extends from the posterior portion of the diencephalon. The pineal body, also known as the pineal gland, is thought to be involved in regulating the body's biological clock; it also produces **melatonin,** which is an important hormone believed to regulate the onset of puberty and the menstrual cycle.

The (10) **brain stem** is the region between the diencephalon and the spinal cord. It consists of the midbrain, pons, and medulla oblongata. The (11) **midbrain** is the upper part of the brain stem. The (12) **pons** is located between the midbrain and the medulla. The (13) **medulla oblongata** is the lowest part of the brain stem and is continuous with the spinal cord. The brain stem serves as a pathway for conduction of impulses between the brain and spinal cord. It controls such vital functions as respiration, blood pressure, and heart rate.

The Spinal Cord

The spinal cord is the pathway for impulses traveling to and from the brain. It carries 31 pairs of spinal nerves that affect the limbs and lower part of the body. The spinal cord is protected by cerebrospinal fluid, the three layers of the meninges, and the bony encasement of the cervical, thoracic, and lumbar vertebrae.

Vocabulary

The following vocabulary words are frequently used when discussing the nervous system.

WORD	DEFINITION
absence seizure (**AB**-senz **SEE**-zyoor)	A small seizure in which there is a sudden, temporary loss of consciousness, lasting only a few seconds.
acetylcholine (ah-seh-till-**KOH**-leen)	A chemical substance in the body tissues that facilitates the transmission of nerve impulses from one nerve to another; it has a stimulant, or excitatory, effect on some parts of the body such as the skeletal muscles, and a depressant, or inhibitory, effect on other parts of the body such as the heart muscle; also known as a neurotransmitter.
afferent nerves (**AFF**-er-ent nerves)	Transmitters of nerve impulses toward the central nervous system; also known as sensory nerves.
agnosia (ag-**NOH**-zee-ah) a- = without, not gnos/o = to know -ia = condition	Loss of mental ability to understand sensory stimuli, such as sight, sound, or touch, even though the sensory organs themselves are functioning properly (e.g., the inability to recognize or interpret the images the eye is seeing is known as optic agnosia).
agraphia (ah-**GRAFF**-ee-ah) a- = without, not graph/o = record -ia = condition	The inability to convert one's thoughts into writing.
alexia (ah-**LEK**-see-ah) a- = without, not -lexia = reading	The inability to understand written words.

analgesia (an-al-**JEE**-zee-ah) an- = without, not -algesia = sensitivity to pain	Without sensitivity to pain.
anesthesia (an-ess-**THEE**-zee-ah) an- = without, not esthesi/o = feeling, sensation -ia = condition	Without feeling or sensation.
aneurysm (**AN**-yoo-rizm)	A localized dilatation in the wall of an artery that expands with each pulsation of the artery; usually caused by hypertension or atherosclerosis.
aphasia (ah-**FAY**-zee-ah) a- = without, not phas/o = speech -ia = condition	Inability to communicate through speech, writing, or signs because of an injury to or disease in certain areas of the brain.
apraxia (ah-**PRAK**-see-ah) a- = without, not -praxia = perform	Inability to perform coordinated movements or use objects properly; not associated with sensory or motor impairment or paralysis.
arachnoid membrane (ah-**RAK**-noyd **MEM**-brayn)	The weblike, middle layer of the three membranous layers surrounding the brain and spinal cord.
astrocyte (**ASS**-troh-sight) astr/o = star-shaped cyt/o = cell -e = noun ending	A star-shaped neuroglial cell found in the central nervous system.
astrocytoma (**ass**-troh-sigh-**TOH**-mah) astr/o = star-shaped cyt/o = cell -oma = tumor	A tumor of the brain or spinal cord composed of astrocytes.
ataxia (ah-**TAK**-see-ah) a- = without, not tax/o = order -ia = condition	Without muscular coordination.
aura (**AW**-rah)	The sensation an individual experiences prior to the onset of a migraine headache or an epileptic seizure; it may be a sensation of light or warmth and may precede the attack by hours or only a few seconds.
autonomic nervous system (aw-toh-**NOM**-ik **NER**-vus **SIS**-tem)	The part of the nervous system that regulates the involuntary vital functions of the body, such as the activities involving the heart muscle, smooth muscles, and the glands. The autonomic nervous system has two divisions: the sympathetic nervous system and the parasympathetic nervous system, which are defined separately.

axon (**AK**-son)	The part of the nerve cell that transports nerve impulses away from the nerve cell body.
blood-brain barrier (**BLUD-BRAIN BAY**-ree-er)	A protective characteristic of the capillary walls of the brain that prevents the passage of harmful substances from the bloodstream into the brain tissue or cerebrospinal fluid.
bradykinesia (**brad**-ee-kih-**NEE**-see-ah) brady- = slow kinesi/o = movement -ia = condition	Abnormally slow movement.
brain stem	The stemlike portion of the brain that connects the cerebral hemisphere with the spinal cord. The brain stem contains the midbrain, the pons, and the medulla oblongata.
Brudzinski's sign	A positive sign of meningitis, in which there is an involuntary flexion of the arm, hip, and knee when the patient's neck is passively flexed.
burr hole	A hole drilled into the skull using a form of drill.
cauda equina (**KAW**-dah ee-**KWY**-nah)	The lower end of the spinal cord and the roots of the spinal nerves that occupy the spinal canal below the level of the first lumbar vertebra; so named because it resembles a horse's tail.
causalgia (kaw-**SAL**-jee-ah) caus/o = burn -algia = pain	A sensation of an acute burning pain along the path of a peripheral nerve, sometimes accompanied by erythema of the skin; due to injury to peripheral nerve fibers.
cell body	The part of the cell that contains the nucleus and the cytoplasm.
central nervous system	One of the two main divisions of the nervous system, consisting of the brain and the spinal cord.
cephalalgia (**seff**-ah-**LAL**-jee-ah) cephal/o = head -algia = pain	Pain in the head; headache.
cerebellum (ser-eh-**BELL**-um)	The part of the brain responsible for coordinating voluntary muscular movement; located behind the brain stem.
cerebral concussion (ser-**REE**-bral con-**KUSH**-shun) cerebr/o = brain; cerebrum -al = pertaining to	A brief interruption of brain function, usually with a loss of consciousness lasting for a few seconds. This transient loss of consciousness is usually caused by blunt trauma (a blow) to the head.
cerebral contusion (seh-**REE**-bral con-**TOO**-zhun) cerebr/o = brain; cerebrum -al = pertaining to	Small scattered venous hemorrhages in the brain; better described as a "bruise" of the brain tissue occurring when the brain strikes the inner skull.

cerebral cortex (seh-**REE**-bral **COR**-teks) cerebr/o = brain; cerebrum -al = pertaining to	The thin outer layer of nerve tissue, known as gray matter, that covers the surface of the cerebrum.
cerebrospinal fluid (ser-eh-broh-**SPY**-nal **FLOO**-id) cerebr/o = brain; cerebrum spin/o = spine -al = pertaining to	The fluid flowing through the brain and around the spinal cord that protects them from physical blow or impact.
cerebrum (seh-**REE**-brum) cerebr/o = brain; cerebrum -um = noun ending	The largest and uppermost part of the brain; it controls consciousness, memory, sensations, emotions, and voluntary movements.
Cheyne-Stokes respirations (**CHAIN-STOHKS** res-pir-**AY**-shun)	An abnormal pattern of breathing characterized by periods of apnea followed by deep, rapid breathing.
coma (**COH**-mah)	A deep sleep in which the individual cannot be aroused and does not respond to external stimuli.
comatose (**COH**-mah-tohs)	Pertains to being in a coma.
contracture (kon-**TRAK**-chur)	A permanent shortening of a muscle causing a joint to remain in an abnormally flexed position, with resultant physical deformity.
convolution (kon-voh-**LOO**-shun)	One of the many elevated folds of the surface of the cerebrum; also called a gyrus.
craniotomy (kray-nee-**OTT**-oh-mee) crani/o = skull -tomy = incision into	A surgical incision into the cranium or skull.
deficit (**DEFF**-ih-sit)	Any deficiency or variation of the normal, as in a weakness deficit resulting from a cerebrovascular accident.
dementia (dee-**MEN**-shee-ah)	A progressive, irreversible mental disorder in which the person has deteriorating memory, judgment, and ability to think.
demyelination (dee-**MY**-eh-lye-**NAY**-shun)	Destruction or removal of the myelin sheath that covers a nerve or nerve fiber.
dendrite (**DEN**-dright)	A projection that extends from the nerve cell body; it receives impulses and conducts them on to the cell body.
diencephalon (**dye**-en-**SEFF**-ah-lon)	The part of the brain that is located between the cerebrum and the midbrain. Its main structures consist of the thalamus, hypothalamus, and pineal gland.
diplopia (dip-**LOH**-pee-ah) dipl/o = double -opia = vision	Double vision; also called ambiopia.

dura mater (**DOO**-rah **MATE**-er)	The outermost of the three membranes (meninges) surrounding the brain and spinal cord.
dyslexia (dis-**LEK**-see-ah) dys- = bad, difficult, painful, disordered -lexia = reading	A condition characterized by an impairment of the ability to read; letters and words are often reversed when reading.
dysphasia (dis-**FAY**-zee-ah) dys- = bad, difficult, painful, disordered phas/o = speech -ia = condition	Difficult speech.
efferent nerves (**EE**-fair-ent nerves)	Transmitters of nerve impulses away from the central nervous system; also known as motor nerves.
embolism (**EM**-boh-lizm)	An abnormal condition in which a blood clot (embolus) becomes lodged in a blood vessel, obstructing the flow of blood within the vessel.
epidural space (**ep**-ih-**DOO**-ral space) epi- = upon	The space immediately outside of the dura mater that contains a supporting cushion of fat and other connective tissues.
epilepsy (**EP**-ih-lep-see)	A neurological condition characterized by recurrent episodes of sudden, brief attacks of seizures; the seizure may vary from mild and unnoticeable to full-scale convulsive seizures.
fissure (**FISH**-er)	A deep groove on the surface of an organ.
fontanelle or **fontanel** (fon-tah-**NELL**)	A space covered by tough membrane between the bones of an infant's cranium, called a "soft spot."
gait (**GAYT**)	The style of walking.
ganglion (**GANG**-lee-on)	A knotlike mass of nerve tissue found outside the brain or spinal cord (plural: ganglia).
gray matter	The part of the nervous system consisting of axons that are not covered with myelin sheath, giving a gray appearance.
gyrus (**JYE**-rus)	See *convolution* (plural: gyri).
hemiparesis (hem-ee-par-**EE**-sis) hemi- = half -paresis = partial paralysis	Slight or partial paralysis of one half of the body (i.e., left or right side).
hemiplegia (hem-ee-**PLEE**-jee-ah) hemi- = half -plegia = paralysis	Paralysis of one half of the body (i.e., left or right side).

herpes zoster (**HER**-peez **ZOSS**-ter)	An acute infection caused by the same virus that causes chickenpox, characterized by painful vesicular lesions along the path of a spinal nerve; also called shingles.
hyperesthesia (**high**-per-ess-**THEE**-zee-ah) hyper- = excessive esthesi/o = feeling, sensation -ia = condition	Excessive sensitivity to sensory stimuli, such as pain or touch.
hyperkinesis (**high**-per-kigh-**NEE**-sis) hyper- = excessive kinesi/o = movement -is = noun ending	Excessive muscular movement and physical activity; hyperactivity.
hypothalamus (**high**-poh-**THAL**-ah-mus)	A part of the brain located below the thalamus that controls many functions such as body temperature, sleep, and appetite.
interneurons (**in**-ter-**NOO**-rons)	Connecting neurons that conduct impulses from afferent nerves to or toward motor nerves.
Kernig's sign (**KER**-nigz sign)	A diagnostic sign for meningitis marked by the person's inability to extend the leg completely when the thigh is flexed upon the abdomen and the person is sitting or lying down.
kinesiology (kih-**nee**-see-**ALL**-oh-jee) kinesi/o = movement -logy = the study of	The study of muscle movement.
lethargy (**LETH**-ar-jee)	A state of being sluggish. See *stupor.*
longitudinal fissure (**lon**-jih-**TOO**-dih-nal **FISH**-er)	A deep groove in the middle of the cerebrum that divides the cerebrum into the right and left hemispheres.
medulla oblongata (meh-**DULL**-ah **ob**-long-**GAH**-tah)	One of the three parts of the brain stem. The medulla oblongata is the most essential part of the brain in that it contains the cardiac, vasomotor, and respiratory centers of the brain.
meninges (men-**IN**-jeez) mening/o = meninges -es = noun ending	The three layers of protective membranes that surround the brain and spinal cord.
microglia (my-**KROG**-lee-ah)	Small, neuroglial cells found in the interstitial tissue of the nervous system that engulf cellular debris, waste products, and pathogens within the nerve tissue.
midbrain	The uppermost part of the brain stem.
motor nerves (**MOH**-tor nerves)	See *efferent nerves.*
myelin sheath (**MY**-eh-lin **SHEETH**)	A protective sheath that covers the axons of many nerves in the body; it acts as an electrical insulator and helps to speed the conduction of nerve impulses.

narcolepsy (**NAR**-coh-**lep**-see) narc/o = sleep -lepsy = seizure, attack	Uncontrolled, sudden attacks of sleep.
nerve	A cordlike bundle of nerve fibers that transmit impulses to and from the brain and spinal cord to other parts of the body; a nerve is macroscopic (i.e., able to be seen without the aid of a microscope).
nerve block	The injection of a local anesthetic along the course of a nerve or nerves to eliminate sensation to the area supplied by the nerve(s); also called conduction anesthesia.
neuralgia (noo-**RAL**-jee-ah) neur/o = nerve -algia = pain	Severe, sharp, spasmlike pain that extends along the course of one or more nerves.
neuritis (noo-**RYE**-tis) neur/o = nerve -itis = inflammation	Inflammation of a nerve.
neuroglia (noo-**ROG**-lee-ah) neur/o = nerve gli/o = gluey substance -a = noun ending	The supporting tissue of the nervous system.
neurologist (noo-**RAL**-oh-jist) neur/o = nerves -logist = one who specializes in the study of	A physician who specializes in treating the diseases and disorders of the nervous system.
neurology (noo-**RAL**-oh-jee) neur/o = nerves -logy = the study of	The study of the nervous system and its disorders.
neuron (**NOO**-ron) neur/o = nerve -on = noun ending	A nerve cell.
neurosurgeon (noo-roh-**SIR**-jun)	A physician who specializes in surgery of the nervous system.
neurosurgery (noo-roh-**SIR**-jer-ee)	Any surgery involving the nervous system (i.e., of the brain, spinal cord, or peripheral nerves).
neurotransmitter (noo-roh-**TRANS**-mit-er)	A chemical substance within the body that activates or inhibits the transmission of nerve impulses between synapses.

nuchal rigidity (**NOO**-kal rih-**JID**-ih-tee)	Rigidity of the neck; the neck is resistant to flexion. This condition is seen in patients with meningitis.
occlusion (oh-**KLOO**-zhun)	Blockage.
oligodendrocyte (all-ih-goh-**DEN**-droh-sight) **olig/o** = few, little, scanty **dendr/o** = tree, branches **cyt/o** = cell **-e** = noun ending	A type of neuroglial cell found in the interstitial tissue of the nervous system; its dendrite projections coil around the axons of many neurons to form the myelin sheath.
palliative (**PAL**-ee-ah-tiv)	Soothing.
paraplegia (pair-ah-**PLEE**-jee-ah) **para-** = near, beside, beyond, two like parts **-plegia** = paralysis	Paralysis of the lower extremities and trunk, usually due to spinal cord injuries.
parasympathetic nerves (**pair**-ah-sim-pah-**THET**-ik)	Nerves of the autonomic nervous system that regulate involuntary, essential body functions such as slowing the heart rate, increasing peristalsis of the intestines, increasing glandular secretions, and relaxing sphincters.
parasympathomimetic (**pair**-ah-**sim**-pah-thoh-mim-**ET**-ik)	Copying or producing the same effects as those of the parasympathetic nerves; "to mimic" the parasympathetic nerves.
paresthesia (pair-ess-**THEE**-zee-ah)	A sensation of numbness or tingling.
peripheral nervous system (per-**IF**-er-al nervous system)	The part of the nervous system outside the central nervous system, consisting of 12 pairs of cranial nerves and 31 pairs of spinal nerves.
phagocytosis (fag-oh-sigh-**TOH**-sis) **phag/o** = to eat **cyt/o** = cell **-osis** = process; condition	The process by which certain cells engulf and destroy microorganisms and cellular debris.
pia mater (**PEE**-ah **MATE**-er)	The innermost of the three membranes (meninges) surrounding the brain and spinal cord.
pineal body (**PIN**-ee-al body)	A small cone-shape structure located in the diencephalon of the brain; thought to be involved in regulating the body's biological clock; produces melatonin; also called the pineal gland.
pineal gland (**PIN**-ee-al gland)	See *pineal body.*
plexus (**PLEKS**-us)	A network of interwoven nerves.

pons (**PONZ**)	The part of the brain that is located between the medulla oblongata and the midbrain; it acts as a bridge to connect the medulla oblongata and the cerebellum to the upper portions of the brain.
quadriplegia (kwod-rih-**PLEE**-jee-ah) **quadri-** = four **-pleg/o** = paralysis **-ia** = condition	Paralysis of all four extremities and the trunk of the body; caused by injury to the spinal cord at the level of the cervical vertebrae.
radiculotomy (rah-dick-you-**LOT**-oh-mee) **radicul/o** = root **-tomy** = process of cutting	The surgical resection of a spinal nerve root; a procedure performed to relieve pain. Also called a rhizotomy.
receptor (ree-**SEP**-tor)	A sensory nerve ending (i.e., a nerve ending that receives impulses and responds to various kinds of stimulation).
rhizotomy (rye-**ZOT**-oh-mee) **rhiz/o** = root **-tomy** = process of cutting	The surgical resection of a spinal nerve root; a procedure performed to relieve pain. Also called a radiculotomy.
sciatica (sigh-**AT**-ih-kah)	Inflammation of the sciatic nerve; characterized by pain along the course of the nerve, radiating through the thigh and down the back of the leg.
sensory (**SEN**-soh-ree)	Pertaining to sensation.
sensory nerves (**SEN**-soh-ree nerves)	See *afferent nerves.*
shingles	See *herpes zoster.*
shunt	A tube or passage that diverts or redirects body fluid from one cavity or vessel to another; may be a congenital defect or may be artificially constructed for the purpose of redirecting fluid, as a shunt used in hydrocephalus.
somatic nervous system (soh-**MAT**-ik nervous system)	The part of the peripheral nervous system that provides voluntary control over skeletal muscle contractions.
stimulus (**STIM**-yoo-lus)	Any agent or factor capable of initiating a nerve impulse.
stupor (**STOO**-per)	A state of lethargy; the person is unresponsive and seems unaware of his or her surroundings.
subarachnoid space (sub-ah-**RAK**-noyd space)	The space located just under the arachnoid membrane that contains cerebrospinal fluid.
subdural space (sub-**DOO**-ral space)	The space located just beneath the dura mater that contains serous fluid.
sulcus (**SULL**-kuss)	A depression or shallow groove on the surface of an organ; as a sulcus that separates any of the convolutions of the cerebral hemispheres (plural: sulci).

sympathetic nerves (sim-pah-**THET**-ik)	Nerves of the autonomic nervous system that regulate involuntary, essential body functions such as increasing the heart rate, constricting blood vessels, and raising the blood pressure.
sympathomimetic (sim-pah-thoh-mim-**ET**-ik)	Copying or producing the same effects as those of the sympathetic nerves; "to mimic" the sympathetic nerves.
synapse (**SIN**-aps)	The space between the end of one nerve and the beginning of another, through which nerve impulses are transmitted.
syncope (**SIN**-koh-pee)	Fainting.
thalamus (**THAL**-ah-mus)	The part of the brain located between the cerebral hemispheres and the midbrain; the thalamus receives all sensory stimuli, except those of smell, and relays them on to the cerebral cortex.
thrombosis (throm-**BOH**-sis) **thromb/o** = clot **-osis** = condition	An abnormal condition in which a clot develops in a blood vessel.
tonic-clonic seizure (**TON**-ik-**CLON**-ic **SEE**-zhur)	A seizure characterized by the presence of muscle contraction or tension followed by relaxation, creating a "jerking" movement of the body.
ventricle, brain (**VEN**-trik-l)	A small hollow within the brain that is filled with cerebrospinal fluid.
whiplash	An injury to the cervical vertebrae and their supporting structures due to a sudden back-and-forth, jerking movement of the head and neck. Whiplash may occur as a result of an automobile being struck suddenly from the rear.
white matter	The part of the nervous system consisting of axons that are covered with myelin sheath, giving a white appearance.

Word Elements

The following word elements pertain to the nervous system. As you review the list, pronounce each word element aloud twice and check the box after you "say it." Write the definition for the example word given for each word element. You may use your medical dictionary.

WORD ELEMENT	PRONUNCIATION	"SAY IT"	MEANING
a- **a**phasia	**AH** ah-**FAY**-zee-ah	☐	without, not
an- **an**encephaly	**AN** an-en-**SEFF**-ah-lee	☐	without, not

Word Part	Pronunciation		Meaning
-algesia an**algesia**	al-**JEE**-zee-ah an-al-**JEE**-zee-ah	☐	sensitivity to pain
alges/o an**alges**ic	**AL**-jee-soh an-al-**JEE**-sik	☐	sensitivity to pain
-algia cephal**algia**	**AL**-jee-ah seff-ah-**LAL**-jee-ah	☐	pain
brady- **brady**esthesia	**BRAD**-ee brad-ee-ess-**THEE**-zee-ah	☐	slow
cerebell/o **cerebell**ospinal	ser-eh-**BELL**-oh ser-eh-bell-oh-**SPY**-nal	☐	cerebellum
cerebr/o **cerebr**itis	ser-**EE**-broh ser-eh-**BRYE**-tis	☐	cerebrum
crani/o **crani**otomy	**KRAY**-nee-oh kray-nee-**OTT**-oh-mee	☐	skull, cranium
encephal/o **encephal**ography	en-**SEFF**-ah-loh en-**SEFF**-ah-**LOG**-rah-fee	☐	brain
-esthesia an**esthesia**	ess-**THEE**-zee-ah an-ess-**THEE**-zee-ah	☐	sensation or feeling
esthesi/o an**esthesi**ologist	ess-**THEE**-zee-oh an-ess-thee-zee-**ALL**-oh-jist	☐	feeling, sensation
gli/o **gli**oma	**GLEE**-oh glee-**OM**-ah	☐	neuroglia or gluey substance
-kinesia brady**kinesia**	kih-**NEE**-see-ah brad-ee-kih-**NEE**-see-ah	☐	movement
kinesi/o **kinesi**ology	kih-**NEE**-see-oh kih-**NEE**-see-**ALL**-oh-jee	☐	movement
-lepsy narco**lepsy**	**LEP**-see **NAR**-coh-**lep**-see	☐	seizure, attack
-lexia dys**lexia**	**LEK**-see-ah dis-**LEK**-see-ah	☐	reading
mening/o **mening**itis	men-**IN**-go men-in-**JYE**-tis	☐	meninges
myel/o **myel**ocele	**MY**-eh-loh **MY**-eh-loh-seel	☐	spinal cord or bone marrow
narc/o **narc**osis	**NAR**-koh nar-**KOH**-sis	☐	sleep

neur/o **neur**opathy	**NOO**-roh noo-**ROP**-ah-thee	☐	nerve
-paresis hemi**paresis**	par-**EE**-sis hem-ee-par-**EE**-sis	☐	partial paralysis
-phasia dys**phasia**	**FAY**-zee-ah dis-**FAY**-zee-ah	☐	speech
-plegia para**plegia**	**PLEE**-jee-ah pair-ah-**PLEE**-jee-ah	☐	paralysis
-praxia a**praxia**	**PRAK**-see-ah ah-**PRAK**-see-ah	☐	perform
-sthenia hypo**sthenia**	**STHEE**-nee-ah high-poss-**THEE**-nee-ah	☐	strength
thec/o intra**thec**al	**THEE**-koh in-trah-**THEE**-kal	☐	sheath
ton/o dys**toni**a	**TON**-oh dis-**TON**-ee-ah	☐	tension, tone
ventricul/o **ventricul**ostomy	ven-**TRIK**-yoo-loh ven-trik-yoo-**LOSS**-toh-mee	☐	ventricle of the heart or brain

Pathological Conditions

As you study the pathological conditions of the nervous system, note that the **basic definition** is in bold print, followed by a detailed description in regular print. The phonetic pronunciation is directly beneath each term, and a breakdown of the component parts of the term when appropriate.

The pathological conditions for the nervous system are listed in alphabetical order for easy reference. The pathological conditions fall into the following categories: **congenital** disorders (those occurring at birth); degenerative, functional, and seizure disorders; infectious disorders; intracranial tumors, traumatic disorders; vascular disorders; peripheral nerve disorders; and disk disorders. As each disorder is discussed, its category is identified.

Alzheimer's disease
(**ALTS**-high-merz dih-**ZEEZ**)

Deterioration of a person's intellectual functioning. Alzheimer's disease (AD) is progressive and extremely debilitating. It begins with minor memory loss and progresses to complete loss of mental, emotional, and physical functioning, frequently occurring in persons over 65 years of age.

This process occurs through three identified stages over a number of years.

Stage 1 lasts for approximately 1 to 3 years and includes loss of short-term memory; decreased ability to pay attention or learn new information;

gradual personality changes such as increased irritability, denial, and depression; and difficulties in depth perception. People with AD in stage 1 often recognize and attempt to adjust or cover up mental errors.

Stage 2 lasts approximately 2 to 10 years, during which time the person loses the ability to write, to identify objects by touch, to accomplish purposeful movements, and to perform simple tasks such as getting dressed. During this progressive deterioration, safety is a major concern. Also during the second stage, the person with AD loses the ability to socially communicate with others; he or she uses the wrong words in conversation, tends to repeat phrases, and may eventually develop total loss of language function, called **aphasia**.

Stage 3 lasts for 8 to 10 years, during which time the person with AD has very little, if any, communication skills due to disorientation to time, place, and person. Bowel and bladder incontinence, posture flexion, and limb rigidity also are noted during this stage. This increasing deterioration tends to render the person with AD dependent on others to provide for basic needs. The individual may be cared for by family members or need placement in a long-term care facility. The person with AD is prone to additional complications such as malnutrition, dehydration, and pneumonia.

It has been identified that both chemical and structural changes in the brain cause the symptoms of AD; however, there is no single clinical test to identify Alzheimer's disease. Before a diagnosis is made, other conditions that mimic the symptoms must be excluded. A clinical diagnosis of Alzheimer's is then based upon tests such as physical, psychological, neurological, and psychiatric examinations plus various laboratory tests. With today's new diagnostic tools and criteria, it is possible for physicians to make a positive clinical diagnosis of Alzheimer's with approximately 90% accuracy. A confirmation of the diagnosis of Alzheimer's disease is not possible until death since biopsy or autopsy examination of the brain tissue is required for a diagnosis.

Treatment for Alzheimer's disease includes the use of tacrine hydrochloride (Cognex), which is approved for use in mild to moderate cases due to its ability to improve memory in approximately 40% of persons with AD. Antidepressants and tranquilizers are also frequently used to treat symptoms.

The persons/families experiencing AD need a great deal of education and support to endure this difficult disease.

---

amyotrophic lateral sclerosis (ALS)
(ah-**my**-oh-**TROFF**-ik **LAT**-er-al skleh-ROH-sis)
a- = without, not
my/o = muscle
troph/o = development
-ic = pertaining to
scler/o = hard; also refers to sclera of the eye
-osis = condition

Amyotrophic lateral sclerosis (ALS) is a severe weakening and wasting of the involved muscle groups, usually beginning with the hands and progressing to the shoulders and upper arms then the legs, caused by decreased nerve innervation to the muscle groups.

This lack of muscle innervation is due to the loss of motor neurons in the brain stem and spinal cord. This is specifically a motor deficit and does not involve cognitive (mental thinking) or sensory (hearing, vision, and sensation) changes. As the muscle masses weaken and lose innervation, the person with ALS begins to complain of worsening fatigue with resulting uncoordinated movements, spasticity, and eventually paralysis.

As the brain stem involvement increases, the person with ALS experiences severe wasting of the muscles in the tongue and face causing speech, chewing, and swallowing difficulties. In addition, other manifestations of ALS include difficulty clearing airway and breathing and loss of temperament control with fluctuating emotions.

Complications of ALS include loss of verbal communication, loss of ability to provide self-care, total immobility, depression, malnutrition, pneumonia, and inevitable respiratory failure.

There is no cure for ALS and the primary care focuses on support of the person and family to meet their physical and emotional needs, especially as this physically debilitating disease progresses. The course of ALS varies according to individual, but approximately 50% die in 3 to 5 years after diagnosis. ALS is also called Lou Gehrig's disease.

---

anencephaly
(**an**-en-**SEFF**-ah-lee)
an- = without, not
encephal/o = brain
-y = noun ending

Anencephaly is an absence of the brain and spinal cord at birth, a congenital disorder.

The condition is incompatible with life. It can be detected through an amniocentesis or ultrasonography early in pregnancy.

Bell's palsy
(**BELLZ PAWL**-zee)

Bell's palsy is a temporary or permanent unilateral weakness or paralysis of the muscles in the face following trauma to the face, an unknown infection, or a tumor pressing on the facial nerve rendering it paralyzed.

Symptoms include drooling, inability to close the eye or regulate salivation on the affected side with a distorted facial appearance, as well as loss of appetite and taste perception.

Treatment includes gentle massage, applying warm moist heat, facial exercises to activate muscle tone, prednisone to reduce swelling, and analgesics to relieve pain. Early treatment is important for a complete recovery.

---

brain abscess
(**BRAIN AB**-sess)

A brain abscess is an accumulation of pus located anywhere in the brain tissue due to an infectious process, either a primary local infection or an infection secondary to another infectious process in the body, such as bacterial endocarditis, sinusitis, otitis, or dental abscess.

The initial symptom is a complaint of a headache which results from the increase in intracranial pressure (ICP). Other symptoms follow according to the location of the abscess. They include vomiting, visual disturbances, seizures, neck stiffness, or unequal pupil size. A computerized tomography (CT) scan and/or an electroencephalogram (EEG) will verify the diagnosis and location.

A brain abscess is treated aggressively with intravenous antibiotics. With signs and symptoms of ICP, mannitol, an osmotic diuretic, may be given as well as steroids to reduce cerebral edema and thus decrease the intracranial pressure. If treatment response is not good in a short period of time and there is an increased intracranial pressure, surgical drainage may be required to preserve cerebral functioning.

carpal tunnel syndrome
(**CAR**-pal **TUN**-el **SIN**-drom)

Carpal tunnel syndrome is a pinching or compression of the median nerve within the carpal tunnel due to inflammation and swelling of the tendons causing intermittent or continuous pain that is greatest at night.

The carpal tunnel is a narrow passage from the wrist to the hand housing blood vessels, tendons, and the median nerve. This tendon inflammation occurs largely as a result of repetitious overuse of the fingers, hands, or wrists.

Treatment involves anti-inflammatory medications, splints, physical therapy, and stopping the repetitive overuse. When medical treatment fails to relieve the pain, surgical intervention may be necessary to relieve pressure on the median nerve.

cerebral concussion
(seh-**REE**-bral con-**KUSH**-un)

Cerebral concussion is a brief interruption of brain function usually with a loss of consciousness lasting for a few seconds.

This transient loss of consciousness is usually caused by blunt trauma (a blow) to the head. With a severe concussion, the individual may experience unconsciousness for a longer period of time, a seizure, respiratory arrest, or hypotension.

The individual experiencing a cerebral concussion will likely have a headache after regaining consciousness and not be able to remember the events surrounding the injury. Other symptoms often associated with a cerebral concussion include blurred vision, drowsiness, confusion, visual disturbances, and dizziness.

The individual will need to be observed for signs of increased intracranial pressure or signs of intracranial bleeding during the period of unconsciousness and for several hours after consciousness is resumed. These signs indicate an injury requiring further treatment.

cerebral contusion
(seh-**REE**-bral con-**TOO**-zhun)

Cerebral contusion is a small, scattered venous hemorrhage in the brain, or better described as a "bruise" of the brain tissue, occurring when the brain strikes the inner skull.

The contusion will likely cause swelling of the brain tissue called cerebral edema. Cerebral edema will be at its height 12 to 24 hours after the injury.

Symptoms vary according to the size and location of the contusion. Some symptoms include increased ICP, combativeness, and altered level of consciousness.

Treatment includes close observation for secondary effects, including signs of increasing intracranial pressure and altered levels of consciousness. Hospitalization is usually required to monitor ICP, maintain cerebral perfusion, and administer corticosteroids and osmotic diuretics.

cerebral palsy
(seh-**REE**-bral **PAWL**-zee)
cerebr/o = brain; cerebrum
-al = pertaining to

Cerebral palsy (CP) is a collective term used to describe congenital (at birth) brain damage that is permanent but not progressive. It is characterized by the child's lack of control of voluntary muscles.

The lack of voluntary muscle control in CP is due to a lack of oxygen to the brain either before birth, during birth, or immediately upon delivery. The specific symptoms and types of CP will vary according to the area of the brain that was without oxygen.

The five major types of CP are as follows:

1. **Spastic** results from damage to the cortex of the brain, causing tense muscles and very irritable muscle tone. A very tense heel cord that forces a child to walk on his or her toes is an example of the spastic type of CP.
2. **Ataxic** results from damage to the cerebellum and causes the equilibrium to be affected. This type of CP will force the child to stagger when walking.
3. **Athetoid** is due to damage to the basal ganglia, which causes sudden jerking. This jerking may result from any stimulus including the increased intensity brought on by stress.
4. **Rigidity** causes the child to be in a continual state of tension. This tension is obvious when resistance is noted in both extensor and flexor muscles.
5. **Mixed** CP is a combination of the four types of CP just discussed.

Approximately 50% to 60% of children with cerebral palsy have mental retardation. Other common handicaps associated with CP include oculomotor impairment, convulsive disorder(s), and hearing and speech impairments.

cerebrovascular accident (CVA)
(seh-**REE**-broh-**VASS**-kyoo-lar **AK**-sih-dent)
cerebr/o = brain; cerebrum

A cerebrovascular accident (CVA) involves death of a specific portion of brain tissue, resulting from a decrease in blood flow (ischemia) to that area of the brain; also called stroke.

Causes of a cerebrovascular accident include cerebral hemorrhage, thrombosis (clot formation), and embolism (dislodging of a clot). Transient ischemic attacks (TIAs) or "mini strokes" often precede a full blown thrombotic CVA.

Transient ischemic attacks (TIAs) are brief periods of ischemia in the brain, lasting from minutes to hours, which can cause a variety of symptoms. TIAs or "mini strokes" often precede a full-blown thrombotic CVA. The neurological symptoms range according to the amount of ischemia and the location of the vessels involved. The person experiencing a TIA may complain of numbness or weakness in the extremities or corner of the mouth, as well as difficulty communicating. The person may also experience a visual disturbance. Sometimes the symptoms are vague and difficult to describe; the person may simply complain of a "funny feeling."

Cerebral thrombosis (clot), also called thrombotic CVA, makes up 50% of all CVAs and occurs largely in individuals older than 50 years of age and often during rest or sleep. The cerebral clot is typically caused by atherosclerosis, which is a thickened, fibrotic vessel wall that causes the diameter of the vessel to be decreased or completely closed off from the buildup of plaque. The thrombotic CVA is often preceded by one or many TIAs. The occurrence of the CVA caused by a cerebral thrombosis is rapid, but the progression is slow. It is often called a "stroke-in-evolution," sometimes taking 3 days to become a "completed stroke," when the maximum neurological dysfunction becomes evident and the affected area of the brain is swollen and necrotic.

Cerebral embolism occurs when an embolus or fragments of a blood clot, fat, bacteria, or tumor lodge in a cerebral vessel and cause an occlusion. This occlusion renders the area supplied by this vessel ischemic. A heart problem may lead to the occurrence of a cerebral embolus such as endocarditis, atrial fibrillation, and valvular conditions. A piece of a clot may break off in the carotid artery and move into the circulation causing a cerebral embolism. A fat emboli can occur from the fracture of a long bone. The cerebral emboli will cause immediate neurological dysfunction. If the embolus breaks up and is consumed by the body, the dysfunction will disappear; if the embolus does not break up, the dysfunction will remain. Even when the embolus breaks up, the vessel wall is often left weakened, increasing the possibility of a cerebral hemorrhage at this site.

Cerebral hemorrhage occurs when a cerebral vessel ruptures, allowing bleeding into the CSF, brain tissue, or the subarachnoid space. High blood pressure is the most common cause of a cerebral hemorrhage. The symptoms occur rapidly and generally include a severe headache along with other neurological dysfunctions (related to the area involved).

Symptoms of a cerebrovascular accident may vary from going unnoticed; to numbness, confusion, dizziness; to more severe disabilities such as impaired consciousness ranging from stupor to coma, paralysis, and aphasia. The symptoms of a cerebrovascular accident will differ widely according to the degree of involvement, the amount of time the blood flow is decreased or stopped, and the region of the brain involved.

Treatment of cerebrovascular accident depends on the cause and effect of the stroke. The prognosis, or predicted outcome, for a stroke victim is dependent upon the degree of damage to the affected area of the brain.

degenerative disk
(deh-**JEN**-er-ah-tiv disk)

Degenerative disk is the deterioration of the intervertebral disk, usually due to constant motion and wearing on the disk.

A vertebral misalignment will result in constant rubbing on the disk with gradual wasting and inflammation that results in degenerative disk disease.

Pain is the primary symptom and occurs in the regions served by the spinal nerves of the disk space involved. The pain is described as burning and continuous, sometimes radiating down the leg(s); there may be some motor function loss as well. The person with degenerative disk disease is often unable to carry on normal daily activities due to the pain and/or motor loss.

Treatment includes bed rest, bracing the back, nonsteroidal anti-inflammatory drugs (NSAIDs), analgesics, transcutaneous electrical nerve stimulation (TENS), and finally surgical interventions (spinal fusion or freeing compressed spinal nerve roots).

encephalitis
(en-**seff**-ah-**LYE**-tis)
encephal/o = brain
-itis = inflammation

Encephalitis is the inflammation of the brain or spinal cord tissue largely caused by a virus that enters the CNS when the person experiences a viral disease such as measles or mumps or through the bite of a mosquito or tick.

Encephalitis may also, but less often, be caused by parasites, rickettsia, fungi, or bacteria. Whatever the causative organism, it becomes invasive and destructive to the brain or spinal cord tissue involved.

Encephalitis is characterized by symptoms similar to meningitis; however, there is no buildup of exudate (as there is with meningitis), but small hemorrhages occur in the CNS tissue causing the tissue to become necrotic.

Symptoms include restlessness, seizure, headache, fever, stiff neck, altered mental function, and decreased level of consciousness. The person with encephalitis may also experience facial weakness, difficulty communicating and understanding verbal communication, a change in personality, or weakness on one side of the body. The deterioration of nerve cells and the increase of cerebral edema may eventually result in permanent neurological problems and/or a comatose state. The outcome varies related to the degree of inflammation, the age and condition of the individual experiencing encephalitis, and the cause.

Treatment for encephalitis includes administering medications, treating symptoms, and preventing complications. Administration of mild analgesics for pain, antipyretics for fever, anticonvulsants for seizure activity, antibiotics for intercurrent infections, and corticosteroids or osmotic diuretics to control cerebral edema are all part of the treatment regimen as indicated according to the symptoms.

epilepsy
(**EP**-ih-**lep**-see)

Epilepsy is a syndrome of recurring episodes of excessive irregular electrical activity of the central nervous system called seizures.

These seizures may occur with a diseased or structurally normal CNS, and this abnormal electrical activity may involve a part or all of the person's brain.

Epileptic seizures may affect consciousness level, skeletal motor function, sensation, and autonomic function of the internal organs. Severe seizures may produce a decrease of oxygen in the blood circulating through the body, as well as acidosis and respiratory arrest. Seizures are classified according to the area of the brain or the focus, the cause, and the clinical signs and symptoms experienced. The categories include:

1. **Partial seizures,** arising from a focal area that may be sensory, motor, or even a diverse complex focus.
2. **Generalized seizures,** commonly resulting in loss of consciousness and involving both cerebral hemispheres. Grand mal and petit mal seizures are the most common types of generalized seizures.

grand mal seizure
(grand **MALL SEE**-zyoor)

A grand mal seizure is an epileptic seizure characterized by a sudden loss of consciousness, and generalized involuntary muscular

contraction, vacillating between rigid body extension and an alternating contracting and relaxing of muscles.

Grand mal seizures, also called **tonic-clonic seizures**, are the most common seizures in adults and children. Persons experiencing tonic-clonic seizures may describe an **aura** or an indication of some kind preceding the onset of the tonic phase of the seizure.

The tonic phase begins with a sudden loss of consciousness, followed by the person's falling to the floor with muscle contractions causing rigid extension of the head, legs, and arms, and clenching of the teeth. The eyes roll back and the pupils are dilated and fixed. As the diaphragm contracts and air is forced through closed vocal chords, a cry is often heard and breathing is stopped. Both urinary and bowel incontinence may happen. This phase may last up to 1 minute, but the average duration is 15 seconds before the clonic phase begins.

The clonic phase is characterized by contraction and relaxation of muscle groups in arms and legs with rapid, shallow breathing called hyperventilation. Excessive salivation occurs during the clonic phase but will subside gradually within an average of 45 to 90 seconds.

The person experiencing a grand mal seizure remains unconscious for up to 30 minutes after the clonic phase has stopped. There is confusion and disorientation as consciousness is regained. The person will not remember the seizure itself, but will feel very tired and complain of muscle soreness and fatigue. If an aura occurs with a seizure, that is usually the last memory recalled.

Protection of the person during the tonic-clonic phase is the priority of care.

---

petit mal seizure
(pet-**EE MALL SEE**-zyoor)

Petit mal seizures are small seizures in which there is a sudden, temporary loss of consciousness, lasting only a few seconds; also known as absence seizures.

The individual may have a blank facial expression and may experience repeated blinking of the eyes during this brief period of time. There is no loss of consciousness and the episode often goes unnoticed by the individual; the duration of the seizure is 5 to 10 seconds. Petit mal seizures occur more frequently in children prior to puberty, beginning largely around the age of 5.

Guillain-Barré syndrome
(**GEE**-yon bah-**RAY SIN**-drom)

Guillain-Barré syndrome is acute polyneuritis ("inflammation of many nerves") of the peripheral nervous system in which the myelin sheaths on the axons are destroyed, resulting in decreased nerve impulses, loss of reflex response, and sudden muscle weakness, which usually follows a viral gastrointestinal or respiratory infection.

This polyneuritis usually begins with symmetric motor and sensory loss in the lower extremities, which ascends to the upper torso, upper extremities, and cranial nerves. The person with Guillain-Barré syndrome retains complete mental ability and consciousness while experiencing pain, weakness, and numbness. Approximately 25% of persons with Guillain-Barré syndrome will experience respiratory dysfunction requiring ventilatory assistance. In most persons this disease begins to resolve itself in several weeks, but the patient may take several months to 2 years to regain complete muscle strength.

Treatment is symptomatic, supportive, and aimed at preventing complications related to extended immobility, pain, anxiety, powerlessness, and respiratory dysfunction.

headache (cephalalgia)
(**seff**-ah-**LAL**-jee-ah)
cephal/o = head
-algia = pain

Cephalalgia involves pain anywhere within the cranial cavity varying in intensity from mild to severe, may be chronic or acute, and may occur as a result of a disease process or be totally benign. The majority of headaches are transient and produce mild pain that is relieved by a mild analgesic.

Disturbances in cranial circulation produces two of the three most common types of headaches: migraines and clusters. Tension headaches caused by muscle contraction comprise the other common type.

migraine headache
(**MY**-grain headache)

Migraine headache is a recurring, pulsating, vascular headache usually developing on one side of the head; characterized by a slow onset that may be preceded by an aura during which a sensory disturbance occurs, such as confusion or some visual interference (i.e., flashing lights).

The pain intensity gradually becomes more severe and may be accompanied by nausea, vomiting, irritability, fatigue, sweating, or chills.

Migraines occur at any age with more frequency in females and those with a positive family history for migraine headaches. There is an increase in migraine headaches during periods of stress and crisis as well as a correlation with the menstrual cycle. Dilation of the vessels in the head along with a drop in the serotonin level (which acts as a vasoconstrictor and a neurotransmitter, aiding in nerve transmission) occur at the onset of the migraine, which may last for hours or for days.

Treatment for migraine headaches includes medications to prevent the onset of the headaches and medications to relieve the headache and diminish or reduce the severity of the symptoms.

cluster headache
(**KLUSS**-ter headache)

A cluster headache occurs typically 2 to 3 hours after falling asleep; described as extreme pain around one eye that wakens the person from sleep.

There are usually no prodromal, or early signs; however, the associated symptoms include a discharge of nasal fluid, tearing, sweating, flushing, and facial edema. The duration of a cluster headache is 30 minutes to several hours, and the episodes are clustered together occurring every day for several days or weeks. Then there may be a period of time with no headaches lasting for months until there is a return of the daily cluster headaches.

tension headache
(**TEN**-shun headache)

A tension headache occurs from long, endured contraction of the skeletal muscles around the face, scalp, upper back, and neck.

Tension headaches make up the majority of headaches and occur in relation to excessive emotional tension such as anxiety and stress. The continued contraction of these skeletal muscles result in pain varying in intensity and duration. The onset of tension headaches is often during adolescence, but occur most often in middle age. The headache is described as viselike, pressing, or tight.

Mild analgesics such as acetaminophen or aspirin are used to relieve the tension headache. Tranquilizers may be used to reduce muscle tension.

hematoma, epidural
(hee-mah-**TOH**-mah, **eh**-pih-**DOO**-ral)
- **epi-** = upon, over
- **dur/o** = dura mater
- **-al** = pertaining to
- **hemat/o** = blood
- **-oma** = tumor

Epidural hematoma is a collection of blood (hematoma) located above the dura mater and just below the skull.

The hematoma is blood collected from a torn artery, usually the middle meningeal artery, or from an injury such as a skull fracture or contusion.

The initial symptom is a brief loss of consciousness. This brief period is followed by a period in which the individual is extremely rational (lucid). This lucid period may last for 1 to 2 hours or up to 1 to 2 days. When the lucid period is over, a rapid decline in consciousness occurs accompanied with one or all of the following: drowsiness, confusion, seizures, paralysis, one fixed pupil, an increase in blood pressure, a decrease in pulse rate, and even coma. This epidural hematoma develops rapidly; therefore, timely treatment is necessary to save the individual's life. The hematoma must be evacuated and the artery ligated. **Burr holes** drilled into the skull can often be used to accomplish the clot evacuation and ligation of the artery.

hematoma, subdural
(hee-mah-**TOH**-mah, **sub**-doo-ral)
- **sub-** = below, under
- **dur/o** = dura mater
- **-al** = pertaining to
- **hemat/o** = blood
- **-oma** = tumor

Subdural hematoma is a collection of blood below the dura mater and above the arachnoid layer of the meninges.

This blood usually occurs as a result of a closed head injury, an acceleration-deceleration injury, a cerebral atrophy noted in older adults, use of anticoagulants, a contusion, and/or chronic alcoholism.

Subdural hematomas largely occur as a result of venous bleeding. They vary in the rate of development from the acute subdural hematoma, which occurs in minutes to hours of an injury, to a chronic subdural hematoma, which can evolve over weeks to months.

Symptoms include agitation, drowsiness, confusion, headache, dilation and sluggishness of one pupil, possible seizures, signs of increased intracranial pressure (IICP), and paralysis.

Treatment for large subdural hematomas is surgical evacuation. The acute subdural hematoma may be removed through burr holes, but the chronic subdural hematoma is usually removed by a craniotomy because the blood collects so slowly it tends to solidify, preventing aspiration through burr holes.

herniated disk
(**HER**-nee-**ay**-ted disk)

Herniated disk is rupture or herniation of the disk center (nucleus pulposus) through the disk wall and into the spinal canal, causing pressure on the spinal cord or nerve roots.

The herniation may be caused by trauma or by sudden straining or lifting in an unusual position. An intervertebral disk is a flexible pad of cartilage located between every vertebrae to provide shock absorption and flexibility for movement.

Herniated intervertebral disks occur most frequently in the lumbosacral area, causing symptoms of sciatica: pain radiating from the back to the hip and down the leg. Herniation of the cervical disks occurs occasionally, causing shoulder pain radiating down the arm to the hand, stiffness of the neck, and sensory loss in the fingers. The diagnosis is usually confirmed with a CT scan, MRI, or a myelogram.

Conservative medical treatment such as bed rest, local application of heat, muscle relaxants, anti-inflammatory agents, and analgesics is usually the initial therapy. If back pain and sciatica are persistent and not relieved by the conservative medical treatment or if neurological dysfunctions are increasing, surgical intervention is indicated.

Huntington's chorea
(**HUNT**-ing-tonz koh-**REE**-ah)

Huntington's chorea is an inherited neurological disease characterized by rapid, jerky, involuntary movements and increasing dementia due to the effects of the basal ganglia on the neurons.

There is no cure for this progressive, degenerative disease.

Beginning around the age of 30 to 40, the early effects include irritability, periods of alternating emotions, posture and positioning problems, protruding tongue, speech problems, restlessness, and complaints of a "fidgety" feeling. These abnormal movements, which gradually increase to involve all muscles and the inability to be still for more than several minutes, are aggravated by attempts to perform voluntary movements, stress, and emotional situations. As the disease progresses, movement of the diaphragm becomes impaired, making the person with Huntington's chorea susceptible to choking, aspiration, poor oxygenation, and malnutrition. Other late effects include loss of mental skills and total dependence on others for care. Death typically occurs approximately 15 to 20 years after the onset of symptoms due to an infectious process or aspiration pneumonia.

Because there is no cure for Huntington's chorea, the supportive care includes education of the disease process for the person and family, along with genetic counseling. The emotional and psychological needs of the person and family are great and require much support.

hydrocephalus
(high-droh-**SEFF**-ah-lus)
hydro- = water
cephal/o = head
-us = noun ending

Hydrocephalus is an abnormal increase of cerebrospinal fluid in the brain that causes the ventricles of the brain to dilate, resulting in an increased head circumference in the infant with open fontanel(s); a congenital disorder.

The increase in cerebrospinal fluid may be due to an increased production of CSF, a decreased absorption of CSF, or a blockage in the normal flow of

CSF. The infant may also show frontal bossing (forehead protrudes out), which may cause the "setting sun" sign in which the sclerae (whites of the eyes) above the irises are visible when the eyes are directed downward. The infant will demonstrate other signs of increased pressure, such as a high-pitched cry, a bulging fontanel, extreme irritability, and an inability to sleep for long periods of time.

Hydrocephalus in the young infant may be indicated by increased head circumference, resulting in an abnormal graphing curve. This may be detected when checking the head circumference of the infant on well-baby checkups in the physician's office. (This procedure is discussed in Chapter 19.) Along with checking head circumference the infant should be assessed for any signs and symptoms of IICP.

When the diagnosis of hydrocephalus is made, treatment to relieve or remove the obstruction is initiated. When there is no obstruction, a **shunt** is generally required to relieve the intracranial pressure. The excess CSF is shunted into another body space, thus preventing permanent damage to the brain tissue. As the child grows, the shunt must be replaced with a longer one.

Hydrocephalus is often a complication of another disease or disorder. The infant with spina bifida cystica may develop hydrocephalus. It can also occur as a result of an intrauterine infection due to diseases such as rubella or syphilis.

---

intracranial tumors
(in-trah-**KRAY**-nee-al **TOO**-morz)
intra- = within
crani/o = skull; cranium
-al = pertaining to

Intracranial tumors occur in any structural region of the brain. They may be malignant or benign, classified as primary or secondary, and are named according to the tissue from which they originate.

An intracranial tumor causes the normal brain tissue to be displaced and compressed, leading to progressive neurological deficiencies. The clinical symptoms of intracranial tumors include headaches, dizziness, vomiting, problems with coordination and muscle strength, changes in personality, altered mental function, seizures, paralysis, and sensory disturbances.

Surgical removal is the desired treatment when possible. Radiation and/or chemotherapy are used according to location, classification, and type.

---

primary intracranial tumors
(**PRIGH**-mah-ree in-trah-**KRAY**-nee-al **TOO**-morz)

Primary intracranial tumors arise from gliomas, malignant glial cells that are a support for nerve tissue, and tumors that arise from the meninges.

Gliomas are classified according to the principal cell type, shape, and size, as follows:

1. *Glioblastoma multiforme* comprises approximately 20% of all intracranial tumors. This type of tumor arises in the cerebral hemisphere and is the most rapidly growing of the gliomas.
2. *Astrocytomas* comprise approximately 10% of all intracranial tumors and are slow-growing primary tumors made up of astrocytes (star-shaped cells). Astrocytomas tend to invade surrounding structures and over time become more anaplastic (i.e., they revert to a more primitive form). A highly malignant glioblastoma may develop within the tumor mass.

3. *Ependymomas* comprise approximately 6% of all intracranial tumors. They commonly arise from the ependymomal cells that line the fourth ventricle wall and often extend into the spinal cord. An ependymoma occurs more commonly in children and adolescents and is usually encapsulated and benign.

4. *Oligodendrogliomas* comprise approximately 5% of all intracranial tumors and are usually slow growing. At times the oligodendrogliomas imitate the glioblastomas with rapid growth. Oligodendrogliomas occur most often in the frontal lobe.

5. *Medulloblastomas* comprise approximately 4% of all intracranial tumors. Medulloblastomas occur most frequently in children between 5 and 9 years of age. They affect more boys than girls and typically arise in the cerebellum, growing rapidly. The prognosis is poor.

Meningiomas comprise approximately 15% of all intracranial tumors. They originate from the meninges, grow slowly, and are vascular. Meningiomas largely occur most often in adults.

metastatic intracranial tumors (secondary)
(met-ah-**STAT**-ik
in-trah-**KRAY**-nee-al
TOO-morz)
intra- = within
crani/o = skull; cranium
-al = pertaining to

Metastatic intracranial tumors occur as a result of metastasis from a primary site such as the lung or breast.

Brain metastasis is a common occurrence, comprising approximately 15% of intracranial tumors. The tissue in the brain reacts intensely to the presence of a metastatic tumor, which usually progresses rapidly. Surgical removal of a single metastasis to the brain can be achieved if the tumor is located in an operable region. The removal may provide the individual with several months or years of life.

meningitis (acute bacterial)
(men-in-**JYE**-tis ah-**KYOOT**
back-**TEE**-ree-al)
mening/o = meninges
-itis = inflammation

Meningitis (acute bacterial) is a serious bacterial infection of the meninges—the covering of the brain and spinal cord—that can have residual debilitating effects or even a fatal outcome if not diagnosed and treated promptly with appropriate antibiotic therapy.

The bacteria enters the meninges by way of the bloodstream from an infection in another part of the body (e.g., an upper respiratory infection) or through a penetrating wound such as an operative procedure, a skull fracture, or a break in the skin covering a structural defect such as a meningomyelocele. Once the bacteria invades the meninges causing inflammation, there is a rapid multiplication of the bacteria leading to swelling in the brain tissue, congestion in the blood circulation of the CNS, and formation of clumps of exudate which may collect around the base of the brain and have the potential to occlude CSF circulation.

These alterations lead to an increase in intracranial pressure as well as the following symptoms: irritability; extremely stiff neck (**nuchal rigidity**); headache in the older infant, child, or adult; fever; pain with eye movement; light sensitivity (photophobia); vomiting; diarrhea; drowsiness; confusion; and possibly seizures. Other specific characteristics in the infant include resistance to being diapered or cuddled, crying with position changes, high-pitched cry, decreased activity, bulging tense fontanel, and poor feeding and sleeping.

Prior to beginning the antibiotic therapy, cultures of CSF, urine, blood, and the nasopharynx are obtained in an attempt to identify the causative bacterial organism. A lumbar puncture (LP) is done to obtain the CSF on infants with open fontanel or others who show no signs of long-standing, increased intracranial pressure (papilledema observed when optic fundi observed). In the individual with bacterial meningitis, the CSF obtained from the lumbar puncture will generally appear cloudy, showing the presence of white blood cells (WBCs), as well as a decrease in glucose and an increase in protein.

The treatment for bacterial meningitis includes intravenous antibiotics for at least 10 days, according to organism(s) identified in cultures. The individual will likely be hospitalized initially and placed on isolation for 24 to 48 hours. The environment should be kept dark and quiet with very little stimuli.

The outcome of bacterial meningitis varies from complete recovery to miscellaneous physical and mental disabilities. These outcomes are related to the age of the individual as well as the interval between onset of symptoms and the beginning of treatment. The diagnosis of bacterial meningitis in the infant is often difficult to identify because of the lack of verbal communication and the vagueness of physiological symptoms (e.g., in the infant less than 1 month of age the temperature may go up or down). The long-term complications include mild learning disabilities to severe mental and physical handicaps, cranial nerve malfunctions, peripheral circulatory collapse, arthritis, and subdural effusion.

---

multiple sclerosis (MS)
(**MULL**-tih-pl **SKLEH**-roh-sis)
scler/o = hard; (also refers to sclera of the eye)
-osis = condition

Multiple sclerosis (MS) is a degenerative inflammatory disease of the central nervous system attacking the myelin sheath in the spinal cord and brain, leaving it sclerosed (hardened) or scarred.

Multiple sclerosis largely affects young adults between the ages of 20 and 40, with females being affected more often than males. The course for this disease varies greatly in that the initial onset can be gradual over weeks, months, or years or it may occur within minutes or hours. The common duration of MS is approximately 30 years, although there are documented cases of persons dying within several months after the beginning of the disease. This disease can follow two types: exacerbation-remitting type in which the exacerbation or onset of symptoms is followed by a complete remission, or the chronic progressive type in which there is a steady loss of neurological function. The scarring of the myelin sheath either slows the transmission of nerve impulses or completely inhibits the transmission of stimuli to the spinal cord and brain. The areas involved affect different systems and cause many symptoms, as evidenced by the following:

1. Unsteady balance, poor coordination with shaky irregular movements, and vertigo
2. Numbness and/or weakness of one or more extremities
3. Speech, visual, and auditory disturbance
4. Urinary tract infections due to difficulty urinating
5. Facial pain or numbness, difficulty chewing and swallowing
6. Fatigue, spasticity, muscular wasting or atrophy

7. Impaired sensation to temperature
8. Impotence in males
9. Emotional disturbances

The person experiencing MS is at risk for the following complications: seizures and dementia, blindness, recurring urinary tract infections (UTIs), bowel and bladder incontinence, respiratory infections, and injuries from falls.

There is no cure for MS; however, specific medications have helped to prolong remissions and decrease the exacerbations of ambulatory persons. The goals of drug therapy are to decrease inflammation, slow the immune response, and promote muscle relaxation. The goal of care for the person with MS is to promote independence as much as possible for as long as possible and to provide symptomatic treatment throughout the disease process, which may last as long as 30 years.

---

myasthenia gravis
(my-ass-**THEE**-nee-ah **GRAV**-iss)
my/o = muscle
-asthenia = loss of strength

Myasthenia gravis is a chronic progressive neuromuscular disorder causing severe skeletal muscle weakness (without atrophy) and fatigue, which occurs at different levels of severity.

The muscles are weak because the nerve impulse is not transmitted successfully to the muscle cell from the nerve cell, and these episodes occur periodically with remissions in between.

Myasthenia gravis is considered to be an autoimmune disease in which antibodies block or destroy some acetylcholine receptor sites. It occurs more often in women than men, with the onset usually between the ages of 20 and 40. In men, the onset is between the ages of 50 and 60.

Symptoms of myasthenia gravis may occur gradually or suddenly. Facial muscle weakness may be the most noticeable symptom, owing to drooping eyelids, difficulty with swallowing, and difficulty speaking. The periods of muscle weakness generally occur late in the day or after strenuous exercise. Rest does refresh the tired weak muscles. The weakness eventually becomes so severe that paralysis occurs.

In addition to medications, treatment for myasthenia gravis may require restricted activity, and a soft or liquid diet. The care provided for the person and family is supportive and symptomatic.

---

neuroblastoma
(**noo**-roh-blass-**TOH**-mah)
neur/o = nerve
blast/o = embryonic stage of development
-oma = tumor

Neuroblastoma is a highly malignant tumor of the sympathetic nervous system.

It most commonly occurs in the adrenal medulla with early metastasis spreading widely to liver, lungs, lymph nodes, and bone.

Parkinson's disease
(**PARK**-in-sons dih-**ZEEZ**)

Parkinson's disease is a degenerative, slowly progressive deterioration of nerves in the brain stem's motor system, characterized by a gradual onset of symptoms, such as a stooped posture with the body flexed forward; a bowed head; a shuffling gait; pill-rolling

gestures; an expressionless, masklike facial appearance; muffled speech; and swallowing difficulty.

The cause of Parkinson's disease is not known; however, a neurotransmitter deficiency (dopamine) has been clinically noted in persons with Parkinson's disease. Parkinson's disease is seen more often in males, with the onset of symptoms beginning between the ages of 50 and 60.

The clinical symptoms can be divided into three groups:

1. **motor dysfunction** demonstrated by the nonintentional tremors (pill rolling), slowed movements, inability to start voluntary movements, speech problems, muscle rigidity, and gait and posture disturbances.
2. **autonomic system dysfunction** demonstrated by mottled skin, problems from seborrhea and excess sweating on the upper neck and face, and absence of sweating on the lower body, abnormally low blood pressure when standing, heat intolerance, and constipation.
3. **mental and emotional dysfunction** demonstrated by loss of memory, declining mental processes, lack of problem-solving skills, uneasiness, and depression.

Treatment for Parkinson's disease, in addition to drug therapy, consists of control of symptoms and supportive measures with physical therapy playing an important role in keeping the person's mobility maximized.

A recent surgical technique utilized for the person with Parkinson's disease is a pallidotomy. This procedure involves the destruction of the involved tissue in the brain to reduce tremors and severe dyskinesia. The goal of this procedure, to restore a more normal ambulatory function to the individual, is not always successful.

peripheral neuritis
(per-**IF**-er-al noo-**RYE**-tis)
neur/o = nerve
-itis = inflammation

Peripheral neuritis is a general term indicating inflammation of one or more peripheral nerves, the effects being dependent upon the particular nerve involved.

The peripheral nerve disorders discussed in this chapter are trigeminal neuralgia or *tic douloureux,* Bell's palsy, and carpal tunnel syndrome. Each has been listed alphabetically.

poliomyelitis
(**poh**-lee-oh-**my**-ell-**EYE**-tis)
poli/o = gray matter, in nervous system
myel/o = spinal cord; bone marrow
-itis = inflammation

Poliomyelitis is an infectious viral disease entering through the upper respiratory tract and affecting the ability of spinal cord and brain motor neurons to receive stimulation. Muscles affected become paralyzed without the motor nerve stimulation (i.e., respiratory paralysis requires ventilatory support).

This once dreaded crippling disease has been nearly eliminated due to the vaccine and immunization programs of Salk and Sabin. The clinical symptoms include excessive nasal secretions, low-grade fever, progressive muscle weakness, nausea and vomiting, stiff neck, and flaccid paralysis of the muscles involved. Muscle atrophy then occurs with decreased reflexes, followed by joint and muscle deterioration.

Treatment for poliomyelitis is supportive with medications for fever and pain relief, bed rest, physical therapy, and respiratory support as indicated. Prevention of this infectious disease is the strategy for today with the use of Sabin trivalent oral vaccine which provides immunity for all three forms of poliomyelitis.

postpolio syndrome
(**POST POH**-lee-oh **SIN**-drom)
syn- = together, joined
drom/o = running
-e = noun ending

Postpolio syndrome is progressive weakness occurring at least 30 years after the initial poliomyelitis attack.

It involves already affected muscles in which there is uncontrolled, uncoordinated twitching. These muscle groups begin to waste and the person experiences extreme weakness. The treatment for postpolio syndrome is supportive.

Reye's syndrome
(**RISE SIN**-drom)
syn- = together, joined
drom/o = running
-e = noun ending

Reye's syndrome is an acute brain encephalopathy along with fatty infiltration of the internal organs that may follow acute viral infections; occurs in children under the age of 18, often with a fatal result. There are confirmed studies linking the onset of Reye's syndrome to aspirin administration during a viral illness.

The symptoms of Reye's syndrome typically follow a pattern through stages:

1. Vomiting, confusion, and lethargy (sluggishness and apathy)
2. Irritability, hyperactive reflexes, delirium, and hyperventilation
3. Changes in level of consciousness progressing to coma, and sluggish pupillary response
4. Fixed, dilated pupils, continued loss of cerebral function, periods of absent breathing
5. Seizures, loss of deep tendon reflexes, and respiratory arrest

The prognosis is directly related to the stage of Reye's syndrome at the time of diagnosis and treatment. Treatment includes decreasing intracranial pressure to prevent seizures, controlling cerebral edema, and closely monitoring the child for changes in level of consciousness. In some cases, respiratory support and/or dialysis is necessary.

shingles (herpes zoster)
(**SHING**-lz **HER**-peez **ZOSS**-ter)

Shingles (herpes zoster) is an acute viral infection seen mainly in adults, characterized by inflammation of the underlying spinal or cranial nerve pathway producing painful, vesicular eruptions on the skin along these nerve pathways. See Figure 8-6.

Of the population, 10% to 20% are affected by herpes zoster with the highest incidence in adults over 50.

Symptoms include severe pain before and during eruption, fever, itching, GI disturbances, headache, general tiredness, and increased sensitivity of the skin around the area. The lesions usually take 3 to 5 days to erupt, and

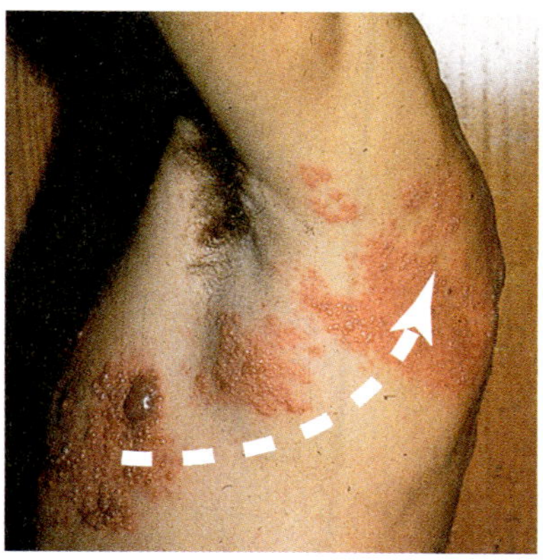

Figure 8-6 Shingles—vesicles follow a nerve pathway (Photo courtesy of Robert A. Silverman, M.D., Clinical Associate Professor, Department of Pediatrics, Georgetown University)

then progress to crusting and drying with recovery in approximately 3 weeks. Treatment with antiviral medications, analgesics, and sometimes corticosteroids aids in decreasing the severity of symptoms.

skull fracture (depressed)
(**SKULL FRAK**-chur, deh-**PREST**)

A broken segment of the skull bone thrust into the brain as a result of a direct force, usually a blunt object, is a skull fracture.

Automobile and industrial accidents are two potential causes of this type of injury.

The manifestations of a depressed skull fracture depend on the section of the brain that is injured and the extent of damage to the underlying vessels. The greater the involvement of vessels, the higher the risk for hemorrhage. Damage to the motor area will likely result in some form of paralysis.

Treatment includes a craniotomy to remove the depressed segment(s) of bone and raise it (them) back into position. Preoperative and postoperative treatment is directed at relieving intracranial pressure (ICP). Postoperative care may include wearing head protection until there is partial healing of the fracture.

spina bifida cystica
(**SPY**-nah **BIFF**-ih-dah **SISS**-tih-kah)

Spina bifida cystica is a congenital defect of the central nervous system in which the back portion of one or more vertebrae is not closed normally and a cyst protrudes through the opening in the back, usually at the level of the fifth lumbar or first sacral vertebrae.

Two types of spina bifida cystica—meningocele and meningomyelocele—are discussed in the following entries.

meningocele
(men-**IN**-goh-seel)
mening/o = meninges
-cele = swelling or herniation

Meningocele is a cystlike sac covered with skin or a thin membrane protruding through the bony defect in the vertebrae containing meninges and CSF. See Figure 8-7.

Some spinal nerve roots may be displaced but their function is still sound. Neurological complications occur rarely and are not as severe as those noted with the meningomyelocele.

Hydrocephalus is a possible complication occurring after surgical closure of the meningocele. Extreme care must be taken to protect the cystlike sac from injury prior to the surgical closure owing to the increased risk of an infection.

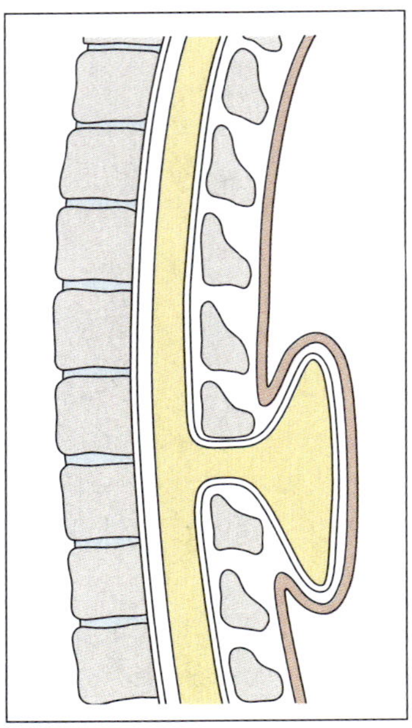

Figure 8-7 Meningocele

meningomyelocele
(men-**in**-goh-my-**ELL**-oh-seel)
mening/o = meninges
myel/o = spinal cord or bone marrow
-cele = swelling or herniation

Meningomyelocele is a cystlike sac covered with skin or a thin membrane protruding through the bony defect in the vertebrae that contains meninges, CSF, and spinal cord segments. See Figure 8-8.

Due to the involvement of the spinal cord segments, there are neurological symptoms such as weakness or paralysis of the legs as well as altered bowel and bladder control. Hydrocephalus is generally present. Extreme care must be taken to protect the sac from injury or rupture prior to surgical closure owing to the increased risk of an infection.

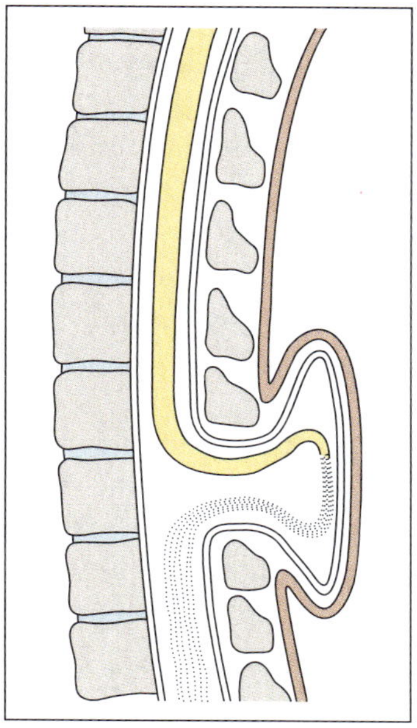

Figure 8-8 Meningomyelocele

spina bifida occulta
(**SPY**-nah **BIFF**-ih-dah oh-KULL-tah)

Spina bifida occulta is a congenital defect of the central nervous system in which the back portion of one or more vertebrae is not closed. A dimpling over the area may occur. See Figure 8-9.

Other symptoms include hair growing out of this area, a port wine **nevus** (pigmented blemish) over the area, and/or a subcutaneous lipoma (fatty tumor) in the area. This defect can occur anywhere along the vertebral column but usually occurs at the level of the fifth lumbar or first sacral vertebrae. There are usually very few neurological symptoms present. Without symptoms there is no treatment recommended.

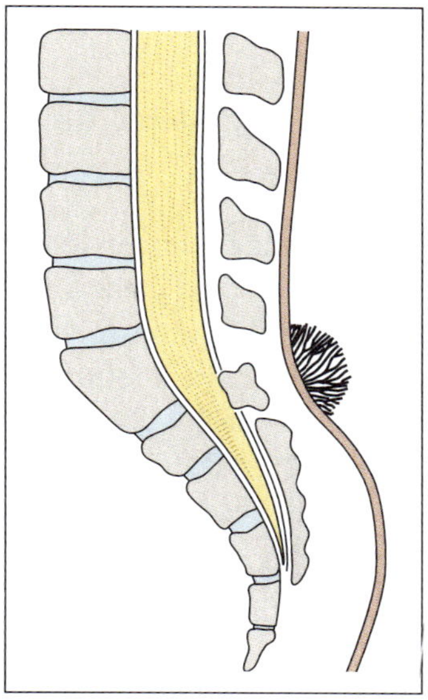

Figure 8-9 Spina bifida occulta

spinal cord injuries (paraplegia and quadriplegia)

Severe injuries to the spinal cord, such as vertebral dislocation or vertebral fractures, resulting in impairment of spinal cord function below the level of the injury.

Spinal cord injuries are generally the result of trauma caused by motor vehicle accidents, falls, diving in shallow water, or accidents associated with contact sports. Spinal cord injuries are seen most often in the male adolescent and young adult population.

Trauma to the spinal cord occurring above the level of the third to fourth cervical vertebrae (C3–C4) often results in a fatality due to the loss of innervation to the diaphragm and intercostal muscles, which maintain respirations.

paraplegia
(pair-ah-**PLEE**-jee-ah)
para- = near, beside, beyond, two like parts
pleg/o = paralysis
-ia = condition

Paraplegia, or paralysis of the lower extremities, is caused by severe injury to the spinal cord in the thoracic or lumbar region, resulting in loss of sensory and motor control below the level of injury.

Other common problems occurring with spinal cord injury to the lumbar and thoracic regions include loss of bladder, bowel, and sexual control.

quadriplegia
(**kwod**-rih-**PLEE**-jee-ah)
quadri- = four
pleg/o = paralysis
-ia = condition

Quadriplegia follows severe trauma to the spinal cord between the fifth and eighth cervical vertebrae, generally resulting in loss of motor and sensory function below the level of injury.

Paralysis in quadriplegia includes the trunk, legs, and pelvic organs with partial or total paralysis in the upper extremities. The higher the trauma the more debilitating the motor and sensory impairments. Quadriplegia may also be characterized by cardiovascular complications, low body temperature, impaired peristalsis, inability to perspire, and loss of control of bladder, bowel, and sexual functions.

Diagnosis and extent of injury with spinal cord injuries is confirmed with physical assessment, spinal x-rays, CT scans, and MRI scans.

Emergency treatment should be started at the scene of the injury to provide stabilization of the normal alignment to prevent additional injury. Further stabilization of the vertebrae will be accomplished at an acute care setting.

Tay-Sachs disease
(**TAY-SACKS** dih-**ZEEZ**)

Tay-Sachs disease is a congenital disorder caused by altered lipid metabolism, resulting from an enzyme deficiency.

An accumulation of a specific type of lipid occurs in the brain and leads to progressive neurological deterioration with both physical and mental retardation. The symptoms of neurological deterioration begin around the age of 6 months. Deafness, blindness with a cherry red spot on each retina, convulsions, and paralysis all occur in the child with Tay-Sachs disease until death occurs around the age of 2 to 4 years. There is no specific therapy for this condition; therefore, supportive and symptomatic care are indicated.

Tay-Sachs disease occurs most frequently in families of Eastern European Jewish origin, precisely the Ashkenazic Jews. This disease can be diagnosed in utero through amniocentesis.

trigeminal neuralgia (*tic douloureux*)
(try-**JEM**-ih-nal noo-**RAL**-jee-ah, tik **DOO**-loh-roo)

Short periods of severe unilateral pain, which radiates along the fifth cranial nerve, is trigeminal neuralgia (*tic douloureux*).

There are three branches of the fifth cranial nerve or the trigeminal nerve, each of which can be affected. Pain in the eye and forehead is experienced when the ophthalmic branch is affected. The mandibular branch causes pain in the lower lip, the section of the cheek closest to the ear, and the outer segment of the tongue. The upper lip, nose, and cheek are painful when the maxillary branch is affected.

Heat, chewing, or touching of the affected area activates the pain. Analgesics are used to control the pain. Persons who smoke are encouraged to quit. The nerve roots can be dissected through a surgical procedure when no other options have relieved the pain.

Diagnostic Techniques and Procedures

Babinski's reflex
(bah-**BIN**-skeez **REE**-fleks)

Babinski's reflex can be tested by stroking the sole of the foot, beginning at midheel and moving upward and lateral to the toes. A positive Babinski's occurs when there is dorsiflexion of the great toe and fanning of the other toes.

Although a normal reflex in newborns, the Babinski's reflex is abnormal when found in children and adults. A positive Babinski's reflex in an adult represents upper motor neuron disease of the pyramidal tract.

brain scan

A brain scan is a nuclear counter scanning of cranial contents 2 hours after an intravenous injection of radioisotopes.

Normally blood does not cross the blood-brain barrier and come in contact with brain tissue; however, in localized pathological situations this barrier is disrupted, allowing isotopes to gather. These isotopes concentrate in abnormal tissue of the brain indicating a pathological process. The scanner can localize any abnormal tissue where the isotopes have accumulated.

The brain scan assists in diagnosing abnormal findings such as an acute cerebral infarction, cerebral neoplasm, cerebral hemorrhage, brain abscess, **aneurysms**, cerebral thrombosis, hematomas, hydrocephalus, cancer metastasis to the brain, and bleeds.

cerebral angiography
(seh-**REE**-bral **an**-jee-**OG**-rah-fee)
- cerebr/o = brain; cerebrum
- -al = pertaining to
- angi/o = vessel
- -graphy = process of recording

Cerebral angiography is visualization of the cerebral vascular system via x-ray after the injection of a radiopaque contrast medium into an arterial blood vessel (carotid, femoral, or brachial).

The arterial, capillary, and venous recording structures are outlined as the contrast medium flows through the brain.

Through the cerebral angiography, cerebral circulation abnormalities such as occlusions or aneurysms are visualized. Vascular and nonvascular tumors can be noted as well as hematomas and abscesses.

cerebrospinal fluid analysis
(ser-eh-broh-**SPY**-nal **FLOO**-id an-**AL**-ah-sis)
- cerebr/o = brain; cerebrum
- spin/o = spine
- -al = pertaining to

Cerebrospinal fluid that is obtained from a lumbar puncture is analyzed for the presence of bacteria, blood, or malignant cells, as well as the amount of protein and glucose present.

Normal CSF is clear and colorless without blood cells, bacteria, or malignant cells. The normal protein level is 15 to 45 mg/dl but may be as high as 70 mg/dl in children and elderly adults. The normal glucose level is 50 to 70 mg/dl.

CT scan of the brain

Computerized tomography is the analysis of a three-dimensional view of brain tissue obtained as x-ray beams pass through successive horizontal layers of the brain.

The images provided are as though you were looking down through the top of the head. The computer detects the radiation absorption and the variation in tissue density in each layer. From this detection of radiation absorption and tissue density, a series of anatomic pictures are produced in varying shades of gray.

When contrast is indicated, intravenous (IV) iodinated dye is injected via a peripheral IV site. If receiving the contrast, the person should have nothing by mouth (n.p.o.) for 4 hours prior to the study because the contrast dye can cause nausea and vomiting.

CT scans are helpful in identifying intracranial tumors, cerebral infarctions, ventricular displacement or enlargement, cerebral aneurysm, intracranial bleeds, multiple sclerosis, hydrocephalus, and brain abscess.

---

chordotomy
(kor-**DOT**-oh-mee)
chord/o = string, cord
-tomy = incision into

Chordotomy is a neurosurgical procedure for pain control accomplished through a laminectomy in which there is surgical interference of pathways within the spinal cord that control pain.

The intent of this surgical procedure is to interrupt tracts of the nervous system that relay pain sensations from their point of origin to the brain in order to relieve pain.

---

cisternal puncture
(sis-**TER**-nal **PUNK**-chur)

Cisternal puncture involves insertion of a short, beveled spinal needle into the cisterna magna (a shallow reservoir of CSF between the medulla and the cerebellum) to drain CSF or obtain a CSF specimen.

The needle is inserted between the first cervical vertebrae and the foramen magnum.

Immediately after the procedure the person should be observed for cyanosis, difficulty breathing, or absence of breathing. Complications are rare.

---

craniotomy
(kray-nee-**OTT**-oh-mee)
crani/o = skull; cranium
-tomy = incision into

Craniotomy is a surgical procedure that makes an opening into the skull.

A craniotomy may be accomplished by creating a bone flap in which one side remains hinged with muscles and other structures to the skull. Another technique to allow entry into the skull is through a free-form flap where a portion of the bone is completely removed from its attachments. A third type of craniotomy is an enlarging burr hole that allows the brain to be exposed for the procedure.

echoencephalography
(**ek**-oh-en-**seff**-ah-**LOG**-rah-fee)
echo- = sound
encephal/o = brain
-graphy = process of recording

Ultrasound used to analyze the intracranial structures of the brain is termed echoencephalography.

Ventricular dilation or a vital shift of midline structures are usually picked up on the echoencephalography. These findings may indicate an enlarging lesion. There is a great chance of error in administering and interpreting the test; therefore, limitations must be considered.

electroencephalography (EEG)
(ee-**lek**-troh-en-**seff**-ah-**LOG**-rah-fee)
electr/o = electricity
encephal/o = brain
-graphy = process of recording

Measurement of electrical activity produced by the brain and recorded through electrodes placed on the scalp is termed electroencephalography.

The electrodes are connected to a machine that amplifies the electrical activity and records it on moving paper.

During the recording of the EEG, the person must remain very still and relaxed. This is usually achieved in a quiet room with subdued lighting. If a sleep EEG recording is ordered, the person is given a sedative and the EEG is recorded as the person falls asleep.

An EEG provides information helpful in evaluating individuals with cranial neurological problems, epileptic seizures, focal damage in the cortex, psychogenic unresponsiveness, and cerebral death.

laminectomy
(**lam**-ih-**NEK**-toh-mee)
lamin/o = lamina
-ectomy = surgical removal

Laminectomy is the surgical removal of the bony arches from one or more vertebrae to relieve pressure from the spinal cord.

This surgical procedure is done under general anesthesia. The pressure on the spinal cord may be caused by a degenerated or a displaced disk or may be from a displaced bone from an injury. If more than one vertebrae is involved, a fusion may be required to maintain stability of the spine.

lumbar puncture
(**LUM**-bar **PUNK**-chur)

Lumbar puncture involves the insertion of a hollow needle and stylet into the subarachnoid space, generally between the third and fourth lumbar vertebrae below the level of the spinal cord under strict aseptic technique.

A lumbar puncture permits CSF to be withdrawn for further examination or to decrease ICP, **intrathecal** injections (material injected into the lumbar subarachnoid space for circulation through the CSF) to be made, and access for further assessment.

A written consent for a lumbar puncture is required in most agencies due to the possible hazards of the procedure. Hazards include discomfort during the procedure, postpuncture headache, possible morbidity or mortality, infection, intervertebral disk damage, and respiratory failure.

A lumbar puncture takes only a few minutes and is performed with the person lying on his or her side with chin tucked down to chest and legs pulled into the abdomen. The person must be completely still to avoid damage by the needle. To decrease discomfort, a local anesthetic is normally injected prior to introduction of the needle and stylet.

A lumbar puncture is valuable in the diagnosis of meningitis, brain tumors, spinal cord tumors, encephalitis, and cerebral bleeding. The lumbar puncture is contraindicated in the presence of greatly increased intracranial pressure due to the potential abrupt release of pressure, which could cause compression of the brain stem and sudden death.

MRI of the brain

This noninvasive scanning procedure provides visualization of fluid, soft tissue, and bony structures without the use of radiation.

The person is placed inside an electromagnetic, tubelike machine where specific radio frequency signals change the alignment of hydrogen atoms in the body. The absorbed radio frequency energy is analyzed by a computer, and an image is projected on the screen.

The MRI provides far more preciseness and accuracy than most diagnostic tools. Those persons with implanted metal devices cannot undergo an MRI due to the strong magnetic field and the possibility of dislodging a chip or rod.

myelography
(my-eh-**LOG**-rah-fee)
myel/o = spinal cord, bone marrow
-graphy = process of recording

Myelography is the introduction of contrast medium into the lumbar subarachnoid space through a lumbar puncture in order to visualize the spinal cord and vertebral canal through x-ray examination.

Roughly 10 ml of CSF are removed, and a radiopaque substance is injected slowly into the lumbar subarachnoid space. Myelography is accomplished on a tilt table in the radiology department in order to visualize the spinal canal in various positions. After a series of films are taken of the vertebral canal viewing various parts, the contrast medium is removed.

Myelography aids in the diagnosis of adhesions and tumors producing pressure on the spinal canal or intervertebral disc abnormalities.

neurectomy
(noo-**REK**-toh-mee)
neur/o = nerve
-ectomy = surgical removal

A neurectomy is a neurosurgical procedure to relieve pain in a localized or small area by incision of cranial or peripheral nerves.

The intent of this surgical procedure is to interrupt tracts of the nervous system that relay pain sensations from their point of origin to the brain in an attempt to relieve pain.

pneumoencephalography
(noo-moh-en-**seff**-ah-**LOG**-rah-fee)
pneum/o = lungs, air
encephal/o = brain
-graphy = process of recording

Pneumoencephalography is used to radiographically visualize one of the ventricles or fluid occupying spaces in the central nervous system.

This process is accomplished by removing CSF through a lumbar puncture and replacing it with injected air, oxygen, or helium prior to the radiograph.

positron emission tomography (PET scan)
(**POZ**-ih-tron ee-**MISH**-un toh-**MOG**-rah-fee)

A positron emission tomography (PET) scan produces computerized radiographic images of various body structures when radioactive substances are inhaled or injected. See Figure 8-10.

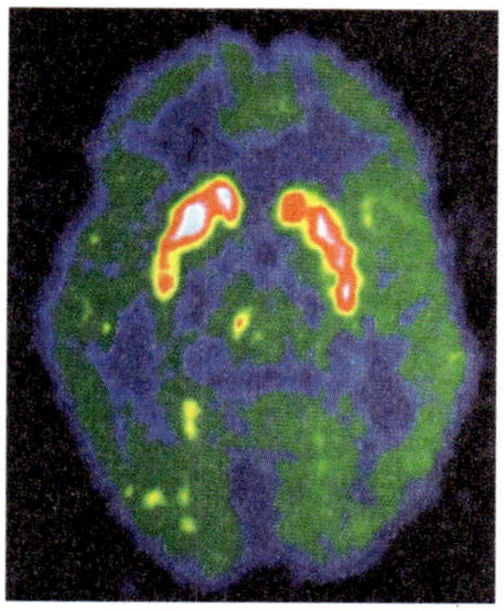

The metabolic activity of the brain and numerous other body structures are shown through computerized color-coded images that indicate the degree and intensity of the metabolic process. The PET scan exposes persons to very little radiation because the radioactive substances used are very short-lived.

PET scans are used in assessing dementia, brain tumors, cerebral vascular disease, and brain tumors. In addition there is a growing employment of the procedure to study biochemical activity of the brain as well as study and diagnose cancer.

Figure 8-10 PET scan shows that cocaine binds to specific brain locations primarily at dopamine-uptake sites (From "Addiction Brain Mechanisms and Their Related Implications," by D. J. Nutt, 1996, *The Lancet,* 347, pp. 33–35)

Romberg test
(**ROM**-berg test)

The Romberg test is used to evaluate cerebellar function and balance.

The person is asked to stand quietly with feet together and hands at the side and to attain equilibrium. The following step is to evaluate if the person can close his or her eyes and maintain equilibrium without swaying or falling. The next part of the evaluation is to assess if the person can lift the hands to shoulder height and then close eyes without hands drifting downward. If these two evaluations are completed successfully, the balance and cerebellar function are intact.

stereotaxic neurosurgery
(**ster**-eh-oh-**TAK**-sik **noo**-roh-**SER**-jer-ee)

Stereotaxic neurosurgery is performed on a precise location of an area within the brain that controls specific function(s) and may involve destruction of brain tissue with various agents such as heat, cold, and sclerosing or corrosive fluids.

This destruction may interrupt pathways of electrical activity or destroy specific nuclei. The precise location is calculated preoperatively. A small hole is drilled in the skull and the tip of a needle or probe is guided accurately to the exact location. The complications of stereotaxic neurosurgery relate to the site of the surgical approach and potential bleeding. It is possible for these tiny lesions to create lasting pain relief.

sympathectomy
(**sim**-pah-**THEK**-toh-mee)

Sympathectomy is a surgical procedure used to interrupt a portion of the sympathetic nerve pathway, for the purpose of relieving chronic pain.

tractotomy
(trak-**TOT**-oh-mee)

A tractotomy involves a craniotomy, through which the anterolateral pathway in the brain stem is surgically divided in an attempt to relieve pain.

Morbidity and mortality rates connected with this procedure are high.

transcutaneous electrical nerve stimulation (TENS)
(**tranz**-kyoo-**TAY**-nee-us ee-**LEK**-trih-kl nerve **stim**-yoo-**LAY**-shun)
trans- = across, through
cutane/o = skin
-ous = pertaining to

Transcutaneous electrical nerve stimulation (TENS) is a form of cutaneous stimulation for pain relief that supplies electrical impulses to the nerve endings of a nerve close to the pain site.

This is accomplished by placing electrodes on the skin and connecting them to a stimulator by flexible wires. Electrical impulses produced are much like the body's impulses, but are distinct enough to hinder transmission of pain signals to the brain.

The person wearing a TENS unit is responsible for controlling the pulsation and voltage of the electrical impulses. The person wearing the TENS must clean the electrodes and skin every 8 hours, along with reapplying the electrode jelly. One use of the TENS is with persons experiencing back pain and/or sciatica.

Common Abbreviations

ABBREVIATION	MEANING
ACTH	adrenocorticotrophic hormone
ALS	amyotrophic lateral sclerosis
ANS	autonomic nervous system
CNS	central nervous system
CSF	cerebrospinal fluid
CT	computerized tomography
CVA	cerebrovascular accident; stroke
EEG	electroencephalogram
EMG	electromyography
EST	electric shock therapy
ICP	intracranial pressure
LOC	level of consciousness
LP	lumbar puncture
MRI	magnetic resonance imaging
MS	multiple sclerosis
NPH	normal-pressure hydrocephalus
NREM	non-rapid eye movement (stage of sleep)
PEG	pneumoencephalogram
PET	positron emission tomography
PNS	peripheral nervous system
REM	rapid eye movement (stage of sleep)
RT	reading test
SNS	somatic nervous system
TENS	transcutaneous electrical nerve stimulation
TIA	transient ischemic attack

Written and Audio Terminology Review

Review each of the following terms from this chapter. Study the spelling of each term and write the definition in the space provided. If you have the Audio CD available, listen to each term, pronounce it, and check the boxes once you are comfortable saying the word. Check definitions by looking up the term in the glossary/index.

TERM	PRONUNCIATION	DEFINITION
absence seizure	☐ **AB**-senz **SEE**-zyoor	____________
acetylcholine	☐ **ah**-seh-till-**KOH**-leen	____________
afferent nerves	☐ **AFF**-er-ent nerves	____________

Term	Pronunciation	
agnosia	☐ ag-**NOH**-zee-ah	______
agraphia	☐ ah-**GRAFF**-ee-ah	______
alexia	☐ ah-**LEK**-see-ah	______
Alzheimer's disease	☐ **ALTS**-high-merz dih-**ZEEZ**	______
amyotrophic lateral sclerosis (ALS)	☐ ah-**my**-oh-**TROFF**-ik **LAT**-er-al skleh-**ROH**-sis	______
analgesia	☐ an-al-**JEE**-zee-ah	______
analgesic	☐ an-al-**JEE**-zik	______
anencephaly	☐ **an**-en-**SEFF**-ah-lee	______
anesthesia	☐ **an**-ess-**THEE**-zee-ah	______
anesthesiologist	☐ an-ess-thee-zee-**ALL**-oh-jist	______
aneurysm	☐ **AN**-yoo-rizm	______
aphasia	☐ ah-**FAY**-zee-ah	______
apraxia	☐ ah-**PRAK**-see-ah	______
arachnoid membrane	☐ ah-**RAK**-noyd **MEM**-brayn	______
astrocyte	☐ **ASS**-troh-sight	______
astrocytoma	☐ **ass**-troh-sigh-**TOH**-mah	______
ataxia	☐ ah-**TAK**-see-ah	______
aura	☐ **AW**-rah	______
autonomic nervous system	☐ aw-toh-**NOM**-ik **NER**-vus **SIS**-tem	______
axon	☐ **AK**-son	______
Babinski's reflex	☐ bah-**BIN**-skeez **REE**-fleks	______
Bell's palsy	☐ **BELLZ PAWL**-zee	______
blood-brain barrier	☐ **BLUD-BRAIN BAIR**-ree-er	______
bradyesthesia	☐ brad-ee-ess-**THEE**-see-ah	______
bradykinesia	☐ **brad**-ee-kih-**NEE**-see-ah	______
brain abscess	☐ **BRAIN AB**-sess	______
Brudzinki's sign	☐ brud-**ZIN**-skis sign	______
burr hole	☐ **BURR HOLE**	______
carpal tunnel syndrome	☐ **CAR**-pal **TUN**-el **SIN**-drom	______
cauda equina	☐ **KAW**-dah ee-**KWY**-nah	______

Term	Pronunciation	
causalgia	☐ kaw-**SAL**-jee-ah	______
cephalalgia	☐ **seff**-ah-**LAL**-jee-ah	______
cerebellospinal	☐ ser-eh-bell-oh-**SPY**-nal	______
cerebellum	☐ ser-eh-**BELL**-um	______
cerebral angiography	☐ **SER**-eh-bral (seh-**REE**-bral) **an**-jee-**OG**-rah-fee	______
cerebral concussion	☐ seh-**REE**-bral con-**KUSH**-shun	______
cerebral contusion	☐ seh-**REE**-bral con-**TOO**-zhun	______
cerebral cortex	☐ seh-**REE**-bral **KOR**-teks	______
cerebral palsy	☐ seh-**REE**-bral **PAWL**-zee	______
cerebritis	☐ ser-eh-**BRYE**-tis	______
cerebrospinal fluid	☐ ser-eh-broh-**SPY**-nal **FLOO**-id	______
cerebrovascular accident (CVA)	☐ seh-**ree**-broh-**VASS**-kyoo-lar **AK**-sih-dent	______
cerebrum	☐ seh-**REE**-brum	______
Cheynes-Stokes respirations	☐ **CHAIN-STOHKS** res-pir-**AY**-shuns	______
chordotomy	☐ kor-**DOT**-oh-mee	______
cisternal puncture	☐ sis-**TER**-nal **PUNK**-chur	______
cluster headache	☐ **KLUSS**-ter headache	______
coma	☐ **COH**-mah	______
comatose	☐ **COH**-mah-tohs	______
contracture	☐ kon-**TRAK**-chur	______
convolution	☐ **kon**-voh-**LOO**-shun	______
craniotomy	☐ kray-nee-**OTT**-oh-mee	______
degenerative disk	☐ dee-**JEN**-er-ah-tiv disk	______
dementia	☐ dee-**MEN**-shee-ah	______
demyelination	☐ dee-**my**-eh-lye-**NAY**-shun	______
dendrite	☐ **DEN**-dright	______
diencephalon	☐ **dye**-en-**SEFF**-ah-lon	______

Term		Pronunciation	
diplopia	☐	dip-**LOH**-pee-ah	________
dura mater	☐	**DOO**-rah **MATE**-er	________
dyslexia	☐	dis-**LEK**-see-ah	________
dysphasia	☐	dis-**FAY**-zee-ah	________
dystonia	☐	dis-**TON**-ee-ah	________
echoencephalography	☐	**ek**-oh-en-**seff**-ah-**LOG**-rah-fee	________
encephalography	☐	en-**seff**-ah-**LOG**-rah-fee	________
efferent nerves	☐	**EE**-fair-ent nerves	________
electroencephalography	☐	ee-**lek**-troh-en-**seff**-ah-**LOG**-rah-fee	________
embolism	☐	**EM**-boh-lizm	________
encephalitis	☐	en-**seff**-ah-**LYE**-tis	________
epidural	☐	**ep**-ih-**DOO**-rall	________
epilepsy	☐	**EP**-ih-**lep**-see	________
fissure	☐	**FISH**-er	________
fontanelles or **fontanel**	☐	**fon**-tah-**NELL**	________
gait	☐	**GAYT**	________
ganglion	☐	**GANG**-lee-on	________
glioma	☐	glee-**OM**-ah	________
grand mal seizure	☐	grand **MALL SEE**-zyoor	________
Guillain-Barré syndrome	☐	**GEE** -yon bah-**RAY SIN**-drom	________
gyrus	☐	**JYE**-rus	________
hematoma	☐	hee-mah-**TOH**-mah	________
hemiparesis	☐	hem-ee-par-**EE**-sis	________
hemiplegia	☐	hem-ee-**PLEE**-jee-ah	________
herpes zoster	☐	**HER**-peez **ZOSS**-ter	________
herniated	☐	**HER**-nee-**ay**-ted	________
Huntington's chorea	☐	**HUNT**-ing-tonz koh-**REE**-ah	________
hydrocephalus	☐	high-droh-**SEFF**-ah-lus	________
hyperesthesia	☐	**high**-per-ess-**THEE**-zee-ah	________
hyperkinesis	☐	**high**-per-kigh-**NEE**-sis	________
hyposthenia	☐	high-poss-**THEE**-nee-ah	________

Term	Pronunciation	
hypothalamus	☐ **high**-poh-**THAL**-ah-mus	________
interneurons	☐ **in**-ter-**NOO**-rons	________
intracranial tumors	☐ in-trah-**KRAY**-nee-al **TOO**-morz	________
intrathecal	☐ in-trah-**THEE**-cal	________
Kernig's sign	☐ **KER**-nigz sign	________
kinesiology	☐ kih-**nee**-see-**ALL**-oh-jee	________
laminectomy	☐ **lam**-ih-**NEK**-toh-mee	________
lethargy	☐ **LETH**-ar-jee	________
longitudinal fissure	☐ **lon**-jih-**TOO**-dih-nal **FISH**-er	________
lumbar puncture	☐ **LUM**-bar **PUNK**-chur	________
medulla oblongata	☐ meh-**DULL**-ah **ob**-long-**GAH**-tah	________
meningitis (acute bacterial)	☐ men-in-**JYE**-tis (ah-**KYOOT** back-**TEE**-ree-al)	________
meninges	☐ men-**IN**-jeez	________
meningocele	☐ men-**IN**-goh-seel	________
meningomyelocele	☐ men-**in**-goh-my-**ELL**-oh-seel	________
metastatic intracranial tumors	☐ **met**-ah-**STAT**-ik in-trah-**KRAY**-nee-al **TOO**-morz	________
microglia	☐ my-**KROG**-lee-ah	________
midbrain	☐ **MID**-brain	________
migraine headache	☐ **MY**-grain headache	________
motor nerves	☐ **MOH**-tor nerves	________
multiple sclerosis (MS)	☐ **MULL**-tih-pl **SKLEH**-roh-sis (MS)	________
myasthenia gravis	☐ my-ass-**THEE**-nee-ah **GRAV**-iss	________
myelin sheath	☐ **MY**-eh-lin **SHEETH**	________
myelocele	☐ **MY**-eh-loh-seel	________
myelography	☐ my-eh-**LOG**-rah-fee	________
narcolepsy	☐ **NAR**-coh-**lep**-see	________

Term	Pronunciation	
narcosis	☐ nar-**KOH**-sis	
neuralgia	☐ noo-**RAL**-jee-ah	
neurectomy	☐ noo-**REK**-toh-mee	
neuritis	☐ noo-**RYE**-tis	
neuroblastoma	☐ **noo**-roh-blass-**TOH**-mah	
neuroglia	☐ noo-**ROG**-lee-ah	
neurologist	☐ noo-**RAL**-oh-jist	
neurology	☐ noo-**RAL**-oh-jee	
neuron	☐ **NOO**-ron	
neuropathy	☐ noo-**ROP**-ah-thee	
neurosurgeon	☐ noo-roh-**SIR**-jun	
neurosurgery	☐ noo-roh-**SIR**-jer-ee	
neurotransmitter	☐ noo-roh-**TRANS**-mit-er	
nuchal rigidity	☐ **NOO**-kal rih-**JID**-ih-tee	
occlusion	☐ oh-**KLOO**-zhun	
oligodendrocytes	☐ all-ih-goh-**DEN**-droh-sights	
palliative	☐ **PAL**-ee-ah-tiv	
paraplegia	☐ pair-ah-**PLEE**-jee-ah	
parasympathetic	☐ **pair**-ah-**sim**-pah-**THET**-ik	
parasympathomimetic	☐ **pair**-ah-**sim**-pah-thoh-mim-**ET**-ik	
paresthesia	☐ pair-ess-**THEE**-jee-ah	
Parkinson's disease	☐ **PARK**-in-sons dih-**ZEEZ**	
peripheral nervous system	☐ per-**IF**-er-al nervous system	
peripheral neuritis	☐ per-**IF**-er-al noo-**RYE**-tis	
petit mal seizure	☐ pet-**EE MALL SEE**-zyoor	
phagocytosis	☐ fag-oh-sigh-**TOH**-sis	
pia mater	☐ **PEE**-ah **MATE**-er	
pineal	☐ **PIN**-ee-al	
plexus	☐ **PLEKS**-us	
pneumoencephalography	☐ noo-moh-en-**seff**-ah-**LOG**-rah-fee	

Term	Pronunciation	
poliomyelitis	☐ **poh**-lee-oh-**my**-ell-**EYE**-tis	______
pons	☐ **PONZ**	______
positron emission tomography (PET)	☐ **POZ**-ih-tron ee-**MISH**-un toh-**MOG**-rah-fee	______
postpolio syndrome	☐ **POST**-**POH**-lee-oh **SIN**-drom	______
primary intracranial tumors	☐ **PRIGH**-mah-ree in-trah-**KRAY**-nee-al **TOO**-morz	______
quadriplegia	☐ **kwod**-rih-**PLEE**-jee-ah	______
receptor	☐ ree-**SEP**-tor	______
Reye's syndrome	☐ **RISE SIN**-drom	______
rhizotomy	☐ rye-**ZOT**-oh-mee	______
Romberg test	☐ **ROM**-berg test	______
sciatica	☐ sigh-**AT**-ih-kah	______
sensory	☐ **SEN**-soh-ree	______
sensory nerves	☐ **SEN**-soh-ree nerves	______
shingles	☐ **SHING**-lz	______
somatic nervous system	☐ soh-**MAT**-ik nervous system	______
spina bifida cystica	☐ **SPY**-nah **BIFF**-ih-dah **SISS**-tih-kah	______
spina bifida occulta	☐ **SPY**-nah **BIFF**-ih-dah oh-**KULL**-tah	______
stereotaxic neurosurgery	☐ **ster**-eh-oh-**TAK**-sik **noo**-roh-**SER**-jer-ee	______
stimulus	☐ **STIM**-yoo-lus	______
stupor	☐ **STOO**-per	______
subarachnoid	☐ sub-ah-**RAK**-noyd	______
subdural	☐ sub-**DOO**-ral	______
sulcus	☐ **SULL**-kuss	______
sympathectomy	☐ **sim**-pah-**THEK**-toh-mee	______
sympathetic	☐ sim-pah-**THET**-ik	______
sympathomimetic	☐ sim-pah-thoh-mim-**ET**-ik	______

Term		Pronunciation	
synapse	☐	**SIN**-aps	______
syncope	☐	**SIN**-koh-pee	______
Tay-Sachs disease	☐	**TAY-SACKS** dih-**ZEEZ**	______
thalamus	☐	**THAL**-ah-mus	______
thrombosis	☐	throm-**BOH**-sis	______
tonic-clonic seizure	☐	**TON**-ik **CLON**-ic **SEE**-zhur	______
tractotomy	☐	trak-**TOT**-oh-mee	______
transcutaneous electrical nerve stimulation (TENS)	☐	**tranz**-kyoo-**TAY**-nee-us ee-**LEK**-trih-kl nerve **stim**-yoo-**LAY**-shun (TENS)	______
trigeminal neuralgia tic douloureux	☐	try-**JEM**-ih-nal noo-**RAL**-jee-ah tik **DOO**-loh-roo	______
ventricle	☐	**VEN**-trik-l	______
ventriculostomy	☐	ven-trik-yoo-**LOSS**-toh-mee	______

Chapter Review Exercises

The following exercises provide a more in-depth review of the chapter material. Your goal in these exercises is to complete each section at a minimum 80% level of accuracy. A space has been provided for your score at the end of each section.

A. Form the Plurals

Write the plural form and definition of each word listed. If you have forgotten how to form plurals, you may wish to refer to the section on forming plurals in Chapter 3. Each correct answer is worth 10 points. Record your score in the space provided at the end of the exercise.

a. ganglion
   1. Plural: ______
   2. Definition: ______

b. gyrus
   3. Plural: ______
   4. Definition: ______

c. dendrite
   5. Plural: ______
   6. Definition: ______

d. stimulus

7. Plural: ______

8. Definition: ______

______

e. sulcus

9. Plural: ______

10. Definition: ______

______

Number correct ______ × 10 points/correct answer: Your score ______%

B. Spelling

Circle the correctly spelled term in each pairing of words. Each correct answer is worth 10 points. Record your score in the space provided at the end of the exercise.

1. aneurysm	anurysm
2. automonic	autonomic
3. cephoalgia	cephalalgia
4. efferent	eferent
5. girus	gyrus
6. narcolepsy	narcrolepsy
7. thalamus	thalmus
8. myalin	myelin
9. nuckle	nuchal
10. sciatica	siatica

Number correct ______ × 10 points/correct answer: Your score ______%

C. Crossword Puzzle

The terms in the following crossword puzzle pertain to the anatomy and physiology of the nervous system. Each correct answer is worth 10 points. When you have completed the puzzle, total your points and enter your score in the space provided.

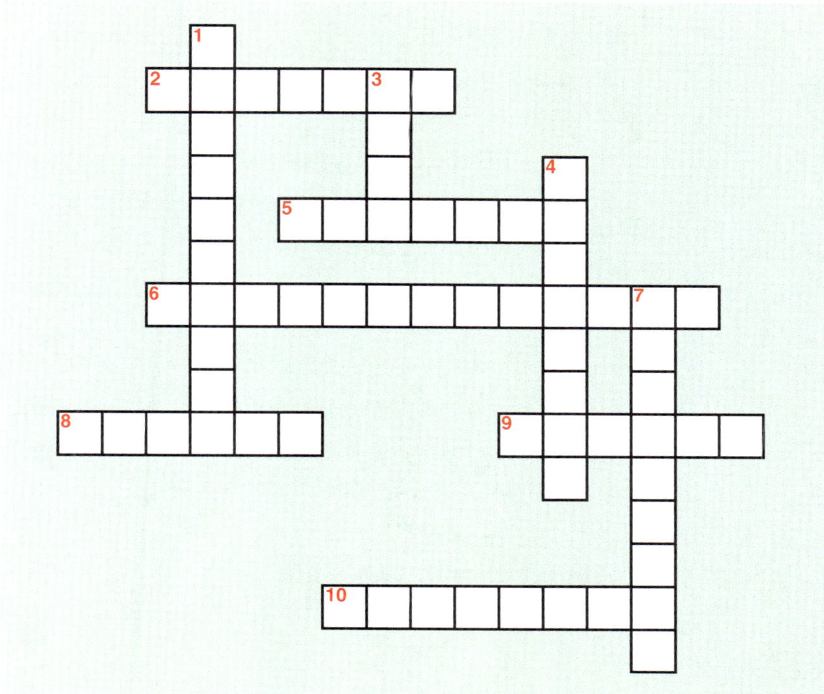

ACROSS

2 Nervous system of brain and spinal cord
5 Space between two nerves
6 Fluid flowing through the CNS
8 Protective sheath covering axons
9 Nerve cell
10 Nerve: transmits toward the CNS

DOWN

1 Nervous system of cranial and spinal nerves
3 Carries impulse away from cell body
4 Three protective membranes of CNS
7 Star-shaped nerve cell

Number correct _______ × 10 points/correct answer: Your score _______%

D. Term to Definition

Define each term by writing the definition in the space provided. Check the box if you are able to complete this exercise correctly the first time (without referring to the answers). Each correct answer is worth 10 points. Record your score in the space provided at the end.

☐ 1. syncope: ______________________________

☐ 2. sciatica: ______________________________

☐ 3. paresthesia: ______________________________

☐ 4. palliative: ______________________________

☐ 5. occlusion: ______________________________

☐ 6. neuritis: ______________________________

☐ 7. lethargy: ______________________________

☐ 8. hemiparesis: ______________________________

☐ 9. fissure: ______________________________

☐ 10. coma: ______________________________

Number correct _______ × 10 points/correct answer: Your score _______%

E. Matching Structures

Match the structures of the central nervous system listed on the left with the most appropriate definition on the right. Each correct answer is worth 10 points. Record your score in the space provided at the end of the exercise.

_____	1. arachnoid membrane	a. a small hollow within the brain that is filled with cerebrospinal fluid
_____	2. brain stem	b. controls body temperature, sleep, and appetite
_____	3. cerebellum	c. stemlike portion of the brain that connects the cerebral hemispheres with the spinal cord
_____	4. cerebrum	d. contains the cardiac, vasomotor, and respiratory centers of the brain
_____	5. diencephalon	e. the weblike, middle layer of the meninges
_____	6. dura mater	f. outermost layer of the meninges
_____	7. medulla oblongata	g. located between the cerebrum and the midbrain (consists of the thalamus, hypothalamus, and pineal gland)
_____	8. hypothalamus	h. responsible for coordinating voluntary muscular movement
_____	9. pons	i. controls consciousness, memory, sensations, etc.
_____	10. ventricle	j. acts as a bridge to connect the medulla oblongata and the cerebellum to the upper portions of the brain

Number correct _______ × 10 points/correct answer: Your score _______%

F. Definition to Term

Use the definitions to identify and provide the appropriate medical word. Write the word in the first space and its combining form in the second space. Each correct answer is worth 5 points. Record your score in the space provided at the end of the exercise.

1. Pain in the head ("headache"):

   _______________________ (word) _______________________ (combining form)

2. A condition in which there is abnormally slow movement:

   _______________________ (word) _______________________ (combining form)

3. Difficult speech:

   _______________________ (word) _______________________ (combining form)

4. The study of the nervous system and its disorders:

   _______________________ (word) _______________________ (combining form)

5. Paralysis of all four extremities of the body:

   _______________________ (word) _______________________ (combining form)

6. An abnormal condition in which a clot develops in a blood vessel:

   _______________________ (word) _______________________ (combining form)

7. Inflammation of the meninges:

_______________ (word) _______________ (combining form)

8. "Without speech":

_______________ (word) _______________ (combining form)

9. Incision into the skull:

_______________ (word) _______________ (combining form)

10. Uncontrolled, sudden attacks of sleep:

_______________ (word) _______________ (combining form)

Number correct _______ × 15 points/correct answer: Your score _______%

G. Labeling

Label the following diagrams by identifying the appropriate structures. Place your answers in the spaces provided. Each correct answer is worth 10 points. Record your score in the space provided at the end of the exercise.

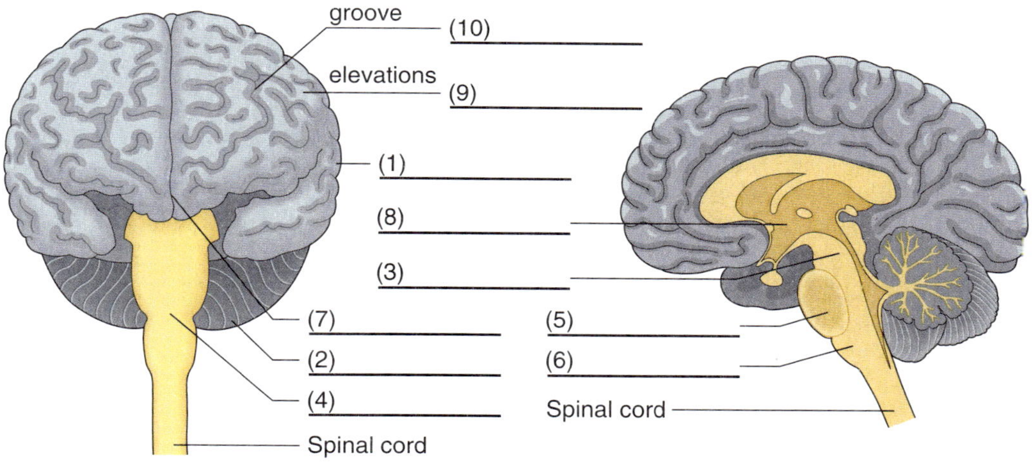

1. _______________
2. _______________
3. _______________
4. _______________
5. _______________
6. _______________
7. _______________
8. _______________
9. _______________
10. _______________

Number correct _______ × 10 points/correct answer: Your score _______%

H. Matching Abbreviations

Match the abbreviations on the left with the appropriate definition on the right. Each correct response is worth 10 points. Record your score in the space provided at the end of the exercise.

_____	1. ANS	a.	electrocardiogram
_____	2. CSF	b.	level of consciousness
_____	3. CVA	c.	computerized tomography
_____	4. EEG	d.	transient ischemic attacks
_____	5. ICP	e.	autonomic nervous system
_____	6. MRI	f.	lumbar puncture
_____	7. REM	g.	cerebrospinal fluid
_____	8. TIA	h.	cardiovascular accident
_____	9. LOC	i.	rapid eye movement
_____	10. LP	j.	magnetic resonance imaging
		k.	intracranial pressure
		l.	adrenocorticotropic hormone serum
		m.	electroencephalogram
		n.	cerebrovascular accident

Number correct _______ × 10 points/correct answer: Your score _______%

I. Definition to Term

Use the following definition to identify and provide the correct procedure. Each correct answer is worth 10 points. Record your score in the space provided at the end of the exercise.

1. Visualization of the cerebrovascular system via x-ray after the injection of a radiopaque contrast medium into an artery.

   ____

2. A noninvasive scanning procedure that provides a computer projected image of fluid, soft tissue, or bony structures without the use of radiation.

   ____

3. Measurement of electrical activity produced by the brain and recorded through electrodes placed on the scalp.

   ____

4. Insertion of a hollow needle and stylet into the subarachnoid space generally between the third and fourth lumbar vertebrae.

   ____

5. A three-dimensional view of brain tissue obtained as x-ray beams pass through successive horizontal layers of the brain.

   ____

6. A surgical procedure that makes an opening into the skull.

   ____

7. A positive finding in an adult represents upper motor neuron disease of the pyramidal tract.

   ____

8. An evaluation of cerebellar function and balance.

____

9. Surgical removal of bony arches from one or more vertebrae in order to relieve pressure from the spinal cord.

____

10. Introduction of contrast medium into the lumbar subarachnoid space through a lumbar puncture in order to visualize the spinal cord and vertebral canal through x-ray examination.

____

Number correct ______ × 10 points/correct answer: Your score ______ %

J. Word Search

Use the following definitions to identify the pathological condition related to the nervous system and then find and circle it in the puzzle. The words may be read up, down, diagonally, across, or backward. Each correct answer is worth 10 points. Record your score in the space provided at the end of the exercise.

Example: The inability to speak.

aphasia

1. This condition is characterized by the child's lack of control of voluntary muscles.

____

2. Many times this condition requires the use of a shunt in order to remove CSF and decrease intracranial pressure.

____

3. An autosomal recessive disorder caused by altered lipid metabolism due to an enzyme deficiency.

____

4. A degenerative disease that progresses through three stages, ending with the deterioration of mental, emotional, and physical functioning.

____

5. A syndrome of recurring episodes of excessive irregular electrical activity of the CNS.

____

6. A type of headache that is often preceded by an aura.

____

7. A degenerative inflammatory disease of the CNS that attacks the myelin sheath.

____

8. Inflammation of the brain or spinal cord tissue.

____

9. A syndrome resulting in decreased nerve impulses, loss of reflex response, and sudden muscle weakness due to acute polyneuritis.

____

10. A syndrome manifested by acute brain encephalopathy, along with the fatty infiltration of the internal organs.

____

Number correct ______ × 10 points/correct answer: Your score ______ %

M	E	A	P	H	A	S	I	A	I	O	N	S	T	I
U	E	R	R	A	B	N	I	A	L	L	I	U	G	S
L	D	B	Y	A	C	U	T	E	I	T	G	E	N	C
T	A	Y	S	A	C	H	S	D	I	S	E	A	S	E
I	A	D	H	R	S	I	F	L	E	X	I	L	N	A
P	C	S	Y	O	I	T	A	N	O	R	P	Z	D	M
L	O	E	D	E	T	H	I	M	B	R	I	H	E	B
E	N	E	R	P	P	L	E	X	I	O	N	E	R	U
S	A	X	O	E	I	N	O	I	T	A	P	I	R	L
C	T	T	C	I	B	N	E	X	T	I	N	M	I	A
L	I	N	E	R	C	R	A	R	L	T	A	E	I	T
E	E	N	P	A	L	Y	A	E	A	D	D	R	C	I
R	N	S	H	D	R	R	P	L	I	P	R	S	N	O
O	S	I	A	I	E	S	U	M	P	O	S	U	P	N
S	O	O	L	S	Y	D	S	H	C	A	S	Y	A	T
I	U	N	U	S	E	P	I	N	A	T	L	N	I	L
S	R	O	S	D	S	R	S	I	F	L	E	S	X	N
P	L	A	N	M	I	G	R	A	I	N	E	O	Y	O

K. Matching Pathological Conditions

Match the pathological conditions on the left with the most appropriate definition on the right. Each correct answer is worth 5 points. Record your score in the space provided at the end of the exercise.

_____ 1. cerebral embolism
_____ 2. meningioma
_____ 3. glioblastoma multiforme
_____ 4. cerebral concussion
_____ 5. epidural hematoma
_____ 6. trigeminal neuralgia
_____ 7. cerebrovascular accident
_____ 8. cerebral contusion
_____ 9. subdural hematoma
_____ 10. depressed skull fracture
_____ 11. cerebral palsy
_____ 12. hydrocephalus
_____ 13. spina bifida occulta
_____ 14. Huntington's chorea
_____ 15. myasthenia gravis

a. The most rapidly growing glioma comprising 20% of all intracranial tumors
b. short periods of severe unilateral pain radiating along the fifth cranial nerve
c. a broken segment of the skull bone thrust into the brain as a result of direct force
d. congenital absence of the brain and spinal cord
e. a brief interruption of brain function, usually with a loss of con sciousness, lasting for a few seconds
f. a collection of venous blood below the dura mater and above the arachnoid layer of the meninges
g. congenital brain damage that is permanent but not progressive
h. fragment of blood clot, fat, bacteria, or tumor that lodges in a cerebral vessel
i. neurological deficits resulting from cerebral ischemia to a specific localized area in the brain

______	16. Parkinson's disease	j.	accumulation of pus located in the brain tissue
______	17. brain abscess	k.	deterioration of nerves in the brain stem's motor system causing stooped posture, a bowed head, shuffling gait, and pill-rolling gestures
______	18. meningitis	l.	an increased amount of CSF in the brain
______	19. poliomyelitis	m.	a congenital defect of the CNS in which the back portion of one or more vertebrae is not closed
______	20. anencephaly	n.	small, scattered, venous hemorrhages in the brain tissue
		o.	a brain tumor occurring largely in adults and originating from the meninges
		p.	an inherited neurological disease characterized by rapid, jerky, involuntary movements with increasing dementia
		q.	considered to be an autoimmune disease in which antibodies block or destroy some acetylcholine receptor sites
		r.	a collection of arterial blood located above the dura mater and just below the skull
		s.	a serious infection of the meninges, usually caused by bacteria
		t.	an infectious viral disease entering through the upper respiratory tract and affecting the ability of the spinal cord and brain motor neurons to receive stimulation

Number correct _______ × 15 points/correct answer: Your score _______%

L. Completion

Complete the following statements with the most appropriate answer. Each correct answer is worth 10 points. Record your score in the space provided at the end of the exercise.

1. A congenital defect of the central nervous system in which the back portion of one or more vertebrae is not closed normally and a cyst protrudes through the opening in the back, usually at the level of L5 or S1.

   ____

   (three words)

2. Also called tonic-clonic, these begin with sudden loss of consciousness, followed by muscle contractions and rigid extension of the head and arms, followed by a brief absence of respirations.

   ____

   (three words)

3. Occurring in any structural region of the brain, these may be malignant or benign, causing normal brain tissue to be displaced and compressed.

   ____

   (two words)

4. This follows severe trauma to the spinal cord between the fifth and eighth cervical vertebrae, generally resulting in loss of motor and sensory function below the level of the injury.

   ____

   (one word)

5. A very brief period of ischemia in the brain lasting from minutes to hours, which can cause a variety of symptoms.

   ____

   (three words)

6. A rupture of the nucleus pulposus through the disk wall and into the spinal canal causing pressure on the spinal cord or nerve roots.

____

(three words)

7. This condition is characterized by intermittent or continuous pain in the hand, wrist, and arm due to the pinching of the median nerve and inflammation and swelling of tendons.

____

(three words)

8. This condition occurs when a cerebral vessel ruptures, allowing blood into the CSF, brain tissue, or subarachnoid space.

____

(two words)

9. This condition is characterized by temporary or permanent unilateral weakness or paralysis to the muscles in the face following trauma to the face, an unknown infection, or a tumor pressing on the facial nerve.

____

(two words)

10. These occur as a result of metastasis from a primary site such as the lung or breast.

____

(three words)

Number correct _______ × 10 points/correct answer: Your score _______%

Answers to Chapter Review Exercises

A. Form the Plurals

1. ganglia
2. knotlike masses of nerve tissue found outside the brain or spinal cord
3. gyri
4. elevations or folds of the surface of the cerebrum
5. dendrites
6. projections extending from the nerve cell body that receive impulses and conduct them on to the cell body
7. stimuli
8. agents or factors capable of initiating nervous impulses
9. sulci
10. depressions or shallow grooves on the surface of an organ

B. Spelling

1. aneurysm
2. autonomic
3. cephalalgia
4. efferent
5. gyrus
6. narcolepsy
7. thalamus
8. myelin
9. nuchal
10. sciatica

C. Crossword Puzzle

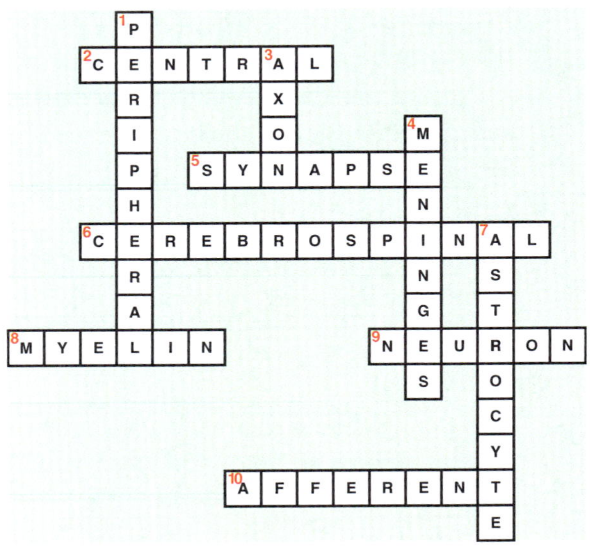

D. Term to Definition

1. fainting
2. inflammation of the sciatic nerve
3. sensation of numbness or tingling
4. soothing
5. blockage
6. inflammation of the nerves
7. sluggishness
8. slight paralysis of half of the body
9. a deep groove on the surface of an organ
10. a deep sleep

E. Matching Structures

1. e	6. f
2. c	7. d
3. h	8. b
4. i	9. j
5. g	10. a

F. Definition to Term

1. cephalalgia	cephal/o
2. bradykinesia	kinesi/o
3. dysphasia	phas/o
4. neurology	neur/o
5. quadriplegia	quadr/i
6. thrombosis	thromb/o
7. meningitis	mening/o
8. aphasia	phas/o
9. craniotomy	crani/o
10. narcolepsy	narc/o

G. Labeling

1. cerebrum	6. medulla oblongata
2. cerebellum	7. longitudinal fissure
3. midbrain	8. thalamus
4. brain stem	9. gyri
5. pons	10. sulcus

H. Matching Abbreviations

1. e	6. j
2. g	7. i
3. n	8. d
4. m	9. b
5. k	10. f

I. Definition to Term

1. cerebral angiography	6. craniotomy
2. MRI	7. Babinski's reflex
3. electroencephalography	8. Romberg test
4. lumbar puncture	9. laminectomy
5. CT scan of the brain	10. myelography

J. Word Search

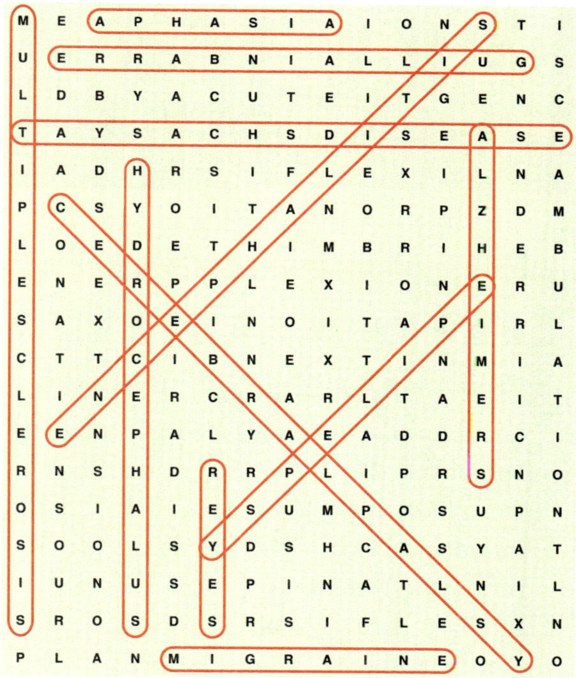

K. Matching Pathological Conditions

1. h	11. g
2. o	12. l
3. a	13. m
4. e	14. p
5. r	15. q
6. b	16. k
7. i	17. j
8. n	18. s
9. f	19. t
10. c	20. d

L. Completion

1. spina bifida cystica
2. grand mal seizures
3. intracranial tumors
4. quadriplegia
5. transient ischemic attack
6. herniated intervertebral disk
7. carpal tunnel syndrome
8. cerebral hemorrhage
9. Bell's palsy
10. metastatic intracranial tumors

CHAPTER 9

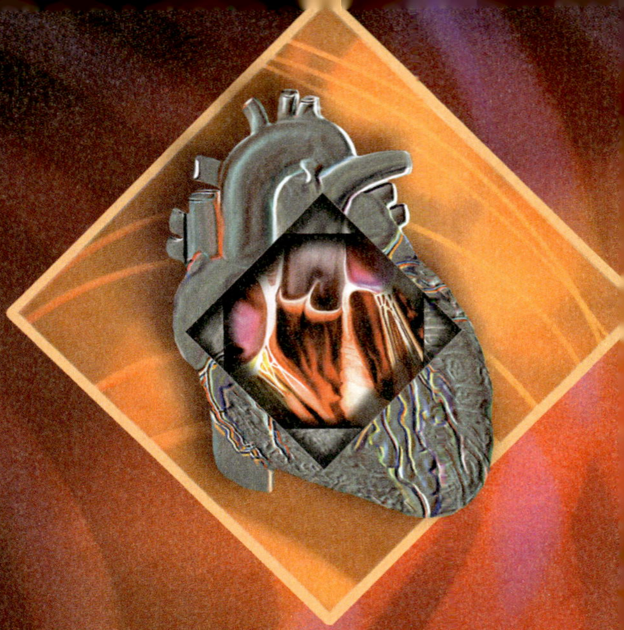

The Blood and Lymphatic Systems

CHAPTER CONTENT

KEY COMPETENCIES

Upon completing this chapter and the review exercises at the end of the chapter, the learner should be able to:

1. List the major functions of the blood and of the lymphatic system as identified in the chapter overview of each system.
2. Identify and define 30 pathological conditions of the blood and lymphatic systems.
3. Identify at least 10 diagnostic techniques used in the diagnosis and treatment of disorders of the blood and lymphatic systems.
4. Correctly spell and pronounce each new term introduced in this chapter using the Activity CD-ROM and Audio CD, if available.
5. Identify and define at least 10 medical terms related to the blood and lymphatic systems.
6. Identify at least 10 abbreviations common to the blood and lymphatic systems.
7. Identify at least 10 combining forms related to the blood and lymphatic systems.

OVERVIEW OF THE BLOOD SYSTEM

The cells of the body are dependent on a steady supply of oxygen and nutrients to carry out their normal metabolic functions. They are also dependent on a means of disposing metabolic waste products to maintain a balanced internal environment. What system does the body use to achieve the transportation of oxygen and nutrients to the body cells and the transportation of waste products away from the body cells? The blood system.

Blood is the liquid pumped by the heart through all the arteries, veins, and capillaries. It is much more than the simple liquid it seems to be; it is composed of a straw-colored fluid called **plasma,** the formed elements (cells and cell fragments), and a series of cell types with different functions. Two major functions of the blood are to transport oxygen and nutrients to the cells and to remove carbon dioxide and other waste products from the cells for elimination. You may have heard of the saying, "blood is thicker than water," when referring to family relationships. The words are true: Blood *is* thicker than water. The term **viscosity** refers to the thickness of a fluid as compared with water; and compared with water, blood is about 4 times thicker. The viscosity of blood remains relatively constant, but it changes if the number of blood cells changes or if the concentration of plasma proteins changes. An example of an increase in the viscosity of blood (e.g., the stickiness of the blood) would be an increase in the number of **erythrocytes** (red blood cells), which would result in the blood becoming more viscous, also causing the blood pressure to increase.

The total blood volume in an average adult male is 5 to 6 liters; in an average adult female, 4 to 5 liters. Blood accounts for approximately 8% of one's total body weight. It is slightly alkaline, having a pH of 7.35 to 7.45 (using water as the standard for a neutral liquid, with a pH of 7.0).

The scientific study of blood and blood-forming tissues is known as **hematology.** A medical specialist in the study of hematology is a **hematologist.**

Anatomy and Physiology (Blood)

The anatomy and physiology section in this chapter will concentrate on the composition of blood (liquid and solid components), the blood types, and the mechanisms of blood clotting.

Composition of Blood

The liquid portion of blood is known as plasma; that is, whole blood minus the formed elements. Plasma is essential for transporting the cellular elements (solid components) of blood throughout the circulatory system. Plasma is a yellow or straw-colored fluid that is about 90% water. The remaining portion consists of the following **solutes** (substances which are dissolved in a solution): electrolytes, proteins, fats, glucose, **bilirubin,** and gases. The most abundant of the solutes are the **plasma proteins.** These plasma proteins, which are manufactured mainly by the liver, are grouped into three major classes: albumins, globulins, and fibrinogen.

1. **Albumins** constitute approximately 60% of the plasma proteins. They help to maintain the normal blood volume and blood pressure. Because of their abundance, albumins attract water into the vessels through the capillaries by **osmosis** (fluid flows from a lesser concentration of solute to a greater concentration of solute). When this happens, the balance between the fluid in the blood and the fluid in the interstitial tissues is maintained; that is, the fluid will remain in the blood vessels as it should and will not leak out into the surrounding tissues. If this balance (osmotic pressure) is upset, then the fluid will leave the blood vessels, seep into the surrounding tissue spaces, and result in swelling of the tissues, or **edema.**
2. **Globulins** constitute approximately 36% of the plasma proteins. There are three types of globulins: alpha, beta, and gamma. The alpha and beta globulins serve primarily to transport lipids (fats) and fat-soluble vitamins in the blood. Gamma globulins are the antibodies that function in immunity.
3. **Fibrinogen** constitutes approximately 4% of the plasma proteins; it is the largest of the plasma proteins. Fibrinogen is essential in the process of blood clotting. The process of blood clotting, or **coagulation,** will be discussed in detail in another section of this chapter.

The solid components of the blood are the formed elements, or the cells and cell fragments, that are suspended in the plasma. The production of the formed elements in the blood is termed **hemopoiesis.** After birth, most of the production of blood cells occurs in the red bone marrow in specific regions of the body (skull, sternum, ribs, vertebrae, pelvis), with all types of blood cells developing from undifferentiated (unspecialized) stem cells called **hemocytoblasts.** As the blood cells develop from the hemocytoblast stage and undergo **differentiation** or become specialized in function, they mature into one of seven different cell lines, with each cell line having a different purpose. These seven different lines of specialized cells are grouped into three classifications: erythrocytes, leukocytes, and thrombocytes. Refer to **Figure 9-1** for a visual reference of the formed elements of the blood as the discussion continues.

Erythrocytes

The **(1) erythrocytes** are tiny biconcave-shaped discs that are thinner in the center than around the edges; they are also known as red blood cells (RBCs). Mature red blood cells do not have a **nucleus;** they have an average life span of approximately 120 days. The main component of the red blood cell is **hemoglobin,** which consists of **heme** (iron) and **globin** (protein). The biconcave shape of the red blood cell provides a maximum surface area for the bonding of oxygen to the hemoglobin to form **oxyhemoglobin.** Oxyhemoglobin is responsible for the bright red color of blood and is formed when the blood circulates through the lungs. Most of the oxygen used by the body cells is transported to the cellular level as oxyhemoglobin.

The primary function of the red blood cell is to transport oxygen to the cells of the body. Once the oxygen has been released to the cells, the biconcave shape of the red blood cell enables it to absorb carbon dioxide (a waste product of cellular metabolism). When this deoxygenated blood is returned to the lungs, the carbon dioxide is released through the process of exhalation and more oxygen is combined with the hemoglobin and distributed to the body cells.

The normal range of erythrocytes for a healthy adult male is 4.5 to 6 million per cubic millimeter of blood, and slightly less for a healthy adult female (about 4.8 million per cubic millimeter of blood). The erythrocytes are the most numerous of the formed elements in the blood.

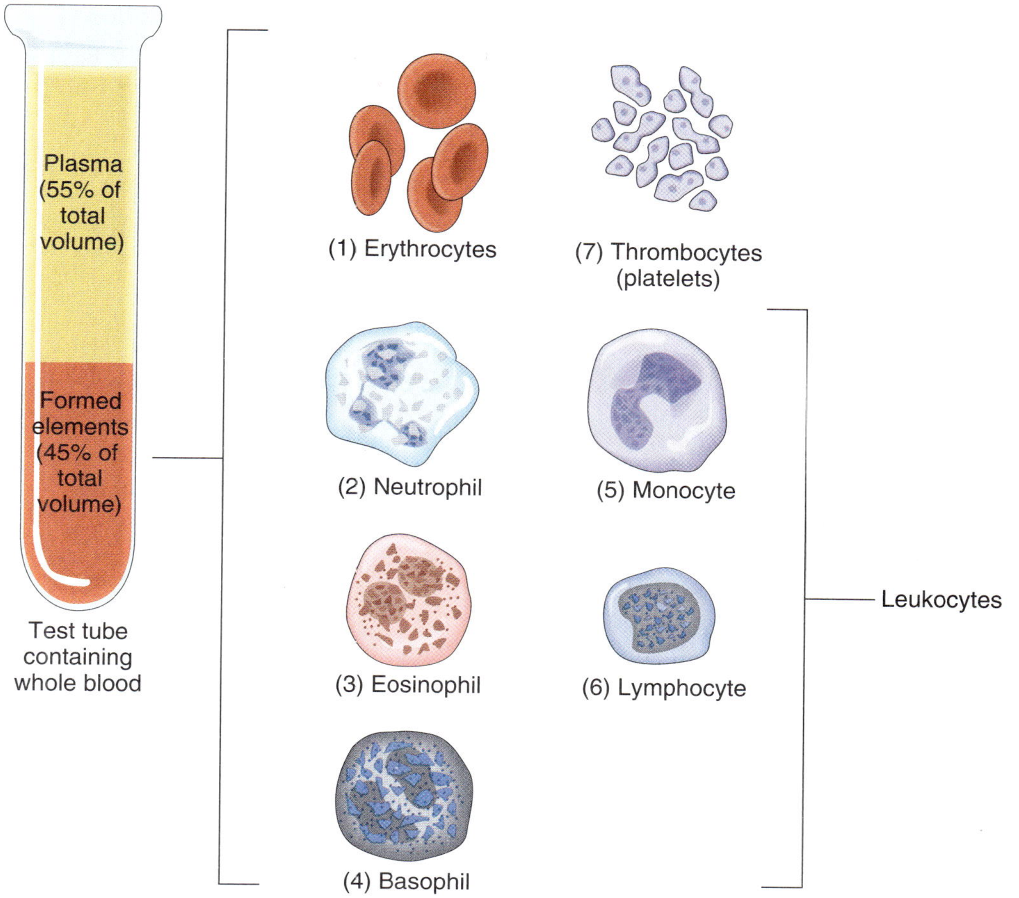

Figure 9-1 Formed elements of the blood

Leukocytes

Leukocytes are larger than erythrocytes, but are fewer in number. They are also called white blood cells (WBCs). A mature leukocyte does not lose its nucleus, and it does not possess hemoglobin. Leukocytes (five different types) are grouped into two categories: granulocytes and agranulocytes.

Granulocytes. **Granulocytes** consist of neutrophils, eosinophils, and basophils. They have granules in their cytoplasm that absorb various dyes when preparing a slide for viewing under the microscope. The various colors, as well as the shapes of the nuclei, help to identify the different white blood cells under the microscope. The **(2) neutrophils** constitute approximately 60% to 70% of all white blood cells; they have multilobed nuclei. Neutrophils are **phagocytic** in nature; that is, they respond to infections and tissue damage by engulfing and destroying bacteria. Neutrophils do not absorb acid or base dye very well; they remain a fairly neutral color. The **(3) eosinophils** constitute approximately 2% to 4% of all white blood cells; they have a nucleus with two lobes. Eosinophils increase in number in response to allergic reactions. Eosinophils will stain a red, rosy color with an acid dye. The **(4) basophils** constitute less than 1% of all white blood cells; they have a nucleus with two lobes. Basophils secrete histamine, which is released during allergic reactions, and **heparin,** which is a natural anticoagulant (prevents clotting). Basophils will stain a dark blue with a base dye.

Agranulocytes. Agranulocytes consist of monocytes and lymphocytes. They do not have granules in their cytoplasm and do not stain a dark color when preparing a slide for viewing under the microscope. Agranulocytes have a large nucleus that is not multi-lobed. The (5) **monocytes** constitute approximately 3% to 8% of all white blood cells; they are the largest of the white blood cells and have a kidney bean–shaped nucleus. Monocytes are phagocytic in nature. The (6) **lymphocytes** constitute approximately 20% to 25% of all white blood cells; they have a large spherical-shaped nucleus. Lymphocytes play an important role in the immune process: Some lymphocytes are phagocytic, in that they attack the bacteria directly, whereas other lymphocytes produce antibodies that destroy bacteria.

Thrombocytes

The (7) **thrombocytes** also known as **platelets,** are small, disc-shaped fragments of very large cells called **megakaryocytes.** Platelets contain no hemoglobin; they are essential for the normal clotting (coagulation) of blood. The average platelet count ranges from 250,000 to 500,000 platelets per cubic milliliter of blood.

Blood Types

When discussing blood types it is important to understand the relationship between antigens and antibodies. An **antigen,** also called an **agglutinogen,** is a substance present on the red blood cell that can stimulate the body to make antibodies. An **antibody** is a substance present in the plasma that reacts in some way with the antigen that stimulated its formation. Once the **antibodies** become established, they will be programmed to recognize the antigen as "foreign to the body" in the future, and will "attack it" if they come in contact with it again. In some cases, the antigen–antibody combination will result in **agglutination,** or clumping of the red blood cells. Because of this, it is critically important to match the antigens and antibodies of the blood donor and the blood recipient to prevent the possibility of agglutination. This is accomplished through clinical laboratory tests called blood typing and cross-matching.

The antigens on the red blood cells are organized into blood groups. Each person's blood belongs to one of the following four blood types: Type A, B, AB, or O. The letter designating the blood type indicates the type of antigen present on the red blood cell; for example, Type A blood has the A antigen present on its red blood cells. This means that the particular individual was born with the A antigen present on his or her red blood cells, and it also means that this individual will not have any anti-A antibodies present in his or her plasma that would destroy the A antigen. The plasma would, however, have anti-B antibodies present that would cause agglutination if the individual received Type B blood instead of its expected Type A. A breakdown of the antigen-antibody combinations for the four ABO blood types is listed in **Table 9-1.**

Table 9-1 ABO Blood Types

BLOOD TYPE	ANTIGEN PRESENT ON RBC	ANTIBODY PRESENT IN PLASMA
A	A	Anti-B antibody
B	B	Anti-A antibody
AB	AB	No antibodies present
O	No antigens present	Both anti-A and anti-B antibodies

The presence, or absence, of a specific antigen on the red blood cell will make a difference in the type of blood that a person can receive in a transfusion. The person who gives blood is called the **donor.** The person who receives the blood is called the **recipient.** For example, Type O blood is considered to be the "universal donor blood," because it does not have A antigens or B antigens present on its red blood cells; consequently, any anti-A or anti-B antibodies present in the recipient's plasma will not cause agglutination of the red blood cells of the donor blood. Type AB blood is considered to be the "universal recipient blood" because it contains no anti-A or anti-B antibodies in its plasma and will not clump any donor blood that contains either A or B antigens on its red blood cells. When blood is transfused from one individual to another, however, it should not be done without first **cross-matching,** that is, mixing the donor blood with the recipient blood and observing the mixture for agglutination of the donor's red blood cells.

Another important antigen located on the surface of the red blood cells is the **Rh factor.** This antigen is named "Rh" because it was first studied in the rhesus monkey. Individuals who have the Rh factor present on their red blood cells are said to be **Rh positive (Rh+)**; people who do not have the Rh factor present on their red blood cells are said to be **Rh negative (Rh−)**. There are two major concerns with Rh− individuals: (1) If an Rh− individual is exposed to Rh+ blood through a transfusion, the Rh− individual will develop anti-Rh antibodies that will cause a transfusion reaction (agglutination) should the Rh− individual receive Rh+ blood a second time. (2) If an Rh− mother gives birth to an Rh+ baby, and the Rh− and Rh+ bloods mix during the birth process (from ruptured vessels in the placenta), the Rh− mother's body will develop anti-Rh antibodies that will cause problems with future pregnancies. Specifically, if the Rh− mother has a subsequent pregnancy with an Rh+ baby, the anti-Rh antibodies that have been formed in her blood will recognize the Rh+ blood as foreign to her body and will pass through the placenta reacting with the Rh antigens on the red blood cells of the fetus. The result will be agglutination and destruction of the fetal red blood cells.

To prevent the possibility of future complications from the Rh negative–Rh positive interaction, the Rh− mother is given an injection of RhoGam after the birth of each Rh+ infant. This special preparation of anti-Rh globulin prevents the development of anti-Rh antibodies in the Rh− mother's blood.

Mechanisms of Blood Clotting

The clotting of blood is known as coagulation; its purpose is to plug ruptured blood vessels to stop bleeding. There are many steps involved in the mechanism of blood clotting. These chemical reactions take place in a definite and rapid sequence, resulting in the formation of a clot that stops the bleeding. The steps involved in the process of blood clotting are as follows:

1. There must be some kind of injury to a blood vessel that creates a roughened area in the vessel.
2. Some of the blood platelets will disintegrate as they flow over the rough spot in the blood vessel, releasing a substance called **thromboplastin.**
3. The thromboplastin will convert **prothrombin** (a blood protein) into the active enzyme, **thrombin.** This occurs in the presence of calcium ions and other clotting factors.
4. The thrombin will convert fibrinogen (another blood protein) into **fibrin.** This also occurs in the presence of calcium ions. The resulting fibrin threads will form a mesh that will adhere to the tissue of the damaged vessel to form a clot.

As mentioned, the normal mechanisms of clotting of blood are designed to stop bleeding. This occurs in response to injury to a blood vessel as described above. Unfortunately, clots sometimes form in uninjured blood vessels. This type of clot formation is abnormal and has the potential for stopping the flow of blood to a vital organ. The abnormal formation of clots can be life threatening. A clot that forms and stays in place in a blood vessel is known as a **thrombus.** The abnormal vascular condition in which a thrombus develops is called **thrombosis.** An abnormal circulatory condition in which a clot dislodges from its place and travels through the bloodstream is called an **embolism.** The dislodged, circulating clot is known as an **embolus.** In addition to a blood clot, an embolus may be a small bit of fatty tissue or air that travels through the bloodstream until it becomes lodged in a vessel.

Vocabulary (Blood)

The following vocabulary words are frequently used when discussing the blood.

WORD	DEFINITION
agglutination (ah-**gloo**-tih-**NAY**-shun)	The clumping together of cells as a result of interaction with specific antibodies called agglutinins. Agglutinins are used in blood typing and in identifying or estimating the strength of immunoglobulins or immune serums.
albumin (al-**BEW**-min)	A plasma protein. Various albumins are found in practically all animal tissues and in many plant tissues. In blood, albumin helps to maintain blood volume and blood pressure.
allergen (**AL**-er-jin)	A substance that can produce a hypersensitive reaction in the body.
allergy (**AL**-er-jee)	A hypersensitive reaction to normally harmless antigens, most of which are environmental.
anaphylaxis (**an**-ah-fih-**LAK**-sis)	An exaggerated, life-threatening hypersensitivity reaction to a previously encountered antigen.
anisocytosis (an-**ih**-soh-sigh-**TOH**-sis) aniso = unequal cyt/o = cell -osis = condition	An abnormal condition of the blood characterized by red blood cells of variable and abnormal size.
antibodies (**AN**-tih-bod-eez)	Substances produced by the body in response to bacteria, viruses, or other foreign substances. Each class of antibody is named for its action.
antigens (**AN**-tih-jenz)	A substance, usually a protein, that causes the formation of an antibody and reacts specifically with that antibody.
ascites (ah-**SIGH**-teez)	An abnormal intraperitoneal (within the peritoneal cavity) accumulation of a fluid containing large amounts of protein and electrolytes.
basophil (**BAY**-soh-fill)	A granulocytic white blood cell characterized by cytoplasmic granules that stain blue when exposed to a basic dye. Basophils represent 1% or less of the total white blood cell count.

bilirubin (bill-ih-**ROO**-bin)	The orange-yellow pigment of bile formed principally by the breakdown of hemoglobin in red blood cells after termination of their normal life span.
coagulation (koh-**ag**-yoo-**LAY**-shun)	The process of transforming a liquid into a solid, especially of the blood.
corpuscle (**KOR**-pus-ehl)	Any cell of the body; a red or white blood cell.
differentiation (**diff**-er-en-she-**AY**-shun)	A process in development in which unspecialized cells or tissues are systemically modified and altered to achieve specific and characteristic physical forms, physiologic functions, and chemical properties.
dyscrasia (dis-**KRAY**-zee-ah)	An abnormal condition of the blood or bone marrow, such as leukemia, aplastic anemia, or prenatal Rh incompatibility.
edema (eh-**DEE**-ma)	The abnormal accumulation of fluid in interstitial spaces of tissues.
electrophoresis (ee-**lek**-troh-for-**EE**-sis) **electr/o-** = electrical; electricity **-phoresis** = transmission	The movement of charged suspended particles through a liquid medium in response to changes in an electric field. Charged particles of a given substance migrate in a predictable direction and at a characteristic speed.
enzyme (**EN**-zime)	An organic substance that initiates and accelerates a chemical reaction.
eosinophil (**ee**-oh-**SIN**-oh-fill) **eosin/o** = red, rosy	A granulocytic, bilobed leukocyte somewhat larger than a neutrophil characterized by large numbers of coarse, refractile, cytoplasmic granules that stain with the acid dye, eosin.
erythremia (**ehr**-rih-**THREE**-mee-ah) **erythr/o** = red **-emia** = blood condition	An abnormal increase in the number of red blood cells.
erythroblast (eh-**RITH**-roh-blast) **erythr/o** = red **-blast** = immature cell	An immature red blood cell.
erythrocyte (eh-**RITH**-roh-sight) **erythr/o** = red **cyt/o** = cell **-e** = noun ending	A mature red blood cell.
erythropoiesis (eh-**rith**-roh-poy-**EE**-sis) **erythr/o** = red **-poiesis** = formation	The process of red blood cell production.
erythropoietin (eh-**rith**-roh-**POY**-eh-tin)	A hormone synthesized mainly in the kidneys and released into the bloodstream in response to anoxia (lack of oxygen). The hormone acts to stimulate and regulate the production of erythrocytes and is thus able to increase the oxygen-carrying capacity of the blood.

fibrin (**FIH**-brin)	A stringy, insoluble protein that is the substance of a blood clot.
fibrinogen (fih-**BRIN**-oh-jen)	A plasma protein that is converted into fibrin by thrombin in the presence of calcium ions.
globin (**GLOH**-bin)	A group of four globulin protein molecules that become bound by the iron in heme molecules to form hemoglobin.
globulin (**GLOB**-yew-lin)	A plasma protein made in the liver. Globulin helps in the synthesis of antibodies.
granulocyte (**GRAN**-yew-loh-sight) **granul/o** = granules **cyt/o** = cell **-e** = noun ending	A type of leukocyte characterized by the presence of cytoplasmic granules.
hematologist (hee-mah-**TALL**-oh-jist) **hemat/o** = blood **-logist** = one who specializes in the study of	A medical specialist in the field of hematology.
hematology (**hee**-mah-**TALL**-oh-jee) **hemat/o** = blood **-logy** = the study of	The scientific study of blood and blood-forming tissues.
heme (**HEEM**)	The pigmented, iron-containing, nonprotein portion of the hemoglobin molecule. Heme binds and carries oxygen in the red blood cells, releasing it to tissues that give off excess amounts of carbon dioxide.
hemoglobin (**hee**-moh-**GLOH**-bin)	A complex protein–iron compound in the blood that carries oxygen to the cells from the lungs and carbon dioxide away from the cells to the lungs.
hemolysis (**hee**-**MALL**-ih-sis) **hem/o** = blood **-lysis** = destruction or destruction breakdown	The breakdown of red blood cells and the release of hemoglobin that occurs normally at the end of the life span of a red cell.
hemorrhage (**HEM**-eh-rij) **hem/o** = blood **-rrhage** = excessive flow or discharge	A loss of a large amount of blood in a short period of time, either externally or internally. **Hemorrhage** may be arterial, venous, or capillary.
hemostasis (**hee**-moh-**STAY**-sis) **hem/o** = blood **-stasis** = stopping or controlling	The termination of bleeding by mechanical or chemical means or by the complex coagulation process of the body, consisting of vasoconstriction, platelet aggregation, and thrombin and fibrin synthesis.
heparin (**HEP**-er-in)	A naturally occurring anticlotting factor present in the body.

hyperalbuminemia (high-per-al-**byoo**-mih-**NEE**-mee-ah) **hyper-** = excessive **albumin/o** = protein, (albumin) **-emia** = blood condition	An increased level of albumin in the blood.
hyperbilirubinemia (high-per-**bill**-ih-roo-bin-**EE**-mee-ah)	Greater than normal amounts of the bile pigment, bilirubin, in the blood.
hyperlipemia (**high**-per-lip-**EE**-mee-ah) **hyper-** = excessive **lip/o** = fat **-emia** = blood condition	An excessive level of blood fats, usually caused by a lipoprotein lipase deficiency or a defect in the conversion of low-density lipoproteins to high-density lipoproteins; also called **hyperlipidemia.**
hyperlipidemia (**high**-per-lip-**id**-**EE**-mee-ah)	See *hyperlipemia.*
ion (**EYE**-on)	An electrically charged particle.
leukocyte (**LOO**-koh-sight) **leuk/o** = white **cyt/o** = cell **-e** = noun ending	A white blood cell, one of the formed elements of the circulating blood system.
leukocytopenia (**loo**-koh-**sigh**-toh-**PEE**-nee-ah) **leuk/o** = white **cyt/o** = cell **-penia** = decrease in; deficiency	An abnormal decrease in number of white blood cells to fewer than 5,000 cells per cubic millimeter.
megakaryocyte (**meg**-ah-**KAIR**-ee-oh-sight) **mega-** = large **kary/o** = nucleus **cyt/o** = cell **-e** = noun ending	An extremely large bone marrow cell.
monocyte (**MON**-oh-sight) **mono-** = one **cyt/o** = cell **-e** = noun ending	A large mononuclear leukocyte.
myeloid (**MY**-eh-loyd) **myel/o** = bone marrow, spinal cord **-oid** = resembling	Of or pertaining to the bone marrow or the spinal cord.

neutrophil (**NOO**-troh-fill)	A polymorphonuclear (multilobed nucleus), granular leukocyte that stains easily with neutral dyes.
pancytopenia (**pan**-sigh-toh-**PEE**-nee-ah) pan- = all cyt/o = cell -penia = deficiency	A marked reduction in the number of the red blood cells, white blood cells, and platelets.
plasma (**PLAZ**-mah)	The watery, straw-colored, fluid portion of the lymph and the blood in which the leukocytes, erythrocytes, and platelets are suspended.
platelet (**PLAYT**-let)	A clotting cell; a thrombocyte.
prothrombin (proh-**THROM**-bin)	A plasma protein precursor of thrombin. It is synthesized in the liver if adequate vitamin K is present.
reticulocyte (reh-**TIK**-yoo-loh-sight)	An immature erythrocyte characterized by a meshlike pattern of threads and particles at the former site of the nucleus.
septicemia (sep-tih-**SEE**-mee-ah)	Systemic infection in which pathogens are present in the circulating bloodstream, having spread from an infection in any part of the body.
seroconversion (**see**-roh-con-**VER**-zhun)	A change in serologic tests from negative to positive as antibodies develop in reaction to an infection or vaccine.
serology (see-**RALL**-oh-jee)	The branch of laboratory medicine that studies blood serum for evidence of infection by evaluating antigen–antibody reactions.
serum (**SEE**-rum)	Also called blood **serum.** The clear, thin, and sticky fluid portion of the blood that remains after coagulation. Serum contains no blood cells, platelets, or fibrinogen.
splenomegaly (**splee**-noh-**MEG**-ah-lee) splen/o = spleen -megaly = enlargement	An abnormal enlargement of the spleen.
stem cell	A formative cell; a cell whose daughter cells may give rise to other cell types.
thrombin (**THROM**-bin)	An enzyme formed from prothrombin, calcium, and thromboplastin in plasma during the clotting process; it causes fibrinogen to change to fibrin, which is essential in the formation of a clot.
thrombocyte (**THROM**-boh-sight) thromb/o = clot cyt/o = cell -e = noun ending	A clotting cell; a platelet.
thrombocytopenia (**throm**-boh-**sigh**-toh-**PEE**-nee-ah) thromb/o = clot cyt/o = cell -penia = decrease in; deficiency	An abnormal hematologic condition in which the number of platelets is reduced.

thromboplastin (throm-boh-**PLAST**-in)	A complex substance that initiates the clotting process by converting prothrombin into thrombin in the presence of calcium ion.
thrombus (**THROM**-bus) **thromb/o** = clot **-us** = noun ending	A clot.

Word Elements (Blood)

The following word elements pertain to the blood system. As you review the list, pronounce each word element aloud twice and check the box after you "say it." Write the definition for the example word given for each word element. You may use your medical dictionary.

WORD ELEMENT	PRONUNCIATION	"SAY IT"	MEANING
agglutin/o **agglutin**ation	ah-**GLOO**-tin-oh ah-**gloo**-tin-**NAY**-shun	☐	to clump
aniso- **aniso**cytosis	**AN**-ih-soh an-**ih**-soh-sigh-**TOH**-sis	☐	unequal
bas/o **baso**phil	**BAY**-soh **BAY**-soh-fill	☐	base
blast/o, -blast **blast**ocyte	**BLAST**-oh, **BLAST** **BLAST**-oh-sight	☐	embryonic stage of development
chrom/o **chromo**philic	**KROH**-moh kroh-moh-**FILL**-ik	☐	color
coagul/o **coagul**ation	koh-**AG**-yoo-loh koh-**ag**-yoo-**LAY**-shun	☐	clotting
cyt/o **cyto**genesis	**SIGH**-toh **sigh**-toh-**JEN**-ess-is	☐	cell
-emia polycyth**emia**	**EE**-mee-ah **pol**-ee-sigh-**THEE**-mee-ah	☐	blood condition
eosin/o **eosino**philia	ee-oh-**SIN**-oh **ee**-oh-**sin**-oh-**FILL**-ee-ah	☐	red, rosy
erythr/o **erythro**cytopenia	eh-**RITH**-roh eh-**rith**-roh-**sigh**-toh-**PEE**-nee-ah	☐	red
-globin hemo**globin**	**GLOH**-bin **hee**-moh-**GLOH**-bin	☐	containing protein
hem/o **hemo**dialysis	**HEE**-moh **hee**-moh-dye-**AL**-ih-sis	☐	blood

hemat/o **hemat**ologist	hee-**MAH**-toh hee-mah-**TALL**-oh-jist	☐	blood
is/o **is**otonic	**EYE**-soh **eye**-soh-**TON**-ik	☐	equal
kary/o **kary**ocyte	**KAR**-ee-oh **KAR**-ee-oh-sight	☐	nucleus
leuk/o **leuk**ocyte	**LOO**-koh **LOO**-koh-sight	☐	white
-lytic hemo**lytic**	**LIT**-ik **hee**-moh-**LIT**-ik	☐	destruction
mono- **mono**cytopenia	**MON**-oh **mon**-oh-**sigh**-toh-**PEE**-nee-ah	☐	one
morph/o **morph**ology	**MOR**-foh mor-**FALL**-oh-jee	☐	form, shape
myel/o **myel**oblast	**MY**-ell-oh **MY**-ell-oh-blast	☐	bone marrow or spinal cord
nucle/o **nucle**us	**NOO**-klee-oh **NOO**-klee-us	☐	nucleus
-oid spher**oid**	**OID** **SFEE**-royd	☐	resembling
-osis erythrocyt**osis**	**OH**-sis eh-**rith**-roh-sigh-**TOH**-sis	☐	condition
-penia pancyto**penia**	**PEE**-nee-ah **pan**-sigh-toh-**PEE**-nee-ah	☐	decrease in; deficiency
-phage macro**phage**	**FAYJ** **MAK**-roh-fayj	☐	to eat
phag/o **phag**ocyte	**FAG**-oh **FAG**-oh-sight	☐	to eat
-philia hemo**philia**	**FILL**-ee-ah **hee**-moh-**FILL**-ee-ah	☐	attraction to
-phoresis electro**phoresis**	for-**EE**-sis ee-**lek**-troh-for-**EE**-sis	☐	transmission
-poiesis erythro**poiesis**	poy-**EE**-sis eh-**rith**-roh-poy-**EE**-sis	☐	formation
poikil/o **poikil**ocytosis	**POY**-kill-oh **poy**-kill-oh-sigh-**TOH**-sis	☐	varied; irregular

sider/o **sider**oblast	**SID**-er-oh **SID**-er-oh-**blast**	☐	iron
spher/o **spher**ocytosis	**SFEE**-roh **sfee**-roh-sigh-**TOH**-sis	☐	round; sphere
-stasis hemo**stasis**	**STAY**-sis **hee**-moh-**STAY**-sis	☐	stopping or controlling
thromb/o **thromb**osis	**THROM**-boh throm-**BOH**-sis	☐	clot

Pathological Conditions (Blood)

As you study the pathological conditions of the blood, note that the **basic definition** is in bold print, followed by a detailed description in regular print. The phonetic pronunciation is directly beneath each term, and a breakdown of the component parts of the term when appropriate.

anemia
(an-**NEE**-mee-ah)
an- = without
-emia = blood condition

Anemia describes a condition in which there is a deficiency of oxygen being delivered to the cells because of a decrease in the quantity of hemoglobin or red blood cells.

There are various classifications of anemias; each is named according to the cause. The following are some clinical manifestations that are similar in all the types of anemia: fatigue, paleness of the skin, headache, fainting, tingling sensations and numbness, loss of appetite, swelling in the lower extremities, and difficulty breathing.

anemia, aplastic
(an-**NEE**-mee-ah, ah-**PLAST**-ik)
an- = without
-emia = blood condition
a- = without
plast/o = formation, development
-ic = pertaining to

Also called bone marrow depression anemia, aplastic anemia is characterized by pancytopenia, an inadequacy of the formed blood elements (RBCs, WBCs, and platelets).

The lack of formation of the blood elements is believed to be due to an insult to the bone marrow's stem cells.

The cause of aplastic anemia is not known in at least two-thirds of the cases. It may develop simultaneously with infections, or following an injury to the bone marrow. Aplastic anemia may occur because of a neoplastic disorder of the bone marrow, chemotherapy drugs, certain antibiotics (chloramphenicol) and other medications, or exposure to radiation or certain toxic chemicals.

The person with aplastic anemia will be treated with blood transfusions until their bone marrow is capable of forming new cells. In some persons, the preferred treatment is a bone marrow transplant from a close tissue match (usually an identical twin or sibling).

anemia, hemolytic
(an-**NEE**-mee-ah, **he**-moh-**LIT**-ik)
an- = without
-emia = blood condition
hem/o = blood
-lytic = destruction

Hemolytic anemia is characterized by the extreme reduction in circulating RBCs due to their destruction.

The destruction of the RBCs may occur because of intrinsic or extrinsic causes. Cell membrane weaknesses and structural defects in the hemoglobin are examples of intrinsic causes. Extrinsic examples include infections, drugs, toxins, chemicals, trauma, and artificial heart valves.

anemia, pernicious
(an-**NEE**-mee-ah, per-**NISH**-us)
an- = without
-emia = blood condition

Pernicious anemia results from a deficiency of mature RBCs and the formation and circulation of megaloblasts (large nucleated, immature, poorly functioning RBCs) with marked poikilocytosis (RBC shape variation), and anisocytosis (RBC size variation).

The formation of these distorted RBCs is due to a lack of vitamin B_{12} absorption necessary for proper maturation of the RBCs. Vitamin B_{12} chemically binds with the intrinsic factor, a protein secreted by the stomach, which protects the vitamin B_{12} until it is absorbed in the ileum. A shortage or absence of the intrinsic factor, normally found in gastric acids, results in an inadequate amount of vitamin B_{12}, erythroblast destruction, and ineffective erythropoiesis. There may also be a mild reduction in the production of mature WBCs and platelets.

Pernicious anemia typically occurs in persons over 60 years of age and is believed to be related to an autoimmune response. Along with loss of appetite, fatigue, irritability, and shortness of breath, the person experiencing pernicious anemia may also complain of a sore tongue. The destruction of the erythroblasts may result in elevated bilirubin levels in the blood and a jaundiced (yellowish) appearance to the skin. Treatment is lifelong vitamin B_{12} administration.

anemia, sickle cell
(an-**NEE**-mee-ah, **SIKL SELL**)
an- = without, not
-emia = blood condition

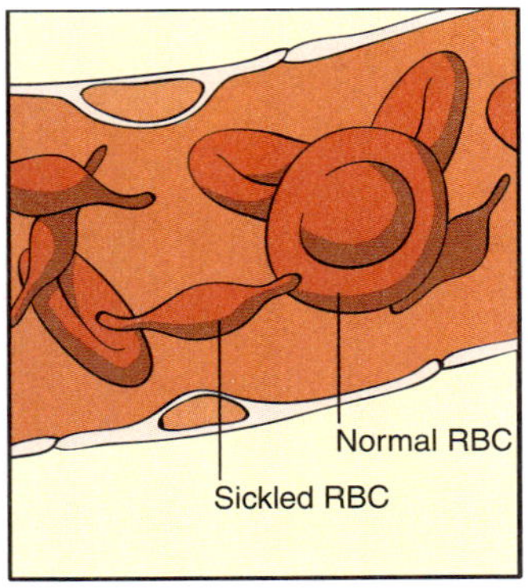

Figure 9-2 Regular and sickled RBCs

Sickle cell is a chronic hereditary form of hemolytic anemia in which the RBCs become shaped like a crescent in the presence of low oxygen concentration. See Figure 9-2.

These elongated, crescent-shaped RBCs clump together forming thromboses (clots), which occlude small blood vessels and cause areas of infarction (loss of oxygen), creating a great deal of pain for the individual. The pain is usually located in the hands, feet, and abdominal cavity. As oxygen concentration is reestablished, the crescent-shaped cells begin to resume their unsickled shape. It is the frequency of the changes in shape that renders the RBCs weakened, which then leads to hemolysis.

This disorder is inherited by the presence of one gene (sickle cell trait) or two genes (sickle cell disease) most typically among persons of African descent. Complications of sickle cell anemia include heart murmurs, congestive heart failure, enlarged liver, jaundice, gallstones, reduced urine concentration, hematuria, osteomyelitis, lower extremity ulcers, and problem with the eyes.

granulocytosis
(**gran**-yew-loh-sigh-**TOH**-sis)
granul/o = granules

Granulocytosis is an abnormally elevated number of granulocytes in the circulating blood as a reaction to any variety of inflammation or infection.

cyt/o = cell
-osis = condition

In particular allergic conditions such as parasitic infections or asthma, there is a spiraling of eosinophilic granulocytes called eosinophilia. In particular types of leukemia, the number of basophilic granulocytes are increased; a condition called basophilia.

---

hemochromatosis
(**hee**-moh-**kroh**-mah-**TOH**-sis)
hem/o = blood
chromat/o = color
-osis = condition

Hemochromatosis is a rare iron metabolism disease characterized by iron deposits throughout the body, usually as a complication of one of the hemolytic anemias.

Typically seen in men over 40, the person with hemochromatosis has an enlarged liver and a bronze skin pigmentation. Congestive heart failure or diabetes mellitus are frequent secondary complications of hemochromatosis. Treatment is multiple blood transfusions.

---

hemophilia
(**hee**-moh-**FILL**-ee-ah)
hem/o = blood
phil/o = attraction to
-ia = condition

Hemophilia involves different hereditary inadequacies of coagulation factors resulting in prolonged bleeding times.

Hemophilia A, also called classic hemophilia, is the most common type (accounts for approximately 83%) and is the result of a deficiency or absence of antihemophilic factor VIII. This factor VIII deficiency results in traumatic or spontaneous bleeding. Nearly all cases are reported in males and are characterized by bleeding in the joints, gums, or mouth. Hematuria is a common characteristic. Repeated joint bleeding produces extreme pain and deformity. The bleeding tendency can be relieved by transfusing factor VIII or fresh plasma.

Hemophilia B, also called Christmas disease, is the deficiency of a coagulation factor called factor IX and accounts for approximately 10% to 15% of the cases of hemophilia. Hemophilia B is only distinguishable from Hemophilia A through laboratory differentiation of factor deficiencies.

Other less common forms of hemophilia are Von Willebrand's disease and Rosenthal's disease.

---

leukemia (ALL, AML, CML)
(loo-**KEE**-mee-ah)
leuk/o = white
-emia = blood condition

Leukemia is an excessive uncontrolled increase of immature WBCs in the blood eventually leading to infection, anemia, and thrombocytopenia (decreased number of platelets).

The course of leukemia is subclassified as acute or chronic.

Acute leukemia has a rapid onset and swiftly progresses to severe thrombocytopenia, progressive anemia, infective lesions in the throat and mouth, high fever, and severe infection. Affecting adults and the elderly, the onset of chronic leukemia is gradual and its progression slower than with the acute form. Leukemia is classified further according to tissue type and cell involvement.

Acute myelogenous leukemia (AML) is predominated by immature granulocytes.

Acute lymphocytic leukemia (ALL) is predominated by immature lymphocytes and develops most frequently in children and adolescents.

Chronic myelogenous leukemia (CML) has immature and mature granulocytes existing in the bloodstream and bone marrow.

Chronic lymphocytic leukemia (CLL) is predominated by exceptional amounts of lymphocytes found in the spleen, bone marrow, and lymph nodes that are abnormal, small, and mature.

The symptoms of all types of leukemia are similar and occur because the bone marrow produces large numbers of nonfunctioning leukocytes and decreased production of platelets and RBCs.

Symptoms characteristic of nonfunctioning leukocytes include nail and skin infections, fever, throat and mouth ulcers, pneumonia, cystitis, and **septicemia.**

Symptoms characteristic of decreased RBCs (anemia) include fatigue, lethargy, pallor, rapid pulse, and difficulty breathing.

Symptoms characteristic of decreased platelets include petechiae (pinpoint hemorrhages), hematuria, bruising, hematomas, scleral or retinal hemorrhage, and gastrointestinal bleeding.

Along with the CBC results and a thorough history, a bone marrow aspiration is completed to confirm the diagnosis of leukemia. Treatment for all forms of leukemia focuses on the relief of symptoms and the achievement of remission through the use of radiation therapy, chemotherapy, and bone marrow transplantation.

---

multiple myeloma (plasma cell myeloma)
(**MULL**-tih-pl my-eh-**LOH**-mah)
myel/o = bone marrow, spinal cord
-oma = tumor

A malignant plasma cell neoplasm, multiple myeloma causes an increase in the number of both mature and immature plasma cells, which often entirely replace the bone marrow and destroy the skeletal structure.

The bones grow so fragile that the slightest movement can result in a fracture.

An abnormal protein, called the Bence Jones protein, is found almost exclusively in the urine of individuals with multiple myeloma. Other characteristics include increased susceptibility to infections, anemia, hypercalcemia, and renal damage. The survival statistics for multiple myeloma are poor and depend strongly on the individual's response to chemotherapy.

---

polycythemia vera
(**pol**-ee-sigh-**THEE**-mee-ah **VAIR**-ah)
poly- = many, much, excessive
-cythemia = condition involving cells of the blood

Polycythemia vera is an abnormal increase in the number of RBCs, granulocytes, and thrombocytes leading to an increase in blood volume and viscosity (thickness).

The exact cause of polycythemia vera is unknown. The increased viscosity of the blood results in congestion of the spleen and liver with RBCs as well as stasis and thrombosis in other areas.

The clinical manifestations of polycythemia vera include light-headedness, headaches, visual disturbances, vertigo, ruddy cyanosis of the face, and eventual congestive failure due to the increased work load on the heart. Treatment includes removal of blood through a phlebotomy to decrease the blood volume and administration of myelotoxic drugs to suppress the bone marrow's production of cells.

purpura
(**PURR**-pew-rah)
purpur/o = purple
-a = noun ending

Purpura is a collection of blood beneath the skin in the form of pinpoint hemorrhages appearing as red-purple skin discolorations.

These small hemorrhages are caused from a decreased number of circulating platelets (thrombocytopenia). The body may produce an antiplatelet factor that will damage its own platelets.

Idiopathic thrombocytopenic purpura is a disorder in which antibodies are made by the individual that destroys his or her own platelets. The cause of the prolonged bleeding time is unknown. Corticosteroids are administered and many times the individuals require the removal of the spleen to stop platelet destruction.

Purpura is also seen in persons with low platelet counts for other associated reasons such as drug reactions and leukemia.

thalassemia
(thal-ah-**SEE**-mee-ah)

Thalassemia is a hereditary form of hemolytic anemia in which the alpha or beta hemoglobin chains are defective and the production of hemoglobin is deficient, creating hypochromic microcytic RBCs.

This form of anemia is most frequently seen in persons of Mediterranean descent.

In the severe form of thalassemia, blood transfusions are necessary to sustain life. As a result of these frequent transfusions there is an accumulation of iron in the liver, heart, and pancreas, which eventually leads to failure of these organs.

Diagnostic Techniques and Procedures (Blood)

direct antiglobulin test (Coomb's test)
(dih-**RECT** an-tih-**GLOB**-yew-lin test)

The direct antiglobulin (blood) test is used to discover the presence of antierythrocyte antibodies present in the blood of an Rh negative woman. The production of these antibodies is associated with an Rh incompatibility between a pregnant Rh negative woman and her Rh positive fetus.

If these antibodies are present in the Rh negative woman's blood, it indicates that her red blood cells, which lack the Rh antigen, will be stimulated to produce the antierythrocyte antibodies if they come in contact with Rh positive blood (which could happen if any of the blood from the fetus should pass through the umbilical cord into maternal circulation during the pregnancy). If this interaction occurs between the Rh positive and Rh negative blood, the maternal antibodies can cause severe hemolysis of the fetal blood resulting in high levels of bilirubin by the time of birth.

A Coomb's test can also be performed on an individual who has suffered from a blood transfusion reaction to determine the causative factor.

bleeding time

Measurement of the time required for bleeding to stop.

The normal bleeding time, according to one of the more common methods to evaluate bleeding time (the Ivy method), is 1 to 9 minutes. Prolonged times may be seen in the following situations: decreased number of platelets, over activity of the spleen, leukemia, bone marrow failure, and bone marrow infiltration with primary or metastatic tumor.

blood transfusion
(blood trans-**FEW**-zhun)

An administration of blood or a blood component to an individual to replace blood lost through surgery, trauma, or disease.

It is critical that antibodies to the donor's RBCs are not present in the recipient and antibodies to the recipient's RBCs are not present in the donor. A hypersensitivity reaction (mild fever to severe hemolysis) will occur if either of the previous situations is present. These types of reactions are kept to a minimum by typing for major Rh and ABO antigens.

In addition to typing, the blood is cross-matched to distinguish mismatches caused by minor antigens. The process of cross-matching includes the mixing of the donor's RBCs and the recipient's serum in saline solution, and performing the indirect Coomb's test by adding Coomb's serum.

When a person receives blood or a blood component that has been previously collected from that person through a reinfusion, it is called an **autologous transfusion.**

bone marrow biopsy
(bone marrow **BY**-op-see)

The microscopic exam of bone marrow tissue, which fully evaluates hematopoiesis by revealing the number, shape, and size of the RBCs and WBCs and platelet precursors.

The bone marrow samples are obtained through aspiration or surgical removal.

The bone marrow biopsy procedure is a valuable tool in assessing and diagnosing abnormal blood conditions such as leukemias, anemias, and conditions involving elevated and/or decreased platelet counts.

bone marrow transplant

After receiving an intravenous infusion of aggressive chemotherapy or total-body irradiation to destroy all malignant cells and to inactivate the immune system, a donor's bone marrow cells are infused intravenously into the recipient.

There must be a close match of the donor's tissue and blood cells to that of the recipient. The desired effect is for the infused marrow to repopulate the marrow space of the recipient with normal cells. This procedure is performed on persons with leukemia and aplastic anemia.

Complications of a bone marrow transplant include serious infections, potential for rejection of the donor's cells by the recipient's cells (graft versus host), and relapse of the original disease. Transplant recipients are placed on immunosuppressant medications to lessen the possibility of bone marrow transplant rejection.

complete blood cell count (CBC)

A series of tests performed on peripheral blood, which inexpensively screens for problems in the hematologic system as well as several other organ systems.

Included in the CBC are:

1. **RBC count** (measures the number of RBCs per cubic millimeter of blood)
2. **Hemoglobin** (measures the number of grams of hemoglobin/ 100 ml of blood)
3. **Hematocrit** (measures the percent volume of the RBCs in whole blood)
4. **RBC indices** (measures erythrocyte size and hemoglobin content)
5. **WBC count** (measures the number of white blood cells in a cubic millimeter of blood)
6. **WBC differential** (determines the proportion of each of the five types of white blood cells in a sample of 100 WBCs)
7. **Blood smear** (an examination of the peripheral blood to determine variations and abnormalities in RBCs, WBCs, and platelets)
8. **Platelet count** (measures the number of platelets in a cubic millimeter of blood)

erythrocyte sedimentation rate (ESR)
(eh-**RITH**-roh-sight **sed**-ih-men-**TAY**-shun **RATE**)
erythr/o = red
cyt/o = cell
-e = noun ending

Erythrocyte sedimentation rate (ESR) is a test performed on the blood, which measures the rate at which red blood cells settle out in a tube of unclotted blood. The ESR is determined by measuring the settling distance of RBCs in normal saline over 1 hour.

The protein content of plasma is increased in the presence of inflammation; therefore, the RBCs tend to clump on top of one another, raising their weight and thus increasing the ESR. The ESR will be increased in the following conditions: pneumonia, acute myocardial infarction (heart attack), severe anemia, and cancer. The ESR will be decreased in congestive heart failure, sickle cell anemia, polycythemia vera, and angina pectoris.

hematocrit
(hee-**MAT**-oh-krit)
hemat/o = blood

An assessment of RBC percentage in the total blood volume.

Typically, the hematocrit point percentage is roughly 3 times the hemoglobin when the RBCs contain average quantities of hemoglobin and are standard size. Certain factors may interfere with the hematocrit values such as hemodilution or dehydration, abnormal RBC size, excessive WBC count, pregnancy, high altitudes, and certain drugs.

Increased levels are seen in congenital heart disease, dehydration, polycythemia vera, burns, shock, surgery, trauma, and severe diarrhea. Decreased levels are seen with anemia, leukemia, hemorrhage, hemolytic anemia, dietary deficiency, bone marrow failure, malnutrition, multiple myeloma, and organ failure.

hemoglobin test
(**hee**-moh-**GLOH**-bin)
hem/o = blood
-globin = containing protein

Concentration measurement of the hemoglobin in the peripheral blood. As a vehicle for transport of oxygen and carbon dioxide, hemoglobin levels provide information about the body's ability to supply tissues with oxygen.

There are increased levels of hemoglobin in congenital heart disease, polycythemia vera, chronic obstructive pulmonary disease (COPD), congestive heart failure, dehydration, and severe burns. Decreased levels of hemoglobin are noted in anemia, hemolysis, sickle cell anemia, enlargement of the spleen (**splenomegaly**), cancer, severe hemorrhage, and nutritional deficiency.

lipid profile
(**LIP**-id profile)
lip/o = fat

A lipid profile measures the lipids in the blood.

The standard concentration of total lipids in the blood is 400–800 mg/dl. triglycerides, 10–90 mg/dl; cholesterol, 150–250 mg/dl; phospholipids, 150–380 mg/dl; fatty acids, 9–15 mmol/l; phospholipid as phosphorus, 9–16 mg/dl; and neutral fat, 0–200 mg/dl. Lipids that are insoluble in water are found in foods and stored in the body where their reserve serves as a concentrated source of energy. High levels of cholesterol and triglycerides are identified with an increased risk for atherosclerosis.

partial thromboplastin time (PTT)
(**throm**-boh-**PLAST**-tin)

A blood test used to evaluate the common pathway and system of clot formation within the body.

The PTT assesses various blood clotting factors such as fibrinogen (factor I), prothrombin (factor II), and factors V, VIII, IX, X, XI, and XII. The PTT is prolonged if there is an insufficient quantity of any of these factors. Heparin will prolong the PTT by inactivating factor II and interfering with the formation of thromboplastin. The PTT is used to monitor the effectiveness of heparin therapy. Normal PTT is 60 to 70 seconds; the critical value is greater than 100 seconds.

Increased PTT levels may be the result of vitamin K deficiency, leukemia, heparin administration, cirrhosis, disseminated intravascular coagulation, or clotting factor deficiencies. Decreased PTT levels are usually the result of disseminated intravascular coagulation in the early stages of extensive cancer.

platelet count
(**PLAYT**-let)

The count of platelets per cubic millimeter of blood.

Counts of 150,000–400,000/mm^3 are deemed normal. Thrombocytopenia is indicated at counts less than 100,000/mm^3. Counts greater than 400,000/mm^3 indicate thrombocytosis. This increase in the number of platelets (thrombocytosis) may cause organ tissue death due to loss of blood supply, and spontaneous hemorrhage can occur with thrombocytopenia (decreased number of platelets).

Thrombocytopenia may occur due to leukemia, liver disease, kidney disease, pernicious anemia, hemolytic anemia, cancer chemotherapy, and hemorrhage. Thrombocytosis typically occurs with malignant disorders, polycythemia vera, leukemia, cirrhosis, and trauma.

prothrombin time (PT)
(proh-**THROM**-bin)

Prothrombin time (PT) is a blood test used to evaluate the common pathway and extrinsic system of clot formation.

The PT assesses the clotting proficiency of factors I and II (fibrinogen and prothrombin), and factors V, VII, and X. If there is an insufficient quantity of any of these factors, the PT is prolonged. Anticoagulants (e.g., coumadin) will prolong the PT. The PT is used to monitor the effectiveness of coumadin therapy. Normal PT is 11.0 to 12.5 seconds; the critical value is greater than 20 seconds.

red blood cell count (RBC)

The measurement of the circulating number of RBCs in 1 mm^3 of peripheral blood.

The standard time that a functioning RBC remains in the peripheral blood is an average of 120 days, during which time the RBCs enable oxygen and carbon dioxide to be transported and exchanged. The spleen extracts the hemolyzed RBCs as well as abnormal RBCs from the circulation. Intravascular trauma to the RBCs caused from atherosclerotic plaques and artificial heart valves will shorten the life span of the RBC. Anemia is present with a 10% decrease in value of the RBCs. The standard concentration of RBCs in whole blood of females is 4.2–6.2 million/cubic millimeters and in males is 4.6–6.2 million/cubic millimeters.

Increased levels of RBCs is seen in persons experiencing dehydration/hemoconcentration, polycythemia vera, high altitudes, pulmonary fibrosis, and congenital heart disease. Decreased levels are found in persons with overhydration/hemodilution, anemia, advanced cancer, antineoplastic chemotherapy, organ failure, dietary deficiency, hemorrhage, and bone marrow fibrosis.

red blood cell morphology
(mor-**FALL**-oh-jee)

Red blood cell morphology is an examination of the RBC on a stained blood smear that enables the examiner to identify the form and shape of the RBCs.

RBCs that are hypochromic (have a reduced hemoglobin content) can be seen, as well as the identification of RBCs that are sickled, abnormally shaped, and have an abnormal size. Poikilocytosis (irregular-shaped red blood cells) and anisocytosis (inequality of red blood cell size) can also be distinguished.

reticulocyte count
(reh-**TIK**-yew-loh-sight)

Reticulocyte count is a measurement of the number of circulating reticulocytes, immature erythrocytes, in a blood specimen.

Reticulocyte count is a direct indication of the bone marrow's production of RBCs.

Increased levels may be caused by hemolytic anemia, leukemias, sickle cell anemia, pregnancy, or 3 to 4 days post hemorrhage. A decreased level of reticulocytes is seen in persons with pernicious anemia, aplastic anemia, cirrhosis of the liver, folic acid deficiency, bone marrow failure, chronic infection, as well as those who have received radiation therapy.

rouleaux
(roo-**LOH**)

Rouleaux is an aggregation of RBCs viewed through the microscope that may be an artifact, or may occur with persons with multiple myeloma as a result of abnormal proteins.

Schilling test

A diagnostic analysis for pernicious anemia.

Orally administered radioactive cobalt is tagged with vitamin B_{12} and the gastrointestinal absorption is evaluated by the radioactivity of the urine samples collected over a 24-hour period. The standard percent of radioactive B_{12} within 24 hours is 8% to 40%. In the person with pernicious anemia, the percentage of radioactive B_{12} will be decreased as a result of the inability to absorb vitamin B_{12}.

white blood cell (WBC) count

The measurement of the circulating number of WBCs in 1 mm^3 of peripheral blood.

An elevated WBC count (leukocytosis) typically indicates inflammation, infection, leukemic neoplasia, or tissue necrosis. Physical or emotional stress or trauma may increase the total WBC count. A reduction in the WBC count (leukopenia) results from bone marrow failure, which may occur following chemotherapy or radiation therapy, with an overwhelming infection, autoimmune diseases, drug toxicity, or dietary deficiencies.

white blood cell differential
(**diff**-er-**EN**-shal)

The white blood cell differential is a measurement of the percentage of each specific type of circulating WBCs present in 1 mm^3 of peripheral blood drawn for the WBC count.

The specific types measured are neutrophils, lymphocytes, monocytes, eosinophils, and basophils. Lymphocytes and neutrophils comprise 75% to 90% of the total WBCs.

The standard time that a functioning neutrophil remains in the peripheral blood is an average of 6 hours during which time it is responsible for digesting and killing bacterial microorganisms. The standard percentage of segmented neutrophils is 50% to 70%. Trauma and acute bacterial infections prompt neutrophil production, which results in an elevated WBC count and sometimes a life span of 2 hours or less. Early immature forms of neutrophils enter the circulation early as a result of the increased production and are called "stab" cells or "band" cells (the standard percentage is only 0 to 5%). This process indicates an ongoing acute bacterial infection, also called a "shift to the left."

The life span of the lymphocytes varies immensely from a few days, months, or years. The lymphocytes are responsible for fighting acute viral infections and chronic bacterial infections. The differential count combines the number of the T cells and the B cells and the normal count is 20% to 40%. The T cells are dedicated to cellular-type immune responses and the B cells are committed to antibody production or taking part in cellular immunity.

Monocytes have a standard life span in the circulation of about 36 hours. These phagocytic cells are capable of fighting bacteria similarly to neutrophils, but are manufactured more rapidly and occupy more time in the circulation. The normal percentage of monocytes is 1% to 6%.

The standard percentage of eosinophils is 1% to 4% and basophils is 0 to 1%. Both of these types of WBCs are involved in the allergic response or parasitic infestations.

Common Abbreviations (Blood)

ABBREVIATION	MEANING	ABBREVIATION	MEANING
Ab	antibody	**HDL**	high-density lipoprotein
Ag	antigen	**Hgb**	hemoglobin (also Hbg)
ABO	blood groups: A, AB, B, and O	**IgA, IgD, IgE, IgG, IgM**	immunoglobulin A, D, E, G, and M, respectively
AHF	antihemophilic factor (blood coagulation factor VIII)	**LDL**	low-density lipoprotein
AHG	antihemolytic globulin	**lymph**	lymphocyte
ALL	acute lymphatic leukemia	**MCH**	mean cell hemoglobin
AML	acute myelogenous leukemia	**MCHC**	mean cell hemoglobin concentration
BMT	bone marrow transplantation	**MCV**	mean cell volume
CBC	complete blood (cell) count	**mono.**	monocyte
CLL	cholesterol-lowering lipid chronic lymphocytic leukemia	**poly.**	polymorphonuclear leukocyte
diff. diag.	differential diagnosis	**PMN**	polymorphonuclear neutrophil (leukocytes)
eos.	eosinophil	**PA**	pernicious anemia
ESR	erythrocyte sedimentation rate	**PT**	prothrombin time
G-CSF	granulocyte colony-stimulating factor	**PTT**	partial thromboplastin time
GM-CSF	granulocyte-macrophage colony-stimulating factor	**RBC**	red blood cell (erythrocyte)
Hb	hemoglobin	**segs**	segmented neutrophils
Hbg	hemoglobin (also Hgb)	**VLDL**	very-low-density lipoprotein
Hct	hematocrit	**WBC**	white blood cell (leukocyte)

OVERVIEW OF THE LYMPHATIC SYSTEM

The lymphatic system is often considered a part of the circulatory system because it consists of a moving fluid—**lymph**—which comes from the blood and returns to the blood by way of vessels (the lymphatic vessels). The lymphatic system consists of **lymph fluid,** which stems from the blood and tissue fluid, **lymph vessels,** which are similar to blood vessels and are designed to return the tissue fluid to the bloodstream, **lymph nodes,** which are located along the path of the collecting vessels, and specialized lymphatic organs such as the **thymus, spleen,** and the **tonsils.** The lymph vessels differ from the vessels of the cardiovascular system in that they do not form a closed circuit as do the vessels of the cardiovascular system; instead, they originate in the intercellular spaces of the soft tissues of the body.

The two most important functions of the lymphatic system are (1) to produce antibodies and lymphocytes that are important to immunity, and (2) to maintain a balance of fluid in the internal environment.

The lymphatic system is an important part of the **immune system,** which protects the body against disease-producing organisms and other foreign bodies. The immune system includes the bone marrow, thymus, lymphoid tissues, lymph nodes, spleen, and lymphatic vessels.

The state of being resistant to or protected from a disease is known as **immunity;** the individual is said to be immune. The process of creating immunity to a specific disease in an individual is known as **immunization.** The study of the reaction of tissues of the immune system of the body to antigenic stimulation is **immunology.** The health specialist whose training and experience is concentrated in immunology is an **immunologist.**

Anatomy and Physiology (Lymphatic)

The anatomy and physiology section on the lymphatic system includes a discussion of the lymph vessels, lymph nodes, thymus, spleen, and tonsils.

Lymph Vessels

The smallest lymphatic vessels are the **lymphatic capillaries.** The capillaries originate in the tissue spaces as blind-ended sacs. Water and solutes continually filter out of capillary blood into the interstitial spaces. As interstitial fluid begins to accumulate, it is picked up by the lymphatic capillaries and is eventually returned to the blood. Once the interstitial fluid enters the lymphatic vessels, it is known as lymph. It is critical that the interstitial fluid be returned to the general circulation and not remain in the tissue spaces because the accumulation of fluid within the tissue spaces would cause swelling, or edema. The lymphatic capillaries transport the lymph into larger vessels known as **lymphatic vessels,** which have valves to prevent the backward flow of fluid. The lymphatic vessels, like the veins of the cardiovascular system, have valves; but unlike the cardiovascular system veins, the lymphatic vessels transport fluid in only one direction, which is away from the tissues, toward the thoracic cavity.

The lymphatic vessels continue to merge to form larger vessels, eventually entering the two **lymphatic ducts:** the right lymphatic duct and the thoracic duct. See **Figure 9-3.**

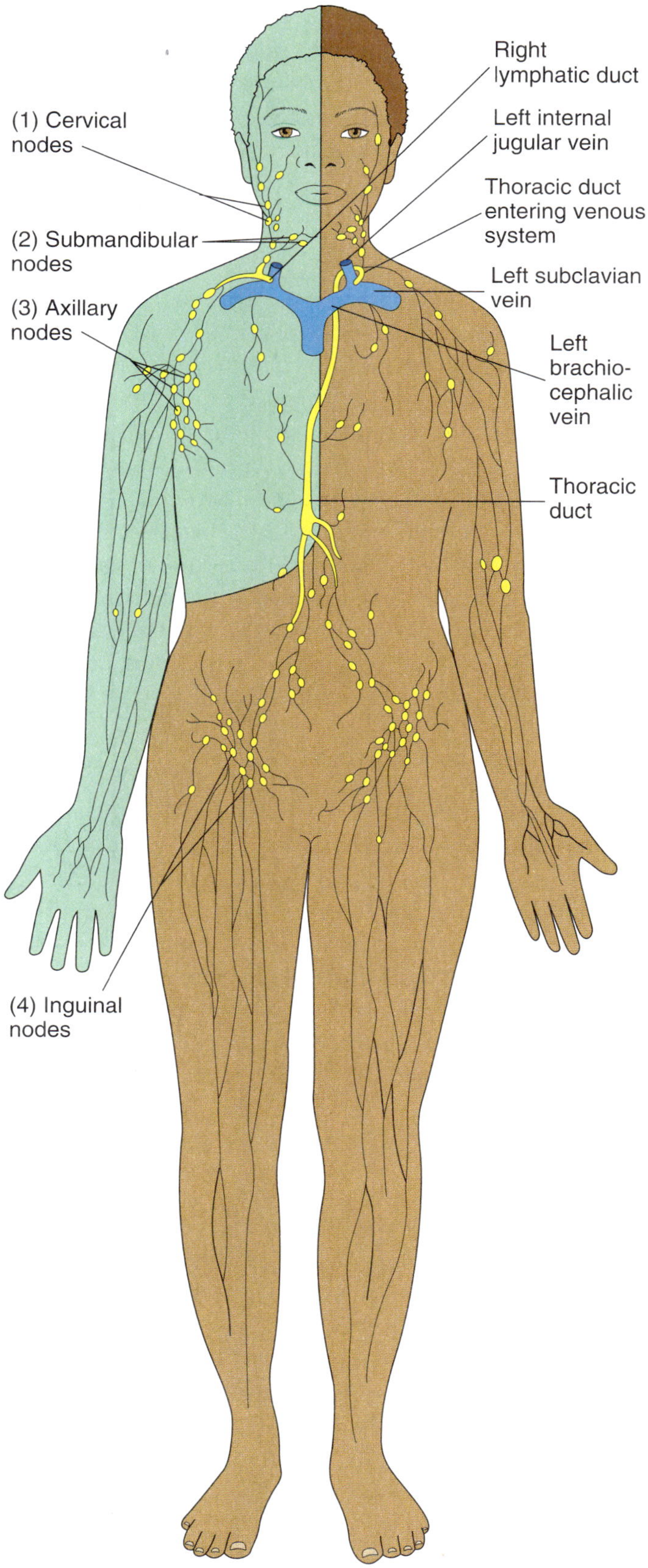

Figure 9-3 Lymphatic ducts and nodes

These two ducts are the only points of entry of the lymph into the blood vessels of the body. Lymph drainage from the right side of the head and neck, the right upper extremity, and the right side of the chest flows into the **right lymphatic duct.** The right lymphatic duct empties into the right subclavian vein. Lymph drainage from the remaining regions of the body flows into the **thoracic duct,** which empties into the left subclavian vein.

Lymph Nodes

Located at various intervals along the course of the lymphatic system vessels are lymph nodes, which are collections of lymphatic tissue; the lymph nodes are also called the lymph glands. The major concentrations of lymph nodes throughout the body are the (1) cervical lymph nodes, (2) submandibular lymph nodes, (3) axillary lymph nodes, and the (4) inguinal lymph nodes. See Figure 9-3. As the lymph passes through the stationary lymph nodes, two processes occur: Old, dead cells and bacteria present in the lymph are filtered out so they will not be emptied into the blood vessels, and phagocytes, called **macrophages,** engulf and destroy the bacteria, which are filtered out. This process of engulfing and destroying the bacteria is known as **phagocytosis.** Macrophages are special phagocytic cells that are involved in the defense against infection and in the disposal of the products of the breakdown of cells. They are found in the lymph nodes, the liver, spleen, lungs, brain, and spinal cord. The lymph nodes also produce antibodies and lymphocytes, which are important to immunity.

Thymus

The **thymus,** also an endocrine gland, is a single gland located in the mediastinum, near the middle of the chest, just beneath the sternum. It secretes a hormone called thymosin, which stimulates the red bone marrow to produce **T lymphocytes** or **T cells,** which are important in the immune response. The T lymphocytes mature in the thymus; upon maturation, they enter the blood and circulate throughout the body providing defense against disease by attacking foreign and/or abnormal cells. The thymus gland completes most of its essential work during childhood, decreasing significantly in size as one ages; it is quite small in older adults.

Spleen

The **spleen,** located in the left upper quadrant of the abdomen just below the diaphragm and behind the stomach, is the largest lymphatic organ in the body. The spleen plays an important role in the immune response by filtering blood in much the same way that the lymph nodes filter the lymph. The macrophages of the spleen remove pathogens of all kinds from circulating blood; they also remove old red blood cells from circulation, breaking them down and forming bile that is returned to the liver to be excreted in bile. The spleen contains venous sinuses that serve as a storage reservoir for blood. In emergencies, such as hemorrhage, the spleen can release blood back into the general circulation. If the spleen should ever have to be removed, its functions can be performed by other lymphatic tissue and the liver. The removal of the spleen is called a **splenectomy.**

Tonsils

The **tonsils** are masses of lymphatic tissue located in a protective ring, just under the mucous membrane, surrounding the mouth and back of the throat. They are divided into three groups:

1. The **pharyngeal tonsils** or **adenoids** are near the opening of the nasal cavity into the pharynx (throat).
2. When we speak of "the tonsils," we are usually referring to the **palatine tonsils** located on each side of the throat, near the opening of the oral cavity into the pharynx.
3. The **lingual tonsils** are located near the base of the tongue.

The tonsils help protect against bacteria and other harmful substances that may enter the body through the nose or mouth. Serving as the first line of defense from the external environment, the tonsils are subject to chronic infection or inflammation known as **tonsillitis.** Removal of the tonsils is known as a **tonsillectomy.**

Vocabulary (Lymphatic)

The following vocabulary words are frequently used when discussing the lymphatic system.

WORD	DEFINITION
acquired immunity (ih-**MEW**-nih-tee)	Immunity that is a result of the body developing the ability to defend itself against a specific agent, as a result of having had the disease or from having received an immunization against a disease.
adenoids (**ADD**-eh-noydz)	Masses of lymphatic tissue located near the opening of the nasal cavity into the pharynx; also called the pharyngeal tonsils.
edema (eh-**DEE**-mah)	The accumulation of fluid within the tissue spaces.
hypersensitivity (**high**-per-**sens**-ih-**TIV**-ih-tee)	An abnormal condition characterized by an excessive reaction to a particular stimulus.
immune reaction (immune response) (im-**YOON**)	A defense function of the body that produces antibodies to destroy invading antigens and malignancies.
immunity (im-**YOO**-nih-tee)	The state of being resistant to or protected from a disease; the individual is said to be "immune."
immunization (**im**-yoo-nigh-**ZAY**-shun)	The process of creating immunity to a specific disease.
immunologist (**im**-yoo-**NALL**-oh-jist)	The health specialist whose training and experience is concentrated in immunology.
immunology (**im**-yoo-**NALL**-oh-jee)	The study of the reaction of tissues of the immune system of the body to antigenic stimulation.
immunotherapy (**im**-yoo-no-**THAIR**-ah-pee)	A special treatment of allergic responses that administers increasingly large doses of the offending allergens to gradually develop immunity.
local reaction	A reaction to treatment that occurs at the site where it was administered.
lymph (**LIMF**)	Interstitial fluid picked up by the lymphatic capillaries and eventually returned to the blood; once the interstitial fluid enters the lymphatic vessels, it is known as lymph.

lymphadenopathy (lim-**fad**-eh-**NOP**-ah-thee) **lymph/o** = lymph **aden/o** = gland **-pathy** = disease	Any disorder of the lymph nodes or lymph vessels.
lymphocyte (**LIM**-foh-sight) **lymph/o** = lymph **cyt/o** = cell **-e** = noun ending	Small, agranulocytic leukocytes, originating from fetal stem cells and developing in the bone marrow.
macrophage (**MACK**-roh-fayj) **macr/o** = large **phag/o** = to eat **-e** = noun ending	Any phagocytic cell involved in the defense against infection and in the disposal of the products of the breakdown of cells. Macrophages are found in the lymph nodes, liver, spleen, lungs, brain, and spinal cord.
natural immunity (ih-**MEW**-nih-tee)	Immunity with which we are born; also called genetic immunity.
pathogens (**PATH**-oh-jenz) **path/o** = disease **-gen** = that which generates	Disease-producing microorganisms.
phagocytosis (**fag**-oh-sigh-**TOH**-sis) **phag/o** = to eat **cyt/o** = cell **-osis** = condition	The process of a cell engulfing and destroying bacteria.
resistance	The body's ability to counteract the effects of pathogens and other harmful agents.
susceptible (suh-**SEP**-tih-bl)	A state of having a lack of resistance to pathogens and other harmful agents; for example, the individual is said to be "susceptible."
T cells (**T SELLS**)	Cells that are important in the immune response; they mature in the thymus. Upon maturation, the T cells enter the blood and circulate throughout the body, providing defense against disease by attacking foreign and/or abnormal cells.
tonsils (**TON**-sills)	Masses of lymphatic tissue located in a protective ring, just under the mucous membrane, surrounding the mouth and back of the throat.

Word Elements (Lymphatic)

The following word elements pertain to the lymphatic system. As you review the list, pronounce each word element aloud twice and check the box after you "say it." Write the definition for the example word given for each word element. You may use your medical dictionary.

WORD ELEMENT	PRONUNCIATION	"SAY IT"	MEANING
cyt/o **cyt**omegalovirus	**SIGH**-toh **sigh**-toh-**meg**-ah-loh-**VY**-rus	☐	cell
hyper- **hyper**splenism	**HIGH**-per high-per-**SPLEN**-izm	☐	excessive
immun/o **immun**odeficiency	im-**YOO**-noh **im**-yoo-noh-deh-**FISH**-en-see	☐	immune, protection
lymph/o **lymph**ocyte	**LIM**-foh **LIM**-foh-sight	☐	lymph
lymphaden/o **lymphaden**itis	lim-**FAD**-en-oh lim-**fad**-en-**EYE**-tis	☐	lymph gland
lymphangi/o **lymphangi**ogram	lim-**FAN**-jee-oh lim-**FAN**-jee-oh-gram	☐	lymph vessel
mon/o **mon**onucleosis	**MON**-oh mon-oh-noo-klee-**OH**-sis	☐	one
sarc/o Kaposi's **sarc**oma	**SAR**-koh **KAP**-oh-seez sar-**KOH**-mah	☐	flesh

Immunity

As we have already learned, the lymphatic system is an important part of the immune system, which protects the body against disease-producing organisms (**pathogens**) and other foreign microorganisms to which it is continually exposed. Immunity is the state of being resistant to or being protected from a disease. This section will discuss both natural and acquired immunity, with a greater concentration on acquired immunity. The purpose of immunity is to develop resistance to a disease or to harmful agents. The body's ability to counteract the effects of pathogens and other harmful agents is called **resistance.** If the body lacks resistance to pathogens and other harmful agents, it is said to be **susceptible.**

Natural immunity is that with which we are born; it is also called genetic immunity. Some pathogens cannot affect certain species; for example, humans do not suffer from canine distemper nor do canines suffer from human measles. Natural immunity is considered to be a permanent form of immunity to a specific disease.

Acquired immunity is immunity indicating that the body has developed the ability to defend itself against a specific agent. This protection can occur as a result of having had the particular disease or from having received immunizations against a disease. Acquired immunity can be divided further into two categories: (1) passive acquired immunity and (2) active acquired immunity.

1. **Passive acquired immunity** is acquired artificially by injecting antibodies from the blood of other individuals or animals into a person's body to protect him or her from a specific disease. This type of immunity is immediate but short lived, lasting only a few

weeks. An example of passive immunity is the administration of **gamma globulin** (a blood protein containing antibodies) to individuals who have been exposed to viruses, such as measles and infectious hepatitis. Another example of passive immunity is the passage of the mother's antibodies through the placenta into the baby's blood. This provides the newborn infant with passive immunity for approximately the first year of life, during which time the infant begins to develop his or her own antibodies.

2. **Active acquired immunity** is either acquired naturally as a result of having had a disease, or is acquired artificially by being inoculated with a vaccine, antigen, or toxoid. With **natural acquired immunity,** an individual who has a full-blown case of a disease such as measles, will usually develop enough antibodies to prevent a recurrence of the disease. Another form of active acquired immunity may be developed over a period of time after repeated exposures to an illness or disease with only mild symptoms. With **artificial acquired immunity,** an individual receives a vaccine, antigen, or toxoid to stimulate the formation of antibodies within his or her body. For example, when a child receives the measles-mumps-rubella vaccine, he or she receives a mild strength of the disease in the form of the vaccine administered. This vaccine then stimulates the production of antibodies within the child's body against measles, mumps, and rubella.

The process of creating immunity to a specific disease is known as immunization. This is accomplished through the administration of vaccines, antigens, or toxoids to stimulate the formation of antibodies within an individual's body. Children receive routine immunizations throughout their early years to provide adequate protection against childhood diseases. These will be discussed in Chapter 19. An individual may receive various immunizations throughout his or her lifetime to provide continued immunity against a disease (as in a tetanus toxoid booster) or to provide immunity against diseases prevalent in other countries (as in overseas travel).

Immune Reaction

The **immune reaction** or **immune response** is a defense function of the body that produces antibodies to destroy invading antigens and malignancies. Antigens trigger the immune response during interaction with innumerable cells within the body. The kinds of immune responses are humoral immune response, involving the B lymphocytes of the body; and cell-mediated immune response, involving the T lymphocytes of the body. Both of these specialized cells have been genetically programmed to recognize specific invading antigens and to destroy them.

B lymphocytes originate from bone marrow stem cells and migrate to the lymph nodes and other lymphoid tissue. In the **humoral immune response,** when the B lymphocytes come in contact with specific invading antigens, they produce antibodies known as **immunoglobulins.** Antibodies belong to a group of blood proteins called gamma globulins. The gamma globulins are divided into five categories of immunoglobulins: immunoglobulin M (IgM), immunoglobulin G (IgG), immunoglobulin E (IgE), immunoglobulin A (IgA), and immunoglobulin D (IgD). Most antibodies are immunoglobulin type G (IgG). These immunoglobulins migrate to the site of the infection, react with the antigen, and destroy it.

T lymphocytes originate from bone marrow stem cells and mature in the thymus gland. Upon maturation, the T lymphocytes enter the blood and circulate throughout the body providing defense against disease by attacking foreign and/or abnormal cells. They migrate to the lymph nodes and lymphoid organs. In the **cell-mediated immune response,** when the T lymphocytes come in contact with specific invading antigens, they multiply rapidly and engulf and digest the antigen. This multiplication of cells produces cells that help to destroy the antigen as well as cells that are called **memory cells.** The memory cells, which remain in circulation for many years, provide the body with resistance to any disease to which it has previously been exposed. When these memory cells face subsequent exposure to the same antigen, they are stimulated to rapidly produce cells that destroy the invading antigen. Immunity is dependent on the action of the memory cells.

Immunology is the study of the reaction of tissues of the immune system of the body to antigenic stimulation. An immunologist is a health specialist whose training and experience is concentrated in immunology. **Immunotherapy** is a special treatment of allergic responses that administers increasingly large doses of the offending allergens to gradually develop immunity.

When something happens to an individual's immune system causing it to function abnormally, the body forms antibodies that react against its own tissues. This is known as an **autoimmune disorder.** Unable to distinguish between internal antigens that are normally present in the cells and external invading antigens, the body reacts against the internal cells to cause localized and systemic reactions. These reactions affect the epithelial and connective tissues of the body causing a variety of symptoms. Autoimmune disorders are divided into two categories: the collagen diseases (connective tissue diseases) and the autoimmune hemolytic disorders. The collagen diseases include disorders such as systemic lupus erythematosus, scleroderma, and rheumatoid arthritis. The autoimmune hemolytic diseases include disorders such as idiopathic thrombocytopenic purpura and acquired hemolytic anemia.

Hypersensitivity

Hypersensitivity is an abnormal condition characterized by an excessive reaction to a particular stimulus. It occurs when the body's immune system fails to protect itself against foreign material. The antibodies formed irritate certain body cells, causing a hypersensitive or allergic reaction. The allergic response is triggered by an **allergen.** Examples of allergens include ingested foods, penicillin and other antibiotics, grass, ragweed pollen, and bee or wasp stings. These allergens stimulate the formation of antibodies that produce the characteristic allergic reactions.

Hypersensitive reactions vary from mild to severe, and from local to systemic. A **local reaction** is one that occurs at the site where treatment or medication was administered. A **systemic reaction** is one that is evidenced by generalized body symptoms such as runny nose, itchy eyes, hives, and rashes.

A severe and sometimes fatal hypersensitive (allergic) reaction is called **anaphylaxis** or **anaphylactic shock.** It is the result of an antigen–antibody reaction that stimulates a massive secretion of histamine. Anaphylaxis can be caused by insect stings, contrast media containing iodide, aspirin, antitoxins prepared with animal serum, allergens used in testing and desensitizing patients who are hypersensitive, and other injected drugs. Penicillin injection is the most common cause of anaphylactic shock.

Health care professionals should always ask patients if they are sensitive to any allergens or drugs to prevent adverse and sometimes fatal allergic responses to treatments or medications. Individuals with known hypersensitivities, or those receiving a first dose of injectable medication or penicillin, should remain in the physician's office for 15 to 20 minutes following the administration of medication or treatment. During this time, the individual should be observed for signs of possible hypersensitivity. Anaphylactic shock may occur within seconds or minutes after exposure to the sensitizing factor (allergen) and is commonly characterized by respiratory distress and vascular collapse. The first symptoms of anaphylactic shock are usually intense anxiety, weakness, sweating, and shortness of breath. This may be followed by hypotension, shock, arrhythmia, and respiratory congestion. Emergency treatment involves the immediate injection of epinephrine, which will raise the blood pressure through its vasoconstrictive action.

Individuals who are known to be hypersensitive to allergens and medications should wear a Medi-Alert tag around the neck or wrist. The presence of this tag will alert the health care professional or first-aid provider to the need for immediate action, informing them of either an allergy or a particular disease, such as diabetes.

Pathological Conditions (Lymphatic)

As you study the pathological conditions of the lymphatic system, note that the **basic definition** is in bold print, followed by a detailed description in regular print. The phonetic pronunciation is directly beneath each term, and a breakdown of the component parts of the term when appropriate.

acquired immunodeficiency syndrome (AIDS)
(ih-**mew**-noh-**dee**-**FIH**-shen-see **SIN**-drom)

Acquired immunodeficiency syndrome (AIDS) involves clinical conditions that destroy the body's immune system in the last or final phase of a human immunodeficiency virus (HIV) infection, which primarily damages helper T cell lymphocytes with CD_4 receptors.

HIV, a slow-growing virus, typically begins with an acute viral infection called the primary infection. This primary infection is systemic (in the bloodstream) and widespread with seeding in the lymphatic system. In approximately 8 weeks after onset, the CD_4 counts (normally 1,000) will have dropped by one-half (500), indicating a deficiency in the body's immune response. The signs and symptoms during this primary stage include headache, stiff neck, malaise, fatigue, fever, night sweats, rash, abdominal cramps, and diarrhea. By the twelfth week, the CD_4 counts will have rebounded to around 700. The measurable aspect of this primary infection is the presence of HIV antibodies. The ELISA and western blot tests are positive for antibodies.

During a latent period of approximately 8 years, the CD_4 count usually declines steadily as the following signs and symptoms become more apparent: measurable presence of generalized lymphadenopathy, chronic diarrhea, weight loss, persistent fever, fatigue, night sweats, and oral thrush. Kaposi's sarcoma or hairy cell leukemia may appear during this latent stage.

When the CD_4 count reaches 200, "acquired immune deficiency" AIDS is clinically apparent. The person may or may not display signs and symptoms or develop an opportunistic neoplasm or infection. The CD_4 count will eventually reach 0 at which time the body has no immune defense and thus opportunistic infections and cancers will occur and affect all the body systems.

Around the tenth or eleventh year after onset, the person will likely die from an overwhelming cancer or infection. HIV can be acquired via a blood transfusion, use of contaminated needles, or during sexual intercourse (especially anal sex). An unborn fetus can acquire HIV from the mother during pregnancy. Medical treatment includes various antiviral drugs.

cytomegalovirus
(**sigh**-toh-**meg**-ah-loh-**VY**-rus)
cyt/o = cell
megal/o = enlarged

Cytomegalovirus is a large species-specific, herpes-type virus with a wide variety of disease effects. It causes serious illness in persons with AIDS, in newborns, and in individuals who are being treated with immunosuppressive drugs (as in individuals who have

received an organ transplant). The virus usually results in retinal or gastrointestinal infection.

hypersensitivity
(**high**-per-**sens**-sih-**TIV**-ih-tee)

Tissue damage resulting from exaggerated immune responses.

The exaggerated responses are caused by one of the following four mechanisms.

1. **IgE-mediated–Type I hypersensitivity response** as occurs in allergic rhinitis, hives, allergic asthma, allergic conjunctivitis, and anaphylactic shock (acute systemic). The acute systemic response occurs as a result of the histamine and mediator release causing increased capillary permeability, bronchial constriction, vasodilation, and smooth muscle contraction, which can lead to hypotension and impaired tissue perfusion, a state known as anaphylactic shock.
2. **Cytoxic–Type II hypersensitivity reaction** develops when antibodies bind to antigens on body cells. Causes of Type II include transfusion reactions, autoimmune hemolytic anemia, and erythroblastosis fetalis.
3. **Immune complex-mediated–Type III sensitivity response** occurs when huge antibody, antigen, and complement proteins interact to form massive complexes, which accumulate in the tissues. Examples of Type III hypersensitivity response include serum sickness, rheumatoid arthritis, systemic lupus erythematosus, and acute poststreptococcal glomerulonephritis.
4. **Delayed–Type IV hypersensitivity responses** are cell mediated rather than antibody mediated and involve T cells. Examples of Type IV hypersensitivity response includes contact dermatitis, graft-versus-host disease, and tuberculin reaction. A collection of skin tests may be used to assess and determine the causes of hypersensitivity.

hypersplenism
(**high**-per-**SPLEN**-izm)
hyper- = excessive
splen/o = spleen
-ism = condition

Hypersplenism is a syndrome involving a deficiency of one or more types of blood cells and an enlarged spleen.

The causes of this syndrome are abundant. A few of the more common causes are hemolytic anemias, portal hypertension, lymphomas, tuberculosis, malaria, and several inflammatory and connective tissue diseases.

Symptoms of hypersplenism include left-sided abdominal pain and the feeling of fullness after a small intake. The enlarged spleen is easily palpated on physical examination. Treatment should begin with concentration on the underlying disorder, which may lead to the cure of the syndrome. A splenectomy is typically performed only for the individual with hemolytic anemia or the person with severe spleen enlargement (at high risk for a vascular accident).

Kaposi's sarcoma
(**KAP**-oh-seez sar-**KOH**-mah)
sarc/o = flesh
-oma = tumor

Kaposi's sarcoma is a locally destructive malignant neoplasm of the blood vessels associated with AIDS typically forming lesions on the skin, visceral organs, or mucous membranes. These lesions appear initially as tiny red to purple macules and evolve into sizable nodules or plaques.

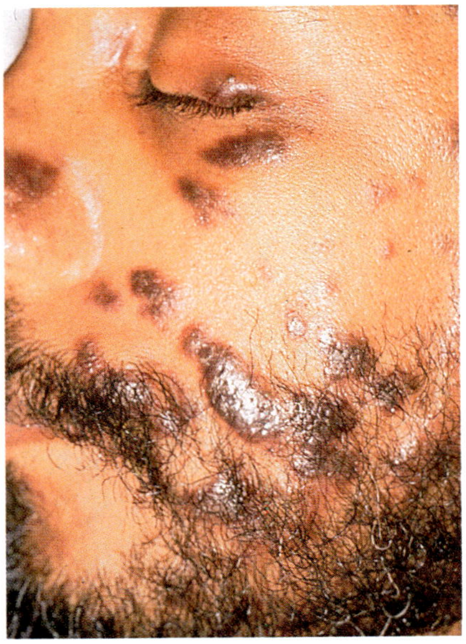

The lesions occur due to an overgrowth of spindle-shaped cells and epithelial cells that result in the narrowing of the diameter of the vessels. The body responds by increasing the number of vessels in that area, thus causing more congestion.

The signs and symptoms of Kaposi's sarcoma will vary but be specific according to the lesion site. Skin lesions are described above. Gastrointestinal lesions may lead to mucosal bleeding, anemia, or obstruction. Pulmonary lesions may result in pulmonary effusion and shortness of breath. If the lesions are located in the lymphatics, there will be swollen lymph nodes and edema.

Kaposi's sarcoma is diagnosed with a biopsy of the lesion. With the pulmonary lesion, a chest x-ray is completed to confirm a pulmonary effusion. The treatment includes radiation therapy, chemotherapy, and or laser cryotherapy. See **Figure 9-4.**

Figure 9-4 Kaposi's sarcoma *(Courtesy of Robert A. Silverman, M.D., Clinical Associate Professor, Department of Pediatrics, Georgetown University)*

---

lymphoma
(**LIM**-foh-mah)
lymph/o = lymph
-oma = tumor

Lymphoma is a lymphoid tissue neoplasm that is typically malignant, beginning with a painless enlarged lymph node(s) and progressing to anemia, weakness, fever, and weight loss.

The spleen and liver usually enlarge with widespread lymphoid tissue involvement. The development of lymphomas has a higher occurrence in the male population. Intensive chemotherapy and radiotherapy are the treatments with a lymphoma.

Burkitt's lymphoma is a malignant neoplasm in the jaw or abdomen and is seen chiefly in Central Africa. Rapid diagnosis and treatment typically results in quick shrinking of the lesion and complete cure of the disease.

Hodgkin's disease is characterized by progressive, painless enlargement of a malignant tumor of the lymph tissue in the lymph nodes and spleen typically noted first in the cervical region. Males are affected twice as often as females. Clinical manifestations include enlarged lymph nodes, splenomegaly, low-grade fever, night sweats, anorexia, anemia, and leukocytosis. Diagnosis is made through the identification of a Reed-Sternberg cell (malignant cell in the lymph nodes). With localized disease, radiotherapy is the choice; however, with more extensive disease, chemotherapy or a combination of chemotherapy and radiation is used.

Non-Hodgkin's lymphoma is the classification of any kind of malignant lymphoma besides Hodgkin's disease, including histiocytic lymphoma and lymphocytic lymphomas. Radiation and chemotherapy are administered to stop the growth and cure this disease.

---

mononucleosis
(mon-oh-**noo**-klee-**OH**-sis)
mono- = one
nucle/o = nucleus
-osis = condition

Usually caused by the Epstein-Barr virus (EBV), mononucleosis typically is a benign, self-limiting acute infection of the B lymphocytes.

Young adults (15 to 20 years old) are primarily affected with this "kissing disease," as it is described due to the main mode of transmission (through saliva).

The body's response to this B lymphocyte infection is the production of antibodies by the unaffected B lymphocytes and the T lymphocytes. As a result of this proliferation of B and T lymphocytes, the lymphoid tissue in the body becomes swollen. This swollen lymphoid tissue is most noted in enlarged tender cervical lymph nodes and sometimes axillary and inguinal lymph nodes, the spleen, and the liver, and typically lasts for 1 to 3 weeks. Other clinical manifestations include fever, chills, malaise, diaphoresis (profuse sweating), sore throat, profound fatigue, headache, red papular rash, and anorexia.

The diagnosis of mononucleosis is confirmed with a physical examination, elevated lymphocyte count and the presence of atypical lymphocytes, and a positive monospot test. Bed rest is the initial treatment with administration of analgesics and corticosteroids, as needed. A 2- to 3-week recovery period is needed and many times the fatigue and debility last for 2 to 3 months.

---

myasthenia gravis
(my-ass-**THEE**-nee-ah **GRAV**-is)
my/o = muscle
-asthenia = loss of strength

Myasthenia gravis is an autoimmune disease in which antibodies block or destroy some acetylcholine receptor sites.

Other structural problems cause the acetylcholine uptake to be decreased and therefore reduce neuromuscular transmissions. In approximately one-fifth of the cases, thymus gland involvement is noted.

Myasthenia gravis occurs more often in women than men. In women, it usually occurs at the age of 20 to 40 years. In men, the onset of myasthenia gravis is between the ages of 50 to 60.

The symptoms may occur gradually or suddenly. Facial muscle weakness may be the most noticeable due to drooping eyelids, difficulty with swallowing, and difficulty speaking. The periods of muscle weakness generally occur late in the day or after strenuous exercise. Rest refreshes the tired, weak muscles. The weakness eventually becomes so severe that paralysis occurs.

Treatment for myasthenia gravis may require restricted activity, a soft or liquid diet, and administration of anticholinesterase drugs (mestinon). Some individuals benefit from corticosteriods.

---

pneumocystis carinii pneumonia (PCP)
(noo-moh-**SIS**-tis kah-**rye**-nee-eye noo-**MOH**-nee-ah)
pneum/o = lungs; air
cyst/o = sac
-is = noun ending
pneumon/o = lungs; air
-ia = condition

Pneumocystis pneumonia is caused by a common worldwide parasite, *Pneumocystis carinii,* for which most people have immunity if they are not severely immunocompromised.

The most frequent opportunistic infection occurring in persons with AIDS, pneumocystis carinii pneumonia (PCP) affects an estimated 75% to 80% of those individuals with AIDS.

Individuals with PCP have severely impaired gas exchange as the disease progresses. The swollen, thickened air sacs of the lungs are filled with a protein-rich, foamy fluid resulting in tachypnea, shortness of breath, fever, and a dry nonproductive cough.

---

sarcoidosis
(**sar**-koyd-**OH**-sis)
sarc/o = flesh
-oid = resembling
-osis = condition

Sarcoidosis is a systemic inflammatory disease resulting in the formation of multiple small, rounded lesions (granulomas) in the lungs (comprising 90%), lymph nodes, eyes, liver, and other organs.

These granulomas can resolve spontaneously or may lead to fibrosis. The occurrence is highest in African American females between 20 and 40.

Although the mortality rate is less than 3%, the disability caused by sarcoidosis of the respiratory, ocular, or other organs can be devastating to the individual. A biopsy of the granuloma may be needed to confirm the diagnosis. Corticosteroids are reserved for those persons experiencing severe manifestations or disabilities caused by the disease.

systemic lupus erythematosus (SLE)
(sis-**TEM**-ik **LOO**-pus **er**-ih-them-ah-**TOH**-sus)

An inflammatory connective tissue disease, chronic in nature, in which immune complexes are formed from the reaction of SLE autoantibodies and their corresponding antigens; these immune complexes are deposited in the connective tissues of lymphatic vessels, blood vessels, and other tissues.

Local tissue damage occurs due to the inflammatory response when the immune complexes are deposited.

These complexes are frequently deposited in the kidneys causing damage to the tissue. Other tissues sometimes affected are the brain, lungs, skin, musculoskeletal system, heart, spleen, GI tract, and peritoneum.

tuberculosis
(too-**ber**-kew-**LOH**-sis)

Tuberculosis is an infectious disease, chronic in nature, primarily affecting the lungs, causing large areas of cavitations and caseous (cheeselike) necrosis.

Typically, tuberculosis has the potential to spread to any organ of the body. Tuberculosis cases in the United States are on the rise. A major contributing factor is the statistic that 4% of persons with AIDS will develop tuberculosis because of their impaired immune function. The disease progresses much more rapidly in persons with AIDS than in an individual who does not have a weakened immune system.

Diagnostic Techniques and Procedures (Lymphatic)

Enzyme-linked immunosorbent assay (ELISA)
(**EN**-zym **LINK'T** **im**-yoo-noh-**SOR**-bent **ASS**-say)

Enzyme-linked immunosorbent assay (ELISA) is a blood test used for screening for an antibody to the AIDS virus.

Positive outcome on this test indicates probable virus exposure but should be confirmed with the western blot test.

western blot

The western blot test detects the presence of the antibodies to HIV, the virus that causes AIDS.

CT (CAT) scan

A collection of x-ray images taken from various angles following injection of a contrast medium.

Diagnosis of abnormalities in lymphoid organs are made in areas such as the spleen, thymus gland, and lymph nodes.

lymphangiogram
(lim-**FAN**-jee-oh-gram)
lymph/o = lymph
angi/o = vessel
-gram = record, picture

Lymphangiogram is an x-ray assessment of the lymphatic system following injection of a contrast medium into the lymph vessels in the hand or foot.

The path of lymph flow is noted moving into the chest region. This procedure is helpful in diagnosing and staging lymphomas.

Common Abbreviations (Lymphatic)

ABBREVIATION	MEANING	ABBREVIATION	MEANING
ARC	AIDS-related complex	**Histo**	histology
AIDS	acquired immunodeficiency syndrome	**HIV**	human immunodeficiency virus
CDC	Centers for Disease Control and Prevention	**HSV**	herpes simplex virus
CMV	cytomegalovirus	**ITP**	idiopathic thrombocytopenic purpura
EBV	Epstein-Barr virus	**KS**	Kaposi's sarcoma
ELISA	enzyme-linked immunosorbent assay	**SLE**	systemic lupus erythematosus

Written and Audio Terminology Review

Review each of the following terms from this chapter. Study the spelling of each term and write the definition in the space provided. If you have the Audio CD available, listen to each term, pronounce it, and check the box once you are comfortable saying the word. Check definitions by looking the term up in the glossary/index.

TERM	PRONUNCIATION	DEFINITION
acquired immunity	☐ acquired ih-**MEW**-nih-tee	______________
acquired immunodeficiency syndrome (AIDS)	☐ acquired ih-**mew**-noh-**dee**-**FIH**-shen-see **SIN**-drom (**AIDS**)	______________
adenoids	☐ **ADD**-eh-noydz	______________
agglutination	☐ ah-**gloo**-tih-**NAY**-shun	______________
albumin	☐ al-**BEW**-min	______________
allergen	☐ **AL**-er-jin	______________

Term	Pronunciation	Definition
allergy	☐ **AL**-er-jee	________
anaphylaxis	☐ **an**-ah-fih-**LAK**-sis	________
anemia	☐ an-**NEE**-mee-ah	________
anisocytosis	☐ an-**ih**-soh-sigh-**TOH**-sis	________
antibodies	☐ **AN**-tih-bod-eez	________
antigens	☐ **AN**-tih-jenz	________
aplastic	☐ ah-**PLAST**-ik	________
ascites	☐ ah-**SIGH**-teez	________
basophil	☐ **BAY**-soh-fill	________
bilirubin	☐ bill-ih-**ROO**-bin	________
blastocyte	☐ **BLAST**-oh-sight	________
chromophilic	☐ kroh-moh-**FILL**-ik	________
coagulation	☐ koh-**ag**-yoo-**LAY**-shun	________
corpuscle	☐ **KOR**-pus-'l	________
cytogenesis	☐ **sigh**-toh-**JEN**-eh-is	________
cytomegalovirus	☐ **sigh**-toh-**meg**-ah-loh-**VY**-rus	________
differentiation	☐ **diff**-er-en-**she**-**AY**-shun	________
direct antiglobulin test	☐ dih-**RECT** **an**-tih-**GLOB**-yew-lin test	________
dyscrasia	☐ dis-**KRAY**-zee-ah	________
edema	☐ eh-**DEE**-ma	________
electrophoresis	☐ ee-**lek**-troh-for-**EE**-sis	________
enzyme-linked immunosorbent assay	☐ **EN**-zym **LINK'T** **im**-yoo-noh-**SOR**-bent **ASS**-say	________
eosinophil	☐ **ee**-oh-**SIN**-oh-fill	________
eosinophilia	☐ **ee**-oh-**sin**-oh-**FEEL**-ee-ah	________
erythremia	☐ **eh**-rih-**THREE**-mee-ah	________
erythroblast	☐ eh-**RITH**-roh-blast	________
erythrocyte	☐ eh-**RITH**-roh-sight	________
erythrocyte sedimentation	☐ eh-**RITH**-roh-sight **sed**-ih-men-**TAY**-shun	________
erythrocytopenia	☐ eh-**rith**-roh-**sigh**-toh-**PEE**-nee-ah	________

Term		Pronunciation	
erythrocytosis	☐	eh-**rith**-roh-sigh-**TOH**-sis	______
erythropoiesis	☐	eh-**rith**-roh-poy-**EE**-sis	______
erythropoietin	☐	eh-**rith**-roh-**POY**-eh-tin	______
fibrin	☐	**FIH**-brin	______
fibrinogen	☐	fih-**BRIN**-oh-jen	______
globin	☐	**GLOH**-bin	______
globulin	☐	**GLOB**-yew-lin	______
granulocytes	☐	**GRAN**-yew-loh-sights	______
granulocytosis	☐	**gran**-yew-loh-sigh-**TOH**-sis	______
hematocrit	☐	hee-**MAT**-oh-krit	______
hematologist	☐	**hee**-mah-**TALL**-oh-jist	______
hematology	☐	**hee**-mah-**TALL**-oh-jee	______
heme	☐	**HEEM**	______
hemochromatosis	☐	**hee**-moh-**kroh**-mah-**TOH**-sis	______
hemodialysis	☐	**hee**-moh-dye-**AL**-ih-sis	______
hemoglobin	☐	**hee**-moh-**GLOH**-bin	______
hemolysis	☐	**hee**-**MALL**-ih-sis	______
hemolytic	☐	**hee**-moh-**LIT**-ik	______
hemophilia	☐	**hee**-moh-**FILL**-ee-ah	______
hemorrhage	☐	**HEM**-eh-rij	______
hemostasis	☐	**hee**-moh-**STAY**-sis	______
heparin	☐	**HEP**-er-in	______
hyperalbuminemia	☐	high-per-al-**byoo**-mih-**NEE**-mee-ah	______
hyperlipemia	☐	**high**-per-lip-**EE**-mee-ah	______
hyperlipidemia	☐	**high**-per-lip-**id**-**EE**-mee-ah	______
hypersensitivity	☐	**high**-per-**sens**-ih-**TIV**-ih-tee	______
hypersplenism	☐	**high**-per-**SPLEN**-izm	______
immune	☐	im-**YOON**	______
immunity	☐	im-**YOO**-nih-tee	______
immunization	☐	im-yoo-nigh-**ZAY**-shun	______

Term	Pronunciation	
immunodeficiency	☐ **im**-yoo-noh-deh-**FISH**-en-see	________
immunologist	☐ **im**-yoo-**NALL**-oh-jist	________
immunology	☐ **im**-yoo-**NALL**-oh-jee	________
immunotherapy	☐ **im**-yoo-no-**THAIR**-ah-pee	________
isotonic	☐ **eye**-soh-**TON**-ik	________
Kaposi's sarcoma	☐ **KAP**-oh-seez sar-**KOH**-mah	________
karyocyte	☐ **KAR**-ee-oh-sight	________
leukemia	☐ loo-**KEE**-mee-ah	________
leukocyte	☐ **LOO**-koh-sight	________
leukocytopenia	☐ **loo**-koh-**sigh**-toh-**PEE**-nee-ah	________
lipid profile	☐ **LIP**-id profile	________
lymph	☐ **LIMF**	________
lymphadenitis	☐ lim-**fad**-en-**EYE**-tis	________
lymphadenopathy	☐ lim-**fad**-eh-**NOP**-ah-thee	________
lymphangiogram	☐ lim-**FAN**-jee-oh-gram	________
lymphoma	☐ **LIM**-foh-mah	________
lymphocyte	☐ **LIM**-foh-sight	________
macrophage	☐ **MACK**-roh-fayj	________
megakaryocyte	☐ **meg**-ah-**KAIR**-ee-oh-sight	________
monocyte	☐ **MON**-oh-sight	________
monocytopenia	☐ **mon**-oh-**sigh**-toh-**PEE**-nee-ah	________
mononucleosis	☐ mon-oh-**noo**-klee-**OH**-sis	________
morphology	☐ mor-**FALL**-oh-jee	________
multiple myeloma	☐ **MULL**-tih-pl my-eh-**LOH**-mah	________
myasthenia gravis	☐ my-ass-**THEE**-nee-ah **GRAV**-is	________
myeloblast	☐ **MY**-ell-oh-blast	________
myeloid	☐ **MY**-eh-loyd	________
natural immunity	☐ natural ih-**MEW**-nih-tee	________

Term	Pronunciation	
neutrophil	☐ **NOO**-troh-fill	
nucleus	☐ **NOO**-klee-us	
pancytopenia	☐ **pan**-sigh-toh-**PEE**-nee-ah	
partial thromboplastin time	☐ **PAR**-sh'l **throm**-boh-**PLAST**-tin time	
pathogens	☐ **PATH**-oh-jenz	
pernicious	☐ per-**NISH**-us	
phagocyte	☐ **FAG**-oh-sight	
phagocytosis	☐ **fag**-oh-sigh-**TOH**-sis	
plasma	☐ **PLAZ**-mah	
platelet	☐ **PLAYT**-let	
pneumocystis pneumonia	☐ **noo**-moh-**SIS**-tis noo-**MOH**-nee-ah	
poikilocytosis	☐ **poy**-kill-oh-sigh-**TOH**-sis	
polycythemia	☐ **pol**-ee-sigh-**THEE**-mee-ah	
polycythemia vera	☐ **pol**-ee-sigh-**THEE**-mee-ah **VAIR**-ah	
prothrombin	☐ proh-**THROM**-bin	
prothrombin time (PT)	☐ proh-**THROM**-bin time (PT)	
purpura	☐ **PURR**-pew-rah	
red blood cell morphology	☐ red blood cell mor-**FALL**-oh-jee	
reticulocyte	☐ reh-**TIK**-yoo-loh-sight	
reticulocyte count	☐ reh-**TIK**-yoo-loh-sight count	
rouleaux	☐ roo-**LOH**	
sarcoidosis	☐ **sar**-koyd-**OH**-sis	
septicemia	☐ sep-tih-**SEE**-mee-ah	
seroconversion	☐ **see**-roh-con-**VER**-zhun	
serology	☐ see-**RALL**-oh-jee	
serum	☐ **SEE**-rum	
sickle cell	☐ **SIKL SELL**	
sideroblast	☐ **SID**-er-oh-**blast**	
spheroid	☐ **SFEE**-royd	

Term	Pronunciation	
spherocytosis	☐ **sfee**-roh-sigh-**TOH**-sis	____
splenomegaly	☐ **splee**-noh-**MEG**-ah-lee	____
stem cell	☐ **STEM SELL**	____
susceptible	☐ suh-**SEP**-tih-bl	____
T cells	☐ **T SELLS**	____
thalassemia	☐ thal-ah-**SEE**-mee-ah	____
thrombin	☐ **THROM**-bin	____
thrombocyte	☐ **THROM**-boh-sight	____
thrombocytopenia	☐ **throm**-boh-**sigh**-toh-**PEE**-nee-ah	____
thromboplastin	☐ **throm**-boh-**PLAST**-in	____
thrombosis	☐ throm-**BOH**-sis	____
thrombus	☐ **THROM**-bus	____
tonsils	☐ **TON**-sulls	____
tuberculosis	☐ too-**ber**-kew-**LOH**-sis	____
western blot	☐ **WEST**-ern **BLOT**	____
white blood cell differential	☐ white blood cell **diff**-er-**EN**-shal	____

Chapter Review Exercises

The following exercises provide a more in-depth review of the chapter material. Your goal in these exercises is to complete each section at a minimum 80% level of accuracy. A space has been provided for your score at the end of each section.

12/12/07 V&

A. Term to Definition

Define each diagnosis or procedure by writing the definition in the space provided. Check the box if you are able to complete this exercise correctly the first time (without referring to the answers). Each correct answer is worth 10 points. Record your score in the space provided at the end of the exercise.

☐ 1. enzyme-linked immunosorbent assay An immunoassay utilizing an antibody labelled with an enzyme maker such as horseradish peroxidase

☐ 2. bleeding time A test with measures the time it takes for small blood vessels to close off and bleeding to stop.

☐ 3. myasthenia gravis The charateristic feature of the disease is easy fatigue of certain voluntary muscle groups on repeated use

☐ 4. mononucleosis An abnormal increase of mononuclear white blood cells in the blood

☐ 5. western blot A technique similar to Southern blotting, through it is used for protein

☐ 6. sickle cell A abnormal red blood cell of crescent shape

☐ 7. lymphangiogram An X-ray picture made by lymphangiography

☐ 8. hemoglobin test Is the protein molecule in red blood cells that carries oxygen from the lungs to the body's tissues

☐ 9. direct anti-globulin test (Coomb's test) Haemagglutination test in which coomb's reagent

☐ 10. Schilling test Band Cell

***Number correct* _______ × *10 points/correct answer: Your score* _______%**

B. Matching Pathological Conditions

Match the following pathological conditions on the left with their descriptions on the right. Each correct answer is worth 10 points. When you have completed the exercise, record your score in the space provided at the end of the exercise.

f 1. hemolytic anemia
d 2. multiple myeloma
e 3. granulocytosis
b 4. leukemia
c 5. purpura
g 6. pernicious anemia
j 7. tuberculosis
a 8. Kaposi's sarcoma
h 9. lymphoma
i 10. PCP

a. A locally destructive malignant neoplasm of the blood vessels associated with AIDS typically forming lesions on the skin, visceral organs, or mucous membranes

b. Excessive uncontrolled increase of immature WBCs in the blood eventually leading to infection, anemia, and thrombocytopenia

c. Collection of blood beneath the skin in the form of pinpoint hemorrhages appearing as red-purple skin discolorations

d. A malignant plasma cell neoplasm causing a proliferation of both mature and immature plasma cells that often entirely replace the bone marrow and destroy the skeletal structure

e. An abnormally elevated number of granulocytes in the circulating blood as a reaction to any variety of inflammation or infection

f. A form of anemia characterized by the extreme reduction in circulating RBCs due to their destruction

g. A form of anemia resulting from a deficiency of mature RBCs and the formation and circulation of megaloblasts (large nucleated, immature, poorly functioning RBCs) with marked poikilocytosis (RBC shape variation), and anisocytosis (RBC size variation)

h. A lymphoid tissue neoplasm that is typically malignant and presents as a painless enlarged lymph node(s) and is followed by anemia, weakness, fever, and weight loss

i. Pneumonia caused by a common worldwide parasite, *Pneumocystis carinii,* for which most people have immunity if they are not severely immunocompromised

j. Infectious disease, chronic in nature, primarily affecting the lungs and causing large areas of cavitations and caseous necrosis

***Number correct* _______ × *10 points/correct answer: Your score* _______%**

C. Crossword Puzzle

Each crossword answer is worth 10 points. When you have completed the crossword puzzle, total your points and enter your score in the space provided at the end of the exercise.

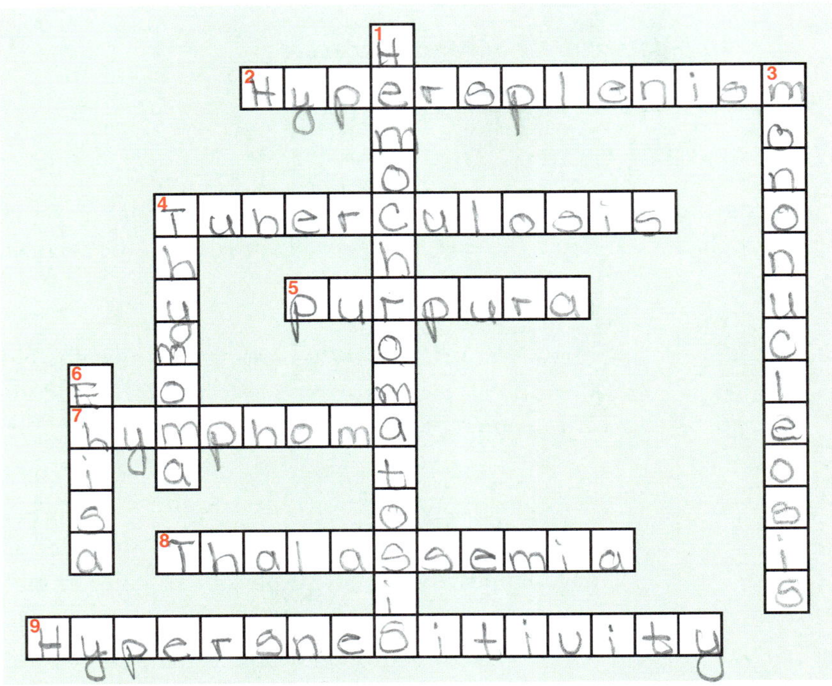

ACROSS

2 Condition of enlargement of the spleen
4 Infection of lungs with cavitations
5 Pinpoint hemorrhages: red-purple
7 Lymphoid tissue neoplasm (tumor)
8 hemolytic anemia = decrease in Hbg.
9 Exaggerated immune response

DOWN

1 Creates a bronze skin pigmentation
3 Acute infection of B lymphocytes
4 Tumor of the thymus gland
6 Test to screen for AIDS antibody

Number correct* _______ × *10 points/correct answer: Your score* _______ *%

D. Definition to Term

Using the following definitions, identify and provide the medical term(s) to match the definition. Each correct answer is worth 10 points. Record your score in the space provided at the end of the exercise.

1. A form of anemia characterized by the extreme reduction in circulating RBCs due to their destruction
hemolytic anemia
(two words)
2. A form of anemia resulting from a deficiency of mature RBCs and the formation and circulation of megaloblasts (large nucleated, immature, poorly functioning RBCs) with marked poikilocytosis (RBC shape variation), and anisocytosis (RBC size variation)
pernicious anemia
(two words)
3. Also called "bone marrow depression anemia," it is a form of anemia characterized by pancytopenia, an inadequacy of all the formed blood elements (RBCs, WBCs, and platelets)
aplastic anemia
(two words)

4. A chronic hereditary form of hemolytic anemia in which the RBCs become shaped like crescents in the presence of low oxygen tension

Sickle cell anemia

(three words)

5. An abnormal proliferation of RBCs, granulocytes, and thrombocytes leading to an increase in blood volume and viscosity (thickness)

polycythemia vera

(two words)

6. A term used to define different hereditary inadequacies of coagulation factors, which result in prolonged bleeding times

hemophilia

(one word)

7. Excessive uncontrolled increase of immature WBCs in the blood eventually leading to infection, anemia, and thrombocytopenia

leukemia

(one word)

8. Collection of blood beneath the skin in the form of pinpoint hemorrhages appearing as red-purple skin discolorations

purpura

(one word)

9. An inflammatory connective tissue disease, chronic in nature, in which immune complexes are formed from the reaction of SLE autoantibodies and their corresponding antigens

Systemic lypus erythematosus

(three words)

10. A syndrome presenting with immunodeficiency in the last or final phase of a human immunodeficiency virus (HIV) infection that primarily damages helper T cell lymphocytes with CD_4 receptors

acquired immunodeficiency syndrome

(three words)

Number correct _______ × 10 points/correct answer: Your score _______%

E. Word Search

Using the definitions provided, identify the term and then find and circle it in the puzzle. The words may be read up, down, diagonally, across, or backward. Each correct answer is worth 10 points. When you have completed the exercise, record your score in the space provided at the end of the exercise.

Example: The name for a red blood cell

erythrocyte

1. A systemic inflammatory disease resulting in the formation of multiple granulomas in the lungs (comprising 90%), lymph nodes, eyes, liver, and other organs

____

2. A locally destructive malignant neoplasm of the blood vessels associated with AIDS typically forming lesions on the skin, visceral organs, or mucous membranes

____

M	K	E	R	Y	T	H	R	O	C	Y	T	E	S	L
Y	A	S	R	E	T	S	O	P	O	R	E	T	N	A
A	P	R	Y	A	H	D	I	P	I	L	G	R	Y	S
S	O	I	S	P	E	C	S	T	S	S	U	T	N	I
T	S	O	I	T	D	I	B	L	E	I	I	T	A	S
H	I	H	Y	O	E	T	H	C	U	S	T	P	D	Y
E	S	R	D	E	R	E	I	M	B	I	I	A	I	L
N	S	M	E	U	I	O	N	X	R	T	N	R	O	A
I	A	O	A	V	U	N	G	C	T	N	P	G	P	N
A	R	M	C	T	Q	N	O	I	A	E	N	O	A	A
G	C	E	E	R	C	T	A	R	S	G	A	I	Q	C
R	O	U	L	E	A	U	X	J	I	O	R	D	U	I
A	M	I	T	M	T	A	E	R	C	N	A	A	E	R
V	A	I	E	I	A	S	R	M	L	I	S	R	V	T
I	J	H	L	S	Y	H	S	H	C	M	S	Y	A	I
S	I	S	O	D	I	O	C	R	A	S	M	Y	R	A
S	O	O	S	S	S	R	S	L	F	D	E	P	X	G
P	C	A	I	M	I	G	A	I	U	B	H	P	Y	A
T	Q	S	D	A	R	E	P	Y	M	A	K	L	T	R

3. An assessment of RBC percentage in the total blood volume

____

4. Immunity that occurs as a result of having had a disease or from having received an immunization against the disease

____

5. An aggregation of RBCs viewed through the microscope that may be an artifact or may occur with persons with multiple myeloma as a result of abnormal proteins

____

6. An abbreviation for a series of tests performed on peripheral blood that determines the number of red and white blood cells per cubic millimeter of blood

____

7. The name of a blood profile that measures triglycerides, cholesterol, phospholipids, fatty acids, and neutral fat

____

8. An autoimmune disease in which antibodies block or destroy some acetylcholine receptor sites decreasing neuromuscular transmissions, with resulting increased muscular weakness, extreme fatigue, and dysphagia

____

9. The abbreviation for the test that measures the rate at which red blood cells settle out in a tube of unclotted blood; the figure is expressed in millimeters per hour

____

10. The abbreviation for a one-stage blood test that detects certain plasma coagulation defects caused by a deficiency of various clotting factors; that is, factors V, VII, or X

Number correct _______ × 10 points/correct answer: Your score _______%

F. Matching Abbreviations

Match the abbreviations on the left with the most appropriate definition on the right. Each correct response is worth 10 points. When you have completed the exercise, record your score in the space provided at the end of the exercise.

_____	1. CMV	a. systemic lupus erythematosus
_____	2. ARC	b. Kaposi's sarcoma
_____	3. EBV	c. human immunodeficiency virus
_____	4. ITP	d. AIDS-related complex
_____	5. AIDS	e. autoimmune deficiency syndrome
_____	6. HSV	f. Epstein-Barr virus
_____	7. HIV	g. idiopathic thrombocytopenic purpura
_____	8. SLE	h. acquired immune deficiency syndrome
_____	9. KS	i. herpes simplex virus
_____	10. ELISA	j. H-influenza virus
		k. cytomegalovirus
		l. enzyme-linked immunosorbent assay

Number correct _______ × 10 points/correct answer: Your score _______%

G. Spelling

Circle the correctly spelled term in each pairing of words. Each correct answer is worth 10 points. Record your score in the space provided at the end of the exercise.

1. anaphylaxis	anaphlaxis
2. acites	ascites
3. basophile	basophil
4. dyscrasia	discrasia
5. fibrinogen	fibrinergen
6. hemorrage	hemorrhage
7. hyperlipemia	hyperlypemia
8. myeloid	myloid
9. nutrophil	neutrophil
10. tonsills	tonsils

Number correct _______ × 10 points/correct answer: Your score _______%

H. Completion

Complete each sentence with the most appropriate answer. Each correct answer is worth 10 points. Record your score in the space provided at the end of the exercise.

1. When someone has a lack of resistance to pathogens and other harmful agents, this individual is said to be: susceptible
2. Immunity with which we are born, also called genetic immunity, is known as: natural immunity
3. An abnormal condition characterized by an excessive reaction to a particular stimulus is known as: hypersensitivity
4. Immunity that is a result of the body's developing the ability to defend itself against a specific agent as a result of having had the disease or from having received an immunization against a disease is known as: acquired immunity
5. Another word for a platelet is: thrombocyte
6. The clear, thin, and sticky fluid portion of the blood that remains after coagulation is known as: serum
7. A systemic infection in which pathogens are present in the circulating bloodstream, having spread from an infection in any part of the body, is known as: septicemia
8. A naturally occurring anticlotting factor present in the body is: heparin
9. The breakdown of red blood cells and the release of hemoglobin that occurs normally at the end of the life span of a red blood cell is known as: hemolysis
10. A hormone that acts to stimulate and regulate the production of erythrocytes is: erythropoietin

Number correct _______ × 10 points/correct answer: Your score _______%

I. Identify the Combining Form

For each word on the left, provide the appropriate combining form and its definition in the blank space provided. Each correct answer is worth 10 points. Record your score in the space provided at the end of the exercise.

	Medical Term	Combining Form	Definition
1.	erythrocytosis	erythr/o	red
2.	hematology	hemat/o	blood
3.	hyperlipemia	lip/o	fat
4.	myeloid	myel/o	bone marrow, spinal cord
5.	pancytopenia	cyt/o	cell
6.	splenomegaly	splen/o	spleen
7.	thrombus	thromb/o	clot

8. pathogens path/o disease
9. electrophoresis electr/o electricity
10. hemolysis hem/o blood

Number correct ______ × 10 points/correct answer: Your score ______%

C. Multiple Choice

Read each statement carefully and select the correct answer from the options listed. Each correct answer is worth 10 points. Record your score in the space provided at the end of the exercise.

1. The watery, straw-colored fluid portion of the lymph and blood, in which leukocytes, erythrocytes, and platelets are suspended, is the:
   a. plasma
   b. fibrin
   c. hemoglobin
   d. thrombin
2. A stringy, insoluble protein that is the substance of a blood clot is:
   a. plasma
   b. fibrin
   c. hemoglobin
   d. thrombin
3. The abnormal accumulation of fluid in interstitial spaces of tissues is known as:
   a. heme
   b. globin
   c. edema
   d. hemostasis
4. An abnormal condition of the blood or bone marrow, such as leukemia, aplastic anemia, or prenatal Rh incompatibility, is termed:
   a. dyscrasia
   b. ascites
   c. erythremia
   d. erythropoiesis
5. A naturally occurring anticlotting factor present in the body is:
   a. hemoglobin
   b. plasma
   c. heparin
   d. serum
6. The abbreviation for hematocrit is:
   a. Hb
   b. Ht
   c. Hct
   d. Hmt

7. A diagnostic analysis for pernicious anemia is the:
   a. white blood cell count
   b. Schilling test
   c. hematocrit
   d. lipid profile
8. An assessment of RBC percentage in the total blood volume is:
   a. white blood cell count
   b. Schilling test
   c. hematocrit
   d. lipid profile
9. An x-ray assessment of the lymphatic system following injection of a contrast medium into the lymph vessels in the hand or foot is known as a:
   a. lymphangiogram
   b. western blot
   c. ELISA
   d. Coomb's test
10. When a person receives blood or a blood component that has been previously collected from that person through a reinfusion it is called a(n):
    a. bone marrow transplant
    b. direct antiglobulin test
    c. autologous transfusion
    d. rouleaux

Number correct _______ × 10 points/correct answer: Your score _______%

Answers to Chapter Review Exercises

A. Term to Definition

1. a blood test used for screening for an antibody to the AIDS virus.
2. measurement of the time required for bleeding to stop. The normal bleeding time according to one of the more common methods to evaluate bleeding time (the Ivy method) is 1 to 9 minutes.
3. an autoimmune disease in which antibodies block or destroy some acetylcholine receptor sites.
4. usually caused by the Epstein-Barr virus (EBV), mononucleosis typically is a benign, self-limiting acute infection of the B lymphocytes.
5. a blood test that detects the presence of the antibodies to HIV; the virus that causes AIDS.
6. a chronic hereditary form of hemolytic anemia in which the RBCs become shaped like crescents in the presence of low oxygen tension causing an abnormal proliferation of RBCs, granulocytes, and thrombocytes, which leads to an increase in blood volume and viscosity (thickness).
7. an x-ray assessment of the lymphatic system following injection of a contrast medium into the lymph vessels in the hand or foot.
8. concentration measurement of the hemoglobin in the peripheral blood. As a vehicle for transport of oxygen and carbon dioxide, hemoglobin levels provide information about the body's ability to supply tissues with oxygen.
9. blood test used to discover autoantibodies opposing RBCs, which can produce cellular damage, typically to ABO Rh antigens.
10. a diagnostic analysis for pernicious anemia.

B. Matching Pathological Conditions

1. f
2. d
3. e
4. b
5. c
6. g
7. j
8. a
9. h
10. i

C. Crossword Puzzle

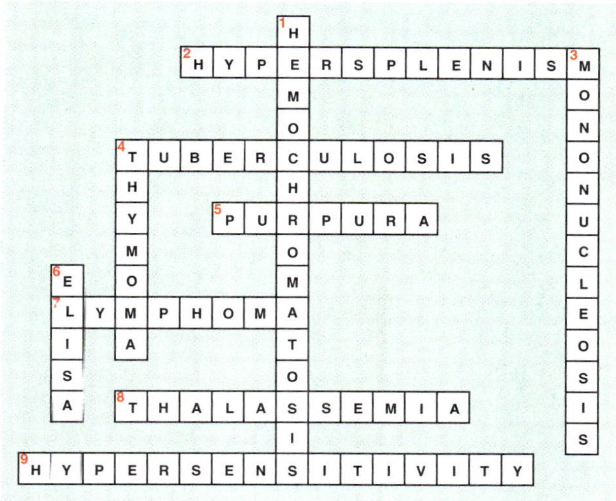

D. Definition to Term

1. hemolytic anemia
2. pernicious anemia
3. aplastic anemia
4. sickle cell anemia
5. polycythemia vera
6. hemophilia
7. leukemia
8. purpura
9. systemic lupus erythematosus
10. acquired immunodeficiency syndrome

E. Word Search

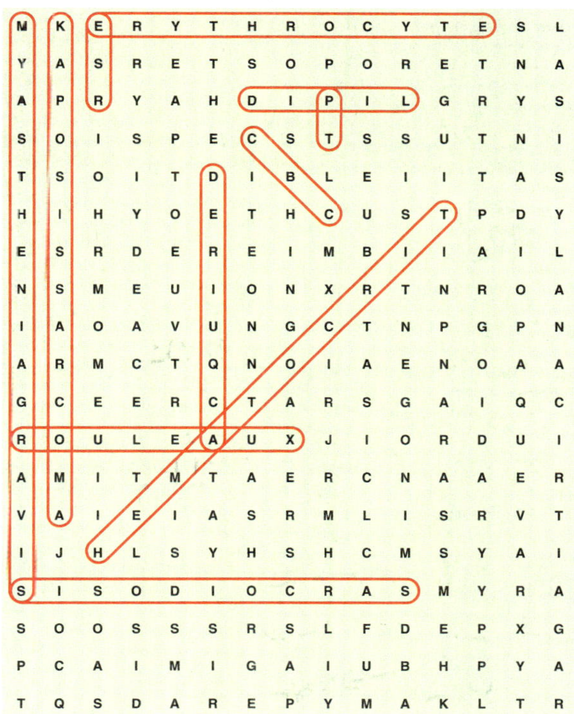

F. Matching Abbreviations

1. k
2. d
3. f
4. g
5. h
6. i
7. c
8. a
9. b
10. l

G. Spelling

1. anaphylaxis
2. ascites
3. basophil
4. dyscrasia
5. fibrinogen
6. hemorrhage
7. hyperlipemia
8. myeloid
9. neutrophil
10. tonsils

H. Completion

1. susceptible
2. natural immunity
3. hypersensitivity
4. acquired immunity
5. thrombocyte
6. serum
7. septicemia
8. heparin
9. hemolysis
10. erythropoietin

I. Identify the Combining Form

1. erythr/o	red
2. hemat/o	blood
3. lip/o	fat
4. myel/o	bone marrow, spinal cord
5. cyt/o	cell
6. splen/o	spleen
7. thromb/o	clot
8. path/o	disease
9. electr/o	electricity
10. hem/o	blood

J. Multiple Choice

1. a
2. b
3. c
4. a
5. c
6. c
7. b
8. c
9. a
10. c

CHAPTER 10

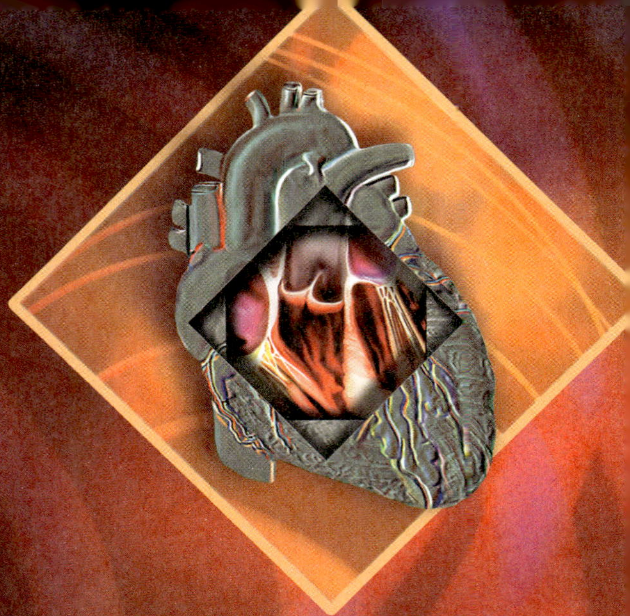

The Cardiovascular System

CHAPTER CONTENT

KEY COMPETENCIES

Upon completing this chapter and the review exercises at the end of the chapter, the learner should be able to:

1. Identify and label the pathway of blood as it travels through the heart, to the lungs, and back through the heart.
2. List two major functions of the cardiovascular system.
3. Identify and label the structures of the heart by completing the exercise at the end of the chapter.
4. Define at least 10 common cardiovascular signs and symptoms.
5. Correctly spell and pronounce each new term introduced in this chapter using the Activity CD-ROM and Audio CD, if available.
6. Define at least 20 common cardiovascular conditions.
7. Proof and correct one transcription exercise relative to the cardiovascular system.
8. Identify at least 20 abbreviations common to the cardiovascular system.
9. Identify four congenital heart diseases.
10. Identify at least three heart arrhythmias.

OVERVIEW

"And the beat goes on. . . ." Isn't it great that the beat of the heart *goes on* without conscious control? As we go about our busy schedules from day to day, the heart and the supporting structures of the cardiovascular system are responsible for pumping blood to the body tissues and cells, supplying these tissues and cells with oxygen and other nutrients, while removing carbon dioxide and other waste products of metabolism from the tissues and cells. The heart and blood vessels conjoin to pump and circulate the equivalent of 7,200 quarts of blood through the heart over a 24-hour period—approximately 5 quarts per minute, or 2.5 ounces per beat, at the rate of 80 beats per minute!

Anatomy and Physiology

Heart

The heart is the center of the circulatory system. It lies within the **mediastinum** (in the thoracic cavity cradled between the lungs, just behind the sternum): Place your hand to the left of the midline of your chest cavity, just above the diaphragm to locate the position of the heart. The area of the chest covering the heart is the **precordium.** Because the heart has a conelike shape, the broader upper portion is called the base, and the narrower lower tip of the heart is called the apex. The apex of the heart is located between the fifth and sixth ribs on a line perpendicular to the midpoint of the left clavicle. This position is usually just below the nipple. See **Figure 10-1.**

Apical pulses are taken on all children under 2 years of age and on patients with possible heart problems (the stethoscope is placed on the chest wall adjacent to the apex of the heart).

The heart is described as being roughly the size of a clenched fist, weighing less than a pound (approximately 10.6 ounces). There are, however, other factors that influence heart weight and size such as age, body weight, gender, frequency of physical activity, and heart disease. Using **Figure 10-2** as a guide, identify the linings and layers of the heart as described next.

The heart is enclosed by a thin, double-walled, membranous sac called the **(1) pericardium**. The outer covering of this sac providing strength to the pericardium is known as the **(2) parietal pericardium.** The inner layer of this membranous sac forms a thin, tight covering over the heart surface and is known as the **(3) visceral pericardium,** also known as the epicardium. Between these two layers is a small space called the **(4) pericardial cavity.** This cavity contains a very small amount of fluid that lubricates the surface of the heart and reduces friction during cardiac muscle contraction. The heart itself is composed of three layers: the outer layer, known as the **(5) epicardium**, the middle, muscular layer, known as the **(6) myocardium**, and the inner layer, known as the **(7) endocardium.**

The heart functions as two pumps working simultaneously to move blood to all sites in the body. Divided into four chambers, the upper chambers, known as the **right** and **left atria** (singular: atrium) are the receiving chambers; the lower chambers, known as the **right** and **left ventricles** (singular: ventricle) are the pumping chambers. The common

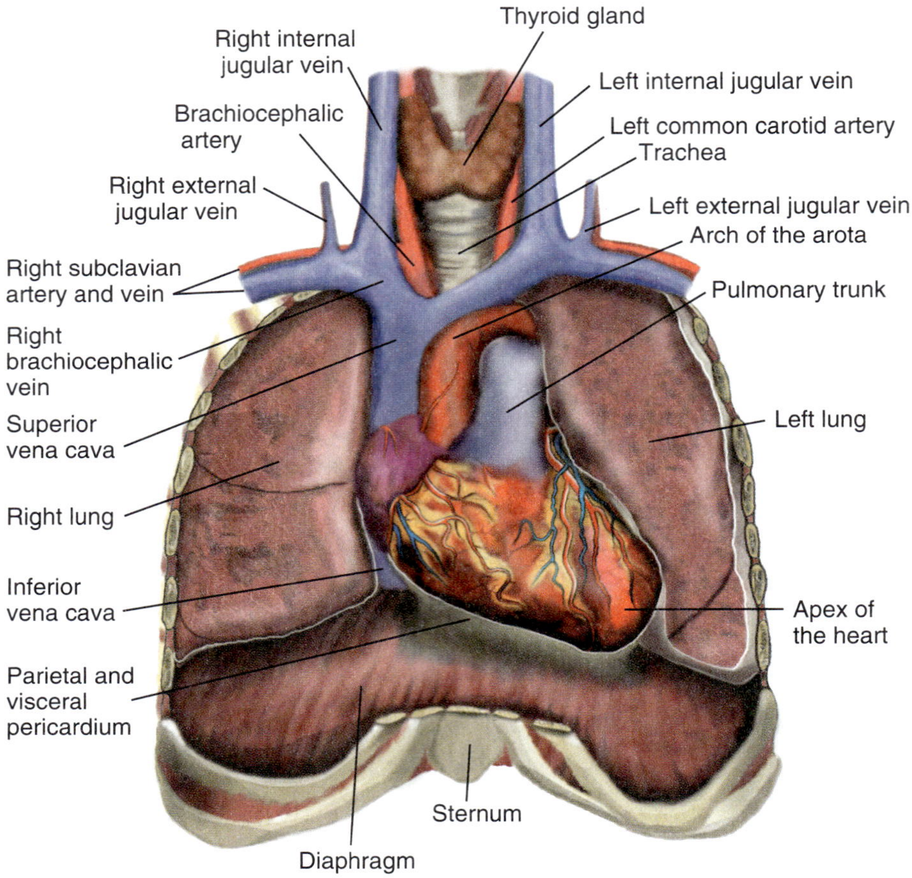

Figure 10-1 Apex/base of the heart

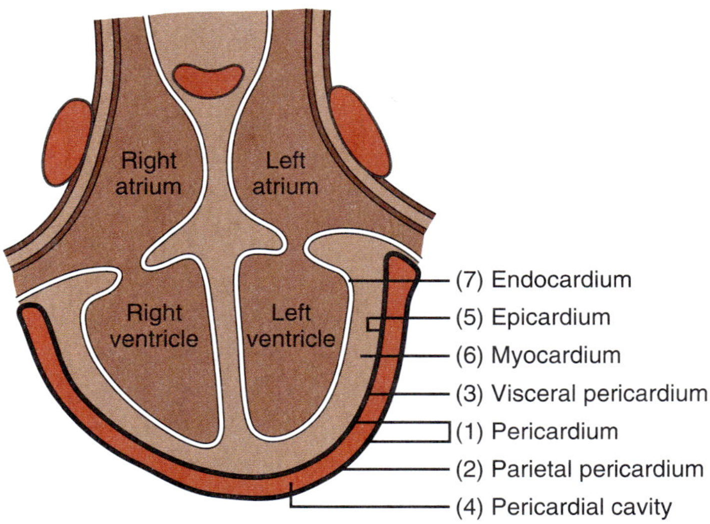

Figure 10-2 Linings and layers of the heart

wall between the right and left side of the heart is known as the septum (with the **interatrial septum** dividing the atria, and the **interventricular septum** dividing the ventricles). The varying thicknesses of the atrial and ventricular walls relate to the workload required by each chamber. The atrial walls are thinner than the ventricular walls because the atria receive blood, routing it on to the ventricles. The ventricular walls are thicker

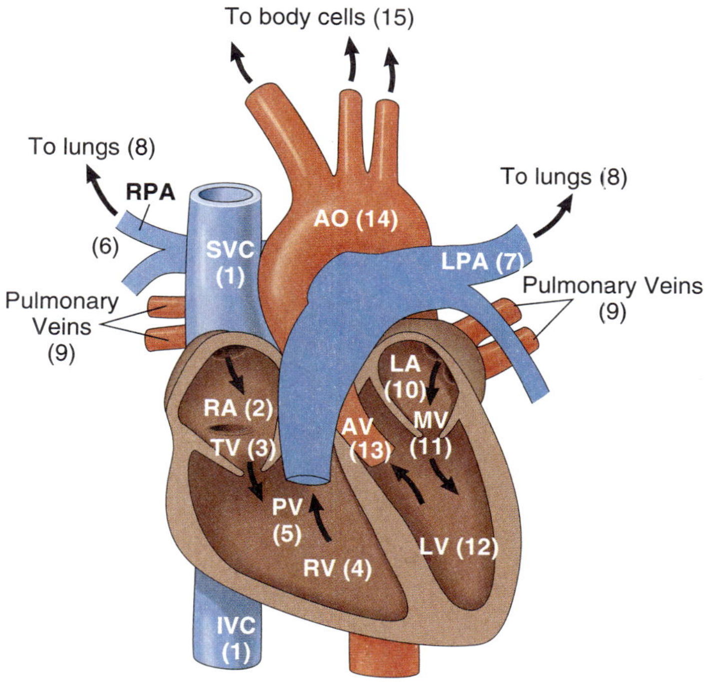

Figure 10-3 Blood flow pattern through the heart

than those of the atria because the ventricles are responsible for pumping the blood through to the lungs (from the right ventricle) and throughout the entire body (from the left ventricle). Because the left ventricle has the greater workload of the two lower chambers, its muscle is approximately 2.5 to 3 times thicker than that of the right ventricle.

Circulation Through the Heart

Figure 10-3 identifies the parts of the heart and the vessels that transport blood. Refer to this figure as we discuss the flow pattern of the blood through the heart.

Deoxygenated blood enters the (2) **right atrium** from the (1) **superior vena cava,** which brings blood from the head, thorax, and upper limbs, and from the (1) **inferior vena cava,** which returns blood from the trunk, lower limbs, and abdominal viscera. From the right atrium, the deoxygenated blood passes through the (3) **tricuspid valve** into the (4) **right ventricle.** The right ventricle then contracts to pump the deoxygenated blood through the (5) **pulmonary valve** into the right and left **(6 and 7) pulmonary arteries**, which carry the oxygen-poor blood to the capillary network of the (8) **lungs**. The pulmonary arteries are the only arteries in the body that carry deoxygenated blood.

It is in the lungs where the exchange of gases takes place. Carbon dioxide leaves the bloodstream by way of the capillaries and passes into the alveoli of the lungs to be eliminated during respiration; oxygen passes from the alveoli of the lungs through the capillaries into the bloodstream, oxygenating the blood. This circulation of the blood from the heart to the lungs for oxygenation and back to the heart is known as **pulmonary circulation.** The oxygenated blood is returned to the (10) **left atrium** of the heart by way of four (9) **pulmonary veins** (two from each lung). The pulmonary veins are the only veins in the body that carry oxygenated blood.

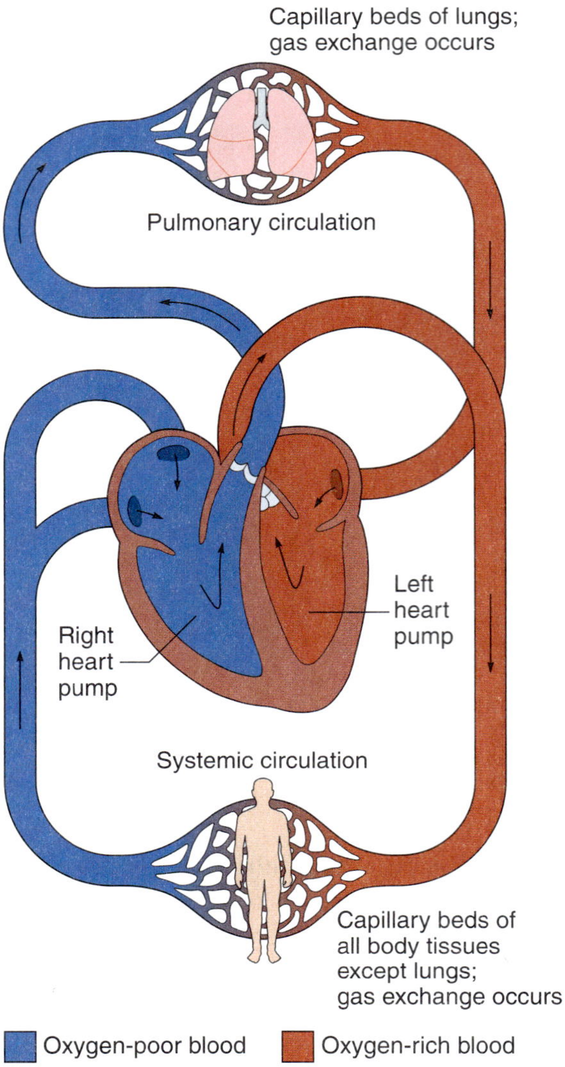

Figure 10-4 Pulmonary and systemic circulation

From the left atrium, the blood passes through the (11) **mitral,** or **bicuspid, valve** into the (12) **left ventricle.** The left ventricle then pumps the blood through the (13) **aortic valve** into the (14) **aorta.** The aorta branches into arteries that distribute the freshly oxygenated blood to (15) **each body part** and region. This circulation of the blood from the heart to all parts of the body and back to the heart is known as systemic circulation. **Figure 10-4** illustrates both pulmonary and systemic circulation.

An important principle that determines the direction of the flow of blood in the heart is that fluid flows from a region of higher pressure to a region of lower pressure. When the left ventricle contracts, it creates increased pressure within the aorta, causing the blood to be forced progressively through the arteries and capillaries and into the veins. Skeletal muscle contractions promote the venous return of blood to the heart through their contraction and relaxation actions, as will be discussed in the section on the supporting blood vessels. The blood eventually returns to the right atrium where the pressure within the right atrium is less than the pressure within the vena cavae.

In addition to circulating blood throughout the body, arteries also provide the blood supply to the heart muscle. The coronary arteries arise from the aorta near its origin at the left ventricle. These vessels supply blood to the heart muscle, which has a great need

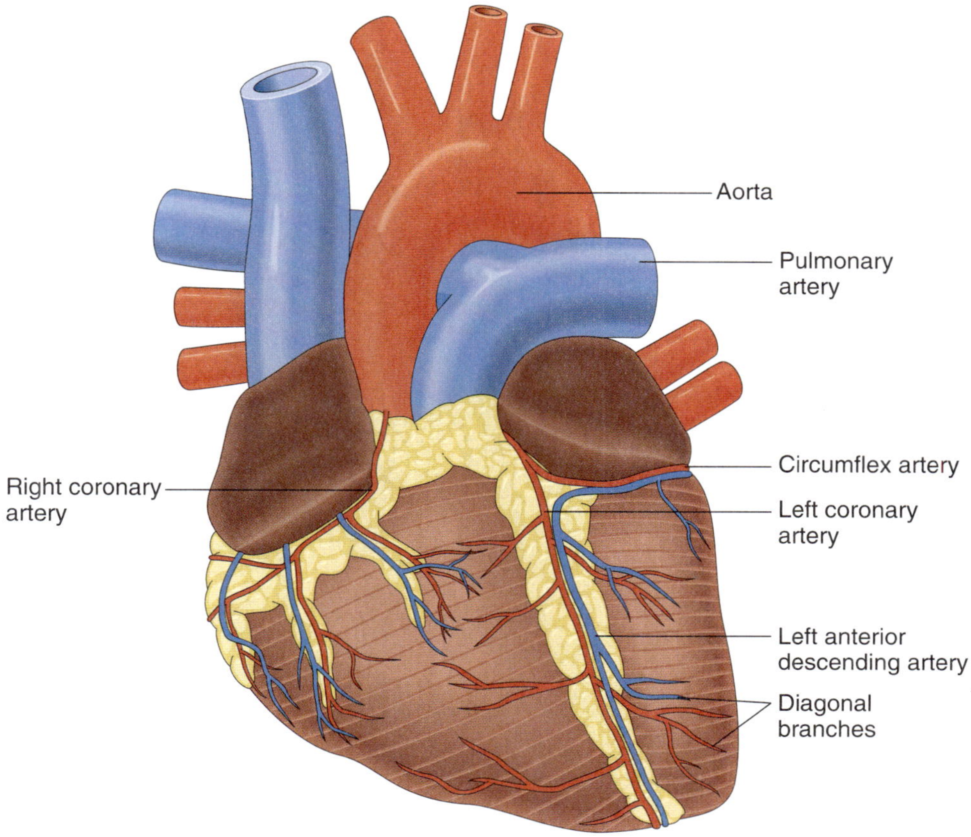

Figure 10-5 The coronary arteries

for oxygen and nutrients. The heart uses approximately 3 times more oxygen than other organs of the body. In this day and time, when there is great discussion of coronary artery disease, it is helpful to visualize the coronary arteries and realize their importance to effective myocardial function. See **Figure 10-5.**

Conduction System of the Heart

As stated earlier, "the beat goes on"; but what is it that causes the heart to contract rhythmically to keep the blood flowing throughout the body? Orderly contraction of the heart occurs because the specialized cells of the conduction system methodically generate and conduct electrical impulses throughout the **myocardium.** The **sinoatrial node (SA node),** a cluster of hundreds of cells, is located at the junction of the superior vena cava and the right atrium. The rate of impulses initiated by the sinoatrial node sets the rhythm for the entire heart; therefore, the sinoatrial node is called the **pacemaker** of the heart. Once the impulse is initiated from the SA node, it travels across the atria, causing them to contract, and forcing the blood into the ventricles of the heart.

The wave of electricity continues traveling through the myocardium to the **atrioventricular node (AV node),** which is located within the interatrial septum just above the junction of the atria and the ventricles. The AV node coordinates the incoming electrical impulses from the atria and relays the impulse to the ventricles through a bundle of specialized muscle fibers called the bundle of His.

The **bundle of His** enters the septum that separates the right and left ventricles (interventricular septum). It divides into **right** and **left bundle branches** that terminate in

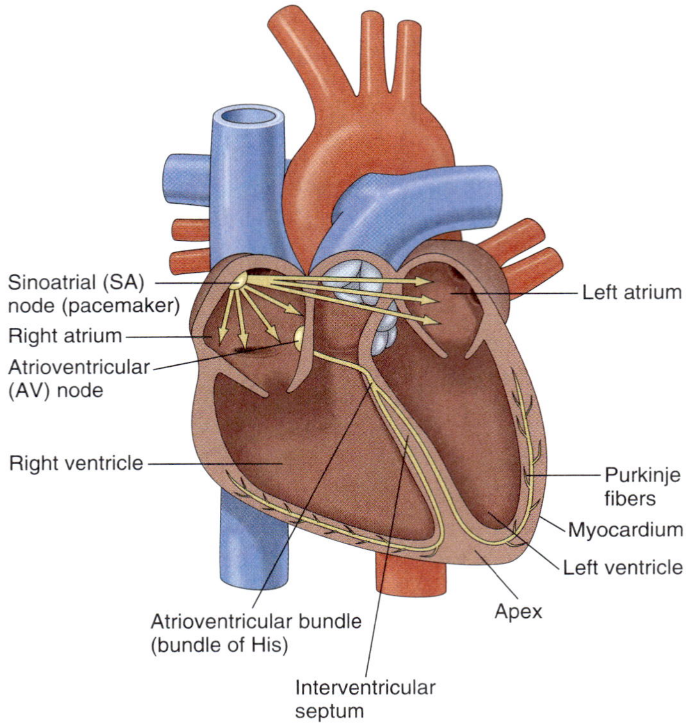

Figure 10-6 Conduction system of the heart

fibers called **Purkinje fibers.** The Purkinje fibers fan out into the muscles of the ventricles, forming the electrical impulse-conducting system of the heart. Receiving the electrical impulse from the bundle of His, the fibers cause the ventricles to contract.

To recap, the normal sequence of electrical impulses through the conduction system of the heart is as follows: SA node, through the atria to the AV node, from the AV node to the bundle of His, from the bundle of His to the bundle branches, and then to the Purkinje fibers. **Figure 10-6** illustrates the conduction system of the heart.

Supporting Blood Vessels

Upon leaving the heart, the blood enters the vascular system, which is composed of many blood vessels. These blood vessels responsible for transporting blood to and from the heart and throughout the body are the arteries, arterioles, veins, venules, and capillaries.

Arteries are large, thick-walled vessels that carry the blood away from the heart. The walls of the aorta and large arteries are thicker than those of the veins, allowing them to withstand the force of the blood as the heartbeat propels it forward throughout the circulatory system. As the arteries continue on their path away from the heart, they branch into smaller vessels called arterioles. The **arterioles** have thinner walls than the arteries and are composed almost entirely of smooth muscle with very little elastic tissue. The arterioles carry the blood on to the minute blood vessels known as capillaries.

Capillaries have extremely thin walls, consisting of a single layer of endothelial cells. The thin walls of the capillaries allow for the exchange of materials between the blood and the tissue fluid surrounding the body cells. The exchange that takes place at the cellular level is one of the cells receiving the oxygen and nutrients for energy and nourishment and the blood vessels receiving the waste products of metabolism (carbon dioxide and urea) for removal from the body cells. These waste products are then transported by way of the cardiovascular system to their appropriate sites for elimination from the body: to the lungs for elimination of carbon dioxide and to the kidneys for elimination of urea. The capillaries connect the ends of the arterioles with the beginnings of the venules.

Venules are the smallest veins that collect the deoxygenated blood from the cells for transport back to the heart. The venules branch into larger vessels known as veins. The **veins** have thinner walls than the arteries, but thicker walls than the capillaries. The veins transport the blood from the venules to the heart. This is achieved by the contraction of the skeletal muscles, which creates a squeezing or "milking" action on the veins, keeping the blood moving in one direction: toward the heart. The valves within the veins support the flow of blood in one direction by closing when the skeletal muscles relax, thereby preventing the backflow of blood.

Cardiac Cycle

One cardiac cycle is equivalent to one complete heartbeat. As the heart carries out the function of propelling the blood through the blood vessels, it repeats two alternating phases: contraction, forcing blood out of the heart (**systole**), and relaxation, allowing the heart to refill with blood (**diastole**).

During the **diastolic phase,** the ventricles relax and fill with blood. Deoxygenated blood enters the right atrium from the vena cavae and passes through the tricuspid valve to the right ventricle. The pulmonary valve is closed during this time, keeping the blood in the right ventricle. Simultaneously, oxygenated blood enters the left atrium from the pulmonary vein and passes through the mitral (bicuspid) valve into the left ventricle. The aortic valve is closed during this time, keeping the blood in the left ventricle.

Following this relaxation and filling period is the **systolic phase,** in which the ventricles contract. The right ventricle contracts to force the blood through the pulmonary valve into the pulmonary artery, which will carry the blood to the lungs for oxygenation. The tricuspid valve is closed at this time to prevent the backflow of blood into the right atrium. Simultaneously, the left ventricle contracts to force the blood through the aortic valve into the aorta, which then circulates the oxygenated blood to all parts of the body. The mitral (bicuspid) valve is closed at this time to prevent the backflow of blood into the left atrium.

With computerlike efficiency, the beat goes on, and the heart contracts every second of every day throughout one's life. The normal, healthy heart beats continuously, resting only 0.4 second between beats.

Blood Pressure

Blood pressure is defined as the pressure exerted by the blood on the walls of the arteries. This pressure reaches its highest values in the left ventricle during systole. The maximum pressure reached within the ventricles is called **systolic pressure,** with the minimum pressure within the ventricles being called the **diastolic pressure.** Recording of these pressure changes within the heart is known as measuring the blood pressure. Blood pressure is measured with a **sphygmomanometer** and a **stethoscope.** The reading is recorded as a fraction, with the systolic reading on the top and the diastolic reading on the bottom: For example, "The patient had a blood pressure reading of 120/80."

Vocabulary

The following vocabulary words are frequently used when discussing the cardiovascular system.

WORD	DEFINITION
analgesic (**an**-al-**JEE**-sik) an- = without algesi/o = sensitivity to pain -ic = pertaining to	Pertaining to relieving pain; a medication that relieves pain.
anastomosis (ah-**nas**-toh-**MOH**-sis)	A surgical joining of two ducts, blood vessels, or bowel segments to allow flow from one to the other; **anastomosis** of blood vessels may be performed to bypass an occluded area and restore normal blood flow to the area.
aneurysm (**AN**-yoo-rihzm) aneurysm/o = aneurysm	Localized dilation of a weakened area of the wall of an artery. The weakened area balloons out with every pulsation of the artery.
aneurysmectomy (**AN**-yoo-riz-**MEK**-toh-mee) aneurysm/o = aneurysm -ectomy = surgical removal	Surgical removal of the sac of an **aneurysm**.
anomaly (ah-**NOM**-ah-lee)	Deviation from normal; birth defect; for example, congenital **anomaly**.
anorexia (an-oh-**REK**-see-ah) an- = without	Lack or loss of appetite, resulting in the inability to eat. **Anorexia** is seen in individuals who are depressed, with the onset of **fever** and illness, with stomach disorders, or as a result of excessive intake of alcohol or drugs.
arthralgia (ar-**THRAL**-jee-ah) arthr/o = joint -algia = pain	Joint pain.
ascites (ah-**SIGH**-teez)	An abnormal collection of fluid within the peritoneal cavity (the peritoneum is the serous membrane that lines the entire abdominal cavity). This fluid contains large amounts of protein and electrolytes; general abdominal swelling occurs with **ascites**.
atherosclerosis (**ath**-er-**oh**-scleh-**ROH**-sis) ather/o = fatty scler/o = hardening -osis = condition	A form of **arteriosclerosis** (hardening of the arteries) characterized by fatty deposits building up within the inner layers of the walls of larger arteries.
benign (bee-**NINE**)	Noncancerous; not progressive.
bruit (brew-**EE**)	An abnormal sound or murmur heard when listening to a carotid artery, organ, or gland with a stethoscope; for example, during auscultation.

carditis (car-**DYE**-tis) **card/o** = heart **-itis** = inflammation	Inflammation of the heart muscles.
claudication (klaw-dih-**KAY**-shun)	Cramplike pains in the calves of the legs caused by poor circulation to the muscles of the legs; commonly associated with **atherosclerosis**.
coronary artery (**KOR**-oh-nah-ree **AR**-ter-ee) **coron/o** = heart **-ary** = pertaining to **arter/o** = artery **-y** = noun ending	One of a pair of arteries that branch from the aorta; the coronary arteries and their branches supply blood and oxygen to the heart muscle (myocardium).
cusp	Any one of the small flaps on the valves of the heart.
dependent edema (dependent eh-**DEE**-mah)	A fluid accumulation in the tissues influenced by gravity; usually greater in the lower extremities than in tissue levels above the level of the heart.
diastole (dye-**ASS**-toh-lee)	The period of relaxation of the heart, alternating with the contraction phase known as systole.
dysrhythmia (dis-**RITH**-mee-ah) **dys-** = bad, difficult, painful, disordered **rhythm/o** = rhythm **-ia** = condition	Abnormal rhythm.
edema (ee-**DEE**-mah)	The localized or generalized collection of fluid within the body tissues, causing the area to swell.
endocarditis (**en**-doh-car-**DYE**-tis) **endo-** = within **cardi/o** = heart **-itis** = inflammation	Inflammation of the inner lining of the heart.
epicardium (**ep**-ih-**CARD**-ee-um) **epi-** = upon, over **cardi/o** = heart **-um** = noun ending	The inner layer of the pericardium, which is the double-folded membrane that encloses the heart.
hepatomegaly (**heh**-pat-oh-**MEG**-ah-lee) **hepat/o** = liver **megal/o** = enlarged **-y** = noun ending	Enlargement of the liver.
Homan's sign	Pain felt in the calf of the leg, or behind the knee, when the examiner is purposely dorsiflexing the foot of the patient (bending the toes upward toward the foot). If the patient feels pain, it is called a positive Homan's sign, indicating **thrombophlebitis**.

hyperlipidemia (**high**-per-lip-ih-**DEE**-mee-ah) hyper- = excessive lip/o = fat -emia = blood condition	An excessive level of fats in the blood.
hypertension (**high**-per-**TEN**-shun) hyper- = excessive	Elevated blood pressure persistently higher than 140/90 mmHg; high blood pressure; also known as arterial hypertension.
hypotension (**high**-poh-**TEN**-shun) hypo- = under, below, beneath, less than normal	Low blood pressure; less than normal blood pressure reading.
infarction (in-**FARC**-shun)	A localized area of necrosis (death) in tissue, a vessel, an organ, or a part, resulting from lack of oxygen (anoxia) due to interrupted blood flow to the area.
ischemia (iss-**KEY**-mee-ah) -emia = blood condition	Decreased supply of oxygenated blood to a body part or organ.
lesion (**LEE**-zhun)	A wound, injury, or any pathological change in body tissue.
lipid (**LIP**-id) lip/o = fat	Any of a group of fats or fatlike substances found in the blood; some examples of lipids are cholesterol, fatty acids, and triglycerides.
lumen (**LOO**-men)	A cavity or the channel within any organ or structure of the body; the space within an artery, vein, intestine, or tube.
malaise (mah-**LAYZ**) mal- = bad, poor	A vague feeling of body weakness or discomfort, often indicating the onset of an illness or disease.
mediastinum (**mee**-dee-ass-**TYE**-num)	The area between the lungs in the chest cavity that contains the heart, aorta, trachea, esophagus, and bronchi.
murmur	A low-pitched humming or fluttering sound, as in a "heart murmur," heard on auscultation.
myocardium (my-oh-**CAR**-dee-um) my/o = muscle cardi/o = heart -um = noun ending	The middle, muscular layer of the heart.
nocturia (nok-**TOO**-ree-ah) noct/o = night ur/o = urine -ia = condition	Urination at night.
occlusion (ah-**KLOO**-shun)	Closure, or state of being closed.

orthopnea (**or-THOP**-nee-ah) **orth/o** = straight **-pnea** = breathing	An abnormal condition in which a person sits up straight or stands up to breathe comfortably.
pacemaker	The SA node (sinoatrial) of the heart located in the right atrium, that is responsible for initiating the heartbeat, influencing the rate and rhythm of the heart beat. The cardiac pacemaker (artificial pacemaker) is an electric apparatus used for maintaining a normal heart rhythm by electrically stimulating the heart muscle to contract.
palpable (**PAL**-pah-bl)	Detectable by touch.
palpitation (pal-pih-**TAY**-shun)	A pounding or racing of the heart, associated with normal emotional responses or with heart disorders.
pericardial	Pertaining to the pericardium.
pericardium (**pair**-ih-**CAR**-dee-um) **peri-** = around **cardi/o** = heart **-um** = noun ending	The double membranous sac that encloses the heart and the origins of the great blood vessels.
petechiae (peh-**TEE**-kee-ee)	Small, purplish, hemorrhagic spots on the skin; may be due to abnormality in the blood-clotting mechanism of the body.
pitting edema (pitting ee-**DEE**-mah)	**Pitting edema** is swelling, usually of the skin of the extremities, that when pressed firmly with a finger will maintain the dent produced by the finger.
prophylactic (proh-fih-**LAK**-tik)	An agent that protects against disease.
pulmfonary artery (**PULL**-moh-neh-ree artery) **pulmon/o** = lungs **-ary** = pertaining to **arter/o** = artery **-y** = noun ending	One of a pair of arteries that transports deoxygenated blood from the right ventricle of the heart to the lungs for oxygenation; the pulmonary arteries are the only arteries in the body to carry deoxygenated blood.
pulmonary circulation (**PULL**-moh-neh-ree) **pulmon/o** = lungs **-ary** = pertaining to	The circulation of deoxygenated blood from the right ventricle of the heart to the lungs for oxygenation and back to the left atrium of the heart; that is, from the heart, to the lungs, back to the heart.
pulmonary vein (**PULL**-moh-neh-ree vein) **pulmon/o** = lungs **-ary** = pertaining to	One of four large veins (two from each lung) that returns oxygenated blood from the lungs back to the left atrium of the heart; the pulmonary veins are the only veins in the body to carry oxygenated blood.
SA node	Sinoatrial node; pacemaker of the heart; see *pacemaker.*
septum (**SEP**-tum)	A wall, or partition, that divides or separates two cavities. The interatrial septum separates the right and left atria; the atrioventricular septum separates the atria and the ventricles; and the interventricular septum separates the right and left ventricles.

serum sickness (**SEE**-rum)	A hypersensitivity reaction that may occur 2 to 3 weeks after administration of an antiserum; symptoms include fever, enlargement of the spleen (splenomegaly), swollen lymph nodes, joint pain, and skin rash.
Sydenham's chorea (**SID**-en-hamz koh-**REE**-ah)	A form of chorea (involuntary muscle twitching) associated with rheumatic fever, usually occurring in childhood.
systemic circulation (sis-**TEM**-ik ser-kew-**LAY**-shun)	The circulation of blood from the left ventricle of the heart, throughout the body, and back to the right atrium of the heart. Oxygenated blood leaves the left ventricle of the heart and is distributed to the capillaries; deoxygenated blood is picked up from the capillaries and is transported back to the right atrium of the heart.
systole (**SIS**-toh-lee)	The contraction phase of the heartbeat forcing blood into the aorta and the pulmonary arteries. Systole is marked by the first sound heard on auscultation, or the first pulse palpated, after the release of the blood pressure cuff (sphygmomanometer).
thrombosis (throm-**BOH**-sis) thromb/o = clot -osis = condition	The formation or existence of a blood clot.
vasoconstriction (**vaz**-oh-con-**STRIK**-shun)	Narrowing of the lumen of a blood vessel.
vegetation (vej-eh-**TAY**-shun)	An abnormal growth of tissue around a valve.

Word Elements

The following word elements pertain to the cardiovascular system. As you review the list, pronounce each word element aloud twice and check the box after you "say it." Write the definition for the example word given for each word element. You may use your medical dictionary.

WORD ELEMENT	PRONUNCIATION	"SAY IT"	MEANING
aneurysm/o **aneurysm**ectomy	an-yoo-**RIZ**-moh **an**-yoo-riz-**MEK**-toh-mee	☐	aneurysm
angi/o **angi**ography	**AN**-jee-oh an-jee-**OG**-rah-fee	☐	vessel
arter/o, arteri/o **arteri**osclerosis	ar-**TEE**-roh, ar-**TEE**-ree-oh ar-tee-ree-oh-skleh-**ROH**-sis	☐	artery
arteriol/o **arteriol**e	ar-**tee**-ree-**OH**-loh ar-**TEE**-ree-ohl	☐	arteriole
ather/o **ather**oma	ah-**THAIR**-oh ah-thair-**OH**-ma	☐	fatty

cardi/o **cardi**ologist	**CAR**-dee-oh car-dee-**ALL**-oh-jist	☐	heart
coron/o **coron**ary arteries	cor-**OH**-no **KOR**-oh-nah-ree **AR**-ter-eez	☐	heart
echo- **echo**cardiogram	**EH**-koh ek-oh-**CAR**-dee-oh-**gram**	☐	sound
electr/o **electr**ocardiogram	ee-**LEK**-troh ee-**lek**-troh-**CAR**-dee-oh-**gram**	☐	electrical, electricity
endo- **endo**carditis	**EN**-doh en-doh-car-**DYE**-tis	☐	within
-graphy electrocardio**graphy**	**GRAH**-fee ee-**lek**-troh-**CAR**-dee-**OG**-rah-fee	☐	process of recording
megal/o **megalo**cardia	**MEG**-ah-loh **meg**-ah-loh-**CAR**-dee-ah	☐	enlarged
my/o **my**ocardium	**MY**-oh my-oh-**CAR**-dee-um	☐	muscle
ventricul/o **ventricul**ar	ven-**TRIK**-yoo-loh ven-**TRIK**-yoo-lar	☐	ventricle of the heart or brain

Common Signs and Symptoms

The following lists common complaints (signs and symptoms) that individuals with cardiovascular problems may describe when talking with the health professional. The observant health professional will listen carefully to all of the descriptions used by the patient. As you study the terms below, write each definition and word a minimum of three times (use a separate sheet of paper), pronouncing the word aloud each time. Note that the word and the **basic definition** are in bold print, if you choose to learn only the abbreviated form of the definition. A more detailed description follows most words. Once you have mastered each word to your satisfaction, check the box provided beside the word.

☐ **anorexia**
(an-oh-**REK**-see-ah)

Loss of appetite.

☐ **anxiety**
(ang-**ZIGH**-eh-tee)

A feeling of apprehension, worry, uneasiness, or dread, especially of the future.

Anxiety is defined as a vague, uneasy feeling, the source of which is often nonspecific or unknown to the individual.

bradycardia
(**brad**-ee-**CAR**-dee-ah)
brady- = slow
cardi/o = heart
-ia = condition

A slow heart rate that is characterized by a pulse rate under 60 beats per minute.

The heart rate normally slows during sleep, and in some physically fit people, the heart rate may be slow.

chest pain

A feeling of discomfort in the chest area.

This may be described as tightness, aching, squeezing, pressing, heaviness, crushing, strangling, indigestion, burning, or as a choking feeling in the throat.

cyanosis
(sigh-ah-**NO**-sis)
cyan/o = blueness
-osis = condition

Slightly bluish, grayish, slatelike, or dark discoloration of the skin due to the presence of abnormal amounts of reduced hemoglobin in the blood.

Bluish discoloration of the skin and mucous membranes, especially the lips, tongue, and fingernail beds.

dyspnea
(**DISP**-nee-ah)
dys- = difficult
pne/o = breathing

Air hunger resulting in labored or difficult breathing, sometimes accompanied by pain (normal when caused by vigorous work or athletic activity).

Audible labored breathing, distressed anxious expression, dilated nostrils, protrusion of abdomen and expanded chest, gasping, and marked cyanosis are among the symptoms of someone with dyspnea; shortness of breath.

edema
(eh-**DEE**-mah)

A local or generalized condition in which the body tissues contain an excessive amount of tissue fluid; swelling; generalized edema is sometimes called dropsy.

Pitting edema is swelling, usually of the skin of the extremities, that when pressed firmly with a finger will maintain the dent produced by the finger. Dependent edema is a fluid accumulation in the tissues influenced by gravity; usually greater in the lower extremities than in tissue levels above the level of the heart.

fatigue
(**FAH**-teeg)

A feeling of tiredness or weariness resulting from continued activity or as a side effect from some psychotropic drug; a state of exhaustion or a loss of strength or endurance.

fever
(**FEE**-ver)

Elevation of temperature above the normal.

The normal temperature taken orally is 98.6°F; however, it may be within the range of normal if it is one degree above or one degree below this value.

headache
(**HED**-ache)

A diffuse pain in different portions of the head and not confined to any nerve distribution area.

May be acute or chronic; may be frontal, temporal, or occipital; may be confined to one side of the head or to the region immediately over one eye.

The pain may be dull and aching or acute and almost unbearable; it may be intermittently intense, throbbing, or a pressure where the head feels as if it will burst. The medical term for a headache is cephalalgia.

☐ **nausea** (**NAW**-see-ah)	**Unpleasant sensation usually preceding vomiting;** intense pain can cause nausea.
☐ **pallor** (**PAL**-or)	**Lack of color; paleness;** an unnatural paleness or absence of color in the skin.
☐ **palpitation** (pal-pih-**TAY**-shun)	**Rapid, violent, or throbbing pulsation, as an abnormally rapid throbbing or fluttering of the heart. The palpitation is felt by the patient.**
☐ **sweat** (**SWET**)	**Perspiration; the liquid secreted by the sweat glands, having a salty taste.** The medical term for profuse sweating is diaphoresis.
☐ **tachycardia** (**tak**-ee-**CAR**-dee-ah) tachy- = rapid cardi/o = heart -ia = condition	**Abnormal rapidity of heart action, usually defined as a heart rate over 100 beats per minute.**
☐ **vomiting** (**VOM**-it-ing)	**Ejection through the mouth of the gastric contents;** the forcible expulsion of the contents of the stomach through the mouth; also called emesis.
☐ **weakness** (**WEEK**-ness)	**Lacking physical strength or vigor (energy).**

Pathological Conditions

As you study the pathological conditions of the cardiovascular system, note that the **basic definition** is in bold print followed by a detailed description in regular print. The phonetic pronunciation is directly beneath each term, and a breakdown of the component parts of the term when appropriate.

The pathological conditions are grouped into four categories: pathological conditions of the heart, pathological conditions of the blood vessels, congenital heart diseases, and arrhythmias.

Pathological Conditions of the Heart

coronary artery disease
(**KOR**-oh-nah-ree **AR**-ter-ee dih-**ZEEZ**)
coron/o = heart
arter/o = artery
-y = noun ending

Coronary artery disease is the narrowing of the coronary arteries to the extent that adequate blood supply to the myocardium is prevented.

The narrowing is usually caused by atherosclerosis; it may progress to the point where the heart muscle is damaged due to lack of blood supply (ischemia), as the lumen of the coronary artery narrows. When the lumen of the artery is narrowed and the wall is rough, there is a great tendency for clots to form, creating the possibility for **thrombotic occlusion** of the vessel.

As a result of the ischemia of the myocardial muscle, the individual experiences a burning, squeezing tightness in the chest that may radiate to the neck, shoulder blade, and left arm; nausea, vomiting, sweating, and anxiety may also accompany the pain.

Accepted treatments for occluded coronary arteries (that reduce or prevent sufficient flow of blood to the myocardium) include medications, percutaneous transluminal coronary angioplasty, directional coronary atherectomy, and coronary bypass surgery.

1. Medications may be used alone or in conjunction with other types of therapy.
2. **Percutaneous transluminal coronary angioplasty** is a nonsurgical procedure in which a catheter, equipped with a small inflatable balloon on the end, is inserted into the femoral artery and is threaded up the aorta (under x-ray visualization) into the narrowed coronary artery. When properly positioned, the balloon is carefully inflated, compressing the fatty deposits against the side of the walls of the artery, thus enlarging the opening of the artery to increase blood flow through the artery. Once the plague is compressed against the walls of the artery, the balloon-tipped catheter is then removed or replaced with a stent (a mesh tube used to hold the artery). Typically, a stent remains in place permanently unless re-occlusion occurs. This procedure is also called a balloon catheter dilation or a balloon angioplasty. See **Figure 10-7.**
3. **Directional coronary atherectomy** uses a catheter (AtheroCath), which has a small mechanically driven cutter that shaves the plaque and stores it in a collection chamber. See **Figure 10-8.**

   The plaque is then removed from the artery when the device is withdrawn. This procedure usually lasts from 1 to 3 hours and requires overnight hospitalization.

   During the atherectomy procedure, the patient remains awake, but sedated. The catheter is inserted into the femoral artery and is advanced into position using x-ray visualization as a guide. Once in place, the catheter balloon is inflated, pressing the cutting device against the plaque on the opposite wall of the artery. This causes the plaque to protrude into the window of the cutting device. As this happens, the rotating blade of the cutting device then shaves off the plaque, storing it in the tip of the catheter until removal from the body. The process is repeated several times using the cutting device, to widen the opening of the artery at the blockage site.

   If the medications, angioplasty, and atherectomy are not successful methods of treatment or the coronary artery disease is severe, coronary bypass surgery will then be the treatment of choice.
4. **Coronary bypass surgery** is designed to increase the blood flow to the myocardial muscle and involves bypass grafts to the coronary arteries

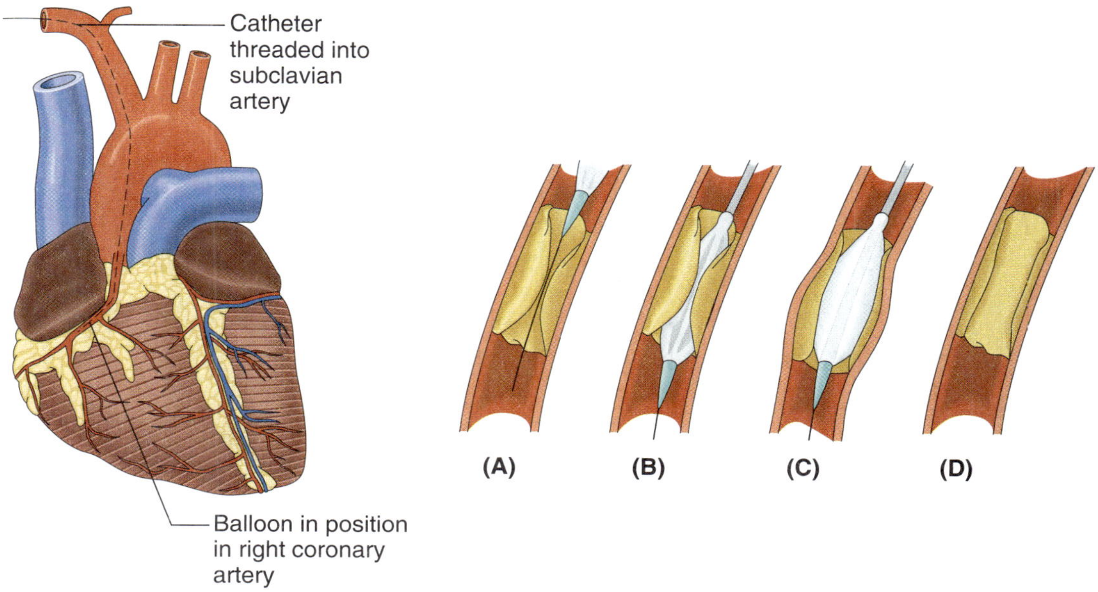

Figure 10-7 Balloon angioplasty (PTCA)

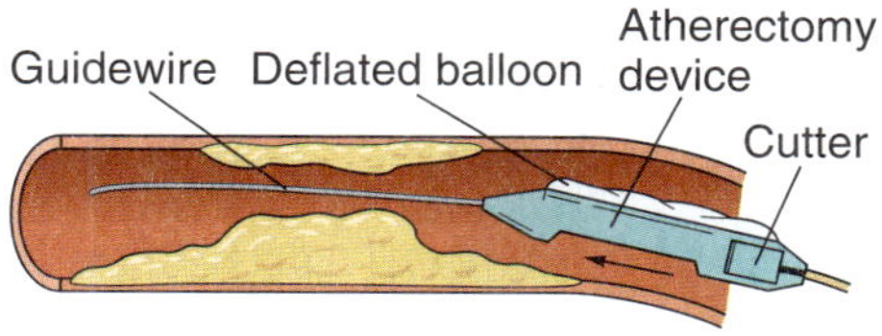

1. In coronary atherectomy procedures, a special cutting device with a deflated balloon on one side and an opening on the other is pushed over a wire down the coronary artery.

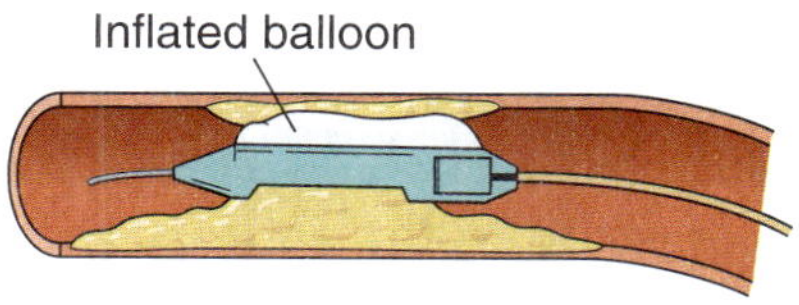

2. When the device is within a coronary artery narrowing, the balloon is inflated, so that part of the atherosclerotic plaque is "squeezed" into the opening of the device.

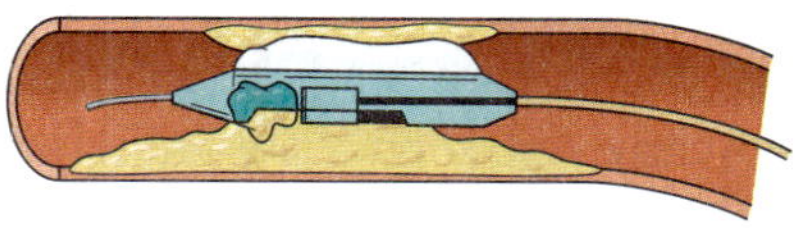

3. When the physician starts rotating the cutting blade, pieces of plaque are shaved off into the device.

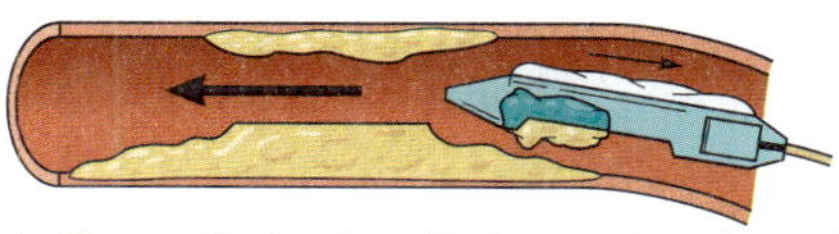

4. The catheter is withdrawn, leaving a larger opening for blood flow.

Figure 10-8 Directional coronary atherectomy

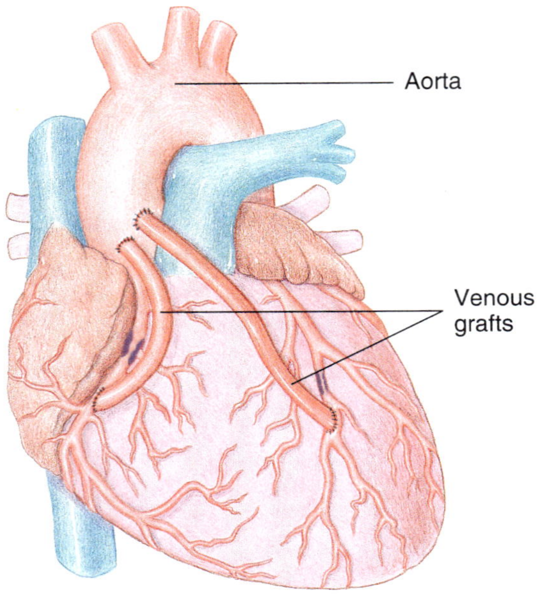

Figure 10-9 Coronary artery bypass surgery

that reroute the blood flow around the occluded area of the coronary artery. See **Figure 10-9.**

Grafts are made from veins taken from other parts of the body (usually the saphenous vein from the leg), and are connected to the coronary artery above and below the occlusion. This anastomosis (plural: anastomoses) joins the two vessels, restoring the normal flow of oxygenated blood to the myocardium.

angina pectoris
(an-**JI**-nah *or* **AN**-jin-nah **PECK**-tor-is)

Angina pectoris is severe pain and constriction about the heart, usually radiating to the left shoulder and down the left arm, creating a feeling of pressure in the anterior chest.

Angina is caused by an insufficient supply of blood to the myocardium. This ischemia produces pain that can vary from substernal pressure to severe, agonizing pain. The person with an angina attack experiences classic signs such as burning, squeezing, and tightness in the chest that may radiate to the neck and left arm and shoulder blade. Nausea and vomiting sometimes accompany the pain. The individual may have a sense of impending death; an apprehension very characteristic of angina.

In susceptible individuals, angina attacks are frequently triggered by conditions that increase the oxygen demand of the myocardium, such as exertion or stress. An important characteristic of anginal pain is that it subsides when the precipitating cause is removed; an attack usually lasts less than 15 minutes and not more than 30 minutes. If the pain persists for more than 30 minutes, the individual should see a physician immediately because these symptoms could also be those of an impending **myocardial infarction** (heart attack).

Treatment of angina consists of improving the oxygen supply to the myocardium by administering vasodilators such as nitroglycerine preparations to relieve the pain. If the individual does not respond to these measures, further testing will be necessary to determine the appropriate method of treatment.

---

myocardial infarction
(my-oh-**CAR**-dee-al in-**FARC**-shun)
my/o = muscle
cardi/o = heart

Heart attack: a condition caused by occlusion of one or more of the coronary arteries. This life-threatening condition results when myocardial tissue is destroyed in areas of the heart that are deprived of an adequate blood supply due to the occluded vessels.

This condition, which is caused by occlusion of one or more of the coronary arteries, is a medical emergency that requires immediate attention. To wait may result in loss of life.

Symptoms of a myocardial infarction include prolonged heavy pressure or squeezing pain in the center of the chest behind the sternum. The pain may radiate to the shoulder, neck, arm, and fourth and fifth fingers of the left hand. The patient may describe the pain as "crushing" or "viselike," and may clench a fist and hold it over the heart to demonstrate the character of the pain.

Pain associated with a myocardial infarction may be similar to anginal pain but usually is severe and is *not* relieved by the same measures that relieve anginal pain. This pain is often accompanied by shortness of breath, pallor, cold, clammy skin, profuse sweating, dizziness, nausea, and vomiting.

Treatment involves measures directed at minimizing myocardial damage. This is accomplished by relieving the pain, providing rest, stabilizing the heart rhythm, and reducing the workload of the heart. The most critical period for a person who has suffered a myocardial infarction is the first 24 to 48 hours after the attack (the area of infarction can increase in size for several hours or days after the onset of the attack). The mortality rate for myocardial infarctions is approximately 35% with most deaths occurring within the first 12 hours after the onset of the attack.

A myocardial infarction may be called an MI, heart attack, or coronary occlusion.

---

congestive heart failure
(kon-**JESS**-tiv heart failure)

Condition characterized by weakness, breathlessness, abdominal discomfort; edema in the lower portions of the body resulting from the flow of the blood through the vessels being slowed (venous stasis) and the outflow of blood from the left side of the heart is reduced; the pumping ability of the heart is progressively impaired to the point that it no longer meets bodily needs; also known as cardiac failure.

The principal feature in congestive heart failure is increased intravascular volume. Congestion of the tissues results from increased arterial and venous pressure due to decreased cardiac output in the failing heart.

Left-sided cardiac failure occurs when the left ventricle is unable to sufficiently pump the blood that enters it from the lungs. This causes increased pressure in the pulmonary circulation, which results in the forcing of fluid into the pulmonary tissues, creating pulmonary edema (congestion). The patient experiences dyspnea, cough (mostly moist sounding), **fatigue**, **tachycardia**, restlessness, and anxiety.

Right-sided cardiac failure occurs when the right side of the heart is unable to sufficiently empty its blood volume and cannot accommodate all of the blood that it receives from the venous circulation. This results in congestion of the viscera and the peripheral tissues. The patient experiences edema of the lower extremities (pitting edema), weight gain, enlargement of the liver (hepatomegaly), distended neck veins, ascites, anorexia, **nocturia**, and weakness.

Treatment involves promoting rest to reduce the workload on the heart, medications to increase the strength and efficiency of the heartbeat, and medications to eliminate the accumulation of fluids within the body. Dietary sodium may also be restricted.

---

endocarditis
(**en**-doh-car-**DYE**-tis)
endo- = within
cardi/o = heart
-itis = inflammation

Inflammation of the membrane lining of the valves and chambers of the heart caused by direct invasion of bacteria or other organisms and leading to deformity of the valve cusps. Abnormal growths called vegetations are formed on or within the membrane.

Endocarditis, also called bacterial endocarditis, is most frequently caused by infection from streptococcal bacteria. Other causative microorganisms include other bacteria such as staphylococci, pneumococci, and enterococci, and fungi and rickettsiae. Patients who have rheumatic heart disease, who have had prosthetic valve surgery, or who have mitral valve prolapse, are at greater risk for bacterial endocarditis.

The onset of bacterial endocarditis is misleading and may imitate many systemic diseases, with no early signs of cardiac involvement. There may be weakness and fatigue, an intermittent fever that persists for weeks, and night sweats. Chills, **malaise**, and **arthralgia** are also frequent complaints. A heart murmur may be heard that was not present initially.

The damage to the heart valves may cause lesions called vegetations that may break off into the bloodstream, forming **emboli** that lodge in other organs. If the emboli lodge in the small vessels of the skin, small pinpoint hemorrhages called **petechiae** may appear. The possibility of emboli lodging in other organs is also present with endocarditis.

Treatment involves the use of antibiotics to destroy the invading microorganism; therapy will likely continue over the course of several weeks.

---

pericarditis
(per-ih-car-**DYE**-tis)
peri- = around
cardi/o = heart
-itis = inflammation

Inflammation of the pericardium (the saclike membrane that covers the heart muscle); it may be acute or chronic.

Pericarditis is usually caused by bacterial infection of the pericardium. Other causes include neoplasms, viruses, rheumatic fever, myocardial infarction, trauma, and tuberculosis.

The characteristic symptom of pericarditis is pain, usually over the precordium (area of the body overlying the heart and part of the lower thorax). The pericardial pain is aggravated by breathing, turning, or twisting of the body; it is relieved by sitting up (**orthopnea**). The characteristic sign of pericarditis is a pericardial friction rub that may be heard on auscultation (a grating sound heard as the heart beats).

Other symptoms include dyspnea, tachycardia, malaise, fever, and accumulation of fluid within the pericardial cavity. If the fluid accumulates rapidly, the pressure against the heart may result in shocklike symptoms: **pallor**; damp, moist skin; and a drop in blood pressure. The patient may appear extremely ill.

Treatment for pericarditis includes determining the underlying cause of pericarditis and treating it; if it is a result of bacterial invasion, treatment with antibiotics is in order. The patient is placed on bed rest until the fever, chest pain, and friction rub have disappeared. **Analgesics** may be prescribed for the pain.

---

myocarditis
(**my**-oh-car-**DYE**-tis)
my/o = muscle
cardi/o = heart
-itis = inflammation

Inflammation of the myocardium; may be caused by viral or bacterial infections or may be a result of systemic diseases such as rheumatic fever; may also be caused by fungal infections, **serum sickness**, or chemical agent.

The signs and symptoms of uncomplicated **myocarditis** may be mild or absent, and are often nonspecific. They may include symptoms such as fatigue, dyspnea, fever, and heart palpitations. A more complicated case of myocarditis can lead to congestive heart failure.

Treatment is specific to the underlying cause of myocarditis, if it is known; analgesics, oxygen, anti-inflammatory agents, and bed rest help until symptoms have disappeared.

---

rheumatic fever
(roo-**MAT**-ic fever)

An inflammatory disease that may develop as a delayed reaction to insufficiently treated Group A beta-hemolytic streptococcal infection of the upper respiratory tract.

This disorder usually occurs in school-age children (primarily ages 5 to 15), and may affect the joints, heart, central nervous system, skin, and other body tissues.

Early symptoms of **rheumatic fever** include fever, joint pains, nosebleeds, abdominal pain, and vomiting. Other symptoms include **polyarthritis**, **carditis**, and sometimes a late symptom of **Sydenham's chorea**. Mild cases of rheumatic fever may last for 3 to 4 weeks; severe cases, which include arthritis and carditis, may last 2 to 3 months. Except for the carditis, all of the symptoms of rheumatic fever usually subside without any permanent consequences.

Treatment includes bed rest and restriction of activities. Antibiotics are usually administered to ensure that no traces of Group A streptococci remain in the body. Salicylates are given to reduce fever, joint pain, and swelling.

The prognosis for rheumatic fever depends on the degree of scarring and deformity that may have occurred to the heart valves if the patient developed carditis. Involvement of the heart may be evident during acute rheumatic fever, or it may be discovered long after the acute disease has subsided. The damage to the heart muscle and heart valves caused by episodes of rheumatic fever is known as **rheumatic heart disease.**

hypertensive heart disease
(high-per-**TEN**-siv heart dih-**ZEEZ**)

Hypertensive heart disease is a result of long-term hypertension. The heart is affected because it must work against increased resistance due to increased pressure in the arteries.

The heart enlarges in an attempt to compensate for the increased cardiac workload. Cardiac failure can occur if the underlying hypertension is not treated. (Hypertension will be discussed later in this chapter.)

mitral valve prolapse
(**MY**-tral valve proh-**LAPS**)

Mitral valve prolapse is drooping of one or both cusps of the mitral valve back into the left atrium during ventricular systole (when the heart is pumping blood), resulting in incomplete closure of the valve and mitral insufficiency. (Normally the mitral valve would completely close to prevent the backflow of blood into the left atrium during systole.) Also known as click-murmur syndrome, Barlow's syndrome, and floppy mitral valve.

Many individuals are symptom-free. The improper closing of the mitral valve produces an extra heart sound referred to as a mitral click, which can be heard on auscultation. Approximately 10% of the population has mitral valve prolapse.

The condition is relatively **benign**, with symptoms including atypical chest pain and palpitations. Treatment is directed at controlling the symptoms the patient is experiencing. Patients should be instructed on the importance of receiving **prophylactic** antibiotic therapy before any invasive procedures, such as dental work.

Pathological Conditions of the Blood Vessels

aneurysm
(**AN**-yoo-rizm)
aneurysm/o = aneurysm

A localized dilatation of an artery formed at a weak point in the vessel wall. This weakened area balloons out with each pulsation of the artery.

Once an aneurysm develops, the tendency is toward an increase in size. The danger of rupture is always a possibility and can lead to hemorrhage and ultimately death.

Aneurysms are most commonly caused by atherosclerosis and hypertension. Other, less frequent, causes include trauma to the wall of the artery, infection, and congenital defects. The most common site for an aneurysm is the aorta, and most of these occur below the renal arteries.

Treatment of choice for a large abdominal, aortic aneurysm is surgery. The **aneurysmectomy** involves resection of the aneurysm and insertion of a bypass graft. During surgery, the aneurysm is removed and circulation is restored by suturing the synthetic graft to the aorta at one end, and to the iliac arteries at the other end. **Figure 10-10** illustrates surgical treatment of a large abdominal aneurysm involving the iliac arteries.

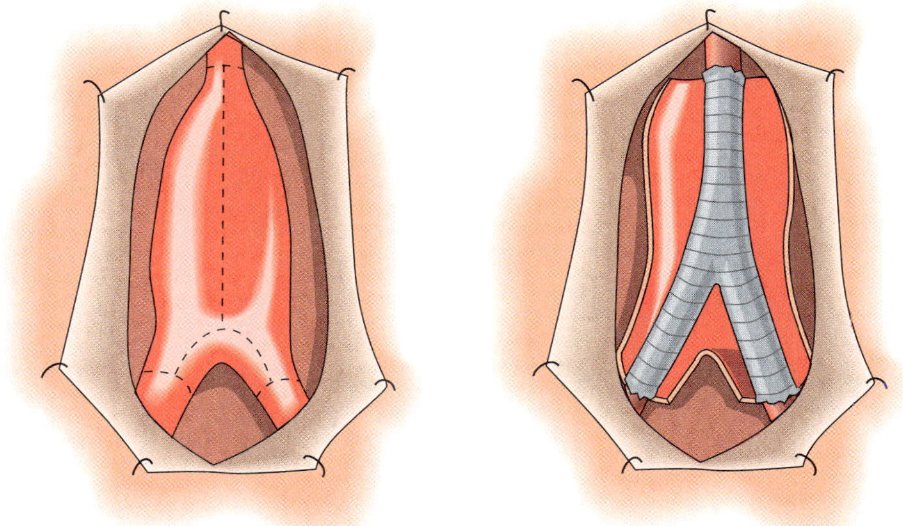

Figure 10-10 Surgical repair of an abdominal aneurysm

arteriosclerosis
(ar-tee-ree-oh-skleh-**ROH**-sis)
arteri/o = artery
scler/o = hard, also refers to sclera of the eye
-osis = condition

An arterial condition in which there is thickening, hardening, and loss of elasticity of the walls of arteries, resulting in decreased blood supply, especially to the lower extremities and cerebrum; hardening of the arteries.

Symptoms include intermittent **claudication**, changes in skin temperature and color, altered peripheral pulses, **bruits** over the involved artery, headache, dizziness, and memory defects (depending on the organ system involved).

Some risk factors for arteriosclerosis include hypertension, increased blood **lipids** (particularly cholesterol and triglycerides), obesity, diabetes, cigarette smoking, inability to cope with stress, and family history of early-onset atherosclerosis.

Treatment options may include a diet low in saturated fatty acids, medications to lower the blood lipid levels (in conjunction with the low-fat diet), proper rest and regular exercise, avoidance of stress, discontinuing cigarette smoking, and additional treatment specific to the condition for factors such as hypertension, diabetes, and obesity.

thrombophlebitis
(throm-boh-fleh-**BY**-tis)
thromb/o = clot
phleb/o = vein
-itis = inflammation

Inflammation of a vein associated with the formation of a thrombus (clot); usually occurs in an extremity, most frequently a leg.

Thrombophlebitis is classified as either superficial or deep. **Superficial thrombophlebitis** is usually obvious and is accompanied by a cordlike or thready appearance to the vessel, which is **palpable**; the vessel is extremely sensitive to pressure; the extremity may be pale, cold, and swollen. **Deep vein thrombosis** (**DVT**) occurs primarily in the lower legs, thighs, and pelvic area. It is not as evident as superficial thrombophlebitis and may be characterized by symptoms such as aching or cramping pain in the legs.

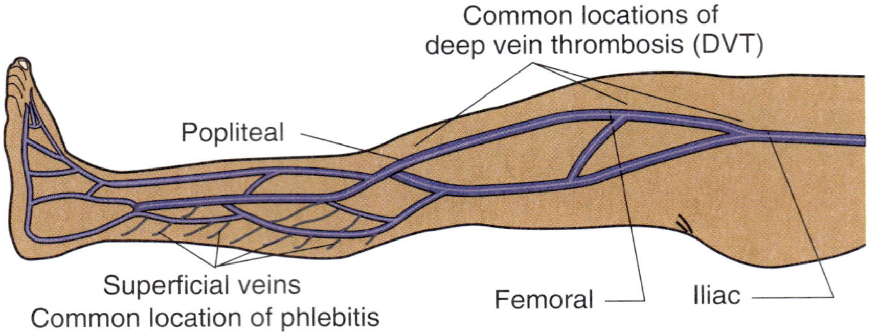

Figure 10-11 Superficial versus deep veins in development of phlebitis and thrombus

Figure 10-11 provides a visual reference for superficial versus deep veins in the development of phlebitis. The pain experienced in the calf of the leg when dorsiflexing the foot is known as a positive Homans' sign.

Thrombophlebitis may be caused by poor venous circulation, which may be due to obesity, congestive heart failure, sitting in one position for long periods of time without exercising (as in riding in an automobile), or immobility of an extremity for long periods of time; damage to the inner lining of the vein caused by trauma to the vessel (e.g., venipuncture); and a tendency of the blood to coagulate more rapidly than normal (hypercoagulability).

Treatment for thrombophlebitis of the leg involves complete bed rest and elevation of the affected extremity until the tenderness has subsided, which is usually 5 to 7 days. Warm moist compresses may be applied to the affected area to help relieve some of the pain and to treat inflammation. Analgesics may be given for the pain. Vital signs are taken frequently and circulation of the affected extremity is checked. Anticoagulants are not routinely used for superficial thrombophlebitis, but are used to treat deep vein thrombophlebitis. Elastic stockings, which support venous circulation (antiembolic stockings), are recommended when the patient becomes ambulatory.

---

varicose veins
(**VAIR**-ih-kohs veins)

Enlarged, superficial veins; a twisted, dilated vein with incompetent valves.

Veins have valves that keep the blood flowing in one direction only. In normal veins, the wall of the vein is strong enough to withstand the lateral pressure of the blood, and the blood flows through the valves in one direction. In varicose veins, however, the dilatation of the vein from long periods of pressure prevents the complete closure of the valves, resulting in backflow of blood in the veins, creating the varicosities. See **Figure 10-12.**

Patients with varicose veins often complain of pain and muscle cramps, with a feeling of heaviness in the legs, moderate swelling, easy fatigability, minimal skin discoloration, and palpable, distended veins (that may have a cordlike feel to them).

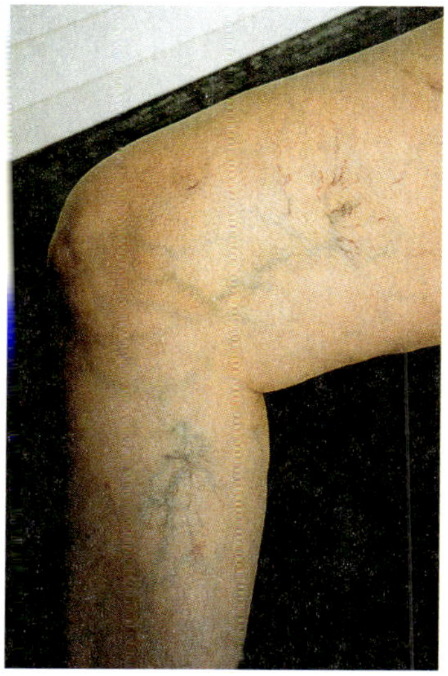

Figure 10-12 Varicose veins (venous star)

Treatment includes conservative measures such as rest and elevation of the affected extremity, along with the use of elastic stockings. Another non-surgical treatment of varicose veins and spider veins is sclerotherapy.

Sclerotherapy is a form of treatment that involves the injection of a chemical irritant (sclerosing agent) into the varicosed vein. The sclerosing agent irritates the inner lining of the vein causing localized inflammation of the vein, followed by formation of fibrous tissue, which closes the vein. Following the injections, compression bandages are applied to the leg (elastic leg wraps), and are worn for approximately 5 days. This is followed with the use of full therapeutic support hose for several weeks.

If the varicosities are severe enough, surgical intervention may become necessary. **Vein stripping** is a surgical procedure that consists of ligation (tying off) of the saphenous vein. A nylon wire is then inserted into the saphenous vein from an incision in the ankle and is threaded up the vein to the groin area. The wire is brought out of the vein in the groin area and is capped. It is then pulled downward to the ankle incision, "stripping" the vein.

The patient may stay in the hospital overnight following vein stripping surgery, or may have this done on an outpatient basis. In either case, bed rest is maintained for 24 hours following surgery. Elastic compression bandages are applied to the leg, from the toe area to the groin, and remain on for approximately 1 week following surgery. It is important to promote exercise and movement of the legs, and to elevate the head of the patient's bed to promote venous circulation. The patient will begin walking for short periods of time 24 to 48 hours after surgery.

---

hypertension
(high-per-**TEN**-shun)
hyper- = excessive

A condition in which the patient has a higher blood pressure than that judged to be normal; characterized by elevated blood pressure persistently exceeding 140/90 mmHg; often asymptomatic.

Essential hypertension, accounting for approximately 90% of all hypertension, has no single known cause. Leading risk factors include hypercholesterolemia (high cholesterol level in the blood), obesity, high serum sodium level (high level of sodium in the blood), and a family history of high blood pressure.

There are also physical conditions that can cause hypertension, including complications of pregnancy and kidney disease. This type of hypertension is known as **secondary hypertension,** accounting for approximately 10% or less of all hypertension. Treatment of the primary condition can reduce the elevated blood pressure in secondary hypertension.

Malignant hypertension is a term given to hypertension that is severe and rapidly progressive. It is most common in African American men under the age of 40. Malignant hypertension is characterized by a diastolic pressure higher than 120 mmHg, severe headaches, confusion, and blurred vision. Unless medical treatment is successful, malignant hypertension may result in a cerebrovascular accident (stroke), fatal uremia (kidney failure), myocardial infarction (heart attack), or congestive heart failure.

Generally, treatment for hypertension includes medications designed to control the blood pressure, and a diet low in sodium and saturated fats;

low calorie diet for obesity. Patients are advised to exercise, avoid stress, and to get proper rest.

Raynaud's phenomenon
(ray-**NOZ**)

Intermittent attacks of vasoconstriction of the arterioles, causing pallor of the fingers or toes, followed by cyanosis, then redness, before returning to normal color; initiated by exposure to cold or emotional disturbance.

The characteristic color change of Raynaud's phenomenon is described as white (pallor), blue (cyanosis), and red (return of color). Numbness, tingling, and burning pain occur as the color changes. Normal color and sensation are restored by heat.

Raynaud's phenomenon can be secondary to physical conditions or it can be idiopathic (cause unknown). It occurs most frequently in young women age 18 to 30, and is usually treated by protecting the body and extremities from exposure to cold and sometimes use of medications to calm the individual and to dilate the blood vessels.

peripheral arterial occlusive disease
(per-**IF**-er-al ar-**TEE**-ree-al)

Obstruction of the arteries in the extremities (predominantly the legs). The leading cause of this disease is atherosclerosis, which leads to narrowing of the lumen of the artery. The classic symptom of peripheral arterial occlusive disease is intermittent claudication, which is a cramplike pain in the muscles brought on by exercise and relieved by rest.

The patient may experience a feeling of coldness or numbness in the affected extremity. The extremity may appear pale when elevated or a ruddy, cyanotic color when allowed to dangle over the side of the bed. Observations of the color of the extremity, the feel (e.g., coolness) of the extremity, and the strength of the pulses is important for proper assessment of this condition. Unequal strength of pulses between extremities and absence of a pulse, which is normally palpable, is a reliable sign of arterial occlusion.

Peripheral arterial disease is usually found in individuals over age 50, and most often in men. The obstructive lesions are essentially confined to segments of the arterial system in the lower extremities; extending from the abdominal aorta, below the renal arteries, to the popliteal artery (behind the knee). See **Figure 10-13.**

Treatment involves exercises designed to promote arterial blood flow in the extremities, avoidance of nicotine, which causes **vasoconstriction**; and measures necessary to control the contributing risk factors such as diabetes, **hyperlipidemia**, and hypertension.

If the condition is severe enough, surgical intervention may become necessary. The most common surgical procedure to improve the blood flow beyond the occlusion is a vascular bypass graft. This is the same type of bypass graft surgery discussed in the section on coronary artery disease, where the occluded area is "bypassed" with a graft attached above and below the blocked area, thus restoring a normal blood flow pattern to the vessel.

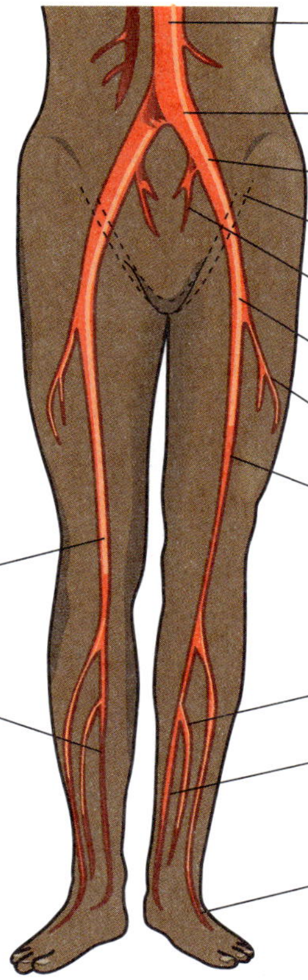

Figure 10-13 Common sites for peripheral arterial occlusive disease

Congenital Heart Diseases

tetralogy of Fallot
(teh-**TRALL**-oh-jee of fal-**LOH**)

A congenital heart anomaly that consists of four defects: pulmonary stenosis, interventricular septal defect, dextraposition (shifting to the right) of the aorta so that it receives blood from both ventricles, and hypertrophy of the right ventricle; named for the French physician, Etienne Fallot, who first described the condition.

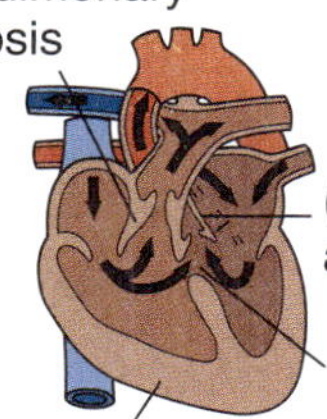

Figure 10-14 Tetralogy of Fallot

Further description of tetralogy of Fallot identifies the four defects in more detail: the (1) pulmonary stenosis (narrowing of the opening into the pulmonary artery from the right ventricle) restricts the flow of blood from the heart to the lungs; the (2) interventricular septal defect creates a right-to-left shunt between the ventricles, allowing deoxygenated blood from the right ventricle to communicate with the oxygenated blood in the left ventricle, which then exits the heart via the aorta; the (3) shifting of the aorta to the right causes it to override the right ventricle and thus communicate with the interventricular septal defect, allowing the oxygen-poor blood to pass more easily into the aorta; and the (4) hypertrophy of the right ventricle occurs because of the increased work required to pump blood through the obstructed pulmonary artery. See **Figure 10-14.**

Most infants born with tetralogy of Fallot display varying degrees of cyanosis, which may typically occur during activities that increase the need for oxygen such as crying, feeding, or straining with a bowel movement. The cyanosis develops as a result of the decreased flow of blood to the lungs for oxygenation, and as a result of the mixing of oxygenated and deoxygenated blood released into the systemic circulation; these babies are termed "blue babies."

Treatment for tetralogy of Fallot involves surgery to correct the multiple defects.

patent ductus arteriosus
(**PAY**-tent **DUCK**-tus ar-**tee**-ree- **OH**-sis)

Patent ductus arteriosus is an abnormal opening between the pulmonary artery and the aorta caused by failure of the fetal ductus arteriosus to close after birth. This defect is seen primarily in premature infants. See Figure 10-15.

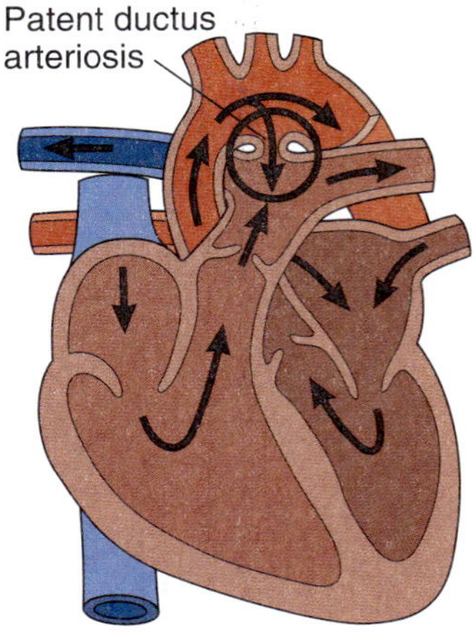

Figure 10-15 Patent ductus arteriosus

During the prenatal period, the ductus arteriosus serves as a normal pathway in the fetal circulatory system. It is a large channel between the pulmonary artery and the aorta, which is open, allowing fetal blood to bypass the lungs, passing from the pulmonary artery to the descending aorta, and ultimately to the placenta. This passageway is no longer needed after birth and usually closes during the first 24 to 72 hours of life, once the normal circulatory pattern of the cardiovascular system is established.

If the ductus arteriosus remains open after birth, blood under pressure from the aorta is shunted into the pulmonary artery, resulting in oxygenated blood *recirculating* through the pulmonary circulation. A strain is placed on the heart due to the pumping of blood a second time through the pulmonary circulation.

Treatment for patent ductus arteriosus is surgery to close the open channel.

coarctation of the aorta
(**koh**-ark-**TAY**-shun)

A congenital heart defect characterized by a localized narrowing of the aorta, which results in increased blood pressure in the upper extremities (area proximal to the defect) and decreased blood pressure in the lower extremities (area distal to the defect). See Figure 10-16.

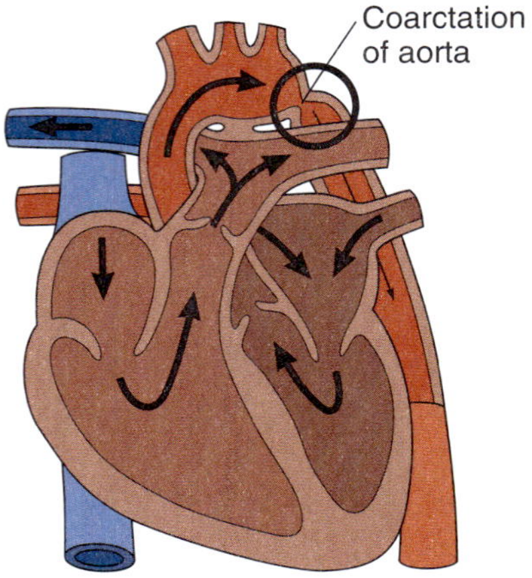

The classic sign of coarctation of the aorta is a contrast in pulsations and blood pressures in the arms and legs. The femoral, popliteal, and pedal pulses are weak or delayed in comparison with the strong, bounding pulses found in the arms and carotid arteries. See **Figure 10-17** for pulse points of the body.

Surgical correction of the defect is curative if the disease is diagnosed early.

Figure 10-16 Coarctation of the aorta

transposition of the great vessels
(tranz-poh-**ZIH**-shun)

A condition in which the two major arteries of the heart are reversed in position, which results in two noncommunicating circulatory systems.

The aorta arises from the right ventricle (instead of the left) and delivers unoxygenated blood to the systemic circulation. This blood is returned from the body tissues back to the right atrium and right ventricle without being oxygenated, because it does not pass through the lungs.

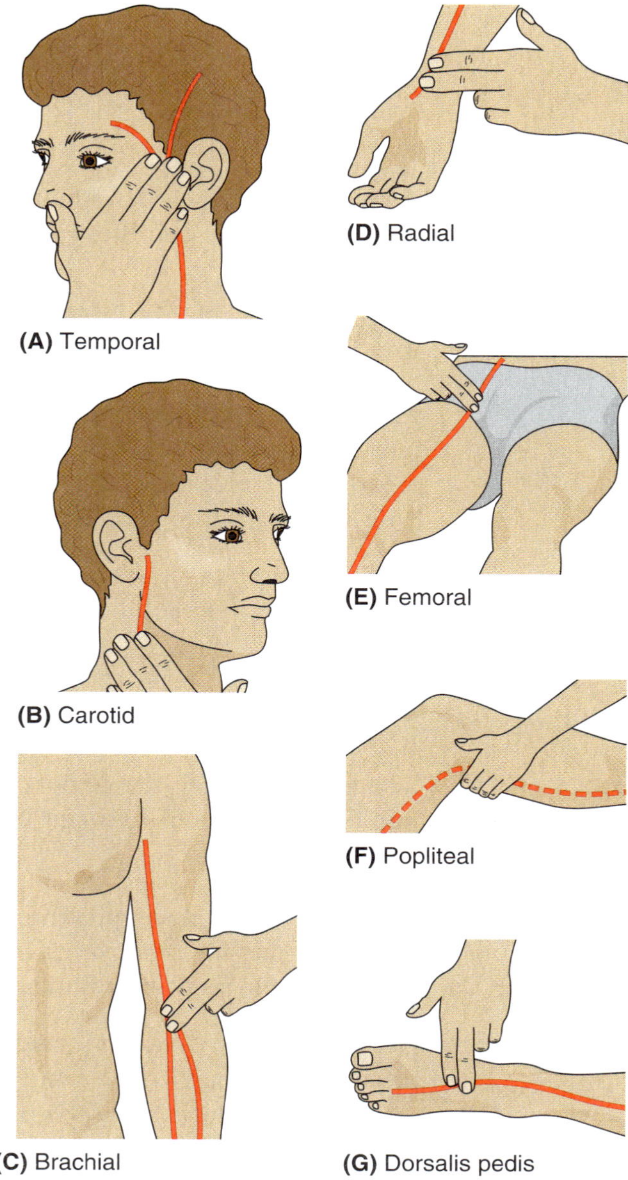

Figure 10-17 Pulse points of the body

The pulmonary artery arises from the left ventricle (instead of the right) and delivers blood to the lungs for oxygenation. The oxygenated blood returns from the lungs to the left atrium and the left ventricle and back to the lungs without sending the oxygenated blood throughout the systemic circulation.

This congenital anomaly creates an oxygen deficiency to the body tissues and an excessive workload on the right and left ventricles. The infant is usually severely cyanotic at birth.

Treatment involves surgical correction of the defect and repositioning of the vessels to reestablish a normal pattern of blood flow through the circulatory system. Surgical correction of the defect is delayed, if possible, until 6 months of age, when the infant can better tolerate the procedure. Immediate **palliative** surgery, aimed at achieving adequate mixing of oxygenated and unoxygenated blood, can enable the child to survive until corrective surgery can be performed.

Arrhythmias

An **arrhythmia** is any deviation from the normal pattern of the heartbeat. The following is a list of some of the more common arrhythmias.

---

heart block (AV)

Heart block is an interference with the normal conduction of electric impulses that control activity of the heart muscle.

In first-degree AV block, the impulse initiated by the SA node is conducted normally through the atria but is slowed when passing through the AV node (i.e., AV block). After the impulse passes through the AV node, it continues normally through the ventricles.

AV block may be a result of organic heart disease or the effect of digitalis; it may also be a complication of a myocardial infarction or rheumatic fever.

There is no specific treatment for first-degree AV block, but it should be watched because it may precede higher degrees of block.

---

atrial flutter
(**AY**-tree-al flutter)

Condition in which the contractions of the atria become extremely rapid, at the rate of between 250 to 400 beats per minute.

An important characteristic of **atrial flutter** is that a therapeutic block occurs at the AV node, preventing some impulse transmission. This, in turn, prevents the rapid firing of the impulses to the ventricles, which could result in ventricular fibrillation, a life-threatening arrhythmia.

Treatment for atrial flutter is medication given to slow and strengthen the heartbeat. If drug therapy is unsuccessful, atrial flutter will often respond to electrical cardioversion (electrical shock), which will slow the heart rate and restore the heart's normal rhythm.

---

fibrillation (atrial/ ventricular)
(fih-brill-**AY**-shun)

Atrial fibrillation is extremely rapid, incomplete contractions of the atria resulting in disorganized and uncoordinated twitching of the atria.

The rate of contractions for the atria may be as high as 350 to 600 beats per minute, with a ventricular response rate of contraction being between 120 to 200 beats per minute. At these rates, the ventricles cannot contract efficiently or recover adequately between contractions. These inefficient contractions of the heart reduce the blood flow, leading to angina and congestive heart failure.

Treatment involves medication directed at decreasing the atrial contraction rate and the ventricular response rate.

Ventricular fibrillation is a condition similar to atrial fibrillation, which results in rapid, tremulous (quivering like a bowl of Jell-O®) and ineffectual contractions of the ventricles; patient has no audible heartbeat, no palpable pulse, no respiration, and no blood circulation; if prolonged, this will lead to cardiac arrest.

Immediate treatment is necessary, consisting of cardiopulmonary resuscitation (CPR) and defibrillation (electrical countershock using defibrillation paddles). Ventricular fibrillation will result in death if an effective rhythm is not reestablished within 3 to 4 minutes.

Diagnostic Techniques and Procedures

angiography
(an-jee-OG-rah-fee)
angi/o = vessel
-graphy = process of recording

X-ray visualization of the internal anatomy of the heart and blood vessels after introducing a radiopaque substance (contrast medium) that promotes the imaging (makes them visible) of internal structures that are otherwise difficult to see on x-ray film. This substance is injected into an artery or a vein.

It is important to perform a hypersensitivity test before the radiographic material is used because the iodine in the contrast material has been known to cause severe allergic reactions in some patients.

Angiography is used to diagnose conditions such as myocardial infarction, occlusion of blood vessels, calcified atherosclerotic plaques, stroke (cerebrovascular accident), hypertension of the vessels leading to the liver (portal hypertension), and narrowing of the renal artery.

cardiac catheterization
(CAR-dee-ak cath-eh-ter-ih-ZAY-shun)
cardi/o = heart
-ac = pertaining to

A diagnostic procedure in which a catheter (a hollow, flexible tube) is introduced into a large vein or artery, usually of an arm or a leg, and is then threaded through the circulatory system to the heart. Cardiac catheterization is used to obtain detailed information about the structure and function of the heart chambers, valves, and the great vessels.

In the case of coronary artery disease, the patient may undergo a cardiac catheterization to determine the amount of occlusion of his or her coronary arteries for the physician to determine the most appropriate treatment; treatment may consist of coronary artery bypass surgery or percutaneous transluminal coronary angioplasty.

cardiac enzymes test
(CAR-dee-ak EN-zyms test)
cardi/o = heart

Cardiac enzymes tests are performed on samples of blood obtained by venipuncture to determine the presence of damage to the myocardial muscle.

Cardiac enzymes are present in high concentrations in the myocardial tissue. Tissue damage causes the release of the cardiac enzymes from their normal intracellular area and creates an elevation of serum cardiac enzyme levels. In addition to indicating the presence of damage to the myocardial muscle, the elevated enzyme levels can disclose the timing of the acute cardiac event.

For example, the enzymes most commonly used to detect myocardial infarction (heart attack) are creatine kinase (CK) and lactic acid dehydrogenase (LDH); these enzyme levels are elevated after a myocardial infarction.

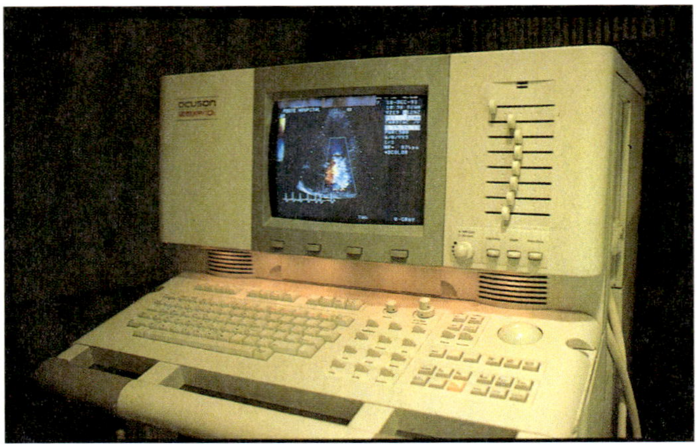

Figure 10-18 Echocardiograph (Photo by Marcia Butterfield. Courtesy of W.A. Foote Memorial Hospital, Jackson, MI)

Another enzyme level, CK-MB, determines muscle damage to the heart. An elevated CK-MB would indicate that there was myocardial muscle damage. (This particular enzyme level would elevate within 4 to 6 hours after the acute attack and would peak within 18 to 24 hours after the attack.)

(CAT) computed axial tomography
(computed **AK**-see-al toh-**MOG**-rah-fee)
tom/o = to cut
-graphy = process of recording

Computed axial tomography (CAT) is a diagnostic x-ray technique that uses ionizing radiation to produce a cross-sectional image of the body. It is often used to detect aneurysms of the aorta. X-ray signals are fed into a computer, which then turns them into a cross-sectional picture of the section of the body being scanned; called CAT scan.

CAT scans are helpful in evaluating areas of the body that are difficult to assess using standard x-ray procedures. As is true with magnetic resonance imaging, patients should be informed that the CAT is a very confining procedure because they are placed within a tubelike structure, and should be asked if they are claustrophobic (fear enclosed spaces).

echocardiography
(ek-oh-car-dee-**OG**-rah-fee)
echo- = sound
cardi/o = heart
-graphy = process of recording

Echocardiography is a diagnostic procedure for studying the structure and motion of the heart. It is useful in evaluating structural and functional changes in a variety of heart disorders. See Figure 10-18.

Ultrasound waves pass through the heart, via a transducer, bounce off tissues of varying densities, and are reflected backward, or echoed, to the transducer, creating an image on the graph.

Uses for echocardiography include, but are not limited to, assessing and detecting atrial tumors, determining the measurement of the ventricular septa and ventricular chambers, and determining the presence of mitral valve motion abnormalities.

electrocardiogram
(ee-**lek**-troh-**CAR**-dee-oh-**gram**)
electr/o = electrical; electricity
cardi/o = heart
-gram = record

An electrocardiogram is a graphic record (visual representation) of the electrical action of the heart as reflected from various angles to the surface of the skin; known as an EKG or ECG.

An EKG is performed with an electrocardiograph, which is the machine that records the electrical activity of the heart to detect transmission of the

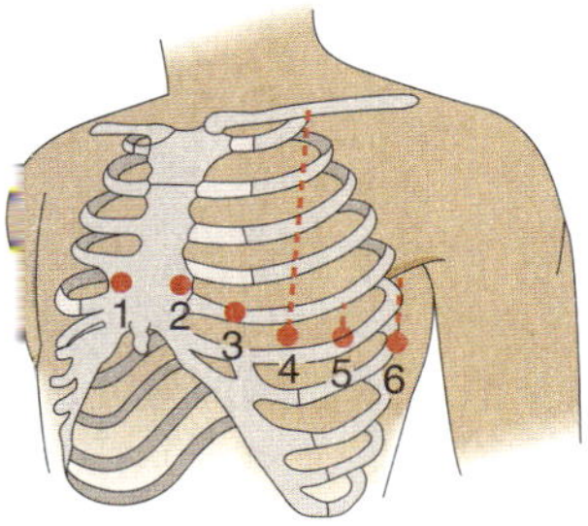

Figure 10-19 Standard chest lead placements for EKG

cardiac impulse throughout the heart muscle. Electrodes are positioned on the chest wall in standardized anatomic positions that will provide the clearest EKG waveforms. See **Figure 10-19.**

The EKG is recorded as a tracing on a strip of graph paper that moves through the machine as the stylus (recording needle) records the impulses. Analysis of the EKG waveforms can assist the physician in identifying disorders of heart rate, rhythm, or conduction, presence of myocardial ischemia, or presence of a myocardial infarction.

exercise stress testing

A means of assessing cardiac function, by subjecting the patient to carefully controlled amounts of physical stress, for example, using the treadmill. See Figure 10-20.

A stress test may be ordered for many reasons, some of which include the following: to determine the cause of chest pain; to screen for ischemic heart problems; to identify any disorders of cardiac rate, rhythm, or conduction; to determine the functional ability of the heart after a myocardial infarction; and to identify any heart irregularities that may occur during physical exercise.

During exercise stress testing, the patient may walk on a treadmill, climb a set of stairs, or pedal a stationary bicycle. The exercise speed is increased as the patient can tolerate it. EKGs are recorded throughout the procedure.

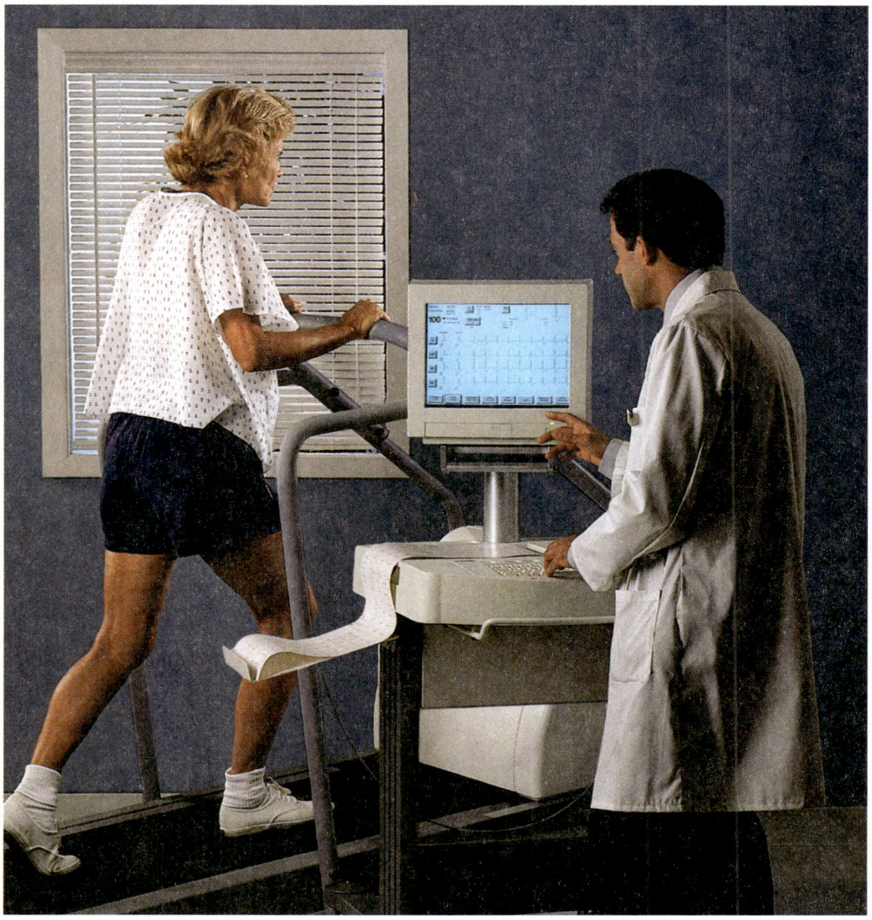

Figure 10-20 Quest Exercise Stress System (Courtesy of Spacelabs Medical, Inc.)

The patient is closely monitored throughout the test and the procedure is discontinued if the patient shows any signs of distress.

Holter monitoring

A small, portable monitoring device that makes prolonged electrocardiograph recordings on a portable tape recorder. The continuous EKG is recorded on a magnetic tape recording while the patient conducts normal daily activities. See Figure 10-21.

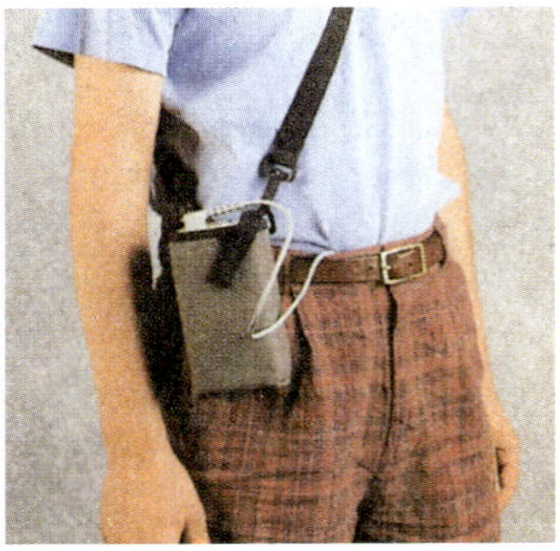

The Holter monitor (not halter) is used to detect heart dysrhythmias or evidence of myocardial ischemia. It weighs about 2 pounds and can be carried over the shoulder, using the shoulder strap.

The patient usually maintains a diary of his or her daily activities, being careful to note the particular time of any unusual activities performed, any symptoms, or any unusual experiences that occur during the day. The monitor is returned the next day and is examined with a special scanner, analyzed, and interpreted by the doctor.

Figure 10-21 Holter monitor

magnetic resonance imaging (MRI)
(mag-**NEH**-tic **REHZ**-oh-nans imaging)

Magnetic resonance imaging (MRI) involves the use of a strong magnetic field and radiofrequency waves to produce imaging that is valuable in providing images of the heart, large blood vessels, brain, and soft tissue.

MRI is used to examine the aorta, to detect masses or possible tumors, and pericardial disease; it can show the flowing of blood and the beating of the heart. The radiofrequency waves are directed at the heart and an image is produced on the screen.

Patients with pacemakers, any recently implanted wires or clips, or prosthetic valves are not eligible for MRI, because of the magnetic field. Patients should be informed that MRI is a very confining procedure because they are placed within a tubelike structure, and should be asked if they are claustrophobic (fear enclosed spaces).

positron emission tomography (PET)
(**PAHZ**-ih-tron *or* **PAWZ**-ih-tron ee-**MISH**-un toh-**MOG**-rah-fee)
tom/o = to cut
-graphy = process of recording

A computerized x-ray technique that uses radioactive substances to examine the blood flow and the metabolic activity of various body structures, such as the heart and blood vessels. The patient is given doses of strong radioactive tracers by injection or inhalation; the radiation emitted is measured by the PET camera.

The PET scanner is helpful in detecting coronary artery disease, assessing the progression of narrowing of the coronary arteries (stenosis), and distinguishing between ischemic, infarcted, and normal cardiac tissue. PET is also used in the study and diagnosis of cancer and in the studies of the biochemical activity of the brain. One major disadvantage of the use of positron emission tomography is its high cost.

serum lipid test
(**SEE**-rum **LIP**-id test)
ser/o = blood serum
lip/o = fat

A serum lipid test measures the amount of fatty substances (cholesterol, triglycerides, and lipoproteins) in a sample of blood obtained by venipuncture.

These fatty substances, which are insoluble in water, play a major role in the development of atherosclerosis. The lipid profile is used to assess the patient's degree of risk for developing coronary artery disease.

thallium stress test
(**THAL**-ee-um stress test)

Thallium stress testing is a combination of exercise stress testing with thallium imaging (myocardial perfusion scan) to assess changes in coronary blood flow during exercise.

Thallium imaging is used with exercise stress testing to determine if the coronary blood flow changes under stressed conditions such as increased activity. When injected intravenously, thallium concentrates in myocardial tissue in direct proportion to the blood flow to various regions of the myocardium. If severe coronary artery narrowing or decreased blood flow to an area (ischemia) is present, the concentration of thallium will be decreased. The area of decreased concentration of thallium is referred to as a "cold spot."

The thallium is injected intravenously 1 minute before the end of the exercise stress test. This allows enough time for adequate distribution of the thallium throughout the myocardium before the end of the test. Images of the myocardial tissue are taken immediately and are repeated 3 to 4 hours later to assess for any cold spots (areas of little or no concentration of thallium).

If a cold spot appears on the initial imaging but disappears on the repeated image, it is referred to as an ischemic area (area of decreased blood flow). If the cold spot continues to show on the repeated imaging, it indicates an area of no blood flow, or an area of infarction.

Common Abbreviations

ABBREVIATION	MEANING	ABBREVIATION	MEANING
AMI	acute myocardial infarction	**CPR**	cardiopulmonary resuscitation
AS	aortic stenosis	**CT (scan) or CAT (scan)**	computed axial tomography (scan)
ASD	atrial septal defect	**CVD**	cardiovascular disease
ASHD	arteriosclerotic heart disease	**DOE**	dyspnea on exertion
AV	atrioventricular	**DVT**	deep vein thrombosis
BBB	bundle branch block	**ECG**	electrocardiogram
BP	blood pressure	**ECHO**	echocardiogram
CABG	coronary artery bypass graft	**EKG**	electrocardiogram
CAD	coronary artery disease	**HCVD**	hypertensive cardiovascular disease
Cath	catheterization	**HDL**	high-density lipoprotein
CC	cardiac catheterization	**LDL**	low-density lipoprotein
CCU	coronary care unit	**MI**	myocardial infarction
CHD	coronary heart disease	**MRI**	magnetic resonance imaging
CHF	congestive heart failure		

MS	mitral stenosis
MVP	mitral valve prolapse
PACs	premature atrial contractions
PAT	paroxysmal atrial tachycardia
PDA	patent ductus arteriosus
PET	positron emission tomography
PTCA	percutaneous transluminal coronary angioplasty
PVCs	premature ventricular contractions
SA	sinoatrial
VSD	ventricular septal defect
VT	ventricular tachycardia

Written and Audio Terminology Review

Review each of the following terms from this chapter. Study the spelling of each term, and write the definition in the space provided. If you have the Audio CD available, listen to each term, pronounce it yourself, and check the box once you are comfortable saying the word. Check definitions by looking the term up in the glossary/index.

TERM	PRONUNCIATION	DEFINITION
analgesic	☐ **an**-al-**JEE**-zik	______________
anastomosis	☐ ah-**nas**-toh-**MOH**-sis	______________
aneurysm	☐ **AN**-yoo-rizm	______________
aneurysmectomy	☐ **an**-yoo-riz-**MEK**-toh-mee	______________
angina pectoris	☐ **AN**-jih-na **PECK**-tor-is *or* an-**JYE**-na **PECK**-tor-is	______________
angiography	☐ an-jee-**OG**-rah-fee	______________
anomaly	☐ ah-**NOM**-ah-lee	______________
anorexia	☐ an-oh-**REK**-see-ah	______________
anxiety	☐ ang-**ZIGH**-eh-tee	______________
arrhythmia	☐ ah-**RITH**-mee-ah	______________
arteriosclerosis	☐ ar-tee-ree-oh-skleh-**ROH**-sis	______________
arthralgia	☐ ar-**THRAL**-jee-ah	______________
ascites	☐ ah-**SIGH**-teez	______________
atherosclerosis	☐ **ath**-er-**oh**-skleh-**ROH**-sis	______________
atrial flutter	☐ **AY**-tree-al flutter	______________
benign	☐ bee-**NINE**	______________
bradycardia	☐ brad-ee-**CAR**-dee-ah	______________

Term	Pronunciation	
bruits	☐ brew-**EE**	______
cardiac catheretization	☐ **CAR**-dee-ak cath-eh-ter-ih-**ZAY**-shun	______
cardiac enzymes test	☐ **CAR**-dee-ak **EN**-zyms test	______
carditis	☐ car-**DYE**-tis	______
claudication	☐ klaw-dih-**KAY**-shun	______
coarctation	☐ koh-ark-**TAY**-shun	______
computed axial tomography (CAT)	☐ computed **AK**-see-al toh-**MOG**-rah-fee	______
congestive heart failure	☐ kon-**JESS**-tiv heart failure	______
coronary artery	☐ **KOR**-ah-nair-ree **AR**-ter-ee	______
coronary artery disease	☐ **KOR**-ah-nair-ree **AR**-ter-ee dih-**ZEEZ**	______
cyanosis	☐ sigh-ah-**NO**-sis	______
diastole	☐ dye-**ASS**-toh-lee	______
dyspnea	☐ **DISP**-nee-ah	______
dysrhythmia	☐ dis-**RITH**-mee-ah	______
echocardiography	☐ ek-oh-car-dee-**OG**-rah-fee	______
edema	☐ eh-**DEE**-mah	______
electrocardiogram	☐ ee-**lek**-troh-**CAR**-dee-oh-**gram**	______
endocarditis	☐ **en**-doh-car-**DYE**-tis	______
epicardium	☐ **ep**-ih-**CARD**-ee-um	______
fatigue	☐ **FAH**-teeg	______
fever	☐ **FEE**-ver	______
fibrillation	☐ **fih**-brill-**AY**-shun	______
hepatomegaly	☐ **heh**-pat-oh-**MEG**-ah-lee	______
hyperlipidemia	☐ **high**-per-lip-ih-**DEE**-mee-ah	______
hypertension	☐ high-per-**TEN**-shun	______
hypertensive heart disease	☐ **high**-per-**TEN**-siv heart dih-**ZEEZ**	______
hypotension	☐ **high**-poh-**TEN**-shun	______
infarction	☐ in-**FARC**-shun	______

Term		Pronunciation	
ischemia	☐	iss-**KEY**-mee-ah	________________
lesion	☐	**LEE**-zhun	________________
lipid	☐	**LIP**-id	________________
lumen	☐	**LOO**-men	________________
magnetic resonance imaging (MRI)	☐	mag-**NEH**-tic **REHZ**-oh-nance imaging (MRI)	________________
malaise	☐	mah-**LAYZ**	________________
mediastinum	☐	**mee**-dee-ass-**TYE**-num	________________
mitral valve prolapse	☐	**MY**-tral valve **PROH**-laps	________________
myocardial infarction	☐	my-oh-**CAR**-dee-al in-**FARC**-shun	________________
myocarditis	☐	my-oh-car-**DYE**-tis	________________
myocardium	☐	my-oh-**CAR**-dee-um	________________
nausea	☐	**NAW**-see-ah	________________
nocturia	☐	nok-**TOO**-ree-ah	________________
occlusion	☐	ah-**KLOO**-shun	________________
orthopnea	☐	**or**-**THOP**-nee-ah	________________
pallor	☐	**PAL**-or	________________
palpable	☐	**PAL**-pah-b'l	________________
palpitation	☐	pal-pih-**TAY**-shun	________________
patent ductus arteriosus	☐	**PAY**-tent **DUCK**-tus ar-tee-ree-**OH**-sis	________________
pericarditis	☐	pair-ih-car-**DYE**-tis	________________
pericardium	☐	**pair**-ih-**CAR**-dee-um	________________
peripheral arterial	☐	per-**IF**-er-al ar-**TEE**-ree-al	________________
petechiae	☐	pee-**TEE**-kee-ee	________________
pitting edema	☐	pitting eh-**DEE**-mah	________________
prophylactic	☐	proh-fih-**LAK**-tik	________________
pulmonary	☐	**PULL**-mon-air-ee	________________
pulmonary artery	☐	**PULL**-mon-air-ee artery	________________
pulmonary vein	☐	**PULL**-mon-air-ee vein	________________
Raynaud's	☐	ray-**NOZ**	________________

rheumatic fever	☐ roo-**MAT**-ic fever	______
septum	☐ **SEP**-tum	______
serum lipid test	☐ **SEE**-rum **LIP**-id test	______
Sydenham's chorea	☐ **SID**-en-hamz koh-**REE**-ah	______
systemic circulation	☐ sis-**TEM**-ik ser-kew-**LAY**-shun	______
systole	☐ **SIS**-toh-lee	______
tachycardia	☐ tak-ee-**CAR**-dee-ah	______
tetralogy of Fallot	☐ teh-**TRALL**-oh-jee of fal-**LOH**	______
thallium stress test	☐ **THAL**-ee-um stress test	______
thrombophlebitis	☐ **throm**-boh-fleh-**BY**-tis	______
thrombosis	☐ throm-**BOH**-sis	______
varicose veins	☐ **VAIR**-ih-kohs veins	______
vasoconstriction	☐ **vass**-oh-con-**STRIK**-shun	______

Chapter Review Exercises

The following exercises provide a more in-depth review of the chapter material. Your goal in these exercises is to complete each section at a minimum 80% level of accuracy. A space has been provided for your score at the end of each section.

A. Labeling

Label the following structures of the heart by writing your answers in the spaces provided. Each correct answer is worth 10 points. When you have completed the exercise, record your score in the space provided.

1. ______________________
2. ______________________
3. ______________________
4. ______________________
5. ______________________
6. ______________________
7. ______________________
8. ______________________
9. ______________________
10. ______________________

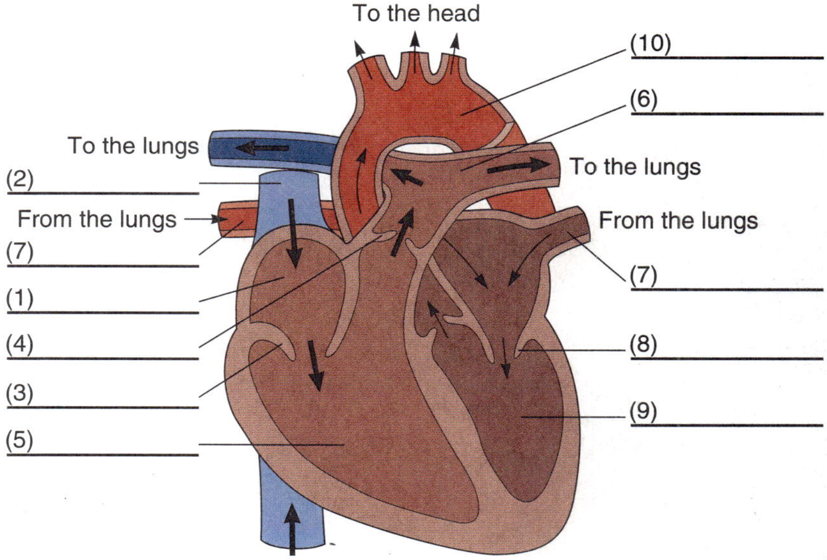

***Number correct* ______ × *10 points/correct answer: Your score* ______%**

B. Follow the Flow

As you read the following review of the flow of blood through the heart, complete the statements below with the most appropriate answer. Each correct answer is worth 10 points. Record your score in the space provided at the end of this exercise.

As blood flows through the heart, deoxygenated blood enters the (1) ______________ atrium from the (2) ______________. It passes through the tricuspid valve into the right ventricle. From the right ventricle, the blood passes through the pulmonary valve into the (3) ______________, which carries the blood to the lungs to receive oxygen. This propelling of the blood from the heart to the lungs and back to the heart is known as (4) ______________ circulation. Oxygenated blood enters the (5) ______________ atrium from the pulmonary veins. The blood passes from the atrium, through the (6) ______________ valve into the left ventricle. The freshly oxygenated blood then passes through the (7) ______________ valve into the (8) ______________, which branches into arteries and then into smaller vessels known as (9) ______________, which then transport the blood throughout the body. This propelling of the blood from the heart to all parts of the body and back to the heart is known as (10) ______________ circulation.

Number correct _______ × 10 points/correct answer: Your score _______%

C. Spelling

Circle the correctly spelled term in each pairing of words. Each correct answer is worth 10 points. Record your score in the space provided at the end of the exercise.

1. sistole — systole
2. diastole — dyastole
3. tachycardia — trachycardia
4. palpatation — palpitation
5. vomiting — vomiking
6. rhumatic — rheumatic
7. Fallot — Fallow
8. aneurism — aneurysm
9. ventriclar — ventricular
10. varicose — vericose

Number correct _______ × 10 points/correct answer: Your score _______%

D. Signs and Symptoms Review

Define each term by writing the definition in the space provided. Check the box if you are able to complete this exercise correctly the first time (without referring to the answers). Each correct answer is worth 10 points. Record your score in the space provided at the end of the exercise.

☐ 1. tachycardia ______________________________

☐ 2. palpitation ______________________________

☐ 3. pallor ______________________________

☐ 4. cyanosis ______________________________

- ☐ 5. edema ______
- ☐ 6. anorexia ______
- ☐ 7. nausea ______
- ☐ 8. vomiting ______
- ☐ 9. anxiety ______
- ☐ 10. fatigue ______

Number correct _______ × 10 points/correct answer: Your score _______%

E. Matching Cardiovascular Conditions

Match the following cardiovascular conditions on the left with the appropriate definitions on the right. Each correct answer is worth 10 points. Record your score in the space provided at the end of the exercise.

_____ 1. myocardial infarction
_____ 2. endocarditis
_____ 3. rheumatic fever
_____ 4. ventricular fibrillation
_____ 5. aneurysm
_____ 6. thrombophlebitis
_____ 7. varicose veins
_____ 8. Raynaud's phenomenon
_____ 9. hypertension
_____ 10. mitral valve prolapse

a. "Click murmur syndrome"
b. A localized dilatation of an artery that balloons out with each pulsation of the artery
c. An inflammatory disease that may develop as a delayed reaction to insufficiently treated Group A beta-hemolytic streptococcal infection of the upper respiratory tract
d. Severe pain and constriction about the heart
e. Blood pressure persistently exceeding 140/90 mmHg
f. "Heart attack"
g. Inflammation of the inner lining of the heart
h. A condition that results in rapid, tremulous (quivering like a bowl of Jell-O®) and ineffectual contractions of this chamber of the heart
i. Intermittent attacks of vasoconstriction of the arterioles, causing pallor of the fingers or toes
j. Enlarged, superficial veins; a twisted, dilated vein with incompetent valves
k. Inflammation of the outer lining of the heart
l. Inflammation of a vein associated with the formation of a clot

Number correct _______ × 10 points/correct answer: Your score _______%

F. Proofreading Skills

Read the following report. For each boldfaced term, provide a brief definition and indicate if the term is spelled correctly. If it is misspelled, provide the correct spelling. Each correct answer is worth 10 points. Record your answer in the space provided at the end.

AUTOPSY REPORT

HILLCREST Medical Center

DATE OF DICTATION: July 27, 2003

DICTATING PHYSICIAN: Dr. R. U. Wright

"This an autopsy on a prematurely born male infant weighing 3 lbs. 2 oz. The body measures 15.26 inches in length. The head, neck, and chest are symmetrical. The abdomen is soft. The genitalia are normal male. The extremities are symmetrical and show no evidence of abnormalities. The abdominal cavity is opened and the liver is enlarged. The spleen also appears to be enlarged. All other organs are in normal position. The pleural cavities are opened, revealing the left lung to be collapsed and lying in the left pleural cavity. The right lung is partially expanded and the pleura is smooth and glistening. The **midiostinum** contains a moderate amount of thymic tissue. The **pericardal** sac is opened, containing a few cc of **serious** fluid. The heart is in normal position and appears to be average in size. Thorough examination of the heart reveals no evidence of congenital anomaly. The foramen ovale has a thin membrane over its surface. The **ductus arteriosis** is **paytent.** There is no defect of the ventricular **septum,** and the **ventrucles** appear to be well developed. There is no evidence of **transposition** of the great vessels. The **pulmonery** artery is noted and appears normal. A few **petechii** are noted on the surface of the **endocardium.**"

R U Wright

Example:

midiostinum *The area between the lungs, in the chest cavity, that contains the heart, aorta, trachea, esophagus, and bronchi.*

Spelled correctly? ☐ Yes ☑ No *mediastinum*

1. **pericardal**

   Spelled correctly? ☐ Yes ☐ No __________

2. **serious**

   Spelled correctly? ☐ Yes ☐ No __________

3. **ductus arteriosis**

   Spelled correctly? ☐ Yes ☐ No __________

4. **paytent**

   Spelled correctly? ☐ Yes ☐ No __________

5. **septum**
   Spelled correctly? ☐ Yes ☐ No ______________________________

6. **ventrucles**
   Spelled correctly? ☐ Yes ☐ No ______________________________

7. **transposition**
   Spelled correctly? ☐ Yes ☐ No ______________________________

8. **pulmonery**
   Spelled correctly? ☐ Yes ☐ No ______________________________

9. **petechii**
   Spelled correctly? ☐ Yes ☐ No ______________________________

10. **endocardium**
    Spelled correctly? ☐ Yes ☐ No ______________________________

Number correct _______ × 10 points/correct answer: Your score _______%

G. Abbreviations Identification

Read the following set of doctor's orders and define the highlighted abbreviations in the spaces provided. Each correct answer is worth 10 points. Record your score in the space provided at the end of this exercise.

John Peach was admitted to Fruitland Memorial Hospital on Saturday, July 29, 2003, with initial diagnoses of **CAD** and **HCVD.** He was placed in the **CCU** and was scheduled for an **MRI** the following morning. The doctor also ordered an **EKG.**

The results of the MRI revealed that Mr. Peach had greater than 60% blockage in two of his coronary arteries. The attending physician considered the treatment options of **PTCA** or directional coronary atherectomy vs surgery for Mr. Peach. Considering the fact that Mr. Peach was at increased risk for an **MI,** his **BP** was 240/120 mmHg, he was experiencing **DOE,** the doctor opted for the **CABG** surgery as soon as all lab work had been completed.

On Tuesday, August 2, 2003, Mr. Peach went to surgery for the coronary artery bypass surgery. He tolerated the procedure well and was returned to CCU for the remainder of the week.

1. CAD: ______________________________
2. HCVD: ______________________________
3. CCU: ______________________________
4. MRI: ______________________________
5. EKG: ______________________________
6. PTCA: ______________________________
7. MI: ______________________________
8. BP: ______________________________
9. DOE: ______________________________
10. CABG: ______________________________

Number correct _______ × 10 points/correct answer: Your score _______%

H. Matching Abbreviations

Match the abbreviations on the left with the correct definition on the right. Each correct answer is worth 10 points. Record your score in the space provided at the end of this exercise.

_____ 1. CHF		a. cardiopulmonary resuscitation
_____ 2. ECHO		b. arteriosclerotic heart disease
_____ 3. MVP		c. sinoatrial
_____ 4. PET		d. echocardiogram
_____ 5. PVCs		e. bundle branch block
_____ 6. SA		f. congestive heart failure
_____ 7. PDA		g. mitral valve prolapse
_____ 8. ASHD		h. computerized tomography
_____ 9. EKG		i. positron emission tomography
_____ 10. CPR		j. premature ventricular contractions
		k. patent ductus arteriosus
		l. electrocardiogram
		m. urinary tract infection

Number correct _______ × 10 points/correct answer: Your score _______%

I. Crossword Puzzle

Each crossword answer is worth 10 points. When you have completed the crossword puzzle, total your points and enter your score in the space provided.

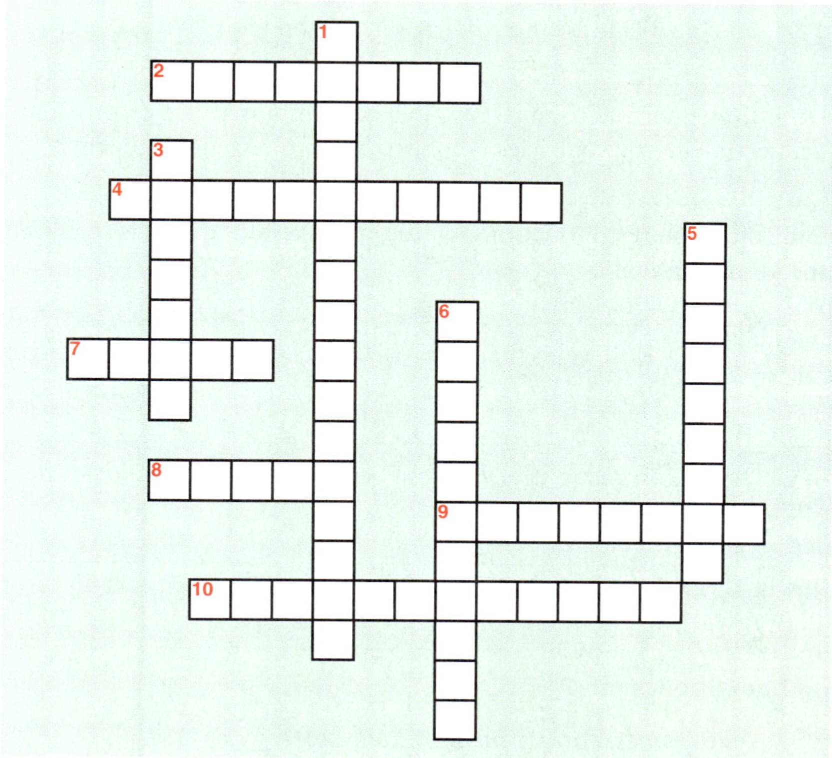

ACROSS
2 Ballooning of weakened artery wall
4 Inflammation of heart muscle
7 Perspiration
8 Temperature elevated above normal
9 Condition of blueness
10 Inflammation/outer lining of heart

DOWN
1 Hardening of the arteries
3 Difficulty breathing
5 Feeling of discomfort in chest area
6 Abnormally slow heartbeat

Number correct _______ × 10 points/correct answer: Your score _______%

J. Completion

Complete the statements below with the most appropriate answer. Each correct answer is worth 10 points. Record your score in the space provided at the end of this exercise.

1. An abnormal opening between the pulmonary artery and the aorta, caused by failure of the ductus arteriosus to close after birth, is known as

   ____

2. A congenital heart anomaly that consists of four defects is known as

   ____

3. The congenital heart disease in which the two major arteries of the heart are reversed in position, resulting in two noncommunicating circulatory systems, is known as

   ____

4. A congenital heart disease characterized by a localized narrowing of the aorta, resulting in increased pressure in the upper extremities and decreased pressure in the lower extremities, is known as

____

5. A condition that results in rapid, tremulous, and ineffective contractions of the ventricles; patient has no audible heartbeat, no palpable pulse, no respiration, and no blood circulation, is known as

____

6. An interference with the normal conduction of electric impulses that control activity of the heart muscle; the conduction time to the ventricles is abnormally prolonged, is known as

____

7. Extremely rapid, incomplete contractions of the atria resulting in disorganized and uncoordinated twitching of the atria is known as

____

8. A form of treatment for varicose veins that involves the injection of a chemical irritant into the varicosed vein is

____

9. A condition in which the contractions of the atria become extremely rapid, at the rate of between 250 to 400 beats per minute, is known as

____

10. A condition in which the arteries of the leg are obstructed is known as

____

Number correct _______ × 10 points/correct answer: Your score _______%

Answers to Chapter Review Exercises

A. Labeling

1. right atrium
2. superior vena cava
3. tricuspid valve
4. pulmonary valve
5. right ventricle
6. pulmonary artery
7. pulmonary vein
8. mitral valve
9. left ventricle
10. aorta

B. Follow the Flow

1. right
2. vena cavae (superior and inferior)
3. pulmonary artery
4. pulmonary
5. left
6. mitral
7. aortic
8. aorta
9. arterioles
10. systemic

C. Spelling

1. systole
2. diastole
3. tachycardia
4. palpitation
5. vomiting
6. rheumatic
7. Fallot
8. aneurysm
9. ventricular
10. varicose

D. Signs and Symptoms Review

1. Abnormally rapid heart action, usually defined as a heart rate over 100 beats per minute.
2. Rapid, violent, or throbbing pulsation, as an abnormally rapid throbbing or fluttering of the heart, the palpitation is felt by the individual.
3. Lack of color; paleness.
4. Slightly bluish, grayish, slatelike, or dark discoloration of the skin due to the presence of abnormal amounts of reduced hemoglobin in the blood.
5. A local or generalized condition in which the body tissues contain an excessive amount of tissue fluid; swelling.
6. Loss of appetite.
7. Unpleasant sensation felt in the abdomen (over the stomach) usually preceding vomiting.
8. Ejection through the mouth of the gastric contents.
9. A feeling of apprehension, worry, uneasiness, or dread, especially of the future.
10. A feeling of tiredness or weariness.

E. Matching Cardiovascular Conditions

1. f
2. g
3. c
4. h
5. b
6. l
7. j
8. i
9. e
10. a

F. Proofreading Skills

1. Pertaining to the pericardium.
   Spelled correctly? No **pericardial**
2. Pertaining to serum, the clear, watery fluid that moistens or lubricates the surfaces of membranes.
   Spelled correctly? No **serous**
3. During the prenatal period the ductus arteriosus serves as a normal pathway in the fetal circulatory system. It is a large channel between the pulmonary artery and the aorta, which is open, allowing fetal blood to bypass the lungs, passing from the pulmonary artery to the descending aorta and ultimately to the placenta.
   Spelled correctly? No **ductus arteriosus**
4. Open.
   Spelled correctly? No **patent**
5. The common wall between the right and left side of the heart.
   Spelled correctly? Yes
6. The two lower chambers of the heart.
   Spelled correctly? No **ventricles**
7. A condition in which the two major arteries of the heart are reversed in position is called transposition of the great vessels and results in two noncommunicating circulatory systems.
   Spelled correctly? Yes
8. Pertaining to the lungs: the pulmonary artery carries the oxygen-poor blood to the capillary network of the lungs from the right ventricle of the heart to receive oxygen; the pulmonary artery is the only artery in the body that carries deoxygenated blood.
   Spelled correctly? No **pulmonary**
9. Small pinpoint hemorrhages.
   Spelled correctly? No **petechiae**
10. The inner layer of the heart.
    Spelled correctly? **Yes**

G. Abbreviations Identification

1. coronary artery disease
2. hypertensive cardiovascular disease
3. coronary care unit
4. magnetic resonance imaging
5. electrocardiogram
6. percutaneous transluminal coronary angioplasty
7. myocardial infarction
8. blood pressure
9. dyspnea on exertion
10. coronary artery bypass graft

H. Matching Abbreviations

1. f	6. c
2. d	7. k
3. g	8. b
4. i	9. l
5. j	10. a

I. Crossword Puzzle

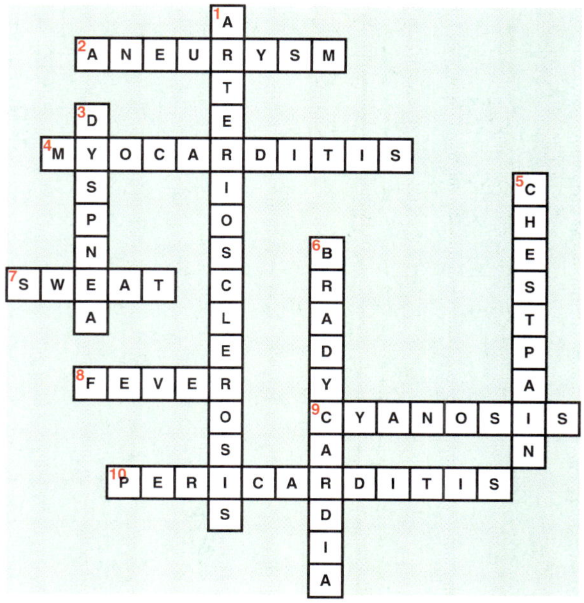

J. Completion

1. patent ductus arteriosus
2. tetralogy of Fallot
3. transposition of the great vessels
4. coarctation of the aorta
5. ventricular fibrillation
6. heart block (AV)
7. atrial fibrillation
8. sclerotherapy
9. atrial flutter
10. peripheral arterial occlusive disease

CHAPTER 11

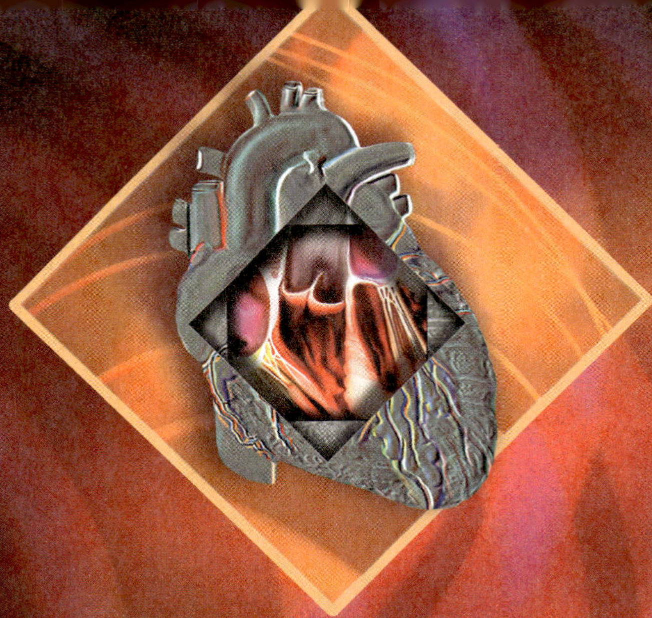

The Respiratory System

CHAPTER CONTENT

KEY COMPETENCIES

Upon completing this chapter and the review exercises at the end of the chapter, the learner should be able to:

1. List two major functions of the respiratory system.
2. State the difference between external respiration and internal respiration.
3. Identify the pathway of air as it travels from the nose to the capillaries of the lungs.
4. Identify 10 structures related to the respiratory system.
5. Define 10 common respiratory signs and symptoms.
6. Identify at least 10 breath sounds.
7. Define 20 common pathological conditions of the respiratory system.
8. Identify at least 10 abbreviations common to the respiratory system.
9. Correctly spell and pronounce each new term introduced in this chapter using the Activity CD-ROM and Audio CD, if available.
10. Correctly define at least 10 word elements relating to the respiratory system.

OVERVIEW

The respiratory system is responsible for the exchange of gases between the body and the air, a process called respiration. The respiratory system, along with the cardiovascular system, provides oxygen to the body cells for energy and removes carbon dioxide (a waste product of cellular metabolism) from the body cells. This is accomplished by two processes: external respiration and internal respiration.

In external respiration, oxygen is inhaled into the lungs (when you breathe in), passing through the capillaries of the lungs (alveoli) into the pulmonary bloodstream, while carbon dioxide passes from the blood through the same capillaries into the lungs and is exhaled (as you breathe out).

In internal respiration, the oxygen that you inhale circulates from the pulmonary bloodstream in the lungs, back through the heart, to the systemic bloodstream (which carries it all the way to the body cells). At the cellular level, the oxygen passes through the capillaries into the individual tissue cells where it is used for energy. In exchange, carbon dioxide passes from the tissue cells into the capillaries and travels through the bloodstream for removal from the body via the lungs (from the tissues, via the bloodstream, to the heart, to the lungs).

In addition to providing for the exchange of gases between the body and the air, the organs of the respiratory system are also responsible for producing sound and assisting in the body's defense against foreign materials.

Anatomy and Physiology

The respiratory system consists of a series of tubes or airways that transport air into and out of the lungs. The respiratory system is divided into the upper respiratory tract (consisting of the nose, pharynx, and larynx) and the lower respiratory tract (consisting of the trachea, bronchi, and lungs). A discussion of these structures, and the processes of respiration they support, follows. See **Figure 11-1.**

Nose

Air enters the body through the **(1) nose** and mouth. The external portion of the nose is composed of cartilage and bone covered with skin. The entrance to the nose is known as the **nostrils** or **nares**. As the air enters through the nose, it passes into the **(2) nasal cavity,** which is divided into left and right chambers by a dividing wall called the **septum**. Air passing through these chambers also passes through the **(3) paranasal sinuses**, which are hollow areas or cavities within the skull that communicate with the nasal cavity. The internal nose and the sinuses are lined with mucous membranes, which help to warm and filter the air as it enters the respiratory system. Hairlike projections on the mucous membranes, called **cilia,** sweep dirt and foreign material toward the throat for elimination. Because the hollow cavities of the paranasal sinuses are air spaces and not solid bone, they also lighten the skull and enhance the sound of the voice.

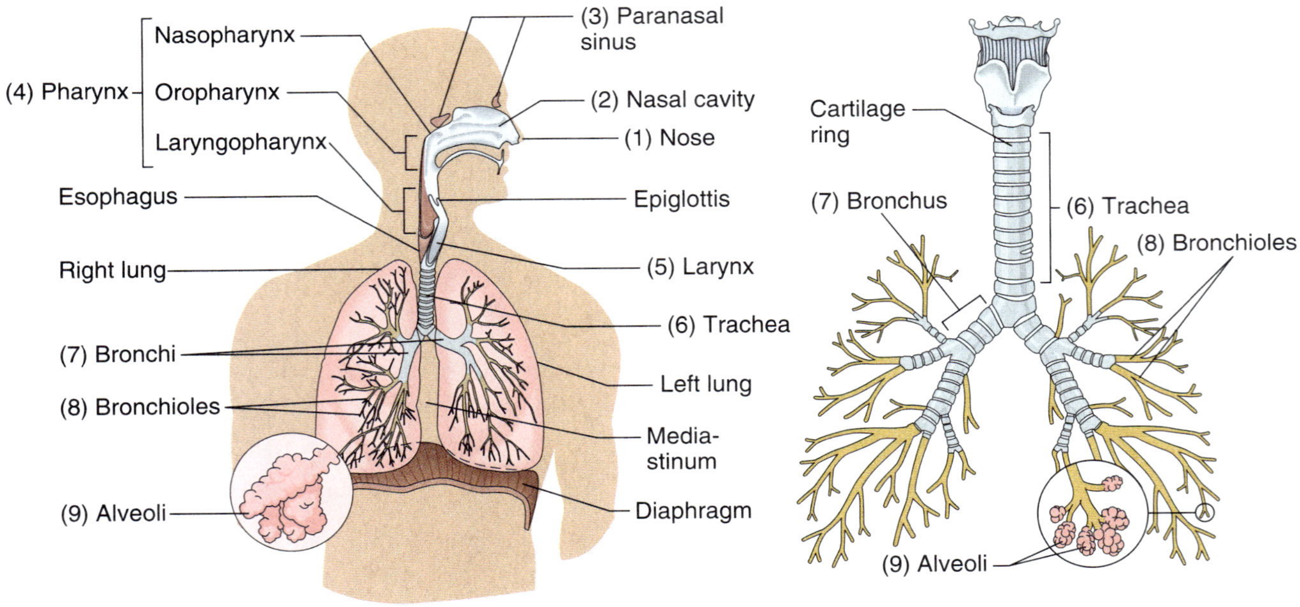

Figure 11-1 Pathway of air from nose to alveoli

Pharynx

Once the air passes through the nasal cavity and paranasal sinuses, it reaches the **(4) pharynx**. The pharynx, or throat, is the airway that connects the mouth and nose to the larynx. Although the pharynx is a single organ, it is commonly divided into three sections: the **nasopharynx**, the upper portion located behind the nose; the **oropharynx**, the middle portion located behind the mouth; and the **laryngopharynx** (also known as the hypopharynx), is the lower portion located just behind the larynx.

Located in the nasopharynx are two rounded masses of lymphatic tissue known as the **adenoids** (also called the pharyngeal tonsils). The adenoids and the tonsils help to filter out bacteria and other foreign matter that pass through the area. Hypertrophy (enlargement) of the adenoids in young children may be great enough to interfere with the child's breathing: The child will have a noisy, snoring sound when breathing. The **palatine tonsils** (more commonly called the tonsils), are located on either side of the soft palate in the oropharynx. The tonsils are normally enlarged in young children.

The pharynx is unique in that it serves as a common passageway for both air and food. As a result of this, there must be a mechanism to prevent food from accidentally entering the respiratory tract. During the act of swallowing, a small flap of cartilage called the **epiglottis** covers the opening of the larynx so that food cannot enter the larynx and lower airways while passing through the pharynx to the lower digestive structures.

Larynx

Also known as the voice box, the **(5) larynx** contains the structures that make vocal sounds possible: the vocal cords. Consisting of two reedlike folds of tissue that stretch across the larynx, the vocal cords vibrate as air passes through the space between them, producing sound (this space is known as the **glottis**). The high or low pitch of the voice depends on how tensely the vocal cords are stretched. The larynx connects the pharynx with the trachea. It is supported by nine cartilages, the most prominent of which is the thyroid cartilage at the front that forms the **Adam's apple.**

Trachea

The **(6) trachea** is commonly known as the windpipe. It extends into the chest and serves as a passageway for air to the bronchi. The trachea lies in front of the esophagus, the tube through which food passes on its way to the stomach. The trachea consists of muscular tissue embedded with 16 to 20 C-shaped rings of cartilage separated by fibrous connective tissue. These rings of cartilage provide rigidity to the trachea, which helps keep the tracheal tube open (you can feel these rings of cartilage if you press your fingers gently against the front of your throat). Without the structural rigidity, the long tracheal tube could collapse against the pressure of other internal tissues.

Bronchi

The trachea branches into two tubes called the **(7) bronchi** (singular: bronchus). Each bronchus leads to a separate lung and divides and subdivides into progressively smaller tubes called **(8) bronchioles**. The bronchioles terminate at the **(9) alveoli**, also known as air sacs. The alveoli, known as the **pulmonary parenchyma**, have very thin walls that allow for the exchange of gases between the lungs and the blood.

Lungs

The lungs are two cone-shaped, spongy organs consisting of alveoli, blood vessels, elastic tissue, and nerves. Each of the two lungs consists of smaller divisions called lobes. The left lung has two lobes, whereas the right lung is divided into three lobes. The uppermost part of the lung is called the **apex**, and the lower part of the lung is called the **base.** The portion of the lung in the midline region where the blood vessels, nerves, and bronchial tubes enter and exit is known as the **hilum.** The lungs are surrounded by a double-folded membrane called the **pleura**. The outer layer of the pleura, which lines the thoracic cavity, is known as the **parietal pleura**. The inner layer of the pleura, which covers the lung, is known as the **visceral pleura**. The small space between these membranes, called the **pleural space,** is filled with a lubricating fluid that prevents friction when the two membranes slide against each other during respiration. The space between the lungs, called the **mediastinum**, contains the heart, aorta, trachea, esophagus, and bronchi. In the lungs, the alveoli are surrounded by a network of tiny blood vessels called **capillaries**. **Figure 11-2** shows the lungs and supporting structures.

Breathing Process

The lungs extend from the collarbone to the **diaphragm** in the thoracic cavity. The diaphragm, a muscular partition that separates the thoracic cavity from the abdominal cavity, aids in the process of breathing. The process of breathing is begun when the **phrenic nerve** stimulates the diaphragm to contract and flatten (descend), thus enlarging the chest cavity. This enlargement of the thoracic cavity that creates a decrease in the

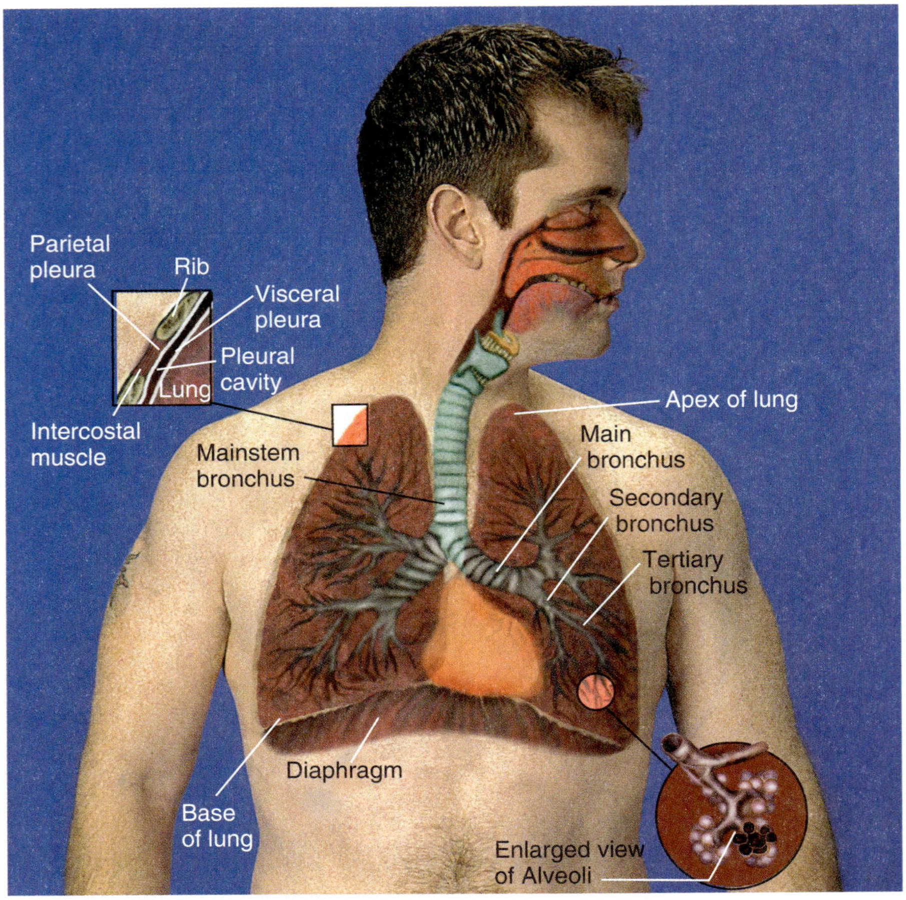

Figure 11-2 The lungs and supporting structures

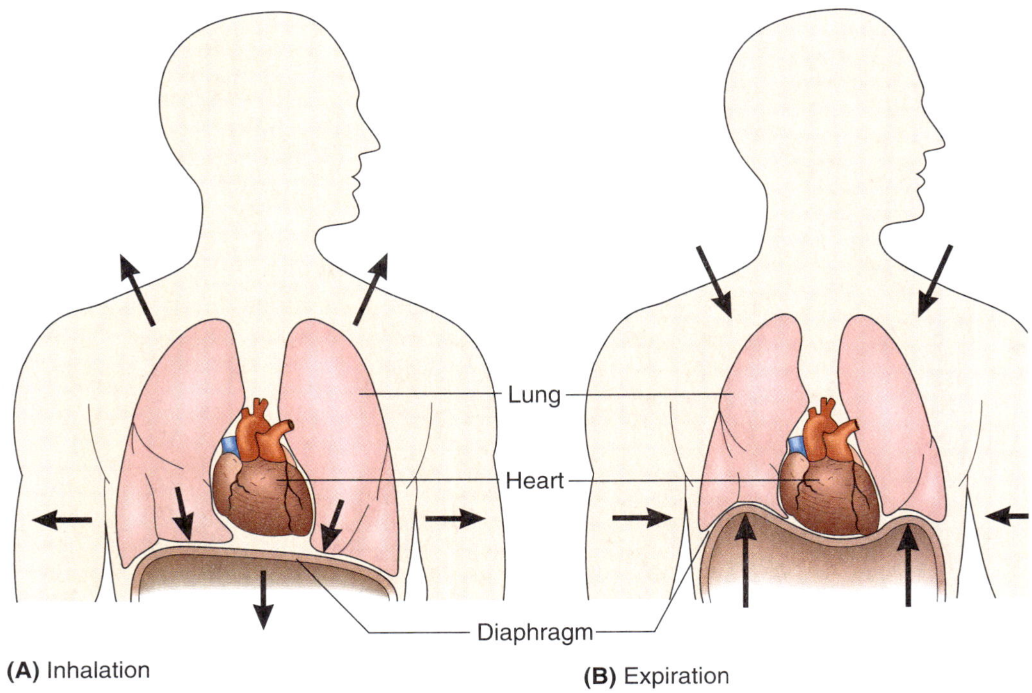

Figure 11-3 Position of diaphragm during (A) inhalation and (B) expiration

pressure within the thorax and draws air into the lungs is called inhalation (inspiration). When the diaphragm relaxes, it rises back into the thoracic cavity, increasing the pressure within the **thorax**. This increase in pressure that causes the air to be forced out of the lungs is called exhalation (expiration). **Figure 11-3** illustrates the increase and decrease of pressure within the thoracic cavity during the breathing process. (As you look at Figure 11-3, take a deep breath and hold it momentarily: Can you feel the enlargement of your chest cavity? As you release your breath, think about the process and how your chest cavity is now decreasing in size as it forces the air back out through the respiratory passages.)

Physical Examination

The following terms relate to techniques used in the physical examination of the respiratory system.

inspection
(in-**SPEK**-shun)

Visual examination of the external surface of the body as well as of its movements and posture.

palpation
(pal-**PAY**-shun)

Palpation is the process of examining by application of the hands or fingers to the external surface of the body to detect evidence of disease or abnormalities in the various organs. See Figure 11-4.

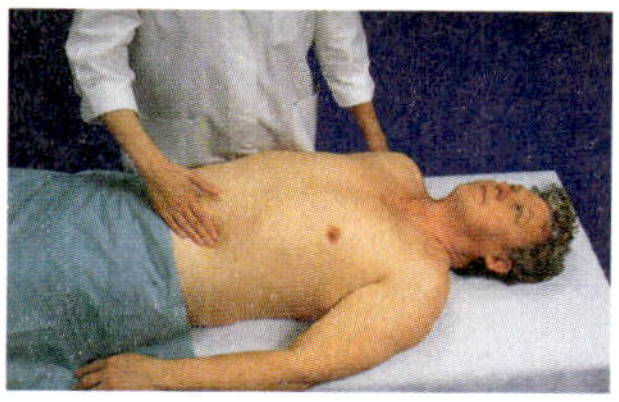

Figure 11-4 Technique of light palpation

auscultation
(oss-kull-**TAY**-shun)

Process of listening for sounds within the body, usually to sounds of thoracic or abdominal viscera, to detect some abnormal condition, or to detect fetal heart sounds. See Figure 11-5.

Auscultation is performed with a stethoscope.

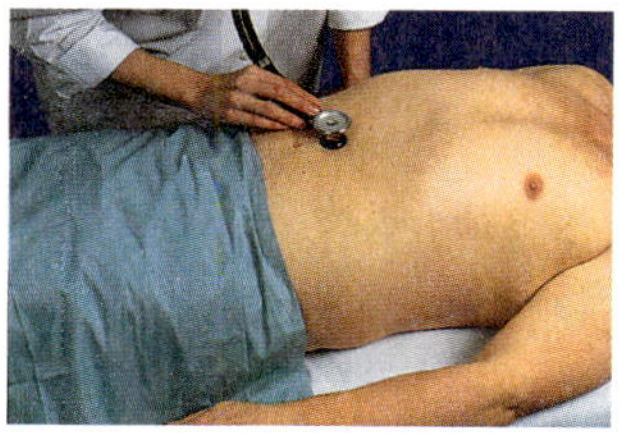

Figure 11-5 Auscultation with bell of stethoscope

percussion
(per-**KUH**-shun)

Use of the fingertips to tap the body lightly but sharply to determine position, size, and consistency of an underlying structure and the presence of fluid or pus in a cavity. See Figure 11-6.

Tapping over a solid organ in the body produces a dull flat sound. Tapping over an air-filled structure, such as the lungs, produces a clear, hollow sound. If the lungs are filled with fluid, as in pneumonia, they will, in turn, take on a dull, flat sound during **percussion**.

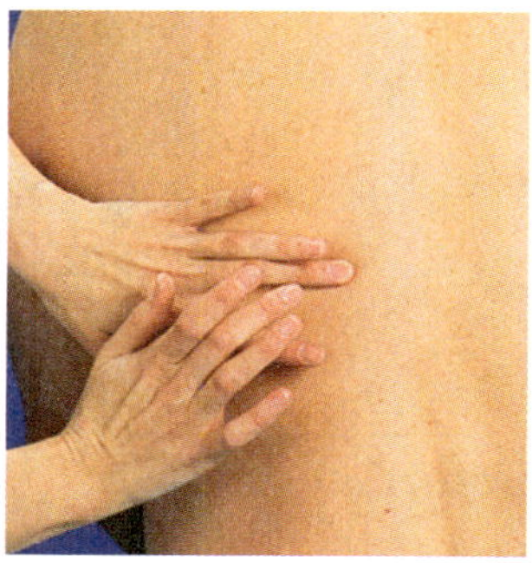

Figure 11-6 Percussion strike

Vocabulary

The following vocabulary words are frequently used when discussing the respiratory system.

WORD	DEFINITION
adenoids (**ADD**-eh-noydz) aden/o = gland -oid = resembling	Lymphatic tissue forming a prominence on the wall of the recess of the nasopharynx.
alveoli (al-**VEE**-oh-lye)	Air cells of the lungs; known as the pulmonary parenchyma (functional units of the lungs).
apex of lung (**AY**-peks of lung)	The upper portion of the lung, rising about 2.5 to 5 cm above the collarbone.
base of lung	The lowest part of the lung, resting on the diaphragm.
bronchi (**BRONG**-kigh) bronch/o = bronchus -i = plural ending	The two main branches leading from the trachea to the lungs, providing the passageway for air movement.
bronchiole (**BRONG**-key-ohl) bronchi/o = bronchiole -ole = small or little	One of the smaller subdivisions of the bronchial tubes.
capillaries (**CAP**-ih-**lair**-eez)	Any of the minute (tiny) blood vessels; the capillaries connect the ends of the smallest arteries (arterioles) with the beginnings of the smallest veins (venules).
diaphragm (**DYE**-ah-fram)	The musculomembranous wall separating the abdomen from the thoracic cavity.
epiglottis (**ep**-ih-**GLOT**-iss)	A thin, leaf-shaped structure located immediately posterior to the root of the tongue; covers the entrance of the larynx when the individual swallows.
glottis (**GLOT**-iss)	The sound-producing apparatus of the larynx consisting of the two vocal folds and the intervening space (the epiglottis protects this opening).
laryngalgia (**lair**-ring-**GAL**-jee-ah)	Pain in the larynx.
laryngopharynx (lah-**ring**-go-**FAIR**-inks) laryng/o = larynx pharyng/o = pharynx	Lower portion of the pharynx that extends from the vestibule of the larynx (the portion just above the vocal cords) to the lowermost cartilage of the larynx.
larynx (**LAIR**-inks) laryng/o = larynx	The enlarged upper end of the trachea below the root of the tongue; the voice box.

mediastinum (mee-dee-ass-**TYE**-num)	The mass of organs and tissues separating the lungs. It contains the heart, aorta, trachea, esophagus, and bronchi.
nares (**NAIRZ**)	External nostrils.
nasopharynx (**nay**-zoh-**FAIR**-inks) nas/o = nose pharyng/o = pharynx	Part of the pharynx located above the soft palate (postnasal space).
oropharynx (**or**-oh-**FAIR**-inks) or/o = mouth pharyng/o = pharynx	Central portion of the pharynx lying between the soft palate and upper portion of the epiglottis.
palatine tonsils (**PAL**-ah-tyne **TON**-sills)	Lymphatic tissue located in the depression of the mucous membrane of fauces (the constricted opening leading from the mouth and the oral pharynx) and the pharynx.
paranasal sinuses (pair-ah-**NAY**-sal **SIGH**-nuss-ez) para- = near, beside, beyond, two like parts nas/o = nose -al = pertaining to	Hollow areas or cavities within the skull that communicate with the nasal cavity.
parietal pleura (pah-**RYE**-eh-tal **PLOO**-rah) pleur/o = pleura -a = noun ending	Portion of the pleura that is closest to the ribs.
pharynx (**FAIR**-inks) pharyng/o = pharynx	Passageway for air from nasal cavity to larynx and food from mouth to esophagus. Serves both the respiratory and digestive systems; the throat.
phrenic nerve (**FREN**-ic nerve) phren/o = mind; also refers to the diaphragm -ic = pertaining to	The nerve that is known as the motor nerve to the diaphragm.
pleura (**PLOO**-rah) pleur/o = pleura -a = noun ending	The double-folded membrane that lines the thoracic cavity.
pleural space (**PLOO**-ral space) pleur/o = pleura -al = pertaining to	The space that separates the visceral and parietal pleurae, which contains a small amount of fluid that acts as a lubricant to the pleural surfaces during respiration.

pulmonary parenchyma (**PULL**-mon-air-ee par-**EN**-kih-mah) pulmon/o = lung -ary = pertaining to	The functional units of the lungs, for example, the alveoli, which have very thin walls that allow for the exchange of gases between the lungs and the blood.
septum (**SEP**-tum)	A wall dividing two cavities.
thorax (**THOH**-raks)	The chest; that part of the body between the base of the neck and the diaphragm.
trachea (**TRAY**-kee-ah) trache/o = trachea -a = noun ending	A cylinder-shaped tube lined with rings of cartilage (to keep it open) that is 4.5 inches long, from the larynx to the bronchial tubes; the windpipe.
visceral pleura (**VISS**-er-al **PLOO**-rah) viscer/o = internal organs	Portion of the pleura that is closest to the internal organs.

Word Elements

The following word elements pertain to the respiratory system. As you review the list, pronounce each word element aloud twice and check the box after you "say it." Write the definition for the example word given for each word element. You may use your medical dictionary.

WORD ELEMENT	PRONUNCIATION	"SAY IT"	MEANING
alveol/o **alveol**ar	al-vee-**OHL**-oh al-**VEE**-oh-lar	☐	alveolus
bronch/o **bronch**opneumonia	**BRONG**-koh **brong**-koh new-**MOH**-nee-ah	☐	bronchus
bronchiol/o **bronchiol**ar	brong-kee-**OH**-loh brong-kee-**OH**-lar	☐	bronchus
epiglott/o **epiglott**itis	ep-ih-**GLOT**-oh ep-ih-glot-**EYE**-tis	☐	epiglottis
laryng/o **laryng**ospasm	lair-**RING**-oh lair-**RING**-go-**spazm**	☐	larynx
nas/o **nas**al	**NAYZ**-oh **NAYZ**-al	☐	nose
orth/o **orth**opnea	**ORTH**-oh **or**-**THOP**-nee-ah	☐	straight

pector/o **pector**al	**PEK**-tor-oh **PEK**-toh-ral	☐	chest
pharyng/o **pharyng**itis	fair-**ING**-oh fair-in-**JYE**-tis	☐	pharynx
phren/o **phreni**c	**FREN**-oh **FREN**-ic	☐	mind; also refers to the diaphragm
pleur/o **pleur**isy	**PLOOR**-oh **PLOOR**-is-ee	☐	pleura
pne/o dys**pne**a	**NEE**-oh disp-**NEE**-ah	☐	breathing
pneum/o **pneum**othorax	**NEW**-moh new-moh-**THOH**-raks	☐	lungs; air
pneumon/o **pneumon**itis	new-**MOHN**-oh new-mohn-**EYE**-tis	☐	lungs; air
pulmon/o **pulmon**ary	pull-**MON**-oh **PULL**-mon-air-ee	☐	lungs
rhin/o **rhin**orrhea	**RYE**-noh rye-noh-**REE**-ah	☐	nose
-scope naso**scope**	**SCOHP** **NAYZ**-oh-scohp	☐	an instrument used to view
sinus/o **sinus**itis	sigh-**NUS**-oh sigh-nus-**EYE**-tis	☐	sinus
thorac/o **thorac**ocentesis	thor-**AK**-oh **thoh**-rah-ko-sen-**TEE**-sis	☐	chest
trache/o **trache**obronchitis	**TRAY**-kee-oh tray-kee-oh-brong-**KIGH**-tis	☐	trachea

Common Signs and Symptoms

Listening carefully to the signs and symptoms presented by the patient and reporting them accurately to the physician will help diagnose and treat the patient more effectively. Although many signs and symptoms are relatively nonspecific (i.e., they occur in several different respiratory conditions), they nevertheless point to certain types of abnormalities and thus provide clues about the patient's illness.

A knowledge of the signs and symptoms along with their definitions will enhance your skills as a history taker. The patient will not necessarily tell you the specific word, but will describe the term in his or her own words. As you study the terms below, write each definition and word a minimum of three times, pronouncing the word aloud each time. Note that the word and the **basic definition** are in bold print. A more detailed description follows most words. Once you have mastered each word to your satisfaction, check the box beside the word.

☐ **apnea**
(ap-**NEE**-ah)
a- = without, not
pne/o = breathing
-a = noun ending

Apnea is a temporary cessation of breathing; "without breathing".

May be a result of reduction in stimuli to the respiratory center, as in overbreathing in which the carbon dioxide content of the blood is reduced, or from failure of respiratory center to discharge impulses, as when the breath is held voluntarily.

☐ **bradypnea**
(**brad**-ip-**NEE**-ah)
brady- = slow
pne/o = breathing
-a = noun ending

Abnormally slow breathing.

Bradypnea is evidenced by a respiratory rate slower than 12 respirations per minute. It could indicate neurological or electrolyte disturbance or infection; or it may indicate a protective response to pain, as in the pain of pleurisy. It may also indicate that the patient is in excellent physical fitness.

☐ **cough**

A forceful and sometimes violent expiratory effort preceded by a preliminary inspiration. The glottis is partially closed, the accessory muscles of expiration are brought into action, and the air is noisily expelled.

Most coughs are due to irritation of the airways (e.g., by dust, smoke, or mucus) or infection.

A cough may be described as brassy, bubbling, croupy, hacking, harsh, hollow, loose, metallic, nonproductive, productive, rasping, rattling, or wracking.

The type of cough and the nature, color, and quantity of any sputum produced can be suggestive of the underlying cause.

Types of Coughs

Nonproductive, unproductive: Not effective in bringing up sputum; "dry cough"

Productive: Effective in bringing up sputum; "wet cough"

Types of Sputum

Mucoid: resembling mucus

Mucopurulent: containing mucus and pus

Purulent: containing pus

Serous: resembling serum; containing a thin, watery fluid

☐ **cyanosis**
(sigh-ah-**NOH**-sis)
cyan/o = blue
-osis = condition

Slightly bluish, grayish, slatelike, or dark purple discoloration of the skin due to presence of abnormal amounts of reduced hemoglobin in the blood.

Bluish discoloration of the skin and mucous membranes, especially the lips, tongue, and fingernail beds.

---

dysphonia
(diss-**FOH**-nee-ah)
dys- = bad, difficult, painful, disordered
phon/o = sound
-ia = condition

Difficulty in speaking; hoarseness.

Occurs when the larynx becomes inflamed as a result of infection or overuse.

---

dyspnea
(disp-**NEE**-ah)
dys- = bad, difficult, painful, disordered
pne/o = breathing
-a = noun ending

Air hunger resulting in labored or difficult breathing, sometimes accompanied by pain.

Normal when due to vigorous work or athletic activity. Audible labored breathing, distressed anxious expression, dilated nostrils, protrusion of abdomen and expanded chest, gasping, and marked cyanosis are among the symptoms of someone with dyspnea.

---

epistaxis
(ep-ih-**STAKS**-is)

Hemorrhage from the nose; nosebleed.

Epistaxis may be caused by a blow to the nose, fragile blood vessels, high blood pressure, dislodging of crusted mucus, or may be secondary to local infections or drying of the nasal mucous membrane.

---

expectoration
(ex-**pek**-toh-**RAY**-shun)

The act of spitting out saliva or coughing up materials from the air passageways leading to the lungs.

The expulsion of mucus or phlegm from the throat or lungs.

---

hemoptysis
(hee-**MOP**-tih-sis)
hem/o = blood
-ptysis = spitting

Hemoptysis is expectoration of blood arising from the oral cavity, larynx, trachea, bronchi, or lungs.

---

hypercapnia
(**high**-per-**KAP**-nee-ah)
hyper- = excessive
-capnia = (condition of) carbon dioxide content in the blood

Increased amount of carbon dioxide in the blood.

Hypercapnia results from inadequate ventilation or from great differences between ventilation and perfusion of the blood.

---

hypoxemia
(**high**-pox-**EE**-mee-ah)
hyp- = under, below, beneath, less than normal
ox/o = oxygen
-emia = blood condition

Insufficient oxygenation of the blood.

Hypoxemia is occasionally associated with decreased oxygen content.

hypoxia
(**high-POX**-ee-ah)
hyp- = under, below, beneath, less than normal
ox/o = oxygen
-ia = condition

Deficiency of oxygen.

Hypoxia is the state of having an inadequate supply of oxygen to the tissues, usually due to hypoxemia.

☐ **Kussmaul respirations**
(**KOOS**-mowl)

Kussmaul respirations are a very deep, gasping type of respiration associated with severe diabetic acidosis.

This hyperventilation (with very deep, but not labored, respirations) represents the body's attempt to decrease acidosis, counteracting the effect of the ketone buildup that occurs with diabetic acidosis.

☐ **orthopnea**
(**or-THOP**-nee-ah)
orth/o = straight
pne/o = breathing
-a = noun ending

Respiratory condition in which there is discomfort in breathing in any but erect, sitting, or standing position.

Symptoms of orthopnea include slow or rapid respiratory rate; sitting or standing posture necessary to breathe properly; muscles of respiration forcibly used; patients feel necessity of bracing themselves to breathe. Anxious expression, cyanotic face; struggle to inhale and exhale.

☐ **pleural rub**
(**PLOO**-ral rub)
pleur/o = pleura
-al = pertaining to

Friction rub caused by inflammation of the pleural space.

The sound is heard on auscultation.

☐ **rales**
(**RALZ**)

An abnormal sound heard on auscultation of the chest, produced by passage of air through bronchi that contain secretion or exudate or that are constricted by spasm or a thickening of their walls.

The sound is a crackling sound similar to that of moisture crackling in a tube as air passes through it. The crackles are heard on auscultation, usually during inhalation. Rales may be described as bibasilar, bubbling, coarse, crackling, crepitant, post-tussive, moist, or sticky.

☐ **rhinorrhea**
(**rye**-noh-**REE**-ah)
rhin/o = nose
-rrhea = discharge; flow

Rhinorrhea is thin, watery discharge from the nose.

☐ **rhonchi**
(**RONG**-kigh)

Rales or rattlings in the throat, especially when it resembles snoring.

Loud, coarse, rattling sounds produced by passage of air through obstructed airways. The sounds are heard on auscultation. Rhonchi may be described as coarse, high pitched, humming, low pitched, musical, post-tussive, sibilant (hissing), sonorous (loud), or whistling.

☐ **sneeze**

To expel air forcibly through the nose and mouth by spasmodic contraction of muscles of expiration due to irritation of nasal mucosa.

The sneeze reflex may be produced by a great number of stimuli. Placing a foot on a cold surface will provoke a sneeze in some people, whereas looking at a bright light or sunlight will cause it in others. Firm pressure applied to the middle of the upper lip and just under the nose will sometimes prevent a sneeze that is about to occur.

☐ **stridor**
(**STRIGH**-dor)

Harsh sound during respiration; high pitched and resembling the blowing of wind, due to obstruction of air passages.

Stridor is heard without the aid of a stethoscope, usually during inhalation.

☐ **tachypnea**
(**tak**-ip-**NEE**-ah)
tachy- = rapid
pne/o = breathing
-a = noun ending

Abnormal rapidity of breathing.

Nervous **tachypnea** is evidenced by a respiratory rate of 40 or more respirations per minute. It occurs in hysteria and neurasthenia. If prolonged, it will cause excess loss of carbon dioxide and the hyperventilation syndrome will develop (fall in blood pressure, vasoconstriction; sometimes fainting). Immediate treatment involves having the patient breathe into a paper bag until the carbon dioxide content of the blood has an opportunity to return to normal. It is important to keep the patient calm and reassured.

☐ **wheeze**
(**HWEEZ**)

A whistling sound or sighing sound resulting from narrowing of the lumen of a respiratory passageway.

The **wheeze** is often heard without the aid of a stethoscope, usually during exhalation. Wheezing occurs in asthma, croup, hay fever, mitral stenosis, and pleural effusion. It may result from presence of tumors, foreign obstructions, bronchial spasm, tuberculosis, obstructive emphysema, or edema.

Pathological Conditions

The pathological conditions are also divided into upper respiratory conditions and lower respiratory conditions. As you study the pathological conditions of the respiratory system, note that the **basic definition** is in bold print, followed by a detailed description in regular print. The phonetic pronunciation is directly beneath each term, and a breakdown of the component parts of the term when appropriate.

Upper Respiratory Conditions

---

coryza
(kor-**RYE**-zuh)

Coryza is inflammation of the respiratory mucous membranes known as the common cold. The phrase "common cold" is usually used when referring to symptoms of an upper respiratory tract infection.

The patient may experience nasal discharge and obstruction, sore throat, sneezing, general malaise, fever, chills, headache, and muscle aches. A cough may also accompany a cold. The symptoms may last a week or more and usually occur without fever.

croup
(**KROOP**)

A childhood disease characterized by a barking cough, suffocative and difficult breathing, stridor, and laryngeal spasm.

The symptoms of **croup** can be dramatic and anxiety-producing to the parent and the child. It is important to approach the child and parents in a calm manner to reduce fears and anxiety. Treatment includes providing a high-humidity atmosphere with cool moisture (cool mist vaporizer) and rest to relieve the symptoms. Croup may result from an acute obstruction of the larynx caused by an allergen, foreign body, infection, or new growth.

diphtheria
(diff-**THEER**-ree-uh)

Serious infectious disease affecting the nose, pharynx, or larynx, usually resulting in sore throat, dysphonia, and fever. The disease is caused by the bacterium *Corynebacterium diphtheriae,* which forms a white coating over the affected airways as it multiplies.

The bacterium releases a toxin into the bloodstream that can quickly damage the heart and nerves, resulting in heart failure, paralysis, and death. **Diphtheria** is uncommon in countries such as the United States, where a vaccine against the disease is routinely given to children. This immunization is one of the components of the DPT immunization.

laryngitis
(**lair**-in-**JYE**-tis)
laryng/o = larynx
-itis = inflammation

Inflammation of the larynx, usually resulting in dysphonia (hoarseness), cough, and difficulty swallowing.

Laryngitis commonly occurs as a result of abuse of the voice (as in laryngitis that often accompanies football games) and as part of an upper respiratory tract infection; but may also be the result of chronic bronchitis or chronic sinusitis. Acute laryngitis includes hoarseness or complete loss of voice (aphonia), as well as severe cough. Treatment for laryngitis includes resting the voice, avoiding irritants such as smoking, and cool mist vaporizer.

pertussis
(per-**TUH**-sis)

An acute upper respiratory infectious disease, caused by the bacterium *Bordetella pertussis;* "whooping cough".

Occurring mainly in children and infants, the early stages of **pertussis** are suggestive of the common cold with slight elevation of fever, sneezing, rhinitis, dry cough, irritability, and loss of appetite.

As the disease progresses (approximately 2 weeks later), the cough is more violent and consists of a series of several short coughs, followed by a long drawn inspiration during which the typical whoop is heard. The coughing episode may be severe enough to cause vomiting. If diagnosed early, pertussis can be treated with oral antibiotics. Otherwise, antibiotics are ineffective and treatment (when needed) consists of supportive care such as the administration of sedatives to reduce coughing and oxygen to facilitate respiration. Pertussis may be prevented by immunization of infants beginning at 3 months of age. This immunization is one of the components of the DPT immunization.

pharyngitis
(**fair**-in-**JYE**-tis)
pharyng/o = pharynx
-itis = inflammation

Inflammation of the pharynx, usually resulting in sore throat. See Figure 11-7.

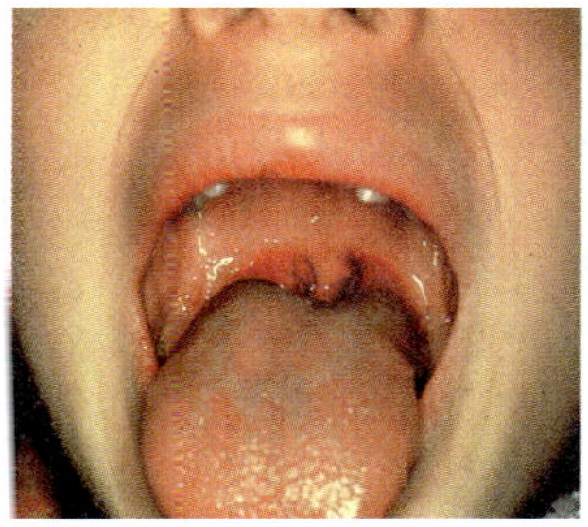

Pharyngitis is usually caused by viral infection, but can also be caused by bacterial infection or other factors. In acute pharyngitis, the patient has fiery red pharyngeal membranes, swollen tonsils flecked with exudate, and the cervical lymph nodes are enlarged and tender. The patient usually experiences fever, malaise, and sore throat. When the causative organism is the group A streptococcus, the acute pharyngitis is termed strep throat.

Figure 11-7 Streptococcal pharyngitis (Courtesy of the Centers for Disease Control and Prevention [CDC])

---

rhinitis
(rye-**NYE**-tis)
rhin/o = nose
-itis = inflammation

Inflammation of the mucous membranes of the nose, usually resulting in obstruction of the nasal passages, rhinorrhea, sneezing, and facial pressure or pain.

Rhinitis is often caused by viral infection, but can also be caused by allergy or other factors.

---

sinusitis
(sigh-nus-**EYE**-tis)
sinus/o = sinus
-itis = inflammation

Inflammation of a sinus, especially a paranasal sinus.

Sinusitis usually results in pain and a feeling of pressure in the affected sinuses; a purulent nasal discharge is also common. Acute sinusitis frequently develops as a result of a common cold, particularly a viral respiratory infection. Treatment of sinusitis includes antibiotics to control the infection, decongestants to decrease the swelling in the nasal mucosa, and analgesics to relieve the pain in the area.

---

tonsillitis
(ton-sill-**EYE**-tis)
tonsill/o = tonsils
-itis = inflammation

Inflammation of the palatine tonsils: located in the area of the oropharynx.

Symptoms include sore throat, fever, snoring, and difficulty in swallowing. The tonsils appear enlarged and red with yellowish exudate. Acute **tonsillitis** has a sudden onset accompanied by fever and chills. The patient may experience malaise and headache in addition to the general symptoms. Treatment includes bed rest, liquid diet, antipyretics, analgesics, and saline gargles. Antibiotic therapy may be indicated depending on the causative organism.

Lower Respiratory Conditions

---

asthma
(**AZ**-mah)

Paroxysmal dyspnea accompanied by wheezing caused by a spasm of the bronchial tubes or by swelling of their mucous membrane.

No age is exempt, but **asthma** occurs most frequently in childhood or early adulthood. Asthma differs from other obstructive lung diseases in that it is a reversible process. The attack may last from 30 minutes to several hours. In some circumstances the attack subsides spontaneously. The asthmatic attack starts suddenly with coughing and a sensation of tightness in the chest. Then slow, laborious, wheezy breathing begins. Expiration is much more strenuous and prolonged than inspiration and the patient may assume a "hunched forward" position in an attempt to get more air. Recurrence and severity of attacks are greatly influenced by secondary factors, by mental or physical fatigue, by exposure to fumes, by endocrine changes at various periods in life, and by emotional situations. Acute attacks of asthma may be relieved by a number of drugs such as epinephrine. Status asthmaticus is a severe asthma attack that is unresponsive to conventional therapy and lasts longer than 24 hours.

---

bronchiectasis
(brong-key-**EK**-tah-sis)
bronchi/o = bronchus

Chronic dilatation of a bronchus or bronchi, with secondary infection that usually involves the lower portion of the lung.

The infection damages the bronchial wall, causing loss of its supporting structure and producing thick sputum that may ultimately obstruct the bronchi. The bronchial walls become permanently distended by severe coughing. Symptoms of **bronchiectasis** include chronic cough, the production of purulent sputum in copious amounts, hemoptysis in a high percentage of patients, and clubbing of the fingers. The patient is also subject to repeated pulmonary infections.

---

bronchitis
(brong-**KIGH**-tis)
bronch/o = bronchus; airway
-itis = inflammation

Inflammation of the mucous membrane of the bronchial tubes. Infection is often preceded by the common cold.

The patient may experience a productive cough, sometimes accompanied by wheezing, dyspnea, and chest pain. Acute **bronchitis** is usually caused by viral infection, but can also be caused by bacterial infection or airborne irritants such as smoke and pollution. In most cases, it resolves without treatment. If a bacterial infection is suspected, the patient may be treated with oral antibiotics, bed rest, increased intake of fluids, antipyretics and analgesics, and cool mist vaporizer.

Chronic bronchitis is primarily associated with cigarette smoking or exposure to pollution. The smoke irritates the airways, resulting in inflammation and hypersecretion of mucus. In chronic bronchitis, the productive cough is present for at least 3 months of 2 consecutive years. Treatment consists of having the patient who smokes stop smoking and treating with antibiotics as necessary.

---

bronchogenic carcinoma
(**brong**-koh-**JEN**-ic car-sin-**OH**-mah)
bronch/o = bronchus, airway
-genic = pertaining to formation; producing
carcin/o = cancer
-oma = tumor

A malignant lung tumor that originates in the bronchi; lung cancer.

Bronchogenic carcinoma is usually associated with a history of cigarette smoking. It is increasing at a greater rate in women than in men and now exceeds breast cancer as the most common cause of cancer deaths in women. Survival rate for lung cancer is low due to usually significant metastasis at the time of diagnosis. More than one-half of the tumors are advanced and inoperable when diagnosed.

---

emphysema
(em-fih-**SEE**-mah)

A chronic pulmonary disease characterized by increase beyond the normal in the size of air spaces distal to the terminal bronchiole, either from dilation of the alveoli or from destruction of their walls. See Figure 11-8.

This nonuniform pattern of abnormal permanent distention of the air spaces appears to be the end stage of a process that has progressed slowly

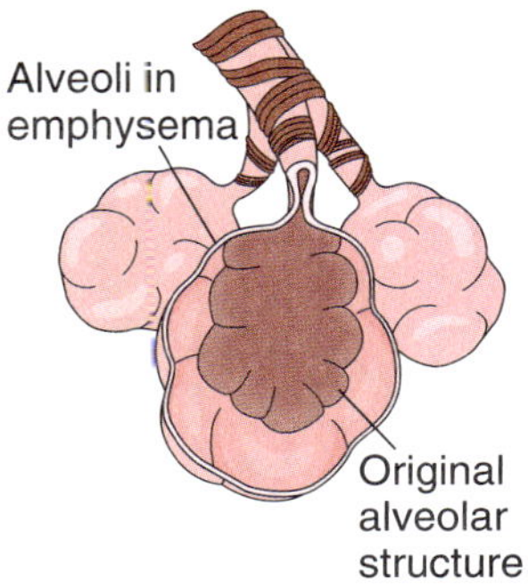

Figure 11-8 Emphysema

for many years. By the time the patient develops the symptoms of emphysema, pulmonary function is often so impaired that it is irreversible.

The major cause of **emphysema** is cigarette smoking. The person with emphysema has a chronic obstruction (increase in airway resistance) to the inflow and outflow of air from the lungs. The lungs lose their elasticity and are in a chronic state of hyperexpansion, making expiration of air more difficult. The act of expiration then becomes one of active muscular movement to force the air out. The patient takes on a "barrel chest" appearance due to the loss of elasticity of lung tissue, becoming increasingly short of breath.

Treatment for emphysema is directed at improving the quality of life for the patient and to slow the progression of the disease. This may involve measures to improve the patient's ventilation (with the use of bronchodilators and medicine to thin the mucous secretions), as well as administration of medications to treat any infection present, and the administration of oxygen to treat the hypoxia that may be present.

---

empyema
(em-pye-**EE**-mah)

Pus in a body cavity, especially in the pleural cavity (pyothorax); usually the result of a primary infection in the lungs.

The patient has fever, night sweats, pleural pain, dyspnea, anorexia, and weight loss. **Empyema** is treated with antibiotic therapy and aspiration of pleural fluid.

---

hyaline membrane disease
(**HIGH**-ah-lighn membrane dih-**ZEEZ**)

Also known as respiratory distress syndrome (RDS) of the premature infant, hyaline membrane disease is severe impairment of the function of respiration in the premature newborn. This condition is rarely present in a newborn of greater than 37 weeks' gestation or in one weighing at least 5 pounds.

Shortly after birth, the premature infant will have a low Apgar score and will develop signs of acute respiratory distress due to atelectasis of the lung; tachypnea, tachycardia, retraction of the rib cage during inspiration, cyanosis, and grunting during expiration will be present.

---

lung abscess
(lung **AB**-sess)

A localized collection of pus formed by the destruction of lung tissue and microorganisms by white blood cells that have migrated to the area to fight infection.

A **lung abscess** usually produces pneumonialike symptoms and a productive cough with blood, purulent, or foul-smelling sputum. Most lung abscesses occur because of aspiration of nasopharyngeal or oropharyngeal material.

---

pleural effusion
(**PLOO**-ral eh-**FYOO**-zhun)
pleur/o = pleura
-al = pertaining to

Accumulation of fluid in the pleural space, resulting in compression of the underlying portion of the lung, with resultant dyspnea. See Figure 11-9.

Pleural effusion is usually secondary to some other disease. Normally, the pleural space contains a small amount of fluid that acts as a lubricant to the pleural surfaces during respiration. With pleural effusion, a significant

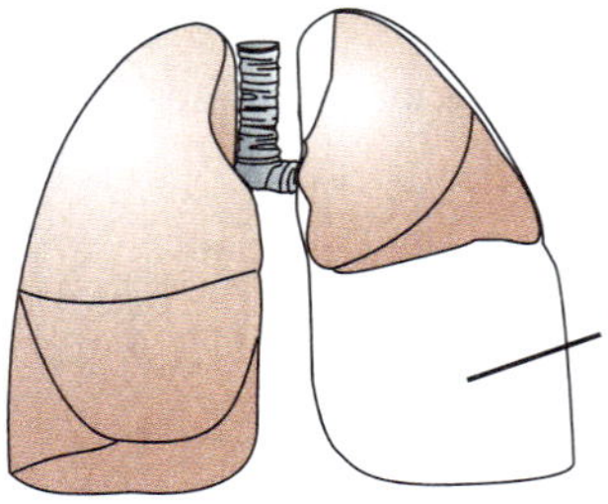

amount of fluid may accumulate in the pleural space. The presence of the fluid is confirmed by chest x-ray, ultrasound, physical examination, and thoracentesis. Treatment is designed to prevent fluid collection from recurring in the pleural space and to relieve the discomfort and dyspnea experienced by the patient.

Figure 11-9 Pleural effusion

---

pleuritis (pleurisy)
(ploor-**EYE**-tis) (**PLOOR**-ih-see)
pleur/o = pleura
-itis = inflammation

Inflammation of both the visceral and parietal pleura.

The pleura is the double-folded membrane that lines the thoracic cavity, with the parietal pleura being the side closest to the ribs and the visceral pleura being the side closest to the internal organs. The pleurae are moistened with a serous secretion that reduces friction during respiratory movements of the lungs.

When these two membranes become inflamed, due to pleurisy, and rub together during respiration (particularly inspiration), the patient experiences a severe, sharp, "knifelike" pain. The pleural rub can be heard on auscultation. Pleuritis may be primary or secondary as a result of some other condition.

---

pneumonia
(new-**MOH**-nee-ah)
pneumon/o = lungs, air
-ia = condition

Inflammation of the lungs caused primarily by bacteria, viruses, and chemical irritants.

The most common bacterial pneumonia, **pneumococcal pneumonia,** is caused by the bacterium *Streptococcus pneumonia.* In certain situations, pneumonia is caused by other microorganisms or by other lung irritants. For example, people with severely impaired immune systems (e.g., those with acquired immune deficiency syndrome [AIDS] or certain types of cancer) are susceptible to **pneumocystis pneumonia,** a type of pneumonia caused by the protozoal parasite *Pneumocystis carinii.* Pneumocystis pneumonia is life threatening in susceptible patients.

Mild cases of pneumonia may resolve without treatment. Moderate cases are often treated with oral antibiotics, whereas severe cases often require hospitalization and treatment with intravenous antibiotics. If the patient has developed complications, these may need to be treated as well.

---

pneumothorax
(new-moh-**THOH**-racks)
pneum/o = lungs, air
-thorax = chest

A collection of air or gas in the pleural cavity. The air enters as the result of a perforation through the chest wall or the pleura covering the lung (visceral pleura). See Figure 11-10.

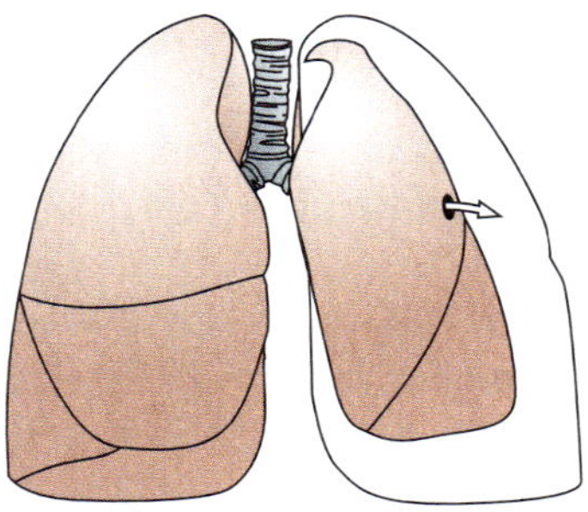

The symptoms of a spontaneous pneumothorax are sudden sharp pain, dyspnea, and cough. Pain may be referred to the shoulder. The majority of cases are mild and require only rest. A pneumothorax, if severe enough, can collapse the lung and shift the heart and the great vessels and trachea toward the unaffected side of the chest, due to the pressure that builds up within the pleural space (tension pneumothorax). This type of pneumothorax would require immediate medical attention to increase the oxygen supply to the patient and to reexpand the lung.

Figure 11-10 Pneumothorax

pulmonary edema
(**PULL**-mon-air-ree eh-**DEE**-mah)
pulmon/o = lung
-ary = pertaining to

Swelling of the lungs caused by an abnormal accumulation of fluid in the lungs, either in the alveoli or the interstitial spaces.

The most common cause of pulmonary edema is cardiac disease. The pulmonary congestion occurs when the pulmonary vessels receive more blood from the right ventricle of the heart than the left ventricle can accommodate and remove. This congestion (or backup of fluid) causes the fluid to leak through the capillary walls and permeate into the airways, creating a sudden onset of breathlessness and a sense of suffocation. The patient's nailbeds become cyanotic and the skin becomes gray. As the condition progresses, breathing is noisy and moist. The patient needs immediate medical attention.

pulmonary embolism
(**PULL**-mon-air-ree **EM**-boh-lizm)
pulmon/o = lung
-ary = pertaining to
embol/i = to throw
-ism = condition

The obstruction of one or more pulmonary arteries by a thrombus (clot) that dislodges from another location, and is carried through the venous system to the vessels of the lung.

The onset of a pulmonary embolism is sudden. The most common symptom is chest pain, followed by dyspnea and tachypnea. A massive embolism blocking the pulmonary artery can produce extreme dyspnea, sudden substernal pain, rapid, weak pulse, shock, fainting (syncope), and sudden death. Massive pulmonary embolism is a true medical emergency because the patient's condition tends to deteriorate rapidly. Most patients who die from a pulmonary embolism do so within the first 2 hours after the embolism.

pulmonary heart disease (cor pulmonale)
(**PULL**-mon-air-ree heart dih-**ZEEZ**)
(cor pull-mon-**ALL**-ee)
pulmon/o = lung
-ary = pertaining to

Pulmonary heart disease (cor pulmonale) is hypertrophy of the right ventricle of the heart (with or without failure) resulting from disorders of the lungs, pulmonary vessels, or chest wall; heart failure resulting from pulmonary disease.

The pulmonary disease reduces proper ventilation to the lungs resulting in increased resistance in the pulmonary circulation. This, in turn, raises the pulmonary blood pressure. Cor pulmonale develops because of the pulmonary hypertension that causes the right side of the heart to work harder to pump the blood against the resistance of the pulmonary vascular circulation, thus creating hypertrophy of the right ventricle of the heart.

Chronic obstructive pulmonary disease (COPD), the most frequent cause of cor pulmonale, produces shortness of breath and cough. The patient develops edema of the feet and legs, distended neck veins, an enlarged liver, pleural effusion, ascites, and a heart murmur.

Treatment is related to treating the underlying cause of cor pulmonale and is often a long-term process. In the case of COPD, treatment involves improving the patient's ventilation (airways must be dilated to improve gas exchange within the lungs). The improved transport of oxygen to the blood and body tissues will reduce the strain on the pulmonary circulation, thus relieving the pulmonary hypertension that leads to cor pulmonale.

sudden infant death syndrome

The completely unexpected and unexplained death of an apparently well, or virtually well, infant. SIDS, also known as crib death, is the most common cause of death between the second week and first year of life.

In the United States, SIDS is responsible for the deaths of approximately 7,000 infants each year. This worldwide syndrome occurs more frequently in the third and fourth months of life, in premature infants, in males, and in infants living in poverty. The deaths usually occur during sleep and are more likely to happen in winter than in summer. These infants are monitored during their sleep and are sometimes placed on an apnea alarm mattress designed to sound an alarm when the infant lying on it ceases to breathe.

tuberculosis
(too-**ber**-kyoo-**LOH**-sis)

An infectious disease caused by the tubercle bacillus, *Mycobacterium tuberculosis*, and characterized by inflammatory infiltrations, formation of tubercles, and caseous (cheeselike) necrosis in the tissues of the lungs.

This necrotic area of the lung, also known as a cavitation, usually appears in the apex of the lung. (It resembles an area shaded by a piece of chalk being rubbed on its side, in a circular motion on a chalkboard.)

In humans, the primary infection usually consists of a localized lesion and regional adenitis. From this state, lesions may heal by fibrosis and calcification and the disease exists in an arrested or inactive state.

Tuberculosis is spread by droplet infection. When bacteria-containing droplets sneezed or coughed into the air by an infected individual are inhaled by an uninfected individual, the bacterium usually settles in the lungs and lies dormant until the immune system is weakened. Then it multiplies, resulting in coughing (productive cough), chest pain, dyspnea, fever, sweating, and poor appetite. The sputum may have a greenish tinge to it.

Diagnosis of tuberculosis usually includes a tuberculin skin test (PPD) and a chest x-ray. A positive skin test will indicate the need for a diagnostic chest x-ray to determine the presence of active lesions. Sputum tests will also be performed to check for the presence of acid-fast bacillus. Tuberculosis is treated with a prolonged (9–12 months) course of antibacterial/antibiotic medications and vitamins.

Work-Related Pathological Conditions

Lung diseases can occur in a variety of occupations as a result of exposure to dusts and gases. The effect of inhaling these materials depends on the nature of the material being inhaled and the length of exposure to the material, as well as the worker's susceptibility. In today's occupational environment, every effort is made by the employer to protect the employee from exposure to hazardous materials. Employees must be informed about all hazardous and toxic substances in their workplace. In addition, they must be educated as to the particular materials to which they will be exposed as well as to the proper methods of protection. The Occupational Safety and Health Act (OSHA) provides guidelines for protecting the safety and health of individuals in industrial and medical settings. There are various other governmental agencies that enforce controls on the workplace for the protection of the employee. The following terms relate to occupational lung diseases.

anthracosis
(an-thrah-**KOH**-sis)
anthrac/o = coal
-osis = condition

Anthracosis is the accumulation of carbon deposits in the lungs due to breathing smoke or coal dust; black lung disease; also called coal worker's pneumoconiosis.

As the disease progresses, the bronchioles and alveoli become clogged with coal dust, which leads to the formation of the "coal macule" (blackish dots on the lung). The macules enlarge causing the weakened bronchiole to dilate, with subsequent development of a focal emphysema (a form of pulmonary emphysema associated with inhalation of environmental dusts, producing dilation of the terminal and respiratory bronchioles).

asbestosis
(as-beh-**STOH**-sis)

Asbestosis is a lung disease resulting from inhalation of asbestos particles.

Exposure to asbestos has been associated with the later development of cancer of the lung, especially mesothelioma. The latency period may be 20 years or more.

byssinosis
(bis-ih-**NOH**-sis)

A lung disease resulting from inhalation of cotton, flax, and hemp; also known as brown lung disease.

Byssinosis is characterized by wheezing and tightness in the chest. The disease does not occur in textile workers who work with cotton after it is bleached.

silicosis
(sill-ih-**KOH**-sis)

Silicosis is a lung disease resulting from inhalation of silica (quartz) dust, characterized by formation of small nodules.

With the passage of time and exposure, the nodules enlarge and grow together forming dense masses. The lung eventually becomes unable to expand fully, and secondary emphysema may develop.

Exposure to silica dust for 10 to 20 years is usually required before silicosis develops and shortness of breath is evident.

Diagnostic Techniques and Procedures

bronchoscopy
(brong-**KOSS**-koh-pee)
bronch/o = bronchus, airway
-scopy = process of viewing

Bronchoscopy is the examination of the interior of the bronchi using a lighted, flexible tube known as a bronchoscope (or endoscope).

The tube is inserted into the bronchi via the nose, pharynx, larynx, and trachea to visually examine the trachea and major bronchi with their branchings. A bronchoscopy may be performed to remove a foreign body, to improve air passage by suctioning out obstructions such as a mucus plug, to obtain a biopsy and/or secretions for examination, and to observe the air passages for signs of disease. As with most endoscopes, tiny forceps or other instruments can be passed through a laryngoscope

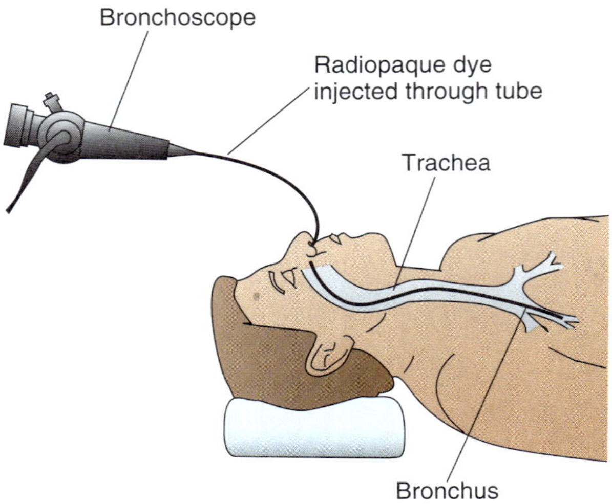

Figure 11-11 Fiberoptic bronchoscopy

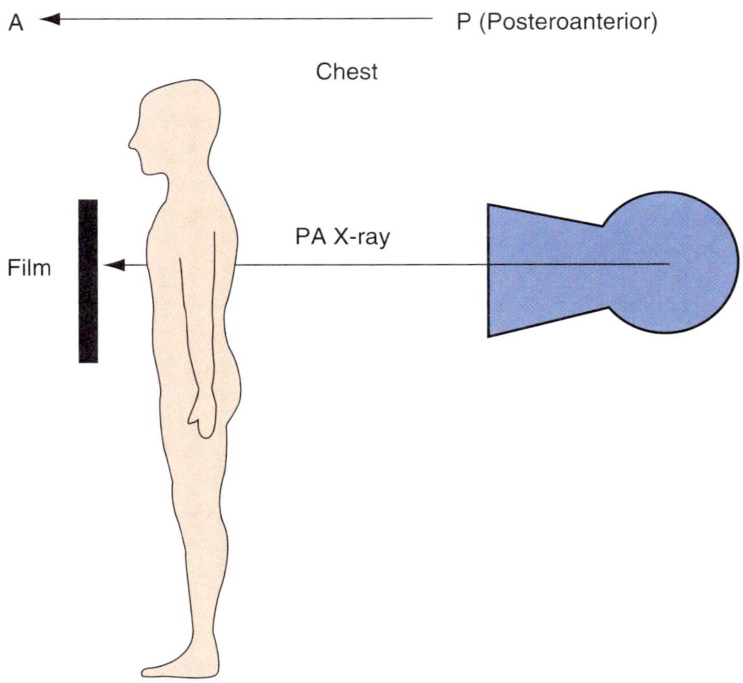

Figure 11-12 Posteroanterior view of chest

or bronchoscope to obtain fluid/tissue specimens for laboratory analysis. See **Figure 11-11.**

---

chest x-ray

The use of high-energy electromagnetic waves passing through the body onto a photographic film, to produce a picture of the internal structures of the body for diagnosis and therapy.

The chest x-ray allows the physician to visualize sites of abnormal density, such as collections of fluid or pus. **Figure 11-12** illustrates the normal posteroanterior (PA) view of the chest.

laryngoscopy
(**lar**-in-**GOSS**-koh-pee)
laryng/o = larynx
-scopy = process of viewing

Laryngoscopy is the examination of the interior of the larynx using a lighted, flexible tube known as a laryngoscope (or endoscope).

The tube is inserted into the larynx via the mouth or nose to visually examine the larynx and associated structures.

lung scan

The visual imaging of the distribution of ventilation or blood flow in the lungs by scanning the lungs after the patient has been injected with or has inhaled radioactive material.

The scanning device records the pattern of pulmonary radioactivity after the patient has received the medication.

pulmonary function tests
pulmon/o = lung
-ary = pertaining to

Physicians use this variety of tests to assess respiratory function.

One of the most common is the use of a measuring device called a **spirometer** to measure the patient's breathing capacity. Measurement of different portions of the patient's lung volume provides an indication of the nature of any breathing impairment, as does measurement of the volume of air a patient can expel during a rapid, vigorous exhalation.

sputum specimen
(**SPEW**-tum specimen)

A specimen of material expectorated from the mouth. If produced after a cough, it may contain, in addition to saliva, material from the throat and bronchi.

The physical and bacterial character of the sputum depend on the disease process involved and the ability of the patient to cough up material. Some bronchial secretions are quite tenacious (adhere to bronchial walls) and are difficult to cough up. When requesting a sputum specimen from the patient, it is important that the patient understands the instructions. He or she should not be collecting saliva from the mouth only, as in spitting. The patient should be instructed to collect a sputum specimen, preferably in the morning before eating or drinking. Encourage the patient to cough deeply (from as far down as possible). The sputum should be placed in the appropriate container and treated as infective until testing proves otherwise.

Sputum may be described as blood streaked, foul tasting, frothy, gelatinous, green, purulent, putrid, stringy, rusty, viscid, viscous, watery, or yellow.

thoracentesis
(**thoh**-rah-sen-**TEE**-sis)
thor/a = chest
-centesis = surgical puncture

Thoracentesis involves the use of a needle to collect pleural fluid for laboratory analysis, or to remove excess pleural fluid or air from the pleural space.

To reach the pleural space, the needle is passed through the patient's skin and chest wall, puncturing these tissues. See **Figure 11-13.** The needle and syringe should be checked carefully to be certain that they fit snugly so that no air is permitted to enter the pleural space.

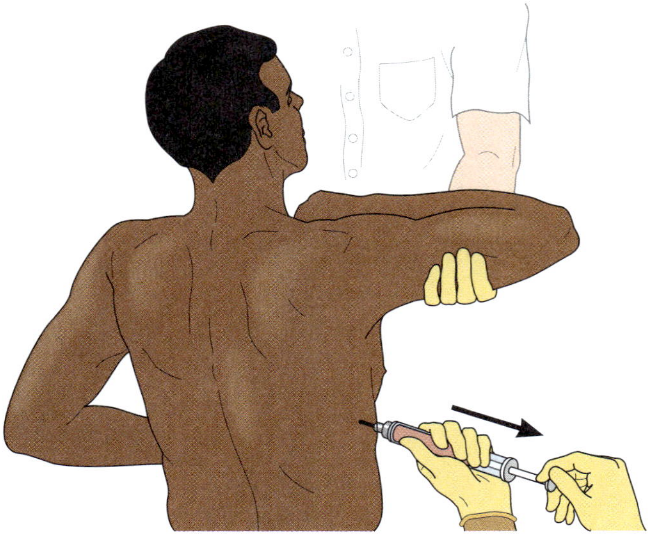

Figure 11-13 Thoracentesis

Common Abbreviations

ABBREVIATION	MEANING
ABG(s)	arterial blood gas(es)
AFB	acid-fast bacilli (The only AFB of clinical significance are organisms of the genus *Mycobacterium,* which cause tuberculosis and leprosy.)
AP	anteroposterior (a directional term, used particularly in x-rays, meaning "from the front to the back"; i.e., anteroposterior view of the chest)
ARD	acute respiratory disease (or distress)
ARDS	adult respiratory distress syndrome
ARF	acute respiratory failure
CO_2	carbon dioxide
COPD	chronic obstructive pulmonary disease (associated with chronic bronchitis and emphysema)
CPR	cardiopulmonary resuscitation
CXR	chest x-ray
DPT	diphtheria, pertussis (whooping cough), and tetanus; an immunization given in childhood to prevent these diseases by providing immunity
IPPB	intermittent positive pressure breathing
LLL	left lower lobe (of the lung)
LUL	left upper lobe (of the lung)
O_2	oxygen
PA	posteroanterior (a directional term, used particularly in x-rays, meaning "from the back to the front"; i.e., posteroanterior view of the chest)
$PaCO_2$	partial pressure of carbon dioxide (CO_2) dissolved in the blood
PaO_2	partial pressure of oxygen (O_2) dissolved in the blood
PCP	*Pneumocystis carinii* pneumonia
PFT(s)	pulmonary function test(s)
PPD	purified protein derivative; substance used in intradermal test for tuberculosis

R	respiration	**SIDS**	sudden infant death syndrome
RDS	respiratory distress syndrome	**SOB**	shortness of breath
RLL	right lower lobe (of the lung)	**TB**	tuberculosis
RML	right middle lobe (of the lung)	**TPR**	temperature, pulse, and respiration
RUL	right upper lobe (of the lung)	**URI**	upper respiratory infection

Written and Audio Terminology Review

Review each of the following terms from the chapter. Study the spelling of each term and write the definition in the space provided. If you have the Audio CD available, listen to each term, pronounce it, and check the box once you are comfortable saying the word. Check definitions by looking the term up in the glossary/index.

TERM	PRONUNCIATION	DEFINITION
adenoids	☐ **ADD**-eh-noydz	____________
alveoli	☐ al-**VEE**-oh-lye	____________
anthracosis	☐ an-thrah-**KOH**-sis	____________
apex	☐ **AY**-peks	____________
apnea	☐ ap-**NEE**-ah	____________
asbestosis	☐ **as**-beh-**STOH**-sis	____________
asthma	☐ **AZ**-mah	____________
auscultation	☐ oss-kull-**TAY**-shun	____________
bradypnea	☐ **brad**-ip-**NEE**-ah	____________
bronchi	☐ **BRONG**-kigh	____________
bronchiectasis	☐ brong-key-**EK**-tah-sis	____________
bronchiole	☐ **BRONG**-key-ohl	____________
bronchitis	☐ brong-**KIGH**-tis	____________
bronchogenic carcinoma	☐ **brong**-koh-**JEN**-ic car-sin-**OH**-mah	____________
bronchoscopy	☐ brong-**KOSS**-koh-pee	____________
byssinosis	☐ bis-ih-**NOH**-sis	____________
capillaries	☐ **CAP**-ih-**lair**-eez	____________
coryza	☐ kor-**RYE**-zuh	____________

Term	Pronunciation	
croup	☐ **KROOP**	______
cyanosis	☐ sigh-ah-**NOH**-sis	______
diaphragm	☐ **DYE**-ah-fram	______
diphtheria	☐ diff-**THEER**-ree-uh	______
dyspnea	☐ disp-**NEE**-ah	______
dysphonia	☐ diss-**FOH**-nee-ah	______
emphysema	☐ em-fih-**SEE**-mah	______
empyema	☐ em-pye-**EE**-mah	______
epiglottis	☐ **ep**-ih-**GLOT**-iss	______
epistaxis	☐ ep-ih-**STAKS**-is	______
expectoration	☐ ex-**pek**-toh-**RAY**-shun	______
glottis	☐ **GLOT**-iss	______
hemoptysis	☐ hee-**MOP**-tih-sis	______
hyaline membrane disease	☐ **HIGH**-ah-lighn membrane dih-**ZEEZ**	______
hypercapnia	☐ **high**-per-**KAP**-nee-ah	______
hypoxemia	☐ **high**-pox-**EE**-mee-ah	______
hypoxia	☐ **high**-**POX**-ee-ah	______
Kussmaul respirations	☐ **KOOS**-mowl respirations	______
laryngitis	☐ **lair**-in-**JYE**-tis	______
laryngopharynx	☐ lair-**ring**-go-**FAIR**-inks	______
laryngoscopy	☐ **lair**-in-**GOSS**-koh-pee	______
larynx	☐ **LAIR**-inks	______
lung abscess	☐ lung **AB**-sess	______
mediastinum	☐ mee-dee-ass-**TYE**-num	______
nares	☐ **NAIRZ**	______
nasopharynx	☐ **nay**-zoh-**FAIR**-inks	______
oropharynx	☐ **or**-oh-**FAIR**-inks	______
orthopnea	☐ **or**-**THOP**-nee-ah	______
palatine tonsils	☐ **PAL**-ah-tyne **TON**-sills	______
palpation	☐ pal-**PAY**-shun	______

Term	Pronunciation
paranasal sinuses	☐ pair-ah-**NAY**-sal **SIGH**-nuss-ez
parietal pleura	☐ pah-**RYE**-eh-tal **PLOO**-rah
percussion	☐ per-**KUH**-shun
pertussis	☐ per-**TUH**-sis
pharyngitis	☐ **fair**-in-**JYE**-tis
pharynx	☐ **FAIR**-inks
phrenic	☐ **FREN**-ic
pleura	☐ **PLOO**-rah
pleural	☐ **PLOO**-ral
pleural effusion	☐ **PLOO**-ral eh-**FYOO**-zhun
pleuritis (pleurisy)	☐ ploor-**EYE**-tis (**PLOOR**-ih-see)
pneumonia	☐ new-**MOH**-nee-ah
pneumothorax	☐ new-moh-**THOH**-racks
pulmonary edema	☐ **PULL**-mon-air-ree eh-**DEE**-mah
pulmonary embolism	☐ **PULL**-mon-air-ee **EM**-boh-lizm
pulmonary heart disease (cor pulmonale)	☐ **PULL**-mon-air-ree heart dih-**ZEEZ** (cor pull-mon-**ALL**-ee)
pulmonary parenchyma	☐ **PULL**-mon-air-ee par-**EN**-kih-mah
rales	☐ **RALZ**
rhinitis	☐ rye-**NYE**-tis
rhinorrhea	☐ **rye**-noh-**REE**-ah
rhonchi	☐ **RONG**-kigh
septum	☐ **SEP**-tum
silicosis	☐ sill-ih-**KOH**-sis
sinusitis	☐ sigh-nus-**EYE**-tis
sputum	☐ **SPEW**-tum
stridor	☐ **STRIGH**-dor

Term		Pronunciation	
tachypnea	☐	**tak**-ip-**NEE**-ah	________
thoracentesis	☐	**thoh**-rah-sen-**TEE**-sis	________
thorax	☐	**THOH**-raks	________
tonsillitis	☐	ton-sill-**EYE**-tis	________
trachea	☐	**TRAY**-kee-ah	________
tuberculosis	☐	too-**ber**-kyoo-**LOH**-sis	________
visceral pleura	☐	**VISS**-er-al **PLOO**-rah	________
wheeze	☐	**HWEEZ**	________

Chapter Review Exercises

The following exercises provide a more in-depth review of the chapter material. Your goal in these exercises is to complete each section at a minimum 80% level of accuracy. A space has been provided for your score at the end of each section.

A. Spelling

Circle the correctly spelled term in each pairing of words. Each correct answer is worth 10 points. Record your score in the space provided at the end of the exercise.

1.	asthma	azthma
2.	thoracentesis	throacentesis
3.	emphysemia	emphysema
4.	pluritis	pleuritis
5.	diphtheria	diptheria
6.	tonsilitis	tonsillitis
7.	rales	rals
8.	apenea	apnea
9.	strydor	stridor
10.	epistaxis	epistacksis

Number correct _______ × 10 points/correct answer: Your score _______%

B. Term to Definition: Signs and Symptoms

Define each term by writing the definition in the space provided. Check the box if you are able to complete this exercise correctly the first time (without referring to the answers). Each correct answer is worth 10 points. Record your score in the space provided at the end of the exercise.

☐ 1. rhinorrhea ________________________________

☐ 2. hemoptysis ________________________________

☐ 3. dysphonia ____

☐ 4. apnea ____

☐ 5. dyspnea ____

☐ 6. orthopnea ____

☐ 7. tachypnea ____

☐ 8. cyanosis ____

☐ 9. hypoxemia ____

☐ 10. hypoxia ____

Number correct _______ × 10 points/correct answer: Your score _______%

C. Matching Breath Sounds

Match the following breath sounds on the left with the correct description on the right. Each correct answer is worth 10 points. Record your score in the space provided at the end of the exercise.

_____ 1. pleural rub

_____ 2. rales

_____ 3. rhonchi

_____ 4. stridor

_____ 5. wheeze

_____ 6. dyspnea

_____ 7. Kussmaul respirations

_____ 8. sneeze

_____ 9. cough

_____ 10. tachypnea

a. crackling sounds heard on auscultation, usually during inhalation

b. loud, coarse, rattling sounds heard on auscultation

c. abnormal rapidity of breathing

d. forceful, sometimes violent expiratory effort preceded by a preliminary inspiration

e. harsh, high-pitched sound heard without a stethoscope, usually during inhalation

f. to expel air forcibly through the nose and mouth by spasmodic contraction of muscles of expiration due to irritation of nasal mucosa

g. air hunger resulting in labored or difficult breathing

h. very deep gasping type of respiration associated with severe diabetic acidosis

i. whistling sound heard without a stethoscope, usually during exhalation

j. rubbing sound heard on auscultation

k. abnormally slow breathing

l. difficulty in speaking; hoarseness

Number correct _______ × 10 points/correct answer: Your score _______%

D. Matching Respiratory Conditions

Match the following respiratory conditions on the left with the most appropriate definition on the right. Each correct answer is worth 10 points. Record your score in the space provided at the end of this exercise.

_____ 1. rhinitis
_____ 2. croup
_____ 3. sudden infant death syndrome
_____ 4. empyema
_____ 5. pleuritis
_____ 6. pneumonia
_____ 7. asthma
_____ 8. emphysema
_____ 9. pneumothorax
_____ 10. bronchiogenic carcinoma

a. lung cancer
b. inflammation of the lungs caused primarily by viruses, bacteria, and chemical irritants
c. a childhood disease characterized by a barking cough, suffocative and difficult breathing, stridor, and laryngeal spasm
d. pus in a body cavity, especially in the pleural cavity
e. a collection of air or gas in the pleural cavity
f. inflammation of the mucous membrane of the nose
g. swelling of the lungs caused by an abnormal accumulation of fluid in the lungs
h. inflammation of both the visceral and parietal pleura; pleurisy
i. crib death
j. a chronic pulmonary disease characterized by increase beyond the normal in the size of the alveoli
k. paroxysmal dyspnea accompanied by wheezing caused by a spasm of the bronchial tubes
l. an infectious disease caused by the tubercle bacillus, *Mycobacterium tuberculosis*

Number correct _______ × 10 points/correct answer: Your score _______%

E. Proofreading Skills

Read the following report. For each boldfaced term, provide a brief definition and indicate if the term is spelled correctly. If it is misspelled, provide the correct spelling. Each correct answer is worth 10 points. Record your answer in the space provided at the end of the exercise.

HILLCREST Medical Center

"Patient presented as a 46-year-old male with signs of **pnumonia**. He appeared acutely ill, with fever, chills, cough, blue-tinged lips, and severe **dispnea.** Fine **wheezes** could be heard on expiration, which he said was not unusual since he suffered from **azthma.** He said his asthma was generally well controlled, but that **pulmonary function tests** usually show reduced lung capacity. Using a **stethascope**, **rawls** could clearly be heard. A chest x-ray confirmed the diagnosis of pneumonia and also revealed a **plural effusion**. Ordered a **sputum culture** to determine the causative pathogen and **arterial blood gases** to assess the extent of **respritory** impairment. Patient was admitted to the hospital for treatment. Treatment plan: intravenous antibiotic beginning immediately, to be adjusted pending results of sputum culture."

Example:

pnumonia *Inflammation of one or both lungs, usually due to infection.*

Spelled correctly? ☐ Yes ☑ No *pneumonia*

1. **dispnea** ______

   Spelled correctly? ☐ Yes ☐ No ______

2. **wheezes** ______

   Spelled correctly? ☐ Yes ☐ No ______

3. **azthma** ______

   Spelled correctly? ☐ Yes ☐ No ______

4. **pulmonary function tests** ______

   Spelled correctly? ☐ Yes ☐ No ______

5. **stethascope** ______

   Spelled correctly? ☐ Yes ☐ No ______

6. **rawls** ______

   Spelled correctly? ☐ Yes ☐ No ______

7. **plural effusion** ______

   Spelled correctly? ☐ Yes ☐ No ______

8. **sputum culture** ______

   Spelled correctly? ☐ Yes ☐ No ______

9. **arterial blood gases** ______

   Spelled correctly? ☐ Yes ☐ No ______

10. **respritory** ______

    Spelled correctly? ☐ Yes ☐ No ______

Number correct ______ × 10 points/correct answer: Your score ______%

F. Matching Abbreviations

Match the abbreviations on the left with the correct definition on the right. Each correct answer is worth 10 points. When you have completed the exercise, record your score in the space provided at the end of the exercise.

_____	1. AFB	a. acute respiratory distress syndrome
_____	2. COPD	b. cardiopulmonary resuscitation

_____ 3. LLL
_____ 4. URI
_____ 5. PFT(s)
_____ 6. SIDS
_____ 7. SOB
_____ 8. IPPB
_____ 9. CPR
_____ 10. PA

c. pulmonary function tests
d. left upper lobe
e. left lower lobe
f. acid-fast bacilli
g. chronic obstructive pulmonary disease
h. upper respiratory infection
i. sudden infant death syndrome
j. shortness of breath
k. intermittent positive pressure breathing
l. posteroanterior
m. urinary tract infection

Number correct _______ × 10 points/correct answer: Your score _______%

G. Crossword Puzzle

Each crossword answer is worth 10 points. When you have completed the crossword puzzle, total your points and enter your score in the space provided.

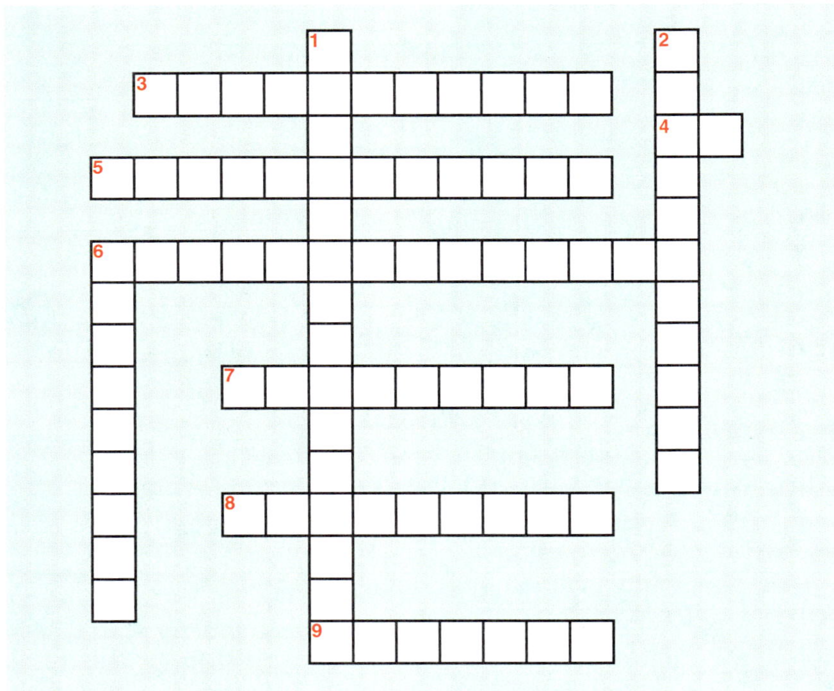

ACROSS
3 Inflammation of pharynx
4 Tuberculosis (abbrev.)
5 Pulmonary heart disease
6 Swelling of the lungs (two words)
7 Pleurisy
8 Whooping cough
9 Pus in a body (pleural) cavity

DOWN
1 Respiratory distress syndrome
2 Black lung disease
6 Viral inflammation of the lungs

Number correct _______ × 10 points/correct answer: Your score _______%

H. Word Element Review

The following words relate to the respiratory system. The prefixes and suffixes have been provided. Read the definition carefully and complete the word by filling in the blank, using the word elements provided in this chapter. If you have forgotten your word building rules, refer to Chapter 1. Each correct word is worth 10 points. Record your score in the space provided at the end of this exercise.

1. Inflammation of the lining of the chest cavity:
   ____________________ / itis
2. An instrument used to view the bronchi:
   ____________________ /o / scope
3. Inflammation of the nose:
   ____________________ / itis
4. Drainage or discharge from the nose:
   ____________________ /o / rrhea
5. Absence of breathing (without breathing):
   a / ____________________ / a
6. Sitting up straight to breathe properly:
   ____________________ /o / pne / a
7. Slow breathing:
   brady / ____________________ / a
8. Rapid breathing:
   tachy / ____________________ / a
9. Inflammation of the voice box:
   ____________________ / itis
10. Pertaining to the air sacs in the lungs:
    ____________________ / ar

Number correct _______ × 10 points/correct answer: Your score _______%

I. Matching

Match the anatomical structures on the right with the most appropriate descriptions on the left. Each correct response is worth 10 points. When you have completed the exercise, record your score in the space provided at the end of the exercise.

_____ 1. Hollow areas or cavities within the skull that communicate with the nasal cavity

_____ 2. Hairlike projections on the mucous membranes, that sweep dirt and foreign material toward the throat for elimination

_____ 3. Another name for this structure is the throat

_____ 4. The two rounded masses of lymphatic tissue located in the nasopharynx are known as this

_____ 5. The two rounded masses of lymphatic tissue located on either side of the soft palate in the oropharynx are known as this

_____ 6. A small flap of cartilage that covers the opening of the larynx so that food cannot enter the larynx and lower airways while passing through the pharynx to the lower digestive structures

_____ 7. Also known as the voice box

_____ 8. Commonly known as the windpipe

_____ 9. These structures branch off from the trachea and lead into the lungs

_____ 10. The outer layer of the pleura that lines the thoracic cavity

a. epiglottis
b. pharynx
c. trachea
d. parietal pleura
e. paranasal sinuses
f. cilia
g. adenoids
h. palatine tonsils
i. larynx
j. bronchi

Number correct _____ × 10 points/correct answer: Your score _____%

J. Word Search

Using the definitions provided, identify the terms related to the respiratory system. After you have identified each term, find and circle it in the word search puzzle. The words may be read up, down, diagonally, across, or backward. Each correct answer is worth 10 points. Record your score in the space provided at the end of the exercise.

Example: Inflammation of the mucous membranes of the nose.

rhinitis

1. The upper portion of the lung.

____

2. The musculomembranous wall separating the abdomen from the thoracic cavity.

____

3. The voice box.

____

4. The external nostrils.

____

5. The double-folded membrane that lines the thoracic cavity.

____

6. The medical term for nosebleed.

____

7. Thin, watery discharge from the nose.

____

8. Temporary cessation of breathing ("without breathing").

____

9. Abnormally slow breathing.

____

10. Abnormally rapid breathing.

____

A	L	O	A	T	I	N	G	Y	S	T	N	M	I	C
P	L	E	U	R	A	O	I	D	A	S	T	T	S	C
E	I	S	K	T	M	N	M	E	T	T	R	N	V	R
X	A	I	N	E	E	L	O	S	D	I	C	C	B	O
I	L	T	T	D	I	A	P	H	R	A	G	M	T	S
M	U	I	O	I	Y	R	O	T	E	L	R	L	T	Z
L	R	N	T	H	L	Y	I	U	A	S	I	P	E	C
P	U	I	R	E	P	N	E	M	A	R	O	F	E	A
P	U	H	O	S	I	X	A	T	S	I	P	E	E	E
E	A	R	C	D	A	D	I	R	D	E	Y	S	M	N
R	R	H	I	N	O	R	R	H	E	A	D	S	R	P
N	I	A	A	A	R	C	H	S	S	S	S	A	I	Y
B	S	S	N	E	R	U	Y	A	I	D	I	S	G	D
P	U	I	T	X	E	S	P	I	N	A	E	N	P	A
L	R	S	E	H	L	O	I	I	U	A	S	C	O	R
T	A	C	H	Y	P	N	E	A	T	U	R	E	S	B
F	R	O	T	T	E	U	R	I	S	M	E	M	I	C
E	X	H	I	B	I	T	D	I	O	M	A	S	E	S

Number correct* _______ × *10 points/correct answer: Your score* _______ *%

Answers to Chapter Review Exercises

A. Spelling

1. asthma
2. thoracentesis
3. emphysema
4. pleuritis
5. diphtheria
6. tonsillitis
7. rales
8. apnea
9. stridor
10. epistaxis

B. Term to Definition: Signs and Symptoms

1. thin watery discharge from the nose
2. expectoration of blood arising from the oral cavity, larynx, trachea, bronchi, or lungs
3. difficulty in speaking; hoarseness
4. temporary cessation of breathing
5. difficult breathing, sometimes accompanied by pain
6. respiratory condition in which there is discomfort in breathing in any but erect, sitting, or standing position
7. abnormal rapidity of breathing
8. slightly bluish, grayish, or slatelike discoloration of the skin due to presence of abnormal amounts of reduced hemoglobin in the blood
9. insufficient oxygenation of the blood
10. deficiency of oxygen

C. Matching Breath Sounds

1. j
2. a
3. b
4. e
5. i
6. g
7. h
8. f
9. d
10. c

D. Matching Respiratory Conditions

1. f
2. c
3. i
4. d
5. h
6. b
7. k
8. j
9. e
10. a

E. Proofreading Skills

1. difficult breathing, sometimes accompanied by pain.
   Spelled correctly? No **dyspnea**
2. whistling sounds or sighing sounds resulting from narrowing of the lumens of respiratory passageways.
   Spelled correctly? Yes
3. paroxysmal dyspnea accompanied by wheezing caused by a spasm of the bronchial tubes or by swelling of their mucous membrane.
   Spelled correctly? No **asthma**
4. a variety of tests to assess respiratory function.
   Spelled correctly? Yes
5. an instrument used to auscultate heart and lung sounds.
   Spelled correctly? No **stethoscope**
6. abnormal sounds heard on auscultation of the chest, produced by passage of air through bronchi that contain secretion or exudate or that are constricted by spasm or a thickening of their walls.
   Spelled correctly? No **rales**
7. accumulation of fluid in the pleural space.
   Spelled correctly? No **pleural effusion**
8. a laboratory test identifying the microorganisms or cells in material coughed up from the lungs.
   Spelled correctly? Yes
9. the measurement of the oxygen and carbon dioxide in arterial blood.
   Spelled correctly? Yes
10. of or pertaining to the process of breathing and gas exchange in the lungs.
    Spelled correctly? No **respiratory**

F. Matching Abbreviations

1. f
2. g
3. e
4. h
5. c
6. i
7. j
8. k
9. b
10. l

G. Crossword Puzzle

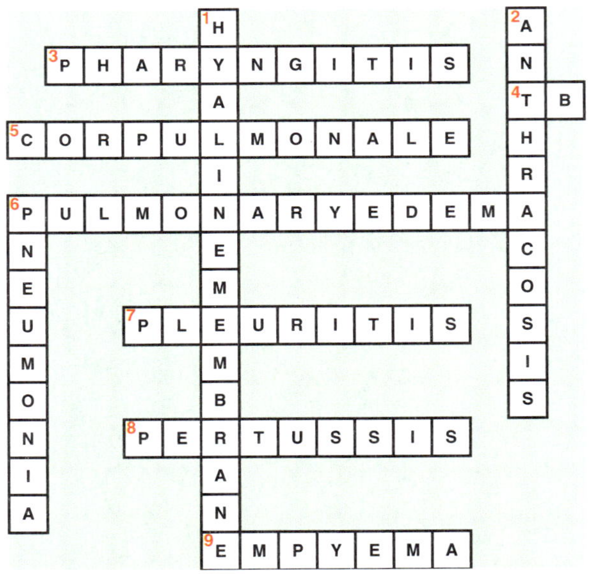

H. Word Element Review

1. **pleur** /itis
2. **bronch** /o/ scope
3. **rhin** /itis
4. **rhin** /o/ rrhea
5. a/ **pne** /a
6. **orth** /o/ pne /a
7. brady /**pne** /a
8. tachy /**pne** /a
9. **laryng/** itis
10. **alveol** /ar

I. Matching

1. e
2. f
3. b
4. g
5. h
6. a
7. i
8. c
9. j
10. d

J. Word Search

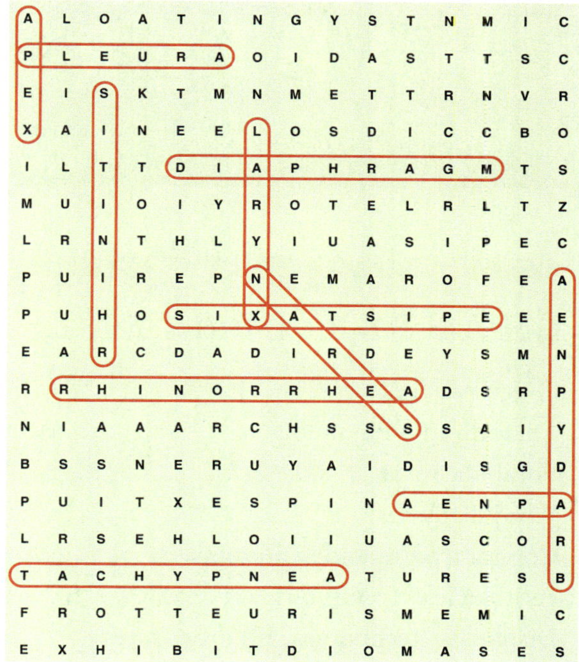

CHAPTER 12

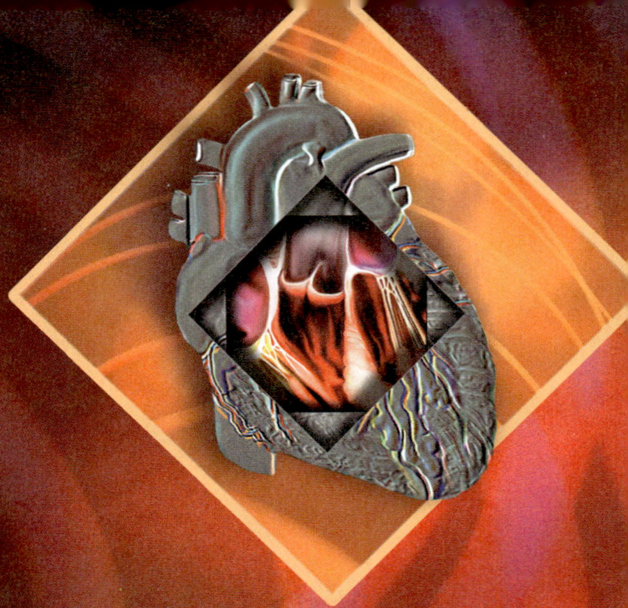

The Digestive System

CHAPTER CONTENT

KEY COMPETENCIES

Upon completing this chapter and the review exercises at the end of the chapter, the learner should be able to:

1. Identify and label the structures of the digestive system.
2. List five basic functions of the digestive system.
3. Identify and define at least 25 pathological conditions of the digestive system.
4. Identify at least 10 diagnostic techniques used in diagnosis and treatment of disorders of the digestive system.
5. Correctly spell and pronounce each new term introduced in this chapter using the Activity CD-ROM and Audio CD, if available.
6. Create at least 10 medical terms related to the digestive system and identify the appropriate combining form(s) for each term.
7. Identify at least 20 abbreviations common to the digestive system.

OVERVIEW

"How many times a day do you eat?" The American tradition is to have breakfast, lunch, and dinner (or supper, in the south). In addition to these three basic meals, count the number of snacks you consume each day, and then answer the question as to how many times a day you eat . . . the answer could be surprising! Foods of little value or a well-balanced diet: What shall it be? The task of the digestive system will remain the same no matter what we choose.

The digestive system is also known as the **gastrointestinal tract, digestive tract**, or the **alimentary canal**. It is approximately 30 feet long, beginning with the mouth (oral cavity) and ending with the anus. The organs of the digestive system work together to prepare foods for **absorption** into the bloodstream and to prepare foods for use by the body cells. In addition to this vital function, the digestive system is also responsible for elimination of solid wastes from the body. Normal functioning of the human body depends on a properly functioning digestive system. Food ingested in a meal or snack must be modified both chemically and physically to be absorbed as nutrients that can be used by the body cells. As the ingested food passes through the gastrointestinal tract, it goes through the many changes necessary for it to be received into the bloodstream and distributed to the body cells as nutrients. The process of altering the chemical and physical composition of food is known as **digestion.**

The physician who specializes in the study of diseases affecting the gastrointestinal tract, including the stomach, intestines, gallbladder, and bile duct, is known as a **gastroenterologist**. The allied health professional who studies and applies the principles and science of nutrition is known as a **nutritionist**. A **dietitian** is an allied health professional trained to plan nutrition programs for sick as well as healthy people; this may involve planning meals for a hospital or large organization or individualized diet counseling with patients.

Anatomy and Physiology

The structures of the digestive system are divided into two sections: the **upper gastrointestinal tract** consists of the oral cavity, pharynx, esophagus, and stomach; the **lower gastrointestinal tract** consists of the large and small intestines. The related organs of the digestive system include the salivary glands, liver, gallbladder, and pancreas.

Oral Cavity

The **oral** cavity is the first part of the digestive tract. It is designed to receive food for ingestion. See **Figure 12-1.**

The oral cavity consists of the (1) **lips,** which surround the opening to the mouth, and the (2) **cheeks,** which form the walls of the oral cavity, are continuous with the lips, and are lined with mucous membrane. The lips and cheeks help hold the food in the mouth and keep it in place for chewing. The oral cavity is also known as the **buccal cavity.** The (3) **hard palate**, which forms the anterior, upper roof of the mouth is supported by

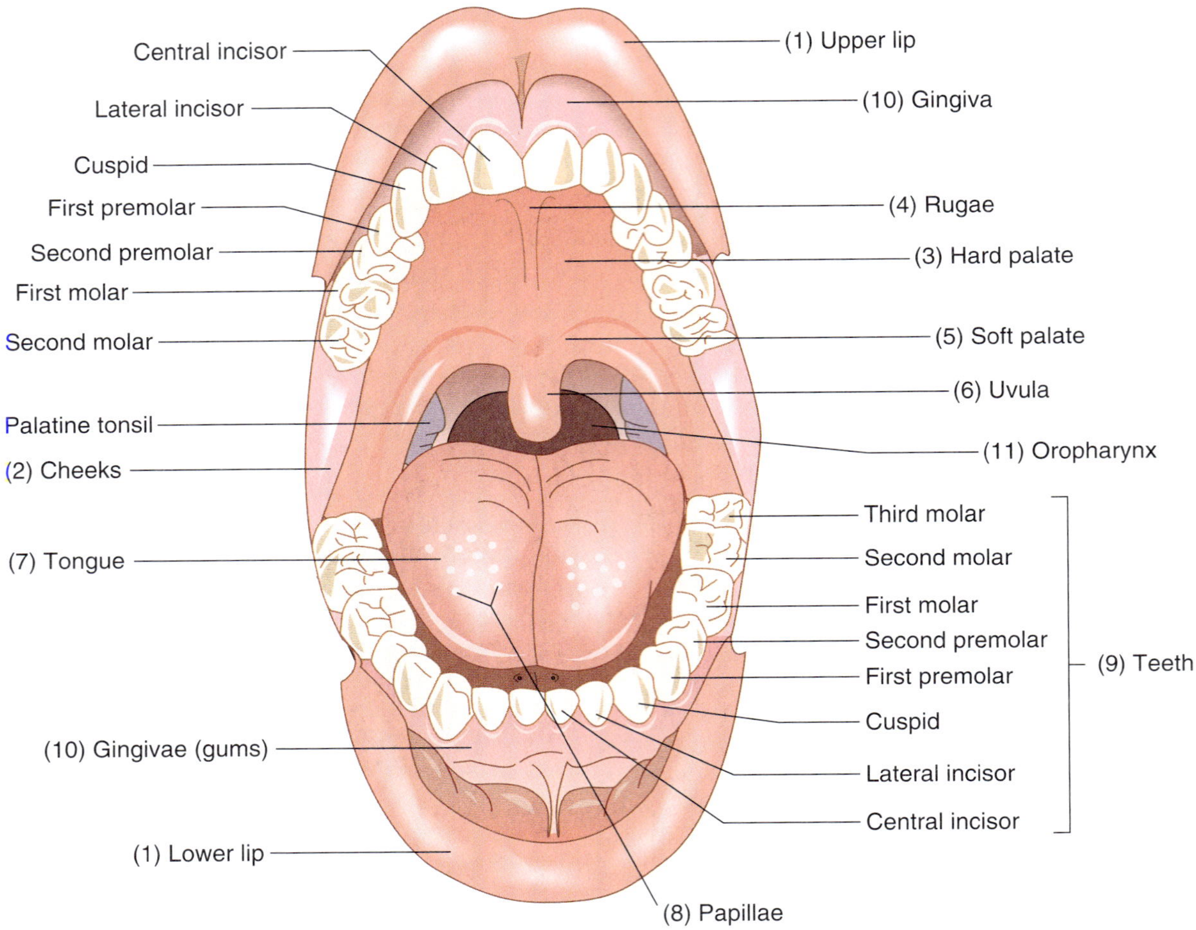

Figure 12-1 The oral cavity

bone. It has irregular ridges or folds in its mucous membrane lining. These ridges are called **(4) rugae**. Rugae are also found in the stomach. The **(5) soft palate,** which forms the posterior portion of the upper roof of the mouth (closer to the throat), is composed of skeletal muscle and connective tissue. The soft palate ends in a small cone-shaped projection called the **(6) uvula**. In addition to aiding in the digestive process, the uvula also helps in producing sounds and speech. The **(7) tongue** is a solid mass of very strong, flexible, skeletal muscle covered with mucous membrane. It is located in the floor of the mouth within the curve of the lower jaw bone (mandible). The tongue is the principal organ of the sense of taste and also assists in the process of chewing (**mastication**) and swallowing (**deglutition**). The upper surface of the tongue is normally moist, pink, and covered with small, rough elevations known as **(8) papillae**. The papillae contain the taste buds that detect sweet, sour, salty, and bitter tastes of food or beverages. During the process of chewing the food, the tongue aids the digestive process by moving the food around to mix it with saliva, shaping it into a ball-like mass called a **bolus,** and moving it toward the throat (**pharynx**) to be swallowed.

Salivary Glands

The three pairs of salivary glands known as the **parotids**, the **submandibulars**, and the **sublinguals** secrete most of the **saliva** produced each day. Saliva is mostly water, but also contains mucus and digestive enzymes that aid in the digestive process. The water in the saliva helps to liquefy the food as it is chewed. The mucus helps to lubricate the food as it passes through the gastrointestinal tract. The digestive **enzymes** help to break the food down into nutrients. Two enzymes contained in saliva are **amylase**, an enzyme that aids in the digestion of carbohydrates, and **lipase**, an enzyme that aids in the digestion of fats. The **salivary glands** are part of the accessory structures of the digestive system. They secrete saliva into the digestive tract by way of ducts.

The process of chewing is primarily the responsibility of the **(9) teeth.** When food enters the mouth, it is ground up by the teeth and softened by saliva. The process of chewing the food is known as mastication. The **(10) gums** surround the necks of the teeth. This fleshy tissue covers the upper and lower jaw bones and is lined with the same mucous membrane covering the interior of the oral cavity. The gums are also known as the **gingivae** (singular: **gingiva**). (A separate discussion of the teeth follows the section on Accessory Organs of Digestion).

Pharynx

The pharynx, also known as the throat, adjoins the oral cavity and is a passageway that serves both the respiratory and the digestive systems. The section of the pharynx leading away from the oral cavity is known as the **(11) oropharynx**. The portion of the pharynx behind the nasal cavity is known as the nasopharynx and the lower portion of the pharynx, which opens into both the esophagus and the larynx, is known as the laryngopharynx. Near the base of the tongue, leading from the mouth into the pharynx (oropharyngeal area) are the tonsils. These masses of lymphatic tissue are located in the depressions of the mucous membrane of the oropharyngeal area.

During the act of swallowing, the soft palate and the uvula move upward to facilitate the movement of the food into the pharynx and to close off the nasal cavity. The tongue forces the food into the pharynx, and the epiglottis drops downward to cover the opening of the larynx, directing the food mass into the esophagus. The bolus of food is propelled through the pharynx into the esophagus by means of peristaltic movements.

Esophagus

The **esophagus** receives the food from the pharynx and propels it on to the stomach. This collapsible muscular tube, which is approximately 10 inches long, passes through an opening in the diaphragm into the abdominal cavity before connecting to the stomach. The passage of the food from the esophagus into the stomach is controlled by a muscular ring known as the **cardiac sphincter**. When the cardiac sphincter relaxes, it opens to allow food to enter the stomach. When the cardiac sphincter contracts and closes, the stomach contents are prevented from reentering the esophagus.

Stomach

The **stomach** is located in the upper left quadrant of the abdomen. It has three major divisions. See **Figure 12-2** for a visual reference of the structures and divisions of the stomach.

The upper rounded portion of the stomach is the **(1) fundus.** It rises to the left and above the level of the opening of the esophagus into the stomach. The **(2) body** is the central part of the stomach and curves to the right. The **(3) pylorus** is the lower tubular part of the stomach that angles to the right from the body of the stomach as it approaches the duodenum (the first part of the small intestines). This area is also referred to as the **gastric** antrum. The **(4) pyloric sphincter** regulates the passage of food from the stomach into the duodenum. The folds in the mucous membrane lining of the stomach are

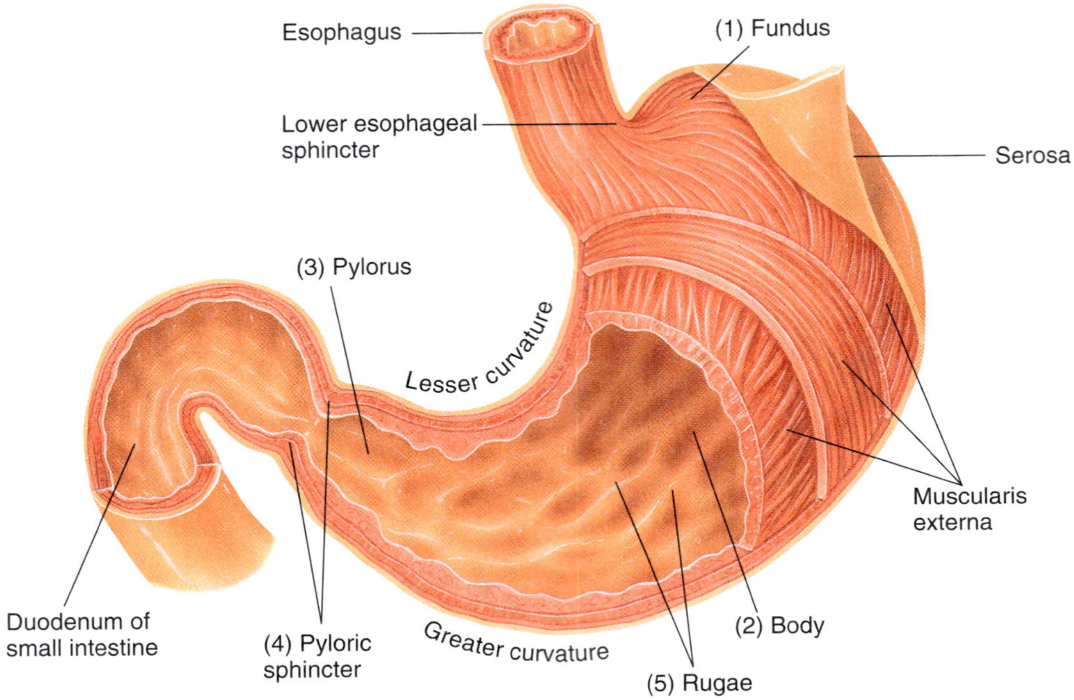

Figure 12-2 The stomach

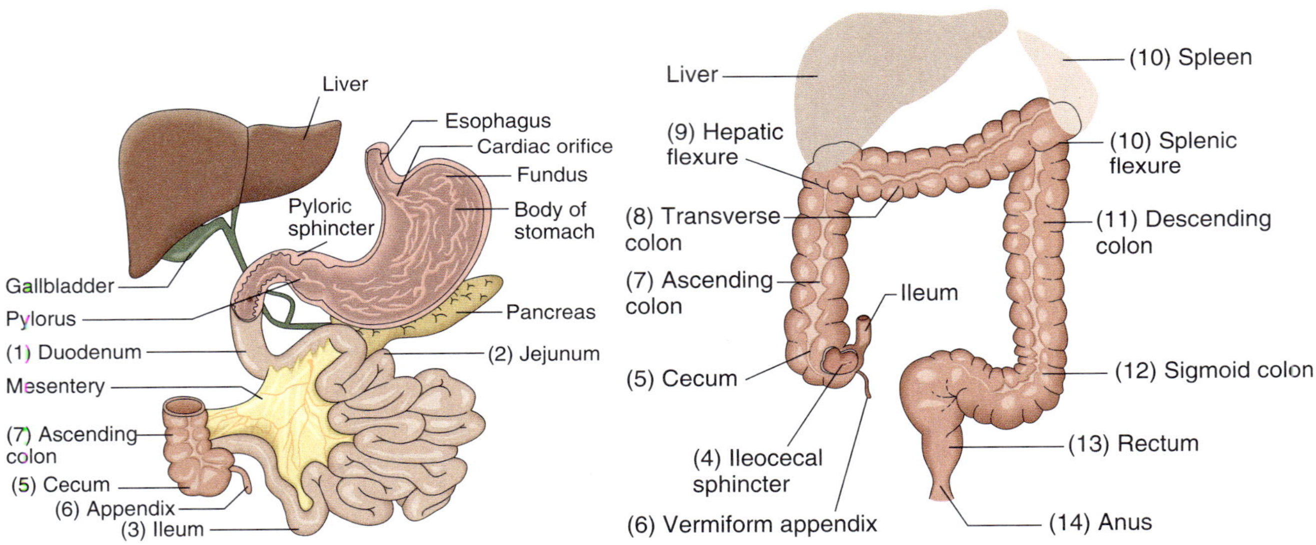

Figure 12-3 The small and large intestines

known as **(5)** rugae. These folds allow the stomach to expand to accommodate its contents. The depressions between the rugae contain the gastric glands that secrete gastric juices containing digestive enzymes and hydrochloric acid. The gastric juices further the digestive process through the chemical breakdown of food, and the muscular action of the stomach causes churning, which mixes the food with the secretions. At this point in the digestive process, the liquidlike mixture of partially digested food and digestive secretions in the stomach is called **chyme**. It is released in small amounts through the pyloric sphincter into the small intestine.

As we continue our discussion of the digestive process, **Figure 12-3** will provide a visual reference for the structures and divisions of the small and large intestines.

Small Intestine

The small intestine is approximately 20 feet long, coiling and looping as it fills most of the abdominal cavity. It is divided into three parts: the duodenum, the jejunum, and the ileum. The **(1) duodenum** is the first part of the small intestine, extending in a C-shaped curve from the pylorus of the stomach to the jejunum and is approximately 12 inches long. The duodenum receives the chyme from the pylorus of the stomach, along with secretions from the liver and the pancreas that further the digestive process. The second portion of the small intestine is the **(2) jejunum**, which connects the duodenum to the ileum. The jejunum is approximately 8 feet long. The third portion of the small intestine is the **(3) ileum**, which is approximately 12 feet long. The ileum is continuous with the jejunum and connects it to the large intestine at the ileocecal sphincter.

The small intestine, also known as the small **bowel**, completes the digestive process through absorption of the nutrients into the bloodstream and passage of the residue (waste products) on to the large intestine for excretion from the body. The mucous membrane lining the small intestine contains millions of tiny, fingerlike projections known as **villi**. The villi surround blood capillaries, which function in the absorption of nutrients.

Large Intestine

The large intestine begins at the **ileocecal** junction and extends to the anus. The ileocecal junction contains a muscular ring called the **(4) ileocecal sphincter,** which prevents the backflow of wastes from the large intestine into the small intestine. The large intestine is divided into the cecum, the colon, and the rectum. The **(5) cecum** is a blind pouch, on the right side of the abdomen, that extends approximately 2 to 3 inches beyond the ileocecal junction to the beginning of the colon. At the lower portion of the cecum hangs a small, wormlike structure known as the **(6) vermiform appendix.** It is approximately 3 to 6 inches in length and is less than 0.5 inch in diameter. The function of the appendix is uncertain, but it appears to serve no specific purpose in the digestive process. The longest portion of the large intestine is the **colon**; it is divided into four sections: the ascending, transverse, descending, and sigmoid colon. The **(7) ascending colon** begins at the ileocecal junction, curving upward toward the liver on the right side of the abdomen. When it reaches the undersurface of the liver it makes a horizontal turn to the left, becoming the **(8) transverse colon.** The point at which the ascending colon turns to the left (just below the liver) is known as the **(9) hepatic flexure.** The transverse colon advances horizontally across the abdomen, below the stomach toward the spleen. When it reaches the area below the spleen, the transverse colon takes a downward turn at a point known as the **(10) splenic flexure.** It then becomes the **(11) descending colon,** passing down toward the pelvis on the left side of the abdomen. At the pelvic brim (the curved top of the hip bones), the descending colon makes an S-shaped curve. This curved portion of the colon is known as the **(12) sigmoid colon**, which connects the descending colon to the rectum. The **(13) rectum**, which is the last 7 to 8 inches of the large intestine, connects the sigmoid colon to the **(14) anus**. The anus is the opening through which **feces** (the solid waste products of digestion) are eliminated from the body. The act of expelling feces from the body is called **defecation**. The anal **sphincter** controls the elimination of waste materials from the rectum.

Accessory Organs of Digestion

The accessory organs of digestion are the salivary glands, liver, gallbladder, and pancreas. The salivary glands have been discussed with the oral cavity. **Figure 12-4** provides a visual reference of the liver, gallbladder, and pancreas.

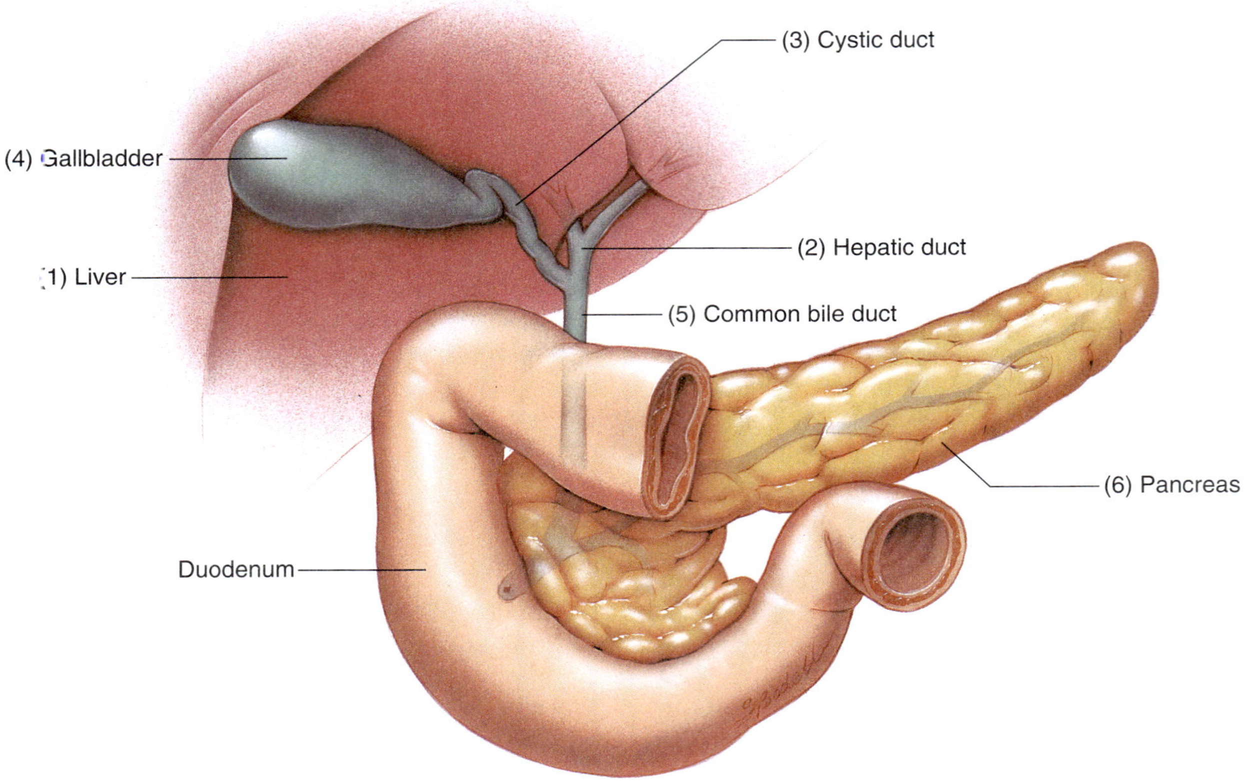

Figure 12-4 The liver, gallbladder, and pancreas

The (1) **liver** is located immediately under the diaphragm, slightly to the right. It is the largest gland in the body and weighs approximately 3 to 4 pounds. The only digestive function of the liver is the production of bile for the emulsification of fats in the small intestine. The liver cells, known as **hepatocytes**, produce a yellowish-green secretion called **bile**. The main components of bile are bile salts, bile pigments, and cholesterol. Bile **emulsifies** (breaks apart) fats, preparing them for further digestion and absorption in the small intestine. Additional functions of the liver are as follows:

- Excretion of bile pigments into bile. The liver recycles the iron and converts the remaining portion into bile pigments, which are excreted with the bile as it is released from the liver. The bile travels down the (2) **hepatic duct** to the (3) **cystic duct** that leads to the gallbladder where the bile is stored. The primary bile pigment is bilirubin, which gives it the yellowish-green color. Bile pigments containing bilirubin are responsible for the color of urine and feces.
- Synthesis of vitamin K–dependent plasma proteins. Albumin, globulin carrier molecules, and the clotting factors.
- **Amino acid** metabolism.
- Carbohydrate metabolism. Mainly glycogenesis and glycogenolysis. The liver converts the excess amounts of circulating blood **glucose** (simple sugar) into a complex form of sugar (starch) for storage in the liver cells, a process known as **glycogenesis**. This complex form of sugar, known as **glycogen**, is preserved in the liver cells for use

when the blood sugar is extremely low. In response to dangerously low blood sugar levels, the liver breaks down the stored glycogen into glucose, releasing it into the circulating blood, a process known as **glycogenolysis**.

- Fat metabolism. Synthesis of cholesterol, lipoproteins for transport of fat to other tissues are synthesized, fatty acids are converted to ketones to be used for energy production.
- Phagocytosis. Phagocytosis of old, worn-out red blood cells (erythrocytes). When the erythrocytes are destroyed in the spleen they are broken down into heme, which contains iron and globin, a blood protein.
- Detoxification. The enzymes produced by the liver convert potentially harmful substances such as ammonia, alcohol, and medications, into less toxic ones.
- Storage of vital nutrients. The liver is responsible for the storage of the vitamins, iron, and copper; fat-soluble vitamins A, D, E, and K; and vitamin B_{12}.

The **(4)** **gallbladder** is a pear-shaped sac, located on the undersurface of the liver. Approximately 3 to 4 inches long, the gallbladder is connected to the liver via the cystic duct. The cystic duct joins the hepatic duct to form the **(5) common bile duct,** which leads to the duodenum. The main function of the gallbladder is to store and concentrate the bile produced by the liver. When food (chyme) enters the duodenum and the presence of fatty contents is detected, the gallbladder is stimulated to release bile. The bile travels from the cystic duct, to the common bile duct, to the duodenum where it serves its purpose as an emulsifier of fats.

The **(6)** **pancreas** is an elongated organ of approximately 6 to 9 inches. It is located in the upper left quadrant of the abdomen, behind the stomach; it extends horizontally across the body, beginning at the first part of the small intestines (duodenum) and ending at the edge of the spleen. The pancreas functions as both an exocrine and an endocrine gland. As an **exocrine** **gland,** the pancreas manufactures the digestive juices containing (1) trypsin, which breaks down proteins, (2) pancreatic lipase, which breaks down fats, (3) pancreatic amylase, which breaks down carbohydrates, and (4) sodium bicarbonate, which neutralizes acidic stomach contents. These digestive juices are secreted into a network of tiny ducts located throughout the gland; the ducts merge into the main **pancreatic duct,** which extends throughout the length of the pancreas. The pancreatic duct joins the common bile duct just before it enters the duodenum. As an **endocrine** **gland,** the pancreas manufactures insulin, which passes directly into the blood capillaries instead of being transported by way of ducts. The specialized group of cells known as the islets of Langerhans are scattered throughout the pancreas. The beta cells of the pancreas secrete **insulin**, a hormone that makes it possible for glucose to pass from the blood through the cell membranes to be used for energy. Insulin also promotes the conversion of excess glucose into glycogen. The alpha cells of the pancreas secrete **glucagon**, a hormone that stimulates the liver to convert glycogen into glucose in time of need.

Teeth

As mentioned, the process of chewing is the primary responsibility of the teeth. **Figures 12-5 A** and **B** provide a visual reference for the teeth.

Each individual has two sets of teeth that develop in the mouth during his or her lifetime. The first set of teeth, or "baby teeth," are called the **primary** or **deciduous** **teeth.** This set

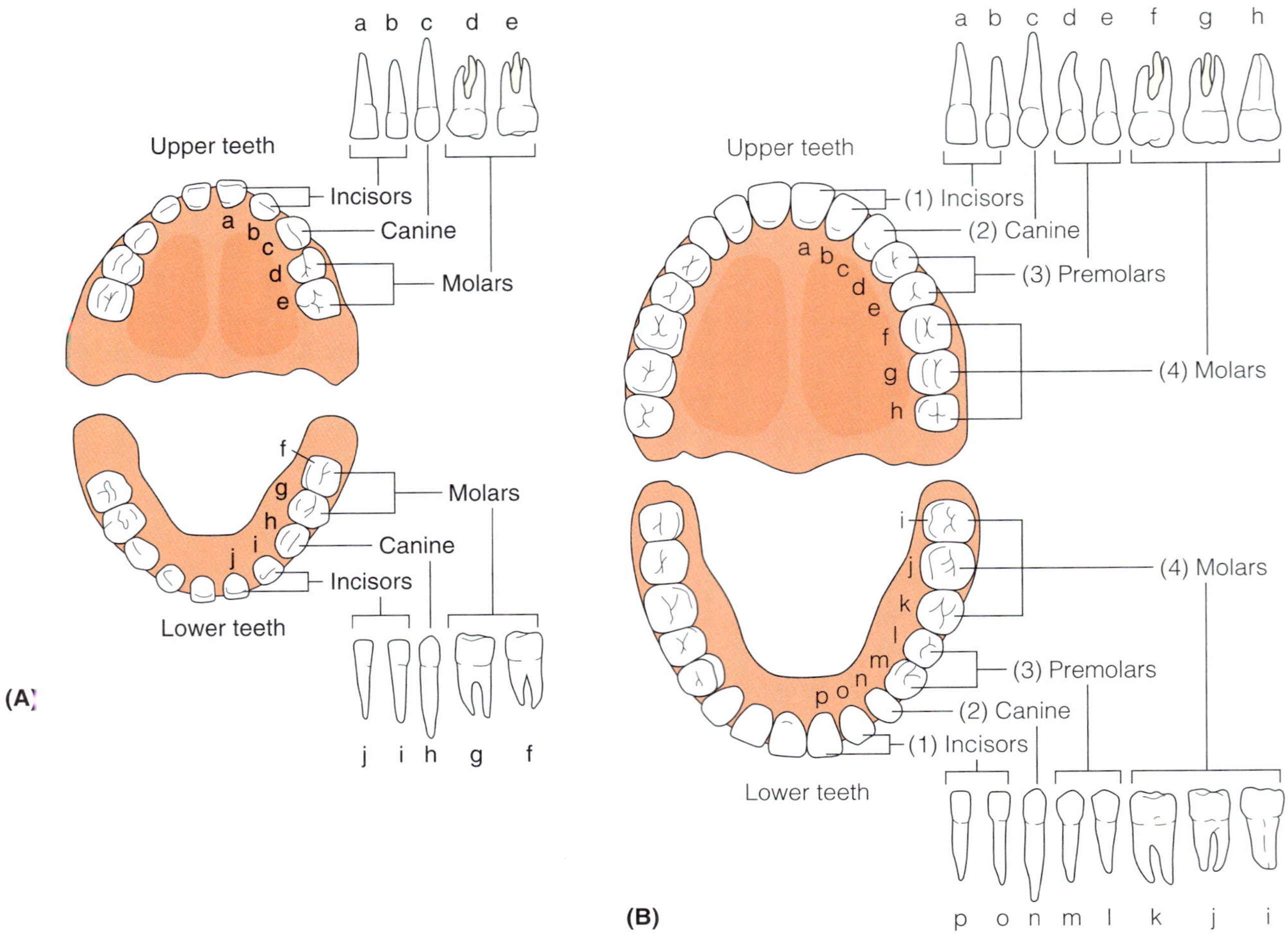

Figure 12-5 (A) Primary teeth; (B) permanent teeth

of 20 teeth (10 in each jaw bone) begins to appear at approximately 6 months of age. The **secondary** or **permanent teeth** begin to appear around the age of 6, replacing the deciduous teeth. The set of permanent teeth consists of 32 teeth (16 in each jaw bone), with the last of the teeth, the third molars (wisdom teeth), usually erupting sometime after the age of 17.

The various teeth are shaped in different ways to aid in the digestion of food. The **(1) incisors** have a chisel shape with sharp edges for biting food. The single point (cusp) of the **(2) canine** or **cuspid** teeth make them useful for grasping and tearing food. The **(3) bicuspids** (**premolars**) and the **(4) molars** have flat surfaces with multiple projections (cusps) for crushing and grinding the food.

The typical tooth has three main parts. See **Figure 12-6.** The visible part of the tooth is known as the **(5) crown;** it is covered with **(6) enamel**, which is the hardest substance in the body. The **(7) neck** of the tooth lies just beneath the gum line and the **(8) root** of the tooth is embedded in the bony socket of the jaw bone. The central core of the tooth is the pulp cavity, or **(9) root canal.** It contains connective tissue, blood and lymphatic vessels, and sensory nerve endings. The pulp cavity is surrounded by **(10) dentin**, which forms the bulk of the tooth shell. The dentin in the neck and root area of the tooth is surrounded by a thin layer of hardened connective tissue known as **(11) cementum.** The dentin in the crown of the tooth is covered by enamel.

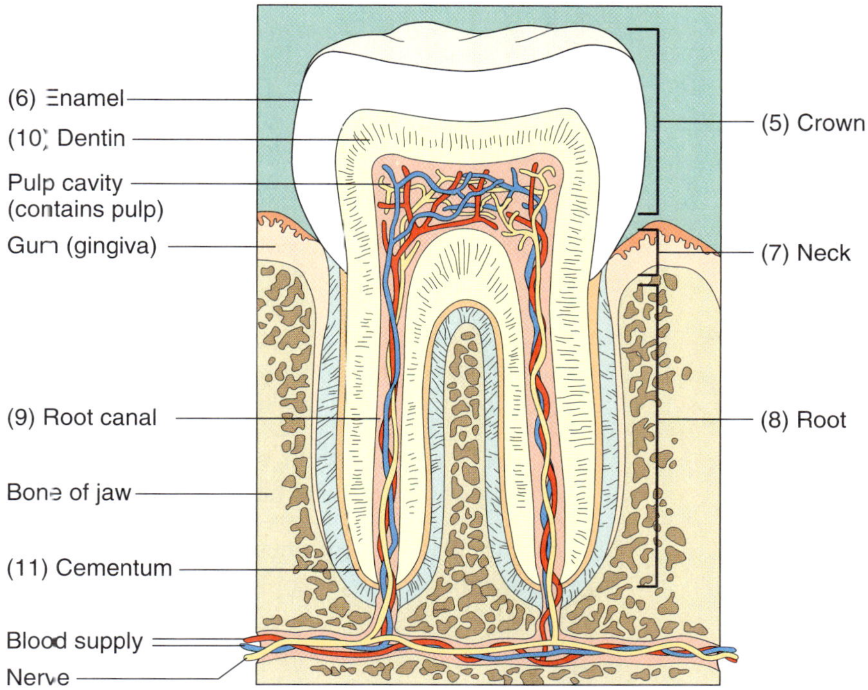

Figure 12-6 Layers of a tooth

Vocabulary

The following vocabulary words are frequently used when discussing the digestive system.

WORD	DEFINITION
absorption (ab-**SORP**-shun)	The passage of substances across and into tissues, such as the passage of digested food molecules into intestinal cells or the passage of liquids into kidney tubules.
alimentary canal (**al**-ih-**MEN**-tar-ee can-**NAL**)	A musculomembranous tube, about 30 feet long, extending from the mouth to the anus and lined with mucous membrane. Also called the digestive tract or the gastrointestinal tract.
amino acids (ah-**MEE**-noh acids)	An organic chemical compound composed of one or more basic amino groups and one or more acidic carboxyl groups.
amylase (**AM**-ih-lays) amyl/o = starch -ase = enzyme	An enzyme that breaks down starch into smaller carbohydrate molecules.
anus (**AY**-nus) an/o = anus -us = noun ending	The opening through which the solid wastes (feces) are eliminated from the body.
ascitic fluid (ah-**SIT**-ik fluid)	A watery fluid containing albumin, glucose, and electrolytes that accumulates in the peritoneal cavity in association with certain disease conditions, such as liver disease.

bicuspid tooth (bye-**CUSS**-pid)	One of the two teeth between the molars and canines of the upper and lower jaw, the bicuspid teeth have a flat surface with multiple projections (cusps) for crushing and grinding food; also known as premolar tooth.
bile (**BYE**-al)	A bitter, yellow-green secretion of the liver.
bilirubin (bill-ih-**ROO**-bin)	The orange-yellow pigment of bile, formed principally by the breakdown of hemoglobin in red blood cells after termination of their normal life span.
bowel (**BOW**-el)	The portion of the alimentary canal extending from the pyloric opening of the stomach to the anus.
canine tooth (**KAY**-nine)	Any one of the four teeth, two in each jaw, situated immediately lateral to the incisor teeth in the human dental arches; also called cuspid tooth.
cardiac sphincter (**CAR**-dee-ak **SFINGK**-ter) cardi/o = heart -ac = pertaining to	The muscular ring (sphincter) in the stomach that controls the passage of food from the esophagus into the stomach.
cecum (**SEE**-kum)	A cul-de-sac containing the first part of the large intestine. It joins the ileum, the last segment of the small intestine.
cholelithiasis (**koh**-lee-lih-**THIGH**-ah-sis) chol/e = bile lith/o = stone; calculus -iasis = presence of an abnormal condition	Abnormal presence of gallstones in the gallbladder.
chyme (**KIGHM**)	The liquidlike material of partially digested food and digestive secretions found in the stomach just before it is released into the duodenum.
colon (**COH**-lon)	The portion of the large intestine extending from the cecum to the rectum.
common bile duct	The duct formed by the joining of the cystic duct and hepatic duct.
crown	The part of the tooth that is visible above the gum line.
cuspid tooth (**CUSS**-pid)	See *canine tooth.*
deciduous teeth (dee-**SID**-you-us)	The first set or primary teeth; baby teeth.
defecation (deff-eh-**KAY**-shun)	The act of expelling feces from the rectum through the anus.
deglutition (**dee**-gloo-**TISH**-un)	Swallowing.
dentin (**DEN**-tin)	The chief material of teeth surrounding the pulp and situated inside of the enamel and cementum.
dietitian (**dye**-ah-**TIH**-shun)	An allied health professional trained to plan nutrition programs for sick as well as healthy people; this may involve planning meals for a hospital or large organization or individualized diet counseling with patients.

digestion (dye-**JEST**-shun)	The process of altering the chemical and physical composition of food so that it can be used by the body cells; this occurs in the digestive tract.
digestive tract (dye-**JESS**-tiv)	See *alimentary canal.*
duodenum (doo-oh-**DEE**-num *or* do-**OD**-eh-num) **duoden/o** = duodenum **-um** = noun ending	The first portion of the small intestine; the duodenum is the shortest, widest, and most fixed portion of the small intestine, taking an almost circular course from the pyloric valve of the stomach so that its termination is close to its starting point.
emulsify (eh-**MULL**-sih-figh)	To disperse a liquid into another liquid, making a colloidal suspension.
enamel (en-**AM**-el)	A hard, white substance that covers the dentin of the crown of a tooth; enamel is the hardest substance in the body.
endocrine gland (**EN**-doh-krin)	A gland that secretes its enzymes directly into the blood capillaries instead of being transported by way of ducts.
enzyme (**EN**-zighm)	A protein produced by living cells that catalyzes chemical reactions in organic matter.
esophagus (eh-**SOF**-ah-gus) **esophag/o** = esophagus **-us** = noun ending	A muscular canal, about 24 cm long, extending from the pharynx to the stomach.
exocrine gland (**EKS**-oh-krin)	A gland that secretes its enzymes into a network of tiny ducts that transport it to the surface of an organ or tissue or into a vessel.
fatty acids	Any of several organic acids produced by the hydrolysis of neutral fats.
feces (**FEE**-seez)	Waste or excrement from the digestive tract that is formed in the intestine and expelled through the rectum.
gallbladder (**GALL**-blad-er)	A pear-shaped excretory sac lodged in a fossa on the visceral surface of the right lobe of the liver.
gastroenterologist (**gas**-troh-**en**-ter-**ALL**-oh-jist) **gastr/o** = stomach **enter/o** = small intestine **-logist** = one who specializes in the study of	A medical doctor who specializes in the study of the diseases and disorders affecting the gastrointestinal tract including the stomach, intestines, gallbladder, and bile duct.
gastrointestinal tract (**gas**-troh-in-**TESS**-tih-nal)	See *alimentary canal.*
gavage (gah-**VAZH**)	A procedure in which liquid or semiliquid food is introduced into the stomach through a tube.
gingivae (jin-**JYE**-vah *or* **JIN**-jih-vah) **gingiv/o** = gums **ae** = noun ending	Gums.

glucagon (**GLOO**-kah-gon)	A hormone produced by the alpha cells of the pancreas that stimulates the liver to convert glycogen into glucose when the blood sugar level is dangerously low.
glucose (**GLOO**-kohs) gluc/o = sugar, sweet -ose = carbohydrate	A simple sugar found in certain foods, especially fruits, and major source of energy occurring in human and animal body fluids.
glycogen (**GLIGH**-koh-jen) glyc/o = sugar, sweet -gen = that which generates	A complex sugar (starch) that is the major carbohydrate stored in animal cells. It is formed from glucose and stored chiefly in the liver and, to a lesser extent, in muscle cells.
glycogenesis (**gligh**-koh-**JEN**-eh-sis) glyc/o = sugar, sweet -genesis = the production of; formation of	The conversion of simple sugar (glucose) into a complex form of sugar (starch) for storage in the liver.
glycogenolysis (**gligh**-koh-jen-**ALL**-ih-sis) glyc/o = sugar, sweet gen/o = to produce -lysis = destruction or detachment	The breakdown of glycogen into glucose by the liver, releasing it back into the circulating blood in response to a very low blood sugar level.
hepatocyte (**HEP**-ah-toh-sight) hepat/o = liver cyt/o = cell -e = noun ending	Liver cell.
hydrochloric acid (**high**-droh-**KLOH**-rik acid)	A compound consisting of hydrogen and chlorine.
ileum (**ILL**-ee-um) ile/o = ileum -um = noun ending	The distal portion of the small intestine extending from the jejunum to the cecum.
incisor (in-**SIGH**-zor)	One of the eight front teeth, four in each dental arch, that first appear as primary teeth during infancy are replaced by permanent incisors during childhood, and last until old age.
insulin (**IN**-soo-lin)	A naturally occurring hormone secreted by the beta cells of the islets of Langerhans in the pancreas in response to increased levels of glucose in the blood.
jejunum (jee-**JOO**-num) jejun/o = jejunum -um = noun ending	The intermediate or middle of the three portions of the small intestine, connecting proximally with the duodenum and distally with the ileum.
lavage (lah-**VAZH**)	The process of irrigating, or washing out an organ, usually the bladder, bowel, paranasal sinuses, or stomach for therapeutic purposes.

lipase (**LIH**-pays *or* **LIGH**-pays) lip/o = fat -ase = enzyme	An enzyme that aids in the digestion of fats.
liver	The largest gland of the body and one of its most complex organs.
lower GI tract	The lower portion of the gastrointestinal tract consisting of the small and large intestines.
mastication (mass-tih-**KAY**-shun)	Chewing, tearing, or grinding food with the teeth while it becomes mixed with saliva.
molar tooth (**MOH**-lar)	Any of 12 molar teeth, 6 in each dental arch, located posterior to the premolar teeth; the molar teeth have a flat surface with multiple projections (cusps) for crushing and grinding food.
nutritionist (noo-**TRIH**-shun-ist)	An allied health professional who studies and applies the principles and science of nutrition.
oropharynx (or-oh-**FAIR**-inks) or/o = mouth	The section of the pharynx leading away from the oral cavity.
palate (**PAL**-at)	A structure that forms the roof of the mouth.
pancreas (**PAN**-kree-ass)	An elongated organ approximately 6 to 9 inches long, located in the upper left quadrant of the abdomen that secretes various substances such as digestive enzymes, insulin, and glucagon.
papillae (pah-**PILL**-ay)	A small, nipple-shaped projection, such as the conoid papillae of the tongue and the papillae of the corium, that extend from collagen fibers, the capillary blood vessels, and sometimes the nerves of the dermis.
parotid gland (pah-**ROT**-id gland)	One of the largest pairs of salivary glands that lie at the side of the face just below and in front of the external ear.
peristalsis (pair-ih-**STALL**-sis)	The coordinated, rhythmic, serial contraction of smooth muscle that forces food through the digestive tract, bile through the bile duct, and urine through the ureters.
permanent teeth	The full set of teeth (32 teeth) that replace the deciduous or temporary teeth.
pharynx (**FAIR**-inks) pharyng/o = pharynx	The throat; a tubular structure about 13 cm long that extends from the base of the skull to the esophagus and is situated just in front of the cervical vertebrae.
premolar tooth	See *bicuspid tooth.*
pulp	Any soft, spongy tissue, such as that contained within the spleen, the pulp chamber of the tooth, or the distal phalanges of the fingers and the toes.
pyloric sphincter (pigh-**LOR**-ik **SFINGK**-ter)	A thickened muscular ring in the stomach that regulates the passage of food from the pylorus of the stomach into the duodenum.

rectum (**REK**-tum) **rect/o** = rectum **-um** = noun ending	The portion of the large intestine, about 12 cm long, continuous with the descending sigmoid colon, just proximal to the anal canal.
rugae (**ROO**-gay)	A ridge or fold, such as the rugae of the stomach that presents large folds in the mucous membrane of that organ.
saliva (sah-**LYE**-vah)	The clear, viscous fluid secreted by the salivary and mucous glands in the mouth.
salivary glands (**SAL**-ih-vair-ee glands)	One of the three pairs of glands secreting into the mouth, thus aiding the digestive process.
secondary teeth	See *permanent teeth.*
sigmoid colon (**SIG**-moyd colon)	The portion of the colon that extends from the end of the descending colon in the pelvis to the juncture of the rectum.
sphincter (**SFINGK**-ter)	A circular band of muscle fibers that constricts a passage or closes a natural opening in the body, such as the hepatic sphincter in the muscular coat of the hepatic veins near their union with the superior vena cava, and external anal sphincter, which closes the anus.
stomach (**STUM**-ak)	The major organ of digestion located in the left upper quadrant of the abdomen and divided into a body and pylorus.
triglycerides (try-**GLISS**-er-eyeds)	A compound consisting of a fatty acid (oleic, palmitic, or stearic) and glycerol.
upper GI tract	The upper part of the gastrointestinal tract consisting of the mouth, pharynx, esophagus, and stomach.
uvula (**YOO**-vyoo-lah)	The small, cone-shaped process suspended in the mouth from the middle of the posterior border of the soft palate.
villi (**VIL**-eye)	One of the many tiny projections barely visible to the naked eye clustered over the entire mucous surface of the small intestine.

Word Elements

The following word elements pertain to the digestive system. As you review the list, pronounce each word element aloud twice and check the box after you "say it." Write the definition for the example word given for each word element. You may use your medical dictionary.

WORD ELEMENT	PRONUNCIATION	"SAY IT"	MEANING
amyl/o **amyl**ase	**AM**-ih-loh **AM**-ih-lays	☐	starch
append/o **append**ectomy	ah-**PEN**-doe ap-en-**DEK**-toh-mee	☐	appendix

appendic/o **appendic**itis	ah-**PEN**-dih-koh ap-**pen**-dih-**SIGH**-tis	☐	appendix
-ase lip**ase**	**AYS** **LYE**-pays	☐	enzyme
bil/i **bil**iary	**BILL**-ee **BILL**-ee-air-ee	☐	bile
bucc/o **bucc**al	**BUCK**-oh **BUCK**-al	☐	cheek
cec/o **cec**ostomy	**SEE**-koh see-**KOSS**-toh-mee	☐	cecum
celi/o **celi**ac rickets	**SEE**-lee-oh **SEE**-lee-ak **RICK**-ets	☐	pertaining to the abdomen
-centesis abdomino**centesis**	sen-**TEE**-sis ab-**dom**-ih-noh-sen-**TEE**-sis	☐	surgical puncture
cheil/o **cheil**osis	**KIGH**-loh kigh-**LOH**-sis	☐	lips
chol/e **chole**cystogram	**KOH**-lee **koh**-lee-**SIS**-toh-gram	☐	bile
cholecyst/o **cholecyst**itis	koh-lee-**SIS**-toh **koh**-lee-sis-**TYE**-tis	☐	gallbladder
cirrh/o **cirrh**osis	sih-**ROH** sih-**ROH**-sis	☐	yellow, tawny
col/o **col**orectal	**KOH**-loh **koh**-loh-**REK**-tal	☐	colon
colon/o **colon**oscopy	koh-**LON**-oh **koh**-lon-**OSS**-koh-pee	☐	colon
dent/o **dent**al hygienist	**DEN**-toh **DEN**-tahl high-**JEE**-nist	☐	tooth
duoden/o **duoden**ostomy	doo-**ODD**-en-oh **doo**-odd-eh-**NOSS**-toh-mee	☐	duodenum (first part of the small intestine)
-ectasia gastr**ectasia**	ek-**TAY**-zhe-ah gas-trek-**TAY**-zhe-ah	☐	stretching or dilatation
-emesis hyper**emesis**	**EM**-eh-sis **high**-per-**EM**-eh-sis	☐	to vomit

enter/o **enter**itis	**EN**-ter-oh en-ter-**EYE**-tis	☐	intestine
esophag/o **esophag**itis	eh-**SOFF**-ah-go eh-soff-ah-**JIGH**-tis	☐	esophagus
gastr/o **gastr**ostomy	**GAS**-troh gas-**TROSS**-toh-mee	☐	stomach
gingiv/o **gingiv**itis	**JIN**-jih-voh jin-jih-**VIGH**-tis	☐	gums
gloss/o **gloss**itis	**GLOSS**-oh gloss-**SIGH**-tis	☐	tongue
gluc/o **gluc**ogenesis	**GLOO**-koh gloo-koh-**JEN**-eh-sis	☐	sugar, sweet
glyc/o **glyc**olysis	**GLIGH**-koh gligh-**KALL**-ih-sis	☐	sugar, sweet
hepat/o **hepat**omegaly	hep-**AH**-toh **hep**-ah-toh-**MEG**-ah-lee	☐	liver
-iasis cholelith**iasis**	**EYE**-ah-sis koh-lee-lih-**THIGH**-ah-sis	☐	presence of an abnormal condition
ile/o **ile**ocecal	**ILL**-ee-oh **ILL**-ee-oh-**SEE**-kahl	☐	ileum
jejun/o **jejun**ostomy	jee-**JOO**-noh jee-joo-**NOSS**-toh-mee	☐	jejunum
lapar/o **lapar**oscopy	**LAP**-ah-roh lap-ar-**OSS**-koh-pee	☐	abdominal wall
lingu/o **lingu**al	**LING**-oo-oh **LING**-gwall	☐	tongue
lip/o **lip**oma	**LIH**-poh lih-**POH**-mah	☐	fat
lith/o **lith**ogenesis	**LITH**-oh **lith**-oh-**JEN**-eh-sis	☐	stone; calculus
-lysis lipo**lysis**	**LIH**-sis lip-**ALL**-ih-sis	☐	destruction or detachment
mandibul/o **mandibul**ar	man-**DIB**-yoo-loh man-**DIB**-yoo-lar	☐	mandible (lower jaw bone)
odont/o ortho**dont**ist	oh-**DON**-toh or-thoh-**DON**-tist	☐	teeth

or/o **or**al	**OR**-oh **OR**-al	☐	mouth
pancreat/o **pancreat**itis	pan-kree-**AH**-toh pan-kree-ah-**TYE**-tis	☐	pancreas
-pepsia dys**pepsia**	**PEP**-see-ah diss-**PEP**-see-ah	☐	state of digestion
-phagia poly**phagia**	**FAY**-jee-ah pall-ee-**FAY**-jee-ah	☐	to eat
pharyng/o **pharyng**oscope	fair-**IN**-goh fair-**IN**-goh-skohp	☐	pharynx
peritone/o **peritone**al	**pair**-ih-toh-**NEE**-oh **pair**-ih-toh-**NEE**-al	☐	peritoneum
-plasty stomato**plasty**	**PLASS**-tee **STOH**-mah-toh-**PLASS**-tee	☐	surgical repair
proct/o **proct**oscopy	**PROK**-toh prok-**TOSS**-koh-pee	☐	anus or rectum
rect/o **rect**ocele	**REK**-toh **REK**-toh-seel	☐	rectum
-rrhagia gastro**rrhagia**	**RAY**-jee-ah **gas**-troh-**RAY**-jee-ah	☐	excessive flow or discharge
-rrhaphy hepato**rrhaphy**	**RAH**-fee hep-ah-**TOR**-ah-fee	☐	suturing
sial/o **sial**ogram	sigh-**AL**-oh sigh-**AL**-oh-gram	☐	salivary gland; saliva
sigmoid/o **sigmoid**oscopy	sig-**MOYD**-oh **sig**-moyd-**OSS**-koh-pee	☐	sigmoid colon
-spasm gastro**spasm**	**SPAZM** **GAS**-troh-spazm	☐	twitching; involuntary contraction
steat/o **steat**orrhea	stee-**AH**-to **stee**-**AH**-toh-**REE**-ah	☐	fat
stomat/o **stomat**itis	stoh-**MAH**-toh stoh-mah-**TYE**-tis	☐	mouth
-tresia a**tresia**	**TREE**-zee-ah ah-**TREE**-zee-ah	☐	perforation
-tripsy litho**tripsy**	**TRIP**-see **LITH**-oh-**trip**-see	☐	intentional crushing

Common Signs and Symptoms

Following are common complaints (signs and symptoms) that individuals with digestive system problems may experience, describe, or express when talking with the health professional. The observant health professional will listen carefully to all of the descriptions used by the patient. As you study the terms below, write each definition and word a minimum of three times, pronouncing the word aloud each time. Note that the word and the **basic definition** are in bold print. Once you have mastered each word to your satisfaction, check the box provided beside the word.

☐ **achlorhydria** (ah-klor-**HIGH**-dree-ah) a- = without, not chlor/o = green hydr/o = water -ia = condition	**Achlorhydria is an abnormal condition characterized by the absence of hydrochloric acid in the gastric juice.**
☐ **anorexia** (an-oh-**REK**-see-ah)	**Lack or loss of appetite, resulting in the inability to eat.**
☐ **aphagia** (ah-**FAY**-jee-ah) a- = without, not phag/o = to eat -ia = condition	**Aphagia is a condition characterized by the loss of the ability to swallow as a result of organic or psychologic causes.**
☐ **ascites** (ah-**SIGH**-teez)	**An abnormal accumulation of fluid within the peritoneal cavity; the fluid contains large amounts of protein and electrolytes.**
☐ **borborygmus** (bor-boh-**RIG**-mus)	**A borborygmus is an audible abdominal sound produced by hyperactive intestinal peristalsis. Borborygmi are rumbling, gurgling, and tinkling noises heard when listening with a stethoscope.**
☐ **constipation** (kon-stih-**PAY**-shun)	**Constipation is difficulty in passing stools, or an incomplete or infrequent passage of hard stools.**
☐ **diarrhea** (dye-ah-**REE**-ah) di/a = through -rrhea = discharge; flow	**The frequent passage of loose, watery stools.**
☐ **dyspepsia** (dis-**PEP**-see-ah) dys- = bad, difficult, painful, disordered peps/o = digestion -ia = condition	**A vague feeling of epigastric discomfort after eating. Dyspepsia involves an uncomfortable feeling of fullness, heartburn, bloating, and nausea.**

dysphagia (dis-**FAY**-jee-ah) dys- = bad, difficult, painful, disordered; phag/o = to eat	**Dysphagia** is difficulty in swallowing, commonly associated with obstructive or motor disorders of the esophagus.
emaciation (ee-**may**-she-**AY**-shun)	Excessive leanness caused by disease or lack of nutrition is **emaciation**.
emesis (**EM**-eh-sis)	The material expelled from the stomach during vomiting; **vomitus**.
eructation (eh-ruk-**TAY**-shun)	**Eructation** is the act of bringing up air from the stomach with a characteristic sound through the mouth; belching.
flatus; flatulence (**FLAY**-tus; **FLAT**-yoo-lens)	**Flatus** or **flatulence** is air or gas in the intestine that is passed through the rectum.
gastroesophageal reflux (gas-troh-eh-soff-ah-**JEE**-al **REE**-flucks) gastr/o = stomach; esophag/o = esophagus; -eal = pertaining to	**Gastroesophageal reflux** is a backflow of contents of the stomach into the esophagus that is often the result of incompetence of the lower esophageal sphincter.
icterus (**ICK**-ter-us)	A yellow discoloration of the skin, mucous membranes, and sclera of the eyes, caused by greater than normal amounts of bilirubin in the blood; also called **jaundice**.
jaundice (**JON**-diss)	See *icterus*.
melena (**MELL**-eh-nah)	**Melena** is an abnormal, black, tarry stool containing digested blood.
nausea (**NAW**-zee-ah)	An unpleasant sensation often leading to the urge to **vomit**.
pruritus ani (proo-**RIGH**-tus **AN**-eye)	**Pruritus ani** is a common chronic condition of itching of the skin around the anus.
steatorrhea (stee-ah-toh-**REE**-ah) steat/o = fat; -rrhea = flow, drainage	Greater than normal amounts of fat in the feces, characterized by frothy, foul-smelling fecal matter that floats, as in celiac disease, some malabsorption syndromes, and any condition in which fats are poorly absorbed by the small intestine.
vomit (**VOM**-it)	To expel the contents of the stomach through the esophagus and out of the mouth.
vomitus (**VOM**-ih-tus)	See *emesis*.

Pathological Conditions

As you study the pathological conditions of the digestive system, note that the **basic definition** is in bold print, followed by a detailed description in regular print. The phonetic pronunciation is directly beneath each term, and a breakdown of the component parts of the term when appropriate.

achalasia
(ak-al-**LAY**-zee-ah)

Decreased mobility of the lower two-thirds of the esophagus along with constriction of the lower esophageal sphincter.

Because of the lack of nerve impulses and the absence of sympathetic receptors, the relaxation of the lower esophageal sphincter (LES) fails to happen with swallowing. Food and fluid accumulate in the lower esophagus due to the decreased mobility in the lower esophagus and its constriction. Among the diagnostic tests used to diagnose achalasia are the barium swallow and endoscopy studies.

anal fistula
(**AY**-nal **FISS**-too-lah)
an/o = anus
-al = pertaining to

An abnormal passageway in the skin surface near the anus usually connecting with the rectum.

The anal fistula may occur as the result of a draining abscess.

aphthous stomatitis
(**AFF**-thus stoh-mah-**TYE**-tis)
stomat/o = mouth
-itis = inflammation

Small inflammatory noninfectious ulcerated lesions occurring on the lips, tongue, and inside the cheeks of the mouth; also called canker sores.

There is no known cause for aphthous stomatitis; however, some of the possible causes are emotional stress, food and drug allergies, endocrine imbalances, viral infections, vitamin deficiency, and stress. The lesions are painful, but heal within 7 to 14 days. See **Figure 12-7.**

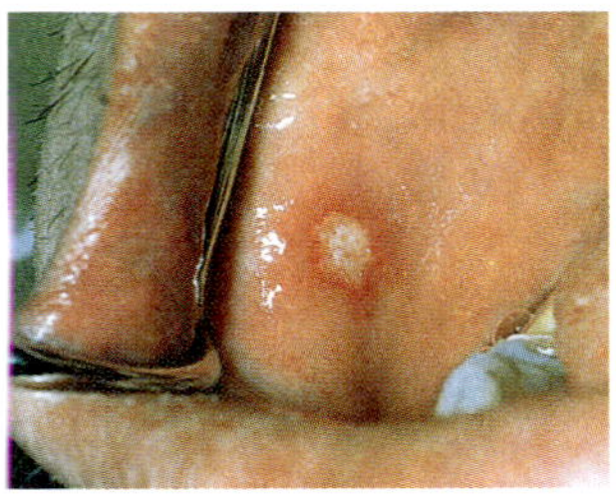

Figure 12-7 Aphthous stomatitis (Courtesy of Dr. Joseph Konzelman, School of Dentistry, Medical College of Georgia)

celiac disease
(**SEE**-lee-ak disease)

Nutrient malabsorption due to damaged small bowel mucosa.

The damage to the small bowel mucosa occurs because of the ingestion of gluten-containing foods such as barley, rye, wheat, and oats. Fat digestion is affected as is vitamin and carbohydrate absorption.

Clinical manifestations of this gluten-sensitive disease of the small intestine, when untreated, include steatorrhea (large foul-smelling stools with unabsorbed fat), abdominal distension, and a malnourished appearance. These symptoms typically begin after the infant begins to ingest cereals around 6 months of age.

Effective treatment is dietary control of gluten ingestion. The person with celiac disease must remain on a gluten-free diet for life.

chronic polyposis (polyps)
(**KRON**-ik pall-ee-**POH**-sis)
(**pall**-ips)
polyp/o = polyps
-osis = condition

Chronic polyposis indicates a large number of polyps in the large bowel. A polyp is a small growth projecting from a mucous membrane.

cirrhosis
(sih-**ROH**-sis)
cirrh/o = yellow, tawny
-osis = condition

A disease of the liver that is chronic and degenerative causing injury to the hepatocytes (functional cells of the liver).

Fat infiltrates the lobules of the liver, the tissue covering the lobes becomes fibrous, and the functions of the liver eventually deteriorate. Multisystem problems result from the liver's obstructed blood flow and inability to metabolize. Cirrhosis is a final common course for numerous liver diseases. It also is a result of malnutrition, alcoholism, infection, or poisons. Cirrhosis ultimately results in portal hypertension and liver failure.

Diagnosis is made through a biopsy of the liver, results of blood tests, and physical examination. Treatment of cirrhosis is to eliminate the cause. When it is possible to eliminate the cause, liver cells will slowly regenerate. If the cause cannot be removed, hepatic failure will occur, leading to death due to the multisystem devastation. Liver transplantation becomes a viable option when an individual's liver is damaged to the point where liver failure is impending and/or the symptoms cannot be otherwise treated. Most liver transplants in adults are performed due to cirrhosis brought about by a variety of causes.

colorectal cancer
(koh-loh-**REK**-tal)
col/o = colon
rect/o = rectum
-al = pertaining to

The presence of a malignant neoplasm in the large intestine.

Most neoplasms in the large intestine are adenocarcinomas and at least 50% originate in the rectum, causing bleeding and pain.

Although the cause of colorectal cancer is unknown, a number of known risk factors have been identified. These risk factors include the ingestion of a high-fat, low-residue diet that is high in refined foods, a history of Crohn's disease, ulcerative colitis, irritable bowel syndrome, or familial polyposis.

Along with the rectal examination, a **barium enema**, **sigmoidoscopy** and/or **colonoscopy**, and stool examination for occult blood will be used for diagnosis.

constipation
(**kon**-stih-**PAY**-shun)

A state in which the individual's pattern of bowel elimination is characterized by a decrease in the frequency of bowel movements and the passage of hard, dry stools. The individual experiences difficult defecation.

Constipation is a common complaint among the older person. Contributing factors include decreased peristalsis in the intestinal tract, decreased appetite, inadequate fluid intake, and lack of exercise. Repeated overuse or abuse of laxatives over the years worsens the problem.

Dietary concerns are important in preventing constipation in the elderly adult. The individual should be encouraged to eat small frequent meals, increase dietary fiber, and to drink plenty of fluids daily.

Crohn's disease
(**KROHNZ** dih-**ZEEZ**)

Digestive tract inflammation of a chronic nature causing fever, cramping, diarrhea, weight loss, and anorexia.

The inflammation of the bowel wall results in extreme swelling, which can lead to an obstruction causing a tender, distended abdomen. The stools and/or vomitus may have blood. With this chronic disease the individual may experience signs of malnutrition.

The exact etiology of Crohn's disease is unknown; however, there have been various implications such as allergies, dietary factors, and immunological factors. A colonoscopy is used to diagnose this chronic inflammation of the digestive tract.

dental caries
(DEN-tal **KAIR**-eez)
dent/o = tooth
-al = pertaining to

Tooth decay caused by acid-forming microorganisms.

These microorganisms are maintained in the mouth by fermentable carbohydrates (most commonly sugars), which create decalcification of the tooth's enamel and dentin. These fermentable carbohydrates and bacteria are prone to accumulate in the form of plaque between the teeth and on the grooves of the chewing surfaces of the teeth. This is where dental caries are likely to form.

Prevention is the treatment of choice. The topical application or ingestion of fluoride helps the tooth enamel to become more resistant to the acids and thus the formation of dental caries. Flossing and brushing will also aid in the removal of the plaque, which leads to dental caries.

diverticular disease
(**dye**-ver-**TIK**-yoo-lar dih-**ZEEZ**)

An expression used to characterize both diverticulosis and diverticulitis. Diverticulosis describes the noninflamed outpouchings or herniations of the muscular layer of the intestine, typically the sigmoid colon. Inflammation of these outpouchings called diverticula is referred to as diverticulitis. See Figure 12-8.

Diverticular disease is an increasingly common occurrence in persons over 45 years of age. Persons eating diets low in fiber predispose themselves to the formation of diverticulum. Inflammation of the diverticulum results in cramping pain, fever, increased flatus, and elevated white blood cell count (leukocytosis). Proctoscopy and barium enemas are used in the diagnostic process.

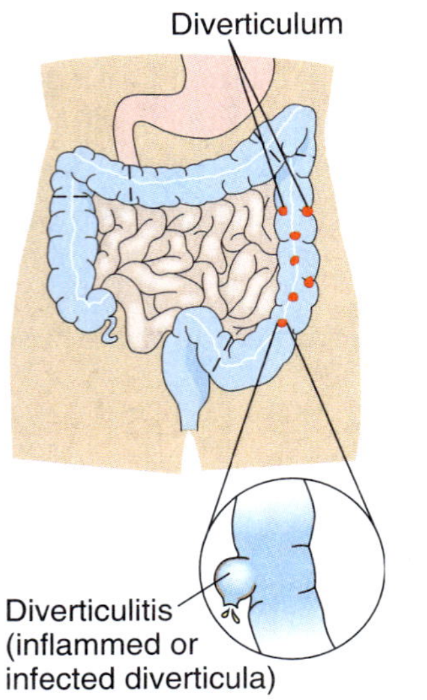

Figure 12-8 Diverticulitis

dysentery
(**DISS**-en-**ter**-ee)
dys- = bad, difficult, painful, disordered
enter/o = intestine
-y = noun ending

A term used to describe painful intestinal inflammation typically caused by ingesting water or food containing bacteria, protozoa, parasites, or chemical irritants.

The person suffering from dysentery has frequent stools that often contain blood. Other symptoms include abdominal pain and intestinal cramping. Dysentery often occurs as a result of unsanitary conditions.

esophageal varices
(eh-soff-ah-**JEE**-al **VAIR**-ih-seez)
esophag/o = esophagus
-eal = pertaining to

Swollen, twisted (tortuous) veins located in the distal end of the esophagus.

Esophageal varices is usually caused by portal hypertension, which occurs as a result of liver disease, in particular, cirrhosis of the liver. Portal hypertension causes the pressure in the veins to increase, making the vessels especially susceptible to hemorrhage.

gallstones (cholelithiasis)
(**koh**-lee-lih-**THIGH**-ah-sis)
chol/e = bile
lith/o = stone
-iasis = presence of an abnormal condition

Pigmented or hardened cholesterol stones formed as a result of bile crystallization.

When the gallstones obstruct the common bile duct or the cystic duct, epigastric and/or upper right quadrant pain develops, sometimes radiating to the upper right back area. This discomfort is generally accompanied by **nausea** and vomiting.

The person's history along with an ultrasound of the gallbladder are usually reliable in diagnosing **cholelithiasis**. With recurring pain, surgical intervention is indicated. When removing a gallbladder, a laparoscopic cholecystectomy may be performed, resulting in a much quicker recovery. Gallstones may be removed through an endoscopic procedure. The medication, chenodiol, is used to disintegrate existing stones and reduce the liver's cholesterol synthesis.

hemorrhoids
(**HEM**-oh-roydz)

A permanently distended vein, called a varicosity, in the distal rectum or anus.

Hemorrhoids arising above the internal sphincter are classified as internal and those emerging outside the sphincter are external hemorrhoids. Internal hemorrhoids become constricted and very painful and may bleed when they enlarge and extrude from the anus. External hemorrhoids do not typically bleed or cause pain.

hepatitis
(**hep**-ah-**TYE**-tis)
hepat/o = liver
-itis = inflammation

Acute or chronic inflammation of the liver due to a viral or bacterial infection, drugs, alcohol, toxins, or parasites.

The resultant inflammation presents itself in the form of abdominal and gastric discomfort, enlarged tender liver, jaundice, **anorexia**, joint pain, and elevated liver enzymes indicative of liver tissue damage. The most common type of **hepatitis** is viral hepatitis.

Viral hepatitis begins in the acute form as a result of:

1. hepatitis A virus frequently transmitted by the fecal–oral route or due to poor hygiene, contaminated water, or shellfish, and in most cases there is a complete recovery.
2. hepatitis B virus, which is transmitted from the blood or body fluid of an infected individual to another individual and has the potential of leading to excessive destruction of liver cells, cirrhosis, or death.
3. hepatitis C virus, which is transmitted through the intravenous route in blood transfusions or when persons share needles, and progresses in about one-half of the cases to a chronic form of hepatitis.

hernia
(**HER**-nee-ah)

An irregular protrusion of tissue, organ, or a portion of an organ through an abnormal break in the surrounding cavity's muscular wall.

Weakness in the muscle walls may be inherited or obtained due to the aging process, heavy lifting, obesity, coughing, or pregnancy. The **hernia** associated with the digestive system is known as a hiatal hernia. Also called a diaphragmatic hernia, this condition occurs as a result of an upward protrusion of the stomach through the diaphragm due to an enlarged cardiac sphincter. See **Figure 12-9.** Individuals with a hiatal hernia may be completely free of symptoms (asymptomatic) or may experience daily symptoms that are usually similar to those of gastroesophageal, the backflow of the acid contents of the stomach into the esophagus.

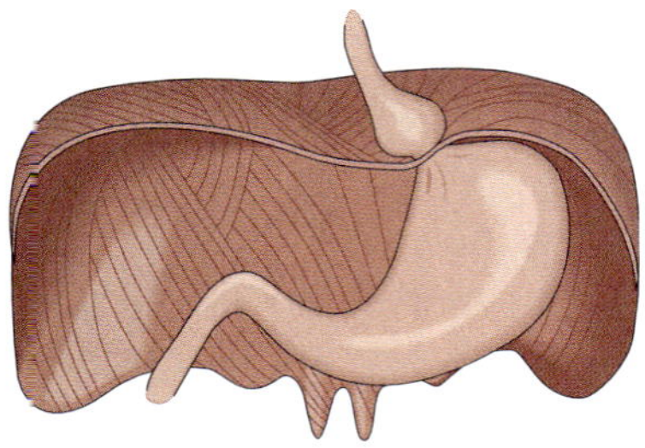

Diagnosis of a hiatal hernia can be made via x-ray films. Treatment is usually directed at relieving the discomfort associated with the reflux through the use of medications such as antacids and histamine receptor antagonists, diet, and proper positioning to decrease pain. Surgical intervention is usually necessary.

Figure 12-9 Hiatal hernia

herpetic stomatitis
(her-**PEH**-tic stoh-mah-**TYE**-tis)
stomat/o = mouth
-itis = inflammation

Inflammatory infectious lesions in or on the oral cavity occurring as a primary or a secondary viral infection caused by herpes simplex.

The primary infection usually occurs during early childhood and is often asymptomatic; other times it appears in the form of ulcerations in the mouth. Secondary **herpetic stomatitis** is a recurrent viral infection believed to lie dormant until it is reactivated by a fever, an upper respiratory infection, or exposure to sunlight. These clear vesicular lesions appear on the lips, palate, tongue, and gingiva of the mouth and are often called "cold sores" or fever blisters.

The lesions from herpetic stomatitis are painful and contagious, but heal without scarring in approximately 7 days. There is no known preventive measure. The treatment includes analgesics, use of local ointments, and anesthetics for the relief of discomfort caused by the lesions. In immunocompromised persons, acyclovir is administered intravenously.

Hirschsprung's disease (congenital megacolon)
(**HIRSH**-sprungz dih-**ZEEZ**)
(kon-**JEN**-ih-tal meg-ah-**KOH**-lon)

Absence at birth of the autonomic ganglia in a segment of the intestinal smooth muscle wall that normally stimulates peristalsis.

With the absence of these autonomic ganglia, the intestinal peristalsis is poor or absent in the aganglionic segment, which results in a buildup of feces and thus the distention of the bowel. This enlarged bowel is sometimes called a megacolon.

Hirschsprung's disease is typically diagnosed during infancy often due to the failure of the newborn to have the first stool, called a meconium ileus. The diagnosis is confirmed with a barium enema and the extent of the affected tissue is determined with biopsies. According to the extent and exact location of the aganglionic segment, surgical repair is done to remove the aganglionic portion.

ileus
(**ILL**-ee-ʊs)
ile/o = ileum
-us = noun ending

A term used to describe an obstruction of the intestine.

There are several reasons an **ileus** may occur such as twisting of the bowel, absence of peristalsis, or presence of adhesions or tumor. An ileus may resolve with medical treatment or require surgical intervention such as an intestinal resection.

intestinal obstruction
(in-**TESS**-tin-al ob-**STRUCK**-shun)

Complete or partial alteration in the forward flow of the contents in the small or large intestines.

An obstruction in the small intestine constitutes a surgical emergency. All **intestinal obstructions** require rapid diagnosis and treatment within a 24-hour period to prevent death.

There are numerous causes of an intestinal obstruction such as:

1. Inflammation causing decreased diameter of the intestinal lumen.
2. Adhesions form after abdominal surgery as bands of fibrous scar tissue, which can become looped over or around the intestine.
3. Tumors may cause an obstruction in the small or large intestine.
4. Hernias may become incarcerated and thus cause an obstruction.
5. **Volvulus** occurs when the bowel becomes twisted or rotated on itself.
6. Intussusception occurs when the proximal bowel telescopes into the distal bowel.
7. Neurogenic factors resulting in lack of peristalsis after abdominal surgery.

The clinical manifestations of an intestinal obstruction include abdominal pain and distension, nausea and vomiting, and altered bowel sounds. Diagnostic tests used to evaluate an intestinal obstruction are flat plate x-ray, barium follow-through, barium enema, CBC, and blood chemistry studies.

The insertion of an intestinal tube is the primary medical treatment for an intestinal obstruction. If the intestinal tube is ineffective in relieving the obstruction, surgery is indicated.

intussusception
(in-tuh-suh-**SEP**-shun)

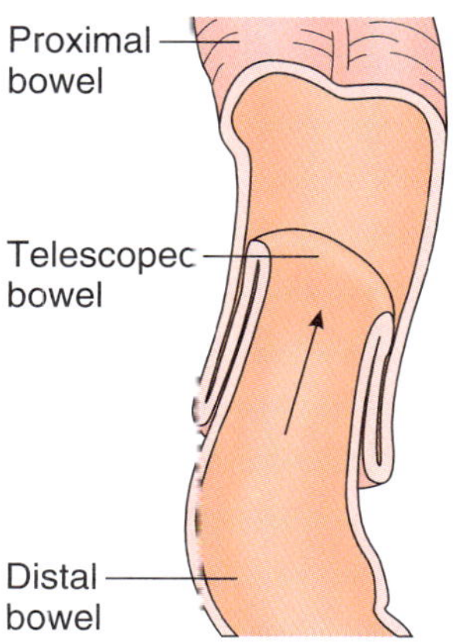

Telescoping of a portion of proximal intestine into distal intestine usually in the ileocecal region causing an obstruction.

Intussusception typically occurs in infants and young children. Clinical manifestations include intermittent severe abdominal pain, vomiting, and a "currant jelly stool," which indicates the presence of bloody mucus. See **Figure 12-10.**

Intussusception is diagnosed and medically treated with a barium enema. During the examination, the telescoping is often reduced with the pressure created with a barium enema. When the obstruction is not reduced with the barium enema, immediate surgical intervention is necessary.

Figure 12-10 Intussusception

irritable bowel syndrome (IBS); spastic colon
(**EAR**-it-ah-b'l **BOW**-el **SIN**-drom)
(**SPAS**-tik **COH**-lon)

Increased motility of the small or large intestinal wall resulting in abdominal pain, flatulence, nausea, anorexia, and the trapping of gas throughout the intestines.

Diarrhea, more often than constipation, may occur. This increased motility is distinctively in response to emotional stress. There are no diagnostic tests to confirm **irritable bowel syndrome (IBS)**, or **spastic colon**, so all other possible causes of the symptoms must be ruled out.

oral leukoplakia
(**OR**-al **loo**-koh-**PLAY**-kee-ah)
or/o = mouth
-al = pertaining to
leuk/o = white
-plakia = a plate; or flat plane

A precancerous lesion occurring anywhere in the mouth.

These elevated gray-white or yellow-white leathery surfaced lesions have clearly defined borders. See **Figure 12-11.**

Etiological factors of **oral leukoplakia** include chronic oral mucosal irritation, which occurs with the use of tobacco and alcohol.

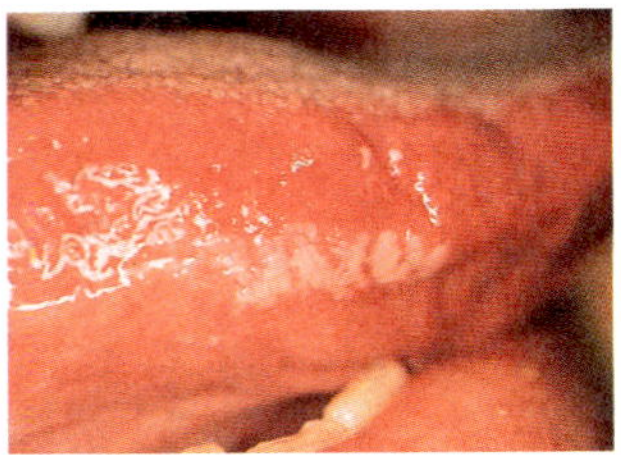

Figure 12-11 Oral leukoplakia (Courtesy of Dr. Joseph Konzelman, School of Dentistry, Medical College of Georgia)

pancreatitis
(pan-kree-ah-**TYE**-tis)
pancreat/o = pancreas
-itis = inflammation

An acute or chronic destructive inflammatory condition of the pancreas.

Acute **pancreatitis** presents itself quickly and creates symptoms, which vary from mild self-limiting pancreatic edema to massive necrotizing hemorrhagic pancreatitis. The initial outstanding symptom is severe continuous epigastric and abdominal pain that radiates to the back and follows the ingestion of excessive alcohol or a fatty meal. Other symptoms include rigid abdominal distension, decreased bowel sounds, nausea and vomiting, hypotension, elevated temperature, and clammy cold skin. After 24 hours, mild jaundice may appear. In addition to alcoholism, other causes of acute pancreatitis include trauma, surgery, metabolic disorders, drugs, infections, or ruptured peptic ulcers.

Serious complications may include development of abscesses or pseudocysts, diabetes mellitus, renal failure, heart failure, hypovolemic shock, multiple organ failure, ascites, and adult respiratory distress syndrome. Treatment is aimed at resolving the immediate problems, relief of pain and avoiding any further GI irritation (NG tube and NPO status), and prevention of serious life-threatening complications.

Chronic pancreatitis is a permanent, progressive destruction of the pancreatic cells identified with fibrosis, atrophy, fatty degeneration, and calcification. The causes of chronic pancreatitis include alcoholism, malnutrition, surgery, or neoplasm. Clinical manifestations include abdominal pain, large fatty stools, weight loss, and signs and symptoms of diabetes mellitus. Treatment includes the administration of pancreatic enzymes, antiemetics, antacids, and insulin if its production is stopped or decreased.

peptic ulcers (gastric, duodenal, perforated)
(**PEP**-tik **ULL**-sir)
(**GAS**-tric, doo-oh-**DEE**-nal, **PER**-foh-ray-ted)

A break in the continuity of the mucous membrane lining of the gastrointestinal tract as a result of hyperacidity or the bacterium, *Helicobacter pylori*.

Peptic ulcers are acute or chronic, singular or clustered, shallow or deep. Acute ulcers are typically multiple and shallow, therefore causing few symptoms and heal without scarring. On the other hand, chronic ulcers are typically singular, deep, symptomatic, persistent, and cause scarring. If an ulcer invades to the point of creating a hole through the complete depth of the stomach or duodenum, it is called a perforating ulcer, which will likely require surgical intervention.

Diagnosis is based on the client's history, upper GI barium studies, and endoscopy. Clinical manifestations of a peptic ulcer include some or all of the following: gnawing epigastric pain, heartburn or indigestion, nausea and vomiting, and bloated feeling after eating. Treatment includes antacids, frequent small meals, medications to decrease the production of hydrochloric acid (Pepcid, Tagamet, Zantac), and antibiotics if the ulcer is due to the *Helicobacter pylori* bacterium.

periodontal disease
(pair-ee-oh-**DON**-tal dih-**ZEEZ**)
peri- = around
odont/o = teeth
-al = pertaining to

A term used to describe a group of inflammatory gum disorders, which may lead to degeneration of teeth, gums, and sometimes surrounding bones.

Periodontal diseases are very common, occurring in at least 90% of the population. The formation and accumulation of plaque due to fermentable carbohydrates and bacteria is the primary cause of periodontal disease.

In the early stages of periodontal disease, minor inflammation of the gums (**gingivitis**) occurs causing discoloration and bleeding. As periodontal disease progresses to the late stages, purulent inflammation of the gums (pyorrhea) develops causing pus to drain from the gum tissue.

thrush
(**THRUSH**)

A fungal infection in the mouth and throat producing sore, creamy white, slightly raised curdlike patches on the tongue and other oral mucosal surfaces. Thrush is caused by *Candida albicans*.

Thrush is common in infants or persons who are debilitated, immunosuppressed, or receiving long-term antibiotic, corticosteroid, and antineoplastic therapy. Treatment consists of an antifungal medication for 2 weeks. See **Figure 12-12**.

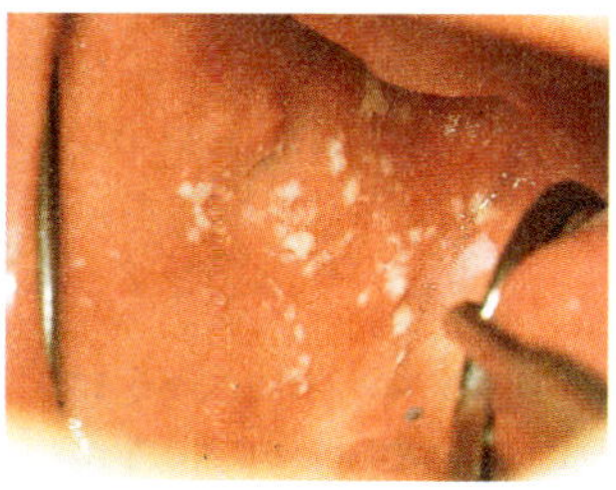

Figure 12-12 Thrush (Courtesy of Dr. Joseph Konzelman, School of Dentistry, Medical College of Georgia)

ulcerative colitis
(**ULL**-sir-an-tiv koh-**LYE**-tis)
col/o = colon
-itis = inflammation

A chronic inflammatory condition resulting in a break in the continuity of the mucous membrane lining of the colon in the form of ulcers. Ulcerative colitis is characterized by large watery diarrheal stools containing mucus, pus, or blood.

The **diarrhea** is accompanied by severe abdominal discomfort and spasms of the intestines. The person will likely experience fever, chills, weight loss, and anemia.

Treatment for ulcerative colitis usually includes corticosteroids or other anti-inflammatory medications. In severe cases that do not respond to medical treatment, surgical intervention is implicated. Ulcerative colitis bears an increased risk of acquiring colon cancer.

volvulus
(**VOL**-vyoo-lus)

A rotation of loops of bowel causing a twisting on itself that results in an intestinal obstruction (see *intestinal obstruction*). See Figure 12-13.

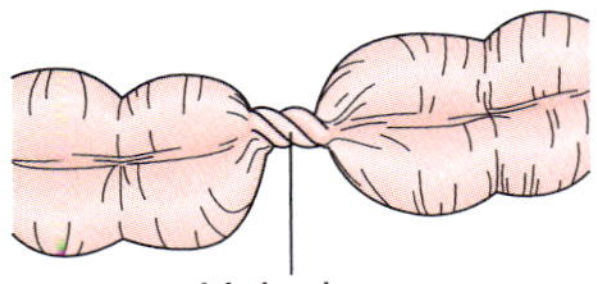

Figure 12-13 Volvulus

Diagnostic Techniques and Procedures

abdominal ultrasound
(ab-**DOM**-ih-nal **ULL**-trah-sound)

The use of very-high-frequency sound waves to provide visualization of the internal organs of the abdomen (liver, gallbladder, bile ducts, pancreas, kidneys, bladder, and ureters).

The **abdominal ultrasound** is a noninvasive diagnostic procedure, which demonstrates normal or abnormal findings of the abdominal organs.

abdominocentesis (paracentesis)
(ab-**dom**-ih-noh-sen-**TEE**-sis)
abdomin/o = abdomen
-centesis = surgical puncture

Abdominocentesis involves insertion of a needle or trochar into the abdominal cavity to remove excess fluid, with the person in a sitting position.

The trochar is attached to a tube and collection bottle. This invasive procedure is typically done to remove large amounts of **ascitic fluid** from the distended abdomen to reduce pressure, which sometimes keeps the person from being able to breathe effectively. A specimen of the **peritoneal** fluid will likely be tested in the laboratory. Increased levels of amylase in the peritoneal fluid is indicative of acute pancreatitis.

After the needle is withdrawn, a small dressing is secured over the puncture site. A physician's order may follow for the administration of salt-poor albumin to replace the lost protein.

alanine aminotransferase (ALT)
(**AL**-ah-neen
ah-mee-no-**TRANS**-fer-ays)

Alanine aminotransferase is a hepatocellular enzyme released in elevated amounts due to liver dysfunction; also known as serum glutamic pyruvic transaminase (SGPT).

The normal serum level of ALT/SGPT is 5 to 35 IU/l. Abnormally high levels occur in hepatitis, cirrhosis, hepatic necrosis, hepatic ischemia, hepatic tumor, hepatotoxic drugs, obstructive jaundice, myositis, and pancreatitis.

alkaline phosphatase (ALP)
(**AL**-kah-line **FOSS**-fah-tays)

Alkaline phosphatase enzyme is found in the highest concentrations in the liver, biliary tract, and bone.

The mucosa of the intestine also contains ALP. A normal level of ALP is 30 to 85 ImU/ml (international milliunits/milliliter). Increased levels of ALP are found in cirrhosis, intrahepatic or extrahepatic biliary obstruction, liver tumors, and intestinal ischemia or infarction. Decreased levels are seen in malnutrition, celiac disease, and excess vitamin B ingestion. The serum ALP level is elevated in obstructive hepatitis or jaundice.

amylase
(**AM**-ih-lays)

An enzyme secreted normally from the pancreatic cells that travels to the duodenum by way of the pancreatic duct and aids in digestion.

When the pancreatic duct is blocked or there is damage to the pancreatic cells that secrete amylase, the enzyme pours into the free peritoneum and intrapancreatic lymph system where blood vessels absorb the excess amylase. A normal blood amylase level is 56 to 190 IU/l. Abnormally increased levels are found in acute pancreatitis, penetrating or perforated peptic ulcers, perforated bowel, necrotic bowel, **duodenal** obstruction, and acute **cholecystitis**.

barium enema (BE)
(lower GI series)
(**BAH**-ree-um **EN**-eh-mah)

Infusion of a radiopaque contrast medium, barium sulfate, into the rectum and held in the lower intestinal tract while x-ray films are obtained of the lower GI tract.

For the most definitive results, the colon should be empty of fecal material. Along with the use of a laxative and/or a cleansing enema, the person having a BE would be without food or drink from the midnight before the procedure. Abnormal findings include malignant tumors, colonic stenosis, colonic fistula, perforated colon, diverticula, and polyps.

barium swallow (upper GI series)
(**BAH**-ree-um swallow)

Barium swallow involves oral administration of a radiopaque contrast medium, barium sulfate, which flows into the esophagus as the person swallows.

X-ray films are obtained of the esophagus and borders of the heart in which varices can be identified, as well as strictures, tumors, obstructions, achalasia, or abnormal motility of the esophagus. As the barium sulfate continues to flow into the upper GI tract (lower esophagus, stomach, and duodenum), x-ray films are taken to reveal ulcerations, tumors, hiatal hernias, or obstruction. Additional information and photo are provided in Chapter 20.

cheiloplasty
(**KYE**-loh-plas-tee)
cheil/o = lip
-plasty = surgical repair

Surgically correcting a defect of the lip is known as cheiloplasty.

cholecystectomy
(**koh**-lee-sis-**TEK**-toh-mee)
cholecyst/o = gallbladder
-ectomy = removal of

The surgical removal of the gallbladder.

The specific technique is based on the location of the stone and the severity of the individual's complications. A simple **cholecystectomy** is performed when the stones are found only in the gallbladder. This simple cholecystectomy may be done through laparascopic laser surgery or conventional surgical methods. When the stones are located or lodged within the ducts, a common bile duct exploration will be needed during surgery and there may also be placement of a T-tube in the duct, which allows the drainage of the bile until the edema of the duct has decreased.

---

cholecystography (oral)
(**koh**-lee-sis-**TOG**-rah-fee)
chol/e = bile
cyst/o = bladder, sac, or cyst
-graphy = process of recording

Visualization of the gallbladder through x-ray following the oral ingestion of pills containing a radiopaque iodinated dye.

The oral cholecystography is not as accurate as the gallbladder ultrasound. Abnormal findings would include gallstones, gallbladder polyps, gallbladder cancer, or cystic duct obstruction.

---

colonoscopy
(**koh**-lon-**OSS**-koh-pee)
colon/o = colon
-scopy = the process of viewing

The direct visualization of the lining of the large intestine using a fiberoptic colonoscope.

A colonoscopy is indicated for individuals with a history of undiagnosed constipation and diarrhea, loss of appetite (anorexia), persistent rectal bleeding, or lower abdominal pain. The procedure is also used to check for colonic polyps or possible malignant tumors.

---

colostomy
(koh-**LOSS**-toh-mee)
col/o = colon
-stomy = the surgical creation of a new opening

The surgical creation of a new opening on the abdominal wall through which the feces will be expelled (an abdominal-wall anus) by bringing the incised colon out to the abdominal surface.

The colostomy may be needed temporarily for the bowel to heal from injury (traumatic or surgical) or inflammation, or it may be needed permanently as the only opening for elimination of feces.

CT of the abdomen
(**CT** of the **AB**-doh-men)

A painless, noninvasive x-ray procedure that produces an image created by the computer representing a detailed cross section of the tissue structure within the abdomen, for example, computerized tomography (CT) of the abdomen.

The CT scan of the abdomen aids in the diagnosis of tumors, abscesses, cysts, inflammation, obstructions, perforation, bleeding, aneurysms, and obstruction. For more information on CT scans, refer to Chapter 20.

---

endoscopic retrograde cholangiopancreatography (ERCP)
(en-doh-**SKOP**-ic **RET**-roh-grayd koh-**lan**-jee-oh-**pan**-kree-ah-**TOG**-rah-fee)
endo- = within
scop/o = to view
-ic = pertaining to
chol/o = bile
angi/o = vessel
pancreat/o = pancreas
-graphy = process of recording

A procedure that examines the size of and the filling of the pancreatic and biliary ducts through direct radiographic visualization with a fiberoptic endoscope.

During the ERCP procedure, a fiberoptic scope (flexible tube with a lens and a light source) is passed through the patient's esophagus and stomach into the duodenum. Passage of the tube is observed on a fluoroscopic screen that makes it possible to view the procedure in action. The doctor locates the ampulla of Vater, a common passageway that connects the common bile duct and the pancreatic duct to the duodenum. Digestive enzymes can be removed from this area for analysis before a contrast medium is injected into the area for visualization upon x-ray.

This procedure requires the person to lie very still during the process. The patient is kept NPO (nothing by mouth) before the procedure and is mildly sedated during the procedure.

Abnormal findings include strictures (narrowing) of the common bile duct, tumors, gallstones, cysts, and anatomic variations of the biliary or pancreatic ducts.

---

extracorporeal shock wave lithotripsy (ESWL)
(**eks**-trah-kor-**POR**-ee-al shock wave **LITH**-oh-**trip**-see)
extra- = outside, beyond
corpor/o = body
-eal = pertaining to
lith/o = stone
-tripsy = intentional crushing

An alternative treatment for gallstones by using ultrasound to align the computerized lithotripter and source of shock waves with the stones, to crush the gallstones and thus enable the contraction of the gallbladder to remove stone fragments.

This contraction of the gallbladder will likely cause discomfort, nausea, and transient hematuria.

---

fluoroscopy
(**FLOO**-or-oh-skop-ee)
-scopy = the process of viewing

Fluoroscopy is a radiological technique used to examine the function of an organ or a body part using a fluoroscope.

There are immediate serial images that are essential in many clinical procedures. For more information see Chapter 20.

---

gastric analysis
(**GAS**-trik analysis)
gastr/o = stomach
-ic = pertaining to

Study of the stomach contents to determine the acid content and to detect the presence of blood, bacteria, bile, and abnormal cells.

The gastric sample is typically obtained through a nasogastric tube and examined. An alternate tubeless method uses the ingestion of Diagnex Blue, a resin dye. The hydrochloric acid in the stomach displaces the dye, which is absorbed by the bowel and excreted in about 2 hours in the urine. The lack of blue color in the urine typically signifies the absence of hydrochloric acid in the stomach.

---

gastric lavage
gastr/o = stomach
-ic = pertaining to

The irrigation, or washing out, of the stomach with sterile water or a saline solution.

A gastric lavage is usually performed before and after surgery to remove irritants or toxic substances from the stomach. It may also be performed before examinations such as endoscopy or gastroscopy.

---

gastrointestinal endoscopy
(**gas**-troh-in-**TESS**-tin-al en-**DOSS**-koh-pee)
gastr/o = stomach
endo- = within
scop/o = to view
-ic = pertaining to

Gastrointestinal endoscopy involves the direct visualization of the esophagus, stomach, and duodenum, using a lighted, fiberoptic endoscope.

An endoscope also has the capability of aspirating fluid, performing a biopsy, and coagulating areas of bleeding. In addition, a laser beam can be passed through the endoscope, which permits endoscopic surgery. Abnormal findings include tumors (malignant and benign), esophagitis, gastroesophageal varices, peptic ulcers, and the source of upper GI bleeding.

herniorrhaphy
(her-nee-**OR**-ah-fee)
-rrhaphy = suturing

Herniorrhaphy is the surgical repair of a hernia by closing the defect using sutures, mesh, or wire.

The person has activity restriction—no heavy labor or lifting for at least 3 weeks after surgery.

liver biopsy
(**LIV**-er **BYE**-op-see)

A piece of liver tissue is obtained for examination by inserting a specially designed needle into the liver through the abdominal wall.

Abnormal findings include hepatitis, abscess, cyst, or infiltrative diseases. There are specific procedures before, during, and after a **liver biopsy**.

liver scan
(**LIV**-er **SCAN**)

A noninvasive scanning technique, which enables the visualization of the shape, size, and consistency of the liver after the IV injection of a radioactive compound.

This compound is readily taken up by the liver's Kupffer cells and later the distribution is recorded by a radiation detector. The **liver scan** can detect cysts, abscesses, tumors, granulomas, or diffuse infiltrative processes affecting the liver.

magnetic resonance imaging (MRI)
(mag-**NEH**-tic **REZ**-oh-nans **IM**-ij-ing)

A noninvasive scanning procedure that provides visualization of fluid, soft tissue, and bony structures without the use of radiation.

The person is placed inside a large electromagnetic, tubelike machine where specific radio frequency signals change the alignment of hydrogen atoms in the body. The absorbed radio frequency energy is analyzed by a computer and an image is projected on the screen.

A strong magnetic field is used and radio frequency waves produce the imaging valuable in providing images of the heart, large blood vessels, brain, and soft tissue. MRI is also used to examine the aorta, to detect masses or possible tumors, and pericardial disease; it can show the flowing of blood and the beating of the heart. The MRI provides far more preciseness and accuracy than most diagnostic tools.

Those persons with implanted metal devices cannot undergo an MRI due to the strong magnetic field and the possibility of dislodging a chip or rod. Thus, persons with pacemakers, any recently implanted wires or clips, or prosthetic valves are not eligible for MRI. Persons should be informed that MRI is a very confining procedure because they are placed within a tube-like structure, and should be asked if they are claustrophobic (fearful of enclosed spaces).

nasogastric intubation
(nay-zoh-**GAS**-trik **in**-too-**BAY**-shun)
nas/o = nose
gastr/o = stomach
-ic = pertaining to

Nasogastric intubation involves tube placement through the nose into the stomach for the purpose of relieving gastric distension by removing gastric secretions, gas, or food.

The nasogastric tube may be the route for instilling medications, fluids, and/or food.

percutaneous transhepatic cholangiography (PTC)
(**per**-kyoo-**TAY**-nee-us trans-heh-**PAT**-ik koh-**lan**-jee-**OG**-rah-fee)
- **per-** = throughout
- **cutane/o** = skin
- **-ous** = pertaining to
- **trans-** = across
- **hepat/o** = liver
- **-ic** = pertaining to
- **chol/e** = bile
- **angi/o** = vessel
- **-graphy** = process of recording

An examination of the bile duct structure using a needle to pass directly into an intrahepatic bile duct to inject a contrast medium; also known as a PTHC.

The bile duct structure can be observed for obstruction, strictures, anatomic variations, malignant tumors, and congenital cysts. If the cause is found to be extrahepatic in persons who are jaundiced, a catheter may be used for external drainage by leaving it in the bile duct.

Abnormal findings include the following:

1. Tumors, gallstones, or strictures of the common bile or hepatic duct
2. Biliary sclerosis
3. Cysts of the common bile duct
4. Tumors, inflammation, or pseudocysts of the pancreatic duct
5. Anatomic biliary or pancreatic duct abnormalities

Although the complication rate after this invasive procedure is low, the patient must be observed closely for symptoms of bleeding, peritonitis (due to leakage of bile), and septicemia. Any signs of these complications and/or pain should be reported to the physician immediately.

serum bilirubin
(**SEE**-rum bill-ih-**ROO**-bin)

A measurement of the bilirubin level in the serum; serum bilirubin levels are a result of the breakdown of red blood cells.

Jaundice is the yellow discoloration of body tissues caused by abnormally high levels of bilirubin. The normal levels of bilirubin in the blood are:

1. Total bilirubin = 0.1–1.0 mg/dl
2. Indirect bilirubin = 0.2–0.8 mg/dl
3. Direct bilirubin = 0.1–0.3 mg/dl

An elevated indirect bilirubin level is seen with hepatic damage, hepatitis, and cirrhosis. An elevated direct bilirubin level is seen with gallstones, extensive liver metastasis, and extrahepatic duct obstruction.

serum glutamic-oxaloacetic transaminase (SGOT)
(**SEE**-rum gloo-**TAM**-ik oks-al-ah-**SEE**-tik trans-**AM**-in-ays)

An enzyme that has very high concentrations in liver cells; also known as aspartate aminotransferase (AST).

An AST/SGOT level measured in the blood that is elevated indicates the extent of disease on the liver cells. AST/SGOT enzyme levels are elevated with damaged hepatocytes. The normal adult level is 8 to 20 U/l.

Abnormally increased levels of AST/SGOT are found in hepatitis, hepatic cirrhosis, drug-induced liver injury, hepatic metastasis, acute pancreatitis, hepatic necrosis, and hepatic infiltrative process (tumor).

small bowel follow-through

Oral administration of a radiopaque contrast medium, barium sulfate, which flows through the GI system. X-ray films are obtained at timed intervals to observe the progression of the barium through the small intestine.

Notable delays in the time for transit may occur with both malignant and benign forms of obstruction or diminished intestinal motility. In hypermotility state, and malabsorption, the flow of barium is much quicker. Small bowel tumors, obstructions, inflammatory disease, malabsorption syndrome, congenital defects, or perforation may be identified with a small bowel follow-through study.

---

stool analysis for occult blood
(stool analysis for uh-**CULT** blood)

The analysis of a stool sample to determine the presence of blood not visible to the naked eye (i.e., hidden or occult blood).

A positive result of blood in the stool would indicate the need for a more thorough gastrointestinal examination. There is normally no occult blood in the stool. Benign and malignant tumors, inflammatory bowel disease, diverticulosis, and ulcers can cause occult blood.

---

stool culture
(**STOOL KULL**-chir)

Stool culture involves collection of a stool specimen placed on one or more culture mediums and allowed to grow colonies of microorganisms to identify specific pathogen(s).

The collector of the specimen should be very careful not to mix the stool specimen with urine because it may inhibit the growth of the bacteria. Abnormal findings include parasitic enterocolitis, protozoan enterocolitis, and bacterial enterocolitis.

---

stool guaiac
(**STOOL GWEE**-ak *or* **GWY**-ak)

Stool guaiac is a test on a stool specimen using guaiac as a reagent, which identifies the presence of blood in the stool.

Also called stool for occult blood or hemoccult test. Abnormal findings that may cause blood to be identified in the stool include GI tumor, polyps, varices, inflammatory bowel disease, ulcer, GI trauma, ischemic bowel disease, hemorrhoids, gastritis, esophagitis, and diverticulosis. See **Figure 12-14.**

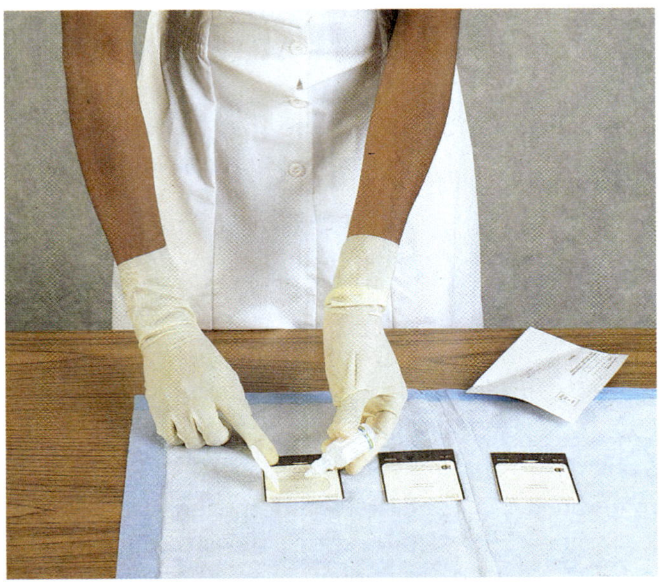

Figure 12-14 Hemoccult test

urinary bilirubin
(YOO-rih-nair-ee bill-ih-ROO-bin)

Urinary bilirubin tests for conjugated or direct bilirubin in a urine specimen.

There should normally be no bilirubin in the urine. Presence of or increased levels of direct bilirubin found in the urine along with the other symptoms specific for the disorders following may be indicative of gallstones, extensive liver metastasis, or extrahepatic duct obstruction.

Common Abbreviations

ABBREVIATION	MEANING
a.c	before meals (ante cibum)
ALT	alanine aminotransferase
AST	aspartate aminotransferase (formerly called serum glutamic-oxaloacetic transaminase [SGOT])
Ba	barium
BE	barium enema
b.i.d.	twice a day
CT SCAN	computerized tomography (scan)
EGD	esophagogastroduodenoscopy
ERCP	endoscopic retrograde cholangiopancreatography
ERS	endoscopic retrograde sphincterectomy
GB	gallbladder
GBS	gallbladder series
GER	gastroesophageal reflux
GERD	gastroesophageal reflux disease
GI	gastrointestinal
GI series	gastrointestinal series
GTT	glucose tolerance test
HAV	hepatitis A virus
HBV	hepatitis B virus
HCl	hydrochloric acid
HCV	hepatitis C virus
IBS	irritable bowel syndrome
IVC	intravenous cholangiography
LES	lower esophageal sphincter
LFTs	liver function tests
MRI	magnetic resonance imaging
N&V	nausea and vomiting
NG	nasogastric
NPO, n.p.o.	nothing by mouth
OCG	oral cholecystogram
p.c.	after meals (post cibum)
PP, pp	postprandial
PPBS	postprandial blood sugar
PPG	postprandial glucose
PTC	percutaneous transhepatic cholangiogram
SBF	small bowel follow-through
SBS	small bowel series
S & D	stomach and duodenum
SGOT	serum glutamic oxaloacetic transaminase; now called aspartate aminotransferase (AST)
SGPT	serum glutamic pyruvic transaminase
TPN	total parenteral nutrition
UGI series	upper gastrointestinal series

Written and Audio Terminology Review

Review each of the following terms from the chapter. Study the spelling of each term and write the definition in the space provided. If you have the Audio CD available, listen to each term, pronounce it, and check the box once you are comfortable saying the word. Check definitions by looking the term up in the glossary/index.

TERM	PRONUNCIATION	DEFINITION
abdominal ultrasound	☐ ab-**DOM**-ih-nal **ULL**-trah-sound	____________
abdominocentesis	☐ ab-**dom**-ih-noh-sen-**TEE**-sis	____________
absorption	☐ ab-**SORP**-shun	____________
achalasia	☐ **ack**-al-**LAY**-zee-ah	____________
achlorhydria	☐ **ah**-klor-**HIGH**-dree-ah	____________
alanine aminotransferase	☐ **AL**-ah-neen ah-mee-no-**TRANS**-fer-ays	____________
alimentary canal	☐ **al**-ih-**MEN**-tar-ee can-**NAL**	____________
alkaline phosphatase	☐ **AL**-kah-line **FOSS**-fah-tays	____________
amino acids	☐ ah-**MEE**-noh acids	____________
amylase	☐ **AM**-ih-lays	____________
anal fistula	☐ **AY**-nal **FISS**-too-lah	____________
anorexia	☐ an-oh-**REK**-see-ah	____________
anus	☐ **AY**-nus	____________
aphagia	☐ ah-**FAY**-jee-ah	____________
aphthous stomatitis	☐ **AFF**-thus stoh-mah-**TYE**-tis	____________
appendectomy	☐ ap-en-**DEK**-toh-mee	____________
appendicitis	☐ ap-**pen**-dih-**SIGH**-tis	____________
ascitic fluid	☐ ah-**SIT**-ik fluid	____________
atresia	☐ ah-**TREE**-zee-ah	____________
barium enema	☐ **BEAR**-ee-um **EN**-eh-mah	____________
barium swallow	☐ **BEAR**-ee-um swallow	____________
bicuspid	☐ bye-**CUSS**-pid	____________
bile	☐ **BYE**-al	____________

Term		Pronunciation	
biliary	☐	**BILL**-ee-air-ee	________
bilirubin	☐	bill-ih-**ROO**-bin	________
borborygmus	☐	**bor**-boh-**RIG**-mus	________
bowel	☐	**BOW**-el	________
buccal	☐	**BUCK**-al	________
canine	☐	**KAY**-nine (tooth)	________
cardiac sphincter	☐	**CAR**-dee-ak **SFINGK**-ter	________
cecostomy	☐	see-**KOSS**-tah-mee	________
cecum	☐	**SEE**-kum	________
celiac disease	☐	**SEE**-lee-ak dih-**ZEEZ**	________
celiac rickets	☐	**SEE**-lee-ak **RICK**-ets	________
cheiloplasty	☐	**KYE**-loh-**plas**-tee	________
cheilosis	☐	kigh-**LOH**-sis	________
cholecystectomy	☐	**koh**-lee-sis-**TEK**-toh-mee	________
cholecystitis	☐	**koh**-lee-sis-**TYE**-tis	________
cholecystogram	☐	**koh**-lee-**SIS**-toh-gram	________
cholecystography	☐	**koh**-lee-sis-**TOG**-rah-fee	________
cholelithiasis	☐	**koh**-lee-lih-**THIGH**-ah-sis	________
chronic polyposis (polyps)	☐	**KRON**-ik **pall**-ee-**POH**-sis **PALL**-ips	________
chyme	☐	**KIGHM**	________
cirrhosis	☐	sih-**ROH**-sis	________
colon	☐	**COH**-lon	________
colonoscopy	☐	**koh**-lon-**OSS**-koh-pee	________
colorectal	☐	**koh**-loh-**REK**-tal	________
colorectal cancer	☐	**koh**-loh-**REK**-tal **CAN**-sir	________
colostomy	☐	koh-**LOSS**-toh-mee	________
constipation	☐	**kon**-stih-**PAY**-shun	________
Crohn's disease	☐	**KROHNZ** dih-**ZEEZ**	________
CT of the abdomen	☐	**CT** of the **AB**-doh-men	________
cuspid	☐	**CUSS**-pid	________

Term	Pronunciation	
deciduous	☐ dee-**SID**-you-us	______
defecation	☐ deff-eh-**KAY**-shun	______
deglutition	☐ **dee**-gloo-**TISH**-un	______
dental caries	☐ **DEN**-tal **KAY**-reez	______
dentin	☐ **DEN**-tin	______
diarrhea	☐ dye-ah-**REE**-ah	______
digestive	☐ dye-**JESS**-tiv	______
diverticular disease	☐ **dye**-ver-**TIK**-yoo-lar dih-**ZEEZ**	______
duodenal	☐ doo-**OD**-en-al	______
duodenostomy	☐ **doo**-od-en-**OSS**-toh-mee	______
duodenum	☐ doo-**OD**-en-um *or* doo-oh-**DEH**-num	______
dysentery	☐ **DISS**-en-**ter**-ee	______
dyspepsia	☐ dis-**PEP**-see-ah	______
dysphagia	☐ dis-**FAY**-jee-ah	______
emaciation	☐ ee-**may**-she-**AY**-shun	______
emesis	☐ **EM**-eh-sis	______
emulsify	☐ eh-**MULL**-sih-figh	______
enamel	☐ en-**AM**-el	______
endocrine	☐ **EN**-doh-krin	______
endoscopic retrograde cholangiopancreatography	☐ en-doh-**SKOP**-ic **RET**-roh-grayd koh-**lan**-jee-oh-**pan**-kree-ah-**TOG**-rah-fee	______
enteritis	☐ **en**-ter-**EYE**-tis	______
enzyme	☐ **EN**-zighm	______
eructation	☐ eh-ruk-**TAY**-shun	______
esophageal varices	☐ eh-**soff**-ah-**JEE**-al **VAIR**-ih-seez	______
esophagitis	☐ eh-soff-ah-**JIGH**-tus	______
esophagus	☐ eh-**SOFF**-ah-gus	______
exocrine	☐ **EKS**-oh-krin	______

Term	Pronunciation	
extracorporeal shock wave lithotripsy	☐ **eks**-trah-kor-**POR**-ee-al shock wave **LITH**-oh-**trip**-see	
feces	☐ **FEE**-seez	
flatus	☐ **FLAY**-tus	
flatulence	☐ **FLAT**-yoo-lens	
fluoroscopy	☐ **FLOU**-or-oh-skop-ee	
gallbladder	☐ **GALL**-blad-er	
gastrectasia	☐ gas-trek-**TAY**-zhe-ah	
gastric	☐ **GAS**-trik	
gastroenterologist	☐ **gas**-troh-**en**-ter-**ALL**-oh-jist	
gastroesophageal reflux	☐ **gas**-troh-eh-**soff**-ah-**JEE**-al **REE**-flucks	
gastrointestinal	☐ **gas**-troh-in-**TESS**-tih-nal	
gastrointestinal endoscopy	☐ **gas**-troh-in-**TESS**-tih-nal en-**DOSS**-koh-pee	
gastrorrhagia	☐ **gas**-troh-**RAY**-jee-ah	
gastrospasm	☐ **GAS**-troh-spazm	
gastrostomy	☐ gas-**TROSS**-toh-mee	
gavage	☐ gah-**VAZH**	
gingiva	☐ **JIN**-jih-vah *or* jin-**JYE**-vah	
gingivitis	☐ jin-jih-**VIGH**-tis	
glossitis	☐ gloss-**SIGH**-tis	
glucagon	☐ **GLOO**-kah-gon	
glucogenesis	☐ **gloo**-koh-**JEN**-eh-sis	
glucose	☐ **GLOO**-kohs	
glycogen	☐ **GLIGH**-koh-jen	
glycogenesis	☐ **gligh**-koh-**JEN**-eh-sis	
glycogenolysis	☐ **gligh**-koh-jen-**ALL**-ih-sis	
glycolysis	☐ gligh-**KALL**-ih-sis	
hemorrhoids	☐ **HEM**-oh-roydz	
hepatitis	☐ **hep**-ah-**TYE**-tis	
hepatocyte	☐ **HEP**-ah-toh-sight	

Term		Pronunciation	
hepatomegaly	☐	**hep**-ah-toh-**MEG**-ah-lee	___
hepatorrhaphy	☐	hep-ah-**TOR**-ah-fee	___
hernia	☐	**HER**-nee-ah	___
herniorrhaphy	☐	her-nee-**OR**-ah-fee	___
herpetic stomatitis	☐	her-**PEH**-tic stoh-mah-**TYE**-tis	___
Hirschsprung's disease	☐	**HIRSH**-sprungz dih-**ZEEZ**	___
hydrochloric acid	☐	**high**-droh-**KLOH**-rik acid	___
hyperemesis	☐	**high**-per-**EM**-eh-sis	___
icterus	☐	**ICK**-ter-us	___
ileocecal	☐	**ill**-ee-oh-**SEE**-kahl	___
ileum	☐	**ILL**-ee-um	___
ileus	☐	**ILL**-ee-us	___
incisor	☐	in-**SIGH**-zor	___
insulin	☐	**IN**-soo-lin	___
intestinal obstruction	☐	in-**TESS**-tih-nal ob-**STRUCK**-shun	___
intussusception	☐	**in**-tuh-suh-**SEP**-shun	___
irritable bowel syndrome (IBS)	☐	**EAR**-it-ah-b'l **BOW**-el **SIN**-drom	___
jaundice	☐	**JAWN**-diss	___
jejunostomy	☐	jee-joo-**NOSS**-toh-mee	___
jejunum	☐	jee-**JOO**-num	___
laparoscopy	☐	lap-ar-**OSS**-koh-pee	___
lingual	☐	**LING**-gwall	___
lipase	☐	**LIH**-pays *or* **LIGH**-pays	___
lipolysis	☐	lip-**ALL**-ih-sis	___
lipoma	☐	lih-**POH**-mah	___
lithogenesis	☐	**lith**-oh-**JEN**-eh-sis	___
lithotripsy	☐	**LITH**-oh-**trip**-see	___
liver biopsy	☐	**LIV**-er **BYE**-op-see	___
liver scan	☐	**LIV**-er **SCAN**	___
mandibular	☐	man-**DIB**-yoo-lar	___

Term		Pronunciation	
mastication	☐	mas-tih-**KAY**-shun	______
melena	☐	**MELL**-eh-nah	______
molar	☐	**MOH**-lar	______
nasogastric intubation	☐	nay-zoh-**GAS**-trik **in**-too-**BAY**-shun	______
nausea	☐	**NAW**-zee-ah	______
nutritionist	☐	noo-**TRIH**-shun-ist	______
oral	☐	**OR**-al	______
oral leukoplakia	☐	**OR**-al **loo**-koh-**PLAY**-kee-ah	______
oropharynx	☐	or-oh-**FAIR**-inks	______
orthodontist	☐	**or**-thoh-**DON**-tist	______
palate	☐	**PAL**-at	______
pancreas	☐	**PAN**-kree-ass	______
pancreatitis	☐	**pan**-kree-ah-**TYE**-tis	______
papillae	☐	pah-**PILL**-ay	______
parotid gland	☐	pah-**ROT**-id gland	______
peptic	☐	**PEP**-tik	______
percutaneous transhepatic cholangiography	☐	**per**-kyoo-**TAY**-nee-us trans-heh-**PAT**-ik koh-**lan**-jee-**OGG**-rah-fee	______
periodontal	☐	pair-ee-oh-**DON**-tal	______
peristalsis	☐	pair-ih-**STALL**-sis	______
peritoneal	☐	**pair**-ih-toh-**NEE**-al	______
pharyngoscope	☐	fair-**IN**-goh-skohp	______
pharynx	☐	**FAIR**-inks	______
polyphagia	☐	**pall**-ee-**FAY**-jee-ah	______
proctoscopy	☐	prok-**TOSS**-koh-pee	______
pruritis ani	☐	proo-**RIGH**-tus **AN**-eye	______
pyloric sphincter	☐	pigh-**LOR**-ik **SFINGK**-ter	______
rectum	☐	**REK**-tum	______
rectocele	☐	**REK**-toh-seel	______
rugae	☐	**ROO**-gay	______
saliva	☐	sah-**LYE**-vah	______

Term	Pronunciation	
salivary glands	☐ **SAL**-ih-vair-ee glands	______
serum bilirubin	☐ **SEE**-rum bill-ih-**ROO**-bin	______
serum glutamic-oxaloacetic transaminase	☐ **SEE**-rum gloo-**TAM**-ik **oks**-al-ah-**SEE**-tik trans-**AM**-in-ays	______
sialogram	☐ sigh-**AL**-oh-gram	______
sigmoid colon	☐ **SIG**-moyd colon	______
sigmoidoscopy	☐ **sig**-moyd-**OSS**-koh-pee	______
spastic colon	☐ **SPAS**-tik **COH**-lon	______
sphincter	☐ **SFINGK**-ter	______
steatorrhea	☐ **stee**-ah-toh-**REE**-ah	______
stomach	☐ **STUM**-ak	______
stomatitis	☐ stoh-mah-**TYE**-tis	______
stomatoplasty	☐ **STOH**-mah-toh-**plass**-tee	______
stool culture	☐ **STOOL KULL**-chir	______
stool guaiac	☐ **STOOL GWEE**-ak	______
thrush	☐ **THRUSH**	______
triglycerides	☐ try-**GLISS**-er-eyeds	______
ulcer	☐ **ULL**-sir	______
ulcerative colitis	☐ **ULL**-sir-ah-tiv koh-**LYE**-tis	______
urinary bilirubin	☐ **YOO**-rih-nair-ee bill-ih-**ROO**-bin	______
uvula	☐ **YOO**-vyoo-lah	______
villi	☐ **VIL**-eye	______
volvulus	☐ **VOL**-vyoo-lus	______
vomit	☐ **VOM**-it	______
vomitus	☐ **VOM**-ih-tus	______

Chapter Review Exercises

The following exercises provide a more in-depth review of the chapter material. Your goal in these exercises is to complete each section at a minimum 80% level of accuracy. A place has been provided for your score at the end of each section.

A. Crossword Puzzle

Read the clues carefully and complete the puzzle. Each crossword answer is worth 10 points. When you have completed the crossword puzzle, total your points and enter your score in the space provided at the end of the exercise.

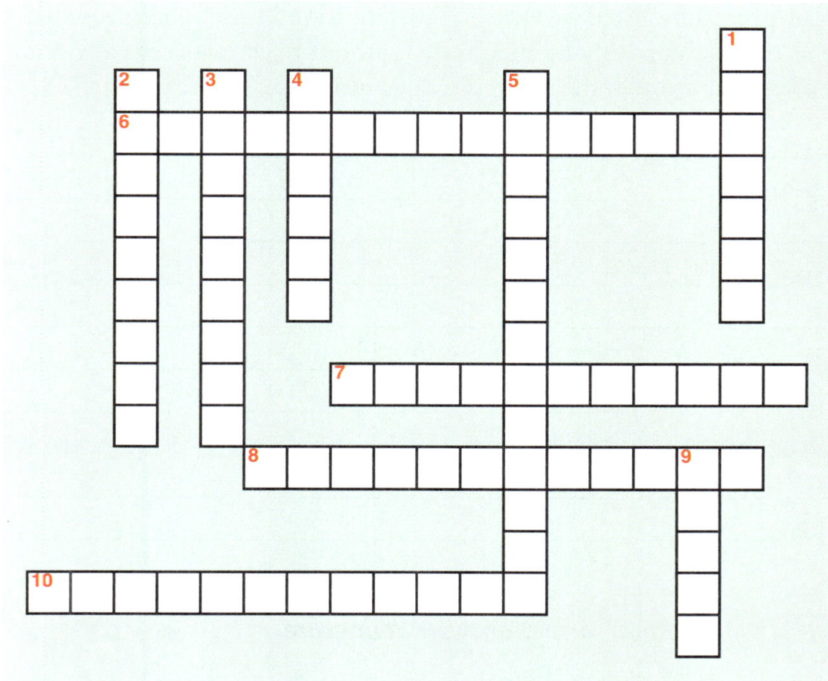

ACROSS

6 Surgical removal of the gallbladder
7 Distended veins in the rectum/anus
8 Inflammation of the pancreas
10 Surgical repair of the lips

DOWN

1 Enzyme that digests sugars
2 Decreased motility of esophagus
3 New opening of colon onto abdomen
4 Protrudes through its cavity wall
5 Surgical repair of a hernia
9 Obstruction of the intestine

Number correct ______ × 10 points/correct answer: Your score ______%

B. Spelling

Circle the correctly spelled term in each pairing of words. Each correct answer is worth 10 points. Record your score in the space provided at the end of the exercise.

1. chyme — chime
2. decidious — deciduous
3. defication — defecation
4. gavage — gevage
5. jejenum — jejunum

6. peristaltsis	peristalsis
7. sphincter	spincter
8. uvula	uvala
9. pharynx	pharynix
10. lipase	lypase

Number correct ______ × 10 points/correct answer: Your score ______%

C. Term to Definition

Define each diagnosis or procedure listed by writing the definition in the space provided. Check the box if you are able to complete this exercise correctly the first time (without referring to the answers). Each correct answer is worth 10 points. Record your score in the space provided at the end of the exercise.

☐ 1. dental caries ______________________________
☐ 2. herpetic stomatitis ______________________________
☐ 3. cirrhosis ______________________________
☐ 4. intussusception ______________________________
☐ 5. paracentesis ______________________________
☐ 6. gastric analysis ______________________________
☐ 7. small bowel follow-through ______________________________
☐ 8. irritable bowel syndrome ______________________________
☐ 9. ERCP ______________________________
☐ 10. oral leukoplakia ______________________________

Number correct ______ × 10 points/correct answer: Your score ______%

D. Matching Pathological Conditions

Match the definitions on the right with the appropriate pathological condition on the left. Each correct answer is worth 10 points. Record your score in the space provided at the end of the exercise.

_____ 1. cholelithiasis
_____ 2. aphthous stomatitis
_____ 3. periodontal disease
_____ 4. celiac disease
_____ 5. achalasia
_____ 6. dysentery
_____ 7. hepatitis
_____ 8. Hirschsprung's disease
_____ 9. peptic ulcer
_____ 10. volvulus

a. A term used to describe a group of inflammatory gum disorders that may lead to degeneration of teeth, gums, and sometimes surrounding bones
b. Nutrient malabsorption due to damaged small bowel mucosa because of gluten sensitivity
c. A rotation of loops of bowel causing a twisting on itself, which results in an intestinal obstruction
d. Pigmented or hardened cholesterol stones formed as a result of bile crystallization
e. Acute or chronic inflammation of the liver due to a viral or bacterial infection, drugs, alcohol, toxins, or parasites
f. Absence at birth of the autonomic ganglia in a segment of the intestinal smooth muscle wall that normally stimulates peristalsis

g. A term used to describe painful intestinal inflammation typically caused by ingesting water or food containing bacteria, protozoa, parasites, or chemical irritants

h. Small inflammatory noninfectious ulcerated lesions occurring on the lips, tongue, and inside the cheeks of the mouth; also called canker sores

i. Decreased mobility of the lower two-thirds of the esophagus along with constriction of the lower esophageal sphincter

j. A break in the continuity of the mucous membrane lining of the GI tract as a result of hyperacidity and/or the bacterium, *Helicobacter pylori*

Number correct _______ × 10 points/correct answer: Your score _______%

E. Definition to Term

Using the following definitions, identify and provide the medical term to match the definition. Each correct answer is worth 10 points. Record your score in the space provided at the end of the exercise.

1. Complete or partial alteration in the forward flow of the contents in the small or large intestines

____

2. Noninflamed outpouchings or herniations through the muscular layer of the intestine, typically the sigmoid colon

____

3. Inflammatory infectious lesions in or on the oral cavity occurring as a primary or a secondary viral infection caused by herpes simplex

____

4. An abnormal passageway in the skin surface near the anus usually connecting with the rectum

____

5. Digestive tract inflammation of a chronic nature causing fever, cramping, diarrhea, weight loss, and anorexia

____

6. A large number of polyps in the large bowel. A polyp is a small growth projecting from a mucous membrane.

____

7. The presence of a malignant neoplasm in the large intestine

____

8. An expression used to characterize both diverticulosis and diverticulitis

____

9. Swollen extended veins located in the esophagus at the distal end in a winding structure. Usually caused by portal hypertension, which occurs as a result of liver disease

____

10. Absence at birth of the autonomic ganglia in a segment of the intestinal smooth muscle wall that normally stimulates peristalsis

____

Number correct _______ × 10 points/correct answer: Your score _______%

F. Word Search

Using the definitions provided, identify the term and then find and circle it in the puzzle. The words may be read up, down, diagonally, across, or backward. Each correct answer is worth 10 points. Record your score in the space provided at the end of the exercise.

Example: A test for conjugated or direct bilirubin in a urine specimen:
urinary bilirubin

1. A permanently distended vein, called a varicosity, in the distal rectum or anus:
____
2. Acute or chronic inflammation of the liver due to a viral or bacterial infection, drugs, alcohol, toxins, or parasites:
____
3. An irregular protrusion of tissue, organ, or a portion of an organ through an abnormal break in the enveloping cavity's muscular wall:
____
4. Surgical creation of an artificial abdominal wall anus by bringing the incised colon out to the abdominal surface:
____
5. Study of the stomach contents to determine the acid content and to detect the presence of blood, bacteria, bile, and abnormal cells:
____
6. Insertion of a needle or trochar into the peritoneal cavity to remove ascitic fluid with the person in a sitting position:
____
7. A disease of the liver that is chronic and degenerative causing injury to the hepatocytes:
____
8. Telescoping of a portion of proximal intestine into distal intestine, usually in the ileocecal region, causing an obstruction:
____
9. A fungal infection in the mouth and throat producing sore, pale yellow, slightly raised lesions or patches:
____
10. An acute or chronic destructive inflammatory condition of the pancreas:
____

U	L	E	X	I	O	N	O	A	T	T	S	I	S	L
R	O	I	R	E	T	S	O	P	O	R	E	T	N	A
I	A	D	Y	A	H	U	T	E	A	A	G	R	Y	S
N	O	I	T	P	E	C	S	U	S	S	U	T	N	I
A	S	O	I	R	P	I	I	L	E	I	I	H	A	S
R	I	H	Y	O	A	T	H	R	U	S	H	P	D	Y
Y	T	R	D	E	T	H	I	M	B	E	I	A	I	L
B	I	R	E	U	I	O	E	X	R	T	N	R	O	A
I	V	O	C	V	T	N	G	N	T	N	P	G	P	N
L	N	M	C	I	I	N	I	I	I	E	N	O	A	A
I	N	E	E	R	S	A	A	R	S	C	A	I	Q	C
R	C	H	O	L	Y	M	A	J	I	O	V	D	U	I
U	S	I	T	I	T	A	E	R	C	N	A	P	E	R
B	U	I	A	I	A	S	R	M	L	I	S	R	P	T
I	J	O	L	S	Y	H	S	H	C	M	S	Y	A	S
N	N	N	U	C	O	L	O	S	T	O	M	Y	R	A
S	O	O	S	S	S	R	S	L	F	D	E	P	X	G
P	C	A	I	M	I	G	A	I	U	B	H	P	Y	A
T	Q	S	D	A	R	E	P	Y	M	A	K	L	T	R

Number correct _______ × 10 points/correct answer: Your score _______%

G. Matching Abbreviations

Match the abbreviations on the left with the correct definition on the right. Each correct answer is worth 5 points. Record your score in the space provided at the end of the exercise.

_____ 1. a.c.	a. total parenteral nutrition
_____ 2. BE	b. small bowel series
_____ 3. GBS	c. postprandial
_____ 4. GERD	d. percutaneous transhepatic cholangiogram
_____ 5. GTT	e. after meals
_____ 6. IBS	f. nasogastric
_____ 7. LES	g. interbowel sphincter
_____ 8. NG	h. nausea and vomiting
_____ 9. PTC	i. magnetic resonance imaging
_____ 10. pp	j. liver function tests
_____ 11. MRI	k. motionless rugae internicus
_____ 12. IVC	l. intravenous colostomy

_____ 13. GI
_____ 14. HBV
_____ 15. HCl
_____ 16. LFTs
_____ 17. N&V
_____ 18. p.c.
_____ 19. SBS
_____ 20. TPN

m. irritable bowel syndrome
n. intravenous cholangiography
o. before meals
p. hepatitis B virus
q. hydrochloric acid
r. barium enema
s. gallbladder series
t. gastroesophageal reflux disease
u. gastrointestinal
v. glucose tolerance test
w. gastric endoscopic retrograde dissection
x. neck and vein
y. lower esophageal sphincter

Number correct _______ × 5 points/correct answer: Your score _______%

H. Identify the Structures

Identify the structures of the oral cavity by writing your answers in the spaces provided. Each correct response is worth 10 points. Record your score in the space provided at the end of the exercise.

1. ______________________________
2. ______________________________
3. ______________________________
4. ______________________________
5. ______________________________
6. ______________________________
7. ______________________________
8. ______________________________
9. ______________________________
10. ______________________________

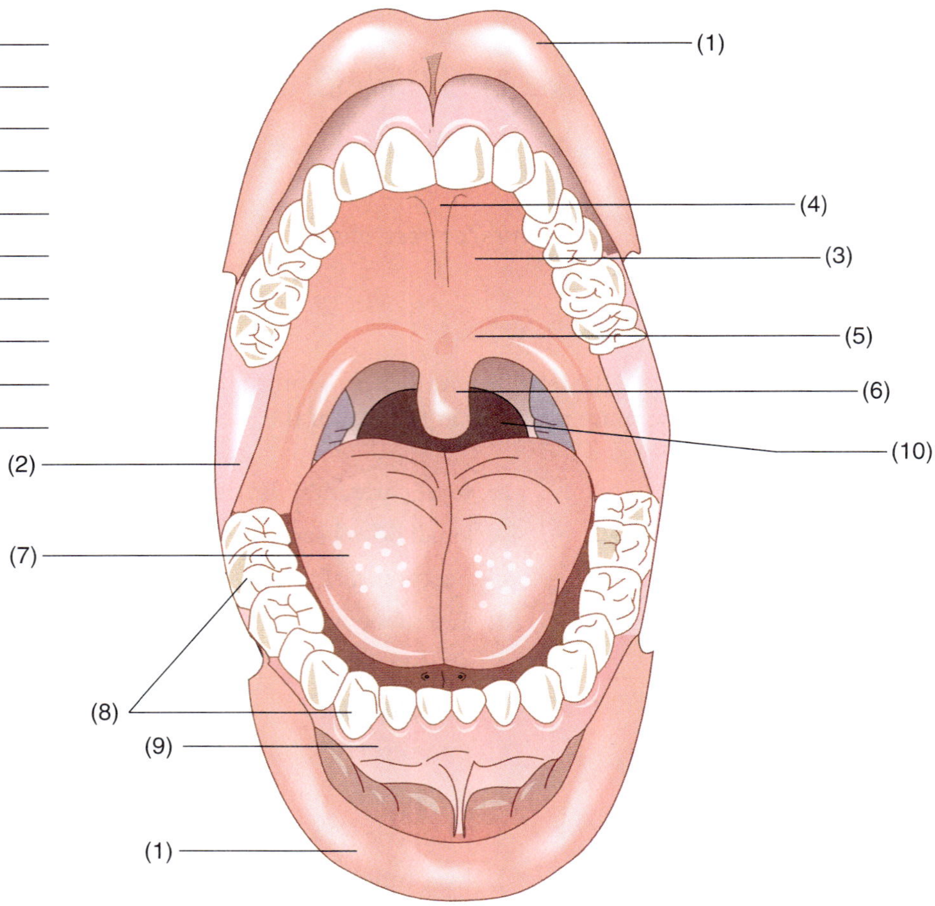

Number correct _______ × 10 points/correct answer: Your score _______%

I. Completion

The following sentences relate to the digestive system. Complete each sentence with the most appropriate word. Each correct answer is worth 10 points. Record your score in the space provided at the end of the exercise.

1. An abnormal condition characterized by the absence of hydrochloric acid in the gastric juice is known as ______________________.
2. A yellow discoloration of the skin, mucous membranes, and sclera of the eyes, caused by greater than normal amounts of bilirubin in the blood, is known as jaundice or ______________________.
3. The material expelled from the stomach during vomiting is known as vomitus or ____________________.
4. An abnormal accumulation of fluid within the peritoneal cavity (the fluid contains large amounts of protein and electrolytes) is known as ______________________.
5. An unpleasant sensation often leading to the urge to vomit is known as ______________________.
6. Decreased mobility of the lower two-thirds of the esophagus along with constriction of the lower esophageal sphincter is called ______________________.
7. A condition known as aphthous stomatitis, in which there are small inflammatory noninfectious ulcerated lesions occurring on the lips, tongue, and inside the cheeks of the mouth called __________________ __________________ (two words).
8. Greater than normal amounts of fat in the feces, characterized by frothy, foul-smelling fecal matter that floats is known as ______________________.
9. A permanently distended vein, called a varicosity, in the distal rectum or anus is known as a ________________.
10. A term used to describe an obstruction of the intestine is ______________________.

Number correct ________ × 10 points/correct answer. Your score ________%

J. True or False

Read each statement carefully and circle the correct answer as true or false. **HINT:** Pay close attention to the word elements written in bold as you make your decision. If the statement is false, identify the meaning of that word element. Each correct answer is worth 10 points. Record your score in the space provided at the end of the exercise.

1. Insertion of a needle or trochar into the peritoneal cavity to remove excess fluid, with the person in a sitting position, is known as an abdomino**centesis.**

   True False

   If your answer is false, what does *-centesis* mean? ____

2. Surgically correcting a defect of the stomach is known as a **cheil**oplasty.

   True False

   If your answer is false, what does *cheil/o* mean? ____

3. The surgical removal of the gallbladder is known as a **chol**ecystectomy.

   True False

   If your answer is false, what does *chol/e* mean? ____

4. The surgical creation of a new opening into the gallbladder is known as a **col**ostomy.

   True False

   If your answer is false, what does *col/o* mean? ______________________

5. The surgical removal of a hernia is known as a hernio**rrhaphy.**

   True False

   If your answer is false, what does *-rrhaphy* mean? ______________________

6. The term **gingiv**ae is another name for the gums.

   True False

   If your answer is false, what does *gingiv/o* mean? ______________________

7. The conversion of simple sugar (glucose) into a complex form of sugar (starch) for storage in the liver is known as glycogeno**lysis.**

   True False

   If your answer is false, what does *-lysis* mean? ______________________

8. A backflow of contents of the duodenum into the esophagus is known as **gastr**oesophageal reflux.

   True False

   If your answer is false, what does *gastr/o* mean? ______________________

9. A condition characterized by the loss of the ability to swallow as a result of organic or psychologic causes is known as a**phag**ia.

   True False

   If your answer is false, what does *phag/o* mean? ______________________

10. The frequent passage of loose, watery stools is known as dia**rrhea.**

    True False

    If your answer is false, what does *-rrhea* mean? ______________________

Number correct* ______ × *10 points/correct answer: Your score* ______*%

Answers to Chapter Review Exercises

A. Crossword Puzzle

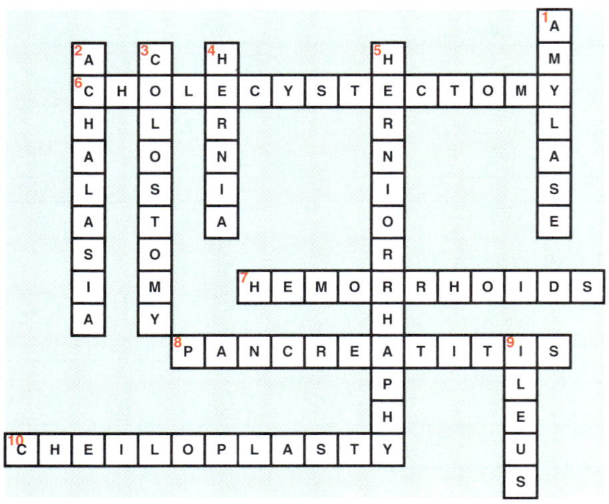

B. Spelling

1. chyme
2. deciduous
3. defecation
4. gavage
5. jejunum
6. peristalsis
7. sphincter
8. uvula
9. pharynx
10. lipase

C. Term to Definition

1. tooth decay caused by acid-forming microorganisms
2. inflammatory infectious lesions in or on the oral cavity occurring as a primary or a secondary viral infection caused by herpes simplex
3. a disease of the liver, which is chronic and degenerative causing injury to the hepatocytes (the functional cells of the liver)
4. telescoping of a portion of proximal intestine into distal intestine usually in the ileocecal region causing an obstruction

5. insertion of a needle or trochar into the peritoneal cavity to remove ascitic fluid with the person in a sitting position
6. study of the stomach contents to determine the acid content and to detect the presence of blood, bacteria, bile, and abnormal cells
7. oral administration of a radiopaque contrast medium, barium sulfate, which flows through the GI system
8. increased motility of the small or large intestinal wall resulting in abdominal pain, flatulence, nausea, anorexia, and the trapping of gas throughout the intestines
9. stands for *e*ndoscopic *r*etrograde which is *c*holangio*p*ancreatography
10. a precancerous lesion occurring anywhere in the mouth

D. Matching Pathological Conditions

1. d
2. h
3. a
4. b
5. i
6. g
7. e
8. f
9. j
10. c

E. Definition to Term

1. intestinal obstruction
2. diverticulosis
3. herpetic stomatitis
4. anal fistula
5. Crohn's disease
6. colonic polyposis
7. colorectal cancer
8. diverticular disease
9. esophageal varices
10. congenital megacolon

F. Word Search

U	L	E	X	I	O	N	O	A	T	T	S	I	S	L
R	O	I	R	E	T	S	O	P	O	R	E	T	N	A
I	A	D	Y	A	H	U	T	E	A	A	G	R	Y	S
N	O	I	T	P	E	C	S	U	S	S	U	T	N	I
A	S	O	I	R	P	I	I	L	E	I	I	H	A	S
R	I	H	Y	O	A	T	H	R	U	S	H	P	D	Y
Y	T	R	D	E	T	H	I	M	B	E	I	A	I	L
B	I	R	E	U	I	O	E	X	R	T	N	R	O	A
I	V	O	C	V	T	N	G	N	T	N	P	G	P	N
L	N	M	C	I	I	N	I	I	I	E	N	O	A	A
I	N	E	E	R	S	A	A	R	S	C	A	I	Q	C
R	C	H	O	L	Y	M	A	J	I	O	V	D	U	I
U	S	I	T	I	T	A	E	R	C	N	A	P	E	R
B	U	I	A	I	A	S	R	M	L	I	S	R	P	T
I	J	O	L	S	Y	H	S	H	C	M	S	Y	A	S
N	N	N	U	C	O	L	O	S	T	O	M	Y	R	A
S	O	O	S	S	S	R	S	L	F	D	E	P	X	G
P	C	A	I	M	I	G	A	I	U	B	H	P	Y	A
T	Q	S	D	A	R	E	P	Y	M	A	K	L	T	R

G. Matching Abbreviations

1. o
2. r
3. s
4. t
5. v
6. m
7. y
8. f
9. d
10. c
11. i
12. n
13. u
14. p
15. q
16. j
17. h
18. e
19. b
20. a

H. Labeling

1. lips
2. cheeks
3. hard palate
4. rugae
5. soft palate
6. uvula
7. tongue
8. teeth
9. gums or gingivae
10. oropharynx

I. Completion

1. achlorhydria
2. icterus
3. emesis
4. ascites
5. nausea
6. achalasia
7. canker sores
8. steatorrhea
9. hemorrhoid
10. ileus

J. True or False

1. True
2. False; cheil/o = lips
3. True
4. False; col/o = colon
5. False; rrhaphy = suturing
6. True
7. False; lysis = destruction or detachment
8. False; gastr/o = stomach
9. True
10. True

CHAPTER 13

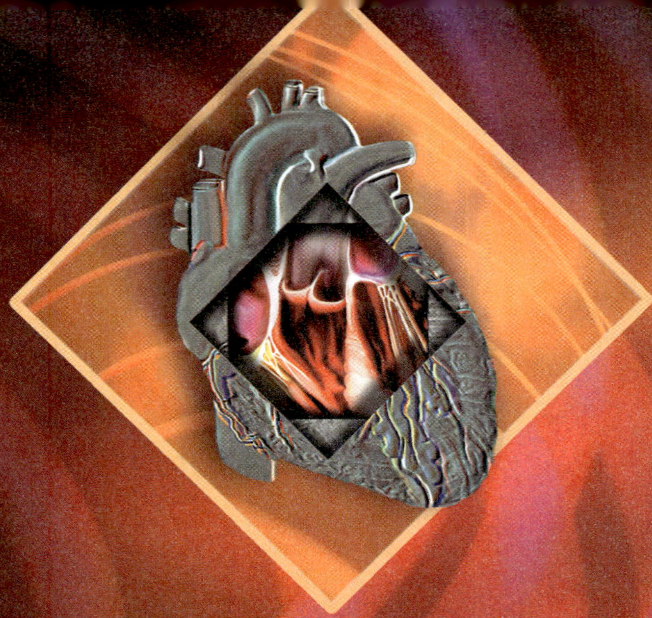

The Endocrine System

CHAPTER CONTENT

KEY COMPETENCIES

Upon completing this chapter and the review exercises at the end of the chapter, the learner should be able to:

1. Define diabetes mellitus, gestational diabetes, and diabetes insipidus and identify the differences among the three conditions.
2. List the nine endocrine glands identified in this chapter.
3. Identify and define at least 20 pathological conditions of the endocrine system.
4. Correctly spell and pronounce each new term introduced in this chapter using the Activity CD-ROM and Audio CD, if available.
5. Create at least 10 medical terms related to the endocrine system and identify the correct combining form for each word.
6. Identify and define at least 10 abbreviations common to the endocrine system.
7. Identify and define at least 10 hormones secreted by the endocrine glands and the gland that secretes each of the hormones.
8. Identify and define at least 20 medical terms defined in the vocabulary section of this chapter.

OVERVIEW

The **endocrine** system consists of a network of ductless glands that secrete chemicals, called hormones, that affect the function of specific organs within the body, thus regulating many of the intricate functions of the body itself. These ductless glands secrete their hormones directly into the bloodstream as opposed to releasing them externally through ducts, as do the sweat glands and the oil glands.

The field of medicine that deals with the study of the endocrine system and the treatment of the diseases and disorders of the endocrine system is known as **endocrinology**. The physician who specializes in the medical practice of endocrinology is known as an **endocrinologist**.

This chapter will concentrate on the following endocrine glands: the pituitary, pineal, thyroid, parathyroid, thymus, adrenal, pancreas, ovaries, and testes. The discussion of each gland will begin with an anatomical description followed by the physiology, or function, of that particular gland and the hormone(s) it secretes.

Anatomy and Physiology

Refer to **Figure 13-1** for a full body view of the endocrine glands discussed as well as other body organs to help identify the location of the glands in the body.

Pituitary Gland

The pituitary gland is a pea-sized gland of minute weight but important responsibility, so much so that it is often referred to as the "master gland." It secretes hormones that control the functions of other glands. It is located beneath the brain in the pituitary fossa (depression) of the sphenoid bone, which is behind and slightly above the nose and throat. Also known as the **hypophysis**, the pituitary gland is connected to the hypothalamus of the brain by a stalklike projection call the **infundibulum**. Although the pituitary gland appears as one gland, it has two distinct lobes: the anterior pituitary gland and the posterior pituitary gland, each with very different functions. **Figure 13-2** shows the pituitary gland.

The **anterior pituitary gland**, also known as the **adenohypophysis**, develops from an upward projection of the pharynx in the embryo, and is composed of regular endocrine tissue. The anterior pituitary gland secretes the following hormones:

1. **Growth hormone (GH),** also known as **somatotropic hormone (STH),** regulates the growth of bone, muscle, and other body tissues.
2. **Adrenocorticotropic hormone** (ACTH) stimulates the normal growth and development of the adrenal cortex and the secretion of corticosteroids (primarily cortisol, corticosterone, and aldosterone).
3. **Thyroid-stimulating hormone** (TSH) promotes and maintains the normal growth and development of the thyroid gland and stimulates the secretions of the thyroid hormones.
4. **Lactogenic hormone** (LTH), also known as **prolactin,** promotes the development of the breasts during pregnancy and stimulates the secretion of milk from the breasts after delivery of the baby.

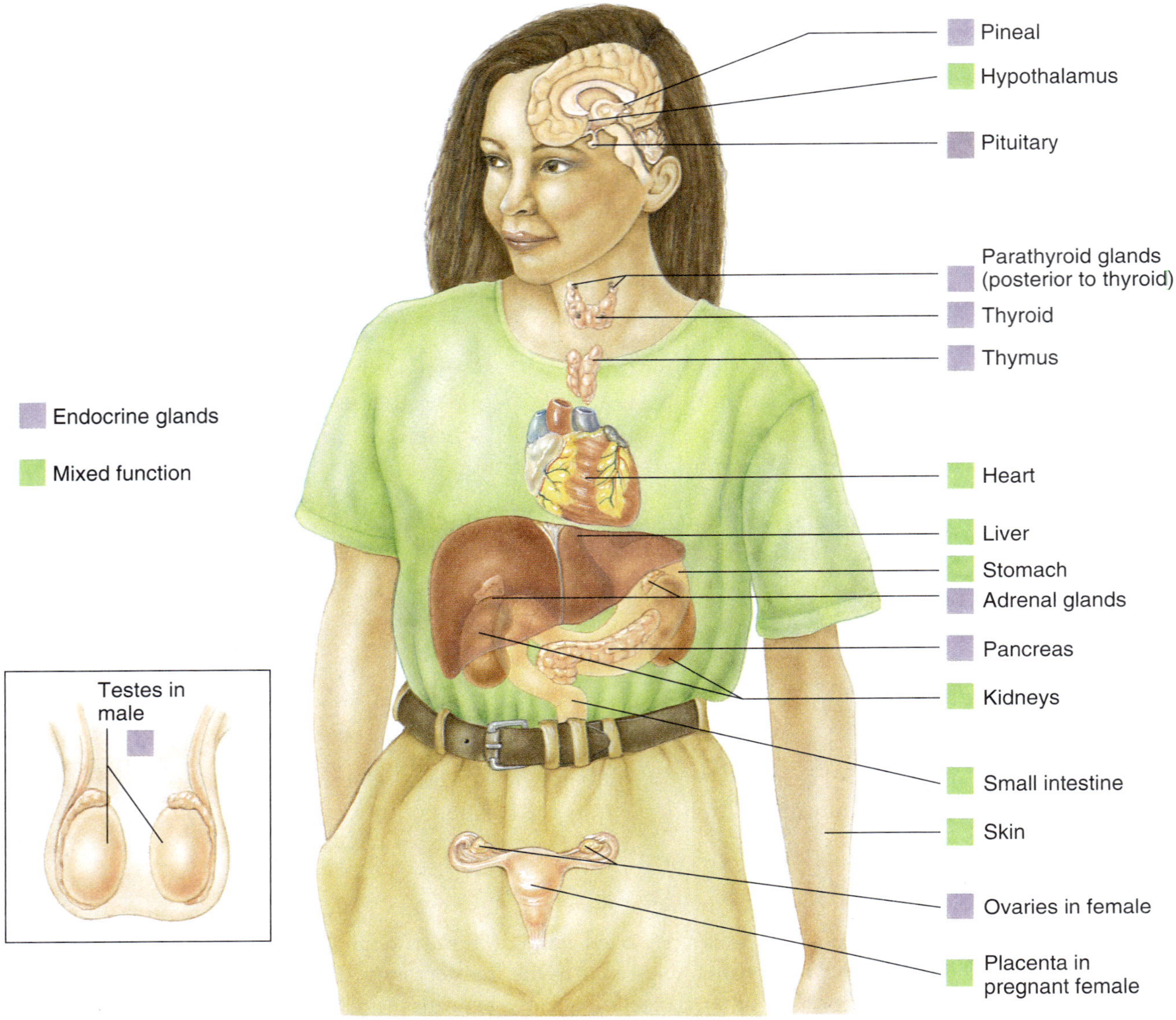

Figure 13-1 The endocrine system

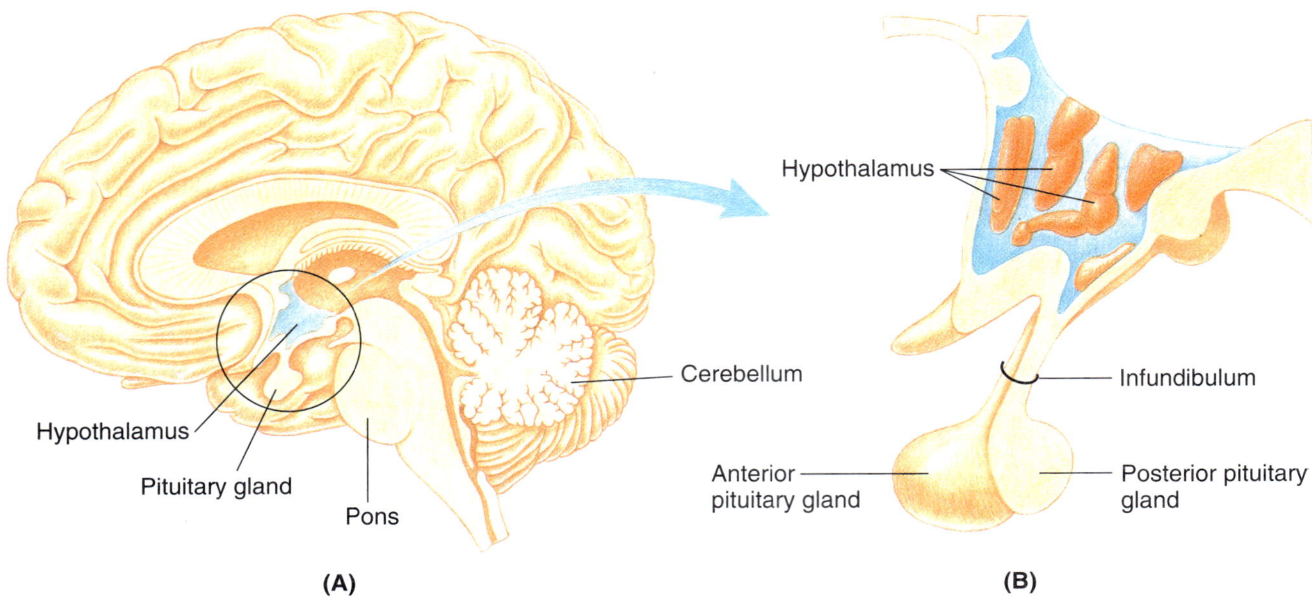

Figure 13-2 Pituitary gland

5. **Follicle-stimulating hormone** (**FSH**) stimulates the secretion of estrogen and the production of eggs (ova) in the female ovaries; also stimulates the production of sperm in the male testes.

6. **Luteinizing hormone** (**LH**) stimulates female ovulation and the secretion of testosterone (male sex hormone) in the male.

7. **Melanocyte-stimulating hormone** (**MSH**) controls the intensity of pigmentation in pigmented cells of the skin.

The **posterior pituitary gland,** also known as the **neurohypophysis,** develops from a downward projection of the base of the brain. The posterior pituitary gland stores and releases the following hormones:

1. **Antidiuretic hormone (ADH),** also called **vasopressin,** decreases the excretion of large amounts of urine from the body by increasing the reabsorption of water by the renal tubules, thus helping to maintain the body's water balance.

2. **Oxytocin** (**OT**) stimulates the contractions of the uterus during childbirth and stimulates the release of milk from the breasts of lactating women (women who breastfeed) in response to the suckling reflex of the infant.

Pineal Gland

The pineal gland is a tiny, pine cone–shaped gland located on the dorsal aspect of the midbrain region. See **Figure 13-3.**

Its exact function is not completely known, but the pineal gland does seem to play a part in supporting the body's "biological clock," that is, the regulation of our patterns of eating, sleeping, and reproduction. The pineal gland is responsible for secreting the hormone, **melatonin,** which is thought to induce sleep.

Thyroid Gland

The **thyroid** gland is located in the front of the neck just below the larynx, on either side of the trachea. It consists of a right and left lobe connected across the front of the trachea by a narrow island-shaped piece called the isthmus. Refer to **Figure 13-4** for a visual reference.

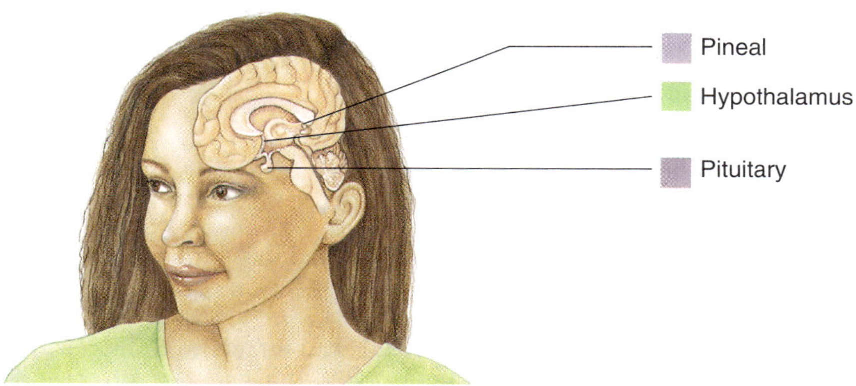

Figure 13-3 Pineal gland

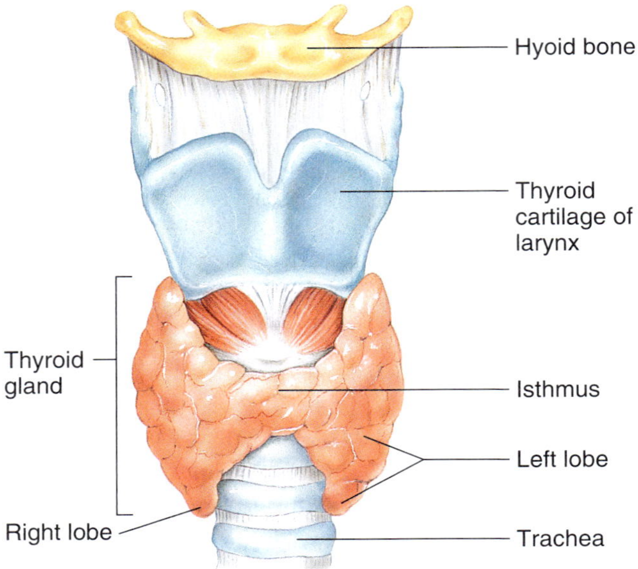

Figure 13-4 Thyroid gland

The thyroid gland secretes the following hormones:

1. **Triiodothyronine (T_3),** which helps regulate growth and development of the body, and helps control **metabolism** and body temperature.
2. **Thyroxine** (T_4), which helps maintain normal body metabolism.
3. **Calcitonin,** which regulates the level of calcium in the blood.

Parathyroid Glands

The parathyroid glands consist of four tiny rounded bodies located on the dorsal aspect of the thyroid gland. See **Figure 13-5.**

The parathyroid glands are responsible for secreting the **parathyroid hormone (PTH),** also known as **parathormone,** which regulates the level of calcium in the blood. Calcium is stored in the bones. If the blood calcium level falls too low (**hypocalcemia**), the parathyroid glands are triggered to secrete more parathyroid hormone, which will draw the calcium from the bones into the bloodstream, restoring the blood calcium level to a normal level. On the other hand, if the blood calcium level is too high (**hypercalcemia**), the parathyroid glands secrete less PTH, which allows the excess calcium to be drawn from the bloodstream into storage in the bones, thus returning the blood calcium back to a normal level.

Thymus

The thymus is a single gland located in the mediastinum near the middle of the chest, just beneath the sternum. See **Figure 13-6** for a visual reference.

The thymus is large in the fetus and infants, and shrinks with increasing age until there is merely a trace of active thymus tissue in older adults. Although it is a gland of the lymphatic system, the thymus is considered to be an endocrine gland because it secretes hor-

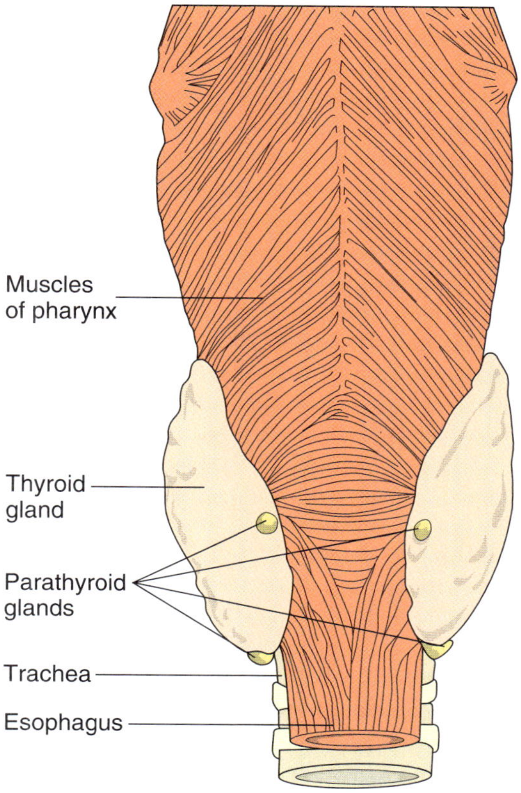

Figure 13-5 Parathyroid glands

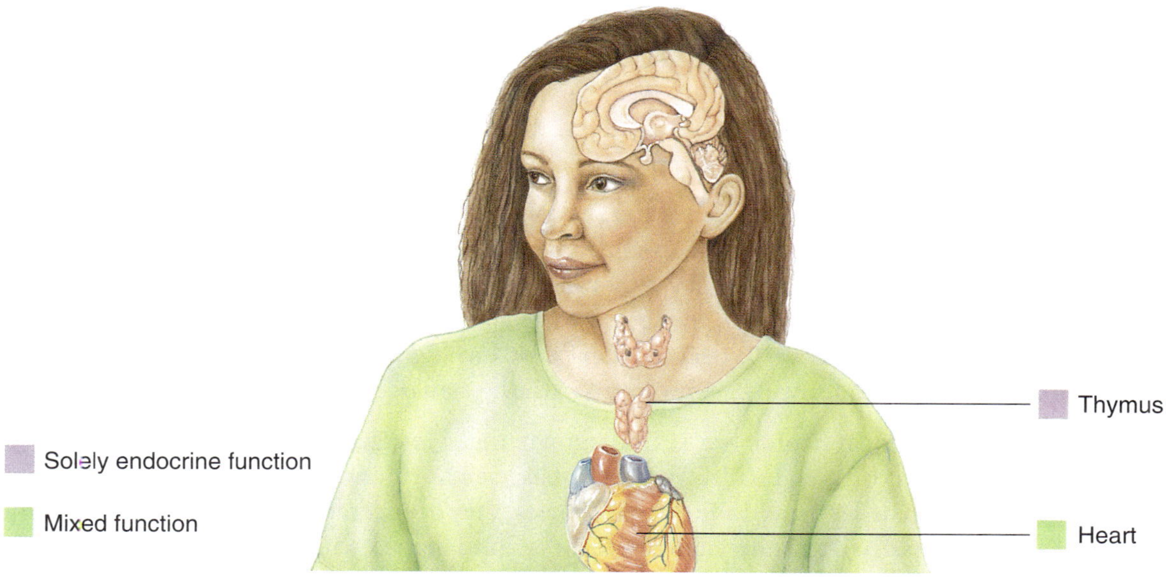

Figure 13-6 Thymus

mones directly into the bloodstream, which have a critical role in the development of the immune system. The hormones secreted by the thymus are:

1. **Thymosin**, thought to stimulate the production of specialized lymphocytes called T cells, which are involved in the immune response.
2. **Thymopoietin**, also thought to stimulate the production of T cells that are involved in the immune response.

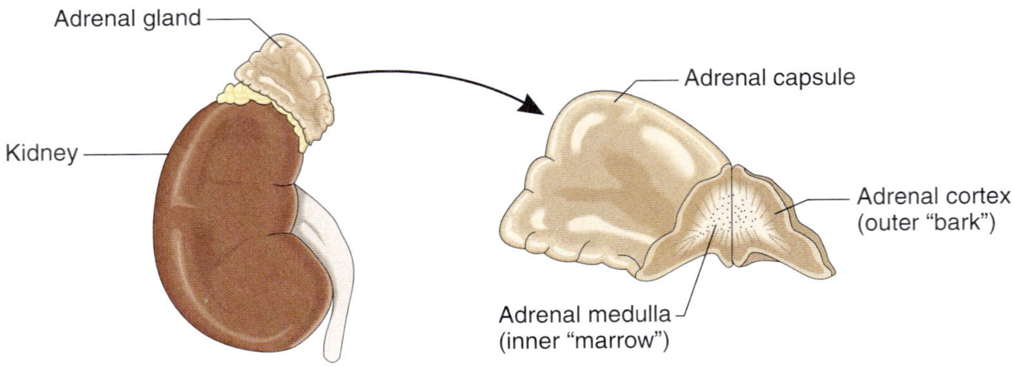

Figure 13-7 Adrenal glands

Adrenal Glands

The adrenal glands consist of two small glands, with one being positioned atop each kidney. Each adrenal gland consists of an **adrenal cortex** or outer portion, and an **adrenal medulla** or inner portion—each part having independent functions. The adrenal glands are also known as the **suprarenal glands. Figure 13-7** provides a visual reference of the adrenal glands.

The adrenal cortex is the outer, greater portion of the adrenal gland. It secretes steroid hormones known as **corticosteroids**. The adrenal cortex secretes the following corticosteroid hormones:

1. **Mineralocorticoids** regulate how mineral salts are processed in the body. Mineral salts are also known as **electrolytes.** The primary mineralocorticoid hormone secreted by the body is **aldosterone**, which is responsible for regulating fluid and electrolyte balance by promoting sodium retention (which promotes water retention) and potassium excretion.
2. **Glucocorticoids** influence the metabolism of carbohydrates, fats, and proteins in the body. In addition, glucocorticoids are necessary in the body for maintaining a normal blood pressure level, they have an anti-inflammatory effect on the body, and during times of stress the increased secretion of glucocorticoids increases the **glucose** available for skeletal muscles needed in "fight-or-flight" responses by the body. The main glucocorticoid secreted in the human body is **cortisol**, or **hydrocortisone.**
3. **Gonadocorticoids** are sex hormones that are released from the adrenal cortex instead of the gonads. Although these sex hormones are produced primarily by the male testes and the female ovaries, they are secreted in small amounts by the adrenal cortex and contribute to secondary sex characteristics in males and females.

The adrenal medulla is the inner portion of the adrenal gland. It secretes nonsteroid hormones called **catecholamines.** The adrenal medulla secretes the following nonsteroid hormones:

1. **Epinephrine**, or **adrenaline,** increases the heart rate and the force of the heart muscle contraction, dilates the bronchioles in the lungs, decreases peristalsis (wavelike movement) in the intestines, and raises blood glucose levels by causing the liver to convert glycogen into glucose. This hormone plays an important role in the body's response to stress by mimicking the actions of the sympathetic nervous system (i.e.,

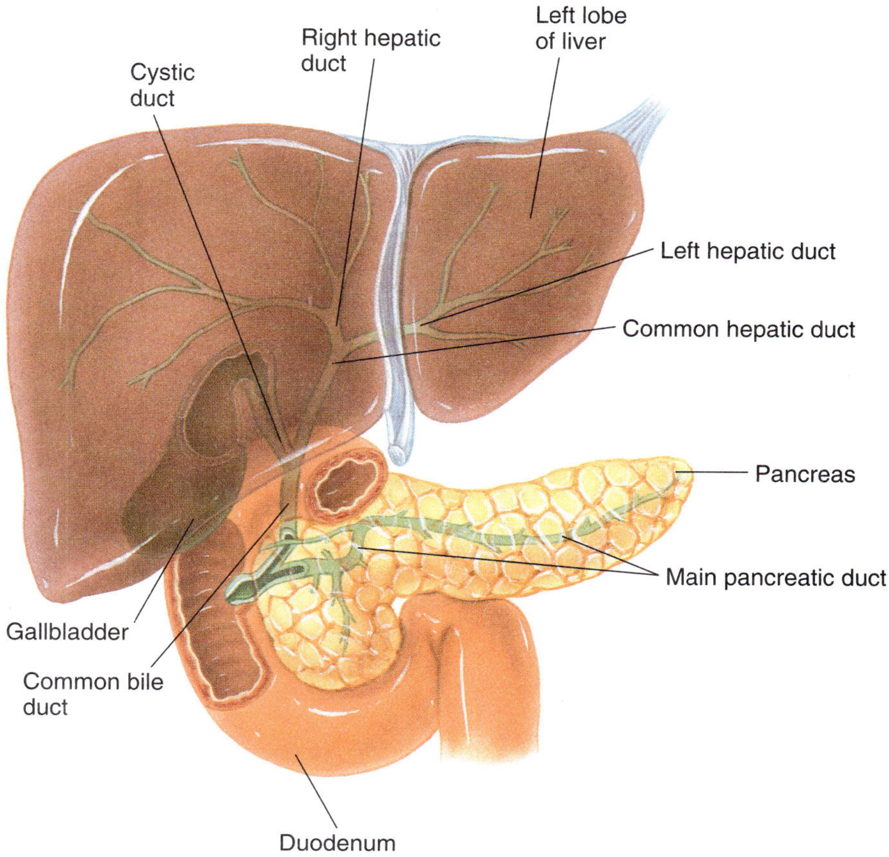

Figure 13-8 Pancreas

increasing the heart rate, dilating the bronchioles, releasing glucose into the bloodstream); epinephrine is therefore known as a **sympathomimetic agent.**

2. **Norepinephrine**, or **noradrenaline,** produces a vasoconstrictor effect on the blood vessels, thereby raising the blood pressure. This hormone also plays an important role in the body's response to stress by mimicking the actions of the sympathetic nervous system (i.e., raising the blood pressure); norepinephrine is also known as a sympathomimetic agent.

Pancreas

The **pancreas** is an elongated gland that is located in the upper left quadrant of the abdomen, behind the stomach. It extends horizontally across the body, beginning at the first part of the small intestines (duodenum) and ending at the edge of the spleen. See **Figure 13-8.**

The pancreas contains specialized groups of cells known as the **islets of Langerhans** that produce important hormones for the body. The islets of Langerhans of the pancreas produce the following hormones:

1. **Glucagon**, produced by the alpha cells of the islets of Langerhans, increases blood glucose levels by stimulating the liver to convert glycogen into glucose. Glycogen is the major carbohydrate stored by the body. It is formed from glucose and is stored chiefly in the liver to be used as needed. When the blood sugar level is extremely low

(**hypoglycemia**), the pancreas is stimulated to release glucagon into the bloodstream, thereby stimulating the liver to convert glycogen to glucose. Glucose is then released into the bloodstream, thereby raising the overall blood glucose level. This process is known as **glycogenolysis**.

2. **Insulin**, produced by the beta cells of the islets of Langerhans, makes it possible for glucose to pass from the blood through the cell membranes to be used for energy. Insulin also promotes the conversion of excess glucose into glycogen for storage in the liver for later use as needed, a process known as **glycogenesis**. When the blood sugar level is high (**hyperglycemia**), the pancreas is stimulated to release insulin into the bloodstream, thereby allowing the cells to use the glucose for energy and converting the excess glucose into a storable form, thereby reducing the overall blood glucose level.

Ovaries

The **ovaries** are the female sex glands, also known as the female **gonads**. Each of the paired ovaries is almond shaped, and is held in place by ligaments. The ovaries are located in the upper pelvic cavity, on either side of the lateral wall of the uterus, near the fimbriated (fringed) ends of the fallopian tubes. See **Figure 13-9.**

The ovaries are responsible for producing mature ova and releasing them at monthly intervals during ovulation. They are also responsible for producing hormones that are necessary for the normal growth and development of the female, and for maintaining pregnancy should it occur. The hormones produced by the ovaries are as follows:

1. **Estrogen** promotes the maturation of the ovum (egg) in the ovary and stimulates the vascularization of the uterine lining each month in preparation for implantation of a fertilized egg. Estrogen also contributes to the secondary sex characteristic changes that occur in the female with the onset of puberty. These changes include development of the glandular tissue in the breasts and deposition of fat in the breasts that give them the characteristic rounded female look, deposition of fat in the buttocks and thighs, creating the rounded adult female curvatures, widening of

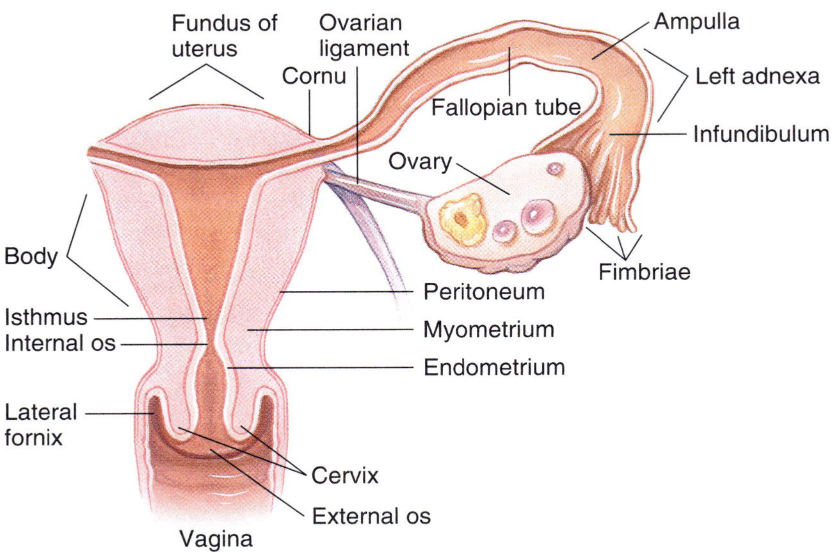

Figure 13-9 Ovaries

the pelvis into a more rounded, basinlike shape that is more appropriate for childbirth, growth of pubic and axillary hair, a general skeletal growth spurt, and a general increase in size of the female reproductive organs. The most evident change during puberty is the onset of menstruation.

2. **Progesterone** is primarily responsible for the changes that occur within the uterus in anticipation of a fertilized ovum, and for development of the maternal placenta after implantation of a fertilized ovum.

Testes

The **testes** or **male gonads** (also known as the **testicles**), are two small ovoid glands that begin their development high in the abdominal cavity, near the kidneys (retroperitoneal cavity), during the gestational period. One to 2 months before, or shortly after birth, the testicles descend through the inguinal canal into the **scrotum** where they remain. See **Figure 13-10.**

The testes are the primary organs of the male reproductive system. They are responsible for production of sperm (the male germ cell) and for the secretion of **androgens**, which are male steroid hormones. The testes produce the male hormone, **testosterone,** which is responsible for the secondary sex characteristic changes that occur in the male with the onset of puberty. These changes include growth of facial hair (beard), growth of pubic hair, deepening of the voice, growth of skeletal muscles, and enlargement of the penis, scrotum, and testes. Testosterone is also responsible for the maturation of sperm.

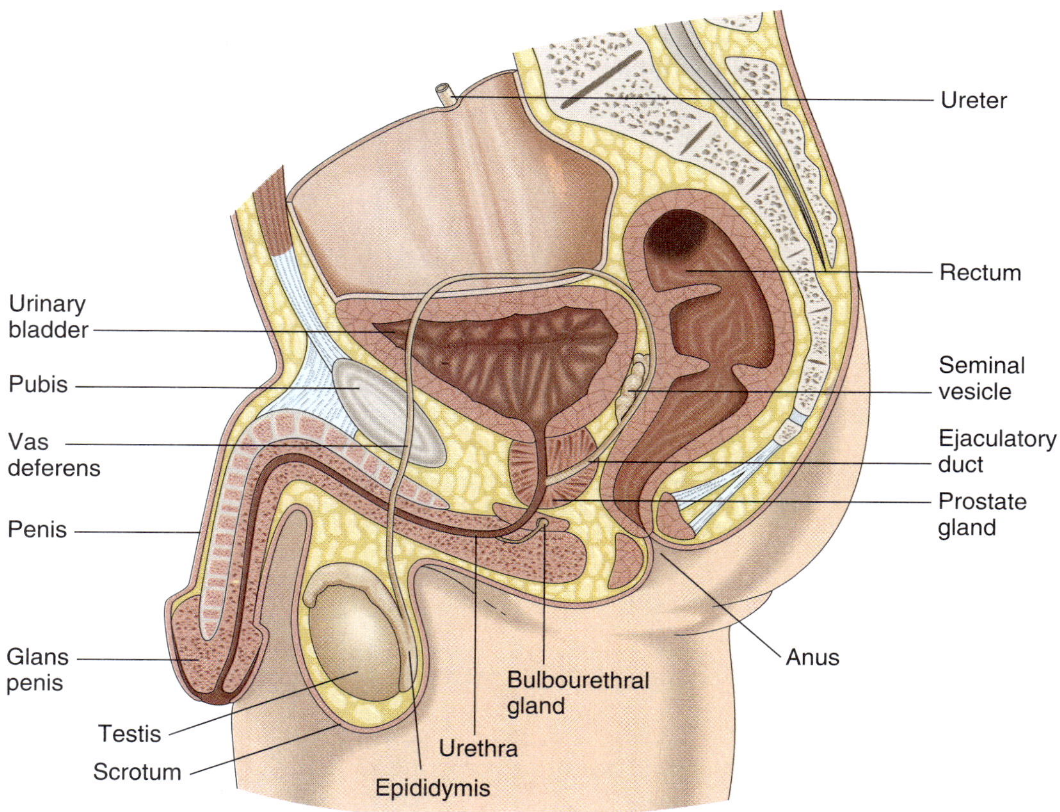

Figure 13-10 Testes

Vocabulary

The following vocabulary words are frequently used when discussing the endocrine system.

WORD	DEFINITION
acromegaly (ak-roh-**MEG**-ah-lee) acr/o = extremities -megaly = enlargement	A chronic metabolic condition characterized by gradual, noticeable enlargement and elongation of the bones of the face, jaw, and extremities, due to oversecretion of the pituitary gland after puberty.
adenohypophysis (ad-eh-noh-high-**POFF**-ih-sis)	The anterior pituitary gland.
adenoma (ad-eh-**NOH**-mah) aden/o = gland -oma = tumor	A glandular tumor.
adenopathy (ad-eh-**NOP**-ah-thee) aden/o = gland -pathy = disease	Any disease of a gland.
adrenalectomy (ad-ree-nal-**EK**-toh-mee) adren/o = adrenal gland -ectomy = surgical removal	Surgical removal of one or both of the adrenal glands.
adrenocortical (ad-ree-noh-**KOR**-tih-kal) adren/o = adrenal gland cortic/o = cortex -al = pertaining to	Pertaining to the cortex of the adrenal gland(s).
aldosterone (al-**DOSS**-ter-ohn)	A hormone secreted by the adrenal cortex that regulates sodium and potassium balance in the blood.
androgen (**AN**-droh-jen)	Any steroid hormone that increases male characteristics for example, testosterone.
antidiuretic (an-tye-dye-yoo-**RET**-ik) anti- = against di/a = through ur/o = urine -etic = pertaining to	Pertaining to the suppression of urine production; an agent given to suppress the production of urine.
cortex (**COR**-tex)	Pertaining to the outer region of an organ or structure.
cortisol (**COR**-tih-sal)	A steroid hormone occurring naturally in the body; also called hydrocortisone.

cretinism (**KREE**-tin-izm)	A congenital condition (one that occurs at birth) caused by a lack of thyroid secretion. This condition is characterized by **dwarfism**, slowed mental development, puffy facial features, dry skin, and large tongue.
diabetes, gestational (dye-ah-**BEE**-teez, jess-**TAY**-shun-al)	A condition occurring in pregnancy that is characterized by the signs and symptoms of **diabetes mellitus** such as impaired ability to metabolize carbohydrates due to insulin deficiency, and elevated blood sugar level. These symptoms usually disappear after delivery of the baby.
diabetes insipidus (dye-ah-**BEE**-teez in-**SIP**-id-us)	A metabolic disorder characterized by extreme **polydipsia** (excessive thirst) and **polyuria** (excessive urination); this is a disorder of the pituitary gland due to a deficiency in secretion of the antidiuretic hormone.
diabetes mellitus (dye-ah-**BEE**-teez **MELL**-ih-tus)	A disorder of the pancreas in which the beta cells of the islets of Langerhans of the pancreas fail to produce an adequate amount of insulin, resulting in the body's inability to appropriately metabolize carbohydrates, fats, and proteins.
dwarfism (**DWARF**-ism)	A condition in which there is an abnormal underdevelopment of the body; this condition is characterized by extremely short height and is usually caused by undersecretion of the pituitary gland (growth hormone).
endocrine gland (**EN**-doh-krin) endo- = within crin/o = secrete -e = noun ending	A ductless gland that produces a chemical substance called a hormone, which is secreted directly into the bloodstream instead of exiting the body through ducts.
endocrinologist (en-doh-krin-**ALL**-oh-jist) endo- = within crin/o = secrete -logist = one who specializes in the study of	A physician who specializes in the medical practice of treating the diseases and disorders of the endocrine system.
endocrinology (en-doh-krin-**ALL**-oh-jee) endo- = within crin/o = secrete -logy = the study of	The field of medicine that deals with the study of the endocrine system and of the treatment of the diseases and disorders of the endocrine system.
epinephrine (ep-ih-**NEF**-rin)	A hormone produced by the adrenal medulla. This hormone plays an important role in the body's response to stress by increasing the heart rate, dilating the bronchioles, and releasing glucose into the bloodstream.
estrogen (**ESS**-troh-jen)	One of the female hormones that promotes the development of female secondary sex characteristics.
euthyroid (yoo-**THIGH**-royd) eu- = well, easily, good, normal thyroid/o = thyroid gland	Pertaining to a normally functioning thyroid gland.

exocrine gland (**EKS**-oh-krin) exo- = outward crin/o = secrete -e = noun ending	A gland that opens onto the surface of the skin through ducts in the epithelium, such as an oil gland or a sweat gland.
exophthalmia (eks-off-**THAL**-mee-ah) ex- = outward ophthalm/o = eye -ia = condition	An abnormal condition characterized by a marked outward protrusion of the eyeballs.
exophthalmos (eks-off-**THAL**-mohs) ex- = outward ophthalm/o = eye -os = a suffix indicating a singular noun	See *exophthalmia.*
gigantism (**JYE**-gan-tism)	An abnormal condition characterized by excessive size and height; this condition is usually due to an oversecretion of the pituitary gland (growth hormone).
glucagon (**GLOO**-kuh-gon)	A hormone secreted by the islets of Langerhans of the pancreas that stimulates the liver to convert glycogen into glucose.
glucogenesis (gloo-koh-**JEN**-eh-sis) gluc/o = sugar, sweet -genesis = production of; formation of	The formation of glycogen from fatty acids and proteins instead of carbohydrates.
glucose (**GLOO**-kohs)	The simplest form of sugar in the body; a simple sugar found in certain foods, especially fruits; also a major source of energy for the human body.
glycogenesis (glye-koh-**JEN**-eh-sis) glyc/o = sugar, sweet -genesis = production of; formation of	The conversion of excess glucose into glycogen for storage in the liver for later use as needed.
glycosuria (glye-kohs-**YOO**-ree-ah) glyc/o = sugar, sweet -uria = urine condition	The presence of sugar in the urine.
goiter (**GOY**-ter)	Enlargement of the thyroid gland due to excessive growth (hyperplasia).
gonads (**GOH**-nadz)	A term used to refer to the female sex glands, or ovaries, and the male sex glands, or testes.
Graves' disease	**Hyperthyroidism**.
growth hormone	See *somatotropic hormone.*
hirsutism (**HER**-soot-izm)	A condition in which there is excessive body hair in a male distribution pattern.

hypercalcemia (high-per-kal-**SEE**-mee-ah) **hyper-** = excessive **calc/i** = calcium **-emia** = blood condition	Elevated blood calcium level.
hyperglycemia (high-per-glye-**SEE**-mee-ah) **hyper-** = excessive **glyc/o** = sugar **-emia** = blood condition	Elevated blood sugar level.
hypergonadism (high-per-**GOH**-nad-izm)	Excessive activity of the ovaries or testes.
hyperinsulinism (high-per-**IN**-soo-lin-izm)	An excessive amount of insulin in the body.
hyperkalemia (high-per-kal-**EE**-mee-ah) **hyper-** = excessive **kal/i** = potassium **-emia** = blood condition	An elevated blood potassium level.
hypernatremia (high-per-nah-**TREE**-mee-ah) **hyper-** = excessive **natr/i** = sodium **-emia** = blood condition	An elevated blood sodium level.
hyperparathyroidism (high-per-pair-ah-**THIGH**-roy-dizm) **hyper-** = excessive **para-** = near, beside **thyroid/o** = thyroid gland **-ism** = condition	Hyperactivity of the four parathyroid glands resulting in an oversecretion of parathyroid hormone.
hyperpituitarism (high-per-pih-**TOO**-ih-tair-izm) **hyper-** = excessive	Overactivity of the anterior lobe of the pituitary gland.
hyperthyroidism (high-per-**THIGH**-roy-dizm) **hyper-** = excessive **thyroid/o** = thyroid gland **-ism** = condition	Overactivity of the thyroid gland; also called Graves' disease.
hypocalcemia (high-poh-kal-**SEE**-mee-ah) **hypo-** = under, below, beneath, less than normal **calc/i** = calcium **-emia** = blood condition	Less than normal blood calcium level.

hypoglycemia (high-poh-glye-**SEE**-mee-ah) hypo- = under, below, beneath, less than normal glyc/o = sugar, sweet -emia = blood condition	Less than normal blood sugar level.
hypokalemia (high-poh-kal-**EE**-mee-ah) hypo- = under, below, beneath, less than normal kal/i = potassium -emia = blood condition	Less than normal blood potassium level.
hyponatremia (high-poh-nah-**TREE**-mee-ah) hypo- = under, below, beneath, less than normal natr/i = sodium -emia = blood condition	Less than normal blood sodium level.
hypophysectomy (high-poff-ih-**SEK**-toh-mee)	Surgical removal of the pituitary gland.
hypothyroidism (high-poh-**THIGH**-roy-dizm) hypo- = under, below, beneath, less than normal thyroid/o = thyroid gland -ism = condition	Less than normal activity of the thyroid gland.
insulin shock (**IN**-soo-lin)	A state of shock due to extremely low blood sugar level caused by an overdose of insulin, a decreased intake of food, or excessive exercise by a diabetic patient who is insulin-dependent.
ketoacidosis (kee-toh-ass-ih-**DOH**-sis) ket/o = ketone bodies acid/o = sour, bitter -osis = condition	Acidosis (increase in the acidity of the blood) due to an accumulation of ketones in the body, resulting from faulty carbohydrate metabolism; this is primarily a complication of diabetes mellitus.
medulla (meh-**DULL**-lah)	The internal part of a structure or organ.
metabolism (meh-**TAB**-oh-lizm)	The sum of all physical and chemical processes that take place within the body.
myxedema (miks-eh-**DEE**-mah)	The most severe form of hypothyroidism in the adult. This condition is characterized by puffiness of the hands and face, coarse, thickened edematous skin, an enlarged tongue, slow speech, loss of and dryness of the hair, sensitivity to cold, drowsiness, and mental apathy.
norepinephrine (nor-ep-ih-**NEH**-frin)	A hormone produced by the adrenal medulla. This hormone plays an important role in the body's response to stress by raising the blood pressure.

oxytocin (**ok**-see-**TOH**-sin) oxy- = rapid, sharp -toc/o = childbirth -in = enzyme	A hormone secreted by the posterior pituitary gland. This hormone stimulates the contractions of the uterus during childbirth and stimulates the release of milk from the breasts of lactating women (women who breastfeed), in response to the suckling reflex of the infant.
polydipsia (pall-ee-**DIP**-see-ah) poly- = many, much, excessive dips/o = thirst -ia = condition	Excessive thirst.
polyphagia (pall-ee-**FAY**-jee-ah) poly- = many, much, excessive phag/o = eating -ia = condition	Excessive eating.
polyuria (pall-ee-**YOO**-ree-ah) poly- = many, much, excessive ur/o = urine -ia = condition	The excretion of excessively large amounts of urine.
progesterone (proh-**JESS**-ter-ohn)	A female hormone secreted by the ovaries. This hormone is primarily responsible for the changes that occur in the endometrium in anticipation of a fertilized ovum, and for development of the maternal placenta after implantation of a fertilized ovum.
somatotropic hormone (soh-mat-oh-**TROH**-pik)	A hormone secreted by the anterior pituitary gland that regulates the cellular processes necessary for normal body growth; also called the growth hormone.
syndrome (**SIN**-drohm) syn- = joined, together -drome = that which runs together	A group of symptoms occurring together, indicative of a particular disease or abnormality.
T cells	Specialized lymphocytes that are involved in the immune response.
tetany (**TET**-ah-nee)	A condition characterized by severe cramping and twitching of the muscles and sharp flexion of the wrist and ankle joints; a complication of hypocalcemia.
thymopoietin (thigh-moh-**POY**-eh-tin)	A hormone secreted by the thymus, thought to stimulate the production of T cells, which are involved in the immune response.
thymosin (thigh-**MOH**-sin)	A hormone secreted by the thymus. This hormone is thought to stimulate the production of specialized lymphocytes, called T cells, which are involved in the immune response.

thyroiditis (thigh-royd-**EYE**-tis) thyroid/o = thyroid gland -itis = inflammation	Inflammation of the thyroid gland.
thyroxine (thigh-**ROKS**-in)	A hormone secreted by the thyroid gland. This hormone helps maintain normal body metabolism.
triiodothyronine (**try**-eye-oh-doh-**THIGH**-roh-neen)	A hormone secreted by the thyroid gland. This hormone helps regulate growth and development of the body, and helps control metabolism and body temperature.
virilism (**VEER**-il-izm)	The development of masculine physical traits in the female such as growth of facial and body hair, increased secretion of the sebaceous glands, deepening of the voice, and enlargement of the clitoris; also called masculinization. This condition may be due to an abnormality or dysfunction of the adrenal gland, as in adrenal virilism.

Word Elements

The following word elements pertain to the endocrine system. As you review the list, pronounce each word element aloud twice and check the box after you "say it." Write the definition for the example word given for each word element. You may use your medical dictionary.

WORD ELEMENT	PRONUNCIATION	"SAY IT"	MEANING
acr/o **acr**omegaly	**AK**-roh ak-roh-**MEG**-ah-lee	☐	extremities
aden/o **aden**opathy	**AD**-en-noh ad-eh-**NOP**-ah-thee	☐	gland
adren/o **adreno**megaly	ad-**REE**-noh ad-ree-noh-**MEG**-ah-lee	☐	adrenal glands
adrenal/o **adrenal**ectomy	ad-**REE**-nal-oh ad-ree-nal-**EK**-toh-mee	☐	adrenal glands
andr/o **andr**ogen	**AN**-droh **AN**-droh-jen	☐	man, male
calc/o hyper**calc**emia	**KAL**-koh high-per-kal-**SEE**-mee-ah	☐	calcium
cortic/o **cortic**osteroid	**KOR**-tih-koh kor-tih-koh-**STAIR**-oyd	☐	cortex
crin/o endo**crin**ology	**KRIN**-oh en-doh-krin-**ALL**-oh-jee	☐	secrete

-crine endo**crine**	**KRIN** **EN**-doh-krin	☐	secrete
dips/o **dips**osis	**DIP**-soh dip-**SOH**-sis	☐	thirst
-dipsia poly**dipsia**	**DIP**-see-ah pall-ee-**DIP**-see-ah	☐	thirst
gonad/o **gonad**otropic	goh-**NAD**-oh goh-nad-oh-**TROH**-pik	☐	sex glands
gluc/o **gluc**oneogenesis	**GLOO**-koh gloo-koh-nee-oh-**JEN**-eh-sis	☐	sugar, sweet
glyc/o **glyc**ogenolysis	**GLYE**-koh glye-koh-jen-**ALL**-eh-sis	☐	sugar, sweet
kal/i hyper**kal**emia	**KAL**-ee high-per-kal-**EE**-mee-ah	☐	potassium
lact/o **lact**ogen	**LAK**-toh **LAK**-toh-jen	☐	milk
myx/o **myx**edema	**MIKS**-oh miks-eh-**DEE**-mah	☐	relating to mucus
natr/o hyper**natr**emia	**NAH**-troh high-per-nah-**TREE**-mee-ah	☐	sodium
oxy- **oxy**tocin	**OK**-see ok-see-**TOH**-sin	☐	sharp, quick
pancreat/o **pancreat**itis	pan-kree-**AH**-toh pan-kree-ah-**TYE**-tis	☐	pancreas
parathyroid/o **parathyroid**ectomy	pair-ah-**THIGH**-royd-oh pair-ah-**thigh**-royd-**EK**-toh-mee	☐	parathyroid glands
somat/o **somat**otropic hormone	soh-**MAT**-oh soh-mat-oh-**TROH**-pik hormone	☐	body
thym/o **thym**oma	**THIGH**-moh thigh-**MOH**-mah	☐	thymus gland
thyr/o **thyr**oxine	**THIGH**-roh thigh-**ROKS**-in	☐	thyroid gland
thyroid/o hyper**thyroid**ism	**THIGH**-royd-oh high-per-**THIGH**-royd-izm	☐	thyroid gland
toxic/o **toxic**ology	**TOKS**-ih-koh toks-ih-**KALL**-ih-jee	☐	poisons

-tropin gonado**tropin**	**TROH**-pin goh-nad-oh-**TROH**-pin	☐	stimulating effect of a hormone
-uria poly**uria**	**YOO**-ree-ah pall-ee-**YOO**-ree-ah	☐	urine condition

Pathological Conditions

As you study the pathological conditions of the endocrine system, note that the **basic definition** is in bold print, followed by a detailed description in regular print. The phonetic pronunciation is directly beneath each term, and a breakdown of the component parts of the term when appropriate.

The pathological conditions will be presented in the same order as the discussion of the endocrine glands; with the exception of the ovaries and testes which are discussed in detail in the chapters on female and male reproductive systems, respectively. Beneath each endocrine gland heading, the pathological conditions will be alphabetized for ease in locating.

Pituitary Gland

acromegaly
(**ak**-roh-**MEG**-ah-lee)
acr/o = extremities
-megaly = enlarged

A chronic metabolic condition characterized by the gradual, noticeable enlargement and elongation of the bones of the face, jaw, and extremities, due to hypersecretion of the human growth hormone after puberty.

The cause of oversecretion of the human growth hormone is most often due to a tumor of the pituitary gland. Treatment for acromegaly is aimed at reducing the size of the pituitary gland through surgery or radiation.

diabetes insipidus
(dye-ah-**BEE**-teez in-**SIP**-ih-dus)

A condition caused by a deficiency in the secretion of antidiuretic hormone (ADH) by the posterior pituitary gland, characterized by large amounts of urine and sodium being excreted from the body.

The person experiencing diabetes insipidus will complain of excessive thirst and will drink large volumes of water. The urine is very dilute with a low specific gravity. ADH is administered as treatment for diabetes insipidus.

dwarfism
(**DWARF**-ism)

Generalized growth retardation of the body due to the deficiency of the human growth hormone; also known as congenital hypopituitarism or hypopituitarism. See Figure 13-11.

The abnormal underdevelopment leaves the child extremely short with a small body. There is an absence of secondary sex characteristics. The condition may have a connection with other defects or varying degrees of mental retardation.

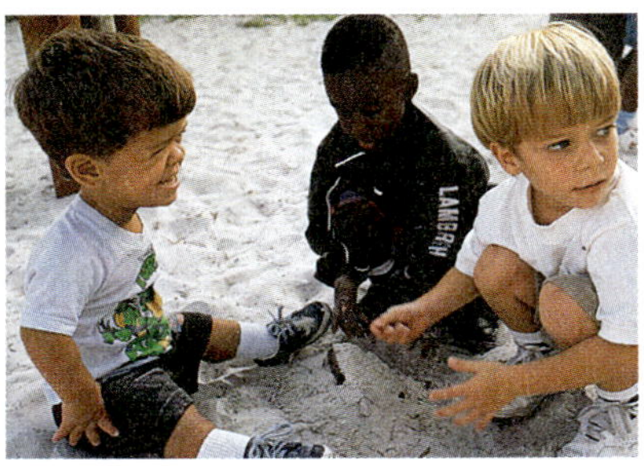

Figure 13-11 Dwarfism

Treatment may include administration of human growth hormone or somatotropin until a height of 5 feet is reached. These children may need replacement of other hormones, especially just before, and during puberty.

gigantism
(**JYE**-gan-tizm)

A proportional overgrowth of the body's tissue due to the hyper-secretion of the human growth hormone before puberty.

The child experiences accelerated abnormal growth chiefly in the long bones.

The cause of oversecretion of the human growth hormone is most often due to an adenoma of the anterior pituitary. Treatment of gigantism is aimed at reducing the size of the pituitary gland through surgery or radiation.

hypopituitarism
(**high**-poh-pih-**TOO**-ih-tah-rizm)

A complex syndrome resulting from the absence or deficiency of the pituitary hormone(s).

Metabolic dysfunction, growth retardation, and sexual immaturity are symptoms of hypopituitarism.

Thyroid Gland

cancer, thyroid gland

Malignant tumor of the thyroid gland, which leads to dysfunction of the gland and thus inadequate or excessive secretion of the thyroid hormone.

The presence of a palpable nodule or lump may be the first indication of thyroid cancer.

A needle aspiration biopsy is used to confirm the diagnosis. A malignant tumor of the thyroid is classified and staged according to the site of origin, size of tumor, amount of lymph node involvement, and the presence of metastasis.

Treatment typically consists of partial or complete removal of the thyroid gland. Lifelong thyroid hormone replacement will be required.

goiter
(simple; nontoxic)
(**GOY**-ter)

Hyperplasia of the thyroid gland.

This condition results from a deficient amount of iodine in the diet, required for the synthesis of T_3 and T_4 thyroid hormones produced by the thyroid gland.

When the body identifies the low levels of thyroid hormone, the anterior pituitary gland secretes the hormone, thyrotropin, which continually stimulates the thyroid gland to produce T_3 and T_4; consequently, the overstimulation increases the number of cells in the thyroid gland and a goiter is produced.

As the goiter increases in size, the person, typically a female, will notice a mass in the anterior aspect of the neck. As this mass or enlarged thyroid gland continuously increases in size, it begins to exert pressure on the trachea and esophagus causing breathing and swallowing difficulties.

Eventually, the goiter may cause the person to experience dizziness and fainting spells.

A goiter is noted on physical examination of the neck and confirmed with blood studies, with evidence of decreased T_3 and T_4 levels and elevated thyrotropin levels. Simple goiters are usually responsive to the administration of potassium iodide. If the goiter is nonresponsive, a subtotal thyroidectomy may be needed. Maintaining iodine in the diet prevents the development of goiter.

Graves' disease (hyperthyroidism)
(**high**-per-**THIGH**-royd-izm)
hyper- = excessive
thyroid/o = thyroid gland
-ism = condition

Hypertrophy of the thyroid gland resulting in an excessive secretion of the thyroid hormone that causes an extremely high body metabolism, thus creating multisystem changes.

Hyperthyroidism occurs most often in the form of Graves' disease, which has three distinguishing characteristics:

1. Hyperthyroidism
2. Thyroid gland enlargement (goiter)
3. Exophthalmia—unnatural protruding of the eyes.

The symptoms of Graves' disease are the result of hyperthyroidism and thus hypermetabolism, which affects all body systems. Hyperthyroidism causes a rapid heartbeat, nervousness, inability to sleep, excitability, increased appetite, weight loss, nausea, vomiting, excessive thirst, and profuse sweating. The speeding up of physical and mental responses result in varied emotional responses from extreme happiness to hyperactivity or delirium. The goiter results from hyperactivity of the thyroid gland, which leads to an increase in the size of the thyroid gland (hypertrophy) and an increase in the number of thyroid cells (hyperplasia). The gland may enlarge up to 3 to 4 times the original size. The person with hyperthyroidism will have decreased levels of serum cholesterol.

Diagnosis is confirmed on the basis of the individual's physical appearance and lack of composure, restlessness, and agitation. The serum levels of T_3 and T_4 are elevated and there is increased uptake of radioiodine in the thyroid scan. Other blood test results may expose elevated levels of particular antithyroid immunoglobulins, thus leaning toward an autoimmune response as a possible cause. The cause is uncertain.

Treatment includes the following therapies: antithyroid medication, radioiodine, and surgery (subtotal thyroidectomy). Graves' disease has three significant complications; (1) exophthalmia, (2) thyroid storm (see thyrotoxicosis), and (3) heart disease.

hypothyroidism
(high-poh-**THIGH**-royd-izm)
hypo- = under, below, beneath, less than normal
thyroid/o = thyroid gland
-ism = condition

A condition in which there is a shortage of thyroid hormone causing an extremely low body metabolism due to a reduced usage of oxygen; also called myxedema in the most severe form.

Hypothyroidism may be the result of:

1. congenital thyroid defects (cretinism)
2. faulty hormone synthesis

3. thyroiditis or iodine deficiency
4. use of antithyroid medications
5. loss of thyroid tissue due to surgery or radioactivity
6. thyroid gland atrophy

Hypothyroidism has a sluggish onset with symptoms developing over months or years. The severity of the disorder varies from mild to severe. In the mild form of hypothyroidism, the person may demonstrate no symptoms or only vague symptoms.

Symptoms, in the more severe cases, include slowed physical and mental function, an obvious apathetic fatigued appearance, bradycardia, anemia, difficulty breathing, decreased urinary output, decreased peristalsis, constipation, transient musculoskeletal pain, dry scaly skin, loss of hair, expressionless face, cold intolerance, and slow movement. A goiter may be a manifestation of hypothyroidism.

The person with hypothyroidism will have increased levels of serum cholesterol and triglycerides as a result of the effect on lipid metabolism.

Myxedema is the most severe form of hypothyroidism identified by water retention all over the body in the connective tissues. The person with myxedema has a puffy appearance and a thick tongue. Myxedema coma occurs with an extreme reduction in metabolic rate and is manifested by hypoventilation, hypotension, and hypothermia.

Diagnosis of hypothyroidism is confirmed with the clinical presentation of the person and an elevated serum TSH level due to the attempt to compensate for the levels of T_3 and T_4, which are low.

With thyroid hormone replacement therapy, the physical and mental symptoms will reverse. To maintain reversal permanently, a thyroid hormone preparation will be needed throughout life. Hypothyroidism occurs more frequently in females with the highest incidence between 30 and 60 years of age.

---

thyroiditis
(thigh-royd-**EYE**-tis)
(Hashimoto's)
(**HASH**-ee-moh-**TOZ**)
thyroid/o = thyroid gland
-itis = inflammation

Chronic inflammation of the thyroid gland, leading to enlargement of the thyroid gland.

This is a disease of the immune system in which the gland tissue is destroyed by antibodies and replaced with fibrous tissue. Chronic inflammation causes massive infiltration of the thyroid gland with plasma cells and lymphocytes. The body recognizes a decrease in the level of thyroid hormone and stimulates the anterior pituitary to secrete thyrotropin, which continually stimulates the thyroid gland to produce T_3 and T_4. Consequently, the stimulation increases the number of cells in the thyroid gland in an attempt to compensate and a goiter is produced. Hashimoto's thyroiditis is a common form of primary hypothyroidism (see *hypothyroidism*).

To confirm the diagnosis, the blood is evaluated for autoantibodies and the function of the thyroid gland is measured with a radioactive iodine uptake (RAIU) test. A needle biopsy in a person with Hashimoto's disease will usually show characteristic changes in the gland tissue.

Treatment is thyroid hormone replacement for life. The replacement will prevent further growth of the goiter.

---

thyrotoxicosis (thyroid storm)
(**thigh**-roh-toks-ih-**KOH**-sis)
thyr/o = thyroid gland
toxic/o = poison
-osis = condition

An acute, sometimes fatal, incident of overactivity of the thyroid gland resulting in excessive secretion of thyroid hormone.

Thyrotoxicosis, or a thyroid storm, is characterized by a critically high fever and pulse rate, dehydration, extreme irritability, and delirium.

A thyroid storm is a medical emergency typically precipitated by infection, surgery, trauma, labor and delivery, a myocardial infarction, medication overdosage, or undiagnosed or untreated hyperthyroidism. Diagnosis is made on the clinical picture of the person.

Parathyroid Gland

---

hyperparathyroidism
(**high**-per-pair-ah-**THIGH**-royd-izm)
(hypercalcemia)
(high-per-kal-**SEE**-mee-ah)
hyper- = excessive
parathyroid/o = parathyroid gland
-ism = condition
hyper- = excessive
calc/i = calcium
-emia = blood condition

Overactivity of any one of the parathyroid glands, which leads to high levels of calcium in the blood and low levels of calcium in the bones.

The accelerated activity of the parathyroid gland in primary hyperparathyroidism is due to the effects of a parathyroid tumor or hyperplasia of the parathyroid gland (excessive increase in the number of cells). Secondary hyperparathyroidism is usually related to renal disease or endocrine disorders.

Symptoms of hyperparathyroidism are due to hypercalcemia and include muscle weakness and atrophy; nausea, vomiting, and gastrointestinal pain; increased irritability of the heart muscle leading to arrhythmias; bone tenderness and fragility leading to bone fractures; and deposits of calcium in soft tissue leading to renal calculi and low back pain.

Diagnostic laboratory results will demonstrate a high level of PTH on the radioimmunoassay, and elevated blood levels of calcium, alkaline phosphatase, and chloride. The blood phosphorus levels will be reduced. The extent of demineralization of the bones can be evaluated on x-ray film.

Treatment for hyperparathyroidism will vary, but will be directly related to the cause. Surgical intervention involves removal of the gland or glands causing the hypersecretion of PTH.

---

hypoparathyroidism
(**high**-poh-pair-ah-**THIGH**-royd-izm)
hypo- = under, below, beneath, less than normal
parathyroid/o = parathyroid gland
-ism = condition

Decreased production of parathyroid hormone resulting in hypocalcemia, characterized by nerve and muscle weakness with muscle spasms or tetany (a state of continual contraction of the muscles).

Symptoms include hair loss, brittle nails, malabsorption, arrhythmias, mood disorders, and hyperactive reflexes. Blood phosphate levels are elevated.

Treatment of hypoparathyroidism is aimed at increasing calcium levels. Immediate administration of intravenous calcium will aid in decreasing tetany. Long-term calcium supplements, an increase of calcium in the diet, and vitamin D therapy are usually helpful to raise the blood calcium level.

Adrenal Glands

Addison's disease
(**Ad**-ih-son's)

A life-threatening disease process due to failure of the adrenal cortex to secrete adequate mineralocorticoids and glucocorticoids resulting from an autoimmune process, a neoplasm, an infection, or a hemorrhage in the gland.

Symptoms include low blood glucose, low blood sodium, weight loss, dehydration, generalized weakness, gastrointestinal disturbances, increased pigmentation of the skin and mucous membranes, cold intolerance, anxiety, and depression.

Diagnosis is confirmed through an ACTH stimulation test. Treatment for **Addison's disease** is replacement of natural hormones with mineralocorticoid and glucocorticoid drugs, to continue for life.

Conn's disease
(primary aldosteronism)
(al-doss-**STAIR**-ohn-izm)

A condition characterized by excretion of excessive amounts of aldosterone, the most influential of the mineralocorticoids, which causes the body to retain extra sodium and excrete extra potassium, leading to an increased volume of blood (hypervolemia) and hypertension.

Other symptoms include headache, nocturia (excessive urination during the night), fatigue, ventricular arrhythmias, tetany, and muscular weakness.

Conn's disease is caused by an aldosteronoma, a benign aldosterone-secreting **adenoma** or adrenal hyperplasia.

Surgical removal of one or both adrenal glands is the preferred treatment for **primary aldosteronism**. Medical treatment involves the administration of the medication aldactone. Early diagnosis and treatment will aid in preventing progressive renal complications and hypertension.

Cushing's syndrome
(**CUSH**-ings **SIN**-drom)

A condition of the adrenal gland in which there is a cluster of symptoms occurring as a result of an excessive amount of cortisol or ACTH circulating in the blood.

The high levels of circulating cortisol have been either secreted from the adrenal cortex or are present because of the administration of very large doses of glucocorticoids for some time.

A benign or malignant adrenal tumor is the cause of primary **Cushing's syndrome** causing the excessive production of cortisol. Secondary Cushing's syndrome occurs as a result of Cushing's disease, a disorder of the pituitary or hypothalamus, which results in the increased release of ACTH. The increased ACTH stimulation leads to hyperplasia of the adrenal cortex and thus increased production of cortisol.

Symptoms of Cushing's syndrome are central obesity, round "moon" face, edema, hypertension, supraclavicular fat pads (buffalo hump), muscular weakness and wasting, skin infection, poor wound healing, low potassium level, and emotional changes. See **Figure 13-12.**

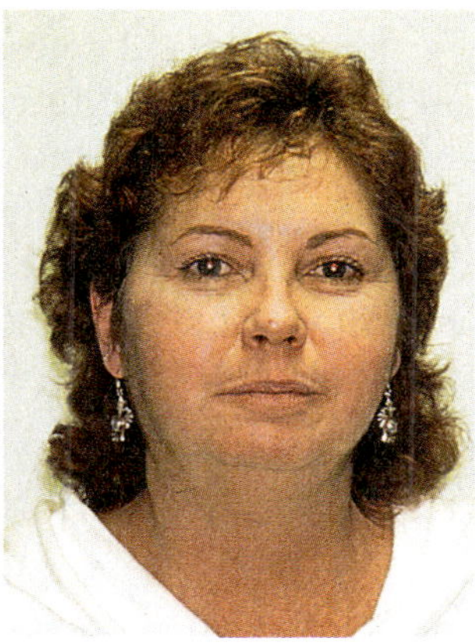

Figure 13-12 Cushing's syndrome (Courtesy of Dr. Matthew Leinung, Acting Head, Division of Endocrinology, Albany Medical College, Albany, NY)

Treatment varies according to the cause. When a tumor is the cause, surgical excision and/or radiation will be used. Drug therapy can be used to suppress ACTH secretions.

---

pheochromocytoma
(fee-oh-**kroh**-moh-sigh-**TOH**-mah)
phe/o = dusky
chrom/o = color
cyt/o = cell
-oma = tumor

A vascular tumor of the adrenal medulla that produces extra epinephrine and norepinephrine, leading to persistent or intermittent hypertension and heart palpitations.

Other symptoms include flushing of the face, sweating, severe headaches, muscle spasms, and high blood glucose.

Possible complications of pheochromocytoma consist of weight loss, cardiac dysrhythmia, and heart failure. With surgical excision of one or both adrenal glands, depending on the tumor involvement, the person can be cured if cardiovascular damage has not become permanent. Early diagnosis and treatment is essential to prevent long-term complications.

---

virilism
(**VEER**-il-izm)

Development of male secondary sex characteristics in the female due to the excessive secretion of adrenocortical androgens from the adrenal cortex.

The overactivity of the adrenal gland may be caused by an adrenal tumor or hyperplasia; virilism typically occurs in adult women 30 to 40 years of age.

Symptoms include excessive hair on the body and face (hirsutism), absence of menstruation (amenorrhea), deepening of the voice, acne, oily skin, muscular hypertrophy, atrophy of the breasts and uterus, and ovarian changes.

Treatment consists of tumor resection, adrenalectomy, and administration of cortisol to suppress androgen production.

Pancreas

---

diabetes mellitus
(dye-ah-**BEE**-teez **MELL**-ih-tus)

A disorder of the pancreas in which the beta cells of the islets of Langerhans of the pancreas fail to produce an adequate amount of insulin, resulting in the body's inability to appropriately metabolize carbohydrates, fats, and proteins.

Two classic characteristics of the disease are hyperglycemia and ketosis. First, the individual will experience abnormally elevated blood glucose levels, known as hyperglycemia, due to the body's inability to use glucose for energy. Insulin is necessary for the body cells to use glucose for energy. Secondly, when the body cannot use glucose for energy, the cells begin to break down fats and proteins for energy. This breakdown of fats and proteins releases waste products known as **ketones** into the bloodstream, which spill over into the urine as a result of abnormal accumulations.

The classic symptoms of diabetes mellitus are glycosuria (sugar in the urine), polydipsia (excessive thirst), and polyuria (excessive urine output). Other symptoms include increased eating (polyphagia) and weight loss, presence of ketones in the urine, itching (pruritus), muscle weakness, and fatigue.

Diabetes mellitus is classified as either insulin-dependent diabetes (type I) or non-insulin-dependent diabetes (type II). Each classification is described below.

Insulin-dependent diabetes mellitus (IDDM), also known as type I diabetes, usually occurs before the age of 30, having a sudden onset. Individuals with IDDM usually have no pancreatic activity and require administration of insulin injections to control the disease. These individuals are prone to developing ketosis.

Non-insulin-dependent diabetes mellitus (NIDDM), also known as type II diabetes, usually appears in adults after the age of 40, having a gradual onset; the majority of these individuals are obese. Individuals with NIDDM usually have some pancreatic activity making it possible to control the disease with diet and exercise. These individuals usually do not rely on insulin to control the disease and they are not prone to developing ketosis. Approximately 80% of all diabetics have NIDDM, which is also known as adult-onset diabetes.

Despite the name, non-insulin-dependent diabetes, a few type II diabetics are insulin dependent. This often makes it difficult for the individual to understand how he or she can be a type II diabetic (non-insulin dependent) and still require insulin injections. These individuals are usually able to control their **diabetes** with diet and exercise in the beginning, but eventually have to convert to the administration of insulin injections for proper control, when the pancreatic activity becomes insignificant or ceases completely. The individual with adult-onset diabetes (type II) who does require insulin injections to control the disease experiences all of the symptoms and problems that accompany type I diabetes or IDDM.

Diagnosis of diabetes mellitus is confirmed with a **glucose tolerance test**. This test is described in detail in the section on diagnostic treatments and procedures.

Treatment of IDDM consists of a balance between diet, exercise, and insulin. Individuals with NIDDM usually control their diabetes with diet and exercise, occasionally requiring the use of oral hypoglycemic agents to stimulate the production of insulin by the pancreas.

Complications of diabetes mellitus vary according to the individual and the type of diabetes. The most common acute complication for the insulin-dependent diabetic is **insulin shock,** which is the result of a drastic drop in the blood sugar level (severe hypoglycemia) due to an overdose of insulin, a decreased intake of food, or excessive exercise. Insulin shock is characterized by cool moist skin (damp skin that is cool to the touch), sweatiness (the clothing will be damp or wet), chilliness (the individual will begin to shiver in response to the shocklike symptoms), nervousness, and irritability, which may lead to disorientation and coma if left untreated.

Treatment for insulin shock requires an immediate dose of glucose orally if the individual is still alert. If the individual is stuporous and beyond the point of ingesting food or liquid by mouth, treatment (if readily available) would include the injection of the hormone glucagon to stimulate the liver to release glucose into the bloodstream, raising the blood glucose level to a normal level within 15 minutes and maintaining that level for approximately 45 minutes. The individual should then ingest a complex carbohydrate and protein snack to maintain the normal blood sugar level. If the individual is unresponsive, and a glucagon emergency kit is not available, emergency help will be necessary.

Other complications of long-term diabetes include poor circulation in the extremities, especially the lower legs and feet, infections that heal poorly due to the decreased circulation, kidney disease and renal failure, **diabetic retinopathy**, which is a leading cause of blindness, involvement of the nervous system (diabetic neuropathy) characterized by numbness (decreased sensitivity of the fingers to touch and grasp), and intermittent but severe episodes of pain in the extremities.

Diabetics who maintain near normal blood glucose levels can reasonably expect to live for many years without major complications.

---

diabetic retinopathy
(dye-ah-**BET**-ik ret-in-**OP**-ah-thee)
retin/o = retina
-pathy = disease

A disorder of the blood vessels of the retina of the eye in which the capillaries of the retina experience localized *areas of bulging* (microaneurysms), hemorrhages, and scarring.

This disorder occurs as a consequence of an 8- to 10-year duration of diabetes mellitus. The scarring, along with the leakage of blood, causes a permanent decline in the sharpness of vision. The inability to get the oxygen and nutrients needed for good vision to the retina eventually will lead to permanent loss of vision. In the United States, diabetic retinopathy is the leading cause of blindness.

---

gestational diabetes
(jess-**TAY**-shun-al dye-ah-**BEE**-teez)

A disorder in which women who are not diabetic before pregnancy develop diabetes during the pregnancy; that is, they develop an inability to metabolize carbohydrates (glucose intolerance), with resultant hyperglycemia.

This disorder develops during the latter part of pregnancy, with symptoms usually disappearing at the end of the pregnancy. Women who have **gestational diabetes** have a higher possibility of developing it with subsequent pregnancies; they are also at higher risk of developing diabetes later in life.

Factors that increase the risk of developing gestational diabetes include, but are not limited to, the following:

1. Obesity
2. Maternal age over 30 years of age
3. History of birthing large babies (usually over 10 pounds)
4. Family history of diabetes
5. Previous, unexplained, stillborn birth
6. Previous birth with congenital anomalies (defects)

Symptoms vary from classic symptoms of diabetes, such as excessive thirst, hunger, and frequent urination, to being asymptomatic (no symptoms present). Because a high number of pregnant women have gestational diabetes without obvious symptoms, all pregnant women are routinely screened for diabetes with a blood test; this usually occurs between weeks 24 and 28 of the pregnancy.

---

pancreatic cancer
(**pan**-kree-**AT**-ik **CAN**-sir)
pancreat/o = pancreas
-ic = pertaining to

A life-threatening primary malignant neoplasm typically found in the head of the pancreas.

Of those diagnosed with pancreatic cancer, 95% lose their lives 1 to 3 years after diagnosis. The occurrence of pancreatic cancer for smokers is twice the number as it is for nonsmokers. Other related risk factors include high-fat diet, pancreatitis, exposure to chemicals and toxins, and diabetes mellitus.

With a slow onset, pancreatic cancer causes nonspecific symptoms such as nausea, anorexia, dull epigastric pain, weight loss, and flatulence. As the tumor grows, the pain worsens. If there is an early diagnosis, surgical removal of the tumor may be possible.

---

pancreatitis
(**pan**-kree-ah-**TYE**-tis)
pancreat/o = pancreas
-itis = inflammation

An acute or chronic destructive inflammatory condition of the pancreas.

Acute pancreatitis presents itself quickly and creates symptoms that vary from mild self-limiting pancreatic edema to massive necrotizing hemorrhagic pancreatitis.

The initial outstanding symptom is severe, continuous epigastric and abdominal pain, which radiates to the back and follows the ingestion of excessive alcohol or a fatty meal. Other symptoms include rigid abdominal distension, decreased bowel sounds, nausea and vomiting, hypotension, elevated temperature, and clammy cold skin. After 24 hours, mild jaundice may appear.

In addition to alcoholism, other causes of acute pancreatitis include trauma, surgery, metabolic disorders, drugs, infections, or ruptured peptic ulcers.

Serious complications may occur, including the development of abscesses or pseudocysts, diabetes mellitus, renal failure, heart failure, hypovolemic shock, multiple organ failure, accumulation of fluid within the abdomen (ascites), and adult respiratory distress syndrome.

Treatment is aimed at resolving the immediate problems, relief of pain and avoiding any further GI irritation, and prevention of serious life-threatening complications.

Chronic pancreatitis is a permanent, progressive destruction of pancreatic cells identified with fibrosis, atrophy, fatty degeneration, and calcification. The causes of chronic pancreatitis include alcoholism, malnutrition, surgery, or neoplasm.

Symptoms include abdominal pain, large fatty stools, weight loss, and signs and symptoms of diabetes mellitus.

Treatment includes the administration of pancreatic enzymes, antiemetics, antacids, and insulin if its production is stopped or decreased.

Diagnostic Techniques and Procedures

thyroid function tests
(**THIGH**-royd)
(T_3, T_4, TSH)
thyr/o = thyroid gland
-oid = resembling

Tests that measure the blood levels of the hormones T_3, T_4, and TSH.

These thyroid hormones aid in maintaining the body's metabolic rate and tissue growth and development. Hormones T_3 and T_4 are secreted in response to TSH.

thyroid-stimulating hormone (TSH) blood test
thyr/o = thyroid gland
-oid = resembling

A test that measures the concentration of TSH in the blood.

This test is used in differentiating primary hypothyroidism (due to a defect in the structure or function of the thyroid gland) from secondary hypothyroidism (due to insufficient stimulation of the normal thyroid gland).

In addition to differentiating primary and secondary hypothyroidism, the serum level of TSH is used to monitor thyroid hormone replacement. It is important to remember that TSH levels are decreased in persons with a severe illness.

fasting blood sugar (FBS)

Blood glucose sample taken usually early in the morning after the person has been without food or drink since midnight.

FBS is a more accurate evaluation of the blood glucose level because of the fasting state of the body.

glucose tolerance test (GTT)
(**GLOO**-kohs **TALL**-er-ans)
gluc/o = sugar, sweet
-ose = carbohydrate

A test that evaluates the person's ability to tolerate a concentrated oral glucose load by measuring the glucose levels:

1. prior to glucose administration
2. 30 minutes after glucose administration
3. 1 hour after glucose administration
4. 2 hours after glucose administration
5. 3 hours after glucose administration

In persons with diabetes mellitus, the serum glucose levels will be markedly increased from 1 to sometimes 5 hours. The person whose insulin response is appropriate will have only a minimal elevation in serum glucose levels during the first hour.

radioactive iodine uptake (RAIU) test
(**ray**-dee-o-**AK**-tiv **EYE**-oh-dine **UP**-tayk)

A thyroid function test that evaluates the function of the thyroid gland by administering a known amount of radioactive iodine and later placing a gamma ray detector over the thyroid gland to determine the percentage or quantity of radioactive iodine absorbed by the gland over specific time periods.

Persons in hyperthyroid states will have an increased uptake of the iodine. A decreased uptake is seen in persons with hypothyroid conditions.

serum glucose tests
(**SEE**-rum **GLOO**-kohs)
gluc/o = sugar, sweet

Serum glucose tests measure the amount of glucose in the blood at the time the sample was drawn.

True serum glucose elevations are indicative of diabetes mellitus; however, the value must be evaluated according to the time of day and the last time the person has eaten. A glucose level can be collected in a tube or evaluated with a finger stick.

thyroid echogram (ultrasound)
(**THIGH**-royd **EK**-oh-gram)
thyr/o = thyroid gland
-oid = resembling
ech/o = sound
-gram = record or picture

An ultrasound examination important in distinguishing solid thyroid nodules from cystic nodules.

The type of nodule will provide information for treatment. In addition to differentiating the type of nodule, the thyroid echogram is used to evaluate the reaction to the medical therapy for a thyroid mass.

thyroid scan
(**THIGH**-royd)
thyr/o = thyroid gland
-oid = resembling

An examination that determines the position, size, shape, and physiological function of the thyroid gland through the use of radionuclear scanning.

An image of the thyroid is recorded and visualized after a radioactive substance is given. Nodules are readily noted with this scan and are classified as hot (functioning) or cold (nonfunctioning). The thyroid scan is helpful in the diagnosis of the following cases:

1. Neck or substernal masses
2. Thyroid nodules (thyroid cancers are typically cold)
3. Cause of hyperthyroidism
4. Evaluating metastatic tumors with an unknown primary site

Common Abbreviations

ABBREVIATION	MEANING	ABBREVIATION	MEANING
ACTH	adrenocorticotropic hormone	**GH**	growth hormone
ADH	antidiuretic hormone	**GTT**	glucose tolerance test
BMR	basal metabolic rate	**HDL**	high-density lipoprotein
Ca	calcium	**IDDM**	insulin-dependent diabetes mellitus
DI	diabetes insipidus	**K**	potassium
DM	diabetes mellitus	**LH**	luteinizing hormone
FBS	fasting blood sugar	**LTH**	Lactogenic hormone
FSH	follicle-stimulating hormone	**MSH**	melanocyte-stimulating hormone

Na	sodium
NIDDM	non-insulin-dependent diabetes mellitus
OT	oxytocin
PBI	protein-bound iodine
PTH	parathyroid hormone
RAI	radioactive iodine
RAIU	radioactive iodine uptake
T_3	triiodothyronine (thyroid hormone)
T_4	thyroxine (thyroid hormone)
TFT	thyroid function test
TSH	thyroid-stimulating hormone
VLDL	very-low-density lipoprotein

Written and Audio Terminology Review

Review each of the following terms from this chapter. Study the spelling of each term and write the definition in the space provided. If you have the Audio CD available, listen to each term, pronounce it, and check the box once you are comfortable saying the word. Check definitions by looking the term up in the glossary/index.

TERM	PRONUNCIATION	DEFINITION
acromegaly	☐ **ak**-roh-**MEG**-ah-lee	______
Addison's disease	☐ **AD**-ih-sons dih-**ZEEZ**	______
adenohypophysis	☐ ad-eh-noh-high-**POFF**-ih-sis	______
adenoma	☐ ad-eh-**NOH**-mah	______
adenopathy	☐ ad-eh-**NOP**-ah-thee	______
adrenalectomy	☐ ad-ree-nal-**EK**-toh-mee	______
adrenocortical	☐ ad-**ree**-noh-**KOR**-tih-kal	______
adrenomegaly	☐ ad-ree-noh-**MEG**-ah-lee	______
aldosterone	☐ al-**DOSS**-te-rohn	______
androgen	☐ **AN**-droh-jen	______
antidiuretic	☐ an-tye-dye-yoo-**RET**-ik	______
Conn's disease	☐ Conn's disease	______
cortex	☐ **COR**-tex	______
corticosteroid	☐ kor-tih-koh-**STAIR**-oyd	______
cortisol	☐ **COR**-tih-sal	______
cretinism	☐ **KREE**-tin-izm	______

Term		Pronunciation	
Cushing's syndrome	☐	**CUSH**-ings **SIN**-drom	____
diabetes	☐	dye-ah-**BEE**-teez	____
diabetes insipidus	☐	dye-ah-**BEE**-teez in-**SIP**-ih-dus	____
diabetes mellitus	☐	dye-ah-**BEE**-teez **MELL**-ih-tus	____
diabetic retinopathy	☐	dye-ah-**BET**-ik ret-in-**OP**-ah-thee	____
dipsosis	☐	dip-**SOH**-sis	____
dwarfism	☐	**DWARF**-ism	____
endocrine	☐	**EN**-doh-krin	____
endocrinologist	☐	en-doh-krin-**ALL**-oh-jist	____
endocrinology	☐	en-doh-krin-**ALL**-oh-jee	____
epinephrine	☐	ep-ih-**NEF**-rin	____
estrogen	☐	**ESS**-troh-jen	____
euthyroid	☐	yoo-**THIGH**-royd	____
exocrine	☐	**EKS**-oh-krin	____
exophthalmia	☐	eks-off-**THAL**-mee-ah	____
exophthalmos	☐	eks-off-**THAL**-mohs	____
gestational diabetes	☐	jess-**TAY**-shun-al dye-ah-**BEE**-teez	____
gigantism	☐	**JYE**-gan-tizm	____
glucagon	☐	**GLOO**-kuh-gon	____
glucogenesis	☐	gloo-koh-**JEN**-eh-sis	____
gluconeogenesis	☐	gloo-koh-nee-oh-**JEN**-eh-sis	____
glucose	☐	**GLOO**-kohs	____
glucose tolerance test	☐	**GLOO**-kohs **TALL**-er-ans test	____
glycogenesis	☐	glye-koh-**JEN**-eh-sis	____
glycogenolysis	☐	glye-koh-jen-**ALL**-eh-sis	____
glycosuria	☐	glye-kohs-**YOO**-ree-ah	____
goiter	☐	**GOY**-ter	____
gonadotropic	☐	goh-nad-oh-**TROH**-pik	____
gonadotropin	☐	goh-nad-oh-**TROH**-pin	____

Term		Pronunciation	
gonads	☐	**GOH**-nadz	______
hirsutism	☐	**HER**-soot-izm	______
hypercalcemia	☐	high-per-kal-**SEE**-mee-ah	______
hyperglycemia	☐	high-per-glye-**SEE**-mee-ah	______
hypergonadism	☐	high-per-**GOH**-nad-izm	______
hyperinsulinism	☐	high-per-**IN**-soo-lin-izm	______
hyperkalemia	☐	high-per-kal-**EE**-mee-ah	______
hypernatremia	☐	high-per-nah-**TREE**-mee-ah	______
hyperparathyroidism (hypercalcemia)	☐	high-per-pair-ah-**THIGH**-royd-izm (high-per-kal-**SEE**-mee-ah)	______
hyperpituitarism	☐	high-per-pih-**TOO**-ih-tair-izm	______
hyperthyroidism	☐	**high**-per-**THIGH**-royd-izm	______
hypocalcemia	☐	high-poh-kal-**SEE**-mee-ah	______
hypoglycemia	☐	high-poh-glye-**SEE**-mee-ah	______
hypokalemia	☐	high-poh-kal-**EE**-mee-ah	______
hyponatremia	☐	high-poh-nah-**TREE**-mee-ah	______
hypoparathyroidism	☐	**high**-poh-**pair**-ah-**THIGH**- royd-izm	______
hypophysectomy	☐	high-poff-ih-**SEK**-toh-mee	______
hypopituitarism	☐	**high**-poh-pih-**TOO**-ih-tah-rizm	______
hypothyroidism	☐	high-poh-**THIGH**-royd-izm	______
insulin	☐	**IN**-soo-lin	______
ketoacidosis	☐	kee-toh-ass-ih-**DOH**-sis	______
lactogen	☐	**LAK**-toh-jen	______
medulla	☐	meh-**DULL**-lah	______
metabolism	☐	meh-**TAB**-oh-lizm	______
myxedema	☐	miks-eh-**DEE**-mah	______
norepinephrine	☐	nor-**EP**-ih-**neh**-frin	______
oxytocin	☐	**ok**-see-**TOH**-sin	______
pancreatic cancer	☐	**pan**-kree-**AT**-ik **CAN**-sir	______

Term		Pronunciation	
pancreatitis	☐	**pan**-kree-ah-**TYE**-tis	______
parathyroidectomy	☐	pair-ah-**thigh**-royd-**EK**-toh-mee	______
pheochromocytoma	☐	fee-oh-**kroh**-moh-sigh-**TOH**- mah	______
polydipsia	☐	pall-ee-**DIP**-see-ah	______
polyuria	☐	pall-ee-**YOO**-ree-ah	______
primary aldosteronism	☐	primary al-doss-**STAIR**-ohn-izm	______
progesterone	☐	proh-**JESS**-ter-ohn	______
radioactive iodine uptake test	☐	ray-dee-oh-**AK**-tiv **EYE**-oh-dine **UP**-take test	______
serum glucose test	☐	**SEE**-rum **GLOO**-kohs test	______
somatotropic hormone	☐	soh-mat-oh-**TROH**-pik hormone	______
syndrome	☐	**SIN**-drom	______
tetany	☐	**TET**-ah-nee	______
thymoma	☐	thigh-**MOH**-mah	______
thymopoietin	☐	thigh-moh-**POY**-eh-tin	______
thymosin	☐	thigh-**MOH**-sin	______
thyroid	☐	**THIGH**-royd	______
thyroid echogram	☐	**THIGH**-royd **EK**-oh-gram	______
thyroiditis	☐	thigh-royd-**EYE**-tis	______
thyroiditis (Hashimoto's)	☐	thigh-royd-**EYE**-tis (**HASH**-ee-moh-toz)	______
thyrotoxicosis	☐	**thigh**-roh-**toks**-ih-**KOH**-sis	______
thyroxine	☐	thigh-**ROKS**-in	______
toxicology	☐	toks-ih-**KALL**-ih-jee	______
triiodothyronine	☐	**try**-eye-**oh**-doh-**THIGH**-roh-neen	______
virilism	☐	**VEER**-il-izm	______

Chapter Review Exercises

The following exercises provide a more in-depth review of the chapter material. Your goal in these exercises is to complete each section at a minimum 80% level of accuracy. A space has been provided for your score at the end of each section.

A. Term to Definition

Define each term by writing the definition in the space provided. Check the box if you are able to complete this exercise correctly the first time (without referring to the answers). Each correct answer is worth 10 points. Record your score in the space provided at the end of the exercise.

☐ 1. acromegaly ____________________

☐ 2. endocrinologist ____________________

☐ 3. exophthalmia ____________________

☐ 4. glucagon ____________________

☐ 5. glycogenesis ____________________

☐ 6. hirsutism ____________________

☐ 7. polydipsia ____________________

☐ 8. polyuria ____________________

☐ 9. tetany ____________________

☐ 10. virilism ____________________

Number correct _______ × 10 points/correct answer: Your score _______%

B. Spelling

Circle the correctly spelled term in each pairing of words. Each correct answer is worth 10 points. Record your score in the space provided at the end of the exercise.

1. acromegally — acromegaly
2. luteinizing — leutenizing
3. islets (of Langerhans) — ilets (of Langerhans)
4. cretanism — cretinism
5. uthyroid — euthyroid
6. hirsutism — hirtsutism
7. myxedema — mixedema
8. virelism — virilism
9. pancreatitis — pancretitis
10. thyroidectomy — throidectomy

Number correct _______ × 10 points/correct answer: Your score _______%

C. Matching Abbreviations

Match the abbreviations on the left with the appropriate definition on the right. Each correct response is worth 10 points. Record your score in the space provided at the end of the exercise.

_____	1. ACTH	a.	thyroid-stimulating hormone
_____	2. BMR	b.	protein-bound iodine
_____	3. FBS	c.	non-insulin-dependent diabetes mellitus
_____	4. GTT	d.	adrenocorticotropic hormone
_____	5. HDL	e.	basal metabolic rate
_____	6. K	f.	hyperdiabetic lipidemia
_____	7. Na	g.	calcium
_____	8. NIDDM	h.	sodium
_____	9. PBI	i.	fasting blood sugar
_____	10. TSH	j.	glucose tolerance test
		k.	high-density lipoprotein
		l.	potassium

Number correct _______ × 10 points/correct answer: Your score _______%

D. Definition to Term

Using the following definitions, identify and provide the medical word to match the definition. Write the word in the first space and the appropriate combining form for the word in the second space. Each correct answer is worth 5 points. Record your score in the space provided at the end.

1. Enlargement of the extremities

_______________________________ _______________________________

(word) (combining form)

2. Surgical removal of one or both adrenal glands

_______________________________ _______________________________

(word) (combining form)

3. More than normal blood calcium level

_______________________________ _______________________________

(word) (combining form)

4. The study of the endocrine system

_______________________________ _______________________________

(word) (combining form)

5. More than normal blood potassium level

_______________________________ _______________________________

(word) (combining form)

6. Inflammation of the pancreas

_______________________________ _______________________________

(word) (combining form)

7. Condition of an overactive thyroid gland

______________________ ______________________

(word) (combining form)

8. The study of poisons and their antidotes

______________________ ______________________

(word) (combining form)

9. More than normal blood sodium level

______________________ ______________________

(word) (combining form)

10. Any disease of a gland

______________________ ______________________

(word) (combining form)

***Number correct* ______ × *5 points/correct answer: Your score* ______%**

E. Crossword Puzzle

Read the clues carefully and complete the puzzle. Each crossword answer is worth 10 points. When you have completed the crossword puzzle, total your points and enter your score in the space provided.

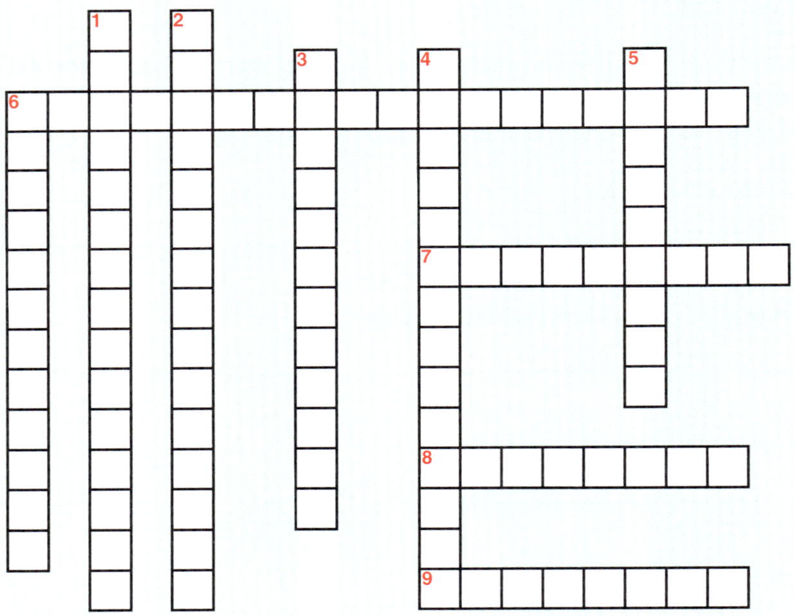

ACROSS

6 Low parathyroid hormone secretion
7 Excessive hair on face and body
8 Low growth hormone secretion
9 Most severe form of hypothyroidism

DOWN

1 Overactive thyroid gland
2 Deficiency of pituitary hormones
3 Inflammation of pancreas
4 Due to shortage of thyroid hormone
5 Hypersecretion of growth hormone
6 Low blood sugar level

***Number correct* ______ × *10 points/correct answer: Your score* ______%**

F. Matching Hormones

Match the hormones on the left with the principal endocrine gland that secretes them on the right. Each correct answer is worth 10 points. Record your score in the space provided at the end of the exercise.

_____	1. growth hormone	a.	pancreas
_____	2. antidiuretic hormone	b.	adrenal cortex
_____	3. thyroxine	c.	anterior pituitary gland
_____	4. parathormone	d.	ovaries
_____	5. thymosin	e.	testes
_____	6. hydrocortisone	f.	thymus gland
_____	7. epinephrine (adrenaline)	g.	parathyroid glands
_____	8. testosterone	h.	thyroid gland
_____	9. estrogen	i.	posterior pituitary gland
_____	10. insulin	j.	adrenal medulla

Number correct _______ × 10 points/correct answer: Your score _______%

G. Proofreading Skills

The following is a portion of a history and physical report. For each boldface term, provide a brief definition and indicate if the term is spelled correctly. If it is misspelled, provide the correct spelling. Each correct answer is worth 10 points. Record your score in the space provided at the end of the exercise.

Example:

polyphagia *excessive eating* ______________________________

Spelled correctly? ☑ Yes ☐ No ______________________________

1. **polyuria** ______________________________
   Spelled correctly? ☐ Yes ☐ No ______________________________

2. **polydispia** ______________________________
   Spelled correctly? ☐ Yes ☐ No ______________________________

3. **glycasuria** ______________________________
   Spelled correctly? ☐ Yes ☐ No ______________________________

4. **hyperglycemia** ______________________________
   Spelled correctly? ☐ Yes ☐ No ______________________________

5. **hypoglycemia** ______________________________
   Spelled correctly? ☐ Yes ☐ No ______________________________

6. **gestational diabetes** ______________________________
   Spelled correctly? ☐ Yes ☐ No ______________________________

7. **diabetes mellitis** ______________________________
   Spelled correctly? ☐ Yes ☐ No ______________________________

8. **hyperthroidism** ______________________________
   Spelled correctly? ☐ Yes ☐ No ______________________________

9. **exopthalmia** ______________________________

Spelled correctly? ☐ Yes ☐ No ______________________________

10. **thyroxine** ______________________________

Spelled correctly? ☐ Yes ☐ No ______________________________

Number correct* _______ × *10 points/correct answer: Your score* _______*%

NAME: Smith, Jane M.

ROOM NO: 1256

HOSPITAL NO: 65231

ATTENDING PHYSICIAN: Dr. U. R. Wright

ADMISSION DATE: 9-12-03

CHIEF COMPLAINT: Tiredness, headaches, increased thirst and hunger, frequency of urination, nervousness, irritability, sleepiness, vague pains, general malaise.

PRESENT ILLNESS: This 42-year-old female was admitted to the hospital because of a 3-week history of **polyuria, polydispia,** and **polyphagia.** She has been very nervous, irritable, very sensitive emotionally, and cries easily. During this time period, she has had frequent headaches, has become very sleepy and tired after eating, and has had leg pains. She was seen in my office 5 days ago and found then to have a blood pressure of 198/98 mmHg and **glycasuria.** (4+). Lab tests revealed **hyperglycemia.**

PAST HISTORY: She has had the common childhood diseases. She states that when she was in college (approximately 7 years ago), she had bouts of **hypoglycemia** that were pretty severe at times. She found that adding protein snacks throughout the day seemed to help the situation. Five years ago when she was pregnant, she was found to have **gestational diabetes,** but this disappeared after delivery. She has no history of surgeries.

FAMILY HISTORY: Strong family history of diabetes. Father and two sisters have **diabetes mellitis.** Mother has **hyperthroidism** with somewhat noticeable **exopthalmia,** but this is well controlled with **thyroxine.** One brother was thought to have diabetes as a child, but GTT revealed that his blood glucose levels were normal.

REVIEW OF SYSTEMS: "Omitted"

PHYSICAL EXAMINATION: "Omitted"

DIAGNOSIS: (1) Diabetes mellitus
(2) Hypertension

H. Completion

Complete each sentence with the most appropriate pathological condition. Each correct answer is worth 10 points. Record your score in the space provided at the end of the exercise.

1. An abnormal overgrowth of the bones in the feet, hands, and face with onset occurring after puberty and epiphyseal closure is known as:

   ____

2. A disease in which there is chronic thyroiditis leading to enlargement of the thyroid. This disease of the immune system in which the gland tissue is destroyed by antibodies and replaced with fibrous tissue is known as:

   ____

3. Hypertrophy of the thyroid gland resulting in an excessive secretion of the thyroid hormone causing an extremely high body metabolism is known as:

   ____

4. An acute, sometimes fatal, incident of overactivity of the thyroid gland resulting in excessive secretion of thyroid hormone is known as:

   ____

5. A cluster of symptoms occurring due to an excessive amount of circulating cortisol or ACTH is termed:

   ____

6. A vascular tumor of the adrenal medulla that produces extra epinephrine and norepinephrine leading to persistent or intermittent hypertension and heart palpitations is known as:

   ____

7. A condition that occurs as a consequence of an 8- to 10-year duration of diabetes mellitus in which the capillaries of the retina experience scarring is known as:

   ____

8. A life-threatening primary malignant neoplasm typically found in the head of the pancreas is known as:

   ____

9. Thyroid function is evaluated by administering a known amount of radioactive iodine and later placing a gamma ray detector over the thyroid gland to determine the percentage or quantity of radioactive iodine absorbed by the gland over specific time. This diagnostic test is called:

   ____

10. An ultrasound examination important in distinguishing solid thyroid nodules from cystic nodules is a:

    ____

Number correct ______ × 10 points/correct answer: Your score ______%

I. Matching Conditions

Read the descriptions on the right and match them with the appropriate pathological conditions on the left. Each correct answer is worth 10 points. Record your score in the space provided at the end of the exercise.

_____ 1. diabetes mellitus
_____ 2. simple goiter
_____ 3. Addison's disease
_____ 4. hyperparathyroidism
_____ 5. primary aldosteronism
_____ 6. diabetic retinopathy
_____ 7. virilism
_____ 8. thyroid cancer
_____ 9. diabetes insipidus
_____ 10. thyrotoxicosis

a. Occurs as a consequence of an 8- to 10-year duration of diabetes mellitus in which the capillaries of the retina experience scarring
b. Excretion of excessive amounts of aldosterone, the most influential of the mineralocorticoids
c. Output of extreme amounts of adrenocortical androgens caused by an adrenal tumor or hyperplasia typically in adult women (30 to 40 years)
d. An acute, sometimes fatal, incident of overactivity of the thyroid gland resulting in excessive secretion of thyroid hormone
e. A life-threatening disease process caused from failure of the adrenal cortex to secrete adequate mineralocorticoids and glucocorticoids resulting from an autoimmune process, a neoplasm, an infection, or a hemorrhage in the gland
f. Escalated activity of the parathyroid that leads to high levels of calcium in the blood and low levels of calcium in the bones as a result of demineralization, the breakdown of bone
g. A deficiency in the secretion of antidiuretic hormone (ADH) by the posterior pituitary gland
h. A disorder of the pancreas in which the beta cells of the islets of Langerhans of the pancreas fail to produce an adequate amount of insulin
i. Hyperplasia, an elevation in the amount of cells of the thyroid gland
j. Malignant tumors of the thyroid gland lead to dysfunction of the gland and thus inadequate or excessive secretion of the thyroid hormone

Number correct _______ × 10 points/correct answer: Your score _______%

J. Definition to Term

Using the following definitions, identify and provide the word for the pathological condition to match the definition. (A clue has been provided for the number of words needed in your answer.) Each correct answer is worth 10 points. Record your score in the space provided at the end of the exercise.

1. Congenital hypopituitarism

   ____

   (one word)
2. Thyroid gland hyperplasia

   ____

   (three words)
3. Chronic enlargement of the thyroid gland

   ____

   (two words)

4. Causes an extremely high body metabolism

____

(one word)

5. Unnatural protruding of the eyes

____

(one word)

6. Results in low levels of calcium in the blood

____

(one word)

7. Occurs when large doses of glucocorticoids are given over a period of time

____

(two words)

8. Excess secretion of the human growth hormone before puberty

____

(one word)

9. Causes an extremely low body metabolism

____

(one word)

10. A result of demineralization in the bones

____

(one word)

Number correct _______ × 10 points/correct answer: Your score _______%

K. Word Search

Using the definitions provided, identify the pathological condition and then find and circle it in the puzzle below. The words may be read up, down, diagonally, across, or backward. Each correct answer is worth 10 points. Record your score in the space provided at the end of the exercise.

Example: Low blood sugar

hypoglycemia

1. Excretion of excessive amounts of aldosterone, the most influential of the mineralocorticoids, is known as primary:

____

2. A vascular tumor of the adrenal medulla that produces extra epinephrine and norepinephrine leading to persistent or intermittent hypertension and heart palpitations

____

3. A life-threatening disease process caused from failure of the adrenal cortex to secrete adequate mineralocorticoids and glucocorticoids resulting from an autoimmune process, a neoplasm, an infection, or a hemorrhage in the gland

____

4. An acute, sometimes fatal, incident of overactivity of the thyroid gland resulting in excessive secretion of thyroid hormones

____

5. An abnormal overgrowth of the bones of the feet, hands, and face with the onset occurring after puberty

____

6. Congenital hypothyroidism

____

7. The most severe form of hypothyroidism

____

8. Increased activity of this gland leading to high levels of calcium in the blood and low levels of calcium in the bones is known as hyperthyroidism

____

9. The development of masculine physical and mental traits in the female such as growth of facial and body hair, increased secretion of the sebaceous glands, deepening of the voice, and enlargement of the clitoris

____

10. Excessive secretion of the thyroid hormone causing extremely high body metabolism

____

A	E	H	Y	P	O	G	L	Y	C	E	M	I	A	O
M	E	Y	D	A	B	N	I	A	L	L	I	U	G	S
O	D	P	Y	D	C	U	A	E	I	C	G	E	N	S
T	A	E	S	A	I	H	C	D	I	R	E	A	N	E
Y	A	R	H	R	S	S	R	L	E	E	I	O	N	A
C	C	T	Y	O	I	T	O	N	O	T	S	Z	D	M
O	C	H	O	C	H	R	M	N	O	I	Y	T	O	M
M	N	Y	R	P	P	L	E	X	D	N	E	R	U	X
O	A	R	E	E	I	N	G	D	T	I	P	I	R	L
R	T	O	C	T	B	N	A	X	T	S	N	M	I	A
H	I	I	E	R	I	R	L	R	L	M	A	E	I	T
C	E	D	P	A	L	N	Y	E	A	D	D	R	C	I
O	N	I	M	S	I	L	I	R	I	V	R	S	N	O
E	S	S	A	I	E	S	U	S	P	O	S	U	P	N
H	O	M	M	Y	X	E	D	E	M	A	S	Y	A	T
P	A	R	A	T	H	Y	R	O	I	D	I	S	M	L
S	M	S	I	N	O	R	E	T	S	O	D	L	A	N
P	S	I	S	O	C	I	X	O	T	O	R	Y	H	T

***Number correct* _______ × *10 points/correct answer: Your score* _______%**

Answers to Chapter Review Exercises

A. Term to Definition

1. enlargement and elongation of the bones of the face, jaw, and extremities due to oversecretion of the pituitary gland after puberty
2. a physician who specializes in the medical practice treating the diseases and disorders of the endocrine system
3. an abnormal condition characterized by a marked outward protrusion of the eyeballs
4. a hormone secreted by the islets of Langerhans of the pancreas that stimulates the liver to convert glycogen into glucose
5. the conversion of excess glucose into glycogen for storage in the liver for later use as needed
6. a condition in which there is excessive body hair in a male distribution pattern
7. excessive thirst
8. the excretion of excessively large amounts of urine
9. a condition characterized by severe cramping and twitching of the muscles, and sharp flexion of the wrist and ankle joints
10. the development of masculine physical and mental traits in the female

B. Spelling

1. acromegaly
2. luteinizing
3. islets of Langerhans
4. cretinism
5. euthyroid
6. hirsutism
7. myxedema
8. virilism
9. pancreatitis
10. thyroidectomy

C. Matching Abbreviations

1. d
2. e
3. i
4. j
5. k
6. l
7. h
8. c
9. b
10. a

D. Definition to Term

1. acromegaly	acr/o
2. adrenalectomy	adrenal/o
3. hypercalcemia	calc/o
4. endocrinology	crin/o
5. hyperkalemia	kal/i
6. pancreatitis	pancreat/o
7. hyperthyroidism	thyroid/o
8. toxicology	toxic/o
9. hypernatremia	natr/i
10. adenopathy	aden/o

E. Crossword Puzzle

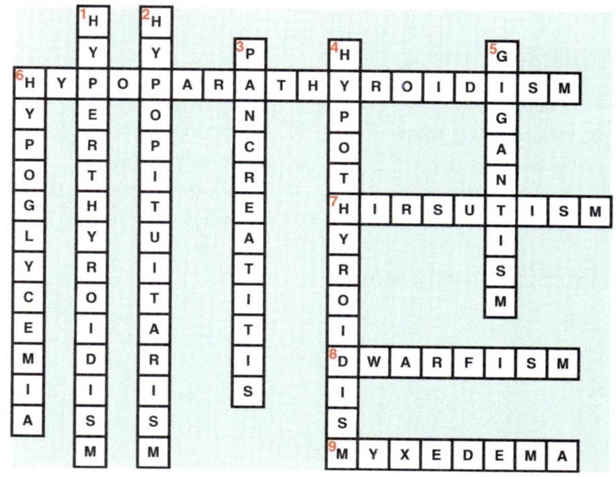

F. Matching Hormones

1. c
2. i
3. h
4. g
5. f
6. b
7. j
8. e
9. d
10. a

G. Proofreading Skills

1. The excretion of excessively large amounts of urine.
   Spelled correctly? Yes
2. Excessive thirst.
   Spelled correctly? No **polydipsia**
3. The presence of sugar in the urine.
   Spelled correctly? No **glycosuria**
4. Elevated blood sugar level.
   Spelled correctly? Yes
5. Less than normal blood sugar level.
   Spelled correctly? Yes
6. A condition occurring in pregnancy that is characterized by the signs and symptoms of diabetes mellitus such as elevated blood sugar level.
   Spelled correctly? Yes
7. A disorder of the pancreas in which the beta cells of the islets of Langerhans of the pancreas fail to produce an adequate amount of insulin, resulting in the body's inability to appropriately metabolize carbohydrates, fats, and proteins.
   Spelled correctly? No **diabetes mellitus**
8. Overactivity of the thyroid gland.
   Spelled correctly? No **hyperthyroidism**

9. An abnormal condition characterized by a marked outward protrusion of the eyeballs.
   Spelled correctly? No **exophthalmia**
10. A hormone secreted by the thyroid gland.
   Spelled correctly? Yes

H. Completion

1. acromegaly
2. Hashimoto's thyroiditis
3. Graves' disease
4. thyroid storm
5. Cushing's syndrome
6. pheochromocytoma
7. diabetic retinopathy
8. pancreatic cancer
9. radioactive iodine uptake test
10. thyroid echogram

I. Matching Conditions

1. h
2. i
3. e
4. f
5. b
6. a
7. c
8. j
9. g
10. d

J. Definition to Term

1. dwarfism
2. simple nontoxic goiter
3. Hashimoto's thyroiditis
4. hyperthyroidism
5. exophthalmus
6. hypoparathyroidism
7. Cushing's syndrome
8. gigantism
9. hypothyroidism
10. hypercalcemia

K. Word Search

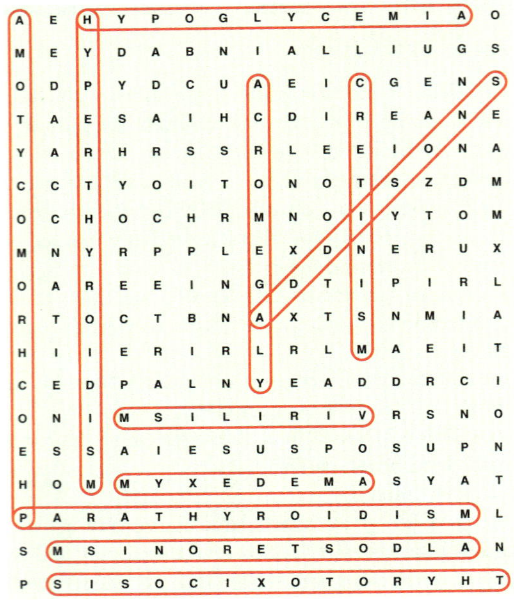

CHAPTER 14

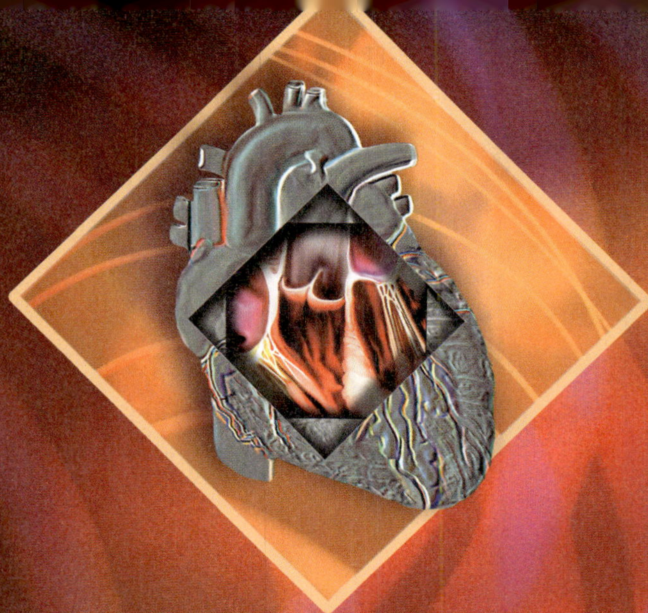

The Special Senses

CHAPTER CONTENT

KEY COMPETENCIES

Upon completing this chapter and the review exercises at the end of the chapter, the learner should be able to:

1. Correctly identify and label the structures of the eye.
2. Identify and define 20 pathological conditions of the eye and ear.
3. Identify at least 10 diagnostic techniques used in treating disorders of the eye and ear.
4. Correctly spell and pronounce each new term introduced in this chapter using the Activity CD-ROM and Audio CD, if available.
5. Create at least 10 medical terms related to the eye and ear and identify the appropriate combining form(s) for each term.
6. Identify at least 20 abbreviations common to the eye and ear.
7. Identify the pathway of sound from the external auditory canal to the cerebral cortex.

OVERVIEW OF THE EYE

Remember the saying, "A picture is worth a thousand words." What a true statement! If you were a camera, you could capture the moment in a photograph by aiming in the right direction, adjusting the lens to bring the object into clear focus, and opening the shutter to allow just the right amount of light to enter upon the sensitive film layer to capture the picture. The processing of the picture, however, would be up to your owner!

You, however, are not a camera; but you do possess the ability to capture the moment with your eyes! As you observe a scene, the lens of your eye will adjust to bring the object into clear focus. The pupil of your eye will constrict to allow less light to enter in a bright setting or will dilate to allow more light to enter in a darker setting. Through several processes of bending the light rays, the image finally reaches the sensitive nerve cell layer of the eye, called the retina. From the retina, the image is transmitted to the brain for interpretation (or processing)—and so you have your picture.

As we discuss the eye, you will gain an understanding of the structure and function of this vital organ that we take for granted but depend on so completely. We will also discuss the corrections for errors of refraction (inability to focus clearly), pathological conditions of the eye, and treatments and procedures common to the eye. As you read, you will see things more clearly!

Anatomy and Physiology (Eye)

The eyes are housed in bony orbits located within the facial bones, at the front of the skull. Embedded in a mass of orbital fat for protection and insulation, each eye is supplied by one of a pair of optic nerves. Most of the eye is contained within the bony orbit, with only the anterior portion of the eye being exposed to view.

We will begin the description of the eye structures based on the frontal view of the eye in **Figure 14-1.**

The **(1)** **sclera** is the white portion of the eye. This tough, fibrous membrane maintains the shape of the eyeball and serves as a protective covering for the eye. The colored portion of the eye is known as the **(2) iris** and may appear to be blue, green, brown, or hazel (yellowish brown). In the center of the iris is an opening called the **(3) pupil.** The pupil controls the amount of light entering the eye, and its diameter is regulated by the relaxing and contracting of the iris.

The **(4) conjunctiva** is a thin mucous membrane layer that lines the anterior part of the eye, which is exposed to air, and the inner part of the eyelids. The conjunctiva is colorless, but appears white because it covers the sclera. If the blood vessels beneath the conjunctiva become dilated due to irritation, it will have a reddish, or "blood-shot" appearance. Crying, smoke, dust, and other eye irritants can cause the blood vessels of the eyes to dilate and give the reddened appearance.

Located at the upper outer edge of each eye (under the upper eyelid) is the **(5)** **lacrimal gland,** which produces tears. The tears flow constantly across the conjunctival surfaces

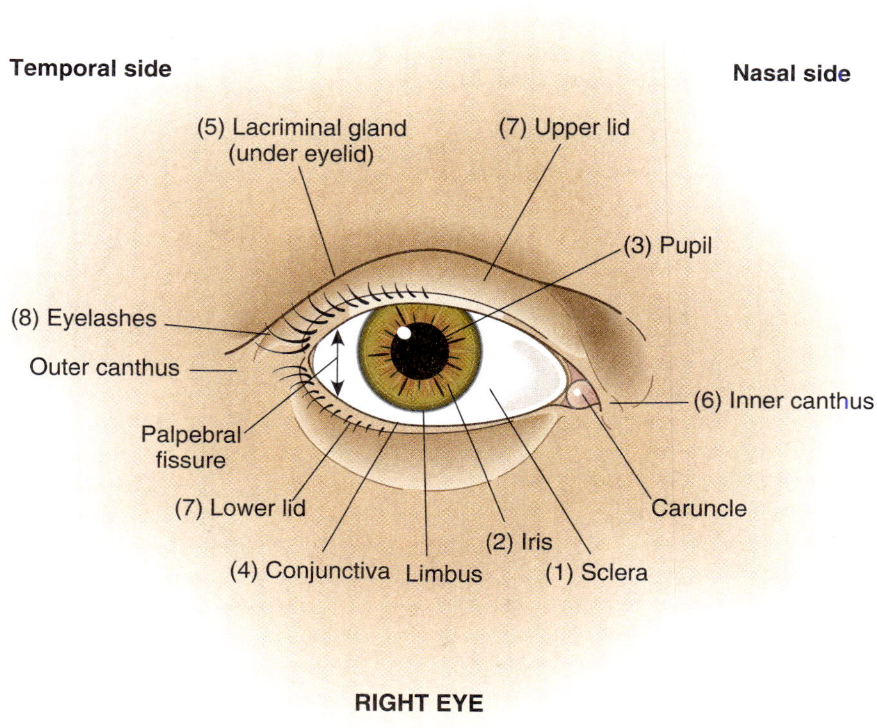

Figure 14-1 Front view of the eye

to cleanse and lubricate them; additionally, tears help to prevent bacterial infections in the eye due to the presence of an antibacterial enzyme called lysozyme, which destroys microorganisms. Tears drain from the eye through the **lacrimal duct**, located at the (6) **canthus (inner edge)** of the eye. In addition to the body's natural production of tears for functional purposes, the human also produces tears in response to an emotional upset in the form of crying.

The upper and lower (7) **eyelids** are continuous with the skin and cover the eyeball, keeping the surface of the eyeball lubricated and protected from dust and debris through their blinking motion. The eyelid skin is very thin. The (8) **eyelashes** are located along the edges of the eyelids. They help to further protect the eyeball by preventing foreign materials and/or insects from coming in contact with the surface of the eyeball.

The lateral cross section of the eye, illustrated in **Figure 14-2,** shows the structures of the eye from front to back. This figure serves as a visual reference as the discussion of the eye continues.

The outermost layer of the eye is the (1) sclera the white portion of the eye. This tough, fibrous membrane maintains the shape of the eyeball and serves as a protective covering for the eye. Also known as the "white of the eye," the sclera is thinnest over the anterior surface of the eye and thickest at the back of the eye near the opening for the entrance of the optic nerve. Continuous with the anterior portion of the sclera is the (2) **cornea**, a transparent, nonvascular layer covering the colored part of the eye, known as the iris. The (3) conjunctiva is the mucous membrane that lines the inner surfaces of the eyelids and the outer surfaces of the eye.

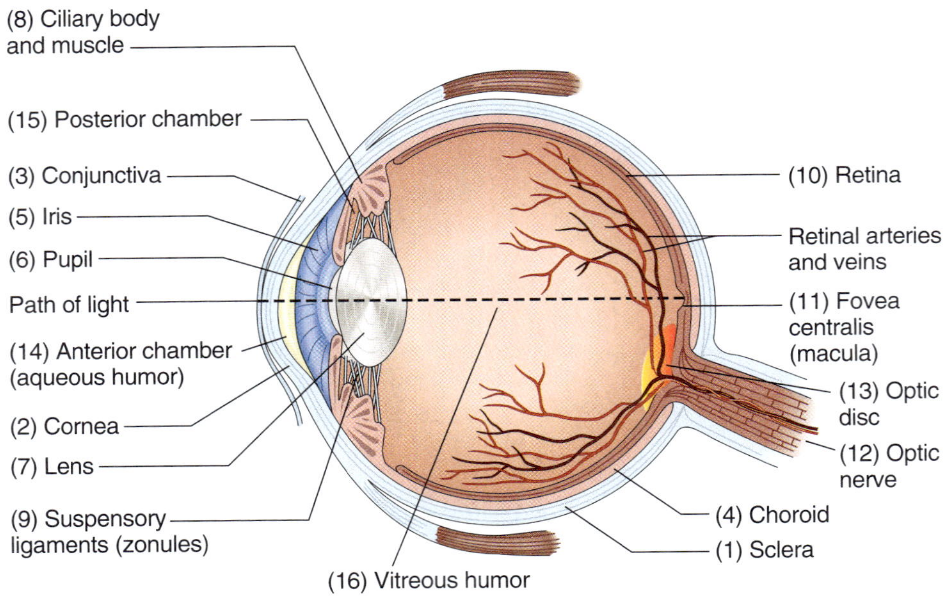

Figure 14-2 Lateral cross section of the eye

The vascular middle layer of the eye contains the **(4) choroid**, a layer just beneath the sclera, which contains extensive capillaries that provide the blood supply and nutrients to the eye. The choroid contains three structures: the iris, ciliary body, and the suspensory ligaments. The **(5)** iris, which is the colored portion of the eye, can be seen through the transparent corneal layer. In the center of the iris is a round opening called the **(6)** pupil.

The pupil controls the amount of light entering the eye by contracting or dilating. This action is actually controlled by two sets of muscles within the iris: the radial muscles within the iris that dilate the pupil in dim light to allow more light to enter the eye, and the circular muscles within the iris that constrict the pupil in bright light to allow less light to enter the eye.

Posterior to the iris is the **(7) lens**, a colorless biconvex structure that aids in focusing the images clearly on the sensitive nerve cell layer called the retina. On each side of the lens is the **(8) ciliary body**, which contains muscles that are responsible for adjusting the lens to view near objects. Radiating from the ciliary body are numerous straight fibrils, called **(9) suspensory ligaments**, that attach to the lens and hold it in place. These ligaments respond to the contraction and relaxation of the ciliary body muscles to adjust the shape of the lens for proper focusing of the eye. The lens becomes thicker or thinner through the relaxation and contraction of these sets of muscles.

The thickening and thinning of the lens causes the light rays to bend appropriately so the image will focus clearly on the sensitive nerve cell layer of the eye. The ability of the lens to clearly focus on objects at various distances is known as **accommodation.** The lens accommodates for the closeness of an object by increasing its curvature (or bulging) to bend the rays more sharply so they will focus directly on the retina, producing a clear image. As one ages, the ability of the lens to accommodate to near vision is lost and correction is needed. This condition is discussed later in the section on pathological conditions.

The third innermost layer of the eye is the **(10) retina**. This sensitive nerve cell layer changes the energy of the light rays into nerve impulses. The nerve impulses are transmitted via the optic nerve to the brain for interpretation of the image seen by the eye. These nerve cells, which are highly specialized for stimulation by light rays, are called **rods** and **cones.** The cones are responsible for visualizing colors, central vision, and vision in bright light. The highest concentration of cones is in the **(11) fovea centralis**, a small depression located within the **macula lutea**. The macula lutea is an oval, yellowish spot near the center of the retina. When the image focuses directly on the fovea centralis, the sharpest image is obtained. This is known as central vision. The rods, located at the outer edges of the retina, are responsible for vision in dim light and for peripheral vision.

The impulses from the retina are transmitted through the **(12) optic nerve** to the brain where they are interpreted as vision. The only part of the retina that is insensitive to light is the **(13) optic disc**, because it contains no rods or cones, and thus is also known as the "blind spot" of the eye. The center of the optic disc serves as a point of entry for the artery that supplies the retina.

The interior of the eye is composed of two cavities: the anterior cavity and the posterior cavity. The anterior cavity contains the **(14) anterior chamber**, located in front of the lens and the **(15) posterior chamber**, located behind the lens. These chambers are filled with a clear, watery fluid known as **aqueous humor**, which flows freely between them. It is constantly produced and is reabsorbed into the venous circulation. The balance between production and absorption of the aqueous humor maintains the proper pressure within the eye.

The posterior cavity is posterior to the lens and is filled with **(16) vitreous humor**, a clear, jellylike substance that gives shape to the eyeball. The vitreous humor is not constantly reproduced. If an injury to the eye causes escape of the vitreous humor, blindness can result. Both the aqueous humor and the vitreous humor aid in the refracting, or bending, of light rays as they pass through these chambers on the way to the retina.

The Process of Vision

When light rays enter the eye, they are transmitted through the cornea, aqueous humor, pupil, lens, and the vitreous humor to the retina where the sensitive nerve cells transmit the image through the optic nerve to the brain where it is interpreted as vision. As the light rays pass through these various structures and fluids, a process of bending occurs that eventually allows the image to focus clearly on the retina, producing a single vision. This bending of the light rays, as they pass through the various structures of the eye to produce a clear image on the retina, is known as **refraction**. If the eye is abnormally shaped or the lens has lost its ability to accommodate to near vision, the individual will have difficulty forming a clear image and will experience blurred vision. These errors of refraction can be adjusted by placing the lenses of glasses in front of the lens of the eye to further refract the light rays, bringing them into focus on the retina. Four errors of refraction will be discussed in the section on pathological conditions: astigmatism, hyperopia, myopia, and presbyopia.

Vocabulary (Eye)

The following vocabulary words are frequently used when discussing the eye.

WORD	DEFINITION
ambiopia (am-bee-**OH**-pee-ah) **ambi-** = both sides **-opia** = visual condition	Double vision caused by each eye focusing separately.
amblyopia (am-blee-**OH**-pee-ah) **ambly/o** = dull, dim **-opia** = visual condition	Dullness or dimness of vision.
anisocoria (an-eye-soh-**KOH**-ree-ah) **aniso-** = unequal **cor/o** = pupil **-ia** = condition	Inequality in the diameter of the pupils of the eyes.
aphakia (ah-**FAY**-kee-ah) **a-** = without, not **phak/o** = lens **-ia** = condition	Absence of the lens of the eye.
aqueous (**AY**-kwee-us)	Watery.
Argyll-Robertson pupil (ar-**GILL ROB**-ert-son pupil)	A pupil that constricts on accommodation but not in response to light.
blepharochalasis (blef-ah-roh-**KAL**-ah-sis) **blephar/o** = eyelid	Relaxation of the skin of the eyelid. The skin may droop over the edge of the eyelid when the eyes are open.
blepharoptosis (blef-ah-roh-**TOH**-sis) **blephar/o** = eyelid **-ptosis** = drooping or prolapse	Drooping of the upper eyelid.
blepharospasm **blephar/o** = eyelid **-spasm** = twitching, involuntary contraction	A twitching of the eyelid muscles; may be due to eyestrain or nervous irritability.
conjunctivitis (kon-junk-tih-**VYE**-tis) **conjunctiv/o** = conjunctiva **-itis** = inflammation	Inflammation of the conjunctiva of the eye; may be caused by a bacterial infection, a viral infection, allergy, or a response to the environment.

corneal (**COR**-nee-al) corne/o = cornea -al = pertaining to	Pertaining to the cornea.
cycloplegia (sigh-kloh-**PLEE**-jee-ah) cycl/o = ciliary body -plegia = paralysis	Paralysis of the ciliary muscle of the eye.
dacryoadenitis (dak-ree-oh-ad-en-**EYE**-tis) dacry/o = tears aden/o = gland -itis = inflammation	Inflammation of the lacrimal (tear) gland.
dacryorrhea (dak-ree-oh-**REE**-ah) dacry/o = tears -rrhea = discharge, flow	Excessive flow of tears.
diplopia (dip-**LOH**-pee-ah) dipl/o = double -opia = vision	Double vision caused by each eye focusing separately. See *ambiopia.*
ectropion (ek-**TROH**-pee-on)	Eversion (turning outward) of the edge of the eyelid.
emmetropia (em-eh-**TROH**-pee-ah)	A state of normal vision; the eye is at rest and the image is focusing directly on the retina.
entropion (en-**TROH**-pee-on)	Inversion (turning inward) of the edge of the eyelid.
episcleritis (ep-ih-skleh-**RYE**-tis) epi- = upon scler/o = hard; also refers to sclera of the eye -itis = inflammation	Inflammation of the outermost layers of the sclera.
esotropia (ess-oh-**TROH**-pee-ah) es/o = within -tropia = to turn	An obvious inward turning of one eye in relation to the other eye; also called crosseyes.
exotropia (eks-oh-**TROH**-pee-ah) ex/o = outward -tropia = to turn	An obvious outward turning of one eye in relation to the other eye; also called walleye.
extraocular (eks-trah-**OCK**-yoo-lar) extra- = outside, beyond ocul/o = eye -ar = pertaining to	Pertaining to outside the eye.

floaters	One or more spots that appear to drift, "or float," across the visual field.
hemianopia (hem-ee-ah-**NOP**-ee-ah) **hemi-** = half **an-** = without **-opia** = visual condition	Blindness in one-half of the visual field.
hemianopsia (hem-ee-ah-**NOP**-see-ah) **hemi-** = half **an-** = without **-opsia** = visual condition	See *hemianopia.*
iriditis (ir-ih-**DYE**-tis) **irid/o** = iris **-itis** = inflammation	Inflammation of the iris; see ***iritis***.
iridocyclitis (ir-id-oh-sigh-**KLEYE**-tis) **irid/o** = iris **cycl/o** = ciliary body **-itis** = inflammation	Inflammation of the iris and ciliary body of the eye.
iritis (ih-**RYE**-tis) **ir/o** = iris **-itis** = inflammation	Inflammation of the iris; see ***iriditis***.
keratoconjunctivitis (ker-ah-toh-kon-junk-tih-**VYE**-tis) **kerat/o** = hard, horny; also refers to cornea of the eye **conjunctiv/o** = conjunctiva **-itis** = inflammation	Inflammation of the cornea and the conjunctiva of the eye.
keratoconus (ker-ah-toh-**KOH**-nus) **kerat/o** = hard, horny; also refers to cornea of the eye	A cone-shaped protrusion of the center of the cornea, not accompanied by inflammation.
keratomycosis (ker-ah-toh-my-**KOH**-sis) **kerat/o** = hard, horny; also refers to cornea of the eye **myc/o** = fungus **-osis** = condition	A fungal growth present on the cornea.

lacrimal (**LAK**-rim-al) lacrim/o = tears -al = pertaining to	Pertaining to tears.
lacrimation (lak-rih-**MAY**-shun)	The secretion of tears from the lacrimal glands.
miosis (my-**OH**-sis) mi/o = smaller -sis = condition	Abnormal constriction of the pupil of the eye.
miotic (my-**OT**-ik) mi/o = smaller -tic = pertaining to	An agent that causes the pupil of the eye to constrict.
mydriasis (mid-**RYE**-ah-sis) mydr/o = widen -iasis = presence of an abnormal condition	Abnormal dilatation of the pupil of the eye.
mydriatic (mid-ree-**AT**-ik) mydr/o = widen -iatic = pertaining to a condition	An agent that causes the pupil of the eye to dilate.
nasolacrimal (nay-zoh-**LAK**-rim-al) nas/o = nose lacrim/o = tears -al = pertaining to	Pertaining to the nose and the lacrimal (tear) ducts.
nystagmus (niss-**TAG**-mus)	Involuntary, rhythmic jerking movements of the eye. These "quivering" movements may be from side to side, up and down, or a combination of both.
ophthalmologist (off-thal-**MALL**-oh-jist) ophthalm/o = eye -logist = one who specializes in the study of	A medical doctor (M.D.) who specializes in the treatment of the diseases and disorders of the eye.
ophthalmology (off-thal-**MALL**-oh-jee) ophthalm/o = eyes -logy = the study of	The branch of medicine that specializes in the study of the diseases and disorders of the eye.
ophthalmopathy (off-thal-**MOP**-ah-thee) ophthalm/o = eye -pathy = disease	Any disease of the eye.

optic (**OP**-tik) opt/o = eye, vision -ic = pertaining to	Pertaining to the eyes or to sight.
optician (op-**TISH**-an) optic/o = eye, vision	A health professional (not an M.D.) who specializes in filling prescriptions for corrective lenses for glasses or for contact lenses.
optometrist (op-**TOM**-eh-trist) opt/o = eye, vision metr/o = to measure -ist = practitioner	A health professional (not an M.D.) who specializes in testing the eyes for visual acuity and prescribing corrective lenses.
palpebral (**PAL**-peh-brahl)	Pertaining to the eyelid.
papilledema (pap-ill-eh-**DEE**-mah)	Swelling of the optic disc, visible on ophthalmoscopic examination of the interior of the eye.
phacomalacia (fak-oh-mah-**LAY**-shee-ah) phac/o = lens malac/o = softening -ia = condition	Softening of the lens of the eye.
photophobia (foh-toh-**FOH**-bee-ah) phot/o = light -phobia = abnormal fear	Abnormal sensitivity to light, especially by the eyes.
presbyopia (prez-bee-**OH**-pee-ah) presby/o = old age -opia = vision	Loss of accommodation for near vision; poor vision due to the natural aging process.
pupillary (**PEW**-pih-lair-ee)	Pertaining to the pupil of the eye.
retinopathy (ret-in-**OP**-ah-thee) retin/o = retina -pathy = disease	Any disease of the retina.
sclerectomy (skleh-**REK**-toh-mee) scler/o = hard; also refers to sclera of the eye -ectomy = surgical removal	Excision, or removal, of a portion of the sclera of the eye.
scotoma (skoh-**TOH**-mah) scot/o = darkness -oma = tumor	An area of depressed vision (blindness) within the usual visual field, surrounded by an area of normal vision.

uveitis
(yoo-vee-**EYE**-tis)

Inflammation of the uveal tract of the eye, which includes the iris, ciliary body, and the choroid.

vitreous
(**VIT**-ree-us)
vitre/o = glassy
-ous = pertaining to

Pertaining to the vitreous body of the eye.

Word Elements (Eye)

The following word elements pertain to the diseases, disorders, signs, symptoms, and diagnostic techniques associated with the eye. As you review the list, pronounce each word element aloud twice and check the box after you "say it." Write the definition for the example word given for each word element. You may use your medical dictionary.

WORD ELEMENT	PRONUNCIATION	"SAY IT"	MEANING
ambi- **ambi**opia	**AM**-bee am-bee-**OH**-pee-ah	☐	both, both sides
ambly/o **ambly**opia	**AM**-blee-oh am-blee-**OH**-pee-ah	☐	dull
aque/o **aque**ous humor	**AY**-kwee-oh **AY**-kwee-us humor	☐	watery
blephar/o **blephar**itis	**BLEF**-ah-roh blef-ah-**RYE**-tis	☐	eyelid
conjunctiv/o **conjunctiv**itis	kon-junk-tih-**VOH** kon-junk-tih-**VYE**-tis	☐	conjunctiva
cor/o aniso**cor**ia	**KOH**-roh an-eye-soh-**KOH**-ree-ah	☐	pupil
corne/o **corne**itis	**COR**-nee-oh cor-nee-**EYE**-tis	☐	cornea
dacry/o **dacry**oadenitis	**DAK**-ree-oh dak-ree-oh-ad-en-**EYE**-tis	☐	tears
dacryocyst/o **dacryocyst**ectomy	dak-ree-oh-**SISS**-toh dak-ree-oh-siss-**TEK**-toh-mee	☐	tear sac
dipl/o **dipl**opia	dip-**LOH** dip-**LOH**-pee-ah	☐	double
epi- **epi**scleritis	**EP**-ih ep-ih-skleh-**RYE**-tis	☐	upon, over

es/o **es**otropia	**ESS**-oh ess-oh-**TROH**-pee-ah	☐	within
ex/o **ex**otropia	**EKS**-oh eks-oh-**TROH**-pee-ah	☐	outward
extra- **extra**ocular	**EKS**-trah eks-trah-**OCK**-yoo-lar	☐	outside, beyond
glauc/o **glauc**oma	**GLAW**-koh glaw-**KOH**-mah	☐	gray, silver
hemi- **hemi**anopia	**HEM**-ee hem-ee-ah-**NOP**-ee-ah	☐	half
ir/o **ir**itis	**IH**-roh ih-**RYE**-tis	☐	iris
irid/o **irid**oplegia	**IR**-id-oh ir-id-oh-**PLEE**-jee-ah	☐	iris
kerat/o **kerat**itis	ker-**AH**-toh ker-ah-**TYE**-tis	☐	hard, horny; also refers to cornea of the eye
lacrim/o **lacrim**al	**LAK**-rim-oh **LAK**-rim-al	☐	tears
mi/o **mi**osis	**MY**-oh my-**OH**-sis	☐	smaller
nas/o **nas**olacrimal	**NAY**-zoh nay-zoh-**LAK**-rim-al	☐	nose
ocul/o **ocul**omotor	**OK**-yoo-loh **ok**-yoo-loh-**MOH**-tor	☐	eye
ophthalm/o **ophthalm**oscope	off-**THAL**-moh off-**THAL**-moh-scohp	☐	eye
-opia dipl**opia**	**OH**-pee-ah dip-**LOH**-pee-ah	☐	visual condition
-opsia hemian**opsia**	**OP**-see-ah hem-ee-ah-**NOP**-see-ah	☐	visual condition
opt/o **opt**ic	**OP**-toh **OP**-tik	☐	eye, vision
optic/o **optic**ian	**OP**-tik-oh op-**TISH**-an	☐	eye, vision

palpebr/o **palpebr**ate	pal-**PEE**-broh pal-**PEE**-brayt	☐	eyelid
phac/o, phak/o **phac**omalacia	**FAK**-oh fak-oh-mah-**LAY**-shee-ah	☐	lens
phot/o **photo**phobia	**FOH**-toh foh-toh-**FOH**-bee-ah	☐	light
-ptosis blepharo**ptosis**	op-**TOH**-sis blef-ah-roh-**TOH**-sis	☐	drooping or prolapse
pupill/o **pupill**ary	**PEW**-pill-oh **PEW**-pill-air-ee	☐	pupil
retin/o **retin**itis	**RET**-in-oh ret-in-**EYE**-tis	☐	retina
scler/o **scler**a	**SKLAIR**-oh **SKLAIR**-ah	☐	hard; also refers to sclera of the eye
scot/o **scot**oma	**SKOH**-toh skoh-**TOH**-mah	☐	darkness
ton/o **ton**ometry	**TOHN**-oh tohn-**OM**-eh-tree	☐	tension
vitre/o **vitre**ous humor	**VIT**-ree-oh **VIT**-ree-us humor	☐	glassy
xer/o **xer**ophthalmia	**ZEE**-roh zee-roff-**THAL**-mee-ah	☐	dry

Pathological Conditions (Eye)

As you study the pathological conditions of the eye, note that the **basic definition** is in bold print, followed by a detailed description in regular print. The phonetic pronunciation is directly beneath each term, and a breakdown of the component parts of the term when appropriate.

astigmatism
(ah-**STIG**-mah-tizm)

A refractive error causing the light rays entering the eye to be focused irregularly on the retina due to an abnormally shaped cornea.

Astigmatism causes blurred vision and discomfort; the individual also may complain of the need to rub the eyes frequently, headaches, and squinting. The diagnosis of astigmatism is verified through an ophthalmoscopic examination. Correction can usually be obtained through contact lenses or eyeglasses, which neutralize the defect.

blepharitis
(blef-ah-**RYE**-tis)
blephar/o = eyelid
-itis = inflammation

Inflammation of the eyelid margins stemming from seborrheic, allergic, or bacterial origin.

Blepharitis is characterized by redness, swelling, burning, and itching of the margin of the eyelid. There is also usually a mucous drainage and sometimes a buildup of scaling, granulation, or crusting on the eyelash margin. In some cases of blepharitis, ulcerations form and eyelashes fall out.

Treatment includes cleansing the eyelid gently with a damp cotton applicator to remove scales, crusts, and granules at least daily; applying warm compresses; and applying an antibiotic ointment to the eyelid margins.

blepharoptosis (ptosis)
(blef-ah-roh-**TOH**-sis)
blephar/o = eyelid
-ptosis = drooping

Occurs when the eyelid partially or entirely covers the eye as a result of a weakened muscle. See Figure 14-3.

Typically only one eye is affected, although both eyes may be involved. This weakened muscle causing drooping of the upper eyelid occurs as a result of damage to the muscle itself or damage to the nerve that controls the muscle raising the eyelid. If severe, **blepharoptosis** can completely obstruct vision. Ptosis may occur at any age and often follows a familial pattern.

There may be an underlying disease process that has caused the weakened eyelid muscle such as myasthenia gravis, muscular dystrophy, diabetes mellitus, or a brain tumor. When treating this condition, an underlying disease must be ruled out so that if one is present, treatment can be started. Blepharoptosis is often corrected with successful treatment of the underlying disease. Other treatment options include surgery to strengthen the eyelid muscle or application of a support device into the individual's glasses, which will keep the eyelid raised.

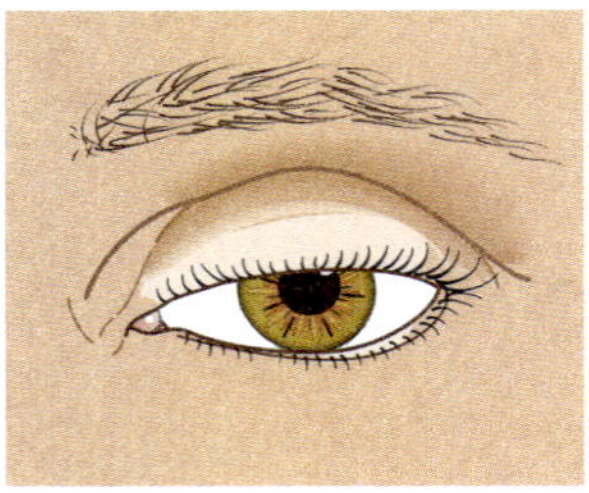

Figure 14-3 Blepharoptosis

blindness

The absence of vision or the need for assistive devices and/or assistance from others to accomplish daily activities due to the inability to see.

The term *blindness* may refer to total blindness in which there is total loss of vision or no light perception, or it may be modified to relate to particular visual limitations. Legal blindness is present when the visual acuity of the better eye is evaluated with the correction of contact lenses or glasses, at best 20/200, or when the visual field (the total area that can be seen with one fixed eye), is less than 20 degrees. Causes of blindness include trauma, cataracts, glaucoma, nutritional deficiencies, trachoma, and onchocerciasis.

color blindness (monochromatism)
(mon-oh-**KROH**-mah-tizm)
mono- = one
chromat/o = color
-ism = condition

An inability to sharply perceive visual colors.

Two examples of forms of **monochromatism** are:

1. **Daltonism**, in which the person is unable to distinguish greens from reds; this is a sex-linked inherited disorder.
2. **Achromatic vision**, in which the person cannot distinguish any color, perceiving only white, gray, and black; this is a defect in the retinal cones or the absence of the retinal cones.

cataract
(**KAT**-ah-rakt)

The lens in the eye becomes progressively cloudy losing its normal transparency and thus altering the perception of images due to the interference of light transmission to the retina.

The occurrence of cataracts can be classified as senile or secondary on the basis of etiology. See **Figure 14-4**.

Senile cataracts typically begin after the age of 50 at which time degenerative changes occur, resulting in the gradual clouding of the crystalline lens due to wear and tear and the change in fibers and protein as it ages. Senile cataracts are common and can be found in an estimated 95% of persons over 65 years of age. Secondary cataracts result from trauma, radiation injury, inflammation, taking certain medications such as corticosteroids, or metabolic diseases such as diabetes mellitus. Congenital cataracts, seen in infants, are usually caused by maternal infection during pregnancy and are also considered secondary cataracts.

Immature cataracts, those in which only a portion of the lens is affected, are diagnosed through ophthalmoscopy and the person's history. Mature cataracts, those in which the entire lens is clouded, can be visualized with the naked eye and appear as a gray-white area behind the pupil. A loss of the red reflex is noted as the cataract matures.

Treatment includes surgical intervention to remove the cataract. Phacoemulsification and extracapsular cataract extraction (ECCE), the two primary ways to remove a cataract, are discussed in the section on Diagnostic Procedures and Techniques at the end of the chapter. Surgery is indicated when the vision loss handicaps the person in the accomplishment of daily activities or when glaucoma or another secondary condition occurs. Surgical intervention for cataract removal is typically completed on an outpatient basis. There is no medical treatment available for cataracts at present.

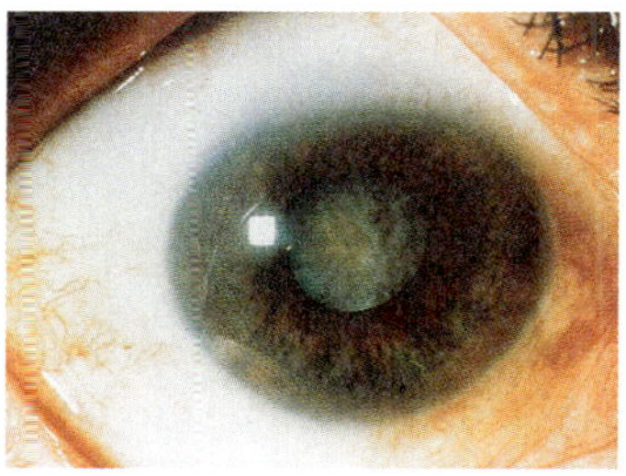

Figure 14-4 Cataract (Courtesy of the National Eye Institute, NIH)

chalazion
(kah-**LAY**-zee-on)

A cyst or nodule on the eyelid resulting from an obstruction of a meibomian gland, which is responsible for lubricating the margin of the eyelid.

A chalazion is diagnosed through a visual examination and the person's history. It may vary in size and will usually disappear spontaneously within 1 to 2 months. When a chalazion does not spontaneously disappear, it can easily be removed through minor surgery in the ophthalmologist's office or as an outpatient.

conjunctivitis, acute
(kon-junk-tih-**VYE**-tis)
conjunctiv/o = conjunctiva
-itis = inflammation

Inflammation of the mucous membrane lining the eyelids and covering the front part of the eyeball.

An inflamed conjunctiva of the eye(s) occurs most commonly as a result of an infection and is also called "pinkeye"; however, it can occur as a result of allergies, environmental irritation, or systemic diseases. Infectious conjunctivitis typically begins in one eye, although if not promptly treated it will readily spread to both eyes.

The clinical manifestations of acute conjunctivitis include redness, tearing, drainage (especially with infectious type), itching (primarily with allergic type), and **photophobia** (extra sensitive to light). The drainage from infectious conjunctivitis is highly contagious and precautions must be taken to prevent spread such as using separate tissues and cloths for each eye, washing hands thoroughly after contact with infected eye(s) (specifically the drainage), and seeking prompt medical treatment. These precautions are especially important when dealing with children because of the close contact with each other and their lack of understanding about spread of infections.

Diagnosis is made on the visual examination of the eye and the cause is determined through the person's history and/or a culture and sensitivity of the drainage. Treatment will vary somewhat according to the cause; however, it may include warm compresses to the eye(s) several times a day, antibiotics for bacterial infections, ophthalmic ointments or drops, antihistamines for allergic conjunctivitis, and avoidance of excessive exposure to light.

---

corneal abrasion
(**COR**-nee-al ah-**BRAY**-zhun)
corne/o = cornea
-al = pertaining to

A disruption of the cornea's surface epithelium commonly caused by an eyelash, a small foreign body, contact lenses, or a scratch from a fingernail.

A **corneal abrasion** may also occur as a result of a chemical irritant and/or dryness of the eye.

Clinical manifestations other than pain include redness, tearing, sensitivity to light, and occasionally visual impairment. Diagnosis of a corneal abrasion is identified by the individual's history and visual examination and then confirmed with **fluorescein** stain, which readily detects abrasions on the cornea.

Treatment of a corneal abrasion will include application of an antibiotic ointment to reduce the chance of infection, and an eye bandage to reduce the motion of the cornea against the eyelid. If there is a small foreign object in the eye it should be carefully removed. Surface abrasions treated promptly usually heal quickly without complication or scarring. If the abrasion is deep enough to damage the deeper supporting tissues, the person should be quickly referred to an **ophthalmologist** because the risks of slower healing, infection, and scar formation are much greater.

---

diabetic retinopathy
(dye-ah-**BET**-ik
reh-tin-**OP**-ah-thee)
retin/o = retina
-pathy = disease

Occurs as a consequence of an 8- to 10-year duration of diabetes mellitus in which the capillaries of the retina experience scarring due to the following:

1. **Abnormal dilation and constriction of vessels**
2. **Hemorrhages**
3. **Microaneurysm**
4. **Abnormal formation of new vessels causing leakage of blood into the vitreous humor**

The scarring and leakage of blood causes a permanent decline in the sharpness of vision. The inability to get the oxygen and nutrients needed for good vision to the retina eventually will lead to permanent loss of vision. In the United States, **diabetic retinopathy** is a leading cause of blindness.

Diagnosis is made from the person's history and a thorough examination of the internal eye via ophthalmoscopy during which the changes in the retinal vasculature can be seen. The person with diabetes mellitus should be followed regularly with ophthalmoscopic examinations to identify the changes taking place because of the available treatment with vitrectomy (removal of vitreous hemorrhages) and laser photocoagulation, normally useful in managing diabetic retinopathy.

ectropion
(ek-**TROH**-pee-on)

"Turning out" or eversion of the eyelash margins (especially the lower eyelid) from the eyeball leading to exposure of the eyelid and eyeball surface and lining. See Figure 14-5.

When an individual is affected by **ectropion**, tears are unable to flow into the tear ducts to keep the eyes moist and therefore flow down the face. This exposure and lack of moisture leads to dryness and irritation of the eye.

Ectropion frequently affects the older population as a result of aging. This occurs with the development of a weakened muscle in the lower eyelid resulting in eversion of the eyelid that causes the outward turning of the eyelid. Facial nerve paralysis and eyelid tissue atrophy are also causes of ectropion as well as scarring of the cheek or eyelid that pulls down on the eyelid.

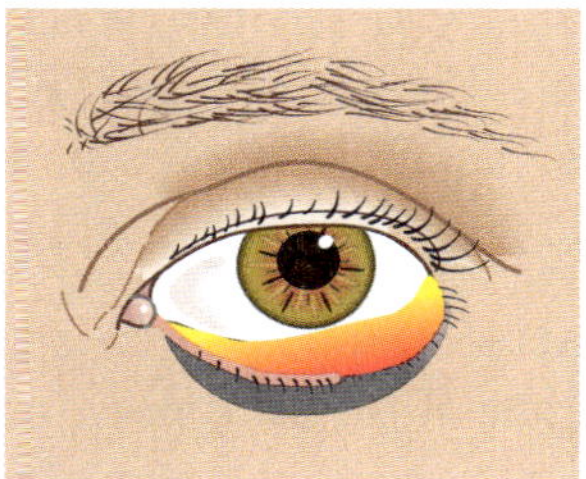

Ectropion is diagnosed through a visual examination. Treatment with a minor surgical process to correct ectropion is usually required because the condition rarely resolves on its own. The dryness and irritation remain a constant threat to the cornea and the development of permanent damage and/or corneal ulcers.

Figure 14-5 Ectropion

entropion
(en-**TROH**-pee-on)

"Turning in" of the eyelash margins (especially the lower margins) resulting in the sensation similar to that of a foreign body in the eye (redness, tearing, burning, and itching). See Figure 14-6.

Entropion may result in damage to the cornea in the form of corneal ulcers due to the constant irritation of the conjunctiva from the rubbing of the lashes.

Entropion frequently affects the older population as a result of aging. This occurs with the development of loose fibrous tissue in the lower eyelid resulting in extreme tightening of the eyelid muscle thus causing the inward turning of the eyelid. This is diagnosed through a visual examination. Treatment with a minor surgical process to correct entropion is required if the condition does not resolve and remains a constant irritant to the conjunctiva and cornea.

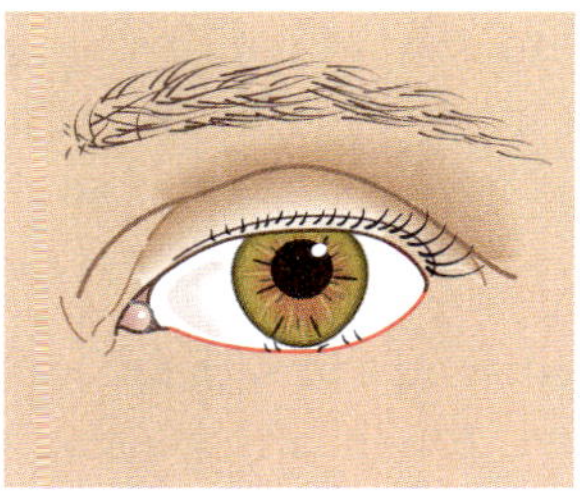

Figure 14-6 Entropion

exophthalmia
(eks-off-**THAL**-mee-ah)
ex- = out, away from, outside
ophthalm/o = eye
-ia = condition

An abnormal protrusion of the eyeball(s) usually with the sclera noticeable over the iris, typically due to an expanded volume of the orbital contents.

The underlying basis of **exophthalmia** may be a tumor, edema associated with inflammation or hemorrhage, or an underlying disease process such as hyperthyroidism (Graves' disease). Typically, both of the eyes are affected and the onset is somewhat gradual. When there is an instant unilateral onset, inflammation and/or hemorrhage are suspected.

The excessive protrusion of the eyeballs results in an inability to close the eyelids and the following symptoms: blurred vision, dryness, complaints of a "gritty feeling," irritation, ulceration, double vision, and restricted eye movement. Diagnosis involves various tests to identify the underlying cause(s) as well as a thorough ophthalmic examination.

Treatment is aimed at relief of the dryness and irritation of the cornea to prevent infections. Specific treatment is determined by the underlying cause. In relentless cases of exophthalmia, surgical decompression of the orbit along with systemic steroids are needed to reduce the pressure and control the swelling.

glaucoma
(glau-**KOH**-mah)

Ocular disorders identified as a group due to the increase in intraocular pressure.

This increase in intraocular pressure may be primary or secondary, acute or chronic, and described as open or closed angle. These disorders occur because of a barrier in the normal outflow of aqueous humor or an increased production of aqueous humor.

Increased intraocular pressure leads to an inhibited blood supply to the optic neurons, which will lead to degeneration and atrophy of the optic nerve and finally total loss of vision. The descriptions of chronic open-angle glaucoma, acute closed-angle glaucoma, and secondary glaucoma are next.

Chronic open-angle glaucoma occurs as a primary disorder with a breakdown in the drainage system of the circulation of aqueous humor. A gradual elevation of internal pressure leads to a decreased blood supply to the optic nerve and the retina. The most common type of **glaucoma**, chronic open-angle is so gradual that the presence in most individuals is long standing before any symptoms are recognized.

When chronic open-angle glaucoma is untreated, peripheral vision is gradually lost. The central vision will eventually be lost as well, rendering the individual completely blind. Routine ophthalmic examinations, which include optic nerve evaluation and readings of intraocular pressure, are important to pick up as well as evaluate the development and presence of chronic open-angle glaucoma.

Along with the person's history and the identified symptoms, the diagnosis of open-angle glaucoma can be confirmed through an ophthalmic examination with **tonometry** (measurement of intraocular pressure). When diagnosis is made and early treatment is started with medication to open the drainage system or reduce the production of aqueous humor, the intraocular pressure is controlled to a certain extent. When medication does not adequately control the intraocular pressure, surgery may be required to bypass the faulty drainage system.

Acute closed-angle glaucoma is a rapid primary occurrence of increased intraocular pressure in a short period of time. It is due to the mouth of the drainage system being narrow and closing completely, allowing no flow of aqueous humor. This rapid occurrence is characterized by severe pain, blurred vision, photophobia, redness, and seeing "halos" around light. Some individuals complain of nausea and vomiting. Within several days, the person with untreated acute closed-angle glaucoma can lose his or her sight.

Treatment is aimed at quickly reducing the pressure inside the eye to avoid vision loss. The creation of a small hole between the posterior and anterior chambers through a procedure called laser iridotomy has been effective in opening the filtering angle, allowing the aqueous humor to flow, and thus decreasing the intraocular pressure. Other surgical interventions for the treatment of glaucoma such as iridectomy, LASIK, trabeculectomy, and trabeculoplasty, are discussed in the Diagnostic Procedures and Techniques section located at the end of the chapter.

Secondary glaucoma occurs as a complication of another disorder, trauma, or surgery. Swelling of eye tissue from the trauma of surgery, injury, or inflammation causes the flow pattern or system to be affected. This leads to obstructed drainage of aqueous humor and increased intraocular pressure.

---

hemianopia
(hem-ee-ah-**NOP**-ee-ah)
hemi- = half
an- = without, not
-opia = visual condition

Hemianopia is abnormal eyesight in one-half of the visual field.

---

hordeolum (stye)
(hor-**DEE**-oh-lum)

Bacterial infection of an eyelash follicle or sebaceous gland originating with redness, swelling, and mild tenderness in the margin of the eyelash. See Figure 14-7.

As a stye progresses, it becomes an acutely tender abscess that will drain after 3 to 4 days.

Treatment of a hordeolum includes warm, hot moist compresses to the eye, application of an antibiotic ointment, and avoiding the temptation to squeeze the stye. Squeezing will spread the infection. An incision and drainage is occasionally necessary.

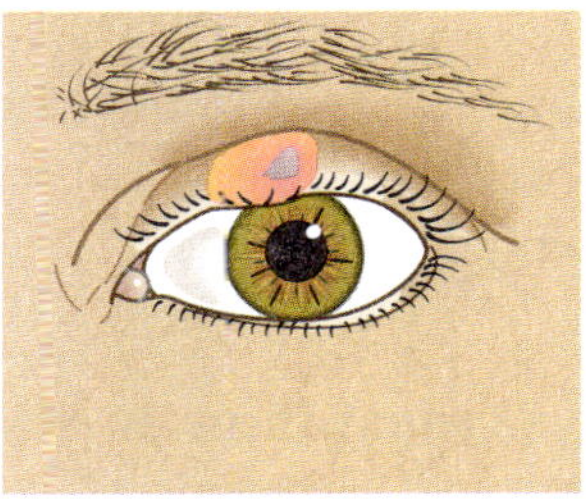

Figure 14-7 Hordeolum (stye)

---

hyperopia
(high-per-**OH**-pee-ah)
hyper- = excessive
-opia = visual condition

A refractive error in which the lens of the eye cannot focus on an image accurately, resulting in impaired close vision that is blurred due to the light rays being focused behind the retina because the eyeball is shorter than normal.

Hyperopia is also called farsightedness due to better clarity of distant objects. See **Figure 14-8.**

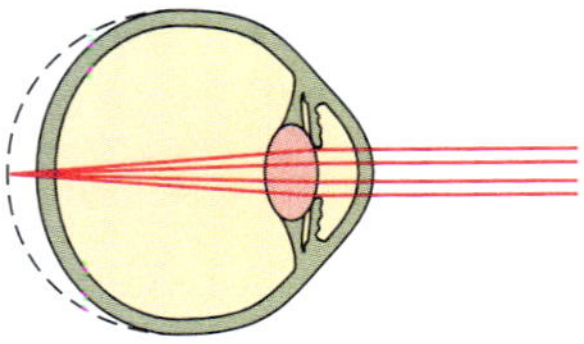

In addition to blurred vision of close objects, the individual may also complain of headaches and frequent squinting. The diagnosis of hyperopia is verified through an ophthalmoscopic examination and corrected through the use of contact lenses or eyeglasses.

Figure 14-8 Hyperopia (farsightedness)

---

hyphema (hyphemia)
(high-**FEE**-mah)

A bleed into the anterior chamber of the eye resulting as a postoperative complication or from a blunt eye injury.

Hyphema is an ocular emergency due to the possibility that the increased pressure of the blood can damage the eye's sensitive structures. As a postoperative occurrence, a hyphema must be reported to the individual's surgeon as soon as possible. An ophthalmologist should treat a hyphema to evaluate the need for evacuation of the blood and/or further use of medications.

Through light observation, blood is visible in the lower portion of the eye when the individual sits upright. Symptoms of hyphema include decreased vision, sudden sharp eye pain, and seeing a reddish tint.

Treatment includes bed rest, with the head of the bed elevated, and administration of a sedative. The blood is usually reabsorbed rapidly. (If intraocular pressure rises, however, an osmotic diuretic, such as mannitol, may be administered to reduce the pressure.)

---

keratitis
(kair-ah-**TYE**-tis)
kerat/o = hard, horny; also refers to cornea of the eye
-itis = inflammation

Corneal inflammation caused by a microorganism, trauma to the eye, a break in the sensory innervation of the cornea, a hypersensitivity reaction, or a tearing defect (may be due to dry eyes or ineffective eyelid closure).

Keratitis is characterized by irritation, decreased visual acuity, tearing, mild redness, photophobia, and possibly pain and superficial ulcerations of the cornea. When keratitis is preceded by an upper respiratory infection with cold sores on the face, herpes simplex is frequently the cause.

Treatment includes administration of ophthalmic eye drops and ointments along with a broad-spectrum antibiotic. An eye patch is sometimes prescribed to decrease the discomfort and photophobia.

---

myopia
(my-**OH**-pee-ah)
my/o = muscle
-opia = visual condition

A refractive error in which the lens of the eye cannot focus on an image accurately, resulting in impaired distant vision that is blurred due to the light rays being focused in front of the retina because the eyeball is longer than normal.

Myopia is also called nearsightedness due to the clarity of close objects. See **Figure 14-9.**

In addition to blurred vision of distant objects, the individual may also complain of headaches and frequent squinting. The diagnosis of myopia is

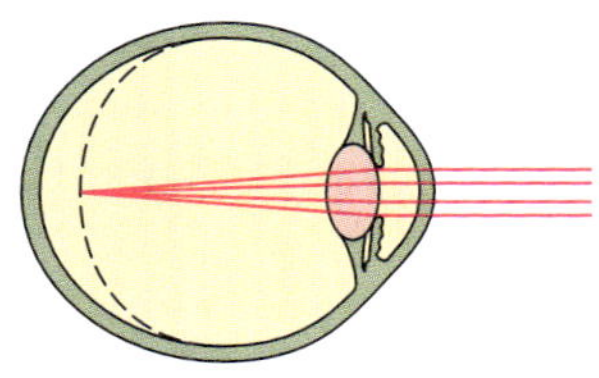

Myopia
(nearsightedness)
Light rays focus in front of the retina

verified through an ophthalmoscopic examination and corrected through the use of contact lenses or eyeglasses. Treatment includes a surgical procedure called a radial keratotomy, which involves creating microscopic incisions in the outside segment of the cornea, making it flatten in specific areas. This procedure has been successful, but it is not without potential complications.

Figure 14-9 Myopia (nearsightedness)

---

nyctalopia
(night blindness)
(nik-tah-**LOH**-pee-ah)
nyct/o = night
-opia = visual condition

Inadequate vision at night or in faint lighting following reduction in the synthesis of rhodopsin, a compound in the rods of the retina that enables the eye to adjust to low-density light.

Retinal deterioration, vitamin A deficiency, or a congenital defect may cause nyctalopia.

---

nystagmus
(niss-**TAG**-mus)

Vertical, horizontal, rotary, or mixed rhythmic involuntary movements of the eye(s) caused by use of alcohol or certain drugs, lesions on the brain or inner ear, congenital abnormalities, nerve injury at birth, or abnormal retinal development. Nystagmus may not be apparent to the patient.

Nystagmus can be acquired when a lesion is produced in the brain or inner ear due to another disease process. With congenital nystagmus, the child often has poor vision that also arises from the congenital abnormalities.

Diagnosis of nystagmus is made from the visualization of the involuntary eye movements. Treatment is aimed at managing the underlying condition, if indicated. Congenital nystagmus often cannot be successfully treated and therefore remains with the individual for life.

---

ophthalmia neonatorum
(off-**THAL**-mee-ah
nee-oh-nay-**TOR**-um)
ophthalm/o = eye
-ia = condition
ne/o = new
nat/i = pertaining to birth

A purulent (contains pus) inflammation of the conjunctiva and/or cornea in the newborn.

The cause of the keratitis and conjunctivitis results from the newborn's exposure to viral, bacterial, chemical, or chlamydial agents.

One category of ophthalmia neonatorum is Neisseria gonorrheal conjunctivitis, which is spread to the neonate while passing through the birth canal. This type is rare in the United States due to the preventive antibiotic ointment applied to the newborn's eyes after birth. Another category of ophthalmia neonatorum is chlamydial conjunctivitis, also transmitted to the newborn while passing through the birth canal.

---

presbyopia
(prez-bee-**OH**-pee-ah)
presby/o = old, elderly
-opia = visual condition

A refractive error occurring after the age of 40, when the lens of the eye(s) cannot focus on an image accurately due to its decreasing loss of elasticity resulting in a firmer and more opaque lens.

This results in decreased color vision and a decline in refraction and accommodation for close vision. Presbyopia is also called farsightedness due to better clarity of distant objects.

In addition to blurred vision of close objects, the individual may also complain of headaches and frequent squinting. The diagnosis of presbyopia is verified through an ophthalmoscopic examination and is corrected through the use of contact lenses or eyeglasses.

pterygium
(ter-**IJ**-ee-um)

An irregular growth developing as a fold in the bulbar conjunctiva on the nasal side of the cornea that can disrupt vision if it extends over the pupil. See Figure 14-10.

Pterygium can be caused by allergies and excessive ultraviolet light exposure.

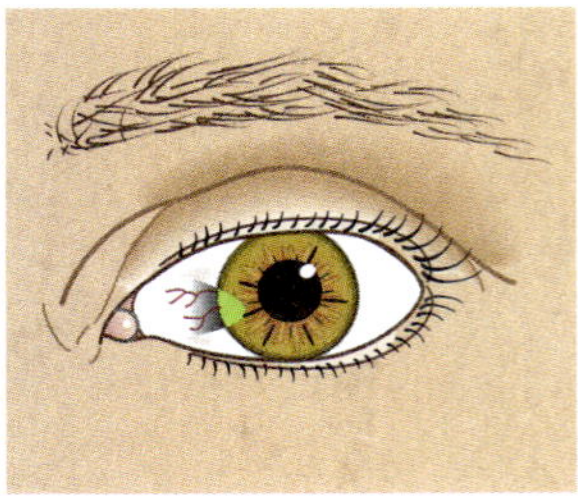

Figure 14-10 Pterygium

retinal detachment
(**RET**-in-al detachment)
retin/o = retina
-al = pertaining to

The partial or complete splitting away of the retina from the pigmented vascular layer called the choroid, allowing the leakage of vitreous humor and thus creating a medical emergency.

Without the attachment to this vascular layer, the neurons of the retina will develop ischemia and die, thus leading to permanent loss of sight. Prompt referral and treatment to an ophthalmologist is indicated.

The causes of a retinal detachment include trauma to the eye and interior changes in the eye's vitreous chamber as a result of aging or inflammation of the inside of the eye. The symptoms include abrupt appearance of floating spots, light flashes, blurred vision, perception of a shade being pulled across the vision field, or increasing loss of vision. Diagnosis is confirmed through an ophthalmoscopic examination.

Surgical intervention to reposition the detached retina as soon as possible is the preferred treatment to prevent permanent loss of vision. The retina will regain most of its function unless the detachment has advanced to the central retina. If the detachment has extended to the macula, there may be decreased central acuity.

retinal tear
(**RET**-in-al tear)
retin/o = retina
-al = pertaining to

An opening in the retina that allows leakage of vitreous humor.

Repair of a retinal tear can be accomplished with cryosurgery or photocoagulation as long as there is no detachment present. Early treatment can prevent a further complication of retinal detachment.

scleritis
(skleh-**RYE**-tis)
scler/o = hard; also refers to sclera of the eye
-itis = inflammation

The presence of inflammation in the white, outside covering of the eyeball, the sclera.

Clinical manifestations of scleritis include intense redness with dull pain and possibly some loss of vision.

When left untreated, scleritis may lead to loss of the eye due to perforation. Treatment includes the use of topical drops and immunosuppressive medications. If there is a perforation in the sclera, a surgical repair called a scleroplasty will be required.

---

scotoma
(skoh-**TOH**-mah)
scot/o = darkness
-oma = tumor

Scotoma is a defined area in one or both eyes, which has a decreased visual function.

---

strabismus
(strah-**BIZ**-mus)

Failure of the eyes to gaze in the same direction due to weakness in the muscles controlling the position of one eye. The most common type of strabismus is nonparalytic strabismus, an inherited defect in which the eye position of the two eyes has no relationship.

The individual with nonparalytic strabismus has to fix with one eye because both eyes cannot be used together. The acuity of vision will begin to dwindle with the decreased use of one eye. Two types of nonparalytic strabismus will be discussed in this section: convergent strabismus or "crosseye" and divergent strabismus or "walleye."

1. **Convergent strabismus or crosseye is also known as esotropia**. In this condition, the affected eye turns inward. Esotropia usually develops in infancy or early childhood. See **Figure 14-11A.**
2. **Divergent strabismus or walleye is also known as exotropia.** In this condition, the affected eye turns outward. See **Figure 14-11B.**

Treatment for strabismus should be started early because loss of vision in the affected eye might result from nonuse of the eye. Treatment includes the use of corrective glasses, orthoptic training in which the normal eye is covered with a patch, forcing the individual to use the affected eye, or surgery to restore the eye muscle balance.

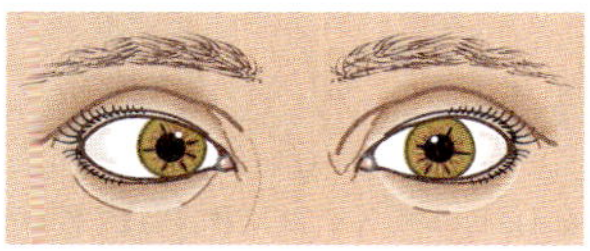

(A)

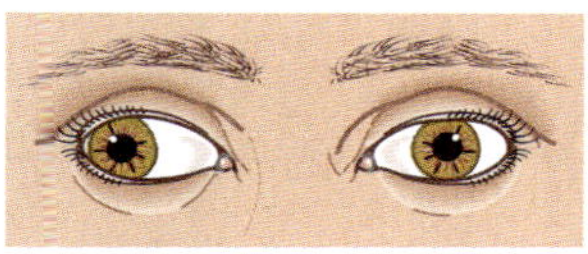

(B)

Figure 14-11 Strabismus: (A) convergent; (B) divergent

---

synechia
(sĭn-**EK**-ee-ah)

An adhesion in the eye that develops as a complication of trauma or surgery, or as a secondary condition of one of the following pathological conditions: cataracts, glaucoma, keratitis, or uveitis.

The adhesion causes the iris to adhere to the lens or the cornea resulting in the blockage of flow of aqueous humor between the posterior and anterior chambers. When aqueous humor flow is blocked, the pressure rises, causing a rapid progression to blindness without immediate treatment. Treatment of synechia initially includes dilation of the pupils using a mydriatic. The subsequent treatment will be directed toward the underlying condition.

---

trachoma
(tray-**KOH**-mah)

An infectious eye disease caused by *Chlamydia trachomatis,* which is chronic and will lead to blindness without effective treatment.

Effective treatment includes the use of topical sulfonamides and administration of erythromycin and tetracycline. Trachoma is contagious.

Early symptoms of trachoma include tearing, pain, photophobia, and inflammation. If the disease progresses without treatment, follicles begin to form on the upper eyelid. With continued development of the follicles and granulation tissue eventually infiltrating the cornea, the result is blindness.

uveitis
(yoo-vee-**EYE**-tis)
-itis = inflammation

Inflammation of all or part of the middle vascular layer of the eye made up of the iris, the ciliary body, and the choroid.

Most frequently **uveitis** is unilateral and is characterized by blurred vision, pain, redness, pupillary constriction, and intense photophobia.

The cause of uveitis is sometimes unknown; however, there are incidences caused by infections and autoimmune disorders. Examination using the slit lamp will confirm the diagnosis.

Treatment includes the use of steroids to combat inflammation, and/or cycloplegic agents which cause paralysis of the ciliary muscle, allowing it to rest. Medications may be administered for pain as needed.

Diagnostic Techniques and Procedures (Eye)

corneal transplant
(**COR**-nee-al)
corne/o = cornea
-al = pertaining to

Surgical transplantation of a donor cornea (cadaver's) into the eye of a recipient usually under local anesthesia.

Young donor corneas are preferred for **corneal transplant** because the endothelial layer of the cornea has a direct relationship to age and health.

electronystagmography
(ee-**lek**-troh-**niss**-tag-**MOG**-rah-fee)
electr/o = electrical, electricity
-graphy = process of recording

A group of tests used in evaluating the vestibulo-ocular reflex.

The vestibulo-ocular reflex is a normal reflex produced by stimulation of the vestibular apparatus (inner ear structures related to position and balance sense) in which eye position compensates for motion of the head. This is done by identifying nystagmus (eye movements) in response to certain stimuli.

Of the **electronystagmography** tests, caloric testing is the best known. It is accomplished by directly installing water into the ear canal, making contact with the tympanic membrane, and simultaneously recording eye movement. In persons with damaged vestibular function, the typical nystagmus reaction is absent or blunted. (Caloric testing should not be performed on persons with a ruptured tympanic membrane.)

electroretinogram (ERG)
(ee-lek-troh-**RET**-ih-noh-gram)
electr/o = electrical, electricity
retin/o = retina
-gram = recording

A recording of the changes in the electrical potential of the retina after the stimulation of light.

This is accomplished with the use of a contact lens electrode, which is placed on the individual's anesthetized cornea. The reading obtained from the **electroretinogram** is an identical response if the electrode was placed directly on the surface of the retina. This process is useful in evaluating retinal disease.

---

extracapsular cataract (eks-trah-**KAP**-syoo-lar) **extraction (ECCE)** (eks-**TRAK**-shun)

Surgical removal of the anterior segment of the lens capsule along with the lens allowing for the insertion of an intraocular lens implant.

The insertion of a posterior chamber intraocular lens has proven to result in less complications during the **extracapsular extraction**.

---

fluorescein staining (floo-oh-**RESS**-ee-in)

Application of a fluorescein-stained sterile filter paper strip moistened with a few drops of sterile saline or sterile anesthetic solution to the lower cul-de-sac of the eye to visualize a corneal abrasion.

Corneal abrasions are stained bright green when fluorescein stain is applied. Fluorescein solution should not be used from a dropper bottle because contamination with *Pseudomonas aeruginosa* is common in these dropper bottles.

---

fundoscopy (fund-**DOSS**-koh-pee)
-scopy = process of viewing

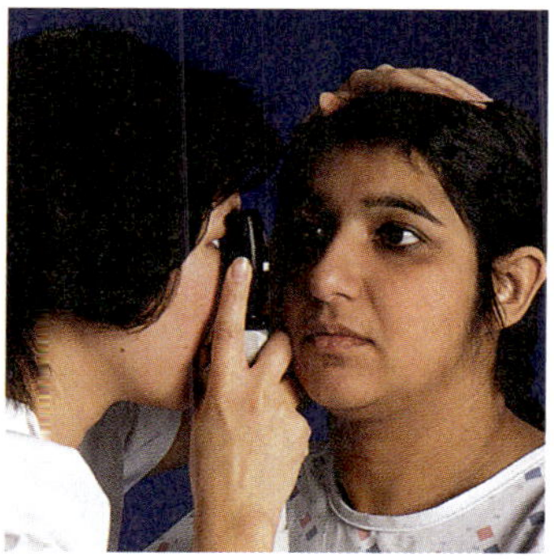

The examination of the fundus of the eye, the base or the deepest part of the eye, with an instrument called an ophthalmoscope through a procedure called ophthalmoscopy. See Figure 14-12.

This process allows the examiner to visualize the interior eye using a focus dial and lenses of differing magnification. The blood vessels in the fundus can be observed directly through this procedure.

Visualizing the fundus can provide the examiner with valuable assessment data about the individual's intracranial and systemic functioning and/or disorders. Disorders that can be detected through a **fundoscopy** include hypertension, brain lesions, or arteriosclerosis.

Figure 14-12 Fundoscopy

---

gonioscopy (**GOH**-nee-oh-skop-ee)
-scopy = process of viewing

Gonioscopy involves using an ophthalmoscope that will establish the anterior chamber angle and display ocular rotation and movement.

---

intraocular lens implant
intra- = within
ocul/o = eye
-ar = pertaining to

Lens implanted during the surgical process of cataract extraction, which restores visual acuity, provides depth perception, light refraction, and binocular vision.

The lens can be implanted in the anterior chamber or the posterior chamber during the **intraocular** implant.

---

iridectomy (ir-id-**EK**-toh-mee)
irid/o = iris
-ectomy = surgical removal

Extraction of a small segment of the iris to open an anterior chamber angle and permit the flow of aqueous humor between the anterior and posterior chambers, thus relieving the person's intraocular pressure.

This is used in the treatment of closed-angle glaucoma.

Laser **iridectomy** is used to create several small openings in the iris, which allow the flow of aqueous humor to the anterior chamber from the posterior chamber.

---

keratoplasty
(**KAIR**-ah-toh-**plass**-tee)
kerat/o = hard, horny; also refers to cornea of the eye
-plasty = surgical repair

The excision of an opaque segment of the cornea during ophthalmologic surgery.

Keratoplasty is indicated in serious conditions involving the cornea such as in corneal dystrophy.

Laser in situ keratomileusis (LASIK)
(**LAY**-sick)

The LASIK procedure (laser in situ keratomileusis) is a form of laser vision correction for nearsightedness (myopia).

A device, called a microkeratome, is used to produce a flap in the cornea by slicing the cornea from the side. The flap is then rolled back to expose the inner layers of the cornea. The doctor then makes the refractive correction on the cornea's inner layer. This procedure is done with a computer-guided excimer laser which delivers a series of cool, ultraviolet light pulses that vaporize the corneal tissue precisely enough to correct the refractive error. Once the correction has been made, the flap is reset in its original position.

---

ophthalmoscopy
(off-thal-**MOSS**-koh-pee)
ophthalm/o = eye
-scopy = process of viewing

Distinct visualization of the structures of the eye at all depths using an ophthalmoscope.

---

phacoemulsification
(**fak**-oh-ee-**MULL**-sih-fih-**kay**-shun)
phac/o = lens

Phacoemulsification is a method of removing a lens by using ultrasound vibrations to split up the lens material into tiny particles that can be suctioned out of the eye.

---

photo refractive keratectomy
(foh-toh ree-**FRAK**-tive kair-ah-**TEK**-toh-mee)
kerat/o = hard, horny; also refers to cornea of the eye
-ectomy = surgical removal

Photo refractive keratectomy is a surgical procedure in which a few layers of corneal surface cells are shaved off by an "excimer laser beam" to flatten the cornea and reduce myopia or nearsightedness.

---

retinal photocoagulation
(**RET**-in-al **foh**-toh-coh-**ag**-yoo-**LAY**-shun)
retin/o = retina
-al = pertaining to
phot/o = light

Retinal photocoagulation is a surgical procedure that uses an argon laser to treat conditions such as glaucoma, retinal detachment, and diabetic retinopathy, in the following ways:

1. Glaucoma: The argon laser destroys portions of the ciliary body to allow flow of aqueous humor.
2. Retinal detachment: The argon laser is used to create an area of inflammation, which will develop adhesions, causing a "welding" of the layers.
3. Diabetic retinopathy: The argon laser is used to seal microaneurysms and to reduce the risk of hemorrhage.

tonometry
(tohn-**OM**-eh-tree)
ton/o = tension, tone
-metry = process of measuring

The process of determining the intraocular pressure by calculating the resistance of the eyeball to an applied force causing indentation.

As the intraocular pressure increases in the eyeball, a greater force is required due to the increased firmness of the eye. The air-puff tonometer, which does not touch the eye, records deflections of the cornea from a puff of pressurized air. The Schiotz impression tonometer, which is placed on the anesthetized eye, records the pressure needed to indent or flatten the cornea.

trabeculectomy
(trah-**bek**-yool-**EK**-toh-mee)
-ectomy = surgical removal

The surgical excision of a portion of corneoscleral tissue to decrease the intraocular pressure in persons with severe glaucoma.

Trabeculectomy will increase the outflow of aqueous humor, thus relieving the pressure of the excess aqueous humor. This procedure normally includes removal of the trabecular meshwork and the canal of Schlemm (a tiny vein that aids in draining aqueous humor).

trabeculoplasty
(trah-**BEK**-yoo-loh-plass-tee)
-plasty = surgical repair

The surgical creation of a permanent fistula used to drain fluid (aqueous humor) from the eye's anterior chamber, usually performed under general anesthesia.

This is used in the treatment of glaucoma to relieve the pressure of the excess aqueous humor.

Laser trabeculoplasty is an outpatient plastic surgery approach used in the management of glaucoma. It involves an argon laser beam to blanch the eye's trabecular meshwork, which allows drainage of the surplus fluid causing elevated pressure within the eyeball.

Common Abbreviations (Eye)

ABBREVIATION	MEANING	ABBREVIATION	MEANING
Acc	accommodation	**OU**	each eye (oculus uterque)
CC	with correction (with glasses)	**PEARL**	pupils equal and reactive to light
ECCE	extracapsular cataract extraction	**PERLA**	pupils equal; react to light and accommodation
EOM	extraocular movement	**PERRLA**	pupils equal; round, react to light, and accommodation
ERG	electroretinogram	**REM**	rapid eye movement
ICCE	intracapsular cataract extraction	**SC**	without correction
IOL	intraocular lens	**VA**	visual acuity
IOP	intraocular pressure	**VF**	visual field
OD	right eye (ocular dexter)		
OS	left eye (ocular sinister)		

OVERVIEW OF THE EAR

The ear has two very important functions: It enables us to hear and it functions as the sensory organ of balance or equilibrium. The location of one ear on each side of the head produces binaural hearing, hearing from both sides. Hearing and balance problems can reduce our ability to communicate with others.

The health professional who specializes in the study of hearing, detects and diagnoses hearing loss, and works to rehabilitate individuals with hearing loss is known as an **audiologist.** The field of research devoted to the study of hearing and impaired hearing is known as **audiology.** The process of checking one's hearing to determine the lowest tones heard by the ear is known as **audiometry**. The chart illustrating the lowest, or faintest, sounds detected by the ear is called an **audiogram**.

Individuals who work in areas of high noise levels are required by Occupational Safety and Health Act (OSHA) to have periodic hearing tests and may be moved to another location in the facility if any deficiencies in the hearing are noted.

Anatomy and Physiology (Ear)

The ear is divided into three distinct sections: the external ear, the middle ear, and the inner ear. Refer to **Figure 14-13** to visualize each section and structure of the ear.

External Ear

The external ear is the visible portion of the ear not contained within the head. It includes the **(1) auricle**, or **pinna**, which is the cartilaginous flap that has a fleshy, lower portion known as the ear lobe. The tube leading from the auricle to the middle ear is

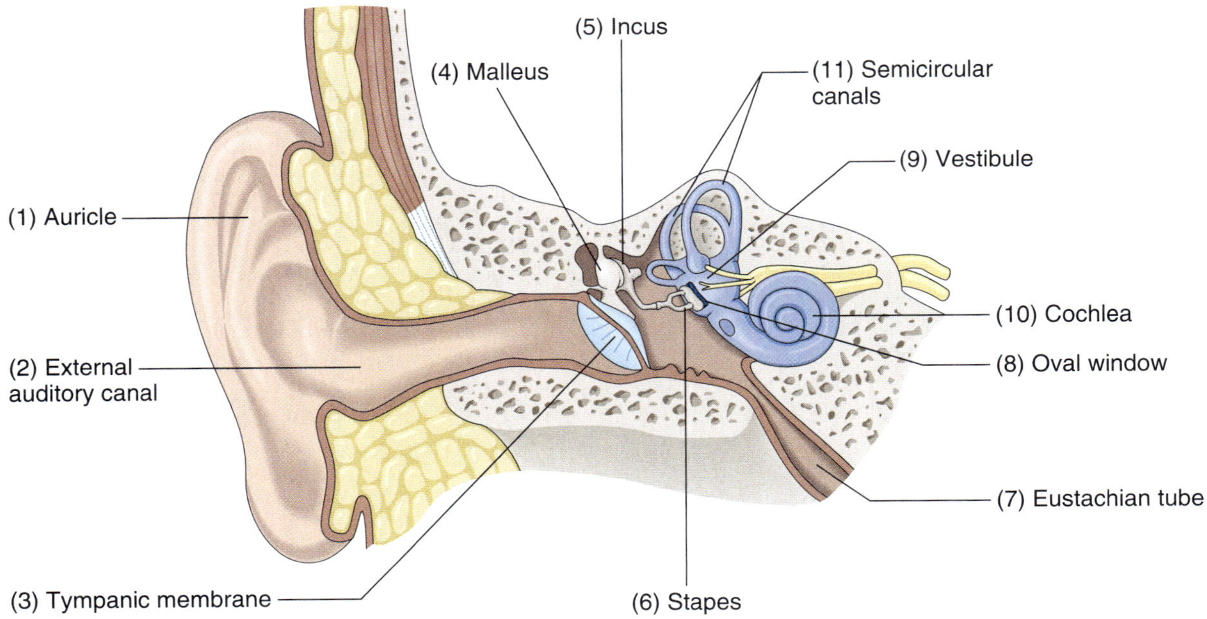

Figure 14-13 Structures of the ear

called the (2) **external** auditory **canal**. The auditory canal is lined with tiny hairs called **cilia,** and modified sweat glands called **ceruminous glands**. The cilia aid in transmitting the sound waves inward. The ceruminous glands secrete a thick, waxy, honey-colored substance that lubricates and protects the ear. This substance is known as earwax, or **cerumen**. The external ear is separated from the middle ear by the tympanic membrane that stretches over the auditory canal. The **(3) tympanic membrane**, also known as the eardrum, is a thin, semitransparent membrane that transmits sound vibrations to the inner ear via the auditory ossicles.

Middle Ear

The middle ear contains three tiny bones known as the **auditory ossicles**. The three auditory ossicles, or tiny bones, are so named for their shape. The first of the three bones is the **(4) malleus**, which resembles the shape of a hammer. It is connected to the tympanic membrane and transmits the sound vibrations to the second auditory ossicle known as the **(5) incus**. The incus resembles the shape of an anvil and transmits the sound vibrations from the malleus to the third auditory ossicle known as the **(6) stapes**. The stapes resembles the shape of a tiny stirrup. It transmits the sound vibrations from the incus to the inner ear. The tube that connects the middle ear to the pharynx, or throat, is the **(7) eustachian tube**, also called the auditory tube. Yawning and swallowing open the eustachian tube to equalize the pressure within the middle ear to that of the atmospheric pressure. The middle ear is separated from the inner ear by an oval-shaped opening called the **(8) oval window**. The base of the stapes fits into the oval window.

Inner Ear

The inner ear is a mazelike structure consisting of the bony structures and membranous structures within the bony structures, which are surrounded by fluid. The bony structures of the inner ear, known as the bony labyrinth, are the vestibule, cochlea, and the semicircular canals. The membranous structures consist of the utricle and saccule (inside the vestibule), the cochlear duct (inside the cochlear), and the membranous semicircular canals (inside the bony semicircular canals). The **(9) vestibule** is the central portion of the inner ear. Located next to the stapes and between the cochlea and the semicircular canals, the vestibule contains the **utricle** and the **saccule,** which are membranous pouches or sacs that aid in maintaining balance. Moving away from and slightly lower than the oval window is the **(10) cochlea**, a snail-shaped bony structure. The cochlea contains **endolymph** and **perilymph**, auditory fluids that aid in the transmission of sound vibrations. The cochlea houses the **organ of Corti**, the true organ of hearing. This spiral structure within the cochlea contains tiny hair cells that are stimulated by sound vibrations. It is here that the sound vibrations are converted into nerve impulses that are transmitted to the brain for interpretation as hearing. The **(11) semicircular canals** are located behind the vestibule. These three bony, fluid-filled loops help to maintain one's balance.

The Process of Hearing

Now that we have reviewed the structures of the ear, let us go back and trace the pathway of sound vibrations as they travel from the external ear to the inner ear and on to the brain for interpretation as hearing. **Figure 14-14** presents a summary of the pathway of sound vibrations through the ear.

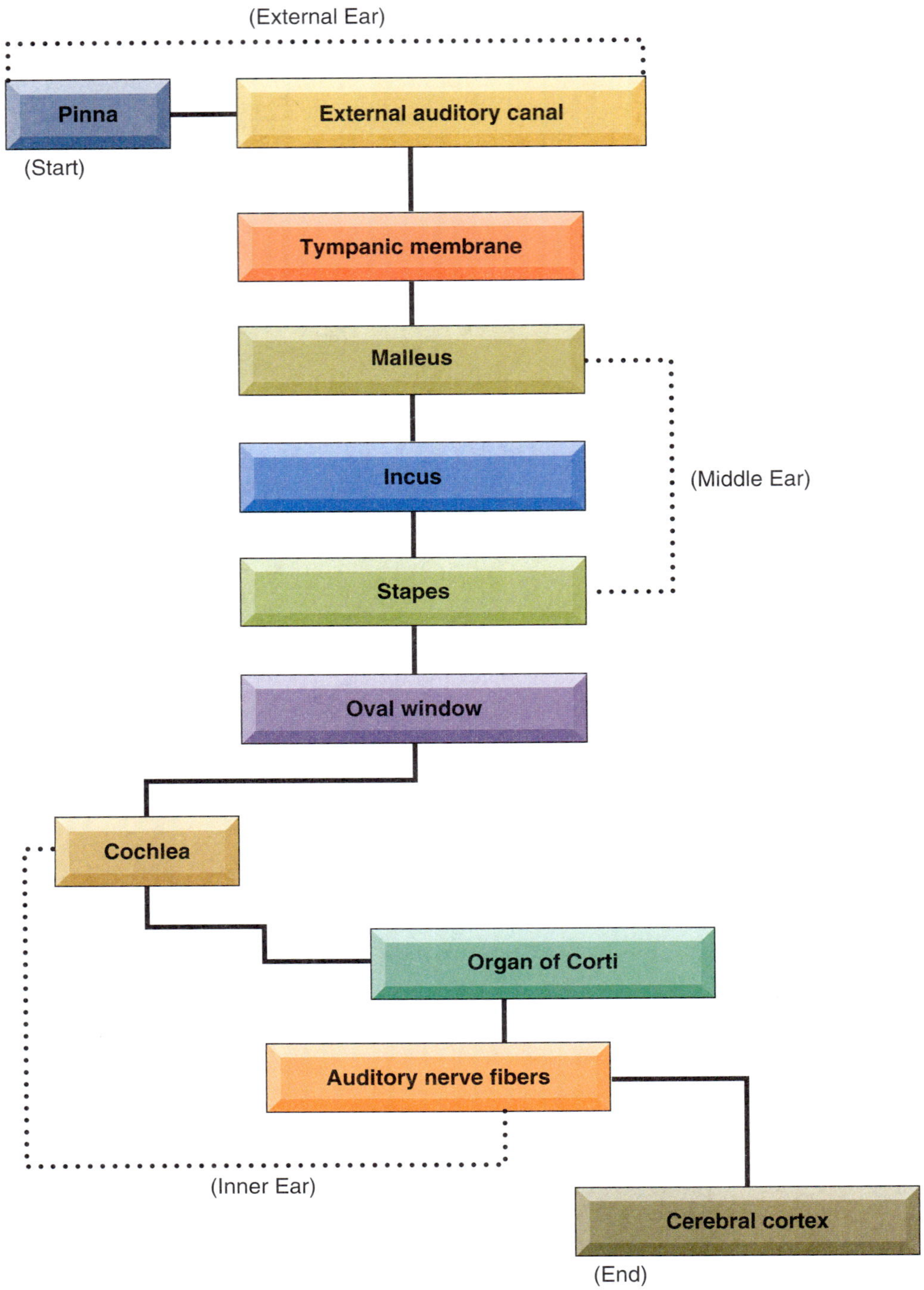

Figure 14-14 Pathway of sound vibrations

The process of hearing begins with the outer ear. The sound vibrations are received by the pinna and are funneled through the external auditory canal to the tympanic membrane. The sound waves strike the tympanic membrane, causing it to vibrate. The vibrations of the tympanic membrane move the three small bones of the middle ear: malleus, incus, and stapes. As the stapes vibrates it causes the oval window to vibrate. The vibration of the oval window transmits the sound waves into the inner ear by causing a "ripple effect" in the endolymph and perilymph fluids within the cochlea. As these fluids fluctuate, they transmit the stimulus to the tiny hair cells of the organ of Corti. The

auditory nerve fibers that lie close to the tiny hair cells of the organ of Corti then pick up the stimulation of the sound waves and transmit it to the **cerebral cortex** of the brain where the impulses are interpreted as hearing.

Vocabulary (Ear)

The following vocabulary words are frequently used when discussing the ear.

WORD	DEFINITION
acoustic (ah-**KOOS**-tik) **acous/o** = hearing **-tic** = pertaining to	Pertaining to sound or hearing.
audiogram (**AW**-dee-oh-gram) **audi/o** = hearing **-gram** = written record	A recording of the faintest sounds an individual is able to hear.
auditory (**AW**-dih-tor-ee) **audi/o** = hearing **-ory** = pertaining to	Pertaining to the sense of hearing.
aural (**AW**-ral) **aur/o** = ear **-al** = pertaining to	Pertaining to the ear.
auriculotemporal (aw-rik-yoo-loh-**TEM**-poh-ral) **auricul/o** = ear **tempor/o** = temple **-al** = pertaining to	Pertaining to the ear and the temporal area.
barotitis media (bar-oh-**TYE**-tis **MEE**-dee-ah) **bar/o** = pressure **ot/o** = ear **-itis** = inflammation **medi/o-** = middle **-a** = noun ending	Inflammation or bleeding of the middle ear caused by changes in atmospheric pressure; the pressure in the middle ear is different from that of the atmosphere. This can happen when there is a sudden change in altitude.
cochlear (**KOE**-lee-ar)	Pertaining to a snail-shaped structure within the middle ear.
labyrinthitis (lab-in-rin-**THIGH**-tis) **labyrinth/o** = inner ear **-itis** = inflammation	Inflammation of the inner ear.

mastoiditis (mass-toyd-**EYE**-tis) **mastoid/o** = mastoid process **-itis** = inflammation process	Inflammation of one of the mastoid processes of the temporal bone; usually an extension of a middle ear infection.
myringoplasty (mir-**IN**-goh-plass-tee) **myring/o** = eardrum **-plasty** = surgical repair	Surgical repair of the eardrum with a tissue graft; this procedure is performed to correct hearing loss. It is also called **tympanoplasty**.
myringotomy (mir-in-**GOT**-oh-mee) **myring/o** = eardrum **-tomy** = incision into	Surgical incision into the eardrum; this procedure is performed to relieve pressure or release fluid from the middle ear. It is also called **tympanotomy**.
otalgia (oh-**TAL**-jee-ah) **ot/o** = ear **-algia** = pain	Pain in the ear; earache. It is also called **otodynia**.
otitis media (oh-**TYE**-tis **MEE**-dee-ah) **ot/o** = ear **-itis** = inflammation **medi/o-** = middle **-a** = noun ending	Inflammation of the middle ear.
otodynia (oh-toh-**DIN**-ee-ah) **ot/o** = ear **-dynia** = pain	See ***otalgia***.
otomycosis (oh-toh-my-**KOH**-sis) **ot/o** = ear **myc/o** = fungus **-osis** = condition	A fungal infection of the external auditory meatus of the ear.
otorrhea (oh-toh-**REE**-ah) **ot/o** = ear **-rrhea** = drainage	Drainage from the ear; usually associated with inflammation of the ear.
presbycusis (prez-bye-**KOO**-sis) **presby/o** = old age	Loss of hearing due to the natural aging process.
purulent (**PEWR**-yoo-lent)	Containing pus.
salpingoscope (sal-**PING**-goh-skohp) **salping/o** = eustachian tubes; also refers to fallopian tubes **-scope** = instrument used to view	An instrument used to examine the nasopharynx and the eustachian tube. (*Note:* The combining form *salping/o* refers to both the eustachian tube and the fallopian tube; when using this combining form, be sure to keep the appropriate body system in mind.)

serous (**SEER**-us) ser/o = blood serum -ous = pertaining to	Pertaining to producing serum.
stapedectomy (stay-pee-**DEK**-toh-mee) staped/o = stapes -ectomy = surgical removal	Surgical removal of the stapes (middle ear) and insertion of a graft and prosthesis.
tinnitus (tin-**EYE**-tus)	A ringing or tinkling noise heard in the ears; may be a sign of injury to the ear, some disease process, or toxic levels of some medications from prolonged use (such as aspirin).
tympanoplasty (tim-pan-oh-**PLASS**-tee) tympan/o = eardrum -plasty = surgical repair	See *myringoplasty*.
tympanotomy (tim-pan-**OT**-oh-mee) tympan/o = eardrum -tomy = incision into	See *myringotomy*.
vertigo (**VER**-tih-goh)	A sensation of spinning around or of having things in the room or area spinning around the person; a result of disturbance of the equilibrium.

Word Elements (Ear)

The following word elements pertain to the diseases, disorders, signs, symptoms, and diagnostic procedures associated with the ear. As you review the list, pronounce each word element aloud twice and check the box after you "say it." Write the definition for the example word given for each word element. You may use your medical dictionary.

WORD ELEMENT	PRONUNCIATION	"SAY IT"	MEANING
acous/o **acous**tic	ah-**KOOS**-oh ah-**KOOS**-tik	☐	hearing
audi/o **audi**ogram	**AW**-dee-oh **AW**-dee-oh-gram	☐	hearing
labyrinth/o **labyrinth**itis	lab-ih-**RIN**-tho lab-ih-rin-**THIGH**-tis	☐	inner ear
myring/o **myring**otomy	mir-**IN**-goh mir-in-**GOT**-oh-mee	☐	eardrum
ot/o **ot**itis media	**OH**-toh oh-**TYE**-tis **MEE**-dee-ah	☐	ear
tympan/o **tympan**oplasty	tim-**PAN**-oh tim-pan-oh-**PLASS**-tee	☐	eardrum

Pathological Conditions (Ear)

As you study the pathological conditions of the ear, note that the **basic definition** is in bold print, followed by a detailed description in regular print. The phonetic pronunciation is directly beneath each term, and a breakdown of the component parts of the term when appropriate.

cholesteatoma
(koh-lee-stee-ah-**TOH**-mah)
chol/e = bile
steat/o = fat
-oma = tumor

A slow-growing cystic mass made up of epithelial cell debris and cholesterol found in the middle ear.

A cholesteatoma occurs as a congenital defect or as a result of chronic otitis media. With chronic otitis media, the epithelial cell debris is formed largely due to marginal tympanic membrane perforations.

The scaly epithelial cells migrate into the middle ear from the ear canal where they accumulate to form a pocket of skin cells, which become an infected cystlike mass. The middle ear lining begins to deteriorate because of the collection of infected material buildup in the cavity. The cholesteatoma can lead to conductive hearing loss, occlusion of the middle ear, destruction of the ossicles, and erosion of the inner ear. Other symptoms include weakness of facial muscles, vertigo, drainage from the affected ear, and an earache.

Diagnosis is confirmed through the person's history, audiometry, otoscopy, and x-ray studies. If drainage is present, the culture results will be helpful in choosing the most effective antibiotic(s).

Treatment is surgical removal of the cholesteatoma. If deterioration of the lining has not begun, the cholesteatoma can be extracted by thoroughly cleaning the middle ear cavity. The removal becomes much more difficult when the cholesteatoma is in advanced stages. Without surgical intervention, the cholesteatoma will deteriorate the roof of the middle ear cavity providing an opportunity for the formation of an abscess or for meningitis to develop.

deafness, conductive
(kon-**DUK**-tiv)

Hearing loss caused by the breakdown of the transmission of sound waves through the middle and/or external ear.

This conductive hearing loss generally occurs when there is a mechanical abnormality in one of the following structures: oval or round windows, tympanic membrane, eustachian tube, ear ossicles, external auditory canal, and/or pinna. These mechanical defects may occur because of otosclerosis, otitis media, ruptured tympanic membrane, or impacted cerumen.

Audiometry is used to assess for and evaluate the extent of conductive hearing loss. Treatment is based on the causative factor or mechanical abnormality. Correcting the mechanical defect should be the beginning point. If the underlying defect cannot be fixed, hearing aids are helpful because of their ability to amplify sound. Hearing aids will improve hearing as long as the inner ear and sound perception organs are functioning normally.

deafness, sensorineural
(sen-soh-ree-**NOO**-ral)
neur/o = nerve
-al = pertaining to

Hearing loss caused by the inability of nerve stimuli to be delivered to the brain from the inner ear due to damage to the auditory nerve or the cochlea.

The results vary from a mild hearing loss to a profound hearing loss. **Sensorineural** hearing loss can occur because of the aging process or damaged hair cells of the organ of Corti, which may result from loud machinery noise, loud music, or medication side effects. Other causes of sensorineural hearing loss include tumors, infections (such as bacterial meningitis), trauma altering the central auditory pathways, vascular disorders, and degenerative or demyelinating diseases. Sensorineural hearing loss makes speech discrimination difficult primarily in noisy surroundings.

Diagnosis is based on the person's history and the results of the audiometry test. The best treatment is prevention when possible, which is accomplished by avoiding exposure to loud noises and being aware of medication with ototoxic effects. If the person cannot totally avoid the loud noises, wearing earplugs will be helpful in preventing or escaping further damage. Hearing aids are helpful in some cases; however, the person with sensorineural hearing loss may require a **cochlear** implant to have sound perception restored.

impacted cerumen
(seh-**ROO**-men)

An excessive accumulation of the waxlike secretions from the glands of the external ear canal.

Excessive hair or dry and scaly skin in the ear canal, or a narrow ear canal, may lead to the accumulation of earwax causing the ear canal to become impacted. The accumulation may cause a hearing loss or an earache. The person may also complain of the ear being "plugged" or **tinnitus** (ringing noise in the ear).

When an ear is found to have impacted cerumen, it must be removed by first softening the wax with oil or hydrogen peroxide. The next step is to irrigate with water until the wax is removed. This condition may recur, so regular ear examinations should be done.

labyrinthitis
(**lab**-ih-rin-**THIGH**-tis)
labyrinth/o = labyrinth
-itis = inflammation

Infection or inflammation of the labyrinth or the inner ear, specifically the three semicircular canals in the inner ear, which are fluid-filled chambers and control balance.

The primary symptom is severe vertigo (dizziness) with altered balance often accompanied by an elevation of temperature and/or nausea and vomiting. Other symptoms include nystagmus (rapid involuntary movements of the eye) and sensorineural hearing loss. A virus is typically the cause; however, bacteria may spread to the inner ear from a middle ear infection.

The diagnosis of **labyrinthitis** is based on blood, audiometry, and neurological studies.

Persons suffering from labyrinthitis are placed on bed rest for several days and prescribed an antiemetic (for the nausea), a tranquilizer, and an antibiotic (for the infection). Labyrinthitis should clear up in 1 to 3 weeks when therapy is carried out properly. If treatment is not initiated appropriately, labyrinthitis may be debilitating because of the sensitivity of the organ.

---

mastoiditis
(mass-toyd-**EYE**-tis)
mastoid/o = mastoid process
-itis = inflammation

Inflammation of the mastoid process, which is usually an acute expansion of an infection in the middle ear (otitis media).

Chronic **mastoiditis** may occur and is usually associated with cholesteatoma. The mastoid process is a round portion of the skull's temporal bone located adjacent to the middle ear and can be felt just behind both ears. The mastoid process is filled with air cavities or mastoid sinuses.

Infections of the middle ear always extend into the mastoid sinuses. These infections are eliminated when the middle ear infection is effectively treated with antibiotics. If the otitis media is not treated effectively with the appropriate antibiotics, the mastoid sinuses remain filled with purulent material, resulting in a bacterial infection of the mastoid process or acute mastoiditis.

The symptoms of acute mastoiditis occur approximately 2 to 3 weeks after the onset of acute otitis media. Symptoms include hearing loss and earache on the affected side, tenderness and swelling over the mastoid process, and constant throbbing pain. The swelling is often so severe that the pinna is displaced interiorly and anteriorly. The affected individual may also have a fever and complain of tinnitus. There is often a profuse drainage from the affected ear.

Diagnosis is confirmed through the person's history, x-ray studies of the mastoid, audiometry, otoscopy, and results of culture studies and blood work. The treatment of acute mastoiditis includes aggressive intravenous antibiotics for a 2-week period. Mastoiditis not responding to the antibiotic treatment may necessitate a surgical procedure to remove the severe infection due to its close proximity to the brain and the possibility of a brain abscess.

Ménière's disease
(may-nee-**ARYZ**)

Chronic inner ear disease in which there is an overaccumulation of endolymph (fluid in the labyrinth) characterized by recurring episodes of vertigo (dizziness), hearing loss, feeling of pressure or fullness in the affected ear, and tinnitus.

Episodes may last for hours or days. Other symptoms include nausea, vomiting, loss of balance, and sweating. Initially only one ear is involved; however, over time both ears are affected.

The cause of **Ménière's** disease is unknown but predisposing factors include head trauma, dysfunction of the autonomic nervous system, middle ear infections, and premenstrual edema.

Diagnosis is usually based on the four major symptoms: vertigo, progressive hearing loss, tinnitus, and a feeling of pressure or fullness in the ear. If these symptoms are not present or are too vague, additional testing with x-ray studies and audiometry will likely be done.

To treat Ménière's disease for the long term, the person may be instructed to modify his or her lifestyle with such details as restricting fluid intake, eating a salt-free diet, and using mild sedatives, antihistamines, and diuretics. Antiemetics are usually prescribed for the acute attacks of Ménière's disease.

otitis externa
(oh-**TYE**-tis eks-**TER**-nah)
(swimmer's ear)
ot/o = ear
-itis = inflammation

Inflammation of the outer or external ear canal, also called "swimmer's ear." This inflammation is produced from the growth of bacteria or fungi in the external ear. In addition to the occurrence after swimming, **otitis externa** can develop due to conditions such as psoriasis or seborrhea, injury to the ear canal when trying to scratch or clean it with a foreign object, and frequent use of earphones or earplugs.

The major symptom is pain, especially when the ear is tugged on, along with a red swollen ear canal. Treatment includes the use of steroid or antibiotic eardrops and systemic antibiotics.

otitis media, acute
(oh-**TYE**-tis **MEE**-dee-ah)
ot/o = ear
-itis = inflammation
medi/o = middle
-a = noun ending

A middle ear infection, which predominately affects infants, toddlers, and preschoolers.

The air-filled middle ear is inflamed causing an accumulation of fluid behind the tympanic membrane. Upper respiratory infections and dysfunction of the auditory tube are associated with both types of **otitis media**. The two types are serous otitis media and suppurative otitis media. A discussion of each type follows.

serous otitis media
(**SEER**-us oh-**TYE**-tis **MEE**-dee-ah)
ot/o = ear
-itis = inflammation
ser/o = blood serum
-ous = pertaining to
medi/o = middle
-a = noun ending

A sterile collection of clear fluid in the middle ear.

Symptoms of **serous otitis media** include complaints of pain, "popping" or "snapping" in the ear, and diminished mobility of the tympanic membrane. When examined, the eardrum or tympanic membrane will look retracted or bulging with air bubbles or fluid visible behind the membrane.

suppurative otitis media
(**SOO**-per-ah-tiv oh-**TYE**-tis **MEE**-dee-ah)
ot/o = ear
-itis = inflammation
medi/o = middle
-a = noun ending

A purulent collection of fluid in the middle ear causing the person to experience pain (possibly severe), an elevation in temperature, dizziness, decreased hearing, vertigo, and tinnitus; also called acute otitis media.

The major concern with **suppurative otitis media** is the potential of a spontaneous rupture of the tympanic membrane as the pressure inside the middle ear rises.

otosclerosis
(oh-toh-sklair-**OH**-sis)
ot/o = ear
scler/o = hard
-osis = condition

A condition in which the footplate of the stapes becomes immobile and secured to the oval window, resulting in a hearing loss.

The hearing loss is due to the inability of the stapes to rock the oval window and thus transmit sound to the inner ear. **Otosclerosis** typically results in conductive hearing loss. Occasionally, individuals experience sensorineural hearing loss or a mixed hearing loss if neural components are involved.

Otosclerosis occurs most commonly in females and Caucasians, resulting in progressive hearing loss. Its onset typically begins between the ages of 11 and 30 with the person having problems with tinnitus and inability to hear soft-spoken tones.

Treatment for otosclerosis includes the use of hearing aids and surgical intervention such as a stapedectomy.

perforation of the tympanic membrane
(per-for-**AY**-shun of the tim-**PAN**-ik)
tympan/o = eardrum
-ic = pertaining to

Rupture of the tympanic membrane or eardrum.

This condition may be due to middle ear trauma such as a severe middle ear infection, direct injury from a sharp object, barotrauma caused by an explosion, or explosive acoustic trauma.

The person experiencing the rupture of the eardrum typically complains of partial hearing loss and slight pain. With some perforations of the tympanic membrane there is drainage from the ear.

The rupture makes a direct opening into the middle ear and the risk for an infection is present until the perforation is closed through the healing process, which requires about 1 to 2 weeks. If needed, a patch can be applied to the eardrum to improve hearing and aid in healing.

Diagnostic Techniques and Procedures (Ear)

audiometry
(aw-dee-**OM**-eh-tree)
audi/o = hearing
metr/i = to measure
-y = noun ending

The process of measuring how well an individual hears various frequencies of sound waves.

Audiometry is more specific than the bone conduction hearing tests (Rinne and Weber) because it provides information on the extent of hearing loss and which frequencies are involved. One form of audiometry that is frequently used to assess hearing acuity is the pure tone audiometry, which uses pure tones that are almost completely free of extraneous noises. The person is placed in a soundproof cubicle with earphones and is instructed to signal or indicate when the sounds are first heard and when the sounds can no longer be heard as the decibels (loudness of the sound) are lowered gradually. The audiometer delivers a single frequency at a time, beginning with low frequency tones and going up to high frequency tones. Each ear is assessed separately and the results are recorded on a graph known as an audiogram.

otoscopy
(oh-**TOSS**-koh-pee)
ot/o = ear
-scopy = process of viewing

The use of an otoscope to view and examine the tympanic membrane and various parts of the outer ear.

The external ear is examined for lesions, cerumen, color, and intactness.

tuning fork test (Rinne test)
(**RIN**-nee test)

An examination that compares bone conduction and air conduction. See Figure 14-15.

When performing the Rinne test, the base of a vibrating tuning fork is placed on the person's mastoid bone and held there until sound can no longer be heard, at which time it is quickly moved in front of the ear near

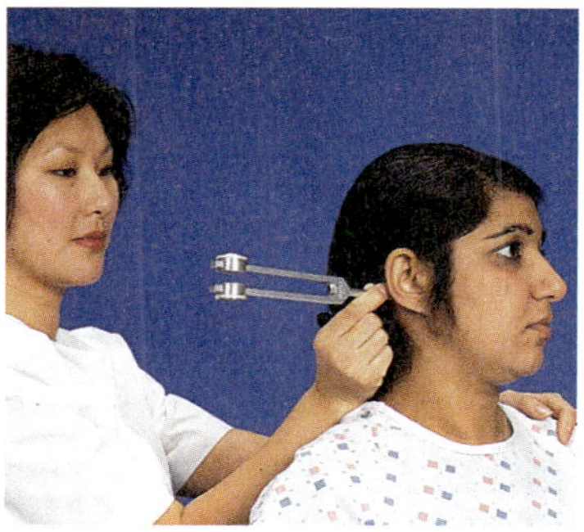

the ear canal. At this time it is determined if the person continues to hear the sound at the ear canal. The person with normal hearing will hear the sound vibrating through the air longer than through bone.

With conduction hearing loss, the sound will be heard longer through bone. With sensorineural hearing loss, air conduction is longer, as is the normal hearing pattern.

Figure 14-15 Rinne tuning fork test

tuning fork test (Weber test)

An examination used to evaluate auditory acuity as well as discover whether a hearing deficit is a conductive loss or a sensorineural loss. See Figure 14-16.

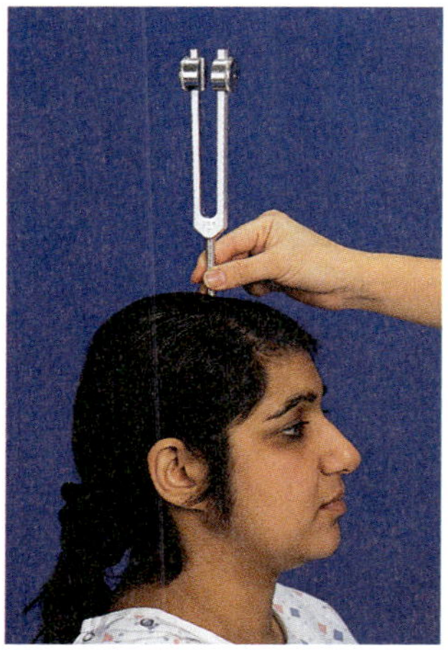

After placing the base of a vibrating tuning fork on the center of the person's forehead, the person is instructed to evaluate the loudness of the sound heard in each ear. Normally the loudness of sound heard is identical in both ears. Hearing the sound more in one ear than in the other is an abnormal finding.

If conductive hearing loss is present, the sound will be heard louder in the affected ear due to the inability to hear normal background sounds conducted through the air. If sensorineural loss is present in one ear, the sound is heard louder in the unaffected ear.

Figure 14-16 Weber tuning fork test

otoplasty
(**OH**-toh-plass-tee)
ot/o = ear
-plasty = surgical repair

Removal of a portion of ear cartilage to bring the pinna and auricle nearer the head.

Otoplasty is accomplished typically for cosmetic purposes through reconstructive plastic surgery.

stapedectomy
(stay-pee-**DEK**-toh-mee)
staped/o = stapes
-ectomy = surgical removal

Microsurgical removal of the stapes diseased by otosclerosis, typically under local anesthesia.

The stapes removal is followed by placement of a tissue graft and prosthesis to reestablish a pathway for vibrations to deliver sound waves through the oval window and to the inner ear. The prosthesis is attached to the incus on one end and to a graft on the oval window on the other end.

The person experiencing hearing loss due to otosclerosis has improved hearing immediately after the stapedectomy. This improved hearing is temporarily diminished after the onset of postoperative swelling and ear packing.

hearing aids

Devices that amplify sound to provide more precise perception and interpretation of words communicated to the individual with a hearing deficit.

This improved interpretation and perception is made possible by the amplification of sound above the individual's hearing threshold as it is introduced to the ear's hearing apparatus.

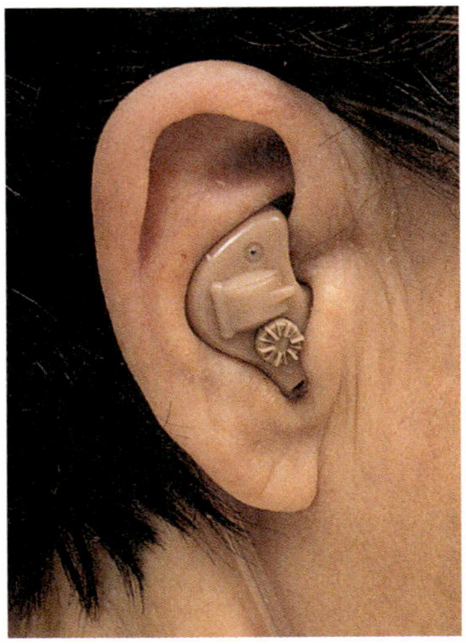

(A)

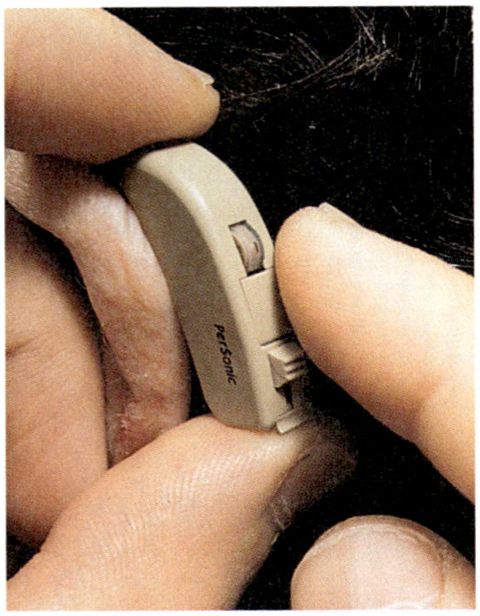

(B)

Hearing aids are accessible in an assortment of styles.

1. The **"in-canal style" hearing aid** is the newest and least conspicuous of the devices, fitting completely into the ear canal and allowing for exercise and talking on the telephone without being obtrusive. The disadvantages of using this style of hearing aid occurs for those individuals who do not have good dexterity with their hands. Because of the size of the hearing aid, the handling, cleaning, and changing of batteries require good manual dexterity, which is difficult for many older individuals. Cleaning is important because of the possible accumulation of earwax, which will plug the small portals and disrupt sound transmission.
2. The **"in-ear style" hearing aid** is worn in the external ear and is larger and more noticeable than the in-canal style. The care of the in-ear style also requires manual dexterity, often a concern for the older individual. Advantages of the in-ear style include a greater degree of amplification and toggle switches that allow for usage of the telephone. Cleaning is important because of the possible accumulation of earwax, which will plug the small portals and disrupt sound transmission. See **Figure 14-17A.**
3. The **"behind-ear style" hearing aid** allows for even greater amplification of sound than the in-ear style and is much easier to manipulate manually for care and control. The predicament presented when one uses this hearing aid with eyeglasses has been addressed with a modification of the hearing aid components fitting into the individual's eyeglasses. See **Figure 14-17B.**
4. A **"body hearing aid"** is used by individuals with profound hearing loss. Sound is delivered to the ear canal by way of a microphone and amplifier clipped on the clothing in a pocket-size container that is connected to a receiver, which is clipped onto the ear mold.

Figure 14-17 Hearing aids: (A) in-ear style; (B) behind-ear style

myringotomy
(mir-in-**GOT**-oh-mee)
myring/o = eardrum
-tomy = incision into

A surgical procedure with insertion of a small ventilation tube introduced into the inferior segment of the tympanic membrane.

These small tubes provide ventilation and drainage of the middle ear when there is a problem with persistent ear infection not responding to antibiotics or persistent severe negative middle ear pressure.

A myringotomy allows drainage of fluid by way of a surgical opening, which aids to:

1. avoid a potential spontaneous rupture of the tympanic membrane
2. relieve pain
3. restore hearing
4. improve speech problems and learning deficits associated with hearing loss
5. equalize pressure in the middle ear

After the middle ear heals, the drainage stops and the small tubes are removed from the tympanic membrane, allowing it to heal. While the tubes are in place, the individual must avoid getting water into the ear canal and potentially into the middle ear.

tympanotomy
(tim-pan-**OT**-oh-mee)
tympan/o = eardrum, tympanic membrane
-tomy = incision into

See *myringotomy*.

myringoplasty
(mir-**IN**-goh-**plass**-tee)
myring/o = eardrum
-plasty = surgical repair

Surgical repair of the tympanic membrane with a tissue graft after a spontaneous rupture that results in hearing loss; also called a tympanoplasty.

The repair surgical procedure is performed under local or general anesthesia. Topical antibiotics and an absorbable packing are applied to the graft site to secure its position.

tympanoplasty
(tim-pan-oh-**PLASS**-tee)
tympan/o = eardrum
-plasty = surgical repair

See *myringoplasty*.

Common Abbreviations (Ear)

ABBREVIATION	MEANING	ABBREVIATION	MEANING
ABLB	alternate binaural loudness balance	**dB**	decibel
ABR	auditory brainstem response	**EENT**	ears, eyes, nose, and throat
AC	air conduction	**ENT**	ears, nose, and throat
AD	right ear (auris dextra)	**PTS**	permanent threshold shift
AS	left ear (auris sinistra)	**TM**	tympanic membrane
AU	each ear (auris unitas)	**TTS**	temporary threshold shift
BC	bone conduction	**BOM**	bilateral otitis media

Written and Audio Terminology Review

Review each of the following terms from this chapter. Study the spelling of each term and write the definition in the space provided. If you have the Audio CD available, listen to each term, pronounce it, and check the box once you are comfortable saying the word. Check definitions by looking the term up in the glossary/index.

TERM	PRONUNCIATION	DEFINITION
acoustic	☐ ah-**KOOS**-tik	________
ambiopia	☐ am-bee-**OH**-pee-ah	________
amblyopia	☐ am-blee-**OH**-pee-ah	________
anisocoria	☐ an-eye-soh-**KOH**-ree-ah	________
aphakia	☐ ah-**FAY**-kee-ah	________
aqueous	☐ **AY**-**kwee**-us	________
aqueous humor	☐ **AY**-kwee-us humor	________
Argyll-Robertson pupil	☐ ar-**GILL ROB**-ert-son pupil	________
astigmatism	☐ ah-**STIG**-mah-tizm	________
audiogram	☐ **AW**-dee-oh-gram	________
audiometry	☐ aw-dee-**OM**-eh-tree	________
auditory	☐ **AW**-dih-tor-ee	________
aural	☐ **AW**-ral	________
auriculotemporal	☐ aw-rik-yoo-loh-**TEM**-poh-ral	________
barotitis media	☐ bar-oh-**TYE**-tis **MEE**-dee-ah	________
blepharitis	☐ blef-ah-**RYE**-tis	________
blepharochalasis	☐ blef-ah-roh-**KAL**-ah-sis	________
blepharoptosis	☐ blef-ah-roh-**TOH**-sis	________
cataract	☐ **KAT**-ah-rakt	________
cerumen	☐ seh-**ROO**-men	________
chalazion	☐ kah-**LAY**-zee-on	________
cholesteatoma	☐ koh-lee-stee-ah-**TOH**-mah	________
cochlear	☐ **COCK**-lee-ar	________
conductive	☐ kon-**DUK**-tiv	________
conjunctivitis	☐ kon-junk-tih-**VYE**-tis	________
cornea	☐ **COR**-nee-a	________
corneal abrasion	☐ **COR**-nee-al ay-**BRAY**-zhun	________
corneal transplant	☐ **COR**-nee-al transplant	________
cycloplegia	☐ sigh-kloh-**PLEE**-jee-ah	________
dacryoadenitis	☐ dak-ree-oh-ad-en-**EYE**-tis	________
dacryocystectomy	☐ dak-ree-oh-sis-**TEK**-toh-mee	________

Term		Pronunciation	
dacryorrhea	☐	dak-ree-oh-**REE**-ah	______
diabetic	☐	dye-ah-**BET**-ik	______
diplopia	☐	dip-**PLOH**-pee-ah	______
ectropion	☐	ek-**TROH**-pee-on	______
electronystagmography	☐	ee-**lek**-troh-niss-tag-**MOG**-rah-fee	______
electroretinogram	☐	ee-lek-troh-**RET**-ih-noh-gram	______
emmetropia	☐	em-eh-**TROH**-pee-ah	______
entropion	☐	en-**TROH**-pee-on	______
episcleritis	☐	ep-ih-skleh-**RYE**-tis	______
esotropia	☐	ess-oh-**TROH**-pee-ah	______
exophthalmia	☐	eks-off-**THAL**-mee-ah	______
extracapsular extraction	☐	eks-trah-**KAP**-syoo-lar eks-**TRAK**-shun	______
extraocular	☐	eks-trah-**OCK**-yoo-lar	______
fluorescein	☐	floo-oh-**RESS**-ee-in	______
fundoscopy	☐	fun-**DOSS**-koh-pee	______
glaucoma	☐	glah-**KOH**-mah	______
gonioscopy	☐	gah-nee-**OSS**-kah-pee	______
hemianopia	☐	hem-ee-ah-**NOP**-ee-ah	______
hemianopsia	☐	hem-ee-ah-**NOP**-see-ah	______
hordeolum	☐	hor-**DEE**-oh-lum	______
hyperopia	☐	high-per-**OH**-pee-ah	______
hyphema	☐	high-**FEE**-mah	______
intraocular	☐	in-trah-**OCK**-yoo-lar	______
iridectomy	☐	ir-id-**EK**-toh-mee	______
iriditis	☐	ir-id-**EYE**-tis	______
iridocyclitis	☐	ir-id-oh-sigh-**KLEYE**-tis	______
iridoplegia	☐	ir-id-oh-**PLEE**-jee-ah	______
iritis	☐	ih-**RYE**-tis	______
keratitis	☐	ker-ah-**TYE**-tis	______

Term		Pronunciation	
keratoconjunctivitis	☐	ker-ah-toh-kon-junk-tih-**VYE**-tis	______
keratoconus	☐	ker-ah-toh-**KOH**-nus	______
keratomycosis	☐	ker-ah-toh-my-**KOH**-sis	______
keratoplasty	☐	**KAIR**-ah-toh-**plass**-tee	______
labyrinthitis	☐	lab-ih-rin-**THIGH**-tis	______
lacrimal	☐	**LAK**-rim-al	______
lacrimation	☐	lak-rih-**MAY**-shun	______
mastoiditis	☐	mass-toyd-**EYE**-tis	______
Ménière's	☐	may-nee-**AIRZ**	______
miosis	☐	my-**OH**-sis	______
miotic	☐	my-**OT**-ik	______
monochromatism	☐	mon-oh-**KROH**-mah-tizm	______
mydriasis	☐	mid-**RYE**-ah-sis	______
mydriatic	☐	mid-ree-**AT**-ik	______
myopia	☐	my-**OH**-pee-ah	______
myringoplasty	☐	mir-**IN**-goh-**plass**-tee	______
myringotomy	☐	mir-in-**GOT**-oh-mee	______
nasolacrimal	☐	nay-zoh-**LAK**-rim-al	______
nyctalopia	☐	nik-tah-**LOH**-pee-ah	______
nystagmus	☐	niss-**TAG**-mus	______
oculomotor	☐	**ok**-yoo-loh-**MOH**-tor	______
ophthalmia neonatorum	☐	off-**THAL**-mee-ah nee-oh-nay-**TOR**-um	______
ophthalmologist	☐	off-thal-**MALL**-oh-jist	______
ophthalmology	☐	off-thal-**MALL**-oh-jee	______
ophthalmoscope	☐	off-**THAL**-moh-scohp	______
ophthalmoscopy	☐	off-thal-**MOSS**-koh-pee	______
optic	☐	**OP**-tik	______
optician	☐	op-**TISH**-an	______
optometrist	☐	op-**TOM**-eh-trist	______
otalgia	☐	oh-**TAL**-jee-ah	______
otitis externa	☐	oh-**TYE**-tis eks-**TER**-nah	______

Term		Pronunciation	
otitis media	☐	oh-**TYE**-tis **MEE**-dee-ah	______
otodynia	☐	oh-toh-**DIN**-ee-ah	______
otomycosis	☐	oh-toh-my-**KOH**-sis	______
otoplasty	☐	**OH**-toh-plass-tee	______
otorrhea	☐	oh-toh-**REE**-ah	______
otosclerosis	☐	oh-toh-sklair-**OH**-sis	______
otoscopy	☐	oh-**TOSS**-koh-pee	______
palpebral	☐	**PAL**-peh-brahl	______
palpebrate	☐	pal-**PEE**-brayt	______
papilledema	☐	pap-ill-eh-**DEE**-mah	______
phacoemulsification	☐	**fak**-oh-ee-**MULL**-sih-fih-**kay**-shun	______
phacomalacia	☐	fak-oh-mah-**LAY**-shee-ah	______
photo refractive keratectomy	☐	**FOH**-toh ree-**FRAK**-tive kair- ah-**TEK**-toh-mee	______
photophobia	☐	foh-toh-**FOH**-bee-ah	______
presbycusis	☐	prez-bee-**KOO**-sis	______
presbyopia	☐	prez-bee-**OH**-pee-ah	______
pterygium	☐	ter-**IJ**-ee-um	______
pupillary	☐	**PEW**-pih-lair-ee	______
purulent	☐	**PEWR**-yoo-lent	______
retinal	☐	**RET**-in-al	______
retinal photocoagulation	☐	**RET**-in-al **foh**-toh-coh-**ag**-yoo-LAY-shun	______
retinitis	☐	ret-in-**EYE**-tis	______
retinopathy	☐	**ret**-in-**OP**-ah-thee	______
Rinne test	☐	**RIN**-nee test	______
salpingoscope	☐	sal-**PING**-goh-skoph	______
sclera	☐	**SKLAIR**-ah	______
sclerectomy	☐	skleh-**REK**-toh-mee	______
scleritis	☐	skleh-**RYE**-tis	______
scotoma	☐	skoh-**TOH**-mah	______
sensorineural	☐	sen-soh-ree-**NOO**-ral	______

serous	☐ **SEER**-us	____
serous otitis media	☐ **SEER**-us oh-**TYE**-tis **MEE**-dee-ah	____
stapedectomy	☐ stay-pee-**DEK**-toh-mee	____
strabismus	☐ strah-**BIZ**-mus	____
suppurative otitis media	☐ **SOO**-per-ah-tiv oh-**TYE**-tis **MEE**-dee-ah	____
synechia	☐ sin-**EK**-ee-ah	____
tinnitus	☐ tin-**EYE**-tus	____
tonometry	☐ tohn-**OM**-eh-tree	____
trabeculectomy	☐ trah-**bek**-yool-**EK**-toh-mee	____
trabeculoplasty	☐ trah-**BEK**-yoo-loh-plass-tee	____
trachoma	☐ tray-**KOH**-mah	____
tympanoplasty	☐ tim-pan-oh-**PLASS**-tee	____
tympanotomy	☐ tim-pan-**OT**-oh-mee	____
uveitis	☐ yoo-vee-**EYE**-tis	____
vertigo	☐ **VER**-tih-goh	____
vitreous	☐ **VIT**-ree-us	____
xerophthalmia	☐ zeer-off-**THAL**-mee-ah	____

Chapter Review Exercises

The following exercises provide a more in-depth review of the chapter material. Your goal in these exercises is to complete each section at a minimum 80% level of accuracy. A space has been provided for your score at the end of each section.

A. Spelling

Circle the correctly spelled term in each pairing of words. Each correct answer is worth 10 points. Record your score in the space provided at the end of the exercise.

1. ophthalmoscope	opthalmoscope
2. ambyopia	ambiopia
3. blepharoptosis	blephroptosis
4. corneitis	corniitis
5. nistagmus	nystagmus
6. cochlear	coclear
7. otorrhea	otorrea
8. serus	serous

9. tinnitus	tinnitis
10. tympanotomy	tempanotomy

Number correct _______ × 10 points/correct answer: Your score _______%

B. Term to Definition

Define each term by writing the definition in the space provided. Check the box if you are able to complete this exercise correctly the first time (without referring to the answers). Each correct answer is worth 10 points. Record your score in the space provided at the end of the exercise.

☐ 1. tinnitus ____________________

☐ 2. vertigo ____________________

☐ 3. presbycusis ____________________

☐ 4. myringoplasty ____________________

☐ 5. labyrinthitis ____________________

☐ 6. blepharoptosis ____________________

☐ 7. optician ____________________

☐ 8. conjunctivitis ____________________

☐ 9. ophthalmologist ____________________

☐ 10. glaucoma ____________________

Number correct _______ × 10 points/correct answer: Your score _______%

C. Matching Abbreviations

Match the abbreviations on the left with the appropriate definition on the right. Each correct answer is worth 10 points. Record your score in the space provided at the end of the exercise.

_____	1. EOM	a. visual acuity
_____	2. OD	b. air conduction
_____	3. PEARL	c. ears, nose, and throat
_____	4. REM	d. pupils equal and reactive to light
_____	5. VA	e. blister on middle ear
_____	6. AC	f. decibel
_____	7. ENT	g. right eye
_____	8. BOM	h. left ear
_____	9. AS	i. rapid eye movement
_____	10. dB	j. extraocular movement
		k. pupils equal and reactive lens
		l. extraorbital mass
		m. bilateral otitis media

Number correct _______ × 10 points/correct answer: Your score _______%

D. Crossword Puzzle

Read the clues carefully and complete the puzzle. Each crossword answer is worth 10 points. When you have completed the crossword puzzle, total your points and enter your score in the space provided.

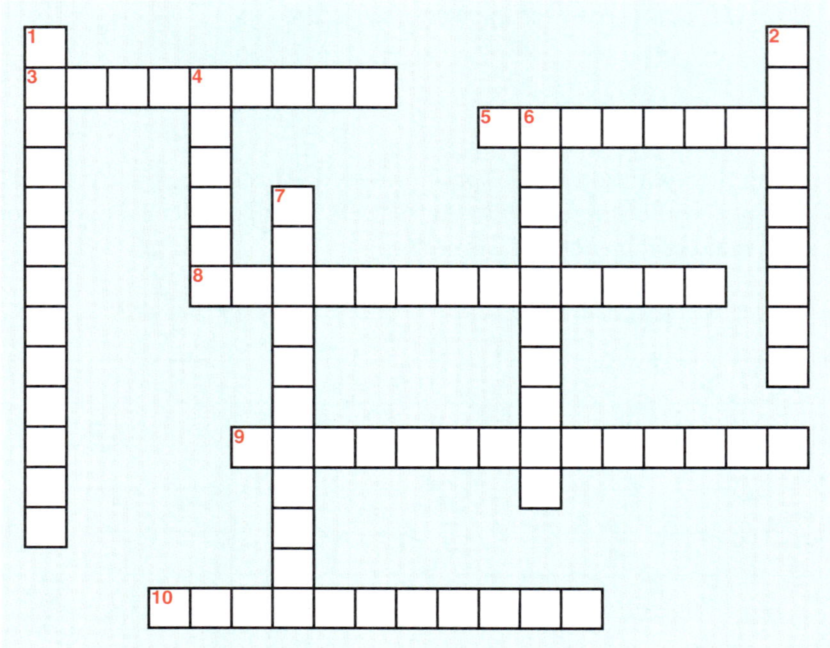

ACROSS

3 Outward turning of the eye
5 Inflammation of the iris
8 Focusing by the lens of the eye
9 Drooping of the upper eyelid
10 Half of visual field blindness

DOWN

1 Fungal growth on the cornea
2 Jerking movements of the eye
4 Sensitive nerve-cell layer of the eye
6 Bending of light rays in the eye
7 Paralysis of the ciliary muscle

Number correct _______ × 10 points/correct answer: Your score _______%

E. Definition to Term

Using the following definitions, identify and provide the medical term to match the definition. Write the word in the first space and the appropriate combining form for the word in the second space. Each correct answer is worth 5 points. Record your score in the space provided at the end of the exercise.

1. drooping of the eyelid

   ____________________ ____________________

   (word) (combining form)

2. double vision

   ____________________ ____________________

   (word) (combining form)

3. paralysis of the ciliary muscle of the eye

   ____________________ ____________________

   (word) (combining form)

4. excessive flow of tears

   ____________________ ____________________

   (word) (combining form)

5. inflammation of the conjunctiva of the eye

   ____________________ ____________________

   (word) (combining form)

6. recording of the faintest sounds an individual is able to hear

   ____________________ ____________________

   (word) (combining form)

7. inflammation of the inner ear

   ____________________ ____________________

   (word) (combining form)

8. incision into the eardrum

   ____________________ ____________________

   (word) (combining form)

9. pertaining to the ear

   ____________________ ____________________

   (word) (combining form)

10. pain in the ear

   ____________________ ____________________

   (word) (combining form)

Number correct ______ × 5 points/correct answer: Your score ______%

F. Labeling

Label the following diagrams by identifying the appropriate structure. Place your answers in the spaces provided. Each correct answer is worth 10 points. Record your score in the space provided at the end of the exercise.

1. ______________________
2. ______________________
3. ______________________
4. ______________________
5. ______________________

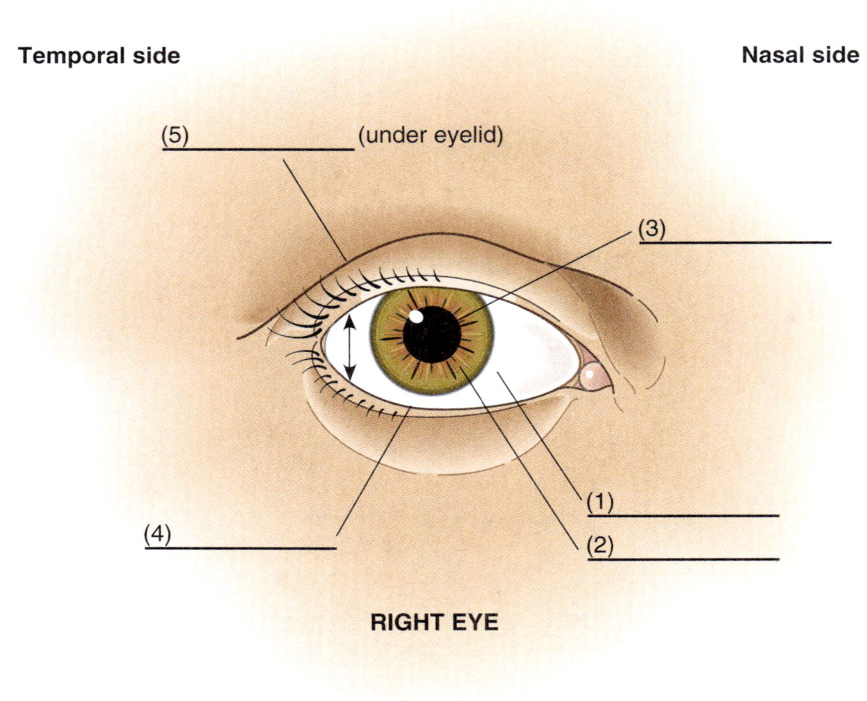

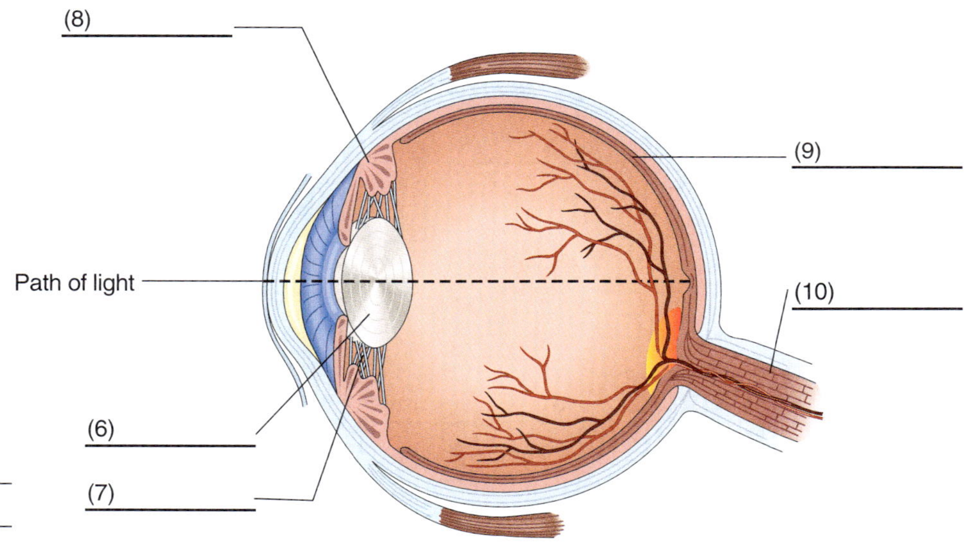

6. ______________________
7. ______________________
8. ______________________
9. ______________________
10. ______________________

***Number correct* _______ × *10 points/correct answer: Your score* _______%**

G. Trace That Sound!

The following completion exercise will trace the sound vibrations through the ear. As you read the discussion, complete the blank spaces with the most appropriate word. Each correct response is worth 10 points. When you have completed the exercise, record your score in the space provided at the end of the exercise.

The process of hearing begins with the outer ear. The sound vibrations are received by the pinna and are funneled through the (1) ____________________ to the (2) ____________________. The sound waves strike the area just mentioned and cause it to vibrate. These vibrations move the three small bones of the middle ear: the (3) ____________________, the (4) ____________________, and the (5) ____________________, each of which is attached to the other. As the last of the three small bones in the middle ear vibrates, it causes the (6) ____________________ to vibrate, setting in motion a "ripple effect" in the fluids within the (7) ____________________. As these fluids fluctuate, they transmit the stimulus on to the tiny hair cells of the (8) ____________________. The stimulation is picked up by the (9) ____________________ that lie close to these tiny hair cells and the stimulation is transmitted on to the (10) ____________________ of the brain where the impulses are interpreted as hearing.

Number correct _______ × 10 points/correct answer: Your score _______%

H. Matching Procedures

Read the descriptions of the diagnostic and treatment procedures on the right and match them with the appropriate answer on the left. Each correct answer is worth 10 points. Record your score in the space provided at the end of the exercise.

_____ 1. stapedectomy
_____ 2. Rinne test
_____ 3. electroretinogram
_____ 4. myringotomy
_____ 5. electronystagmography
_____ 6. myringoplasty
_____ 7. tonometry
_____ 8. fundoscopy
_____ 9. laser iridectomy
_____ 10. photorefractive keratectomy

a. A group of tests used in evaluating the vestibulo-ocular reflex
b. Determines the intraocular pressure by calculating the resistance of the eyeball to an applied force causing indentation
c. A recording of the changes in the electrical potential of the retina after the stimulation of light
d. Examination of the fundus of the eye
e. Creating several small openings in the iris to allow aqueous humor to flow to the anterior chamber from the posterior chamber
f. Shaving off a few layers of the corneal surface to reduce myopia
g. An examination that compares bone conduction and air conduction in an individual
h. Microsurgical removal of the stapes
i. Insertion of a small ventilation tube into the inferior segment of the tympanic membrane through surgery
j. Surgical repair of the tympanic membrane with a tissue graft

Number correct _______ × 10 points/correct answer: Your score _______%

I. Completion

The following statements describe various pathological conditions of the eye and ear. Read each statement carefully and complete the sentences with the most appropriate pathological condition. Each correct answer is worth 10 points. Record your score in the space provided at the end of the exercise.

1. The accumulation of waxlike secretions in the external ear canal that may cause a hearing loss is called:

   ____

2. An inflammatory process usually an acute expansion of a middle ear infection is called:

   ____

3. A refractive error resulting in impaired close vision due to the eyeball being shorter than normal is known as:

   ____

4. A refractive error resulting in impaired distant vision due to the eyeball being longer than normal is known as:

   ____

5. A condition in which the eyelid partially or completely covers the eye as a result of a weakened muscle is known as:

   ____

6. Progressive vision loss due to clouding of the lens is:

   ____

7. A condition in which there is scarring of the retinal capillaries and leakage of blood, which result in a decline in the sharpness of vision is known as:

   ____

8. Inversion (turning inward) of the edge of the eyelid is called:

   ____

9. An ocular disorder characterized by an increase in intraocular pressure is known as:

   ____

10. Inflammation of the cornea is called:

    ____

***Number correct* ______ × *10 points/correct answer: Your score* ______%**

J. Word Search

Using the definitions listed, identify the pathological condition related to the eye and ear and then find and circle it in the following puzzle. The words may be read up, down, diagonally, across, or backward. Each correct answer is worth 10 points. Record your score in the space provided at the end of the exercise.

Example: Drooping of the upper eyelid

blepharoptosis

1. A chronic disease of the inner ear characterized by vertigo, hearing loss, a feeling of fullness in the affected ear, and tinnitus

   ____

2. Causes a hearing loss due to the footplate of the stapes becoming immobile and secured to the oval window

   ____

3. A refractive error causing the light rays entering the eye to be focused irregularly due to an abnormally shaped cornea

____

4. Inflammation of the eyelid margins

____

5. A cyst or nodule on the eyelid due to an obstruction of a meibomian gland

____

6. Inflammation of the mucous membrane lining the eyelids and covering the front of the eyeball

____

7. "Turning out" of the eyelashes

____

8. Bacterial infection of an eyelash follicle or sebaceous gland

____

9. An "ocular emergency" due to a bleed into the anterior chamber of the eye

____

10. Involuntary movements of the eyes

____

Number correct _______ × 10 points/correct answer: Your score _______%

B	L	E	P	H	A	R	O	P	T	O	S	I	S	I
B	E	R	R	A	S	N	I	A	L	T	I	U	N	S
L	L	B	Y	A	T	U	T	E	I	O	G	E	Y	C
T	A	E	S	A	I	H	S	D	I	S	E	A	S	E
I	S	D	P	R	G	I	F	L	E	C	I	E	T	A
P	I	S	Y	H	M	T	A	N	O	L	R	Z	A	M
L	T	E	D	E	A	H	I	M	B	E	I	H	G	B
E	I	E	R	P	T	R	E	X	I	R	N	E	M	U
S	V	X	O	E	I	N	I	N	T	O	P	I	U	L
C	I	T	C	I	S	N	E	T	T	S	N	M	S	M
L	T	N	E	R	M	M	A	R	I	I	A	E	I	U
E	C	H	A	L	A	Z	I	O	N	S	D	R	C	L
R	N	O	I	P	O	R	T	C	E	P	R	S	N	O
O	U	I	A	I	E	S	U	M	P	O	S	U	P	E
S	J	O	L	S	Y	D	S	H	C	A	S	Y	A	D
I	N	N	U	S	E	P	I	N	A	T	L	N	I	R
S	O	O	S	D	S	R	S	I	F	L	E	S	X	O
P	C	A	N	M	I	G	A	I	M	E	H	P	Y	H

Answers to Chapter Review Exercises

A. Spelling

1. ophthalmoscope
2. ambiopia
3. blepharoptosis
4. corneitis
5. nystagmus
6. cochlear
7. otorrhea
8. serous
9. tinnitus
10. tympanotomy

B. Term to Definition

1. a ringing or tinkling noise heard in the ears
2. a sensation of spinning around or of having things in the room or area spinning around the person
3. loss of hearing due to the natural aging process
4. surgical repair of the tympanic membrane (eardrum) with a tissue graft
5. inflammation of the inner ear
6. drooping of the upper eyelid
7. an individual (nondoctor) who specializes in filling prescriptions for corrective lenses for glasses or for contact lenses
8. inflammation of the conjunctiva of the eye
9. a physician who specializes in the treatment of the diseases and disorders of the eye
10. a condition in which there is increased intraocular pressure

C. Matching Abbreviations

1. j
2. g
3. d
4. i
5. a
6. b
7. c
8. m
9. h
10. f

D. Crossword Puzzle

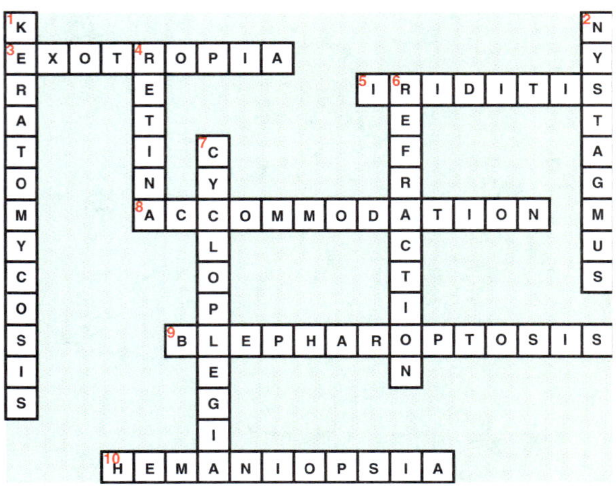

E. Definition to Term

1. blepharoptosis	blephar/o
2. diplopia	dipl/o
3. cycloplegia	cycl/o
4. dacryorrhea	dacry/o
5. conjunctivitis	conjunctiv/o
6. audiometry	audi/o
7. labyrinthitis	labyrinth/o
8. myringotomy	myring/o
tympanotomy	tympan/o
9. aural	aur/o
10. otodynia	ot/o
otalgia	ot/o

F. Labeling

1. sclera
2. iris
3. pupil
4. conjunctiva
5. lacrimal gland
6. lens
7. suspensory ligament
8. ciliary body
9. retina
10. optic nerve

G. Trace That Sound!

1. external auditory canal
2. tympanic membrane
3. malleus
4. incus
5. stapes
6. oval window
7. cochlea
8. organ of Corti
9. auditory nerve fibers
10. cerebral cortex

H. Matching Procedures

1. h
2. g
3. c
4. i
5. a
6. j
7. b
8. d
9. e
10. f

I. Completion

1. impacted cerumen
2. mastoiditis
3. hyperopia
4. myopia
5. blepharoptosis
6. cataract
7. diabetic retinopathy
8. entropion
9. glaucoma
10. keratitis

J. Word Search

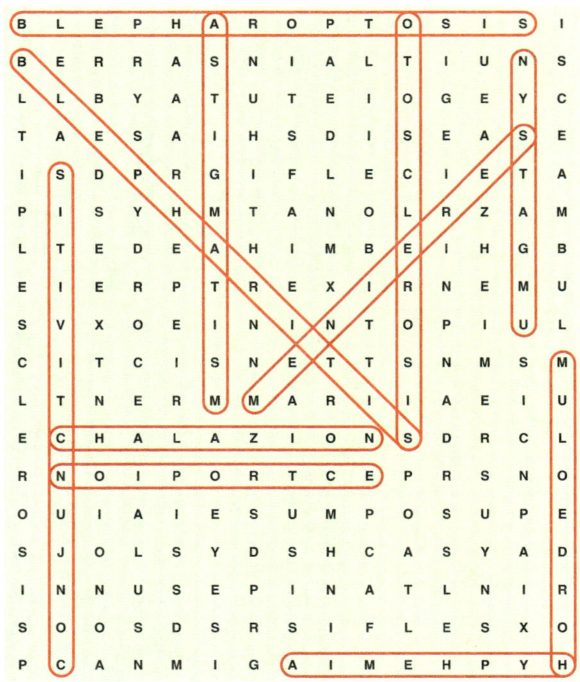

CHAPTER 15

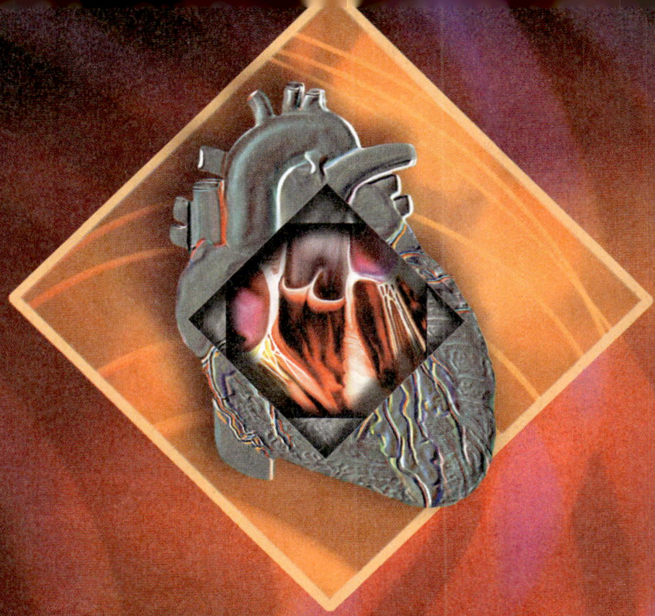

The Urinary System

CHAPTER OUTLINE

KEY COMPETENCIES

Upon completing this chapter and the review exercises at the end of the chapter, the learner should be able to:

1. Identify and label the internal structure of the kidney.
2. List four major functions of the urinary system.
3. Using a flow chart, identify the appropriate structures involved in the process of forming and expelling urine.
4. Define at least 15 common signs and symptoms that indicate possible urinary system problems.
5. Correctly spell and pronounce each new term introduced in this chapter using the Activity CD-ROM and Audio CD, if available.
6. Define 10 urinary system conditions.
7. Proof and correct the transcription exercise relative to the urinary system.
8. Identify at least 10 abbreviations common to the urinary system.
9. Identify the characteristics of normal urine.

OVERVIEW

The urinary system plays a major role in the elimination of waste from the body. In addition to removing waste products from the blood, the kidneys perform the vital function of regulating the volume and chemical composition of blood by selectively adjusting the amounts of water and electrolytes in the body. While some substances are eliminated into the urine, other needed substances are retained in the bloodstream.

When the blood passes through the kidneys, waste products such as urea, uric acid, and creatinine are filtered out, while appropriate amounts of water and other dissolved substances (**solutes**) are reabsorbed into the bloodstream. Excess amounts of water and solutes are excreted as urine. This filtering-reabsorption process is necessary to maintain the balance of substances required for a relatively stable internal body environment. This stable internal body environment is known as **homeostasis** (home/o = same; stasis = control), and is necessary for the cells of the body to survive and carry out their functions effectively.

If the kidneys fail, there is no way the substances they excrete can be eliminated from the body. Consequently, the substances accumulate in the blood to **toxic** (poisonous) levels, upsetting the internal environment of the body to the point that the cells can no longer function. Death will ultimately follow unless the nonfunctioning kidney is replaced with a healthy kidney through kidney transplant, or the impurities are filtered out of the blood by means of an artificial kidney known as kidney dialysis. Kidney transplant and kidney dialysis (artificial kidney) will be discussed later in this chapter.

In addition to producing and eliminating urine, the kidneys act as endocrine glands by secreting substances into the bloodstream that produce specific effects on the body. Erythropoietin (EPO), a hormone that stimulates the production of red blood cells within the bone marrow, is produced by the kidneys. Renin, an enzyme that aids in raising the blood pressure by causing the constriction of blood vessels, is also produced by the kidneys.

Anatomy and Physiology

The **urinary** system (urinary tract) consists of two kidneys, two ureters, one bladder, and one urethra. See **Figure 15-1.**

Kidneys

The **kidneys** are reddish-brown, bean-shaped organs located on either side of the vertebral column at the back of the upper abdominal cavity. The kidneys lie **retroperitoneal**, or behind the peritoneal membrane, resting between the muscles of the back and the peritoneal cavity. If you place your hand just above your waistline on your back, to either side of your spine, you will be touching the general vicinity of the kidneys within the abdominal cavity.

Each kidney is surrounded by a thick cushion of fatty tissues (adipose tissue), which is covered with a fibrous, connective tissue layer. These tissue layers offer protection and support to the kidney and anchor it to the body wall. See **Figure 15-2.**

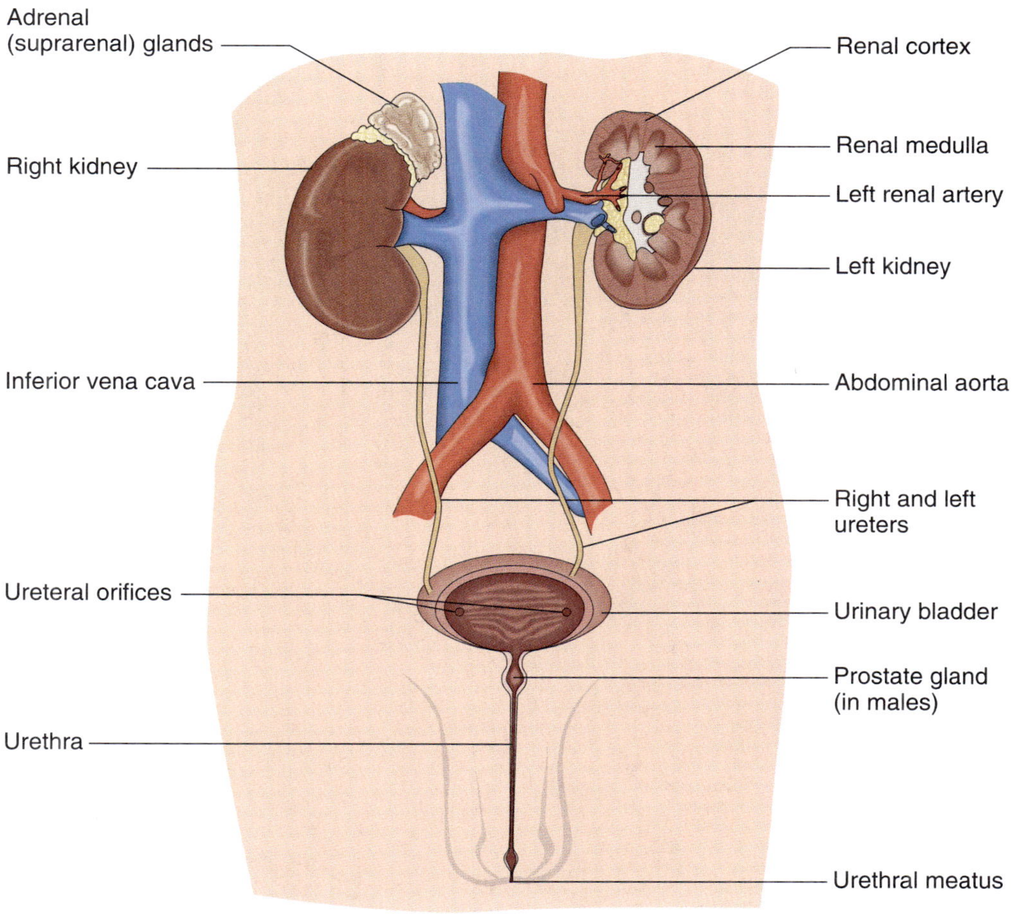

Figure 15-1 The urinary system

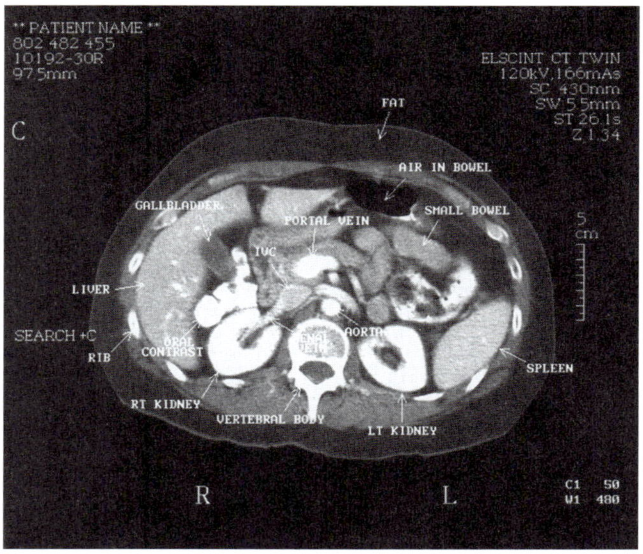

Figure 15-2 CT of the renal system, which shows the location of the urinary system organs

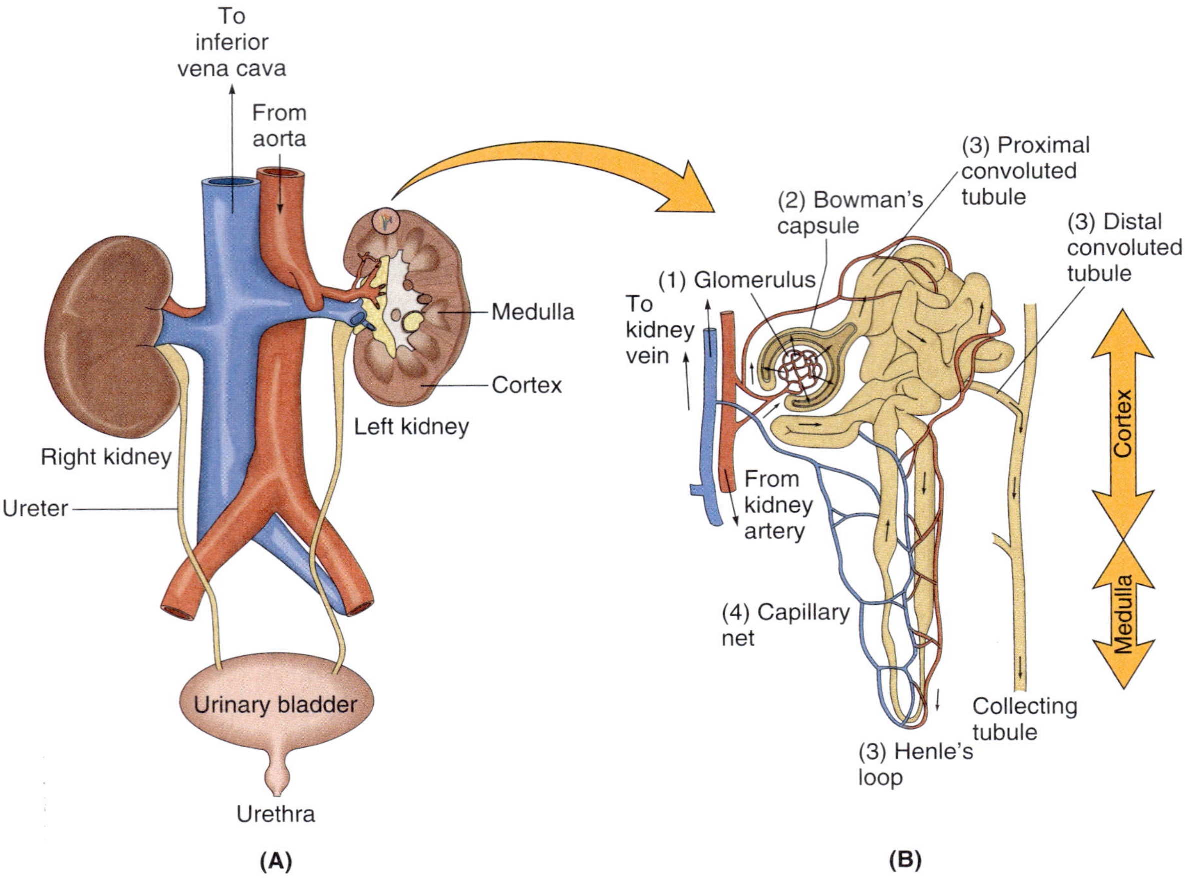

Figure 15-3 Nephron

The adult kidney measures approximately 4 inches (10 cm) long, 2.2 inches (5.5 cm) wide, and 1.2 inches (3 cm) thick, weighing approximately 5.5 ounces (150 g). The size of the adult kidney varies little with differences in body build and weight.

The outer layer, or **cortex**, of the kidney contains millions of microscopic units called **nephrons.** The nephrons are the functional units of the kidneys, carrying on the essential work of forming urine by the process of filtration, reabsorption, and secretion. Each nephron consists of (1) a **glomerulus** (a ball-shaped collection of very tiny, coiled, and intertwined capillaries), (2) a **renal capsule,** or **Bowman's capsule** (a double-walled cup surrounding the glomerulus), (3) the **renal tubule**, and (4) the **peritubular capillaries.** The first portion of the renal tubule is called the proximal convoluted (coiled) tubule; the second portion is called the loop of Henle; and the third portion is called the distal convoluted tubule, which empties into the collecting tubule and leads to the inner portion of the kidney. See **Figure 15-3.**

The inner region, or **medulla,** of the kidney consists of triangular tissues called **renal pyramids.** The pyramids contain the loops and collecting tubules of the nephron. The tip of each pyramid extends into a cuplike urine collection cavity called the minor **calyx**, with several of the minor calyces merging to form a major calyx. The major calyces, in turn, merge to form the central collecting area of the kidney, known as the **renal pelvis**. The urine secreted by the nephrons finally collects in this basinlike structure before entering the ureters. See **Figure 15-4.**

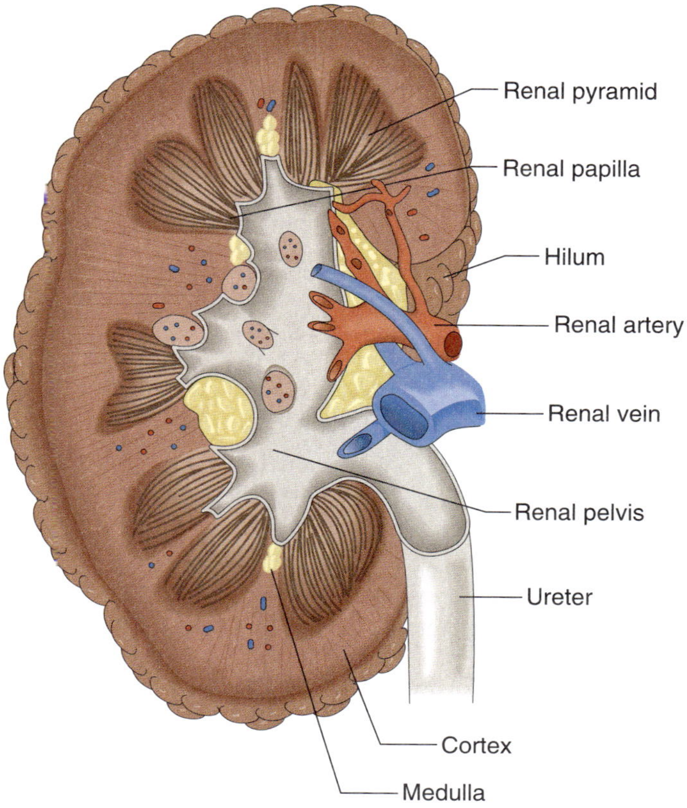

Figure 15-4 Internal anatomy of the kidney

Ureters

The **ureters** are muscular tubes lined with mucous membrane, one leading from each kidney down to the urinary bladder. Each ureter is approximately 12 inches (30 cm) in length. Urine is propelled through the ureters by wavelike contractions known as peristalsis. The paths taken by the ureters in men and women are somewhat different because of variations in the nature, size, and position of the reproductive organs.

Bladder

The **urinary bladder** is a hollow, muscular sac in the pelvic cavity that serves as a temporary reservoir for the urine. The dimensions of the bladder vary, depending on the amount of urine present, but a full urinary bladder can hold approximately a liter (L) of urine (about 1 quart). When full, the bladder is spherical in shape (egg shaped), but when empty, it resembles an inverted pyramid.

The bladder lies between the pubic symphysis and the rectum in men. In women, the bladder lies between the pubic symphysis and the uterus and vagina. See **Figure 15-5.**

Urethra

The urine exits the bladder through the **urethra**. The urethra is a mucous membrane–lined tube that leads from the bladder to the exterior of the body. The external opening of the urethra is called the **urinary meatus**. The external sphincter, located

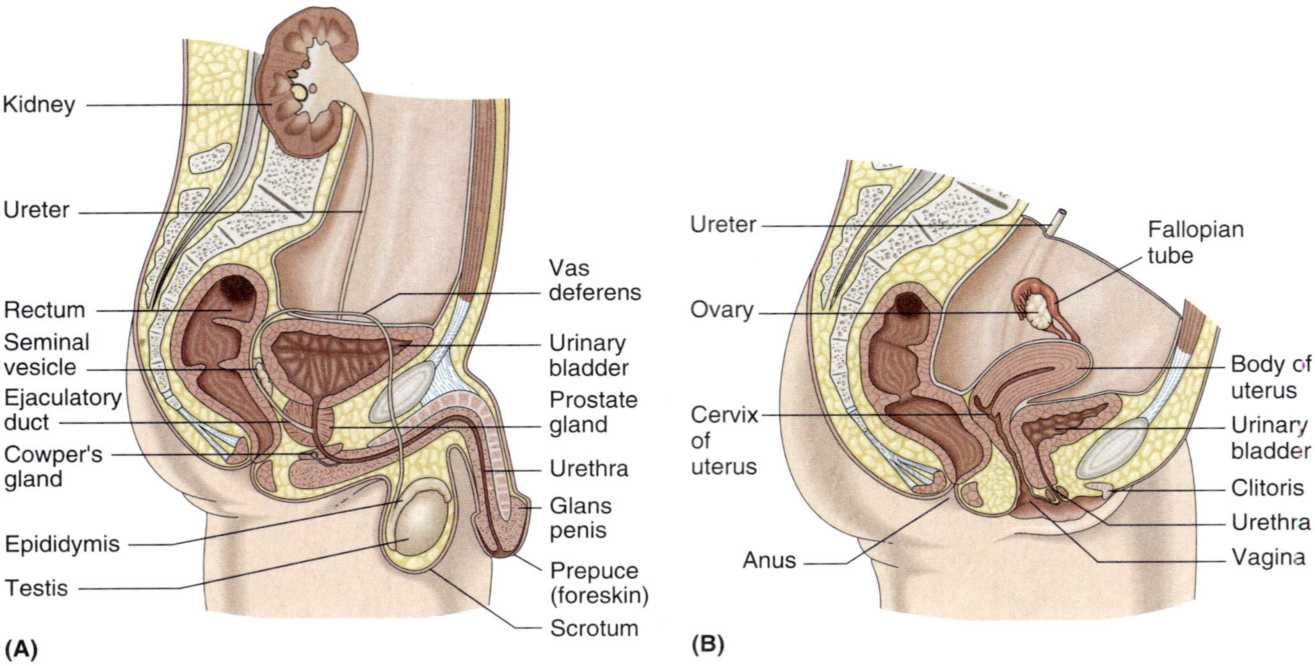

Figure 15-5 Location of urinary bladder: (A) male and (B) female

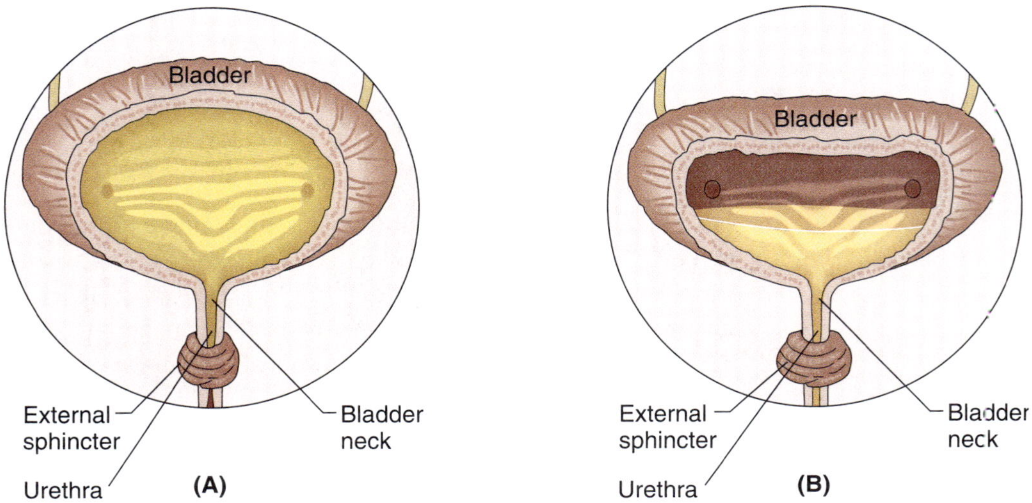

Figure 15-6 Urethra and urinary meatus

below the neck of the bladder, controls the release of urine from the bladder. When the sphincter contracts, it closes the urethra and sends a message to the bladder to relax, releasing no urine. See **Figure 15-6A.** To void, or urinate, the sphincter relaxes and sends a message to the bladder to contract, opening the bladder neck and releasing urine from the body. See **Figure 15-6B.**

The female urethra carries only urine and is approximately 1 to 2 inches (3 to 5 cm) long. The male urethra is approximately 7 to 8 inches (18 to 20 cm) long, and serves both the urinary and male reproductive systems. It transports urine and also carries semen during ejaculation. The relationship of the male urethra to the male reproductive system will be discussed in Chapter 16.

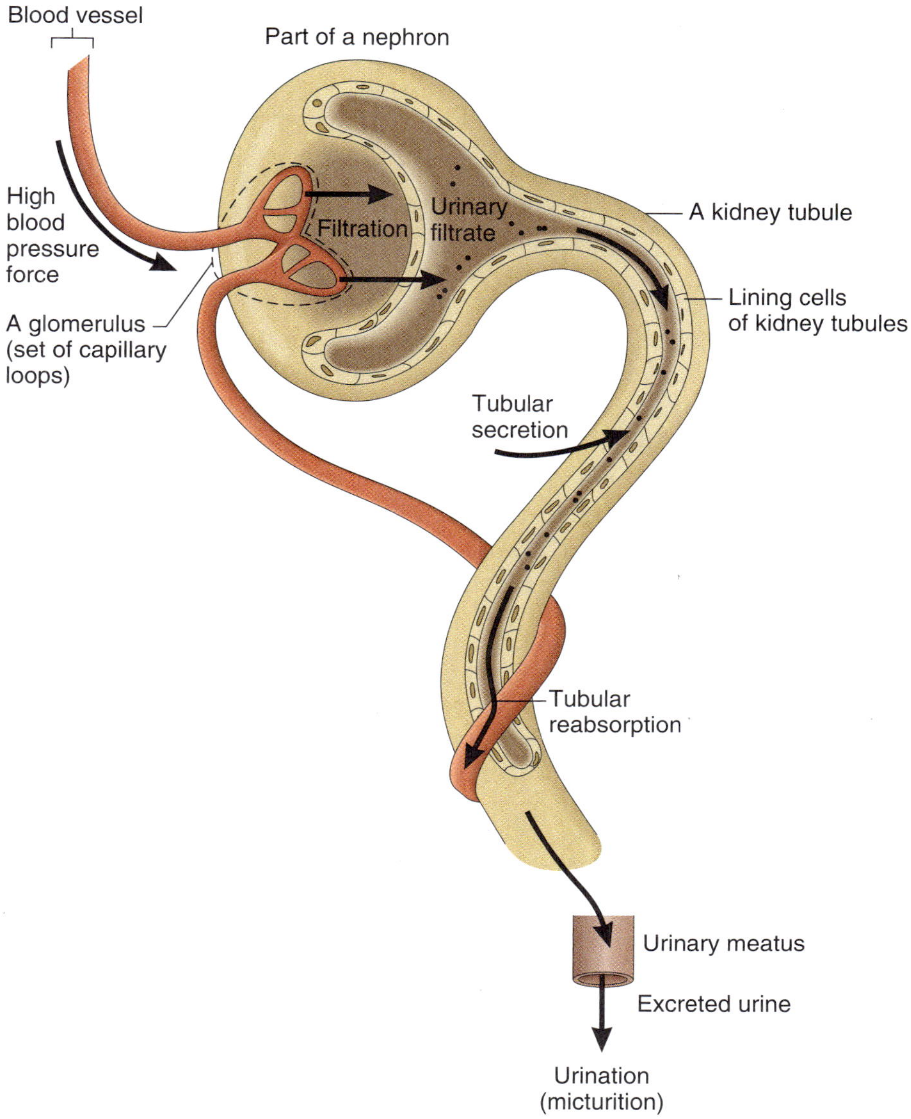

Figure 15-7 Major processes of urine formation

The Formation of Urine

The formation of urine consists of three distinct processes: glomerular filtration, tubular reabsorption, and tubular secretion. Blood enters the kidneys by way of the left and right **renal arteries** and leaves the kidneys by way of the left and right **renal veins**. The blood entering the kidneys comes directly from the abdominal aorta, passing through the renal arteries into the hilum of the kidney. The **hilum** is the depression, or pit, of the kidney where the vessels and nerves enter. Refer to Figure 15-4.

After entering the kidney, the renal arteries branch out into smaller vessels throughout the kidney tissue until the smallest arteries, or **arterioles**, reach the cortex of the kidney. Each arteriole leads to a glomerulus. It is here, in the glomerulus, that the formation of urine begins. See **Figure 15-7.**

As blood slowly but constantly passes through the thousands of glomeruli within the cortex of the kidneys, the blood pressure forces materials through the glomerular walls and into the Bowman's capsule; this process is known as **glomerular filtration.** Water, sugar, salts, and nitrogenous waste products such as urea, creatinine, and uric acid filter out of the blood through the thin walls of the glomeruli. These filtered products are called **glomerular filtrate**. Larger substances, such as proteins and blood cells, cannot press through the glomerular walls; they remain in the blood.

The filtered waste products and toxins (glomerular filtrate) are collected in the cup-shaped Bowman's capsule to be eliminated through the urine. Most of the water, electrolytes, and nutrients will be returned to the blood to maintain the balance of substances required for a relatively stable internal body environment.

The glomerular filtrate passes through the Bowman's capsule into the renal tubule (kidney tubule). As the glomerular filtrate passes through the renal tubules, the water, sugar, and salts are returned to the bloodstream through the network of capillaries that surround them; this process is known as **tubular reabsorption.** If it were not for this process of reabsorption, the body would be depleted of its fluid. Approximately 180 l (18 quarts) of glomerular filtrate pass through the tubules daily. As the filtrate passes through, some acids such as potassium and uric acid are secreted into the tubules directly from the bloodstream.

Tubular secretion occurs in the renal tubules when materials are selectively transferred from the blood into the filtrate to be excreted in the urine. These materials include substances that were unable to pass through the filtering tissues of the glomerulus, as well as substances that may be present in the blood in excessive amounts. Examples of substances that may be secreted into the tubules for excretion through the urine include potassium, hydrogen, and certain drugs.

By the time the glomerular filtrate reaches the end of its journey through the renal tubules, the reabsorption of the essential components has been completed and only the remaining waste products, some water, some salts (electrolytes), and some acids are left to be excreted as **urine.** Normally only 1% of the glomerular filtrate is excreted as urine. Urine, therefore, consists of water and other materials that were filtered or secreted into the tubules but were not reabsorbed.

Considering the fact that only 1% of the 180 l of glomerular filtrate passing through the renal tubules is actually excreted as urine, the amount of urine excreted daily by healthy kidneys is approximately 1.8 l (2 quarts), consisting of 95% water and 5% urea, creatinine, acids, and salts.

From the renal tubules, the urine is emptied into the renal pelvis. Refer to Figure 15-4. Each renal pelvis narrows into the large upper end of the ureter. The urine passes down the ureters into the urinary bladder, a temporary reservoir for the urine. Urine is stored in the bladder until fullness stimulates a reflex contraction of the bladder muscle and the urine is expelled through the urethra. The release of urine is called **urination** or **micturition.** It is regulated by the sphincters (circular muscles) that surround the urethra. A flow chart depicting the formation of urine to the expelling of urine is shown in **Figure 15-8.** The illustrations in the figure are numbered to match those in the flow chart for better visual reference.

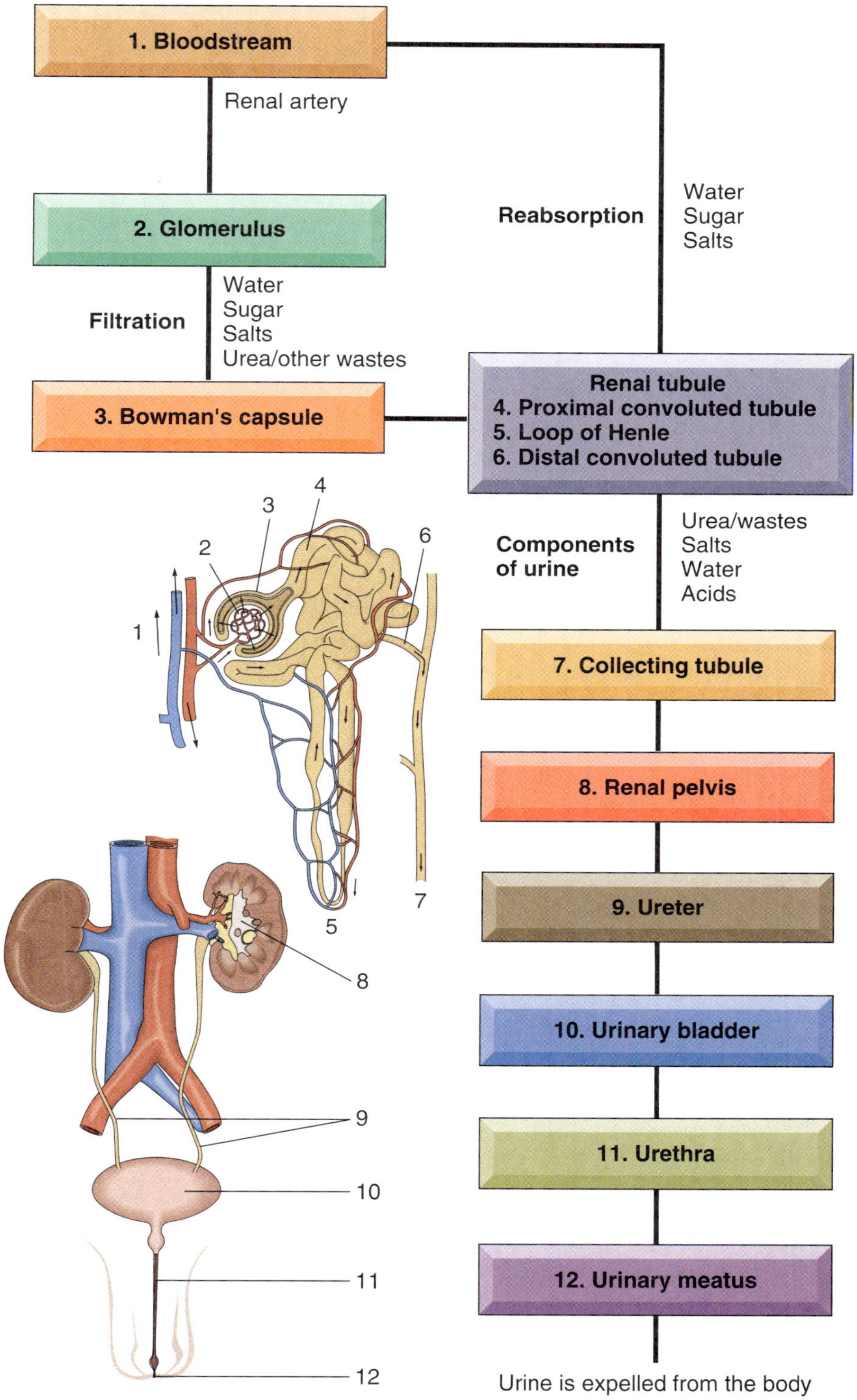

Figure 15-8 Flow chart of urine formation

Vocabulary

The following vocabulary words are frequently used when discussing the urinary system.

WORD	DEFINITION
antiseptic (**an**-tih-**SEP**-tik) anti- = against sept/o = infection -ic = pertaining to	A substance that tends to inhibit the growth and reproduction of microorganisms.
arteriole (ar-**TEE**-ree-ohl) arteri/o = artery -ole = small or little	The smallest branch of an artery.
aseptic technique (ay-**SEP**-tic tek-**NEEK**) a- = without, not sept/o = infection -ic = pertaining to	Any health care procedure in which precautions are taken to prevent contamination of a person, object, or area by microorganisms.
asymptomatic (ay-sim-toh-**MAT**-ic)	Without symptoms.
azotemia (**azz**-oh-**TEE**-mee-ah) azot/o = nitrogen -emia = blood condition	The presence of excessive amounts of waste products of metabolism (nitrogenous compounds) in the blood caused by failure of the kidneys to remove urea from the blood. Azotemia is characteristic of uremia.
Bowman's capsule (**BOW**-manz **CAP**-sool)	The cup-shaped end of a renal tubule containing a glomerulus; also called glomerular capsule.
calculus (**KAL**-kew-lus)	An abnormal stone formed in the body tissues by an accumulation of mineral salts; usually formed in the gallbladder and kidney. See *renal calculus.*
calyx (**KAY**-liks)	The cup-shaped division of the renal pelvis through which urine passes from the renal tubules.
catheter (**CATH**-eh-ter)	A hollow, flexible tube that can be inserted into a body cavity or vessel for the purpose of instilling or withdrawing fluid.
cortex (**KOR**-teks)	The outer layer of a body organ or structure.
cystometer (siss-**TOM**-eh-ter) cyst/o = bladder, sac, or cyst -meter = an instrument used to measure	An instrument that measures bladder capacity in relation to changing pressure.

cystoscope (**SISS**-toh-skohp) **cyst/o** = bladder, sac, or cyst **-scope** = instrument for viewing	An instrument used to view the interior of the bladder, ureter, or kidney. It consists of an outer sheath with a lighting system, a scope for viewing, and a passage for catheters and devices used in surgical procedures.
dialysate (dye-**AL**-ih-**SAYT**) **dia-** = through **lys/o** = breakdown **-ate** = something that...	Solution that contains water and electrolytes that passes through the artificial kidney to remove excess fluids and wastes from the blood; also called "bath."
dialysis (dye-**AL**-ih-sis) **dia-** = through **-lysis** = destruction or detachment	The process of removing waste products from the blood when the kidneys are unable to do so. **Hemodialysis** involves passing the blood through an artificial kidney for filtering out impurities. **Peritoneal dialysis** involves introducing fluid into the abdomen through a catheter. Through the process of osmosis, this fluid draws waste products out of the capillaries into the abdominal cavity; it is then removed from the abdomen via a catheter.
dwell time	Length of time the dialysis solution stays in the peritoneal cavity during peritoneal dialysis.
fossa (**FOSS**-ah)	A hollow or depression, especially on the surface of the end of a bone; in kidney transplantation the donor kidney is surgically placed in the iliac fossa of the recipient.
glomerular filtrate (glom-**AIR**-yoo-lar **FILL**-trayt) **glomerul/o** = glomerulus **-ar** = pertaining to	Substances that filter out of the blood through the thin walls of the glomeruli (e.g., water, sugar, salts, and nitrogenous waste products such as urea, creatinine, and uric acid).
glomerulus (glom-**AIR**-yoo-lus) **glomerul/o** = glomerulus **-us** = noun ending	A ball-shaped collection of very tiny, coiled, and intertwined capillaries, located in the cortex of the kidney.
hilum (**HIGH**-lum)	The depression, or pit, of an organ where the vessels and nerves enter.
hydrostatic pressure	The pressure exerted by a liquid.
meatus (mee-**AY**-tus)	An opening or tunnel through any part of the body, as in the urinary meatus, which is the external opening of the urethra.
medulla (meh-**DULL**-ah)	The most internal part of a structure or organ.
micturition	The act of eliminating urine from the bladder; also called *voiding* or *urination.*
nephrolith (**NEF**-roh-lith) **nephr/o** = kidney **-lith** = stone	A kidney stone; also called a *renal calculus.*

nephrolithiasis (**nef**-roh-lith-**EYE**-ah-sis) nephr/o = kidney lith/o = stone, calculus -iasis = presence of an abnormal condition	A condition of kidney stones; also known as renal calculi.
palpable (**PAL**-pah-b'l)	Distinguishable by touch.
peritoneum (pair-ih-toh-**NEE**-um) peritone/o = peritoneum -um = noun ending	A specific, serous membrane that covers the entire abdominal wall of the body and is reflected over the contained viscera; the inner lining of the abdominal cavity.
peritonitis (**pair**-ih-ton-**EYE**-tis) peritone/o = peritoneum -itis = inflammation	Inflammation of the **peritoneum** (the membrane lining the abdominal cavity).
pyelitis (pye-eh-**LYE**-tis) pyel/o = renal pelvis -itis = inflammation	Inflammation of the renal pelvis.
radiopaque (ray-dee-oh-**PAYK**)	Not permitting the passage of x-rays or other radiant energy; radiopaque areas appear white on an exposed x-ray film.
renal artery (**REE**-nal **AR**-teh-ree) ren/o = kidney -al = pertaining to arter/o = artery y = noun ending	One of a pair of large arteries branching from the abdominal aorta that supplies blood to the kidneys, adrenal glands, and the ureters.
renal calculus	A stone formation in the kidney (plural: renal calculi); also called a *nephrolith.*
renal pelvis (**REE**-nal **PELL**-viss) ren/o = kidney -al = pertaining to pelv/i = pelvis -is = noun ending	The central collecting part of the kidney that narrows into the large upper end of the ureter; it receives urine through the calyces and drains it into the ureters.
renal tubule (**REE**-nal **TOOB**-yool) ren/o = kidney -al = pertaining to	A long, twisted tube that leads away from the glomerulus of the kidney to the collecting tubules. As the glomerular filtrate passes through the renal tubules, the water, sugar, and salts are reabsorbed into the bloodstream through the network of capillaries that surround them.
renal vein (**REE**-nal **VAYN**) ren/o = kidney -al = pertaining to	One of two vessels that carries blood away from the kidney.

residual urine (rih-**ZID**-yoo-al **YOO**-rin)	Urine that remains in the bladder after urination.
solute (**SOL**-yoot)	A substance dissolved in a solution, as in the waste products filtered out of the kidney into the urine.
specific gravity (speh-**SIH**-fik **GRAV**-ih-tee)	The weight of a substance compared with an equal volume of water, which is considered to be the standard. Water is considered to have a specific gravity of 1.000 (one); therefore, a substance with a specific gravity of 2.000 would be twice as dense as water.
toxic (**TOKS**-ik) tox/o = poison -ic = pertaining to	Poisonous.
turbid (**TER**-bid)	Cloudy.
uremia (yoo-**REE**-mee-ah) ur/o = urine -emia = blood condition	The presence of excessive amounts of urea and other nitrogenous waste products in the blood; also called *azotemia*.
ureter (**YOO**-reh-ter) ureter/o = ureter	One of a pair of tubes that carries urine from the kidney to the bladder.
urethra (yoo-**REE**-thrah) urethr/o = urethra -a = noun ending	A small tubular structure that drains urine from the bladder to the outside of the body.
urethritis (yoo-ree-**THRIGH**-tis) urethr/o = urethra -itis = inflammation	Inflammation of the urethra. Urethritis, characterized by dysuria, is usually the result of an infection of the bladder or kidneys.
urinary incontinence (**YOO**-rih-**nair**-ee in-**CON**-tin-ens) urin/o = urine -ary = pertaining to	Inability to control urination; the inability to retain urine in the bladder.
urinary retention (**YOO**-rih-**nair**-ee ree-**TEN**-shun) urin/o = urine -ary = pertaining to	An abnormal, involuntary accumulation of urine in the bladder; the inability to empty the bladder.
urination (**YOO**-rih-**NAY**-shun) urin/o = urine	The act of eliminating urine from the body; also called *micturition* or *voiding*.
urine (**YOO**-rin)	The fluid released by the kidneys, transported by the ureters, retained in the bladder, and eliminated through the urethra. Normal urine is clear, straw colored, and slightly acid.

voiding (VOYD-ing) The act of eliminating urine from the body; also called *micturition* or *urination.*

Word Elements

The following word elements pertain to the urinary system. As you review the list, pronounce each word element aloud twice and check the box after you "say it." Write the definition for the example word given for each word element. You may use your medical dictionary.

WORD ELEMENT	PRONUNCIATION	"SAY IT"	MEANING
albumin/o **albumin**uria	al-**BYOO**-min-oh al-byoo-min-**YOO**-ree-ah	☐	albumin, protein
azot/o **azot**emia	azz-**OH**-toh **azz**-oh-**TEE**-mee-ah	☐	nitrogen
bacteri/o **bacteri**uria	bak-**TEE**-ree-oh bak-**tee**-ree-**YOO**-ree-ah	☐	bacteria
cali/o, calic/o **calic**eal	**KAL**-ih-oh, kah-**LICK**-oh **kal**-ih-**SEE**-al	☐	calyx, calyces
cyst/o **cyst**oscope	**SISS**-toh **SISS**-toh-skohp	☐	bladder, sac, or cyst
dips/o poly**dips**ia	**DIP**-soh pol-ee-**DIP**-see-ah	☐	thirst
glomerul/o **glomerul**ar	glom-**AIR**-yoo-loh glom-**AIR**-yoo-lar	☐	glomerulus
ket/o, keton/o **keton**uria	**KEE**-toh, kee-**TOH**-noh kee-toh-**NOO**-ree-ah	☐	ketone bodies
meat/o **meat**otomy	mee-**AH**-toh mee-ah-**TOT**-oh-mee	☐	meatus
nephr/o **nephr**itis	**NEH**-froh neh-**FRY**-tis	☐	kidney
noct/i **noct**uria	**NOK**-tih nok-**TOO**-ree-ah	☐	night
olig/o **olig**uria	ol-**IG**-yoh ol-ig-**YOO**-ree-ah	☐	few, little, scanty
pyel/o **pyel**itis	**PYE**-eh-loh **pye**-eh-**LYE**-tis	☐	renal pelvis

py/o **py**uria	**PYE**-yoh pye-**YOO**-ree-ah	☐	pus
ren/o **ren**al	**REE**-noh **REE**-nal	☐	kidney
ureter/o **ureter**ostenosis	yoo-**REE**-ter-oh yoo-**ree**-ter-oh-sten-**OH**-sis	☐	ureter
urethr/o **urethr**itis	yoo-**REE**-throh yoo-ree-**THRIGH**-tis	☐	urethra
ur/o, urin/o **urin**ometer	**YOO**-roh, yoo-**RIN**-oh **yoo**-rih-**NOM**-eh-ter	☐	urine
-uria hemat**uria**	**YOO**-ree-ah hee-mah-**TOO**-ree-ah	☐	urine condition
vesic/o **vesic**ocele	**VESS**-ih-koh **VESS**-ih-koh-**seel**	☐	urinary bladder

Characteristics of Urine

The examination of urine is an important screening test that provides valuable information about the status of the urinary system. The routine urinalysis is a test that involves the collection of a random sample of urine. The urine is examined to determine the presence of any abnormal elements that might indicate various pathological (disease-producing) conditions. The following characteristics of urine are determined by observation of the specimen (known as physical examination of urine) and by chemical examination using a reagent strip.

Color

Normal urine varies in color, from pale yellow to a deep golden color, depending on the concentration of the urine. The darker the urine, the greater the concentration. A very pale, almost colorless urine indicates a large amount of water in the urine and less concentration. Certain medications and foods can change the color of urine; for example, certain foods, such as beets, can produce red hues in the urine, and certain medications, such as vitamin B complex, can produce a lemon yellow hue to the urine. The presence of blood in the urine (**hematuria**) can range from a reddish hue, to a cherry red, to a smoky red or brown color. The latter two colors would indicate a large amount of blood in the urine.

Clarity

Normal urine is clear. A cloudy, **turbid** appearance to the urine may be due to the presence of pus (**pyuria**), bacteria (**bacteriuria**), or a specimen that has been standing for more than an hour. The cloudy urine may also indicate the presence of a bladder or kidney infection.

Odor

Normal urine is aromatic; that is, it has a strong but agreeable odor. A foul or putrid odor is common in some infections. Also, urine specimens that are not refrigerated may develop a foul odor after standing for a long period of time. A fruity odor to the urine is found in diabetes mellitus, starvation, or dehydration. Certain medications can also cause a change in the odor of urine.

Specific Gravity

Normal urine has a **specific gravity** of 1.003 to 1.030. The specific gravity is the measurement of the amount of solids in the urine. The lower the specific gravity, the less solids; the higher the specific gravity, the more solids present in the urine. Distilled water is used as the standard of comparison for liquids when measuring the specific gravity. A low specific gravity can be found in kidney diseases indicating that the urine has a greater concentration of water than solids. The water was not reabsorbed into the bloodstream as usual; thus, the urine has been greatly diluted, resembling the specific gravity of water more than that of normal urine. A high specific gravity can be found in diabetes mellitus due to the presence of sugar in the urine.

pH

Normal urine has a pH range of 4.5 to 8.0, with the slightly acid reading of 6.0 being the norm. The pH represents the relative acidity (or alkalinity) of a solution in which a value of 7.0 is neutral, below 7.0 is acid, and above 7.0 is alkaline (base). The urine pH may be alkaline when a urinary tract infection is present.

Protein

Normal urine may have small amounts of protein present, but only in insignificant amounts, that is, in amounts too small to be detected by the reagent strip method. Albumin is the major protein present in renal (kidney) diseases. Because albumin does not normally filter out through the glomerular membrane, the presence of large amounts of protein in the urine (proteinuria or **albuminuria**) may indicate a leak in the glomerular membrane.

Glucose

Normal urine does not contain glucose. There are some normal conditions that can cause glucose to appear in the urine such as having eaten a high-carbohydrate meal, pregnancy, emotional stress, or ingestion of certain medications. If glucose does appear in the urine, the cause must be determined by further studies because the appearance of sugar in the urine can be an indicator of diabetes mellitus. In diabetes mellitus, the hyperglycemia (high blood sugar level) leads to the presence of sugar in the urine because the renal tubules are unable to reabsorb the total quantity of sugar filtered through the glomerular membrane.

Ketones

Normal urine does not contain ketone bodies. Ketones result from the breakdown of fats. In poorly controlled diabetes mellitus, the body is unable to use sugar for energy;

therefore, fat is broken down and used as energy for the body cells. When this happens, ketones accumulate in large quantities in the blood and the urine. It is important to note that the presence of ketones in the urine may also be a result of starvation, dehydration, or excessive ingestion of aspirin; therefore, the cause of ketones in the urine must be determined by further testing.

Common Signs and Symptoms

The following is a list of common signs and symptoms that indicate possible urinary system problems. The patient may actually complain of these symptoms, or the results of the physical, chemical, or microscopic urinalysis may reveal the signs of urinary system problems. As your experience grows in listening carefully to the patient's description of his or her reasons for coming to the doctor, you will become more perceptive in determining which medical term the patient is describing. As you study the terms below, write each definition and word a minimum of three times (use a separate sheet of paper), pronouncing the word aloud each time. Note that the word and the **basic definition** are in bold print, if you choose to learn only the abbreviated form of the definition. A more detailed description follows most words. Once you have mastered each word to your satisfaction, check the box provided beside the word.

☐ **albuminuria**
(al-byoo-min-**YOO**-ree-ah)
albumin/o = albumin, protein
-uria = urine condition

The presence in the urine of abnormally large quantities of protein, usually albumin. (Albuminuria is the same thing as proteinuria.)

Healthy adults excrete less than 250 mg of protein per day. Persistent proteinuria is usually a sign of renal (kidney) disease or renal complications of another disease, such as hypertension or heart failure.

☐ **anuria**
(an-**YOO**-ree-ah)
an- = without
ur/o = urine
-ia = condition

The cessation (stopping) of urine production, or a urinary output of less than 100 ml per day.

Anuria may be caused by kidney failure or dysfunction, a decline in blood pressure below that required to maintain filtration pressure in the kidney, or an obstruction in the urinary passages.

☐ **bacteriuria**
(back-**tee**-ree-**YOO**-ree-ah)
bacteri/o = bacteria
-uria = urine condition

The presence of bacteria in the urine.

The presence of more than 100,000 pathogenic (disease-producing) bacteria per milliliter of urine is usually considered significant and diagnostic of urinary tract infection.

☐ **dysuria**
(diss-**YOO**-ree-ah)
dys- = bad, difficult, painful
ur/o = urine
-ia = condition

Painful urination.

Dysuria is usually the result of a bacterial infection or obstructive condition in the urinary tract. The patient will complain of a burning sensation when passing urine; lab results may reveal the presence of blood, bacteria, or white blood cells.

enuresis
(en-yoo-**REE**-sis)
ur/o = urine
-esis = condition of

A condition of urinary incontinence, especially at night in bed; bedwetting.

fatigue
(fah-**TEEG**)

A state of exhaustion or loss of strength or endurance, such as may follow strenuous physical activity.

Fatigue may be indicative of emotional conflicts, boredom, the result of excessive activity, or a sign of some underlying physical cause.

frequency

The number of repetitions of any phenomenon within a fixed period of time such as the number of heartbeats per minute; or in the case of urinary frequency, urination at short intervals (frequently) without increase in the daily volume of urinary output due to reduced bladder capacity.

Urinary frequency can be a sign of bladder infection.

glycosuria
(**glye**-kohs-**YOO**-ree-ah)
glyc/o = sugar, sweet
-uria = urine condition

Abnormal presence of a sugar, especially glucose, in the urine.

Glycosuria can result from the ingestion of large amounts of carbohydrates, or it may be the result of endocrine or renal disorders. It is a finding most routinely associated with diabetes mellitus.

hematuria
(he-mah-**TOO**-ree-ah)
hemat/o = blood
-uria = urine condition

Abnormal presence of blood in the urine.

Hematuria is symptomatic of many renal diseases and disorders of the genitourinary system.

ketonuria
(kee-toh-**NOO**-ree-ah)
keton/o = ketone bodies
ur/o = urine
-ia = condition

Presence of excessive amounts of ketone bodies in the urine.

Ketonuria occurs as a result of uncontrolled diabetes mellitus, starvation, or any other metabolic condition in which fats are rapidly broken down; also called ketoaciduria.

lethargy
(**LETH**-ar-jee)

The state or quality of being indifferent, apathetic (without emotion), or sluggish.

malaise
(mah-**LAYZ**)

A vague feeling of bodily weakness or discomfort, often marking the onset of disease or infection.

nocturia
(nok-**TOO**-ree-ah)
noct/o = night
-uria = urine condition

Urination, especially excessive, at night; also called nycturia.

Nocturia may be a symptom of renal disease; it may also occur in the absence of disease in people who drink large amounts of fluids, particularly alcohol or coffee, before bedtime or in people with prostatic disease.

☐ **oliguria**
(ol-ig-**YOO**-ree-ah)
olig/o = few, little, scanty
ur/o = urine
-ia = condition

Secretion of a diminished amount of urine in relation to the fluid intake; scanty urine output.

The individual excretes less than 500 ml of urine in every 24 hours, thus the end products of metabolism cannot be excreted efficiently.

Oliguria is usually caused by imbalances in bodily fluids and electrolytes, by renal lesions, or by urinary tract obstruction.

☐ **polydipsia**
(pol-ee-**DIP**-see-ah)
poly- = many, much, excessive
dips/o = thirst
-ia = condition

Excessive thirst.

Polydipsia may be indicative of renal problems; it is also characteristic of diabetes mellitus and diabetes insipidus which are endocrine gland problems.

☐ **polyuria**
(pol-ee-**YOO**-ree-ah)
poly- = many, much, excessive
ur/o = urine
-ia = condition

Excretion of abnormally large amounts of urine.

Several liters in excess of normal may be excreted each day. Polyuria occurs in conditions such as diabetes mellitus, diabetes insipidus, and chronic kidney infections.

☐ **pyuria**
(pye-**YOO**-ree-ah)
py/o = pus
ur/o = urine
-ia = condition

The presence of pus in the urine, usually a sign of an infection of the urinary tract.

☐ **urgency**
(**ER**-jen-see)

A feeling of the need to void urine immediately.

Urgency may accompany a bladder infection.

Pathological Conditions

As you study the pathological conditions of the urinary system, note that the **basic definition** is in bold print followed by a more detailed description in regular print. The phonetic pronunciation is directly beneath each term, and a breakdown of the component parts of the term when appropriate.

cystitis
(siss-**TYE**-tis)
cyst/o = bladder, sac, or cyst
-itis = inflammation

Inflammation of the urinary bladder.

Cystitis is characterized by urgency and frequency of urination, and by hematuria. It may be caused by a bacterial infection, kidney stone, or tumor.

Treatment for cystitis may include antibiotics, increased fluid intake (particularly water), bed rest, and medications to control the bladder spasms. If the cause is due to a stone or tumor, surgery may be necessary.

glomerulonephritis (acute)
(gloh-**mair**-yoo-loh-neh-**FRYE**-tis)
glomerul/o = glomerulus
nephr/o = kidney
-itis = inflammation

An inflammation of the glomerulus of the kidneys.

This condition is characterized by proteinuria, hematuria, and decreased urine production. The specific gravity of the urine will be elevated because of scanty urine output, and the urine may appear as dark as the color of a cola beverage, that is, dark and smoky. The patient frequently experiences headaches, moderate to severe hypertension, and generalized edema, particularly facial and periorbital (around the eye socket) swelling.

Glomerulonephritis (acute) is usually caused by a beta-hemolytic streptococcal infection elsewhere in the body. It may also be caused by other microorganisms, or be the result of some other systemic disorder. Poststreptococcal glomerulonephritis typically occurs around 3 weeks after a streptococcal infection.

Treatment includes the use of antibiotics, such as penicillin, to protect against the recurrence of infection. Sodium and fluid intake are restricted to control the hypertension and general fluid overload. Bed rest is continued until the clinical signs of nephritis have disappeared.

Most patients with acute glomerulonephritis recover within a few weeks of the onset of symptoms. Approximately 90% of the children recover fully from this illness; about 30% of adults acquire this illness, progressing to chronic glomerulonephritis.

hydronephrosis
(high-droh-neh-**FROH**-sis)
hydro- = water
nephr/o = kidney
-osis = condition

Distension of the pelvis and calyces of the kidney caused by urine that cannot flow past an obstruction in a ureter. See Figure 15-9.

Urine production continues but the urine is trapped at the point of the obstruction in the ureter. Obstruction in a single ureter will affect only one kidney; however, if the obstruction is in the bladder or urethra, both kid-

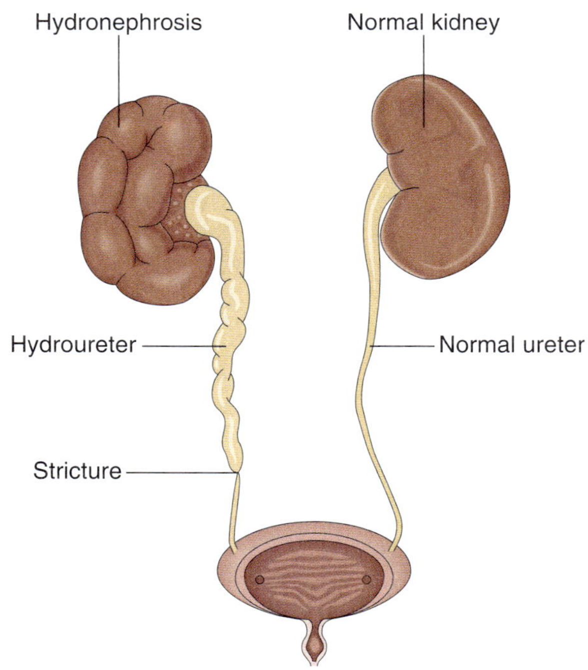

Figure 15-9 Hydronephrosis

neys will be affected. The primary cause of obstruction in adults is kidney stones (renal calculi).

The patient with **hydronephrosis** may complain of intense flank pain, nausea, vomiting, scanty or no urine output, and the presence of blood in the urine (hematuria). Treatment is directed at removing the obstruction to urine flow and preventing infection.

nephrotic syndrome
(neh-**FROT**-ic **SIN**-drohm)
nephr/o = kidney
-tic = pertaining to
syn- = together, joined
drom/o = running

A group of clinical symptoms occurring when damage to the glomerulus of the kidney is present and large quantities of protein are lost through the glomerular membrane into the urine, resulting in severe proteinuria (presence of large amounts of protein in the urine); also called nephrosis.

The excessive loss of protein (albumin) results in a low blood albumin level. These changes create the resultant edema that accompanies the **nephrotic syndrome**; the patient will experience massive generalized edema.

Most cases of nephrotic syndrome result from some form of glomerulonephritis. The syndrome may also occur as a result of systemic diseases such as diabetes mellitus.

Medical treatment for nephrotic syndrome is directed at controlling the edema and reducing the albuminuria, as well as treating the underlying cause.

polycystic kidney disease
(pol-ee-**SISS**-tic kidney disease)
poly- = many, much, excessive
cyst/o = bladder, sac, or cyst
-ic = pertaining to

A hereditary disorder of the kidneys in which grapelike, fluid-filled sacs or cysts, replace normal kidney tissue. See Figure 15-10.

The kidneys are larger than normal and are filled with cysts of various sizes. As the cysts continue to develop, the pressure from the expanding cysts slowly destroys the healthy kidney tissue and renal function deteriorates.

This disease is usually symptom-free until midlife. Once symptoms begin to appear, the patient may complain of pain in one or both kidneys,

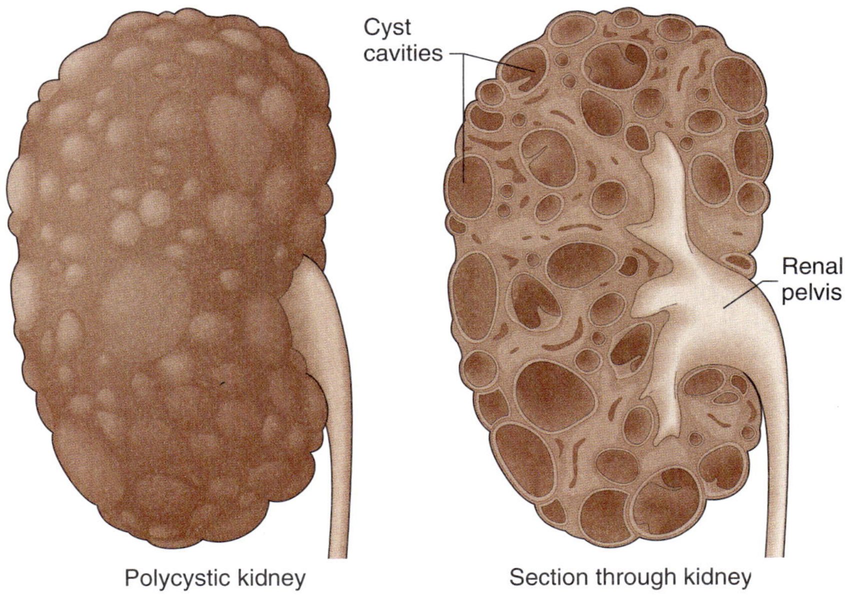

Figure 15-10 Polycystic kidney disease

described as a dull aching, a stabbing-type pain, or a vague sense of heaviness in the area of the kidneys. Hematuria is present in about half the cases and hypertension is common.

Polycystic kidney disease is a slowly progressive disease that ultimately leads to uremia (kidney failure); a process that may take 15 to 30 years from the onset of symptoms. Treatment is directed at preventing urinary tract infections and controlling the secondary hypertension.

---

pyelonephritis (acute)
(pye-eh-loh-neh-**FRY**-tis)
pyel/o = renal pelvis
nephr/o = kidney
-itis = inflammation

A bacterial infection of the renal pelvis of the kidney.

Pyelonephritis is one of the more common diseases of the kidney and usually occurs because of an ascending urinary tract infection, that is, one that begins in the bladder and travels up (ascends) the ureters to the renal pelvis.

Acute pyelonephritis often occurs after bacterial contamination of the urethra or after some instrumentation procedure such as cystoscopy or catheterization. It is characterized by fever, chills, nausea, flank pain on the affected side, headache, and muscular pain. The urine may be cloudy or bloody, have a marked increase in white blood cells and white cell casts, and have a foul-smelling odor.

Treatment includes the use of antibiotics.

---

renal calculi

Stone formations in the kidney.

If the stone is large enough to lodge in the ureter, the individual experiences a sudden, severe attack of pain in the region of one kidney and toward the thigh (known as renal colic). This may be accompanied by chills, fever, hematuria (blood in the urine), and frequency of urination.

Conservative treatment of renal calculi is directed at relief of pain and passage of the stone. Fluids are forced unless the ureter is completely blocked by the calculus. Smooth muscle relaxants and pain relievers are administered. If the stone is completely blocking the ureter and cannot be passed by conservative means, surgery is indicated to remove the stone or the stone may be disintegrated by ultrasound.

---

renal cell carcinoma
(**REE**-nal **SELL** car-sin-**OH**-mah)
ren/o = kidney
-al = pertaining to
carcin/o = cancer
-oma = tumor

A malignant tumor of the kidney occurring in adulthood.

The patient is asymptomatic (symptom free) until the latter stages of the disease. The most common symptom of renal cell carcinoma is painless hematuria, with later development of flank pain and intermittent fever. Once the diagnosis is confirmed, the treatment of choice is surgery to remove the tumor before it can invade adjacent tissue, or metastasize. Chemotherapy and radiation treatment may also follow surgery.

---

renal failure, chronic
(**KRON**-ik **REE**-nal **FAIL**-yoor)
(uremia)
(yoo-**REE**-mee-ah)
ren/o = kidney
-al = pertaining to

Progressively slow development of kidney failure occurring over a period of years. The late stages of chronic renal failure are known as end-stage renal disease (ESRD).

In chronic renal failure there is a progressive, irreversible deterioration in renal function in which the body's ability to maintain metabolic, fluid, and

ur/o = urine
-emia = blood condition

electrolyte balance fails. A gradual progression toward **uremia** occurs. Waste products of metabolism (urea and creatinine) that would normally filter out of the kidney into the urine remain in the bloodstream; that is, "urine constituents are present in the blood." The accumulation of these end products of protein metabolism in the blood is known as **azotemia**. The most common causes of chronic renal failure are hypertension and diabetes.

The numerous symptoms of end-stage renal failure include nausea, vomiting, anorexia, and hiccups. Numbness and burning sensations in both legs and feet are common, with prickly sensations being more intense at night. Anemia is present due to the kidney's suppressed secretion of erythropoietin, which stimulates the production of red blood cells in the bone marrow. Hypertension is usually present and may require antihypertensive therapy to control the blood pressure. The patient may also experience pruritus (itching of the skin), polyuria, weight loss, lack of energy, pale skin with a sallow or brownish hue, and mental confusion. The point at which the patient displays obvious signs of renal failure occurs when approximately 80% to 90% of the renal function has been lost.

Initial treatment is directed at controlling or relieving the symptoms to prevent further complications. Medications may be given to relieve the nausea and the hypertension. The patient may be placed on a protein, sodium, and potassium restricted diet due to the impaired kidney function. Injectable erythropoietin (Epogen) may be administered three times per week to improve the anemic state. As the patient's condition deteriorates, dialysis may be used to "take over as a functioning artificial kidney," prolonging the patient's life until a kidney transplant becomes available.

---

vesicoureteral reflux
(**vess**-ih-koh-yoo-**REE**-ter-al **REE**-fluks)
vesic/o = urinary bladder
ureter/o = ureter
-al = pertaining to

An abnormal backflow (reflux) of urine from the bladder to the ureter.

Vesicoureteral reflux may result from a congenital defect, a urinary tract infection, or obstruction of the outlet of the bladder. The reflux of urine may result in bacterial infection of the upper urinary tract and damage to the ureters and kidney due to increased **hydrostatic pressure.**

Symptoms include abdominal or flank pain, recurrent urinary tract infections, dysuria, frequency, and **urgency**. Pyuria, hematuria, proteinuria, and bacteriuria may also be present. Treatment is directed at correcting the underlying cause of the reflux.

Wilm's tumor

A malignant tumor of the kidney occurring predominately in childhood.

The most frequent finding is a **palpable** mass in the abdomen. The child may also be experiencing abdominal pain, fever, anorexia, nausea, vomiting, and hematuria. Secondary hypertension may also occur.

Once diagnosis is confirmed, the treatment of choice is surgery to remove the tumor, followed by chemotherapy and radiation. With treatment and no evidence of spreading to other areas, the cure rate is high for patients with Wilm's tumors.

Treatment of Renal Failure

The following is a discussion of the various methods of treatment for renal failure.

peritoneal dialysis
(**pair**-ih-toh-**NEE**-al dye-**AL**-ih-sis)
peritone/o = peritoneum
-al = pertaining to
dia- = through
-lysis = destruction or detachment

Dialysis is a mechanical filtering process used to cleanse the blood of waste products, draw off excess fluids, and regulate body chemistry when the kidneys fail to function properly. Instead of using the hemodialysis machine as a filter, the peritoneal membrane (also called the peritoneum) is used as the filter in peritoneal dialysis.

The peritoneal membrane is a thin membrane that lines the abdominal cavity. It is richly supplied with tiny blood vessels, thus providing a continuous supply of blood to be filtered.

Prior to the first peritoneal dialysis exchange, an **access tube,** or catheter (known as a Tenchkoff peritoneal catheter), is surgically placed in the lower abdomen. See **Figure 15-11.**

The access tube is used for the infusion of the dialysate solution and draining of the fluid from the abdomen. The dialysate solution is a mixture of

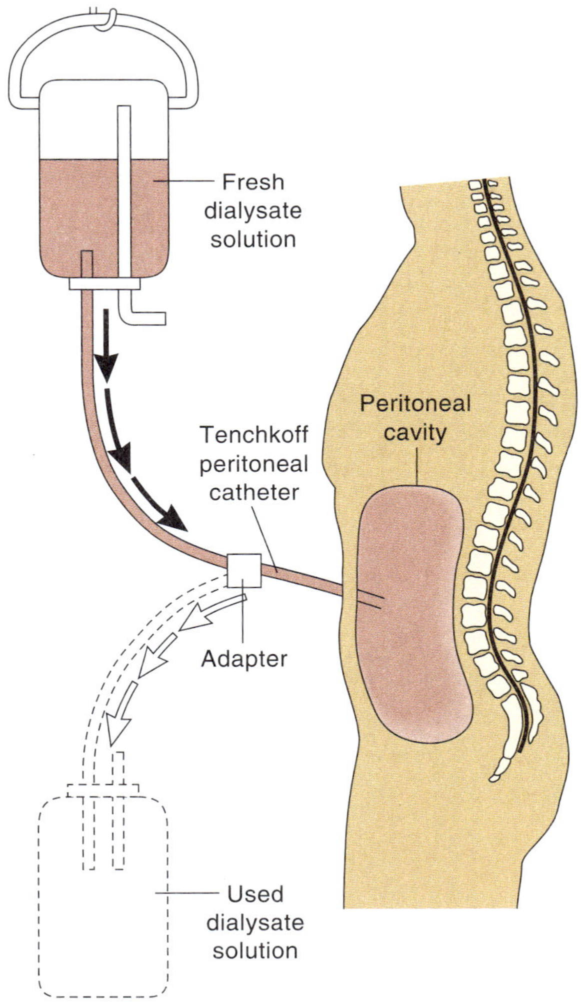

Figure 15-11 Peritoneal dialysis

water and electrolytes that will draw the excess fluid and toxins from the blood, across the peritoneal membrane, into the abdominal cavity.

This process of draining and infusing of dialysate solution is called an exchange. There are two types of peritoneal dialysis exchanges that can be performed at home: continuous ambulatory peritoneal dialysis (CAPD) or continuous cycling peritoneal dialysis (CCPD).

CAPD can be performed by the patient and does not require a machine. Sterile plastic tubing, called a transfer set, is connected to a bag of approximately 2 quarts of slightly warmed dialysate solution. After the proper connections are made with the tubing and the patient's access tube, the dialysate bag is raised above the shoulder and the solution slowly flows into the abdomen.

During a peritoneal dialysis exchange, the dialysate solution remains in the abdomen for approximately 4 hours.

This process is repeated three to five times every day, with the residual fluid from the previous exchange being drained first, followed by the infusion of the dialysate. The last exchange of the day is performed just before bedtime and the dialysate is left in the abdomen overnight.

Training for continuous CAPD procedures takes approximately 1 to 2 weeks. Patients are taught the procedure, the signs and symptoms of infection, and how to make decisions about using the appropriate dialysate solution strength to obtain optimal results. The advantage of CAPD is that a machine is not used and the procedure is convenient for traveling.

CCPD, on the other hand, uses a machine that warms the solution and cycles it in and out of the peritoneal cavity at evenly spaced intervals at night while the patient sleeps. This process takes 8 to 10 hours.

The initial exchange begins with the infusion of a prescribed amount of dialysate into the abdominal cavity. Upon completion, the patient's access tube is clamped and removed from the infusion tubing. The dialysate fluid then remains in the abdomen during the day for approximately 12 to 15 hours.

Before the patient goes to sleep at night, the access catheter is reconnected to the dialysis machine and the residual fluid is drained out of the abdomen. This is followed by the nighttime exchanges: a series of four or more cycles of infusion of dialysate, retention of the solution in the abdominal cavity (known as dwell time), and draining of the fluid from the abdomen. The cyclic exchanges are controlled by the machine as the patient sleeps. See **Figure 15-12.**

When the final cycle of draining is completed, the abdomen is once again infused with dialysate solution that will remain in the abdomen throughout the day. This process is repeated daily. The advantage of CCPD is that exchanges are done at night by the machine, instead of several times throughout the day by the patient, as in ambulatory dialysis.

The major concern with the peritoneal dialysis is the possibility of the patient developing **peritonitis** (inflammation of the peritoneum). Patients are instructed to report any signs of fever, tenderness around the access site, nausea, weakness, or cloudy appearance of the dialysate solution that drains from the abdominal cavity. If peritonitis develops, it is treated with antibiotics.

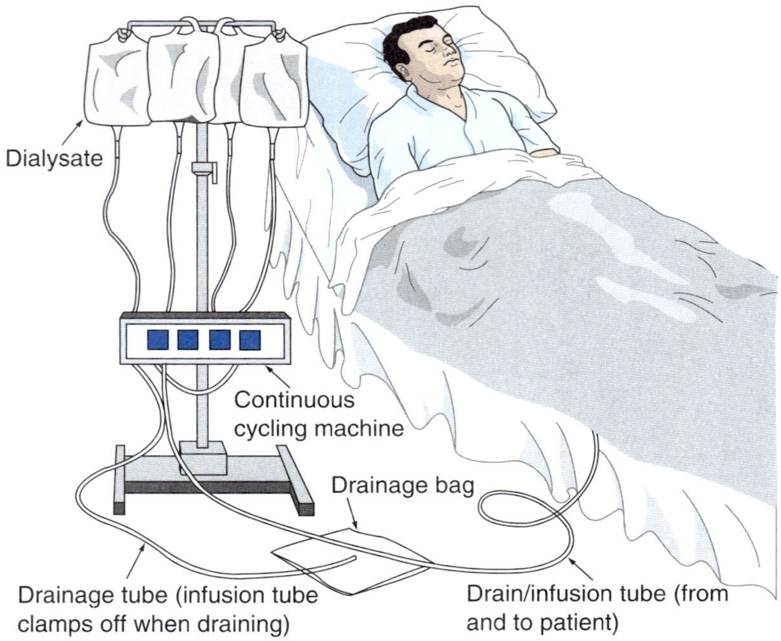

Figure 15-12 Continuous cyclic peritoneal dialysis

hemodialysis
(**hee**-moh-dye-**AL**-ih-sis)
hem/o = blood
dia- = through
-lysis = destruction or detachment

The process of removing excess fluids and toxins from the blood by continually shunting the patient's blood from the body into a dialysis machine for filtering, and then returning the clean blood to the patient's bloodstream.

While the patient's blood flows through the dialyzer, the toxins and excess fluid are drawn across the semipermeable membrane into the dialysate solution, which is circulating on the other side of the membrane. The filtered blood is then routed back into the body while the waste products are channeled out of the machine via the dialysate. See **Figure 15-13.**

To be able to shunt blood from the body to the hemodialyzer and back, a large vessel with a good blood flow is necessary, so an "access" vessel is created. The access of choice for chronic hemodialysis is the internal **arteriovenous fistula** in which an opening, or fistula, has been created between an artery and a vein in the forearm. See **Figure 15-14.**

The flow of the arterial blood into the venous system at the point of the fistula causes the vein to become distended, providing a large enough vessel with a strong blood flow for the hemodialysis connection. The arteriovenous fistula needs approximately 2 to 6 weeks to "mature" so that it is strong enough and large enough for needle insertion during dialysis. The mix of arterial and venous blood, created by the arteriovenous fistula, is so insignificant that it does not cause a problem with the oxygen concentration of the blood.

Patients usually receive hemodialysis treatments three times a week. The length of time for a single hemodialysis treatment may vary from 4 to 6 hours, depending on the type of dialyzer used and the patient's condition. The average length of time for treatments is 3 to 4 hours. Hemodialysis may be performed at home or at the dialysis center.

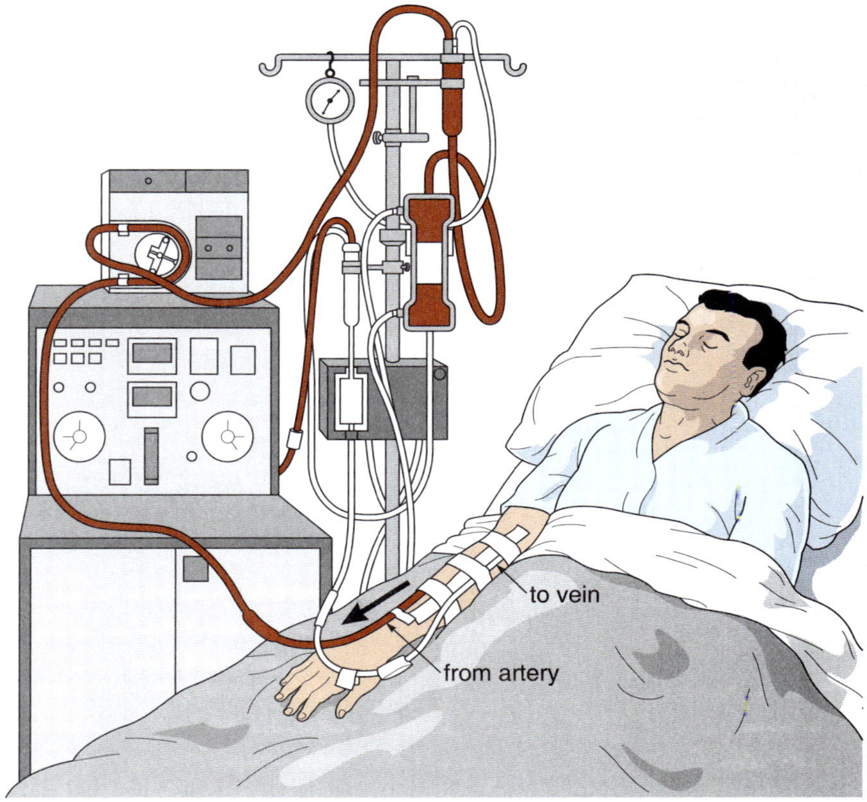

Figure 15-13 Hemodialysis

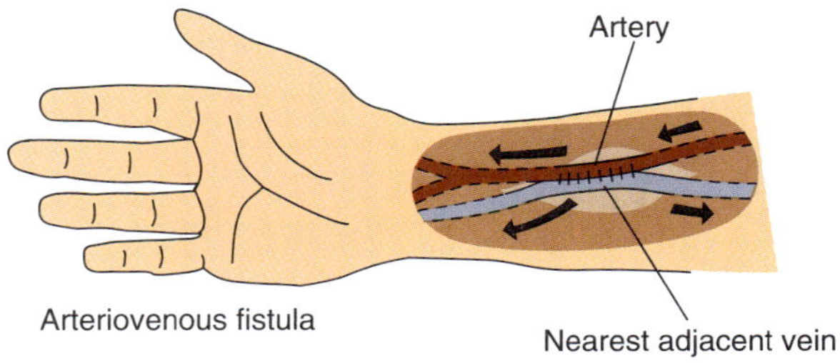

Figure 15-14 Arteriovenous fistula for hemodialysis

---

kidney transplantation
(kidney tranz-plan-**TAY**-shun)

Involves the surgical implantation of a healthy, human donor kidney into the body of a patient with irreversible renal failure. Kidney function is restored with a successful transplant and the patient is no longer dependent on dialysis.

There are two sources used in kidney transplantation: living donors (usually blood relatives) and nonliving (cadaver) donors. Advances in tissue matching and antirejection medications (immunosuppressive drugs) have made transplantation a viable alternative for treating end-stage renal failure.

Only one kidney is needed for transplantation. Generally, the recipient's kidneys are not removed. The donor kidney is surgically placed in the recipient's iliac fossa. The blood supply to the recipient's natural kidneys remains intact. See **Figure 15-15.**

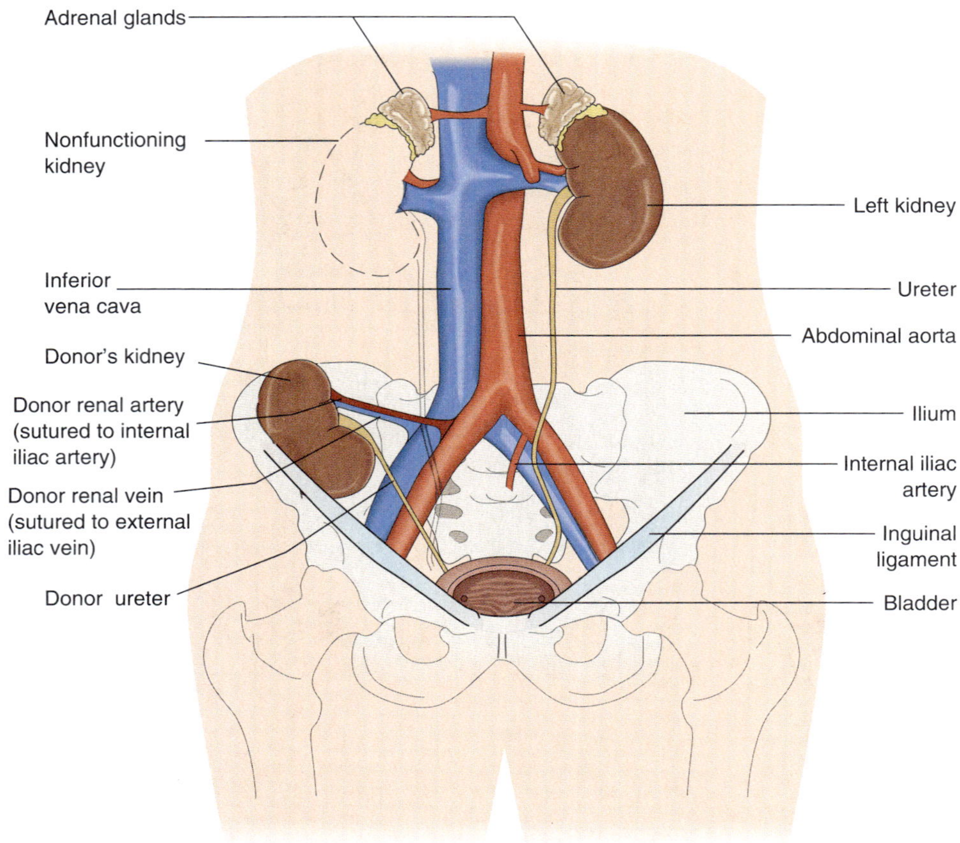

Figure 15-15 Kidney placement for renal transplant

The renal artery of the donor kidney is connected to the recipient's iliac artery, and the iliac vein of the donor kidney is connected to the recipient's iliac vein. Once the transplanted kidney is in place, it usually begins to function immediately. If adequate function is delayed for a few days, a return to dialysis may be necessary until good kidney function is established.

Survival rates (i.e., kidney not being rejected) 1 year after transplantation are 80% to 90% for living, related donor transplants and 70% to 90% for cadaver donor transplants.

Diagnostic Techniques and Procedures

blood urea nitrogen (BUN)
(blud yoo-**REE**-ah **NIGH**-troh-jen)

A blood test performed to determine the amount of urea and nitrogen (waste products normally excreted by the kidney) present in the blood.

The **blood urea nitrogen** level is usually increased with impaired glomerular filtration.

catheterization
(**kath**-eh-ter-**EYE**-zay-shun)

The introduction of a catheter (flexible, hollow tube) into a body cavity or organ to instill a substance or remove a fluid.

The most common type of catheterization is the insertion of a catheter into the urinary bladder for the purpose of removing urine.

A urinary catheterization may be performed to obtain a sterile specimen of urine for testing, to provide relief for urinary retention, to empty the bladder completely before surgery, or to instill a contrast medium into the bladder for the purpose of visualizing the structures of the urinary system on x-ray.

---

creatinine clearance test
kree-**AT**-in-in clearance test)

A diagnostic test for kidney function that measures the filtration rate of creatinine, a waste product (of muscle metabolism), which is normally removed by the kidney.

Creatinine levels are determined on a 24-hour urine specimen collection and on a sample of blood drawn during the same 24-hour period of time. Impaired glomerular function will result in a decrease in creatinine clearance rate and an increase in serum creatinine levels.

---

cystometrography
(**siss**-toh-meh-**TROG**-rah-fee)
cyst/o = bladder, sac, or cyst
metr/o = measure
-graphy = process of recording

An examination performed to evaluate bladder tone; measuring bladder pressure during filling and voiding.

At the beginning of the cystometrography, the patient is asked to empty his or her bladder. A catheter is then inserted through the urethra into the bladder. Any residual urine present will be removed through the catheter and the amount is recorded.

Saline solution or water is then instilled into the bladder, at a constant rate, through the catheter. The patient is asked to report when the urge to urinate is first felt, when the bladder feels full, and when it is impossible to hold any more fluid in the bladder without voiding.

Bladder pressure is measured with the cystometer that is attached to the catheter. The measurement of the pressure that the bladder musculature exerts on the fluid being instilled is recorded after the instillation of every 50 ml of solution.

---

cystoscopy
(siss-**TOSS**-koh-pee)
cyst/o = bladder, sac, or cyst
-scopy = process of viewing

The process of viewing the interior of the bladder using a cystoscope.

The cystoscope is a hollow metal or flexible tube that is introduced into the bladder through the urinary meatus. Visualization of the inside of the bladder is made possible by a light source and magnifying lenses, which are a part of the cystoscope. See **Figure 15-16.**

Cystoscopy is useful in detecting tumors, inflammation, renal calculi, and structural irregularities. It can also be used as a means for obtaining biopsy specimens.

---

extracorporeal lithotripsy
(**ex**-trah-cor-**POR**-ee-al **LITH**-oh-trip-see)
extra- = outside, beyond
lith/o = stone, calculus
-tripsy = intentional crushing

Also known as extracorporeal shock-wave lithotripsy. This is a non invasive mechanical procedure for breaking up renal calculi so they can pass through the ureters.

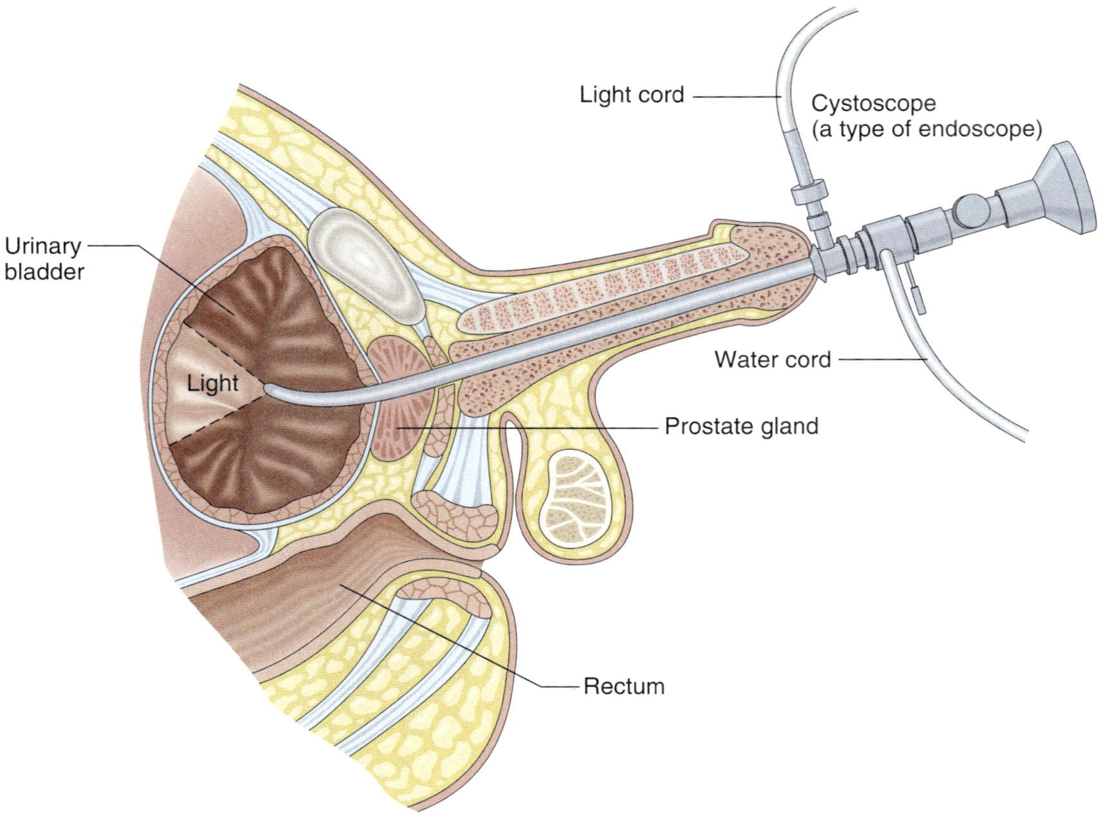

Figure 15-16 Cystoscopy

intravenous pyelogram
(in-trah-**VEE**-nus **PYE**-eh-loh-gram)
- **intra-** = within
- **ven/o** = vein
- **-ous** = pertaining to
- **pyel/o** = renal pelvis
- **-gram** = a record

Also known as intravenous pyelography or excretory urogram; this radiographic procedure provides visualization of the entire urinary tract: kidneys, ureters, bladder, and urethra.

A contrast dye is injected intravenously and multiple x-ray films are taken as the medium is cleared from the blood by the glomerular filtration of the kidney.

Intravenous pyelogram (IVP) is useful in diagnosing renal tumors, cysts, stones, structural or functional abnormalities of the bladder, and ureteral obstruction.

KUB (kidneys, ureters, bladder)

An x-ray of the lower abdomen that defines the size, shape, and location of the kidneys, ureters, and bladder. A contrast medium is not used with this x-ray.

The KUB is useful in identifying malformations of the kidney, soft tissue masses, and calculi (stones).

renal angiography
(**REE**-nal **an**-jee-**OG**-rah-fee)
- **ren/o** = kidney
- **-al** = pertaining to
- **angi/o** = vessel
- **-graphy** = process of recording

X-ray visualization of the internal anatomy of the renal blood vessels after injection of a contrast medium.

A **radiopaque** catheter is inserted into the femoral artery. Using fluoroscopy, the catheter is guided up the aorta to the level of the renal arteries. A contrast dye is then injected, and a series of x-rays are taken to visualize the renal vessels.

Renal angiography is used to detect narrowing of the renal vessels, vascular damage, renal vein thrombosis (clots), cysts, or tumors.

---

renal scan
(**REE**-nal scan)
reno = kidney
-al = pertaining to

A procedure in which a radioactive isotope (tracer) is injected intravenously, and the radioactivity over each kidney is measured as the tracer passes through the kidney.

A renal scan procedure is useful in evaluating renal function and shape of the kidney.

The radioactivity emitted from the tracer rises rapidly as the material concentrates in the kidney and then declines as it leaves the kidney; this produces a characteristic curve. The information is recorded in graph form, with various patterns in the curve being associated with specific conditions.

The patient should be reassured that only a small amount of the radioactive tracer will be administered and the material is completely excreted from the body within 24 hours.

---

retrograde pyelogram (RP)
(**RET**-roh-grayd **PYE**-eh-loh-gram)
retro = backward, behind
pyel/o = renal pelvis
-gram = a record

A radiographic procedure in which small-caliber catheters are passed through a cystoscope into the ureters to visualize the ureters and the renal pelvis.

A contrast medium is injected through the catheters into the ureters and renal pelvis and x-ray pictures are taken to define the structures of the collecting system of the kidneys. X-ray pictures are taken to record the outline of these structures.

The retrograde pyelogram is useful in determining the degree of ureteral obstruction and is used when the IVP does not satisfactorily visualize the renal collecting system and the ureters. It is also used when patients are allergic to the intravenous dye used in the IVP, because the contrast medium is not absorbed through the mucous membranes.

---

ultrasonography
(ul-trah-son-**OG**-rah-fee)
ultra = beyond
son/o = sound
-graphy = process of recording

Also called ultrasound; this is a procedure in which sound waves are transmitted into the body structures as a small transducer is passed over the patient's skin.

The area to be examined is lubricated before applying the transducer. As the sound waves are reflected back into the transducer, they are interpreted by a computer which, in turn, presents the composite in a picture form.

An ultrasound of the kidneys is useful in distinguishing between fluid-filled cysts and solid masses, detecting renal calculi, identifying obstructions, and evaluating transplanted kidneys. Ultrasonography is a noninvasive procedure that requires no contrast medium.

---

urinalysis
(**yoo**-rih-**NAL**-ih-sis)
urin/o = urine
-lysis = breaking down; destruction

Urinalysis is a physical, chemical, or microscopic examination of urine.

The physical examination of urine includes examining the specimen for color, turbidity (cloudiness), specific gravity, and pH. Chemical analysis of urine may involve checking the specimen for presence of sugar, ketones, protein, or blood. This may be accomplished with reagent tablets or reagent strips. See **Figure 15-17.**

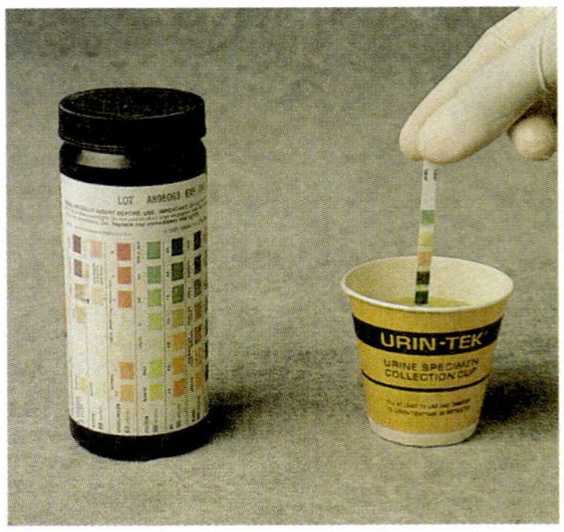

Microscopic examination of urine involves examining the urine specimen for the presence of blood cells, casts, crystals, pus, and bacteria. A microscopic examination is performed after the urine specimen has been spun in a centrifuge to allow for collection of a small amount of sediment that is placed on the microscope slide for examination.

Figure 15-17 Reagent strip immersed in urine sample

---

urine culture
(**YOO**-rin)
urin/o = urine
-e = noun ending

A procedure used to cultivate the growth of bacteria present in a urine specimen, for proper microscopic identification of the specific pathogen (disease-producing microorganism).

A sample of the urine specimen is swabbed onto a culture medium plate and placed into an incubator for 24 to 72 hours. The plate is then examined for growth on the culture medium. A sample is obtained from any colony of growth and examined under the microscope to identify the name and quantity of the specific organism present.

Once the bacterium has been identified, sensitivity testing is performed. This test involves exposing the identified organism to various antibiotics to determine which specific antibiotic will most effectively destroy the pathogen. Identifying the most effective antibiotic for optimum results through urine culture and sensitivity will avoid longer than necessary treatment with a less effective medication.

Urine culture and sensitivity testing has become more and more important as the number of resistant organisms increase. It is best to use the first voided specimen of the day for the urine culture because the bacteria will be more numerous in this specimen. A clean-catch urine specimen is usually collected, although a catheterized specimen may be obtained. The specimen should be cultured within 30 minutes because bacteria will multiply more rapidly at room temperature. If this is not possible, the specimen should be refrigerated.

24-hour urine specimen
(24-hour **YOO**-rin
SPEH-sih-men)

A collection of all of the urine excreted by the individual over a 24-hour period. The urine is collected in one large container. This urine specimen is also called composite urine specimen.

When the 24-hour urine collection begins, the individual should void and discard the first specimen. Each time after that, during the next 24 hours, all of the urine voided should be collected and placed in the container. The large container should be refrigerated. At the end of the 24-hour period (24 hours after the first voiding), the individual should void one last time, adding this urine to the specimen in the large container.

Composite urine specimens, such as the 24-hour urine specimen, provide information on the ability of the kidneys to excrete and/or retain various solutes such as creatinine, sodium, urea, or phosphorus. The amount of these solutes excreted in the urine during a 24-hour period will be compared with their concentration in a blood sample taken at the end of the 24-hour period. The comparisons of urine level to blood concentration will be disproportionate in the presence of kidney disorders.

voiding cystourethrography
(**VOY**-ding **siss**-toh-yoo-ree-**THROG**-rah-fee)
cyst/o = bladder, sac, or cyst
urethr/o = urethra
-graphy = process of recording

X-ray visualization of the bladder and urethra during the voiding process, after the bladder has been filled with a contrast material.

A radiopaque dye is instilled into the bladder via a urethral catheter. The catheter is then removed and the patient is asked to void. X-ray pictures are taken as the patient is expelling the urine. The **voiding cystourethrography** is helpful in diagnosing urethral lesions, bladder and urethral obstructions, and vesicoureteral reflux.

Urine Specimen Collections

In addition to the 24-hour urine specimen collection, there are other methods of obtaining urine specimens for laboratory testing. It is important that the urine is collected and stored properly for optimum testing results. If a specimen will not be tested immediately, it must be refrigerated to lessen the potential for growth of bacteria. The usual amount of urine collected is 50 ml. The following methods for collecting a urine specimen are defined for your convenience and understanding: catheterized specimen, clean-catch specimen (midstream), first-voided specimen, random specimen, and residual urine specimen.

catheterized specimen
(**CATH**-eh-ter-eyezd **SPEH**-sih-men)
(sterile specimen)

Using aseptic techniques, a very small, straight catheter is inserted into the bladder via the urethra to withdraw a urine specimen. The urine flows through the catheter into a sterile specimen container.

This specimen may be obtained for a urine culture.

clean-catch specimen
(**CLEAN-CATCH SPEH**-sih-men)
(midstream specimen)

This collection is used to avoid contamination of the urine specimen from the microorganisms normally present on the external genitalia.

The patient cleanses the external genitalia with an **antiseptic** wipe. After expelling a small amount of urine into the toilet, the patient collects a specimen in a sterile container. The remaining amount of urine is expelled in the toilet. This specimen may be obtained for a urine culture or to determine the presence of a urinary tract infection.

first-voided specimen
(**FIRST-VOYD**-ed **SPEH**-sih-men)
(early-morning specimen)

The patient is instructed to collect the first-voided specimen of the morning and to refrigerate it until it can be taken to the medical office or laboratory.

This specimen may be obtained for pregnancy testing or for any other test that requires more concentrated urine, because it contains the greatest concentration of dissolved substances.

random specimen
(**RAN**-dom **SPEH**-sih-men)

A urine specimen that is collected at anytime.

Freshly voided urine, which is a random specimen, is most often used for testing in the medical office. After the patient collects the urine specimen, it is tested immediately.

residual urine specimen
(ree-**ZID**-yoo-ahl)

A residual urine specimen is obtained by catheterization after the patient empties the bladder by voiding. The amount of urine remaining in the bladder after voiding is noted as the residual amount.

Common Abbreviations

ABBREVIATION	MEANING	ABBREVIATION	MEANING
ADH	antidiuretic hormone	**GFR**	glomerular filtration rate
AGN	acute glomerular nephritis	**HD**	hemodialysis
ARF	acute renal failure	**IVP**	intravenous pyelogram
BUN	blood urea nitrogen	**KUB**	kidneys, ureters, bladder
CAPD	continuous ambulatory peritoneal dialysis	**pH**	abbreviation for the degree of acidity or alkalinity of a solution; pH means potential hydrogen
CCPD	continuous cycling peritoneal dialysis	**RP**	retrograde pyelogram
CRF	chronic renal failure	**sp.gr.**	specific gravity
Cysto	cystoscopy	**UA**	urinalysis
EPO	erythropoietin	**UTI**	urinary tract infection
ESRD	end-stage renal disease	**VCUG**	voiding cystourethrogram
ESWL	extracorporeal shock-wave lithotripsy		

Written and Audio Terminology Review

Review each of the following terms from this chapter. Study the spelling of each term and write the definition in the space provided. If you have the Audio CD available, listen to each term, pronounce it, and check the box once you are comfortable saying the word. Check definitions by looking the term up in the glossary/index.

TERM	PRONUNCIATION	DEFINITION
albuminuria	☐ al-byoo-min-**YOO**-ree-ah	________________
antiseptic	☐ **an**-tih-**SEP**-tik	________________
anuria	☐ an-**YOO**-ree-ah	________________
arteriole	☐ ar-**TEE**-ree-ohl	________________

Term	Pronunciation
aseptic	☐ ay-**SEP**-tik
asymptomatic	☐ ay-simp-toh-**MAT**-ik
azotemia	☐ **azz**-oh-**TEE**-mee-ah
bacteriuria	☐ back-**tee**-ree-**YOO**-ree-ah
blood urea nitrogen	☐ blud-yoo-**REE**-ah **NIGH**-tro-jen
Bowman's capsule	☐ **BOW**-manz **CAP**-sool
calculi	☐ **KAL**-kew-lye
calyx	☐ **KAY**-liks
catheter	☐ **CATH**-eh-ter
catheterization	☐ **kath**-eh-ter-ih-**ZAY**-shun
catheterized specimen	☐ **CATH**-eh-ter-eyezd **SPEH**-sih-men
chronic renal failure (uremia)	☐ **KRON**-ik **REE**-nal **FAIL**-yoor (yoo-**REE**-mee-ah)
cortex	☐ **KOR**-teks
creatinine clearance test	☐ kree-**AT**-in-in clearance test
cystitis	☐ siss-**TYE**-tis
cystometer	☐ siss-**TOM**-eh-ter
cystometrography	☐ **siss**-toh-meh-**TROG**-rah-fee
cystoscope	☐ **SISS**-toh-skohp
cystoscopy	☐ siss-**TOSS**-koh-pee
dialysate	☐ dye-**AL**-ih-sayt
dialysis	☐ dye-**AL**-ih-sis
dysuria	☐ diss-**YOO**-ree-ah
extracorporeal lithotripsy	☐ **ex**-trah-cor-**POR**-ee-al **LITH**-oh-trip-see
fatigue	☐ fah-**TEEG**
fossa	☐ **FOSS**-ah
glomerular filtrate	☐ glom-**AIR**-yoo-lar **FILL**-trayt
glomerulonephritis	☐ glom-**air**-yoo-loh-neh-**FRYE**-tis

Term		Pronunciation	
glomerulus	☐	glom-**AIR**-yoo-lus	________
glycosuria	☐	**glye**-kohs-**YOO**-ree-ah	________
hematuria	☐	hee-mah-**TOO**-ree-ah	________
hemodialysis	☐	hee-moh-dye-**AL**-ih-sis	________
hilum	☐	**HIGH**-lum	________
hydronephrosis	☐	high-droh-neh-**FROH**-sis	________
intravenous pyelogram	☐	in-trah-**VEE**-nus **PYE**-eh-loh-gram	________
ketonuria	☐	kee-toh-**NOO**-ree-ah	________
lethargy	☐	**LETH**-ar-jee	________
malaise	☐	mah-**LAYZ**	________
meatotomy	☐	mee-ah-**TOT**-oh-mee	________
meatus	☐	mee-**AY**-tus	________
nephrolithiasis	☐	**nef**-roh-lith-**EYE**-ah-sis	________
nephrotic syndrome	☐	neh-**FROT**-ik **SIN**-drohm	________
nocturia	☐	nok-**TOO**-ree-ah	________
oliguria	☐	ol-ig-**YOO**-ree-ah	________
palpable	☐	**PAL**-pah-b'l	________
peritoneal dialysis	☐	**pair**-ih-**TOH**-nee-al dye-**AL**-ih-sis	________
peritonitis	☐	**pair**-ih-ton-**EYE**-tis	________
polycystic	☐	pol-ee-**SISS**-tik	________
polydipsia	☐	pol-ee-**DIP**-see-ah	________
polyuria	☐	pol-ee-**YOO**-ree-ah	________
pyelitis	☐	**pye**-eh-**LYE**-tis	________
pyelonephritis	☐	pye-eh-loh-neh-**FRYE**-tis	________
pyuria	☐	pye-**YOO**-ree-ah	________
radiopaque	☐	ray-dee-oh-**PAYK**	________
renal	☐	**REE**-nal	________
renal angiography	☐	**REE**-nal an-jee-**OG**-rah-fee	________
renal artery	☐	**REE**-nal **AR**-teh-ree	________
renal cell carcinoma	☐	**REE**-nal sell car-sin-**OH**-mah	________
renal pelvis	☐	**REE**-nal **PELL**-viss	________

Term		Pronunciation	
renal scan	☐	**REE**-nal scan	______
renal tubule	☐	**REE**-nal **TOOB**-yool	______
renal vein	☐	**REE**-nal **VEIN**	______
residual urine	☐	rih-**ZID**-yoo-al **YOO**-rin	______
retrograde pyelogram	☐	**RET**-roh-grayd **PYE**-eh-loh-gram	______
solute	☐	**SOL**-yoot	______
specific gravity	☐	speh-si-**FIK GRAV**-ih-tee	______
toxic	☐	**TOKS**-ik	______
turbid	☐	**TER**-bid	______
ultrasonography	☐	ul-trah-son-**OG**-rah-fee	______
uremia	☐	yoo-**REE**-mee-ah	______
ureter	☐	**YOO**-reh-ter	______
ureterostenosis	☐	yoo-**ree**-ter-oh-sten-**OH**-sis	______
urethra	☐	yoo-**REE**-thrah	______
urethritis	☐	yoo-ree-**THRIGH**-tis	______
urgency	☐	**ER**-jen-see	______
urinalysis	☐	**yoo**-rih-**NAL**-ih-sis	______
urinary	☐	**YOO**-rih-nair-ee	______
urination	☐	yoo-rih-**NAY**-shun	______
urinometer	☐	**yoo**-rih-**NOM**-eh-ter	______
vesicocele	☐	**VESS**-ih-koh-**seel**	______
vesicoureteral reflux	☐	**vess**-ih-koh-yoo-**REE**-ter-al **REE**-fluks	______
voiding	☐	**VOYD**-ing	______
voiding cystourethrography	☐	**VOYD**-ing **siss**-toh-yoo-ree-**THROG**-rah-fee	______

Chapter Review Exercises

The following exercises provide a more in-depth review of the chapter material. Your goal in these exercises is to complete each section at a minimum 80% level of accuracy. If you score below 80% in any area, return to the appropriate section in the chapter and read the material again. A place has been provided for your score at the end of each section.

A. Trace the Flow

As you trace the flow of urine from the kidney to the urethra, fill in the missing word(s). Each correct answer is worth 10 points. When you have completed this exercise, record your score in the space provided at the end of the exercise.

Blood flows into the kidney via the (1) renal arteries and leaves the kidneys via the (2) renal veins. After entering the kidney, the renal arteries branch out into smaller vessels throughout the kidney until the smallest arteries, known as (3) arterioles, reach the cortex of the kidney. Each of these small arteries lead to a ball-shaped collection of very tiny, coiled capillaries known as the (4) glomerulus. It is here that the formation of urine begins. As blood slowly, but constantly, passes through the thousands of glomeruli within the cortex of the kidney, the blood pressure forces water, salts, sugar, and nitrogenous waste products through the glomeruli walls into the (5) Bowman's. This process is known as (6) filtration. The glomerular filtrate, as it is now called, passes from the Bowman's capsule into a long, twisted tube called the (7) renal tubles. It is here in these tubules that water, sugar, and salts are returned to the bloodstream through the network of capillaries that surround them; this process is known as (8) tublar reabsorption. From the renal tubules, the urine is emptied into the central part of the kidney known as the (9) renal pelvis. The central part of the kidney narrows into the large upper end of a tubular structure known as the (10) ureter, which transports the urine from the kidney to the bladder. Urine is stored in the bladder until fullness stimulates its expulsion through the urethra.

***Number correct* ______ × *10 points/correct answer: Your score* ______%**

B. Spelling

Circle the correctly spelled term in each pairing of words. Each correct answer is worth 10 points. Record your score in the space provided at the end of the exercise.

1. hilum — hylum
2. olyguria — oliguria
3. micturition — micturation
4. palpable — palpitable
5. residule — residual
6. urether — urethra
7. urinary — uronary
8. dysuria — disuria
9. hemeturia — hematuria
10. hydronephrosis — hidronephrosis

***Number correct* ______ × *10 points/correct answer: Your score* ______%**

C. Crossword Puzzle

Read the clues carefully and complete the puzzle. Each crossword answer is worth 10 points. When you have completed the crossword puzzle, total your points and enter your score in the space provided.

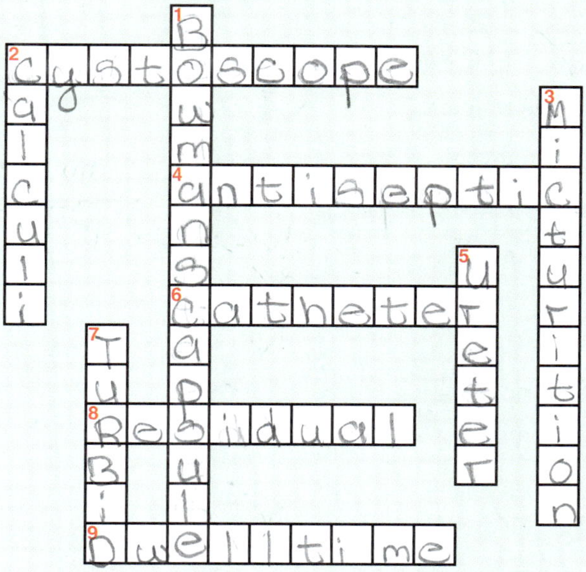

ACROSS

2 Instrument for viewing bladder
4 Inhibits growth of microorganisms
6 Hollow, flexible tube
8 Amount remaining; what is left over
9 Time solution stays in body cavity

DOWN

1 Cup-shaped end of renal tubule
2 Abnormal stones formed in body
3 Urination; voiding
5 Connects the kidneys to the bladder
7 Cloudy

***Number correct* _______ × *10 points/correct answer: Your score* _______%**

D. Term to Definition

Define each of the following sign and symptom terms by writing the definition in the space provided. Check the space provided if you are able to complete this exercise correctly the first time (without referring to the answers). Each correct answer is worth 10 points. Record your score in the space provided at the end of the exercise.

☐ 1. albuminuria The presence of abnormally large quantities of protein in the urine
☐ 2. polyuria Excretion of abnormally large amounts of urine.
☐ 3. anuria Absence of urine output
☐ 4. urgency A feeling of to void urine immediately
☐ 5. dysuria Painful urination
☐ 6. pyuria Pus in urine
☐ 7. frequency Urination at short intervals
☐ 8. glycosuria The presence of the glucose in the urine
☐ 9. nocturia Excessive urination at night
☐ 10. oliguria Secretion of a decreased amount of urine in relation to fluid intake, that is scanty urine output

***Number correct* _______ × *10 points/correct answer: Your score* _______%**

E. Is It Normal?

In this exercise, you will read descriptions of urine samples. Decide whether the description indicates if the urine is normal or abnormal. If it is normal, check the appropriate area. If it is abnormal, identify the condition. Each correct answer is worth 10 points. Record your score in the space provided at the end of this exercise.

SPECIMEN SAMPLE NUMBER	DESCRIPTION OF URINE SAMPLE	CHECK (✓) IF NORMAL FINDINGS	ABNORMAL FINDINGS: IDENTIFY POSSIBLE CONDITION
1	Pale yellow color	✓	
2	Smoky red color		presence of blood in the urine
3	Cloudy appearance		presence of pus (pyuria)
4	Specific gravity of 1.020	✓	
5	pH of 7.4	✓	
6	Reagent strip negative for protein	✓	
7	Reagent strip negative for glucose	✓	
8	Reagent strip negative for ketones	✓	
9	Reagent strip 4+ for glucose		Can be an indicator of diabetes mellitus
10	Reagent strip 3+ for ketones		

Number correct ______ × 10 points/correct answer: Your score ______%

F. Matching Conditions

Match the following urinary system conditions on the left with the most appropriate definitions on the right. Each correct answer is worth 10 points. Record your score in the space provided at the end of the exercise.

i 1. cystitis
j 2. pyelonephritis
d 3. hydronephrosis
h 4. glomerulonephritis
g 5. polycystic kidney
b 6. vesicoureteral reflux
e 7. Wilm's tumor
c 8. renal cell carcinoma
f 9. renal failure
a 10. nephrotic syndrome

a. Large amounts of protein are lost through glomerular membrane into the urine, resulting in severe proteinuria; patient experiences massive generalized edema
b. Abnormal backflow of urine from the bladder to the ureter
c. Malignant tumor of the kidney, occurring in adulthood
d. Distention of the pelvis and calyces of the kidney caused by urine that cannot flow past an obstruction in a ureter
e. Malignant tumor of the kidney, occurring in childhood
f. Uremia
g. A hereditary disorder of the kidneys in which grapelike, fluid-filled sacs replace normal kidney tissue

h. An inflammation of the glomerulus of the kidneys
i. Inflammation of the urinary bladder
j. A bacterial infection of the renal pelvis of the kidney

Number correct _______ × 10 points/correct answer: Your score _______ %

G. Proofreading Skills

Read the following report. For each boldface term, provide a brief definition and indicate if the term is spelled correctly. If it is misspelled, provide the correct spelling. If the boldface term is an abbreviation, provide the definition of the abbreviation. Each correct answer is worth 10 points. Record your score in the space provided at the end of the exercise.

The following is a report on an IVP.

HILLCREST Medical Center

"The preliminary film of the abdomen revealed Pantopaque in the extra-arachnoid space from a previously attempted myelogram. The bony structures were unremarkable.

An **intervenous pyelogram** was performed on this patient on 2-9-03. After injection of 50 cc. of **radiopake** dye, there was visualization of both kidneys at 30 seconds. The **nefrogram** phase revealed, bilaterally, symmetrical kidneys of normal size and density. At five minutes there was excretion bilaterally and there was normal concentrating ability. No evidence of abnormality within the **calyxes** was noted. The upper portion of the left **ureter** revealed a 4 mm. **calculis**; the distal portion, however, was not well visualized. The right ureter did actually appear to be visualized in the post-**voiding** film in its most distal portion and it appeared normal.

The bladder appeared to be normal with a minimal **residule.** Post-**micturition** films were obtained and revealed normal emptying. There was a vague suggestion of a small mass density superior to the bladder which could represent the uterus.

IMPRESSION: Evidence of **renul** calculi; left ureter."

Example:

nefrogram *x-ray record of the kidney*

Spelled correctly? ☐ Yes ☑ No *nephrogram*

1. **intervenous** ______________________

____

Spelled correctly? ☐ Yes ☑ No intravenous

2. **pyelogram** ______

Spelled correctly? ☑ Yes ☐ No ______

3. **radiopake** ______

Spelled correctly? ☐ Yes ☑ No radiopaque

4. **calyxes** ______

Spelled correctly? ☐ Yes ☑ No calyces

5. **ureter** ______

Spelled correctly? ☑ Yes ☐ No ______

6. **calculis** ______

Spelled correctly? ☐ Yes ☑ No calculus

7. **voiding** ______

Spelled correctly? ☑ Yes ☐ No ______

8. **residule** ______

Spelled correctly? ☐ Yes ☑ No residual

9. **micturition** ______

Spelled correctly? ☑ Yes ☐ No ______

10. **renul** ______

Spelled correctly? ☐ Yes ☑ No renal

***Number correct* ______ × *10 points/correct answer: Your score* ______%**

H. Completion

Complete each sentence by identifying the appropriate diagnostic technique. Each correct answer is worth 10 points. Record your score in the space provided at the end of the exercise.

1. A physical, chemical, or microscopic examination of urine is known as a
Urinalysis

2. A procedure that uses sound waves to produce composite pictures is known as

   ultrasongraphy

3. A procedure used to cultivate the growth of bacteria present in a urine specimen for proper microscopic identification of the specific pathogen is a

   urine culture

4. An examination performed to evaluate bladder tone; measuring bladder pressure during filling and voiding is known as a

   Cystometrography

5. The introduction of a flexible, hollow tube into the bladder to instill a substance or to remove urine is known as a

   Catheterization

6. The radiographic procedure that provides visualization of the urinary tract by injecting a contrast dye intravenously into the body is called

   intravenous pyelogram

7. The x-ray visualization of the internal anatomy of the renal blood vessels after injection of a contrast medium is called a

   renal angiography

8. A collection of all of the urine excreted by the individual over a 24-hour period of time is called a

   24-hour urine speciman

9. X-ray visualization of the bladder and urethra during the voiding process after the bladder has been filled with a contrast medium is a

   voiding cystourethrography

10. The introduction of a radiopaque dye through a cystoscope into the ureters and renal pelvis for the purpose of taking x-ray pictures of the collecting structures is known as a

   retrograde pyelogram

Number correct _______ × 10 points/correct answer: Your score _______%

I. Matching Abbreviations

Match the abbreviations on the left with the correct definition on the right. Each correct answer is worth 10 points. Record your score in the space provided at the end of the exercise.

Answer	Abbreviation		Definition
d	1. KUB	a.	blood, urea, nitrogen
g	2. IVP	b.	erythropoietin
i	3. CCPD	c.	continuous ambulatory peritoneal dialysis
h	4. GFR	d.	kidneys, ureters, bladder
j	5. ESRD	e.	urinalysis
b	6. EPO	f.	voiding cystourethrogram
k	7. ADH	g.	intravenous pyelogram
e	8. UA	h.	glomerular filtration rate
f	9. VCUG	i.	continuous cyclic peritoneal dialysis
a	10. BUN	j.	end-stage renal disease
		k.	antidiuretic hormone
		l.	cystoscopy

Number correct _______ × 10 points/correct answer: Your score _______%

J. Word Search

Using the definitions listed, identify the terms related to the urinary system. After you have identified each term, find and circle it in the word search puzzle. The words may be read up, down, diagonally, across, or backward. Each correct answer is worth 10 points. Record your score in the space provided at the end of the exercise.

Example: The smallest branch of an artery.

arteriole

1. A substance that tends to inhibit the growth and reproduction of microorganisms ("pertaining to against infection").

   ____

2. The depression, or pit, of an organ where the vessels and nerves enter.

   ____

3. Another name for the act of eliminating urine from the bladder, other than voiding or urination.

   ____

4. Inflammation of the peritoneum (the membrane that lines the abdominal cavity).

   ____

5. The central collecting part of the kidney that narrows into the large upper end of the ureter.

   ____

6. Urine that remains in the bladder is known as ______________________________ urine.
7. The medical term for *cloudy.*

   ____

8. One of a pair of tubes that carries urine from the kidney to the bladder.

   ____

9. Inability to control urination; the inability to retain urine in the bladder is known as urinary

   ____

10. The medical term for *poisonous* ("pertaining to poison").

    ____

F	L	O	A	R	T	E	R	I	O	L	E	M	I	C
A	C	Y	N	G	E	S	M	S	I	D	A	S	T	T
M	I	H	T	T	M	N	M	E	T	T	R	N	V	R
C	A	O	I	E	E	O	O	S	D	I	C	C	B	O
I	L	C	S	L	T	N	L	I	E	O	O	I	T	S
N	U	H	E	I	U	T	T	O	T	E	L	N	L	T
C	R	O	P	H	L	M	B	I	U	A	E	C	O	E
O	U	S	T	N	P	N	E	M	A	R	O	O	E	O
N	U	I	I	P	O	I	P	I	A	T	E	N	E	C
T	A	V	C	D	A	I	I	N	D	E	Y	T	M	Y
I	A	L	H	G	R	L	T	O	X	I	C	P	E	T
N	I	E	A	A	R	C	H	I	S	I	S	A	I	R
E	S	P	N	D	R	U	Y	A	R	D	I	S	G	S
N	U	L	T	I	R	E	S	I	D	U	A	L	D	T
C	R	A	E	B	L	O	I	I	U	A	T	C	O	A
E	E	N	R	R	H	C	S	U	T	U	R	C	S	A
F	R	E	T	U	U	R	I	S	M	E	M	N	I	C
P	E	R	I	T	O	N	I	T	I	S	A	S	E	M

Number correct ______ × 10 points/correct answer: Your score ______%

Answers to Chapter Review Exercises

A. Trace the Flow

1. renal arteries
2. renal veins
3. arterioles
4. glomerulus
5. Bowman's capsule
6. filtration
7. renal tubules
8. tubular reabsorption
9. renal pelvis
10. ureter

B. Spelling

1. hilum
2. oliguria
3. micturition
4. palpable
5. residual
6. urethra
7. urinary
8. dysuria
9. hematuria
10. hydronephrosis

C. Crossword Puzzle

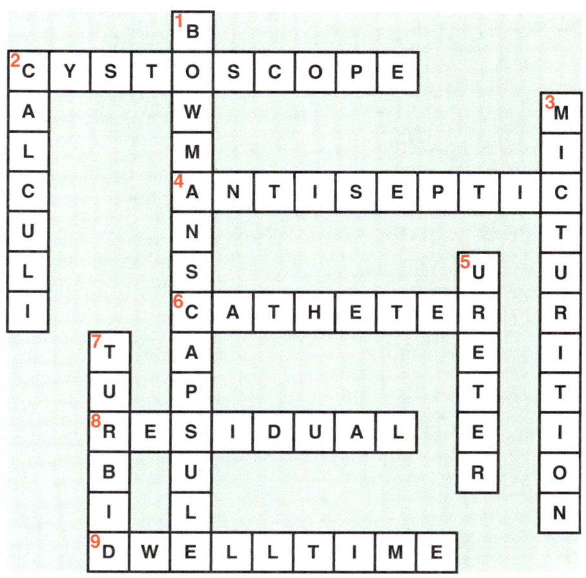

D. Term to Definition

1. the presence of abnormally large quantities of protein in the urine
2. excretion of abnormally large amounts of urine
3. absence of urine output
4. a feeling of the need to void urine immediately
5. painful urination
6. pus in the urine
7. urination at short intervals (frequently) without increase in the daily volume of urinary output due to reduced bladder capacity
8. the presence of glucose in the urine
9. excessive urination at night
10. secretion of a decreased amount of urine in relation to the fluid intake, that is, scanty urine output

E. Is It Normal?

1. normal
2. abnormal—presence of blood in the urine (hematuria)
3. abnormal—presence of pus (pyuria)
4. normal
5. normal
6. normal
7. normal
8. normal
9. abnormal—can be an indicator of diabetes mellitus
10. abnormal—caused from the breakdown of fats, the presence of ketones in the urine may be a result of high blood sugar (uncontrolled diabetes mellitus), starvation, dehydration, or excessive ingestion of aspirin

F. Matching Conditions

1. i
2. j
3. d
4. h
5. g
6. b
7. e
8. c
9. f
10. a

G. Proofreading Skills

1. Pertaining to the inside of a vein.
   Spelled correctly? No **intravenous**
2. A radiographic procedure that provides visualization of the entire urinary tract: kidneys, ureters, bladder, and urethra.
   Spelled correctly? Yes
3. Does not allow the crossing of x-rays or radiant energy.
   Spelled correctly? No **radiopaque**
4. The cuplike divisions through which each tubule empties into the renal pelvis.
   Spelled correctly? No **calyces**
5. Muscular tubes lined with mucous membrane, one leading from each kidney down to the urinary bladder.
   Spelled correctly? Yes
6. Kidney stone.
   Spelled correctly? No **calculus**
7. The process of elimination of urine from the body.
   Spelled correctly? Yes
8. Amount of urine remaining in the bladder after voiding.
   Spelled correctly? No **residual**
9. The act of eliminating urine from the bladder.
   Spelled correctly? Yes
10. Pertaining to the kidney.
    Spelled correctly? No **renal**

H. Completion

1. urinalysis
2. ultrasonography
3. urine culture
4. cystometrography
5. catheterization
6. intravenous pyelogram
7. renal angiography
8. 24-hour urine specimen
9. voiding cystourethrography
10. retrograde pyelogram

I. Matching Abbreviations

1. d
2. g
3. i
4. h
5. j
6. b
7. k
8. e
9. f
10. a

J. Word Search

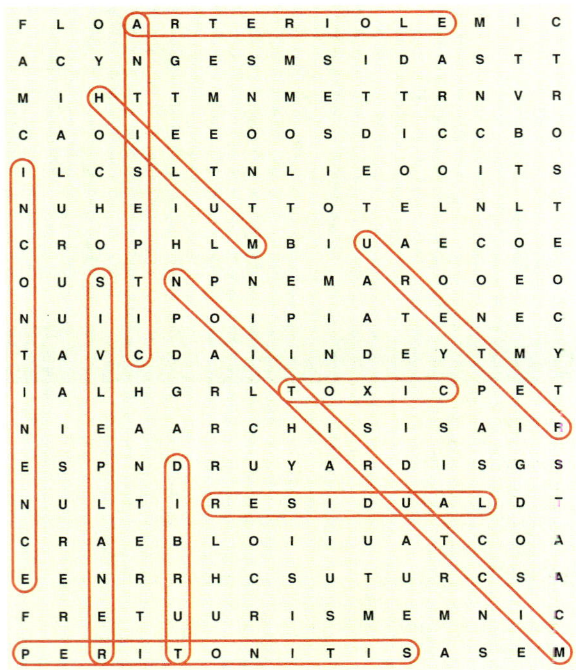

CHAPTER 16

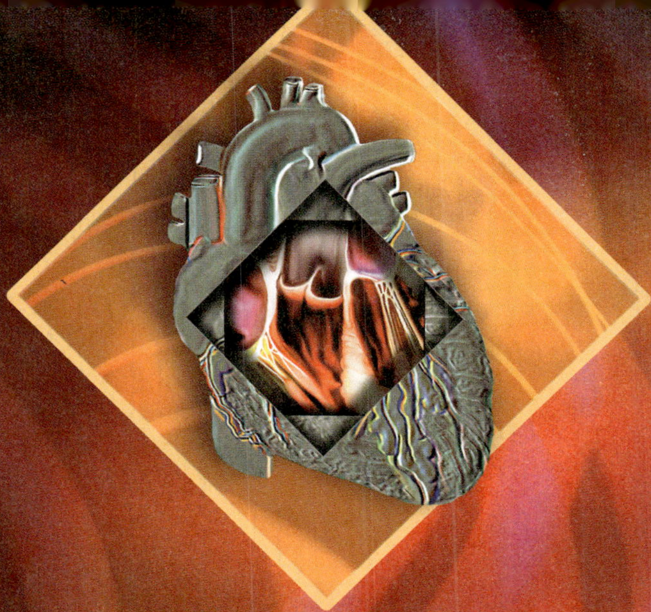

The Male Reproductive System

CHAPTER CONTENT

KEY COMPETENCIES

Upon completing this chapter and the review exercises at the end of the chapter, the learner should be able to:

1. Correctly label the structures of the male reproductive system.
2. Correctly spell and pronounce each new term introduced in this chapter using the Activity CD-ROM and Audio CD, if available.
3. Identify and define at least 10 pathological conditions of the male reproductive system.
4. Identify at least 10 diagnostic techniques used in treating disorders of the male reproductive system.
5. Proof and correct the transcription exercise relative to the male reproductive system provided at the end of this chapter.
6. Demonstrate the ability to correctly construct words relating to the male reproductive system by completing the appropriate exercise at the end of the chapter.
7. Identify three secondary sex characteristic changes that occur in the male body at the onset of puberty.
8. Identify six sexually transmitted diseases.

OVERVIEW

The male reproductive system functions to produce, sustain, and transport sperm, to propel the sperm from the penis into the female vagina during sexual intercourse (**copulation**), and to produce the male hormone, **testosterone**. The primary organs of the male reproductive system are the **gonads**, or male sex glands, which are called the **testes** (singular: testis or **testicle**). The testes are responsible for production of **spermatozoa** (the male germ cell) and for the secretion of testosterone. Testosterone is responsible for the secondary sex characteristic changes that occur in the male with the onset of puberty. These changes include growth of facial hair (beard), growth of pubic hair, and deepening of the voice.

The accessory organs of the male reproductive system are a series of ducts that transport the sperm to the outside of the body (i.e., the epididymis, vas deferens, seminal vesicle, ejaculatory duct, the urethra, and the prostate gland). The supporting structures of the male reproductive system are the scrotum, the penis, and a pair of spermatic cords.

Anatomy and Physiology

As you study the anatomy and physiology of the male reproductive system, refer to **Figure 16-1** for a visual reference.

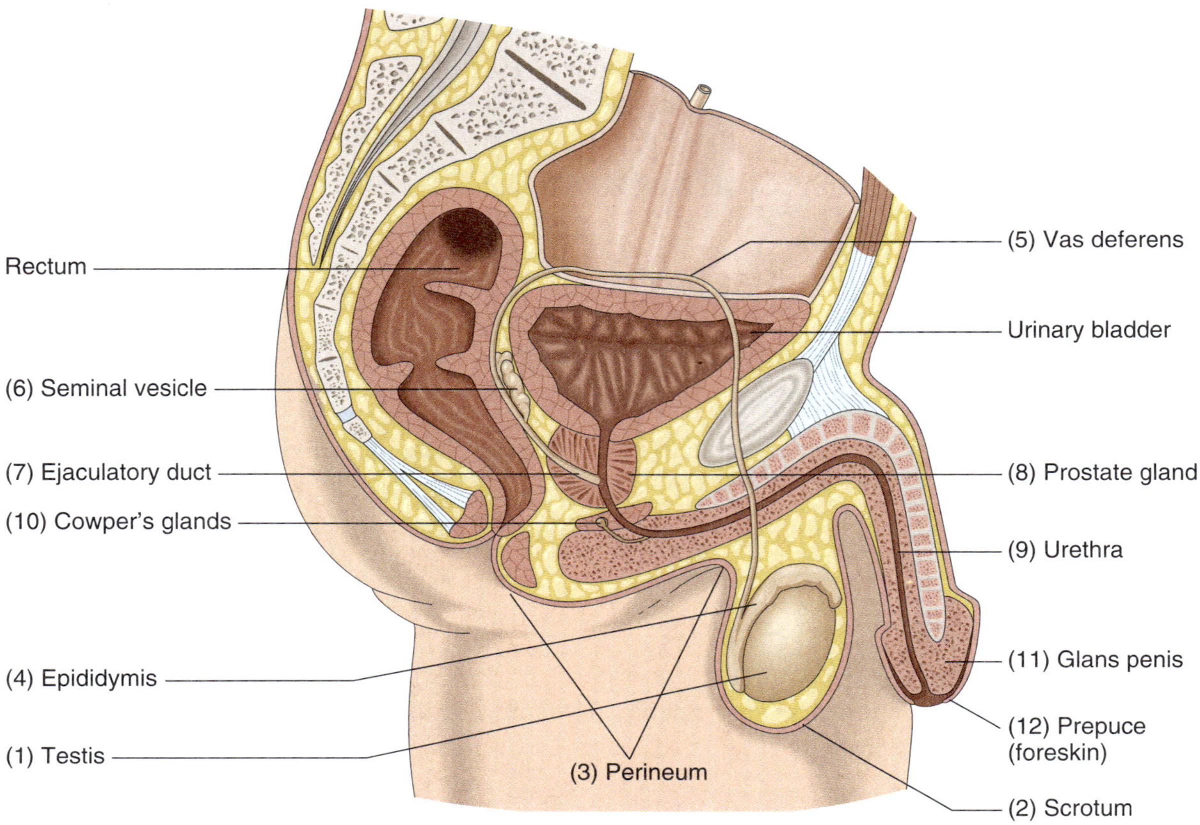

Figure 16-1 Male reproductive system

Primary Organs

The male gonads, or **(1)** testicles, are small ovoid glands that begin their development high in the abdominal cavity, near the kidneys (retroperitoneal cavity), during the gestational period. A month or two before, or shortly after birth, the testicles descend through the inguinal canal into the **(2)** **scrotum** where they remain. The scrotum is a sac located posterior to the penis and is suspended from the **(3)** **perineum**; the perineum is the area between the scrotum and the anus in the male. Each testicle remains suspended in the scrotal sac by a spermatic cord that contains blood and lymphatic vessels, nerves, and the vas deferens. If the testicles are to function normally, they must remain suspended in the scrotal sac.

The scrotum is divided into two compartments, or sacs. Each scrotal sac contains one testicle. Each testicle consists of specialized coils of tiny tubules that are responsible for production of sperm; these tubules are known as the **seminiferous tubules**. The specialized interstitial tissue located between the tubules of the testes is responsible for secreting the male hormone, testosterone.

Accessory Organs

After being produced, sperm are transported through the network of tubules within the male reproductive system to reach the outside of the body. When they leave the seminiferous tubules, the sperm pass through the **(4)** **epididymis**, which is a tightly coiled tubule that resembles a comma. It is here in the epididymis that the sperm mature, becoming fertile and motile (capable of movement). Mature sperm are stored in the lower portion of the epididymis.

The epididymis leads to the **(5)** **vas deferens**, also called the ductus deferens. This straight tube, which is continuous with the epididymis, takes a sharp upward turn and ascends through the scrotum into the abdominopelvic cavity. Passing along the lateral pelvic wall, the vas deferens crosses over the top of the ureter, and then descends along the posterior surface of the urinary bladder toward the prostate gland. At this location, just before the prostate gland, the vas deferens enlarges to form an **ampulla,** a saclike dilation. The vas deferens merges with the adjacent **(6)** **seminal vesicle**, to form the **(7)** **ejaculatory duct**.

The seminal vesicles secrete a thick, yellowish fluid that is known as seminal fluid; this constitutes a large part of the volume of the **semen**. The semen is a combination of sperm and various secretions that is expelled from the body, through the urethra, during ejaculation or sexual intercourse. The process of ejecting, or expelling, the semen from the male urethra is known as **ejaculation**. Each ejaculatory duct (one from each side) passes through the **(8)** **prostate gland**.

The prostate gland lies just below the urinary bladder, where it surrounds the base of the urethra as it leaves the bladder. Ducts from the prostate gland transport its secretions to the urethra. These thin, milky colored, alkaline secretions enhance the motility of the sperm and help to neutralize the secretions within the vagina. The muscular action of the prostate gland also aids in expelling the semen from the body. The ducts from the prostate gland empty into the **(9)** **urethra**, which serves both the urinary system and the male reproductive system. The urethra transports urine from the bladder, and the semen, when ejaculated, to the outside of the body. Just below the prostate gland are a pair of small, pea-sized glands called the **bulbourethral glands** or **(10)** **Cowper's glands**. The ducts from the bulbourethral glands empty into the urethra just before it extends through the penis. During sexual intercourse, the glands are stimulated to secrete an alkaline, mucouslike fluid that provides lubrication during sexual intercourse.

The seminal vesicles, prostate gland, and bulbourethral glands each secrete fluids that nourish the sperm and enhance their **motility.** These fluids also make up the total volume of the semen, with the largest amount being secreted by the seminal vesicles. During sexual intercourse, the volume of semen in a single ejaculation may vary from 1.5 to 6.0 ml, with each milliliter of semen containing between 50 to 150 million sperm. Sperm counts below 10 to 20 million per milliliter are usually indicative of fertility problems.

The **penis** is the male organ of copulation. It consists of a base that attaches it to the pubic arch, a body that is the visible pendant portion, and a tip called the **(11)** glans penis. The glans penis is covered by a loose, retractable fold of skin called the **(12)** prepuce, or foreskin. Shortly after birth, the foreskin is usually removed; this procedure is known as a circumcision. The urethra extends the length of the penis and ends as an opening at the tip of the glans penis; this opening is called the **external urinary meatus.**

The penis is made of a spongelike tissue containing many blood spaces that are relatively empty in the absence of sexual arousal, and the penis is **flaccid.** During sexual arousal, however, these spaces fill with blood, causing the penis to become rigid and enlarge in diameter and length. This process, known as **erection,** allows the penis to remain rigid enough to enter the female vagina during sexual intercourse. The urethra serves as passageway for the exit of the semen following ejaculation, allowing deposit of sperm in the vagina.

Vocabulary

The following vocabulary words are frequently used when discussing the male reproductive system.

WORD	DEFINITION
anorexia (an-oh-**REX**-ee-ah)	Loss of appetite.
asymptomatic (ay-simp-toh-**MAT**-ik)	Without symptoms.
balanoplasty (**BAL**-ah-noh-**plas**-tee) balan/o = glans penis -plasty = surgical repair	Surgical repair of the glans penis.
bulbourethral glands (**buhl**-boh-yoo-**REE**-thral glands) urethr/o = urethra -al = pertaining to	A pair of small, pea-sized glands that empty into the urethra just before it extends through the penis; also known as Cowper's glands.
chancre (**SHANG**-ker)	A skin lesion, usually of primary syphilis, that begins at the site of infection as a small raised area and develops into a red, painless ulcer with a scooped-out appearance; also known as a venereal sore.

Cowper's glands (**KOW**-perz)	See *bulbourethral glands.*
cryosurgery (**kry**-oh-**SER**-jer-ee) cry/o = cold	Use of subfreezing temperature to destroy tissue. The coolant is circulated through a metal probe, chilling it to as low as −160°C. When the probe touches the tissues of the body, the moist tissues adhere to the cold metal of the probe and freeze.
debridement (day-breed-**MON**)	The removal of dirt, damaged tissue, and cellular debris from a wound or a burn to prevent infection and to promote healing.
dormant (**DOOR**-mant)	Inactive.
dysuria (dis-**YOO**-ree-ah) dys- = bad, difficult, painful, disordered ur/o = urine -ia = noun ending	Painful urination.
ejaculation (ee-jack-yoo-**LAY**-shun)	The process of ejecting, or expelling, the semen from the male urethra.
epididymectomy (**ep**-ih-**did**-ih-**MEK**-toh-mee) epididym/o = epididymis -ectomy = surgical removal	Surgical removal of the epididymis.
epididymis (**ep**-ih-**DID**-ih-mis) epididym/o = epididymis -is = noun ending	A tightly coiled tubule that resembles a comma; its purpose is that of housing the sperm until they mature, becoming fertile and motile. Mature sperm are stored in the lower portion of the epididymis.
epididymitis (**ep**-ih-**did**-ih-**MY**-tis) epididym/o = epididymis -itis = inflammation	Inflammation of the epididymis. This condition can be the result of a chlamydial infection in the male.
exudate (**EKS**-yoo-dayt)	Fluid, pus, or serum that is slowly discharged from cells or blood vessels through small pores or breaks in cell membranes.
flaccid (**FLAK**-sid)	Weak; lacking normal muscle tone.
foreskin (**FOR**-skin)	A loose, retractable fold of skin covering the tip of the penis; also called the prepuce.
glans penis (**GLANS PEE**-nis)	The tip of the penis.
gonad (**GOH**-nad)	The male sex glands, which are called the testes (singular: testicle). These are the primary organs of the male reproductive system.
Kaposi's sarcoma (**KAP**-oh-seez sar-**KOH**-mah)	A malignant growth that begins as soft, brownish or purple raised areas on the feet and slowly spreads in the skin, spreading to the lymph nodes and internal organs. It occurs most often in men and is associated with AIDS.

malaise (mah-**LAYZ**)	A vague feeling of bodily weakness or discomfort, often marking the onset of disease.
malodorous (mal-**OH**-dor-us)	Foul smelling; having a bad odor.
motility (moh-**TILL**-ih-tee)	The ability to move spontaneously.
mucopurulent (mew-koh-**PEWR**-yoo-lent) muc/o = mucus	Characteristic of a combination of mucus and pus.
opportunistic infections (op-or-**TOON**-is-tik in-**FEK**-shuns)	An infection caused by normally nondisease-producing organisms that sets up in a host whose resistance has been decreased by surgery, illnesses, and disorders such as AIDS.
orchidopexy (**OR**-kid-oh-peck-see) orchid/o = testicle -pexy = surgical fixation	Surgical fixation of an undescended testicle.
orchiopexy (or-kee-oh-**PECK**-see) orchi/o = testicle -pexy = surgical fixation	See *orchidopexy.*
palpation (pal-**PAY**-shun)	A technique used in physical examinations that involves feeling parts of the body with the hands.
pelvic inflammatory disease (**PELL**-vik in-**FLAM**-mah-tor-ee)	Inflammation of the fallopian tubes; also known as salpingitis; may be associated with sexually transmitted diseases.
perineum (pair-ih-**NEE**-um)	The area between the scrotum and the anus in the male.
prepuce (**PRE**-pus)	See *foreskin.*
prophylactic (proh-fih-**LAK**-tik)	Any agent or regimen that contributes to the prevention of infection and disease.
prostate gland (**PROSS**-tayt gland) prostat/o = prostate gland -e = noun ending	A gland that surrounds the base of the urethra, which secretes a milky colored secretion into the urethra during ejaculation. This secretion enhances the motility of the sperm and helps to neutralize the secretions within the vagina.
prostatectomy (**pross**-tah-**TEK**-toh-mee) prostat/o = prostate gland -ectomy = surgical removal	Removal of the prostate gland. A discussion of two approaches to removing the prostate gland is presented in the section on diagnostic techniques.
purulent (**PEWR**-yoo-lent)	Producing or containing pus.

rectoscope (**REK**-toh-skohp) rect/o = rectum -scope = instrument for viewing	An instrument used to view the rectum that has a cutting and cauterizing (burning) loop.
resectoscope (ree-**SEK**-toh-skohp)	An instrument used to surgically remove tissue from the body; it has a light source and lens attached for viewing the area.
residual urine (rih-**ZID**-yoo-al **YOO**-rin)	Urine that remains in the bladder after urination.
residual urine test	Obtaining a catheterized specimen after the patient has emptied the bladder by voiding, to determine the amount of urine remaining in the bladder; known as a residual specimen.
salpingitis (sal-pin-**JYE**-tis) salping/o = eustachian tubes; also refers to fallopian tubes -itis = inflammation	Inflammation of the fallopian tubes; also known as **pelvic inflammatory disease**; included in this section because it is associated with sexually transmitted diseases.
scrotum (**SKROH**-tum)	An external sac that houses the testicles; it is located posterior to the penis and is suspended from the perineum.
semen (**SEE**-men)	A combination of sperm and various secretions that is expelled from the body through the urethra during sexual intercourse.
seminal vesicles (**SEM**-in-al **VESS**-ih-kls)	Glands that secrete a thick, yellowish fluid, known as seminal fluid, into the vas deferens.
seminiferous tubules (**SEM**-in-**IF**-er-us **TOO**-byoo-ls)	Specialized coils of tiny tubules that are responsible for production of sperm; located in the testes.
spermatozoan (**sper**-mat-oh-**ZOH**-ahn)	A mature male germ cell; also known as **spermatozoon** (plural: spermatozoa).
spermatozoon (**sper**-mat-oh-**ZOH**-on)	See *spermatozoan.*
testicles (**TESS**-tih-kls) **(testes)**	The male gonads, or male sex glands, responsible for production of spermatozoa (the male germ cell), and for the secretion of the male hormone, testosterone.
testosterone (tess-**TOSS**-ter-own)	A male hormone secreted by the testes, responsible for the secondary sex characteristic changes that occur in the male with the onset of puberty. These changes include growth of facial hair (beard), growth of pubic hair, and deepening of the voice.
truss	An apparatus worn to prevent or block the herniation of the intestines or other organ through an opening in the abdominal wall.
urethra (**YOO**-ree-thrah) urethr/o = urethra -a = noun ending	A small tubular structure extending the length of the penis that transports urine from the bladder, and the semen, when ejaculated, to the outside of the body.

urethritis (yoo-ree-**THRY**-tis) **urethr/o** = urethra **-itis** = inflammation	Inflammation of the urethra.
vas deferens (vas **DEF**-er-enz)	The narrow, straight tube that transports sperm from the epididymis to the ejaculatory duct.
vesicles (**VESS**-ih-kls)	Blisters; small raised skin lesions containing clear fluid.

Word Elements

The following word elements pertain to the male reproductive system. As you review the list, pronounce each word element aloud twice and check the box after you "say it." Write the definition for the example word given for each word element. You may use your medical dictionary.

WORD ELEMENT	PRONUNCIATION	"SAY IT"	MEANING
andr/o **andr**oid	**AN**-droh **AN**-droyd	☐	man, male
balan/o **balan**itis	bal-**AH**-noh bal-ah-**NYE**-tis	☐	glans penis
cry/o **cryo**surgery	**KRY**-oh kry-oh-**SIR**-jeer-ee	☐	cold
crypt/o **crypt**orchidism	**KRIPT**-oh kript-**OR**-kid-izm	☐	hidden
epididym/o **epididym**itis	ep-ih-**DID**-ih-moh **ep**-ih-**did**-ih-**MY**-tis	☐	epididymis
hydr/o **hydr**ocele	**HIGH**-droh high-**DROH**-seel	☐	water
orch/o **orch**itis	**OR**-koh or-**KIGH**-tis	☐	testicle
orchi/o **orchi**opexy	or-**KEE**-oh or-kee-oh-**PECK**-see	☐	testicle
orchid/o **orchid**oplasty	**OR**-kid-oh **OR**-kid-oh-plass-tee	☐	testicle
prostat/o **prostat**itis	pross-**TAH**-toh pross-tah-**TYE**-tis	☐	prostate gland

semin/i **semin**al vesicles	**SEM**-ih-neye **SEM**-ih-nal **VESS**-ih-kls	☐	semen
sperm/o **sperm**olysis	**SPERM**-oh sperm-**ALL**-ih-sis	☐	sperm
spermat/o **spermat**ogenesis	sper-**MAT**-oh **sper**-mat-oh-**JEN**-eh-sis	☐	sperm
test/o **test**icular	**TESS**-toh tess-**TIK**-yoo-lar	☐	testis, testes
vas/o **vas**ectomy	**VAS**-oh vas-**EK**-toh-mee	☐	vessel; also refers to vas deferens
zo/o a**zo**ospermia	**ZOH**-oh ah-zoh-oh-**SPER**-mee-ah	☐	animal (man)

Pathological Conditions

As you study the pathological conditions of the male reproductive system, note that the **basic definition** is in bold print followed by a more detailed description in regular print. The phonetic pronunciation is directly beneath each term, and with a breakdown of the component parts of the term when appropriate.

anorchism
(an-**OR**-kizm)
an- = without
orchi/o = testicle
-ism = condition

Anorchism is the absence of one or both testicles.

balanitis
(bal-ah-**NYE**-tis)
balan/o = glans penis
-itis = inflammation

Inflammation of the glans penis and the mucous membrane beneath it.

Balanitis is caused by irritation and invasion of microorganisms. Treatment with antibiotics will help control the localized infection. Good hygiene and thorough drying of the penis when bathing are important preventive measures.

benign prostatic hypertrophy
(bee-**NYEN** pross-**TAT**-ik high-**PER**-troh-fee)
prostat/o = prostate gland
-ic = pertaining to
hyper- = excessive
troph/o = development, growth
-y = noun ending

A benign (noncancerous) enlargement of the prostate gland, creating pressure on the upper part of the urethra or neck of the bladder, causing obstruction of the flow of urine.

Benign prostatic hypertrophy is a common condition occurring in men over the age of 50.

Men with hypertrophy of the prostate gland may complain of symptoms such as difficulty in starting urination, a weak stream of urine (not being able to maintain a constant stream), the inability to empty the bladder completely, or "dribbling" at the end of voiding.

Diagnosis is usually confirmed by thorough patient history and a rectal examination by the physician to confirm prostatic enlargement. The physician may order a urinalysis and culture of the urine to check for urinary tract infection or any abnormalities in the urine, such as blood. Other diagnostic tests may be a **cystourethroscopy** to visualize the interior of the bladder and the urethra, a **KUB** (kidneys, ureters, bladder) **x-ray** to visualize the urinary tract, or a **residual urine test** to check for incomplete emptying of the bladder. If a malignancy (cancer) is suspected, a biopsy of the prostatic tissue may be ordered.

Treatment for benign prostatic hypertrophy is dependent on the degree of urinary obstruction noted. For patients with mild cases of prostatic enlargement (which is normal as the male ages), the condition may simply be monitored. For patients with recurrent and obstructive problems due to hyperplasia of the prostate gland, surgery is usually indicated to remove the prostate gland. Two types of surgery used are **transurethral resection of the prostate** (**TURP**) and **suprapubic prostatectomy**, each of which will be discussed in the diagnostic procedures section of this chapter.

---

carcinoma of the prostate
(**car**-sin-**OH**-mah of the **PROSS**-tayt)
carcin/o = cancer
-oma = tumor

Malignant growth within the prostate gland, creating pressure on the upper part of the urethra.

Cancer of the prostate is the most common cause of cancer among men, and the most common cause of death due to cancer in men over the age of 55. Unfortunately, symptoms are not usually present in the early stages of cancer of the prostate. By the time symptoms are evident, the cancer may have already metastasized (spread) to other areas of the body.

When symptoms of prostate cancer do occur, they may include any of the following:

1. A need to urinate frequently (i.e., urinary frequency) especially at night
2. Difficulty starting or stopping urine flow
3. Inability to urinate
4. Weak or interrupted flow of urine when urinating (patient may complain of "dribbling" instead of having a steady stream of urine)
5. Pain or burning when urinating
6. Pain or stiffness in the lower back, hips, or thighs
7. Painful ejaculation

Because the presence of symptoms usually means that the disease is more advanced, early detection of cancer of the prostate is essential to successful treatment. All men over the age of 40 should have a yearly physical examination that includes a digital rectal examination of the prostate gland. The rectal examination can reveal a cancerous growth before symptoms appear. A PSA blood test may be performed during the examination to detect increased growth of the prostate (the growth could be benign or malignant). The PSA test measures a substance called prostate-specific antigen. The level of PSA in the blood may rise in men who have prostate cancer or benign prostatic hypertrophy. If the level is elevated, the physician will order additional tests to confirm a diagnosis of cancer of the prostate.

The most common procedure used to treat or relieve the urinary obstruction resulting from cancer of the prostate is surgery to remove the prostate tissue that is pressing against the upper part of the urethra. This procedure is also used to treat benign prostatic hypertrophy. This surgery, called transurethral resection of the prostate (TUR or TURP), will be discussed in the diagnostic procedures section of the chapter.

Other methods of treatment include a radical prostatectomy (removal of the prostate gland), radiation therapy, hormone therapy, or chemotherapy. The treatment of choice is dependent on the patient's age, medical history, risks and benefits of treatment, and the stage of the disease.

carcinoma of the testes
(car-sin-**OH**-mah of the **TESS**-teez)
carcin/o = cancer
-oma = tumor

A malignant tumor of the testicle that appears as a painless lump in the testicle; also called testicular cancer.

This type of tumor is rare and usually occurs in men under the age of 40. The cause is unknown.

The diagnosis of testicular cancer is usually confirmed by biopsy, after the physician has palpated the lump in the testicle. The treatment of choice is surgery to remove the diseased testicle, followed by radiation therapy and chemotherapy. The healthy testicle is not removed, thus fertility and potency should not be altered in the male. Chances for complete recovery are excellent if the malignancy is detected in the early stages.

Testicular cancer can spread throughout the body via the lymphatic system if not treated in the early stages. Early treatment is essential for complete recovery; therefore, it is recommended that all men perform monthly testicular self-examinations. See **Figure 16-2.** If a lump is discovered, it should be reported immediately to the man's personal physician.

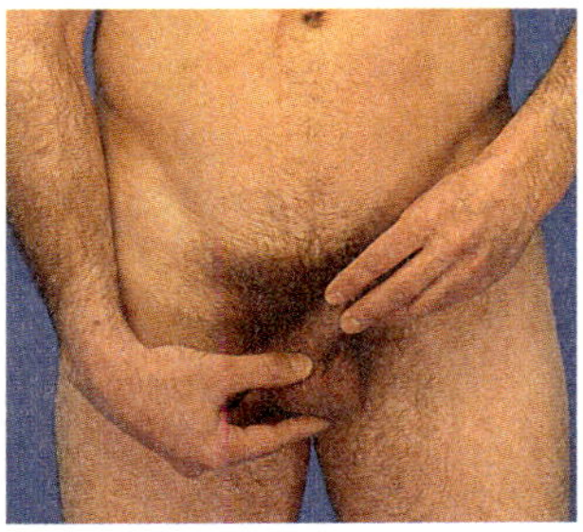

(A)

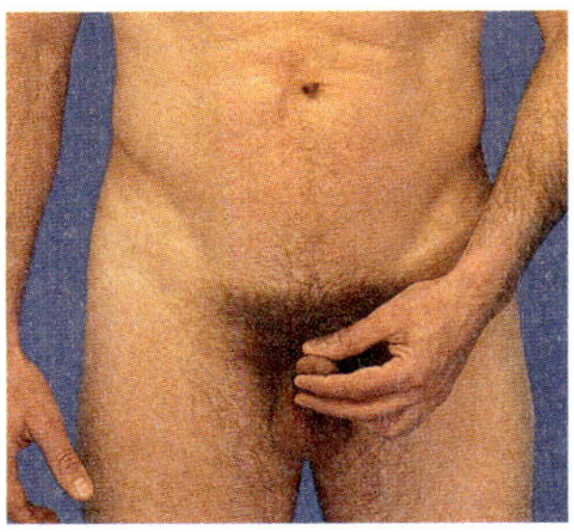

(B)

Figure 16-2 (A) Palpating the testis; (B) assessing for penile discharge

cryptorchidism
(kript-**OR**-kid-izm)
crypt/o = hidden
orchid/o = testicle
-ism = condition

Condition of undescended testicle(s); the absence of one or both testicles from the scrotum.

In cryptorchidism, the testicle may be located in the abdominal cavity or in the inguinal canal. If the testicle does not descend on its own, surgery will be necessary to correct the position. The surgery, known as an orchiopexy, involves making an incision into the inguinal canal, locating the testicle, and bringing it back down into the scrotal sac. This surgery is usually done on an outpatient basis, with normal physical activity being restored within a few weeks to a month.

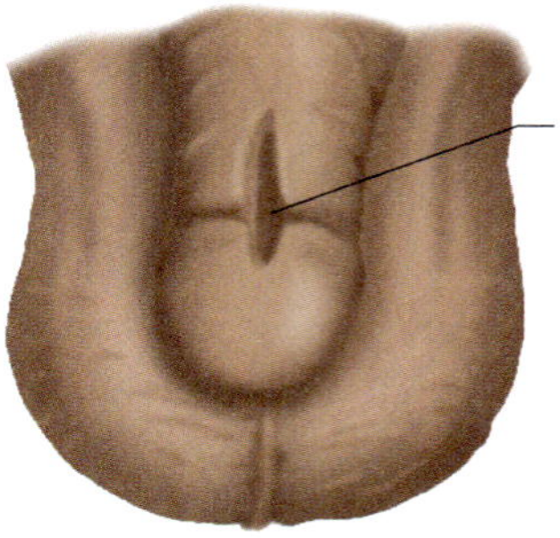

Figure 16-3 Epispadias

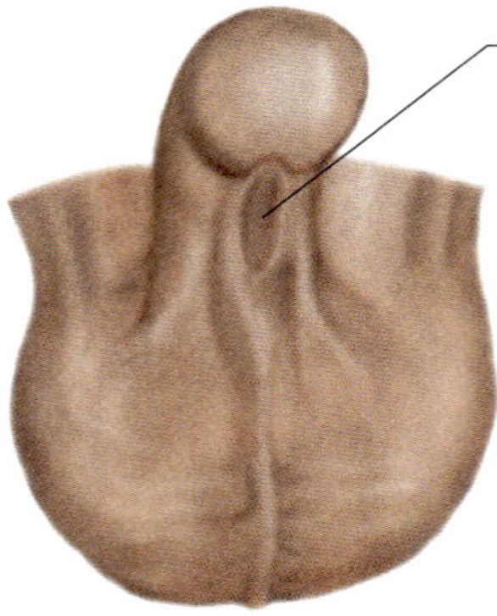

Figure 16-4 Hypospadias

---

epispadias
(**ep**-ih-**SPAY**-dee-as)
epi- = upon, over

A congenital defect (birth defect) in which the urethra opens on the upper side of the penis at some point near the glans. See Figure 16-3.

The treatment for **epispadias** is surgical correction with redirection of the opening of the urethra to its normal position at the end of the penis.

---

hydrocele
(high-**DROH**-seel)
hydro- = water
-cele = swelling or herniation

An accumulation of fluid in any saclike cavity or duct, particularly the scrotal sac or along the spermatic cord.

This condition is caused by inflammation of the epididymis or testis, or by obstruction of lymphatic or venous flow within the spermatic cord. The treatment for a **hydrocele** is surgery to remove the fluid pouch.

---

hypospadias
(high-poh-**SPAY**-dee-as)
hypo- = under, below

A congenital defect in which the urethra opens on the underside of the penis instead of at the end. See Figure 16-4.

Treatment for **hypospadias** involves surgery to redirect the opening of the urethra to its normal location at the end of the penis.

---

impotence
(**IM**-poh-tens)

The inability of a male to achieve or sustain an erection of the penis.

The cause of **impotence** may be psychological (due to anxiety or depression) or physiological (due to some physical disorder such as diabetes, spinal cord injury, or maybe a response to medications). Individuals who are experiencing impotence may be sexually aroused with the inability to sustain an erection, or they may lose their sexual appetite.

A thorough physical examination, along with a complete medical and sexual history, will help the physician determine the underlying cause of impotence. If the cause is determined to be psychological, counseling and/or psychotherapy may be prescribed. If the cause of impotence is determined to be physiological in nature, treatment of the underlying condition may restore normal sexual function. If the underlying physiological cause of impotence is due to an untreatable condition (such as irreversible nerve and/or vascular problems), the patient may choose to have a penile prosthesis surgically implanted.

inguinal hernia
(**ING**-gwih-nal **HER**-nee-ah)

A protrusion of a part of the intestine through a weakened spot in the muscles and membranes of the inguinal region of the abdomen; the intestine pushes into, and sometimes fills, the entire scrotal sac in the male. See Figure 16-5.

The patient may notice a bulge in the inguinal area, particularly when standing; he may also experience a sharp, steady pain in the groin area.

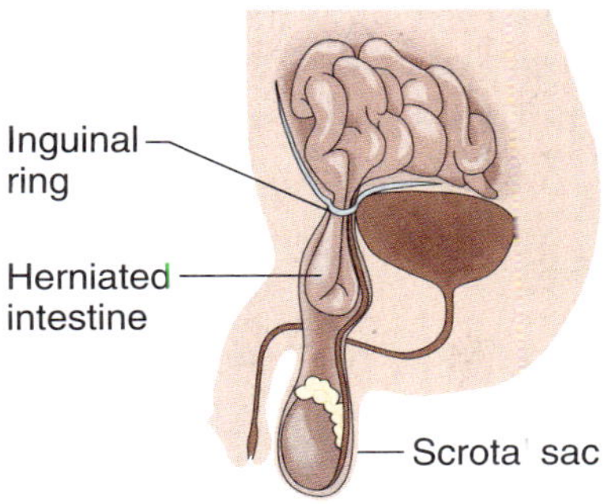

Conservative treatment of an **inguinal hernia** may involve nonsurgical intervention. If the patient is able to press the hernia back into the abdomen, it may be treated with a type of support, called a truss, until the muscle wall strengthens again. If the bulge cannot be gently pressed back into the abdomen, there is a possibility of the herniated intestine being trapped, or strangulated. In this case, surgery will be necessary to return the herniated intestine to its normal environment and to correct the weakened muscle wall. The surgery for a hernia repair is called a herniorrhaphy.

Figure 16-5 Indirect inguinal hernia

orchitis
(or-**KIGH**-tis)
orch/o = testicle
-itis = inflammation

Inflammation of the testes due to a virus, bacterial infection, or injury. The condition may affect one or both testes. Orchitis typically results from the mumps virus.

If the inflammation is severe enough it can result in atrophy (wasting away) of the affected testicle. If severe inflammation involves both testicles, sterility results.

The patient may experience swelling, tenderness, and acute pain in the area. He may also experience fever, chills, nausea and vomiting, and a general feeling of discomfort (**malaise**).

Treatment for orchitis due to bacterial invasion is antibiotics. There is no specific treatment for orchitis caused by the mumps virus other than bed rest and medications to reduce the swelling and fever. All adult men who have never had the mumps virus should take the mumps vaccine as a preventive measure.

phimosis
(fih-**MOH**-sis)

A tightness of the foreskin (prepuce) of the penis that prevents it from being pulled back. The opening of the foreskin narrows due to the tightness and may cause some difficulty with urination.

Phimosis is usually congenital but may be the result of edema and inflammation. Parents of the uncircumcised male infant and adult males who have not been circumcised should understand the importance of proper cleansing of the glans penis. The foreskin should be gently pulled back from the glans penis to clean the area properly. Failure to do this may result in the accumulation of normal secretions and subsequent inflammation of the glans penis (balanitis).

Treatment for phimosis is circumcision (surgery to remove the foreskin).

premature ejaculation
(premature ee-jak-you-**LAY**-shun)

The discharge of seminal fluid prior to complete erection of the penis or immediately after the penis has been introduced into the vaginal canal.

The cause of **premature ejaculation** may be psychological (due to anxiety) or physiological (due to some physical disorder such as diabetes, prostatitis, or urethritis).

A thorough physical examination, along with a complete medical and sexual history, will help the physician determine the underlying cause of premature ejaculation. If the cause is determined to be psychological, counseling and/or psychotherapy may be prescribed. If the cause of premature ejaculation is determined to be physiological in nature, treatment of the underlying condition may restore normal sexual function.

prostatitis
(pross-tah-**TYE**-tis)
prostat/o = prostate gland
-itis = inflammation

Inflammation of the prostate gland.

Prostatitis may be acute (sudden flare-up) or it may be chronic (recurring flare-ups), and may be due to bacterial invasion.

The patient with prostatitis will usually complain of low back pain, fullness or pain in the perineal area, urinary frequency, and discharge from the urethra. An examination of the prostate gland, by **palpation**, will reveal an enlarged, tender prostate gland.

Diagnosis of prostatitis is confirmed with urinalysis, urine culture, and palpation of the prostate gland (via a rectal examination). Treatment involves the use of medications to destroy the bacteria (antimicrobial), medications for pain (analgesics), and medications for fever (antipyretics).

varicocele
(**VAIR**-ih-koh-seel)
-cele = swelling or herniation

An abnormal dilation of the veins of the spermatic cord leading to the testicle.

Each testicle is suspended into the scrotum by a spermatic cord. This stringlike structure is located in the inguinal canal between the scrotum and the abdominal cavity. Each spermatic cord is comprised of arteries, veins, lymphatics, nerves, and the vas deferens of the testis.

A **varicocele** usually causes more discomfort than actual pain. The dilated veins cause some swelling around the testicle. See **Figure 16-6.**

This condition is more common in men between the ages of 15 and 25 and more often affects the left spermatic cord than the right. A varicocele can lower the sperm count because the heat generated from the venous congestion near the testicle may significantly reduce the production of sperm by the testicle.

Treatment for a varicocele consists of relieving the discomfort experienced because of the condition. The patient may be instructed to wear tight-fitting underwear or to use an athletic scrotal supporter until the swelling subsides. If the varicocele causes a great deal of pain, the treatment of choice would be a varicocelectomy to remove the varicocele.

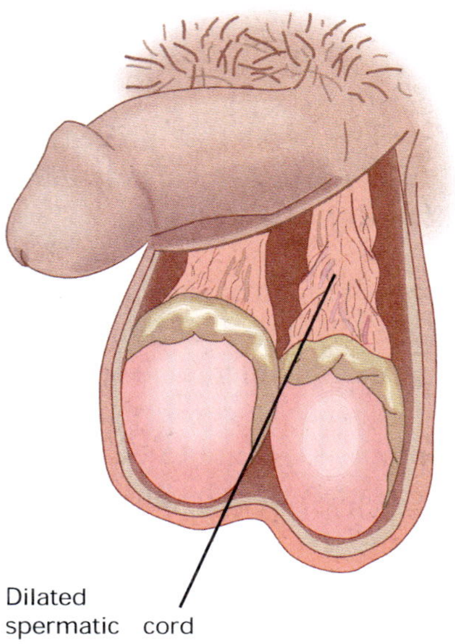

Figure 16-6 Varicocele

Male and Female Sexually Transmitted Diseases

Sexually transmitted diseases (STDs) in the male are the same as those in the female. These contagious diseases are spread from one person to another through contact with body fluids such as blood, semen, and vaginal secretions. STDs may be spread during vaginal, anal, or oral sex, or they may be spread by direct contact with infected skin.

AIDS, which is a sexually transmitted disease, can also be transmitted through blood and blood products, through sharing of needles (as in intravenous drug users), through the placenta of an infected mother to the baby (during the birth process), and through the breast milk of an infected mother to the baby (when nursing the baby).

The incidence of sexually transmitted diseases is alarmingly high in the United States; it has greatly increased in recent years, especially among young people. The following section is a discussion of the more common sexually transmitted diseases.

acquired immunodeficiency syndrome (AIDS)

AIDS is a deadly virus that destroys the body's immune system by invading the helper T lymphocytes (T cells), which play an important part in the body's immune response. The human immunodeficiency virus (HIV) replicates itself within the T cells, destroys the lymphocyte, and then invades other lymphocytes.

HIV is transmitted from person to person through sexual contact, the sharing of HIV-contaminated needles and syringes, and transfusion of infected blood or its components. (The risks of receiving HIV-infected blood through transfusion have been greatly reduced since screening procedures have been improved.) Breastfeeding by HIV-infected women can transmit infection to their infants.

Symptoms are not easily detectable in someone who has been infected with HIV; the condition may lie dormant for years with the individual appearing to be in good health.

Within 1 to 2 weeks after exposure to HIV, the patient may experience a sore throat with fever and body aches. The time period from infection with HIV to the development of detectable antibodies in the blood is usually 1 to 3 months. HIV is transmissible (capable of being passed from one person to another) early after the onset of infection and continues throughout life.

As the disease progresses, the patient may experience enlargement of the lymph glands, fatigue, weight loss, diarrhea, and night sweats. With further progression the body's immune system continues to deteriorate; the patient is susceptible to frequent infections, pneumonia, fever, and malignancies. The most common type of malignancy associated with AIDS is Kaposi's sarcoma, which is an aggressive malignancy of the blood vessels characterized by rapidly growing, purple lesions appearing on the skin, in the mouth, or anywhere in the body.

The time from HIV infection to a diagnosis of AIDS ranges from 1 to 10 years or longer; about half of the HIV-infected adults develop AIDS within 10 years after infection. In the latter stages of AIDS, the patient will eventually die as a result of the repeated bouts of opportunistic infections and/or cancer.

The only sure way to avoid HIV infection through sex is to abstain from sexual intercourse, or to engage in mutually monogamous (only one partner) sexual intercourse with someone known to be uninfected. Latex condoms with water-based lubricants have been shown to reduce the risk of sexual transmission of HIV; it is essential that latex condoms be used correctly each time individuals engage in vaginal, anal, or oral sex.

Both education of the public and health education classes in the schools should stress the facts that having multiple sexual partners and sharing drug paraphernalia increase the risk of infection with HIV. Health care workers should use precautions, known as Standard Precautions, when caring for all patients. These precautions include the wearing of latex gloves, eye protection, and other personal protective equipment to avoid contact with blood and other fluids that are visibly bloody, and taking particular care in handling, using, and disposing of needles.

Selected antiviral agents may prolong life and reduce the risk of the AIDS patient developing opportunistic **infections.** Even though these drugs are used as part of the treatment for AIDS patients, there is no known cure for AIDS and no known treatment for the underlying immune deficiency.

---

chlamydia
(klah-**MID**-ee-ah)

A sexually transmitted bacterial infection that causes inflammation of the cervix (cervicitis) in women and inflammation of the urethra (urethritis) and the epididymis (epididymitis) in men.

Symptoms of chlamydia in men appear 1 to 3 weeks after exposure. These symptoms include a discharge from the penis with burning and itching, along with a burning sensation on urination.

Unfortunately, symptoms do not often appear in women until complications occur as a result of the chlamydial infection.

Early symptoms, however, include a thick vaginal discharge consisting of a combination of mucus and pus (mucopurulent), accompanied by burning and itching. If left untreated, a chlamydial infection can result in pelvic inflammatory disease, which can lead to sterility in the female.

Preventative measures against the spread of chlamydial infections include the use of latex condoms during sexual intercourse. The infection is effectively treated with antibiotic therapy and the patient should refrain from sexual intercourse until the treatment is completed.

---

genital herpes
(**JEN**-ih-tal **HER**-peez)

A highly contagious viral infection of the male and female genitalia; also known as venereal herpes. Caused by the herpes simplex virus (usually HSV-2), genital herpes is transmitted by direct contact with infected body secretions (usually through sexual intercourse). Genital herpes differs from other sexually transmitted

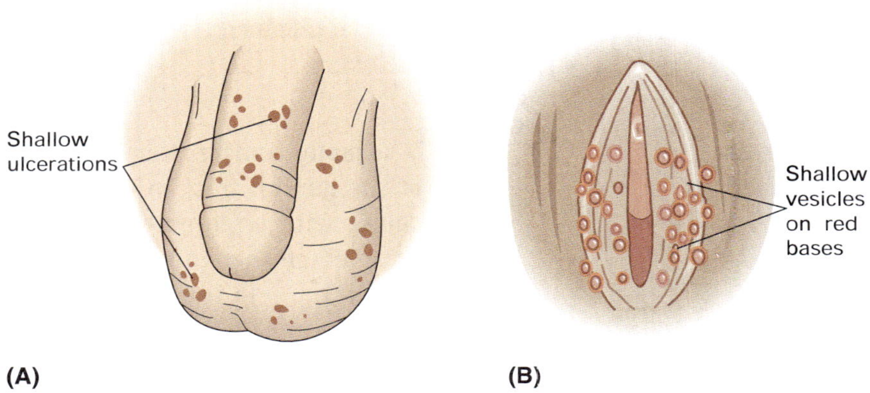

Figure 16-7 Genital herpes (A) in the male; (B) in the female

diseases in that it can recur spontaneously once the virus has been acquired.

This virus is characterized by two phases: the active phase and the dormant phase. The active phase is when the symptoms are present and the virus can be spread. The dormant phase is when the individual is free of symptoms. Unfortunately, some individuals can still transmit the virus during this stage.

Symptoms include multiple shallow ulcerations and/or reddened vesicles of the cervix and vulva in women, and ulcerations of the glans penis, prepuce, or scrotal sac in men. The ulcerations are similar to cold sores, can be very painful, and may be accompanied by itching. See **Figure 16-7.** In addition, the individual may experience flulike symptoms such as fever, headache, malaise, muscle pain (myalgia), swollen glands, and painful urination.

Treatment for genital herpes is symptomatic (the symptoms are treated); that is, medications are given to reduce the swelling and pain. There is no cure for genital herpes. Women who have been diagnosed with genital herpes should be advised to have a Pap smear every 6 months because the virus is known to be associated with cervical cancer.

genital warts
(**JEN**-ih-tal warts)

Small, cauliflower-like, fleshy growths usually seen along the penis in the male and in or near the vagina in women. Genital warts are transmitted from person to person through sexual intercourse; they are caused by the human papillomavirus (HPV). The time span from initial contact with the virus to occurrence of symptoms can be from 1 to 6 months.

The characteristic appearance and location of the genital warts is usually significant enough for a diagnosis. A biopsy may be indicated in some cases for a definitive diagnosis.

Treatment for genital warts is not particularly effective because recurrence is common; however, treatment may include the application of a topical medication to destroy the warts or surgical removal (by cryosurgery or debridement). In some cases, the warts may disappear spontaneously.

Although using latex condoms may reduce the transmission of genital warts, individuals are advised to avoid sexual contact with anyone who has the lesions.

gonorrhea
(**gon**-oh-**REE**-ah)

A sexually transmitted bacterial infection of the mucous membrane of the genital tract in men and women. It is spread by sexual intercourse with an infected partner, and can also be passed on from an infected mother to her infant during the birth process (as the baby passes through the vaginal canal). *Neisseria gonorrhoeae* is the causative organism.

Symptoms of **gonorrhea** differ in the male and female, being much more obvious in the male than in the female. The male may display symptoms such as a greenish-yellow drainage of pus from the urethra (**purulent** drainage), painful urination (**dysuria**), and frequent urination within 2 to 7 days after becoming infected with gonorrhea.

The female infected with gonorrhea may be **asymptomatic** (without symptoms) or she may display symptoms such as a greenish-yellow purulent vaginal discharge, dysuria, urinary frequency. As the infection spreads in the female, inflammation of the fallopian tubes (**salpingitis**) may develop.

Diagnosis is confirmed by culturing the infected body secretions and by microscopic examination of a Gram-stained specimen of the **exudate** (drainage).

Treatment with antibiotics is an effective cure for gonorrhea. Generally, patients with gonorrhea infections should be treated at the same time for presumed chlamydial infections, because their symptoms are often similar and they can occur concurrently. Newborn infants routinely receive an instillation of erythromycin ophthalmic ointment in their eyes immediately after birth as a **prophylaxis** (prevention) against contracting a serious eye infection during the birthing process, due to the presence of gonorrhea or chlamydia in the vaginal canal.

syphilis
(**SIF**-ih-lis)

A sexually transmitted disease characterized by lesions that may involve any organ or tissue. It is spread by sexual intercourse with an infected partner, and can also be passed through the placenta from an infected mother to her unborn infant. The spirochete, *Treponema pallidum*, is the causative organism of this highly contagious disease. If left untreated, this disease progresses through three stages, each with characteristic signs and symptoms: primary syphilis, secondary syphilis, and tertiary syphilis.

1. Primary syphilis is characterized by the appearance of a small, painless, red pustule on the skin or mucous membrane. This highly contagious lesion, known as a **chancre**, appears within 10 days to a few weeks after exposure. The chancre usually develops on the penis of the male and on the labia of the vagina of the female. Primary syphilis can be treated effectively with antibiotics (penicillin G). See **Figure 16-8.**
2. Secondary syphilis occurs approximately 2 months later, if the primary phase of syphilis is left untreated (the spirochetes have had time

to multiply and spread throughout the body). The dominant sign of secondary syphilis is the presence of a nonitching rash on the palms of the hands and the soles of the feet. The individual may also experience symptoms such as headache, sore throat, fever, and a generally poor feeling (malaise), loss of appetite (anorexia), and bone and joint pain. The disease is still highly contagious during the secondary stage, but can be treated effectively with penicillin.

Following the secondary stage of syphilis, the disease (if left untreated) may lie **dormant** (inactive) for 5 to 20 years before reappearing in its final stage.

3. Tertiary syphilis is the final and most serious stage of the disease (in cases of untreated syphilis). Evidence of tertiary syphilis may appear from 2 to 7 years after the initial infection. By this time, the lesions have invaded body organs and systems. The lesions of tertiary syphilis are not reversible, do not respond to treatment with penicillin, and can lead to life-threatening disorders of the brain, spinal cord, and heart.

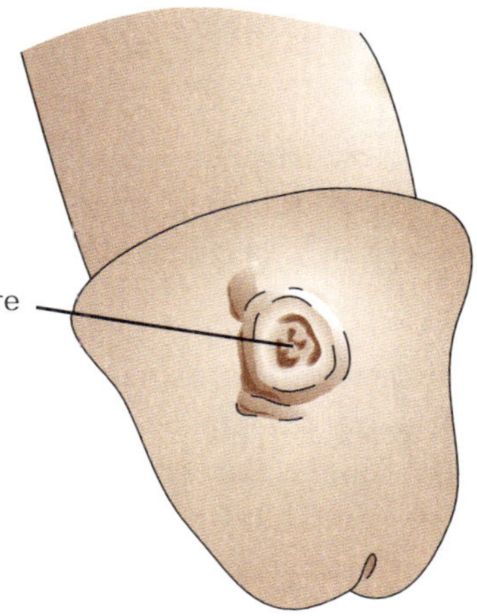

Diagnosis of syphilis is confirmed with microscopic examination of a smear taken from the primary lesion and screening tests for the presence of antibodies in the individual's blood (such as the FTA-ABS or the VDRL).

Treatment of choice for syphilis is administration of penicillin G in the early stages (primary or secondary) before irreversible damage to the body occurs. Following adequate treatment with penicillin, the individual is usually noncontagious within 48 hours.

Individuals who are sexually active should be advised to use latex condoms during sexual intercourse to lessen the chances of contracting syphilis.

Figure 16-8 Primary syphilis: Male

trichomoniasis
(**trik**-oh-moh-**NYE**-ah-sis)

A sexually transmitted protozoal infection of the vagina, urethra, or prostate. It is usually spread by sexual intercourse and affects approximately 15% percent of all sexually active people. The causative organism is *Trichomonas vaginalis*.

Most men are asymptomatic, but some will experience dysuria (painful urination), urinary frequency, and urethritis (inflammation of the urethra).

Women who have **trichomoniasis** will experience symptoms such as itching and burning, and a strong-smelling (**malodorous**) vaginal discharge that is frothy and greenish-yellow. They may also complain of having to change underwear frequently throughout the day due to the drainage and odor.

Diagnosis of trichomoniasis is confirmed by microscopic examination of fresh vaginal secretions from the female or fresh urethral discharge from the male (wet prep).

Treatment of choice for trichomoniasis is an anti-infective drug called Flagyl (metronidazole). It is important that both sexual partners be treated concurrently to prevent passing the infection back and forth.

Diagnostic Techniques and Procedures

castration
(kass-**TRAY**-shun)

The surgical removal of the testicles in the male (or the ovaries in the female); also known as an orchidectomy or orchiectomy in the male, and as an oophorectomy in the female.

Castration is usually performed to reduce the production and secretion of certain hormones that may encourage the growth of malignant (cancerous) cells in either the male or female. An individual who has been castrated is sterile.

cystoscopy
(sis-**TOSS**-koh-pee)
cyst/o = bladder
-scopy = process of viewing

Cystoscopy is the process of visualizing the urinary tract through a cystoscope that has been inserted in the urethra.

circumcision
(sir-kum-**SIH**-shun)

A surgical procedure in which the foreskin (prepuce) of the penis is removed.

Circumcision is widely performed on newborn boys for religious or sociocultural reasons; it may also be performed on adult males who suffer from phimosis (tightness of the foreskin). It is usually performed on the infant during the first or second day of life.

With the infant lying flat on his back and restrained, the penis is exposed and the area is cleansed and draped. A clamp designed especially for circumcisions is placed over the end of the penis, stretching the foreskin tightly. Some physicians apply a local anesthetic to numb the area before excising the foreskin.

After the circumcision is performed, the foreskin can be easily retracted and the glans penis is fully exposed. See **Figure 16-9.**

FTA-ABS test

A serological test for syphilis (performed on blood serum). The acronym stands for fluorescent treponemal antibody-absorption test.

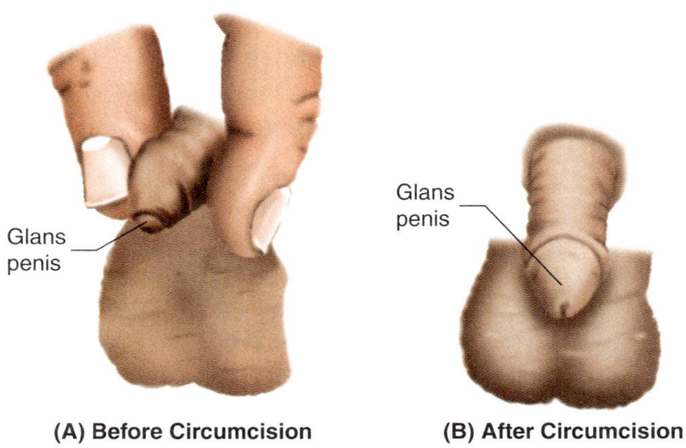

Figure 16-9 Circumcision (A) before and (B) after the procedure

This test uses a fluorescent dye to stain antibodies (as in the treponemal antibody in syphilis) for identification in specimens; the dyed organisms glow visibly when examined under a fluorescent microscope, thus making identification of the causative organism easier. If the test is nonreactive there will be no fluorescence noted.

---

intravenous pyelogram
(in-trah-**VEE**-nuss **PYE**-el-oh-gram)
(IVP)
- **intra-** = within
- **ven/o** = vein
- **-ous** = pertaining to
- **pyel/o** = renal pelvis
- **-gram** = a record

Also known as intravenous pyelography or excretory urogram; this radiographic procedure provides visualization of the entire urinary tract (kidneys, ureters, bladder, and urethra). A contrast dye is injected intravenously and multiple x-ray films are taken as the medium is cleared from the blood by the glomerular filtration of the kidney.

Intravenous pyelogram is useful in diagnosing renal tumors, cysts, or stones, structural or functional abnormalities of the bladder, and ureteral obstruction.

---

orchidectomy
(or-kid-**EK**-toh-mee)
(orchiectomy)
(or-kee-**EK**-toh-mee)
- **orchi/o** = testicle
- **orchid/o** = testicle
- **-ectomy** = surgical removal

The surgical removal of a testicle.

Orchidectomy may be performed when it is determined that an undescended testicle is no longer functional, or as a palliative (relieves the intensity of the symptoms) surgery for cancer of the prostate gland. When used as a palliative surgery, the intent is not to cure the cancer but to halt its spread by removing the hormone, testosterone (which is produced by the testicles).

---

orchidopexy
(**OR**-kid-oh-peck-see)
(orchiopexy)
(or-kee-oh-**PECK**-see)
- **orchi/o** = testicle
- **orchid/o** = testicle
- **-pexy** = surgical fixation

A surgical fixation of a testicle.

This procedure involves making an incision into the inguinal canal, locating the testicle and bringing it back down into the scrotal sac. The surgery is usually done on an outpatient basis, with normal physical activity being restored within a few weeks to a month.

---

semen analysis
(**SEE**-men ah-**NAL**-ih-sis)

An assessment of a sample of semen for volume, viscosity, sperm count, sperm motility, and percentage of any abnormal sperm.

A semen analysis may be performed as part of the evaluation process in attempting to determine the cause of infertility in couples, and is often the first test performed. Also, a semen analysis is performed after a vasectomy to confirm the success of the procedure (male sterility).

A fresh specimen of semen should be collected after a period of abstaining from sexual intercourse for at least 2 to 5 days. The specimen should be delivered to the physician's office within 2 hours after ejaculation and should be protected from the cold.

Examination of a fresh specimen of semen should reveal a very viscous, opaque, grayish-white substance. Examination of a semen specimen after a period of approximately 45 minutes should reveal a more translucent, turbid, and viscous, but more liquid, substance.

The volume of a normal ejaculated specimen should be approximately 3 to 5 ml. A sperm count of more than 20 million sperm/milliliter of semen is considered to be normal; also, approximately 70% of the sperm in a normal specimen should be motile (show movement). The normal semen specimen should contain no more than 25% abnormal sperm forms.

suprapubic prostatectomy
(**soo**-prah-**PEW**-bik **pross**-tah-**TEK**-toh-mee)
supra- = above, over
pub/o = pubis
-ic = pertaining to
prostat/o = prostate gland
-ectomy = surgical removal

The surgical removal of the prostate gland by making an incision into the abdominal wall, just above the pubis.

A small incision is then made into the bladder, which has been distended with fluid. The prostate gland is removed through the bladder cavity.

Suprapubic prostatectomy is done when the surgeon believes that the prostate gland is too enlarged to be removed through the urethra.

transurethral resection of the prostate (TUR or TURP)
(**trans**-you-**REE**-thral **REE**-sek-shun of the **PROSS**-tayt)
trans- = across, through
urethr/o = urethra
-al = pertaining to

The surgical removal of the prostate gland by inserting a resectoscope (an instrument used to remove tissue from the body) through the urethra and into the bladder to remove small pieces of tissue from the prostate gland.

vasectomy
(vas-**EK**-toh-mee)
vas/o = vas deferens; vessel
-ectomy = surgical removal

A surgical cutting and tying of the vas deferens to prevent the passage of sperm, consequently preventing pregnancy; male sterilization. See Figure 16-10.

The vas deferens is the tube that carries the sperm from the testes to the penis. A vasectomy involves making an incision into each side of the scrotal sac, exposing the vas deferens, and cutting it. The ends are tied separately, and may then be cauterized for additional blockage. Because sperm may remain in the vas deferens for a month or more after the vasectomy, it is important for the man and his sex partner to remember that additional protection during sexual intercourse will be necessary until his physician verifies that all of the sperm have been eliminated from the vas deferens. The man will have to submit periodic semen samples to be examined for presence of sperm. When two separate semen samples show no evidence of sperm, the man is considered to be sterile.

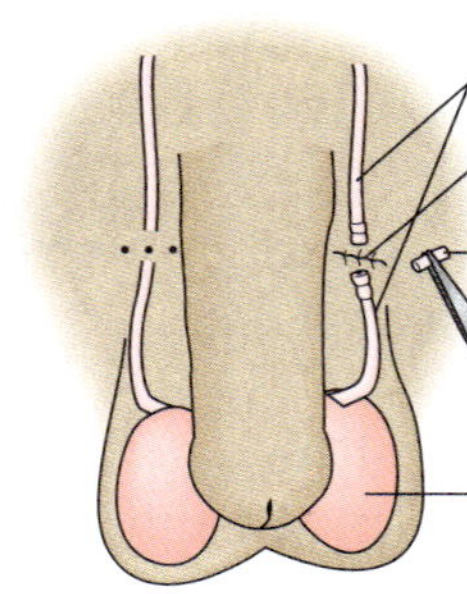

Figure 16-10 Vasectomy

VDRL test

A serological test for syphilis (test performed on blood serum); widely used to test for primary and secondary syphilis. The acronym stands for venereal disease research laboratory test.

The VDRL test generally becomes positive in 1 to 3 weeks after the appearance of a chancre. This test examines the patient's serum under the microscope (after it has been heat-treated and mixed with the VDRL antigen) for the presence of clumping, which indicates a reaction. The results are reported as reactive (medium to large clumps present), weakly reactive (small clumps noted), or nonreactive (no clumping noted). Reactive and weakly reactive results on the VDRL test are considered to be positive for syphilis. If positive, further testing is done to confirm the presence of the spirochete, *Treponema pallidum.*

wet mount; wet prep

The microscopic examination of fresh vaginal or male urethral secretions to test for the presence of living organisms.

A specimen of vaginal or urethral secretions is placed on two separate clean microscopic slides and a drop of normal saline is placed on top of one specimen (to check for the presence of trichomoniasis), while a drop of potassium hydroxide is placed on top of the other specimen (to check for yeast or fungi). After the specimen is mixed with the solution, a cover slip is placed on the slide and the organisms are immediately observed under the microscope.

Common Abbreviations

ABBREVIATION	DEFINITION	ABBREVIATION	DEFINITION
BPH	benign prostatic hypertrophy	**KUB**	kidneys, ureters, bladder; an x-ray of the urinary tract using no contrast medium
FTA-ABS	fluorescent treponemal antibody-absorption test; a serological test for syphilis	**NGU**	nongonococcal urethritis
GC	gonorrhea; gonococcus	**STS**	serological test for syphilis
GU	genitourinary	**TUR, TURP**	transurethral resection of the prostate gland
HSV-2	herpes simplex virus, strain 2	**VDRL**	venereal disease research laboratory
IVP	intravenous pyelogram		

Written and Audio Terminology Review

Review each of the following terms from this chapter. Study the spelling of each term and write the definition in the space provided. If you have the Audio CD available, listen to each term, pronounce it, and check the box once you are comfortable saying the word. Check definitions by looking the term up in the glossary/index.

TERM	PRONUNCIATION	DEFINITION
android	☐ **AN**-droyd	________________
anorchism	☐ an-**OR**-kizm	________________
asymptomatic	☐ ay-simp-toh-**MAT**-ik	________________

Term		Pronunciation	
azoospermia	☐	ah-zoh-oh-**SPER**-mee-ah	______
balanitis	☐	bal-ah-**NYE**-tis	______
balanoplasty	☐	**BAL**-ah-noh-**plas**-tee	______
benign prostatic hypertrophy	☐	bee-**NYEN** pross-**TAT**-ik high-**PER**-troh-fee	______
castration	☐	kass-**TRAY**-shun	______
chancre	☐	**SHANG**-ker	______
chlamydia	☐	klah-**MID**-ee-ah	______
circumcision	☐	sir-kum-**SIH**-shun	______
Cowper's glands	☐	**KOW**-perz glands	______
cryosurgery	☐	kry-oh-**SER**-jer-ee	______
cryptorchidism	☐	kript-**OR**-kid-izm	______
cystoscopy	☐	sis-**TOSS**-koh-pee	______
debridement	☐	day-breed-**MON**	______
dormant	☐	**DOOR**-mant	______
dysuria	☐	dis-**YOO**-ree-ah	______
ejaculation	☐	ee-jack-yoo-**LAY**-shun	______
epididymectomy	☐	**ep**-ih-**did**-ih-**MEK**-toh-mee	______
epididymis	☐	**ep**-ih-**DID**-ih-mis	______
epididymitis	☐	**ep**-ih-**did**-ih-**MYE**-tis	______
epispadias	☐	**ep**-ih-**SPAY**-dee-as	______
exudates	☐	**EKS**-yoo-dayt	______
foreskin	☐	**FOR**-skin	______
genital herpes	☐	**JEN**-ih-tal **HER**-peez	______
genital warts	☐	**JEN**-ih-tal warts	______
glans penis	☐	**GLANS PEE**-nis	______
gonad	☐	**GOH**-nad	______
gonorrhea	☐	**gon**-oh-**REE**-ah	______
hydrocele	☐	**HIGH**-droh-seel	______
hypospadias	☐	high-poh-**SPAY**-dee-as	______
impotence	☐	**IM**-poh-tens	______
inguinal hernia	☐	**ING**-gwih-nal **HER**-nee-ah	______

Term		Pronunciation	
intravenous pyelogram	☐	in-trah-**VEE**-nuss **PYE**-el-oh-gram	____
malaise	☐	mah-**LAYZ**	____
malodorous	☐	mal-**OH**-dor-us	____
mucopurulent	☐	mew-koh-**PEWR**-yoo-lent	____
opportunistic	☐	op-or-toon-**IS**-tik	____
orchidectomy	☐	or-kid-**EK**-toh-mee	____
orchiectomy	☐	or-kee-**EK**-toh-mee	____
orchidopexy	☐	**OR**-kid-oh-peck-see	____
orchiopexy	☐	or-kee-oh-**PECK**-see	____
orchidoplasty	☐	**OR**-kid-oh-plass-tee	____
orchitis	☐	or-**KIGH**-tis	____
palpation	☐	pal-**PAY**-shun	____
pelvic inflammatory disease	☐	**PELL**-vik in-**FLAM**-mah-tor-ee dih-**ZEEZ**	____
perineum	☐	pair-ih-**NEE**-um	____
phimosis	☐	fih-**MOH**-sis	____
premature ejaculation	☐	premature ee-jak-you-**LAY**-shun	____
prepuce	☐	**PRE**-pus	____
prophylaxis	☐	proh-fih-**LAK**-sis	____
prostate	☐	**PROSS**-tayt	____
prostatectomy	☐	pross-tah-**TEK**-toh-mee	____
prostatitis	☐	pross-tah-**TYE**-tis	____
purulent	☐	**PEWR**-yoo-lent	____
rectoscope	☐	**REK**-toh-skohp	____
resectoscope	☐	ree-**SEK**-toh-skohp	____
residual urine	☐	rih-**ZID**-yoo-al **YOO**-rin	____
salpingitis	☐	sal-pin-**JYE**-tis	____
scrotum	☐	**SKROH**-tum	____
semen	☐	**SEE**-men	____
semen analysis	☐	**SEE**-men ah-**NAL**-ih-sis	____

Term		Pronunciation	
seminal vesicles	☐	**SEM**-ih-nal **VESS**-ih-kls	______
seminiferous tubules	☐	sem-in-**IF**-er-us **TOO**-byoo-ls	______
spermatogenesis	☐	**sper**-mat-oh-**JEN**-eh-sis	______
spermatozoa	☐	**sper**-mat-oh-**ZOH**-ah	______
spermatozoon	☐	**sper**-mat-oh-**ZOH**-on	______
spermolysis	☐	sperm-**OL**-ih-sis	______
suprapubic prostatectomy	☐	**soo**-prah-**PEW**-bik **pross**-tah-**TEK**-toh-mee	______
syphilis	☐	**SIF**-ih-lis	______
testicle	☐	**TES**-tih-kl	______
testicular	☐	tess-**TIK**-yoo-lar	______
testosterone	☐	tess-**TOSS**-ter-own	______
transurethral resection	☐	**trans**-you-**REE**-thral **REE**-sek-shun	______
trichomoniasis	☐	**trik**-oh-moh-**NYE**-ah-sis	______
urethra	☐	**YOO**-ree-thrah	______
urethritis	☐	yoo-ree-**THRYE**-tis	______
varicocele	☐	**VAIR**-ih-koh-seel	______
vas deferens	☐	vas **DEF**-er-enz	______
vasectomy	☐	vas-**EK**-toh-mee	______
vesicles	☐	**VESS**-ih-kls	______

Chapter Review Exercises

The following exercises provide a more in-depth review of the chapter material. Your goal in these exercises is to complete each section at a minimum 80% level of accuracy. If you score below 80% in any area, return to the appropriate section in the chapter and read the material again. A place has been provided for your score at the end of each section.

A. Spelling

Circle the correctly spelled term in each pairing of words. Each correct answer is worth 10 points. Record your score in the space provided at the end of the exercise.

1. epididymis   epididymus
2. azospermia   azoospermia

3. seminal	seminel
4. orchipexy	orchiopexy
5. prostatectomy	prostratectomy
6. syphilis	syphillis
7. variocele	varicocele
8. vas deferens	vas defrens
9. epispadias	episapdius
10. impotent	imputent

***Number correct* ______ × *10 points/correct answer: Your score* _____%**

B. Matching

Match the terms on the left with the appropriate definition on the right. Each correct answer is worth 10 points. Record your score in the space provided at the end of the exercise.

______ 1. balanitis	a. Blisters
______ 2. chancre	b. The process of expelling the semen from the male urethra
______ 3. glans penis	c. Congenital defect in which the urethra opens on the upper side of the penis at some point near the glans
______ 4. prepuce	d. A skin lesion, usually of primary syphilis, that begins at the site of infection as a small raised area and develops into a red, painless ulcer with a scooped-out appearance; also known as a venereal sore
______ 5. hypospadias	e. A loose, retractable fold of skin covering the tip of the penis
______ 6. epispadias	f. Sac that houses the testicles
______ 7. spermatogenesis	g. Inflammation of the glans penis
______ 8. ejaculation	h. The tip of the penis
______ 9. scrotum	i. The formation of sperm
______ 10. vesicles	j. A congenital defect in which the urethra opens on the underside of the penis instead of at the end

***Number correct* ______ × *10 points/correct answer: Your score* _____%**

C. Definition to Term

Using the following definitions, provide the medical term to match the definition. Each correct answer is worth 10 points. Record your score in the space provided at the end of this exercise.

Create a word that means:

1. Pertaining to male

   ____

2. Condition of undescended testicles

   ____

3. Inflammation of the testicles

____

4. Destruction of sperm

____

5. Surgical removal of the vas deferens

____

6. Inflammation of the glans penis

____

7. Formation of sperm

____

8. Surgical fixation of the testicles

____

9. Inflammation of the prostate gland

____

10. Surgery involving the rapid freezing of tissue

____

Number correct ______ × 10 points/correct answer: Your score _____%

D. Matching Procedures

Match the procedures on the left with the appropriate description on the right. Each correct answer is worth 10 points. Record your score in the space provided at the end of the exercise.

_____ 1. cryosurgery
_____ 2. circumcision
_____ 3. semen analysis
_____ 4. castration
_____ 5. TURP
_____ 6. vasectomy
_____ 7. suprapubic prostatectomy
_____ 8. orchiopexy
_____ 9. VDRL
_____ 10. PSA-2 test

a. A serological test for syphilis, performed on blood serum
b. A test in which elevated levels indicate significant prostatic hypertrophy; used to confirm or rule out a diagnosis of cancer of the prostate
c. The surgical removal of the testicles in the male
d. A surgical procedure in which the foreskin of the penis is removed
e. The destruction of tissue by rapid freezing with substances such as liquid nitrogen
f. A surgical fixation of a testicle
g. Assessment of a sample of semen for volume, viscosity, sperm count, motility, and percentage of any abnormal sperm
h. The surgical removal of the prostate gland by making an incision into the abdominal wall, just above the pubis
i. The surgical removal of the prostate gland by inserting a resectoscope through the urethra and into the bladder
j. Surgically cutting and tying the vas deferens to prevent the passage of sperm

Number correct ______ × 10 points/correct answer: Your score _____%

E. Crossword Puzzle

Read the clues carefully and complete the puzzle. Each crossword answer is worth 10 points. When you have completed the crossword puzzle, total your points and enter your score in the space provided.

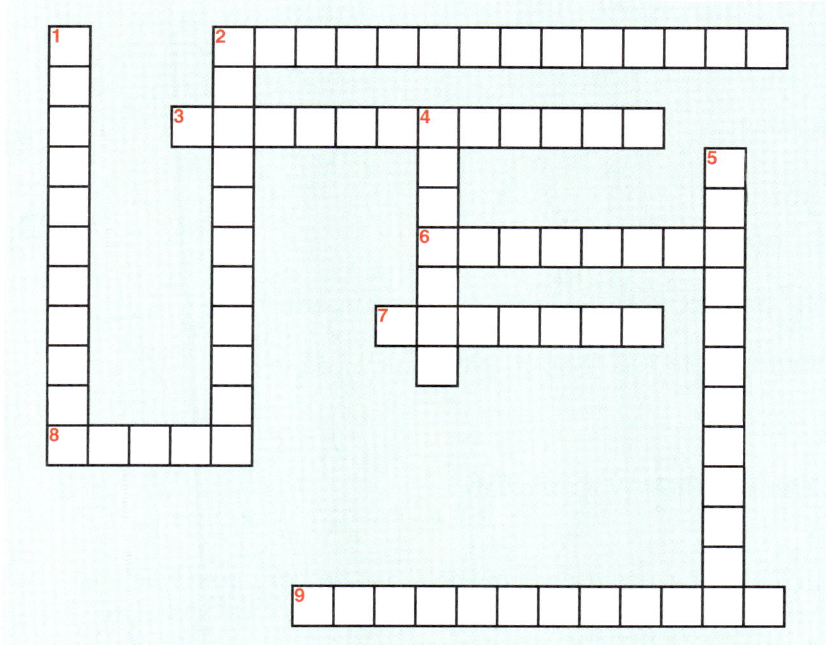

ACROSS

2 Removal of the epididymis
3 Surgical repair of the glans penis
6 Gland that surrounds male urethra
7 Sac that houses the testicles
8 Combination of sperm and secretions
9 Male hormone

DOWN

1 Tube that transports sperm
2 Expulsion of semen from urethra
4 Foreskin
5 Mature male germ cell

Number correct ______ × 10 points/correct answer: Your score _____%

F. Proofreading Skills

Read the following report. For each boldface term, provide a brief definition and indicate if the term is spelled correctly. If it is misspelled, provide the correct spelling. Each correct answer is worth 10 points. Record your score in the space provided at the end of this exercise.

HILLCREST Medical Center

NAME: Walker, Adam

ROOM NO: 4275

HOSPITAL NO: 186902

PREOPERATIVE DIAGNOSIS: Benigne Prostatic **Hyperthrophy**

POSTOPERATIVE DIAGNOSIS: Benign **Prostratic** Hypertrophy

ANESTHESIA: Spinal

OPERATION: Transurethral Prostatectomy

PROCEDURE: With the patient in lithotomy position, the **perineum** was prepared and draped in the usual manner. The **glands penis** and the **urether** were lubricated and dilated with the appropriate sound. A **resectoscope** was inserted through the urethra and was advanced with ease into the bladder. No abnormalities were noted within the bladder. The enlarged portion of the prostate gland was then **resected** out in small pieces and was irrigated out through the resectoscope without any difficulty. **Hemastasis** was achieved with electrocoagulation. A No. 26 Foley catheter was inserted into the **bladder** with the 30 cc balloon being inflated to capacity. Blood loss was minimal at 100 cc, with no replacement necessary.

The patient was returned to the recovery room in stable condition with 1000 cc. Ringer's Lactate infusing at a slow drip.

DICTATED BY: Dr. Yesia Amm

DATE OF DICTATION: 10-27-03

______________________________ MD

Signature of Surgeon

Example:

resected Surgically cut out; removed

Spelled correctly? ☑ Yes ☐ No ______

1. **benigne** ______

   Spelled correctly? ☐ Yes ☐ No ______

2. **hyperthrophy** ______

   Spelled correctly? ☐ Yes ☐ No ______

3. **prostratic** ______

   Spelled correctly? ☐ Yes ☐ No ______

4. **transurethral** ______

   Spelled correctly? ☐ Yes ☐ No ______

5. **perineum** ______

   Spelled correctly? ☐ Yes ☐ No ______

6. **glands penis** ______

   Spelled correctly? ☐ Yes ☐ No ______

7. **urether** ______

   Spelled correctly? ☐ Yes ☐ No ______

8. **resectoscope** ______

   Spelled correctly? ☐ Yes ☐ No ______

9. **hemastasis** ______

   Spelled correctly? ☐ Yes ☐ No ______

10. **bladder** ______

    Spelled correctly? ☐ Yes ☐ No ______

Number correct ______ × 10 points/correct answer: Your score _____%

G. Word Search

Using the definitions listed, identify the appropriate word and then find and circle it in the puzzle. The words may be read up, down, diagonally, across, or backward. Each correct answer is worth 10 points. Record your score in the space provided at the end of the exercise.

```
C O L P O S C O P Y A I D S L A R O S C O H
O R E E N D C M A N B R U R E T H R I T I S
N A Y C A R H I N O M S T F R I A B L U J S
I E Z O V K L I E N T I S I C P E L M I S T
Z R S I S E A N E C O L L U C I N V A S I E
A C C D E U M P O P I I A P E R Y A I P O R
T N I M E S Y Y O T R H P S O U N D Y E A O
I A O M M A D G R S E P R E H L A T I N E G
O H E V A S I X E N I Y R I E S P Y A V I A
N C I H A T A O X R S S O T Y H V E N I L L
C R Y O R U R G I N Y U A A R C O N I C U P
A S P I R R T U L V E M C R B I O L O U G I
S A W E T M O U N T C E O R C H A P H L Y N
T Y P O G R A N I C U N P A R O O L U T E G
A D V E N T T U O E O S Y I N T M R M R L O
M E D I C A W E L G E N I T A L W A R T S G
R I G H E N D O M E T R I A L B I O P S Y R
Y O U R A N S W E I R I S C O R R U J O I A
T E R M I B O L O G V I N T R A U T E U R P
I N T R I C H O M O N I A S I S R O N N M H
C L A S S I F I C B R A E N D O S C O D U Y
P A P K A P O S I S S A R C O M A U R E T H
```

Example: Men who contract trichomoniasis may experience dysuria and inflammation of the urethra, which is known as

urethritis ________________________________

1. Also known as acquired immunodeficiency syndrome

____

2. An aggressive malignancy of the blood vessels characterized by rapidly growing, purple lesions appearing on the skin, in the mouth, or anywhere in the body

____

3. A sexually transmitted bacterial infection that can cause cervicitis and pelvic inflammatory disease in women, and urethritis and epididymitis in men

____

4. A highly contagious viral infection caused by the herpes simplex virus; it can recur spontaneously once the virus has been acquired

____

5. Small, cauliflower-like, fleshy growths usually seen along the penis in the male and in or near the vagina in women; sexually transmitted

____

6. Diagnosis of this sexually transmitted bacterial infection (of the mucous membrane of the genital tract in men and women) is confirmed by culturing the infected body secretions and by examination of a Gram-stained specimen of the drainage

____

7. If left untreated, this sexually transmitted disease progresses through three stages, each with characteristic signs and symptoms

____

8. A sexually transmitted pear-shaped, protozoal infection that causes a profuse vaginal discharge in the female (greenish-yellow)

____

9. A procedure in which a fresh sample of vaginal or urethral secretions are examined under the microscope for presence of active organisms

____

10. A highly contagious lesion that appears within 10 days to a few weeks after exposure to syphilis

____

Number correct ______ × 10 points/correct answer: Your score _____%

H. Matching Conditions

Match the pathological conditions on the left with the appropriate definition on the right. Each correct answer is worth 10 points. Record your score in the space provided at the end of the exercise.

_____ 1. phimosis
_____ 2. epispadias
_____ 3. cryptorchidism
_____ 4. anorchism
_____ 5. cancer of the prostate
_____ 6. hypospadias
_____ 7. impotence
_____ 8. cancer of the testes
_____ 9. inguinal hernia
_____ 10. orchitis

a. The absence of one or both testicles
b. Malignant growth of the gland that surrounds the base of the urethra in the male
c. A congenital defect in which the urethra opens on the underside of the penis instead of at the end
d. Inflammation of the testes due to a virus, bacterial infection, or injury
e. The inability of a male to achieve or sustain an erection of the penis
f. Condition of undescended testicles
g. A congenital defect in which the urethra opens on the upper side of the penis at some point near the glans
h. A tightness of the foreskin of the penis of the male infant that prevents it from being pulled back
i. A protrusion of a part of the intestine through a weakened spot in the muscles and membranes of the inguinal region of the abdomen
j. A malignant tumor of the primary organs of the male reproductive system; malignancy of the male gonads

Number correct ______ × 10 points/correct answer: Your score _____%

I. Completion

Complete the following definitions by filling in the blanks with the most appropriate word. Each correct answer is worth 10 points. Record your score in the space provided at the end of the exercise.

1. Loss of appetite is known as ____________________.
2. A pair of small, pea-sized glands that empty into the urethra just before it extends through the penis (known as Cowper's glands) are called the ____________________ glands.
3. When a disease, such as syphilis, remains inactive for a period of time it is said to be _____________.
4. A tightly coiled tubule that houses the sperm until they mature is known as the _____________.
5. A loose, retractable fold of skin covering the tip of the penis is the foreskin, or ____________________.
6. A vague feeling of bodily weakness or discomfort, often marking the onset of disease or illness is known as ____________________.
7. An infection that sets up in a host whose resistance has been decreased is known as an _____________.
8. The area between the scrotum and the anus in the male is known as the ____________________.
9. The specialized coils of tiny tubules that are responsible for production of sperm and are located in the testes are known as the ____________________.
10. A male hormone secreted by the testes responsible for the secondary sex characteristic changes that occur in the male with the onset of puberty is ____________________.

Number correct ______ × 10 points/correct answer: Your score _____%

J. Multiple Choice

Read each statement carefully and select the correct answer from the options listed. Each correct answer is worth 10 points. Record your score in the space provided at the end of the exercise.

1. The medical term for surgical repair of the glans penis is:
   a. balanoplasty
   b. debridement
   c. cryosurgery
   d. prostatectomy
2. Inflammation of the urethra is known as:
   a. ureteritis
   b. salpingitis
   c. balanoplasty
   d. urethritis
3. The medical term for painful urination is:
   a. pyuria
   b. dysuria
   c. hematuria
   d. oliguria
4. The area between the scrotum and the anus in the male is called the:
   a. prepuce
   b. peritoneum
   c. perineum
   d. truss

5. The absence of one or both testicles is termed:
   a. balanitis
   b. prostatitis
   c. orchitis
   d. anorchism
6. A congenital defect in which the urethra opens on the underside of the penis instead of at the end is known as:
   a. hypospadias
   b. epispadias
   c. cryptorchidism
   d. orchitis
7. The surgical removal of the testicles in the male is known as:
   a. circumcision
   b. castration
   c. orchidopexy
   d. vasectomy
8. A surgical procedure in which the foreskin (prepuce) of the penis is removed is known as:
   a. circumcision
   b. castration
   c. orchidopexy
   d. vasectomy
9. An x-ray of the urinary tract using no contrast medium is known as a:
   a. HSV-2
   b. VDRL
   c. KUB
   d. NGU
10. A male sterilization is called a:
   a. vasectomy
   b. circumcision
   c. orchidopexy
   d. semen analysis

Number correct ______ × 10 points/correct answer: Your score ______%

Answers to Chapter Review Exercises

A. Spelling

1. epididymis
2. azoospermia
3. seminal
4. orchiopexy
5. prostatectomy
6. syphilis
7. varicocele
8. vas deferens
9. epispadias
10. impotent

B. Matching

1. g
2. d
3. h
4. e
5. j
6. c
7. i
8. b
9. f
10. a

C. Definition to Term

1. android
2. cryptorchidism
3. orchiditis
4. spermolysis
5. vasectomy
6. balanitis
7. spermatogenesis
8. orchiopexy
9. prostatitis
10. cryosurgery

D. Matching Procedures

1. e
2. d
3. g
4. c
5. i
6. j
7. h
8. f
9. a
10. b

E. Crossword Puzzle

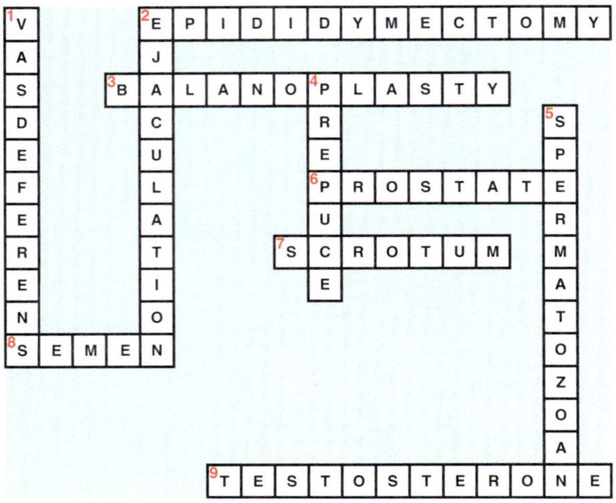

F. Proofreading Skills

1. Noncancerous.
   Spelled correctly? No **benign**
2. Increase in size of an organ by the growth or increase in the size of its cells rather than an increase in the number of cells.
   Spelled correctly? No **hypertrophy**
3. Pertaining to the prostate gland.
   Spelled correctly? No **prostatic**
4. By way of or through (across) the urethra.
   Spelled correctly? Yes
5. The area between the scrotum and the anus in the male.
   Spelled correctly? Yes
6. The distal end or the tip of the penis where the urethral orifice is usually located.
   Spelled correctly? No **glans penis**
7. In the male, a small tubular structure that begins at the bladder, advances through the middle of the prostate gland, and finally proceeds through the urinary meatus of the penis. The urethra transports urine from the bladder, and semen when ejaculated, to the outside of the body.
   Spelled correctly? No **urethra**
8. An instrument used to remove tissue.
   Spelled correctly? Yes
9. The cessation, or stopping, of bleeding.
   Spelled correctly? No **hemostasis**
10. A membranous sac that serves as a receptacle for urine.
    Spelled correctly? Yes

G. Word Search

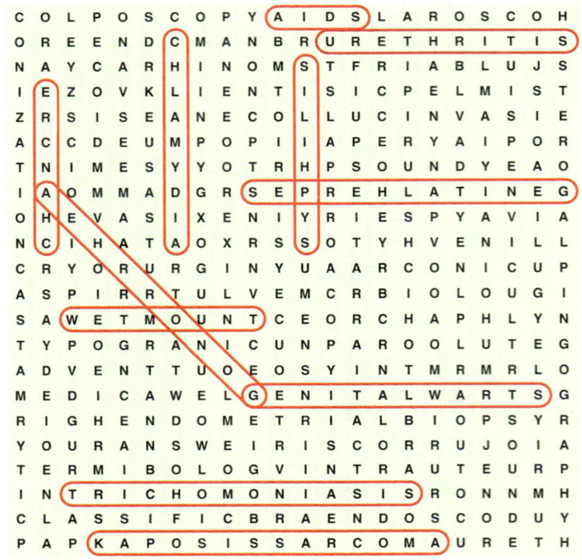

H. Matching Conditions

1. h
2. g
3. f
4. a
5. b
6. c
7. e
8. j
9. i
10. d

I. Completion

1. anorexia
2. bulbourethral
3. dormant
4. epididymis
5. prepuce
6. malaise
7. opportunistic infection
8. perineum
9. seminiferous tubules
10. testosterone

J. Multiple Choice

1. a
2. d
3. b
4. c
5. d
6. a
7. b
8. a
9. c
10. a

CHAPTER 17

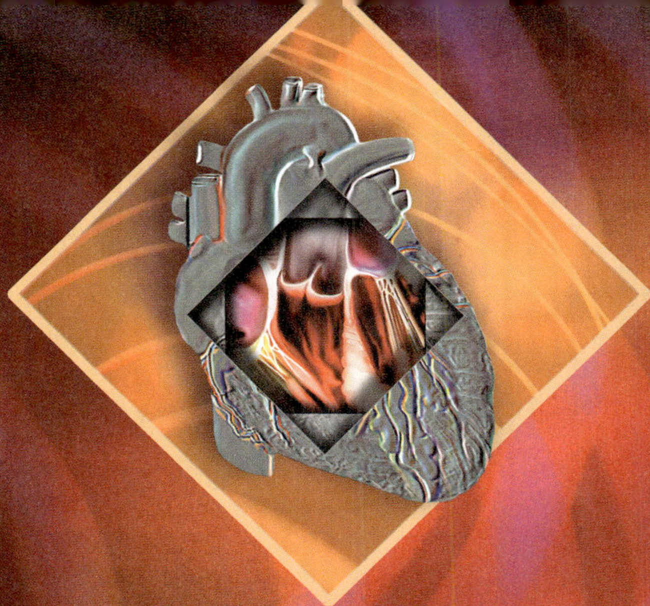

The Female Reproductive System

CHAPTER CONTENT

KEY COMPETENCIES

Upon completing this chapter and the review exercises at the end of the chapter, the learner should be able to:

1. Identify the four phases of the menstrual cycle.
2. Correctly spell and pronounce each new term introduced in this chapter using the Activity CD-ROM and Audio CD, if available.
3. Identify 10 abbreviations common to the female reproductive system.
4. Identify and define at least 10 pathological conditions of the female reproductive system.
5. Identify at least 10 diagnostic techniques used in treating disorders of the female reproductive system.
6. Demonstrate the ability to proof and correct a transcription exercise relative to the female reproductive system by completing the appropriate exercise at the end of the chapter.
7. Demonstrate the ability to correctly identify and label the internal genitalia of the female reproductive system, using the diagram provided at the end of the chapter.
8. Identify five secondary sex characteristic changes that occur in the female body at the onset of puberty.
9. Identify and define four surgical approaches to removing a malignant growth from the female breast.
10. Identify the steps involved in breast self-examination.
11. Identify the five traditional classifications of Pap smear findings.

OVERVIEW

To understand medical care basic to women and the childbearing process, the health care professional must be knowledgeable of the structures and function of the female reproductive system. The medical specialty that deals with diseases and disorders of the female reproductive system is known as **gynecology** (gynec/o = woman + logy = the study of). The physician who specializes in the field of gynecology is known as a **gynecologist** (gynec/o = woman + logist = one who specializes in the study of). This chapter is devoted to the study of the anatomy and physiology of the female reproductive system and gynecology. The study of obstetrics (childbirth) is covered in Chapter 18.

As complex as it may seem, the female reproductive system serves a very basic purpose: that of reproduction. After the onset of puberty, the female reproductive system begins the monthly repetition of providing an environment suitable for **fertilization** of the **ovum** (female egg) and then implantation of that ovum. **Puberty** is the period of life at which the ability to reproduce begins and the development of secondary sex characteristic changes, such as breast development, growth of pubic hair, and menstruation, occur.

The structures of the female reproductive system provide the environment for **coitus** (sexual intercourse), also known as copulation. If fertilization and implantation of the ovum occur, the female reproductive system then sustains the **pregnancy**, providing for the growth, development, and birth of the baby. If fertilization does not occur, the receptive environment changes with the shedding of the uterine lining through a bloody discharge (**menstruation**). This cyclic process repeats itself each month throughout the female's reproductive years. The end of the reproductive period is marked by the cessation, or stopping, of the menstrual cycles. This is known as **menopause**, or **climacteric**, and is characterized by a decrease in hormone production.

Anatomy and Physiology

In this section we will discuss the external and internal genitalia of the female reproductive system, the breasts (accessory organs), and the shape of the female pelvis and its relationship to childbearing. The **mammary** glands are considered accessory organs of the female reproductive system because they play a part in the overall process, by producing milk for nourishing the infant (lactation).

External Genitalia

The **external genitalia** consists of the mons pubis, labia majora, clitoris, labia minora, vestibule, urinary meatus, vaginal orifice, Bartholin's glands, and the perineum. Collectively, the external genitalia is referred to as the **vulva** or **pudendum.** See **Figure 17-1.** As you continue to read about the external genitalia, refer to this figure for a visual reference.

The **(1) mons pubis** is the fatty tissue that covers and cushions the symphysis pubis. The triangular pattern of hair that covers the mons pubis appears after the onset of puberty.

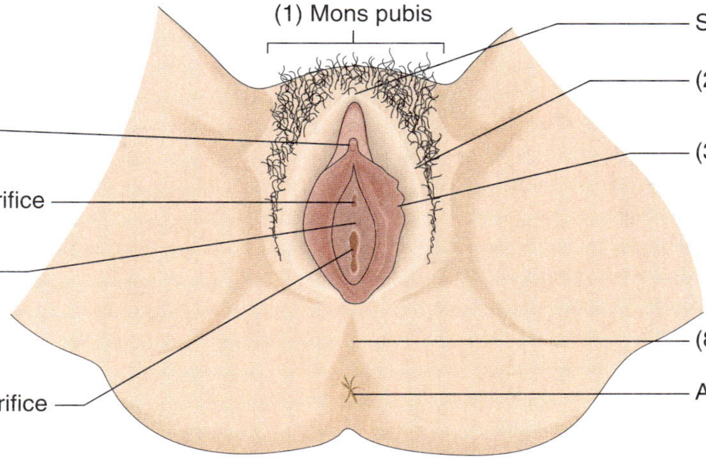

Figure 17-1 External genitalia, female reproductive system

The (2) **labia majora** consists of two folds of skin containing fatty tissue and covered with hair that lie on either side of the vaginal opening, extending from the mons pubis to the perineum. The outer surface of the labia majora is covered by pubic hair; the inner surface is smooth and moist. The (3) **labia minora** consists of two thin folds of tissue located within the folds of the labia majora. The labia minora extends from the clitoris, downward toward the perineum. The point at which the labia minora comes together at the lower or posterior edge of the vaginal opening is known as the **fourchette**. The vestibule is an oval-shaped area between the labia minora containing the urinary meatus, the vaginal orifice, and the **Bartholin's glands**. The Bartholin's glands are located one on each side of the vaginal orifice. They secrete a mucous substance that lubricates the vagina. The labia minora encloses the vestibule and its structures.

The (4) **clitoris** is a short, elongated organ composed of erectile tissue. It is located just behind the upper junction of the labia minora and is homologous to the penis in the male. The (5) **urinary orifice** is not a true part of the female reproductive system, but is mentioned here because it is included as a part of the vulva. The urinary meatus is located just above the vaginal orifice. The (6) **vaginal orifice** is located in the lower portion of the vestibule, below the urinary meatus. The vaginal orifice (opening) is also known as the **vaginal introitus.**

A thin layer of elastic, connective tissue membrane, known as the (7) **hymen**, forms a border around the outer opening of the vagina and may partially cover the vaginal opening. The hymen may remain intact or may be stretched and torn during sexual intercourse or by other means, such as physical activity or using tampons. Therefore, although some cultures still believe that an intact hymen is proof of virginity, its presence does not prove or disprove virginity. If the hymen remains intact and completely covers the vaginal opening, it is termed an **imperforate hymen,** and must be surgically perforated (punctured) before menstruation begins, thus allowing the menstrual flow to escape.

The (8) **perineum** is the area between the vaginal orifice and the anus. It consists of muscular and fibrous tissue and serves as support for the pelvic structures. This thick muscular area thins out during the labor process and is sometimes torn during the stress of childbirth. The physician may choose to surgically incise the area to enlarge the vaginal opening for delivery. If this is done, the incision is called an episiotomy. This term will be discussed more in Chapter 18.

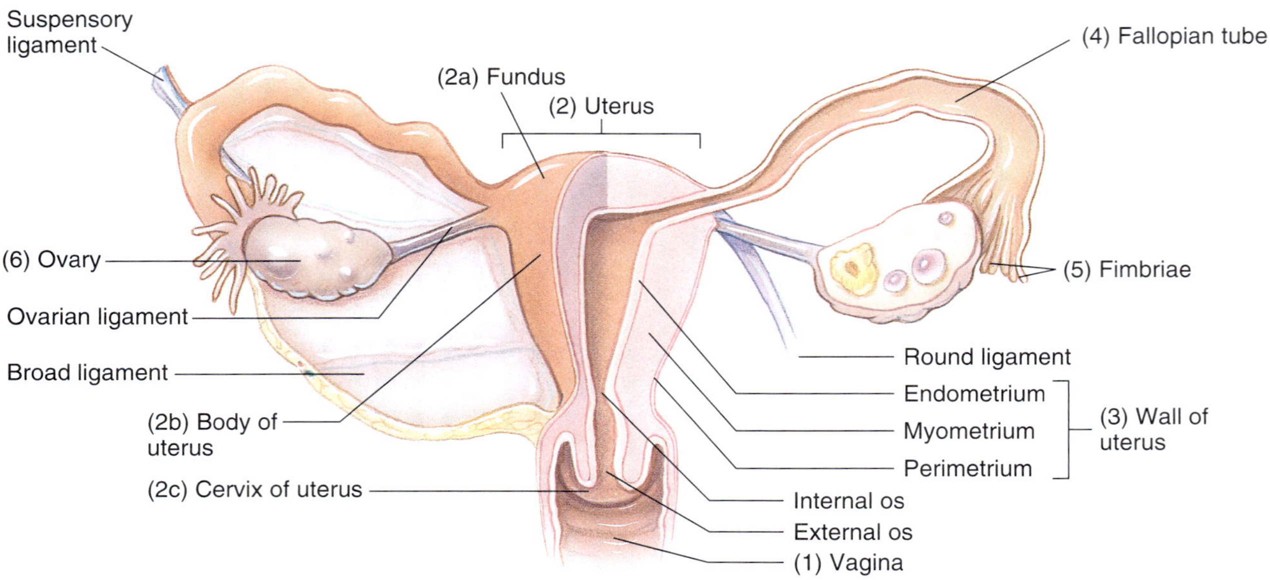

Figure 17-2 Internal genitalia, female reproductive system

Internal Genitalia

The **internal genitalia** of the female reproductive system consists of the vagina, uterus, fallopian tubes, and the ovaries. See **Figure 17-2.**

The **(1)** vagina is the muscular tube that connects the uterus with the vulva. It is approximately 3 inches in length, and rests between the bladder (anteriorly) and the rectum (posteriorly). The folds of the inner lining of the vagina resemble corrugated cardboard. The stretchable folds are called **rugae.** The rugae allow the vagina to expand during childbirth to permit the passage of the baby's head without tearing the lining. In addition to functioning as part of the birth canal, the vagina is the female organ of copulation (coitus, sexual intercourse) and serves as the passageway for the menstrual flow.

The **(2)** uterus is a pear-shaped, hollow, muscular organ that houses the fertilized, implanted ovum as it develops throughout pregnancy. It is also the source of the monthly menstrual flow if pregnancy does not occur. The uterus tilts forward over the urinary bladder and is anterior to the rectum. Also called the womb, the uterus has three identifiable portions: the **(2a)** fundus is the small, dome-shaped portion that rises above the area where the fallopian tubes enter the uterus, the **(2b) body of the uterus** is the wider, central portion (near the bladder), and the **(2c)** cervix **of the uterus** is the narrower, necklike portion at the lower end of the uterus.

The **(3) wall of the uterus** consists of three layers: the **perimetrium,** which is the outermost serous membrane layer, the myometrium, which is the middle muscular layer, and the endometrium, which is the innermost layer. The endometrium is the highly vascular layer that builds up each month in anticipation of receiving a fertilized egg. If pregnancy does not occur, this inner layer of the uterus is shed through a bloody discharge known as menstruation. Two lower segments of the uterus are strictures, or openings, known as the internal cervical os, or **internal os,** which separates the body of the uterus from the cervix and the external cervical os, or **external os,** at the lower end of the cervical canal, which opens into the vagina.

The **(4)** fallopian tubes, also known as the uterine tubes or the oviducts, serve as a passageway for the ova (eggs) as they exit the ovary en route to the uterus. The tubes are approximately 5 inches in length and are lined with mucous membrane and **cilia** (small hairlike projections) that assist in propelling the ovum toward the uterus. One end of each tube is attached to either lateral side of the fundus of the uterus and the other end of each tube ends in fingerlike projections called **(5)** **fimbriae**. The fimbriated ends, which open into the peritoneal cavity, do not actually connect with the ovaries but are able to draw the ovum into the tube through wavelike motions when the ovum is released from the ovary. Once the ovum is drawn into the fallopian tube, the sweeping motion of the cilia and the rhythmic contractions (peristalsis) of the tubes propel the ovum toward the uterus. It takes the ovum approximately 5 days to pass through the fallopian tube on its way to the uterus. It is in the fallopian tubes that fertilization takes place.

The **(6)** **ovaries** are the female sex cells, also known as the female **gonads**. Each of the paired ovaries is almond shaped, and is held in place by ligaments. The ovaries are located in the upper pelvic cavity, on either side of the lateral wall of the uterus, near the fimbriated ends of the fallopian tubes. The ovaries are responsible for producing mature ova (eggs) and releasing them at monthly intervals (**ovulation**). They are also responsible for producing hormones that are necessary for the normal growth and development of the female, and for maintaining pregnancy should it occur. The process of ovulation and hormone production will be discussed later in this chapter.

A woman has all of the ova that she will have for a lifetime when she is born. At birth, the ovaries contain over 700,000 immature ova. Throughout a woman's reproductive years, usually one ovum matures enough to be released from either ovary each month. Considering that a woman's reproductive years may span 30 or more years, approximately 400 ova may become mature enough to be fertilized during this time. The remaining ova reach various stages of development without reaching full maturity.

Mammary Glands (Breasts)

Although the mammary glands (breasts) do not actually play a part in the reproductive process, they are considered to be a part of the female reproductive system because they are responsible for the production of milk (lactation). As we discuss the anatomy and physiology of the mammary glands, **Figure 17-3** and **Figure 17-4** will provide a visual

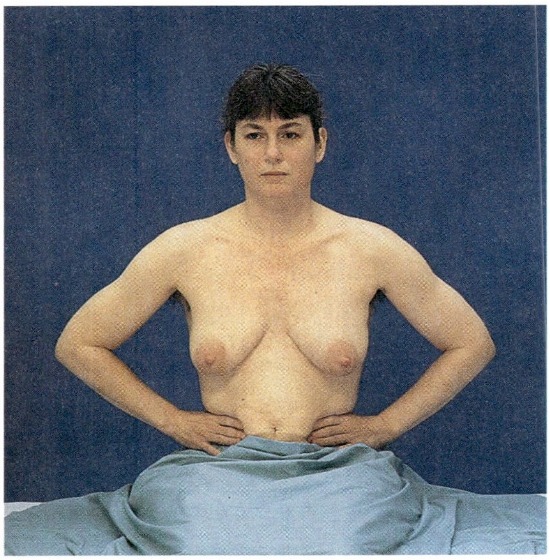

Figure 17-3 Visual appearance of the breast

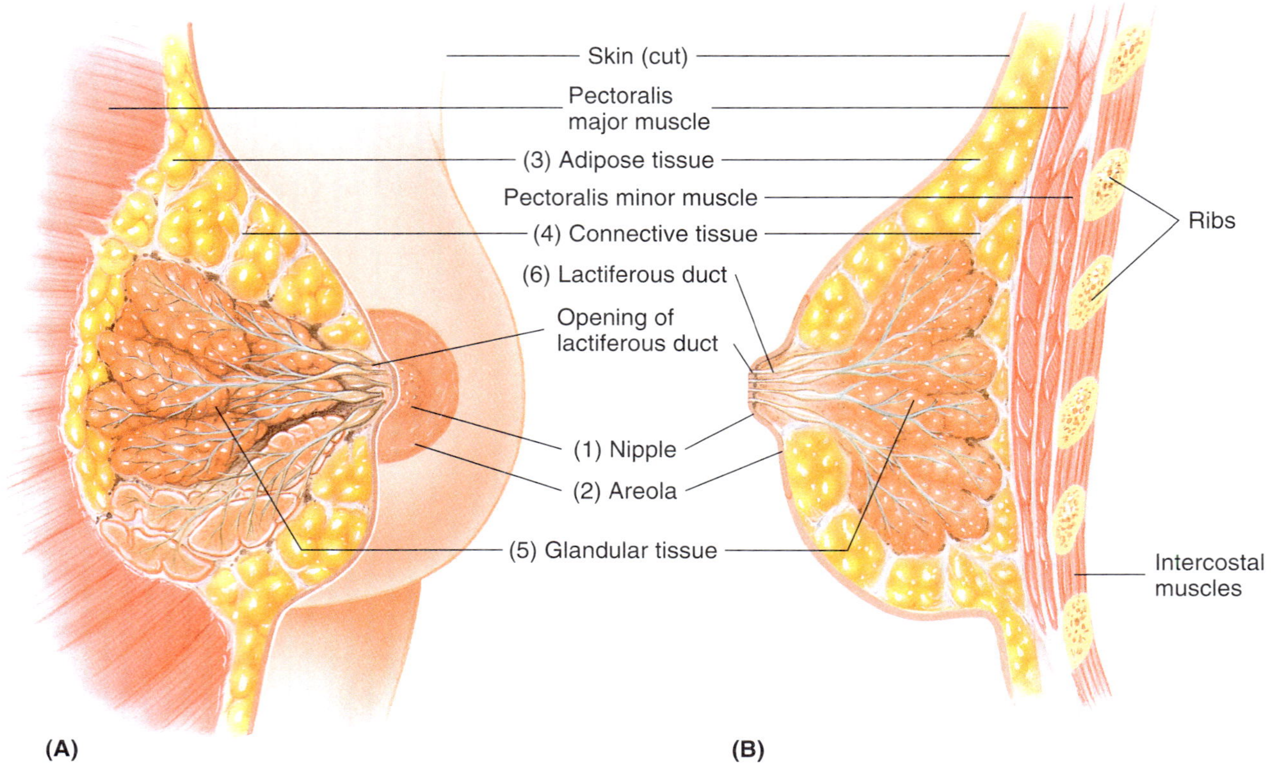

Figure 17-4 Structure of the breast: (A) anterior view; (B) sagittal view

reference of the breast appearance and structure. The breasts are located on the anterior chest wall, over the pectoral muscles. They consist of glandular tissue, with supporting adipose (fatty) tissue and fibrous connective tissue, and are covered with skin. Observation of the female breasts will reveal similarity in size and shape, but not completely equal size and shape. Size and shape of the breast will also vary from individual to individual, depending on the amount of adipose tissue present in the breast. See Figure 17-3.

At the center of each breast is a **(1) nipple,** which consists of sensitive erectile tissue. The nipple can be stimulated, through touch, to become erect. The darker pigmented area surrounding the nipple is known as the (2) **areola**. The areola has a roughened appearance due to the presence of small sebaceous glands known as **Montgomery's tubercles** or **glands.** These glands are active only during pregnancy and lactation. Their purpose is to produce a substance (waxy secretion) during this time that will keep the nipple soft and prevent dryness and cracking of the nipple during nursing.

The internal structure of the breast reveals **(3) adipose tissue** located around the outer edges. The adipose tissue (fatty tissue) is supported by **(4) connective tissue.** The central portion of the breast contains **(5) glandular tissue** that radiates outward around the nipple, like beams of light shining outward all around a central point. There are 15 to 20 glandular lobes that are responsible for the production of milk during lactation. After these glands produce the milk, it travels through a network of passageways, or narrow tubular structures, called **(6) lactiferous ducts** to the nipple for breastfeeding the infant. The amount of glandular tissue is the same in all women; therefore, breast size is not a factor in the ability to produce and secrete milk. The amount of adipose tissue present in the breast determines individual breast size.

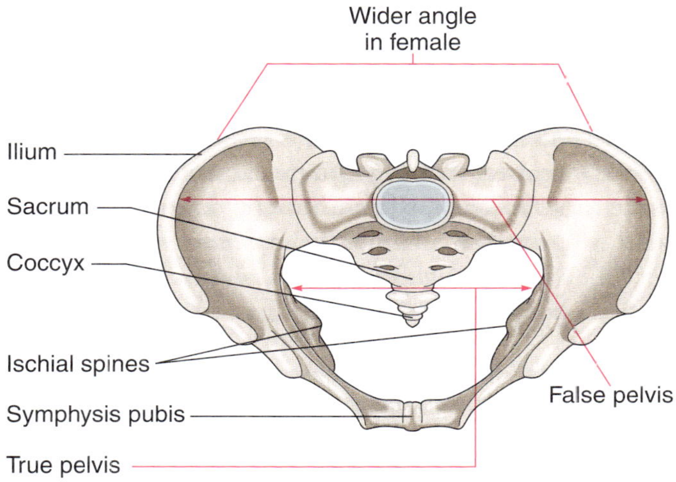

Figure 17-5 The female pelvis

The Female Pelvis

As you read about the female pelvis, refer to **Figure 17-5** for a visual reference. The female pelvis has a slightly oval **pelvic** inlet. The ischial spines are not prominent and the pubic arch is wide. The pelvic outlet has a well-rounded appearance.

Several landmarks of the pelvis play an important role in the successful passage of the fetus from the uterus, through the bony pelvic ring, to the outside of the body. These landmarks are found in the "true" pelvis. The boundaries of the true pelvis are defined by the sacrum, coccyx, and pubic bone as well as by the ischial spines. These bones serve as reference points for measuring across the pelvic outlet from varying angles, to determine the size of the outlet and its adequacy for passage of the fetus. The measurement of the pelvis is known as **pelvimetry**. The goal of pelvimetry is to determine if the head of the fetus can pass through the bony pelvis during the delivery process. Measurement of the pelvis is usually determined by **pelvic ultrasound** during the early part of pregnancy. X-ray pelvimetry may be performed late in the pregnancy or during labor if more precise measurements are needed. The size of the pelvic outlet will determine if the baby is delivered vaginally or by cesarean section.

Puberty and the Menstrual Cycle

Puberty is defined as the period of life at which the ability to reproduce begins; that is, the period when the female reproductive organs are fully developed. The onset of puberty marks the beginning of the reproductive years, which span some 30 or more years in the female.

Puberty is also the time during which the female experiences some secondary sex characteristic changes. These changes include development of the glandular tissue in the breasts and deposition of fat in the breasts that give them the characteristic rounded female look; deposition of fat in the buttocks and thighs, creating the rounded adult female curvatures; widening of the pelvis into a more rounded, basinlike shape that is more appropriate for childbirth; growth of pubic and axillary hair; a general skeletal growth spurt; and a general increase in size of the female reproductive organs. The most evident change during puberty is the onset of menstruation. The first menstrual period is called the **menarche**.

The **menstrual cycle** is also known as the female reproductive cycle. Influenced by hormones (**estrogen** and **progesterone**), the menstrual cycle is a regularly occurring set of changes that occur in the female body in preparation for pregnancy. If pregnancy does not occur, the nurturing environment that develops within the uterus in anticipation of a fertilized ovum is no longer needed. The hormone levels drop and the uterine lining is shed through the menstrual flow. Also known as **menses,** the menstrual flow lasts for approximately 3 to 7 days. The average menstrual cycle occurs every 28 days. The range, however, may vary from 24 to 35 days. The length of the cycle begins with the first day of the current menstrual period and ends with the first day of the menstrual period for the following month. Ovulation (the release of the mature ovum from the ovary) occurs approximately 14 days prior to the beginning of menses.

The menstrual cycle is divided into four time intervals, or phases, which comprise the complete cycle. These four phases consist of the menstrual phase (days 1 to 5), the postmenstrual phase (days 6 to 12), the ovulatory phase (days 13 to 14), and the premenstrual phase (days 15 to 28). A more complete description of each phase follows.

Menstrual Phase

The menstrual phase consists of days 1 to 5. The menstrual flow occurs on day one and lasts for 3 to 5 days.

Postmenstrual Phase

The postmenstrual phase consists of days 6 to 12. This is the interval between the menses and ovulation. As the estrogen level rises, several ova begin to mature in the **graafian follicles** with usually only one ovum reaching full maturity.

Ovulatory Phase

The ovulatory phase consists of days 13 to 14. This phase is known as ovulation: The graafian follicle ruptures, releasing the mature ovum into the pelvic cavity. The ovum is swept up into the fallopian tubes by the fimbriated ends of the tubes. Ovulation usually occurs on day 14 of a 28-day cycle.

Premenstrual Phase

The premenstrual phase consists of days 15 to 28. This phase occurs between the ovulatory phase and the onset of the menstrual flow. Following the rupture of the graafian follicle and the release of the ovum, the empty graafian follicle fills with a yellow substance called lutein, which is high in progesterone with some estrogen; thus the empty graafian follicle is transformed into the **corpus luteum**.

Functioning as an endocrine gland, the corpus luteum secretes high levels of estrogen and progesterone, preparing the uterine lining to receive a fertilized ovum. If fertilization does not occur, hormone levels decrease, the corpus luteum shrinks, and the uterine lining breaks down and sloughs off in the menstrual flow.

In some women, the drop in hormone levels creates a group of symptoms known as **premenstrual syndrome** (**PMS**). Symptoms include irritability, fluid retention, tenderness of the breasts, and a general feeling of depression.

Vocabulary

The following vocabulary words are frequently used when discussing the female reproductive system.

WORD	DEFINITION
adnexa (add-**NEK**-sah)	Tissues or structures in the body that are next to or near another; as in the uterus, the **adnexa** consists of the fallopian tubes, ovaries, and ligaments of the uterus.
areola (ah-**REE**-oh-lah)	The darker pigmented, circular area surrounding the nipple of each breast; also known as the areola mammae or the areola papillaris.
Bartholin's glands (**BAR**-toh-linz glands)	Two small, mucus-secreting glands located on the posterior and lateral aspects of the entrance to the vagina.
cervix (**SER**-viks)	The part of the uterus that protrudes into the cavity of the vagina; the neck of the uterus.
climacteric (kly-**MAK**-ter-ik)	The cessation of menstruation; see *menopause.*
clitoris (**KLIT**-oh-ris)	The vaginal erectile tissue (structure) corresponding to the male penis.
coitus (**KOH**-ih-tus)	The sexual union of two people of the opposite sex in which the penis is introduced into the vagina; also known as sexual intercourse or copulation.
corpus luteum (**KOR**-pus **LOO**-tee-um)	A yellowish mass that forms within the ruptured ovarian follicle after ovulation containing high levels of progesterone and some estrogen. It functions as a temporary endocrine gland for the purpose of secreting estrogen and large amounts of progesterone, which will sustain pregnancy, should it occur, until the placenta forms. If pregnancy does not occur, the corpus luteum will degenerate approximately 3 days prior to the beginning of menstruation.
cul-de-sac (kull-dih-**SAK**)	A pouch that is located between the uterus and rectum within the peritoneal cavity. This pouch is formed by one of the ligaments that serves as support to the uterus. Because it is the lowest part of the abdominal cavity, blood, pus, and other drainage collect in the **cul-de-sac**.
diaphragm (**DYE**-ah-fram)	A term used in gynecology to represent a form of contraception.
endometrium (en-doh-**MEE**-tree-um) **endo-** = within **metri/o** = uterus **-um** = noun ending	The inner lining of the uterus.

estrogen (**ESS**-troh-jen)	One of the female hormones that promotes the development of the female secondary sex characteristics.
fallopian tubes (fah-**LOH**-pee-an **TOOBS**)	One of a pair of tubes opening at one end into the uterus and at the other end into the peritoneal cavity, over the ovary.
fertilization (fer-til-eye-**ZAY**-shun)	The union of a male sperm and a female ovum.
fimbriae (**FIM**-bree-ay)	The fringelike end of the fallopian tube.
fourchette (foor-**SHET**)	A tense band of mucous membranes at the posterior rim of the vaginal opening: the point at which the labia minora connect.
fundus (**FUN**-dus)	The dome-shaped central, upper portion of the uterus between the points of insertion of the fallopian tubes.
gamete (**GAM**-eet)	A mature sperm or ovum.
gonads (**GOH**-nads)	A gamete-producing gland, such as an ovary or a testis.
graafian follicles (**GRAF**-ee-an **FALL**-ik-kls)	A mature, fully developed ovarian cyst containing the ripe ovum.
gynecology (gigh-neh-**KOL**-oh-jee) gynec/o = woman -logy = the study of	The branch of medicine that deals with the study of diseases and disorders of the female reproductive system.
hymen (**HIGH**-men)	A thin layer of elastic, connective tissue membrane that forms a border around the outer opening of the vagina and may partially cover the vaginal opening.
labia majora (**LAY**-bee-ah mah-**JOR**-ah)	Two folds of skin containing fatty tissue and covered with hair that lie on either side of the vaginal opening, extending from the mons pubis to the perineum. The outer surface of the labia majora is covered by pubic hair; the inner surface is smooth and moist.
labia minora (**LAY**-bee-ah mih-**NOR**-ah)	Two folds of hairless skin located within the folds of the labia majora. The labia minora extend from the clitoris, downward toward the perineum.
lumpectomy (lum-**PEK**-toh-mee)	Surgical removal of only the tumor and the immediate adjacent breast tissue; a method of treatment for breast cancer when detected in the early stage of the disease.
mammary glands (**MAM**-ah-ree glands) mamm/o = breast -ary = pertaining to	The female breasts.
mastectomy (mass-**TEK**-toh-mee) mast/o = breast -ectomy = surgical removal	Surgical removal of the breast as a treatment method for breast cancer; can be simple (breast only), modified radical (breast plus lymph nodes in axilla), or radical (breast, lymph nodes, and chest muscles on affected side).

mastitis (mass-**TYE**-tis) mast/o = breast -itis = inflammation	Inflammation of the breast.
menarche (men-**AR**-kee) men/o = menstruation -arche = beginning	Onset of menstruation; the first menstrual period.
menopause (**MEN**-oh-pawz) men/o = menstruation	The permanent cessation (stopping) of the menstrual cycles.
menorrhea (men-oh-**REE**-ah)	Menstrual flow; menstruation.
menstruation (men-stroo-**AY**-shun)	The periodic shedding of the lining of the nonpregnant uterus through a bloody discharge that passes through the vagina to the outside of the body. It occurs at monthly intervals and lasts for 3 to 5 days.
myometrium (my-oh-**MEE**-tree-um) my/o = muscle metri/o = uterus -um = noun ending	The muscular layer of the uterine wall.
ovary (**OH**-vah-ree) ov/o = egg -ary = pertaining to	One of a pair of female gonads responsible for producing mature ova (eggs) and releasing them at monthly intervals (ovulation); also responsible for producing the female hormones, estrogen and progesterone.
ovulation (ov-you-**LAY**-shun) ov/o = egg	The release of the mature ovum from the ovary, occurring approximately 14 days prior to the beginning of menses.
ovum (**OH**-vum) ov/o = egg -um = noun ending	The female reproductive cell; female sex cell or egg.
perineum (pair-ih-**NEE**-um)	The area between the vaginal orifice and the anus that consists of muscular and fibrous tissue and serves as support for the pelvic structures.
pregnancy (**PREG**-nan-see)	The period of intrauterine development of the fetus from conception through birth. The average pregnancy lasts approximately 40 weeks; also known as the gestational period.
premenstrual syndrome (pre-**MEN**-stroo-al **SIN**-drom)	A group of symptoms that include irritability, fluid retention, tenderness of the breasts, and a general feeling of depression occurring shortly before the onset of menstruation; also called PMS.
progesterone (proh-**JESS**-ter-own)	One of the female hormones secreted by the corpus luteum and the placenta. It is primarily responsible for the changes that occur in the endometrium in anticipation of a fertilized ovum, and for development of the maternal placenta after implantation of a fertilized ovum.

puberty (**PEW**-ber-tee)	The period of life at which the ability to reproduce begins; that is, in the female, it is the period when the female reproductive organs are fully developed.
sperm	A mature male germ cell; spermatozoon.
testes (**TESS**-teez)	The paired male gonads that produce sperm. They are suspended in the scrotal sac in the adult male.
uterus (**YOO**-ter-us)	The hollow, pear-shaped organ of the female reproductive system that houses the fertilized, implanted ovum as it develops throughout pregnancy; also the source of the monthly menstrual flow from the nonpregnant uterus.
vagina (vah-**JEYE**-nah)	The muscular tube that connects the uterus with the vulva. It is approximately 3 inches long, and rests between the bladder (anteriorly) and the rectum (posteriorly).
vulva (**VULL**-vah)	The external genitalia that consists of the mons pubis, labia majora, clitoris, labia minora, vestibule, urinary meatus, vaginal orifice, Bartholin's glands, and the perineum; also known as the pudendum.

Word Elements

The following word elements pertain to the female reproductive system. As you review the list, pronounce each word element aloud twice and check the box after you "say it." Write the definition for the example word given for each word element. You may use your medical dictionary.

WORD ELEMENT	PRONUNCIATION	"SAY IT"	MEANING
ante- **ante**flexion	**AN**-tee an-tee-**FLEK**-shun	☐	before; in front
-arche men**arche**	**AR**-kee men-**AR**-kee	☐	beginning
cervic/o **cervic**itis	**SER**-vih-koh ser-vih-**SIGH**-tis	☐	neck; cervix
colp/o **colp**odynia	**KOL**-poh kol-poh-**DIN**-ee-ah	☐	vagina
dys- **dys**menorrhea	**DIS** **dis**-men-oh-**REE**-ah	☐	bad, difficult, painful, disordered
endo- **endo**metrium	**EN**-doh en-doh-**MEE**-tree-um	☐	within
gynec/o **gynec**ologist	**GIGH**-neh-kon gigh-neh-**KOL**-oh-jist	☐	woman

Word Part / Example	Pronunciation		Meaning
hyster/o **hyster**ectomy	**HISS**-ter-oh hiss-ter-**EK**-toh-mee	☐	uterus
in- **in**competent cervix	**IN** in-**COMP**-eh-tent **SIR**-viks	☐	in, inside, within, not
intra- **intra**uterine device	**IN**-trah in-trah-**YOO**-ter-in dee-**VICE**	☐	within
mamm/o **mamm**ography	**MAM**-oh mam-**OG**-rah-fee	☐	breast
mast/o **mast**ectomy	**MASS**-toh mass-**TEK**-toh-mee	☐	breast
men/o a**men**orrhea	**MEN**-oh ah-men-oh-**REE**-ah	☐	menstruation
metr/o **metr**orrhagia	**MET**-roh **met**-roh-**RAY**-jee-ah	☐	uterus
metri/o endo**metri**osis	**MEE**-tree-oh **en**-doh-**MEE**-tree-**OH**-sis	☐	uterus
my/o **my**ometrium	**MY**-oh my-oh-**MEE**-tree-um	☐	muscle
o/o **o**ogenesis	**OH**-oh oh-oh-**JEN**-eh-sis	☐	egg, ovum
oophor/o **oophor**itis	oh-**OFF**-oh-roh oh-off-oh-**RIGH**-tis	☐	ovary
ov/o **ov**ulation	**OV**-oh **ov**-yoo-**LAY**-shun	☐	ovum, egg
ovari/o **ovari**opexy	oh-**VAY**-ree-oh oh-vay-ree-oh-**PEK**-see	☐	ovary
-rrhea meno**rrhea**	**REE**-ah men-oh-**REE**-ah	☐	discharge, flow
retro- **retro**version	**RET**-roh ret-roh-**VER**-shun	☐	backward, behind
salping/o **salping**itis	sal-**PING**-oh sal-pin-**JIGH**-tis	☐	eustachian tubes; also refers to fallopian tubes
uter/o **uter**otomy	**YOO**-ter-oh yoo-ter-**OTT**-oh-mee	☐	uterus

vagin/o **vagin**itis	**VAJ**-ih-oh vaj-in-**EYE**-tis	☐	vagina
vulv/o **vulv**ovaginitis	**VULL**-voh **vull**-voh-**VAJ**-in-eye-tis	☐	vulva

Common Signs and Symptoms

The following is a list of complaints or concerns that the female patient might express or describe. These signs or symptoms may be the only reason she wishes to be seen by the physician. These symptoms may be easily treated, or they may be signs of more serious conditions. Be sure to gather your data carefully when interviewing the patient.

As you study the terms below, write each definition and word a minimum of three times (use a separate sheet of paper), pronouncing the word aloud each time. You will notice that the word and the **basic definition** are written in bold print if you choose to learn only the abbreviated form of the definition. A more detailed description follows most words. Once you have mastered each word to your satisfaction, check the box provided beside each word.

☐ **amenorrhea**
(ah-men-oh-**REE**-ah)
a- = without, not
men/o = menstruation
-rrhea = discharge, flow

Absence of menstrual flow.

Amenorrhea is normal before puberty, during pregnancy, and after menopause. Some individuals experience temporary amenorrhea after discontinuing birth control pills. Amenorrhea can also be due to stress, strenuous exercising (as in competitive exercise), and eating disorders such as anorexia nervosa.

☐ **dysmenorrhea**
(**dis**-men-oh-**REE**-ah)
dys- = bad, difficult, painful, disordered
men/o = menstruation
-rrhea = discharge, flow

Painful menstrual flow.

Dysmenorrhea is extremely common, occurring at least occasionally in all women. If the episode of pain during menstruation is brief and mild, it is considered normal and requires no particular treatment. In approximately 10% of all women, dysmenorrhea may be severe enough to disable them temporarily.

☐ **menorrhagia**
(**men**-oh-**RAY**-jee-ah)
men/o = menstruation
-rrhagia = excessive flow or discharge

Abnormally long or very heavy menstrual periods.

Chronic **menorrhagia** can result in anemia, due to recurrent excessive blood loss. Menorrhagia can also be caused by the presence of benign uterine fibroid tumors.

☐ **metrorrhagia**
(**met**-roh-**RAY**-jee-ah)
metr/o = uterus
-rrhagia = excessive flow or discharge

Uterine bleeding at times other than the menstrual period.

Abnormal uterine bleeding may be due to numerous causes such as diseases of the thyroid gland, diabetes mellitus, cervical polyps, fibroid tumors of the uterus, excessive buildup of the inner lining of the uterus, and endometrial cancer. Any woman who experiences prolonged **metror-**

rhagia that is not associated with normal menstrual periods should seek medical advice.

oligomenorrhea
(ol-ih-goh-**men**-oh-**REE**-ah)
olig/o = few, little, scanty
men/o = menstruation
-rrhea = discharge, flow

Oligomenorrhea is abnormally light or infrequent menstruation.

Other symptoms of possible female reproductive system disorders include, but are not limited to, the following: lower abdominal or pelvic pain, abnormal vaginal discharge or itching, breast changes such as pain and tenderness, abnormalities in the nipple, and feeling a mass or lump in the breast. If a female patient presents with any of these symptoms, they need to be brought to the attention of the physician during the visit.

Family Planning

The term "family planning" encompasses choosing *when to have* children and choosing *when not to have* children. It involves various forms of contraception to prevent pregnancy, as well as methods that will help the couple achieve pregnancy. This segment will be devoted to the discussion of **contraception,** methods used to prevent pregnancy. Methods used to achieve pregnancy will be discussed in Chapter 18.

Considering the fact that the female reproductive years span some 30 or more years, the female may actually be faced with making decisions about which form of birth control she chooses to use for over 30 years. If it is her choice to bear a limited number of children (the national average is two), effective contraceptive methods are essential. Most forms of contraception used by women can be terminated when pregnancy is desired, and resumed after pregnancy.

The decision as to which form of contraception to use primarily rests with the female. The advantages and disadvantages of each type should be considered as she selects the particular form that best suits her body, her health, and her lifestyle. The number of sex partners she has will also affect the female's decision on birth control methods, particularly because of acquired immunodeficiency syndrome (AIDS) and other sexually transmitted diseases. If contraception is a planned decision and not a spontaneous one, the female may seek counsel from her physician as she determines her approach to family planning. Literature on the various methods of contraception should be available through her physician's office.

Forms of Contraception

Each form of contraception discussed in this chapter will be defined as to how it is used, followed by a listing of the advantages and disadvantages of its use. Contraindications (reasons for not using) are listed, when applicable. Although many of these forms of contraception are 99% to 100% effective in preventing pregnancy when used correctly, it must be remembered that they do not protect the female against sexually transmitted diseases. Women who are sexually active should also have their sexual partner(s) use a condom for added protection.

abstinence
(**AB**-stih-nens)

Abstinence means to abstain from having vaginal intercourse.

Abstinence is 100% effective as a means of birth control. Various religious groups support abstinence among unmarried people. With the rise in AIDS and other sexually transmitted diseases, an increased push for abstinence among unmarried people is becoming more evident. Many television commercials may now be seen promoting the "I'm worth waiting for" concept among teenagers.

oral contraceptives
(**ORAL** con-trah-**SEP**-tivz)

Oral contraceptives, or birth control pills, contain synthetic forms of the hormones, estrogen and progesterone, and are taken daily by mouth.

The hormonal influence of oral contraceptives prevents ovulation in the female; this can be reversed when the female ceases to take them. Birth control pills have a nearly 100% effectiveness rate when taken correctly.

The advantages of taking birth control pills include but are not limited to the following:

1. Convenience of taking a pill by mouth at the same time every day
2. Decreased incidence of dysmenorrhea and premenstrual syndrome while taking birth control pills
3. Decreased menstrual flow, making iron-deficiency anemia less of a problem than in nonpill users
4. Regulation of menorrhagia and elimination of menstrual irregularity

The disadvantages of taking birth control pills include but are not limited to the following:

1. Nausea
2. Headaches
3. Weight gain
4. Breakthrough bleeding (i.e., spotting between periods)
5. Mild hypertension

Contraindications or reasons for not taking oral contraceptives include but are not limited to the following:

1. History of thromboembolic disorders, breast cancer, estrogen-fed tumors, or coronary artery disease
2. Migraine headaches
3. Women over the age of 35, who are heavy smokers
4. Women who are breast feeding (the estrogen decreases the milk supply)

Birth control pills are packaged in convenient dispensers, making them easy to carry when traveling. See **Figure 17-6.** Most are packaged in 21- or 28-pill packs. Many women prefer the 28-day pill package because no days are skipped, making it easier to stay on schedule.

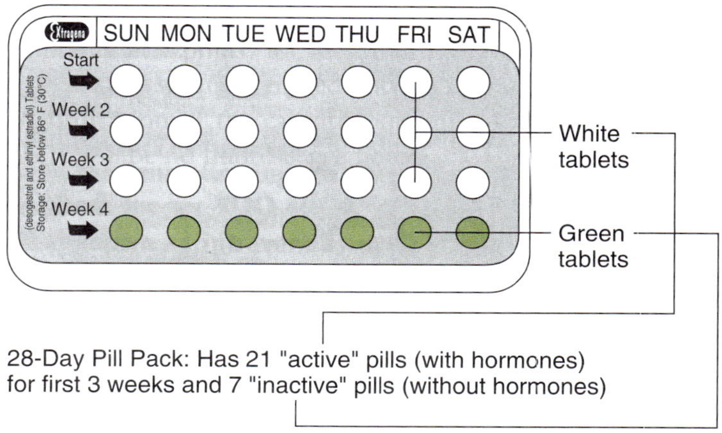

Figure 17-6 Oral contraceptive packaging

Depo-Provera injection
(**DEP**-oh proh-**VAIR**-ah)

Depo-Provera injection is a form of contraception administered intramuscularly, approximately once every 12 weeks.

Depo-Provera acts by preventing ovulation and is considered to be about 99% effective. This injectable form of birth control is also reversible.

The advantages of using Depo-Provera injections as a means of birth control are as follows:

1. The user does not have to remember to take pills daily or to insert a contraceptive just before intercourse.
2. The sexual act can be more spontaneous and more meaningful for some.
3. The medication is taken once every 12 weeks.

The disadvantages of using Depo-Provera injections include but are not limited to the following:

1. Menstrual spotting
2. Weight gain
3. Headaches
4. Decrease in bone mineral stored in the body
5. Women must return to their physician every 12 weeks for the injections.

Contraindications for use of Depo-Provera injections as a means of birth control include but may not be limited to the following:

1. Pregnancy
2. Women who have or have had breast cancer
3. Women who have thromboembolic disease
4. Women who have liver disease

Lunelle injection
(loo-**NELL**)

Lunelle is a monthly contraceptive injection.

The Lunelle injection is given once a month and is effective in preventing pregnancy during the month in which it is given. It is considered to be about 99% effective. This injection form of birth control is reversible.

Advantages of using the Lunelle injections as a means of birth control are as follows:

1. The user does not have to remember to take pills daily or to insert a contraceptive just before intercourse.
2. The sexual act can be more spontaneous and more meaningful for some.
3. The medication is taken every 28 to 30 days.

The disadvantages of using the Lunelle injections include but are not limited to the following:

1. Menstrual spotting
2. Weight gain
3. Fluid retention
4. Women must return to their physician every 28 to 30 days for injections, and no later than 33 days after the previous injection.

---

intrauterine device
(**in**-trah-**YOO**-ter-in)
intra- = within
uter/o = uterus

The intrauterine device is a small plastic T-shaped object with strings attached to the leg of the "T." It is inserted into the uterus, through the vagina, and remains in place in the uterus.

Also known as an IUD, the intrauterine device acts by preventing implantation of an ovum into the uterus. Although the exact action of the IUD is not understood, it is thought that the presence of the foreign body in the uterus prevents the implantation of the ovum. IUDs are not as popular as they were 20 years ago, due to complications with certain brands used at that time.

The advantages of using an IUD as a form of birth control include the following:

1. Once the IUD is inserted, the female only has to check periodically for the strings, which should be suspended in the vagina.
2. The user does not have to remember to take pills daily or to insert a contraceptive just before intercourse.
3. The sexual act can be more spontaneous and more meaningful for some.
4. The IUD can be removed at any time, but is usually left in place for 1 to 4 years, depending on the brand selected.

The disadvantages of the IUD include but may not be limited to the following:

1. **Pelvic inflammatory disease** is the most serious complication of using an IUD.
2. Spotting or uterine cramping for the first few weeks.
3. Some women experience heavier than normal menstrual periods for the first few months after insertion of an IUD.
4. Higher risk of tubal pregnancy.

Contraindications for using the intrauterine device as a means of birth control include, but are not limited to, the following:

1. Women who have never been pregnant, or who are known to have an abnormally shaped uterus (their small uterus could be punctured during insertion)
2. Women who have a history of dysmenorrhea or metrorrhagia
3. History of pelvic infections
4. History of ectopic pregnancy

---

barrier methods

Methods of birth control that place physical barriers between the cervix and the sperm so the sperm cannot pass the cervix and enter the uterus, and thus the fallopian tubes.

Barrier methods are used only during sexual intercourse. Because they function the same way, only three of the more commonly used barrier methods of birth control will be discussed.

1. **Spermicidal** jellies and creams are inserted into the vagina. They increase the acidity of the vaginal secretions, causing the death of the sperm before they can reach the cervix.

   The advantages include the fact that they can be purchased without a prescription.

   The disadvantages include the inconvenience of having to insert the spermicide no more than 1 hour before sexual intercourse and having to leave it in for at least 6 hours after, for optimal effects. The other disadvantage is the higher failure rate of the products.

   Contraindications for use of spermicidal jellies and creams as a means of birth control include women nearing menopause and those with inflammation of the cervix.

2. **Condoms** are thin latex sheaths worn on the penis of the male during sexual intercourse (male condoms), or loose fitting latex sheaths that are inserted into the female vagina before sexual intercourse (female condoms). Both types of condoms are designed to collect semen that leaks or is expelled from the penis during ejaculation; both are designed for one-time use only.

   The advantages of the male condom are that they are readily available without a prescription and they provide good protection against sexually transmitted diseases and the AIDS virus. The advantages of the female condom are the same as those for the male condom; in addition, they are less likely to break or tear than male condoms. The female condoms also allow vaginal penetration before the penis is completely erect.

   The disadvantages are limited mainly to the male condom and include the possibility of the condom becoming dislodged from the penis during sexual intercourse, and the need for the penis to be erect to apply the condom. There are basically no contraindications for the use of condoms as a means of birth control.

3. **Diaphragms** are flexible, circular rubber discs that fit over the cervix after being inserted through the vagina. They prevent the sperm from entering the uterus and thus the fallopian tubes. They are primarily

used in conjunction with spermicidal creams and jellies for added protection. Initial fitting of the diaphragm is performed by the physician to ensure a proper fit; the female inserts the diaphragm thereafter.

Advantages include the fact that the diaphragm can be inserted up to 6 hours before intercourse and can be left in place for 24 hours.

Disadvantages include **cervicitis** (inflamation of the cervix) and the possibility of increased incidence of urinary tract infections due to the pressure of the diaphragm on the urethra.

Permanent Methods of Birth Control

Permanent methods of birth control include surgical sterilization of either the female (**tubal ligation**) or the male (vasectomy). After having children, many people choose sterilization as a permanent means of birth control. Occasionally, they will decide to have the procedure reversed, but this is much more complicated than the sterilization itself and is not always successful. When individuals are considering permanent methods of birth control they should weigh the pros and cons carefully. Even though they may not wish to do so, men and women who have children at a young age should consider the possibilities of divorce, remarriage, or even death of a spouse or a child before deciding on permanent means of birth control.

tubal ligation
(**TOO**-bal lye-**GAY**-shun)

Tubal ligation is surgically cutting and tying the fallopian tubes to prevent passage of ova or sperm through the tubes, consequently preventing pregnancy; female sterilization. See Figure 17-7.

The surgery for a tubal ligation may be performed the day after giving birth, or it may be scheduled as an outpatient. One surgical method involves making a small incision into the abdomen (mini-laparotomy) and bringing the tubes up through the incision. A piece of each tube is then cut away and the ends are tied separately.

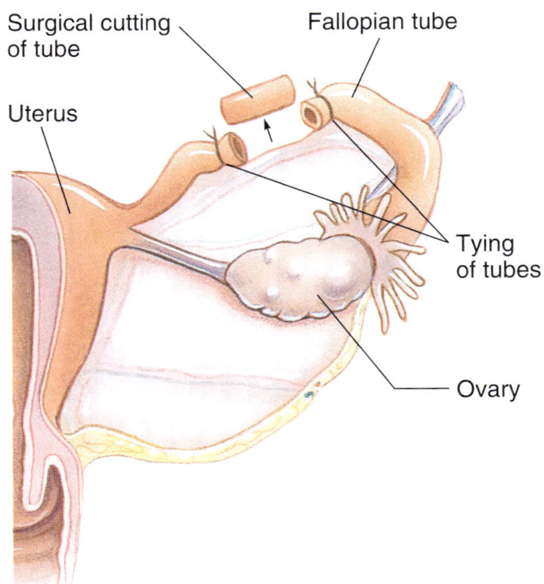

Figure 17-7 Tubal ligation

vasectomy
(vas-**EK**-toh-mee)
vas/o = vessel, vas deferens
-ectomy = surgical removal

Also known as a male sterilization, a vasectomy is surgically cutting and tying the vas deferens to prevent the passage of sperm, consequently preventing pregnancy. Refer to Chapter 16 for more detailed information on a vasectomy.

Pathological Conditions

As you study the pathological conditions of the female reproductive system, note that the **basic definition** is in bold print followed by a more detailed description in regular print. The phonetic pronunciation is directly beneath each term, and a breakdown of the component parts of the term when appropriate.

carcinoma of the breast
(car-sin-**OH**-mah)
carcin/o = cancer
-oma = tumor

A malignant (cancerous) tumor of the breast tissue; the most common type (ductal carcinoma) originates in the mammary ducts. This tumor has the ability to invade surrounding tissue if not detected early enough. Once the cancer cells penetrate the duct, they will metastasize (spread) through the surrounding breast tissue, eventually reaching the axillary lymph nodes. Through the lymph vessels, the cancer cells can spread to distant parts of the body.

Cancer of the breast is the most common malignancy in women in the United States today. It is estimated that one in eight women in the United States will develop breast cancer during their lifetime, based on a 100-year life expectancy. Most breast lumps are discovered by the woman and are felt as a movable mass, generally in the upper outer quadrant of the breast. In some cases, the woman's husband or sexual partner will feel the lump in the breast first. Many women, however, fail to follow through with seeking medical attention when they discover a lump in their breast. Any lump, no matter how small, should be reported to a physician immediately!

Factors that place some women in a higher risk category than others include a family history of breast cancer, nulliparity (having borne no children), early menarche, late menopause, hypertension, obesity, diabetes, chronic cystic breast disease, exposure to radiation, and possibly postmenopausal estrogen therapy.

Once a lump has been discovered in the female breast and has been palpated (felt) by the physician, a mammogram is ordered to confirm the presence of a suspicious mass. This is usually followed with a biopsy of the lump, to confirm the diagnosis.

Most women with early-stage breast cancer are successfully treated. Treatment involves surgical removal of the lump and any diseased tissue surrounding it. If the lump is detected in the early stage of the disease, a **lumpectomy** may be the only surgery necessary. This involves removal of only the tumor and the immediate adjacent breast tissue. Other treatment options include a simple mastectomy in which only the breast is removed, a modified radical mastectomy in which the breast is removed and the lymph nodes in the axilla (armpit), and a radical mastectomy in which the breast, the chest muscles on the affected side, and the lymph nodes in the axilla are removed. Surgery is usually followed by a series of radiation treatments (radiation therapy), chemotherapy, or sometimes both.

Some women opt to have reconstructive breast surgery following a mastectomy. The types of material used to reconstruct the breast include implants and tissue transplanted from one part of the patient's body (such as the hips or thighs) to the breast. Patients considering breast reconstruction should discuss this thoroughly with the physician to ensure their understanding of breast reconstruction.

Early detection and treatment is of utmost importance when the diagnosis is cancer. Women should be encouraged to perform breast self-examinations monthly, to have yearly physical examinations by their physicians, to have a baseline mammogram done at age 35, or to have mammograms as recommended by their physician. The procedure for breast self-examination will appear in the section on diagnostic techniques.

---

cervical carcinoma
SER-vih-kal car-sin-**OH**-ma)
cervic/o = cervix
-al = pertaining to
carcin/o = cancer
-oma = tumor

A malignant tumor of the cervix. Cervical cancer is one of the most common malignancies of the female reproductive tract. Symptoms include bleeding between menstrual periods, after sexual intercourse, after menopause, and an abnormal Pap smear.

Cervical cancer appears to be most frequent in women from ages 30 to 50. Factors that increase the risk of developing cervical cancer at a later age including the following:

1. First sexual intercourse before the age of 20
2. Having many sex partners
3. Having certain sexually transmitted diseases
4. History of smoking

In the earliest stage of cervical cancer, the cancer remains in place without spreading. This early stage is known as carcinoma in situ; that is, "it just sits there." The progression into a more advanced stage that can metastasize to other parts of the body is usually slow. This particular quality of cervical cancer makes the prognosis excellent if the disease is detected in its earliest stage.

The **Papanicolaou smear** (**Pap smear**) is used to detect early changes in the cervical tissue that may indicate cervical cancer. The Pap test consists of obtaining scrapings from the cervix and examining them under a microscope to detect any abnormalities in cervical tissue; approximately 90% percent of the early changes in the cervical tissue are detected by this test. The diagnosis of cervical cancer is confirmed with a tissue biopsy.

Treatment for cervical cancer includes surgery to remove the diseased tissue and a margin of healthy tissue. This may involve removing the cervix or may be more extensive, involving removal of the uterus, fallopian tubes, and ovaries as well. Surgery may be followed with radiation therapy.

cervicitis
(ser-vih-**SIGH**-tis)
cervic/o = cervix
-itis = inflammation

An acute or chronic inflammation of the uterine cervix.

Symptoms may include a thick, foul-smelling vaginal discharge, pelvic pressure or pain, scant bleeding after sexual intercourse, and itching or burning of the external genitalia. Upon examination, the cervix will appear red and swollen; bleeding may occur on contact.

Cervicitis is usually caused by the following microorganisms: *Trichomonas vaginalis, Candida albicans, Haemophilus vaginalis,* or *Chlamydia trachomatis.* Diagnosis is confirmed by a Pap smear with a culture of the area. A biopsy may be taken to rule out the possibility of cervical cancer. Once the causative organism is identified, medication specific to the organism is prescribed.

Cervicitis can also cause cervical erosion. Upon visual examination of the cervix, the cervical mucosa appears "raw" (ulcerated) with red patches on the mucosa. This abrasion, or ulceration, of the cervix is caused by irritation from the infection; it can also be a result of trauma such as childbirth.

Symptoms of cervical erosion include a white or yellowish mucous discharge from the vagina. This is known as leukorrhea.

Once the diagnosis of cervical erosion is confirmed by Pap smear and tissue biopsy, the treatment of choice is **cryosurgery** or cryocautery. Each procedure involves freezing the eroded tissue. Antibiotic therapy may follow.

cystocele
(**SIS**-toh-seel)
cyst/o = bladder, sac, or cyst
-cele = swelling or herniation

Herniation or downward protrusion of the urinary bladder through the wall of the vagina. See Figure 17-8.

This condition develops over a period of years as a result of weakening of the anterior wall of the vagina, often after the woman has given birth to several babies. The weakened anterior wall of the vagina can no longer support the weight of the urine in the bladder, thus the bladder protrudes downward into the vagina. Complete emptying of the bladder becomes a problem because the **cystocele** sags below the neck of the bladder when it protrudes into the vagina. Cystitis may also become a problem as a result of the incomplete emptying of the bladder.

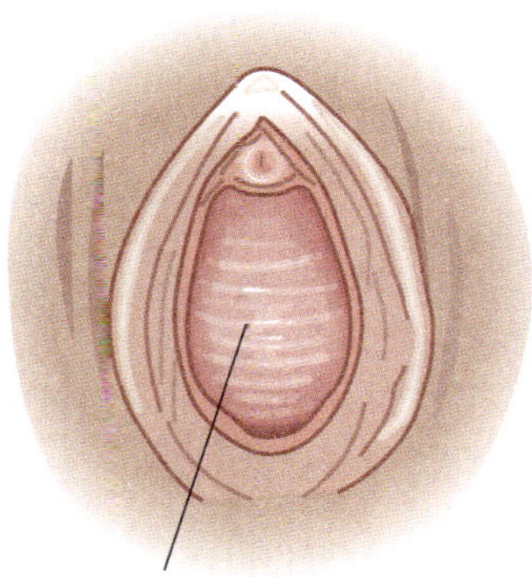

Figure 17-8 Cystocele

endometrial carcinoma
(en-doh-**MEE**-tree-al car-sin-**OH**-ma)
endo- = within
metri/o = uterus
-al = pertaining to
carcin/o = cancer
-oma = tumor

Malignant tumor of the inner lining of the uterus; also known as adenocarcinoma of the uterus.

This is the most common cancer of the female reproductive tract, occurring in women during or after menopause (peak incidence between the ages of 50 and 60).

The classic symptom of **endometrial** cancer is inappropriate uterine bleeding. This includes any postmenopausal bleeding or recurrent metrorrhagia in the premenopausal patient. An abnormal discharge (mucoid or watery discharge) may precede the bleeding by weeks or months.

Diagnosis is usually confirmed with an endometrial biopsy, or **dilatation and curettage** with microscopic examination of the tissue sample. Dilatation involves enlarging the cervical opening, and curettage involves scraping tissue cells from the uterine lining for sampling.

Treatment involves a total abdominal **hysterectomy** (removal of the uterus, fallopian tubes, and ovaries) followed by radiation.

---

endometriosis
(**en**-doh-**mee**-tree-**OH**-sis)
endo- = within
metri/o = uterus
-osis = condition

The presence and growth of endometrial tissue in areas outside the endometrium (lining of the uterus). See Figure 17-9.

The ectopic (out of place) endometrial tissue is generally found within the abdominal cavity. It may be found in the wall of the uterus or on its surface, in the peritoneum of the pelvis, on the small intestine, in or on the fallopian tubes, and ovaries.

Symptoms of **endometriosis** include dysmenorrhea with constant pain and discomfort in the lower abdomen, back, and vagina. The pain may begin before menstruation and continue for several days after the end of menstruation. The woman with endometriosis may also experience heavy menstrual periods and pelvic pain during sexual intercourse. The

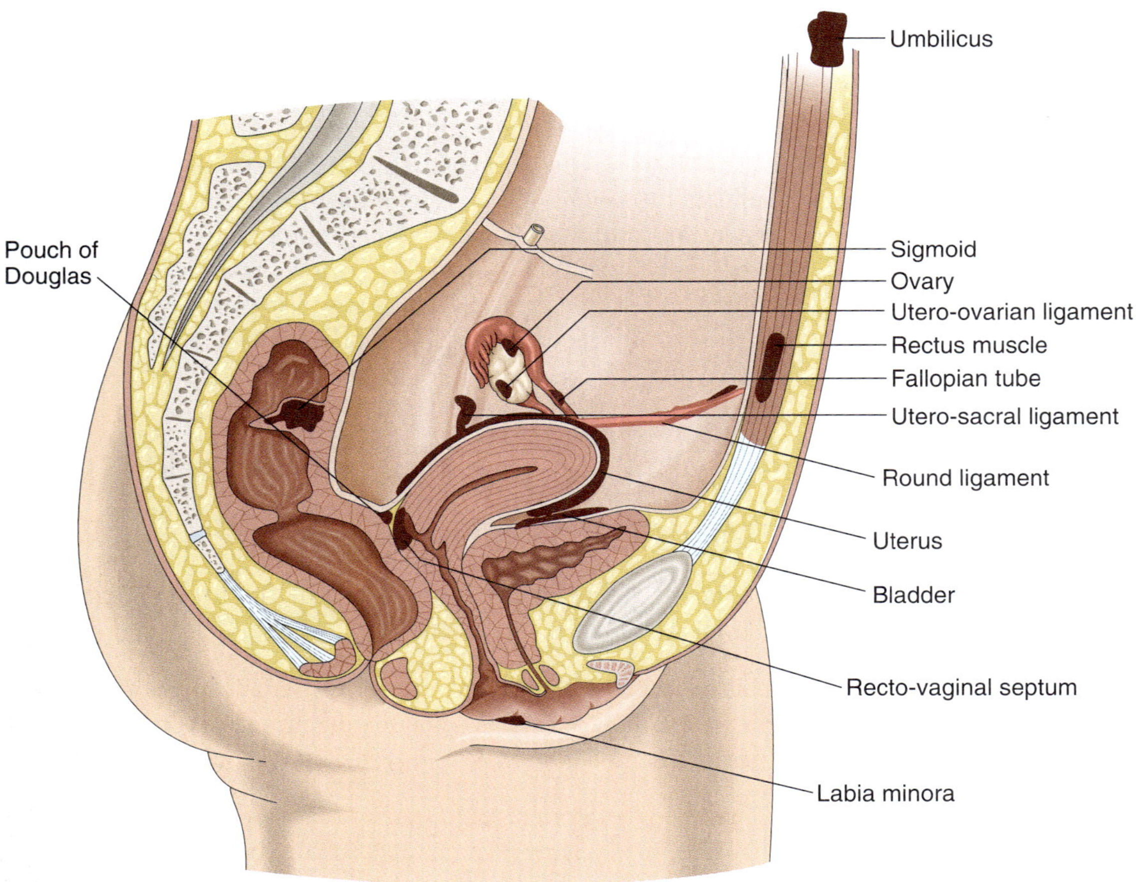

Figure 17-9 Common sites of endometriosis

pain and discomfort are due to the buildup of scar tissue and adhesions resulting from the endometrial tissue thickening and bleeding in unnatural places.

Diagnosis of endometriosis is usually confirmed by visualization of the endometrial deposits in the abdominal cavity through a laparoscope. The physician may also note areas of tenderness within the pelvis while performing a bimanual examination.

There is no known cure for endometriosis other than the removal of the uterus, fallopian tubes, and ovaries. Treatment, therefore, is based on the severity of the condition and can range from regular monitoring of the condition, to analgesics for mild pain and discomfort, to hormonal therapy (use of birth control pills) to shrink the endometrial tissue for those experiencing severe pain.

fibrocystic breast disease
(figh-broh-**SIS**-tik)
fibr/o = fiber
cyst/o = bladder, sac, or cyst
-ic = pertaining to

The presence of single or multiple fluid-filled cysts that are palpable in the breasts.

The cysts are benign (not malignant) and they fluctuate in size with the menstrual period, becoming tender just before menstruation. Often, the woman will not experience any symptoms but will seek medical attention after she discovers a lump in her breast.

Diagnosis is confirmed with a biopsy of the cyst, especially for deeper cysts that are indistinguishable by palpation from carcinoma. Mammography, coupled with the patient's symptoms of pain, fluctuation in size of the cysts, and lumpiness in the breast, is helpful but is not conclusive.

Treatment for **fibrocystic** breast disease includes use of a good support bra to lessen the pain, restriction of caffeine in the diet, and use of mild analgesics. Monthly breast self-examinations are advised because the cysts may continue to recur until menopause, after which time they will subside.

fibroid tumor
(**FIGH**-broyd tumor)
fibr/o = fiber
-oid = resembling

A benign, fibrous tumor of the uterus.

This is one of the most common types of benign tumors of the female reproductive system. **Fibroid** tumors vary in number, size, and location within the uterus, occurring only in premenopausal women.

Symptoms range from none to pelvic pain and pressure accompanied by menorrhagia or metrorrhagia.

Patient history and ultrasonography are used to confirm the diagnosis. Treatment ranges from surgery to remove the tumors, to a hysterectomy, depending on the severity of the symptoms.

leiomyoma
(**ligh**-oh-my-**OH**-mah)
lei/o = smooth
my/o = muscle
-oma = tumor

A benign, smooth muscle tumor of the uterus. Uterine leiomyomas are often mislabeled as fibroid tumors, when in fact they are not.

Leiomyomas do, however, present the same type of symptoms and are treated in the same manner as fibroid tumors. This may account for the interchangeable terminology.

Leiomyomas and fibroid tumors are the most common types of benign tumors of the female reproductive system. Leiomyomas also vary in number, size, and location within the uterus, occurring only in premenopausal women.

Symptoms range from none to pelvic pain and pressure accompanied by menorrhagia or metrorrhagia.

Patient history and ultrasonography are used to confirm the diagnosis. Treatment ranges from surgery to remove the tumors, to a hysterectomy, depending on the severity of the symptoms.

---

ovarian carcinoma
(oh-**VAY**-ree-an car-sin-**OH**-ma)
ovari/o = ovary
-an = characteristic of
carcin/o = cancer
-oma = tumor

A malignant tumor of the ovaries, most commonly occurring in women in their 50s. It is rarely detected in the early stage and is usually far advanced when diagnosed.

Symptoms usually do not appear with **ovarian** cancer until the disease is well advanced. The earliest symptoms of ovarian cancer are swelling, bloating, or discomfort in the lower abdomen, and mild digestive complaints (loss of appetite, feeling of fullness, indigestion, nausea, and weight loss). As the tumor increases in size it may create pressure on adjacent organs, such as the urinary bladder or the rectum, causing frequent urination and dysuria or constipation. Later developments in the course of the disease include an accumulation of fluid within the abdominal cavity (ascites), resulting in swelling and discomfort.

Diagnosis is confirmed with examination of a sample of the tumor tissue under a microscope. This is achieved through surgical removal of the affected ovary. If the ovary is diseased with cancer, the surgeon will then remove the other ovary, the uterus, and the fallopian tubes. A process called staging is important to determine the amount of metastasis, if any. This process involves taking samples (biopsy) of nearby lymph nodes and the diaphragm and sampling the fluid from the abdomen.

Treatment involves the use of surgery, chemotherapy, or radiation therapy. It may involve one or a combination of the treatment choices, depending on the extent of the disease.

---

ovarian cysts
(oh-**VAY**-ree-an **SISTS**)
ovari/o = ovary
-an = characteristic of

Benign, globular sacs (cysts) that form on or near the ovaries. These cysts may be fluid filled or they may contain semisolid material.

An **ovarian cyst** may develop from an unruptured graafian follicle (follicular cyst), or it may develop when the corpus luteum fails to regress, becoming cystic (lutein cyst).

Symptoms vary but may include the following: painless swelling in the lower abdomen that feels firm to touch, pain during sexual intercourse, pelvic pain, low back pain, or an acute, colicky, abdominal pain.

A pelvic examination will usually detect an ovarian cyst. In some cases, however, a pelvic ultrasound is necessary to verify the ovarian cyst. Most ovarian cysts will disappear by themselves. If the cyst does not disappear within a few months, **laparoscopy** with direct visualization may be necessary to rule out the possibility of other causes, such as malignancy; the cyst may be removed surgically for biopsy.

pelvic inflammatory disease (PID)
(**PELL**-vik in-**FLAM**-mah-toh-ree dih-**ZEEZ**)
(salpingitis)
salping/o = eustachian tubes; also refers to fallopian tubes
-itis = inflammation

Infection of the fallopian tubes; also known as salpingitis.

PID occurs predominantly in women under the age of 35 who are sexually active. The most frequent causative organisms of pelvic inflammatory disease are *Chlamydia trachomatis* and *Neisseria gonorrhoeae;* both are sexually transmitted. There is also a higher incidence of PID in women who use IUDs (intrauterine devices used as a means of birth control).

Pelvic inflammatory disease begins with a cervical infection that spreads by surface invasion along the uterine lining (endometrium) and then out to the fallopian tubes and ovaries.

Symptoms of acute PID include fever, chills, malaise, abdomen tender to touch with sudden release (rebound), backache, and a foul-smelling vaginal discharge. As with any active infection, the white blood cell count will be elevated.

Diagnosis is confirmed by obtaining a specimen of the uterine secretions for culture and sensitivity. Once the causative organism is isolated, an antibiotic that is specific in action to the particular bacteria can be prescribed. Medications to relieve pain (analgesics) and bed rest are also prescribed. Early treatment is necessary to prevent complications, such as peritonitis, from the spread of the inflammation throughout the abdominal cavity.

toxic shock syndrome

A potentially fatal condition caused by toxin-producing strains of the bacteria, *Staphylococcus aureus*.

This condition occurs in menstruating females who use tampons, particularly the superabsorbency strength. The presence of the tampon in the warm, moist vaginal canal for extended periods of time creates the ideal environment for the bacteria to grow. The bacteria may have been introduced into the vagina when inserting the tampon, or in a small percentage of women, they may be normally present in the vaginal canal. The toxin that is produced leads to hypovolemia (decreased blood volume in the blood vessels), hypotension (decreased blood pressure), and shock.

Symptoms of toxic shock syndrome include a sudden high fever and flu-like symptoms, hypotension, and a generalized rash resembling sunburn. Within 1 to 2 weeks after the onset of the illness, the skin from the palms of the hands and the soles of the feet may peel.

Diagnosis is based on the patient's symptoms, history of tampon use, and elevated liver enzyme level. Treatment includes intravenous replacement of the lost fluids to counteract the shock, and administration of antibiotics to treat the infection. This therapy should be initiated as soon as possible to prevent serious complications from the shock.

vaginitis
(vaj-in-**EYE**-tis)
vagin/o = vagina
-itis = inflammation

Inflammation of the vagina and the vulva.

This is a common disease that affects women when there is a disturbance in the normal flora or pH of the vagina that allows the microorganisms to flourish. The three most common types of vaginitis are candidiasis, trichomoniasis, and bacterial vaginosis.

1. Candidiasis is also known as moniliasis or as a yeast (fungal) infection. It is the most common form of vaginitis. It occurs when the normal vaginal flora and pH (environment) are disturbed and the conditions are right for accelerated growth of the causative organism, *Candida albicans,* commonly found on the skin and in the digestive tract. The use of certain antibiotics, diabetes, or pregnancy can cause a change in the environment of the vagina that promotes the growth of *Candida albicans.*

   Symptoms of candidiasis include a foul-smelling vaginal discharge accompanied by itching, burning, and soreness of the area. The discharge has a typical "cottage cheese" appearance, and the vulvar and vaginal walls have a red, inflamed appearance.

   Diagnosis is confirmed with visual inspection through pelvic examination, and microscopic examination of a wet mount of the vaginal secretions.

   Treatment consists of applications of vaginal creams designed to destroy yeast/fungal infections. These medications can now be purchased without a prescription. The female should seek medical attention if the symptoms do not disappear after treatment with a vaginal cream. If the discharge is yellow or green and has a bad odor, it may be indicative of another causative microorganism and will require medical attention.

2. Trichomoniasis is caused by the protozoan, *Trichomonas vaginalis,* which thrives in an alkaline environment and is usually transmitted by sexual intercourse. In some cases, infection can be introduced through fecal material due to improper wiping after elimination.

   Symptoms include a greenish-yellow vaginal discharge that has a bad odor. Itching, swelling, and redness of the vulva are usually present.

   Diagnosis for trichomoniasis is confirmed by microscopic examination of the vaginal secretions by wet mount preparation.

   Treatment includes the use of an antibacterial/antiprotozoal medication. It is advisable to treat the female's sex partner to prevent reinfection because men often harbor the protozoan without symptoms.

3. Bacterial vaginosis or Gardnerella vaginitis is caused by the bacillus, *Gardnerella vaginalis,* which normally inhabits the vagina. It is not definite what causes the conditions that set the stage for the overgrowth of bacteria that occurs with bacterial vaginosis, but it does produce an extremely contagious vaginitis.

   The main symptom is an increased vaginal discharge, which is usually thin, watery, and a grayish white or yellow color. The discharge usually has a strong fishy odor, which may be more noticeable after sexual intercourse. Redness and itching of the vulva are not usually present with bacterial vaginosis.

Diagnosis is confirmed by microscopic examination of the vaginal secretions by a saline wet mount preparation.

Treatment includes the use of antibiotics or antibacterial medications. It may also be advisable to treat the female's sex partner.

Diagnostic Techniques and Procedures

aspiration biopsy
(as-pih-**RAY**-shun **BYE**-op-see)

An invasive procedure in which a needle is inserted into an area of the body, such as the breast, to withdraw a tissue or fluid sample for microscopic examination and diagnosis.

Aspiration biopsy is usually performed using a local anesthetic. After the area is anesthetized, a fine needle is inserted into the site to be aspirated. Suction is applied by pulling the plunger of the syringe back until the sample of fluid or tissue is drawn up into the syringe through the needle. The sample is then affixed to a slide and sent to the laboratory for diagnosis.

breast self-examination

A procedure in which the woman examines her breasts and surrounding tissue for evidence of any changes that could indicate the possibility of malignancy.

By the age of 20, women should perform the breast self-examination every month, approximately 7 to 10 days after the menstrual period. At this time of the month the breasts are usually their softest, making the examination easier. Furthermore, women who are familiar with their own normal breast characteristics can notice the development of any abnormalities at an earlier point. They should also be taught the importance of breast self-examinations on a monthly basis and should understand that early detection, if a malignancy is found, increases the survival rate significantly.

A good time of day to do a breast self-examination is just before taking a shower. The breast self-examination consists of inspecting and palpating both breasts in a consistent pattern to detect any abnormalities or lumps. If any abnormalities are detected, they should be reported to a physician immediately. The steps for breast self-examination follow. See **Figure 17-10.**

1. The woman should stand before a mirror to observe the appearance of her breasts. She should check both breasts for any abnormalities; that is, dimpling or puckering of the nipples, unusual scaling of the skin of the breasts, or any unusual discharge from the nipples. She should then observe the breasts for similarity in contour and shape by placing her hands on her hips and tightening her chest muscles as she observes the shape of her breasts. See Figure 17-10A and B.
2. The female should check the nipples for discharge by squeezing each nipple to see if discharge is present. See Figure 17-10C.
3. The female should palpate each breast for the presence of lumps, in an orderly pattern; beginning at the armpit of the left breast, she should

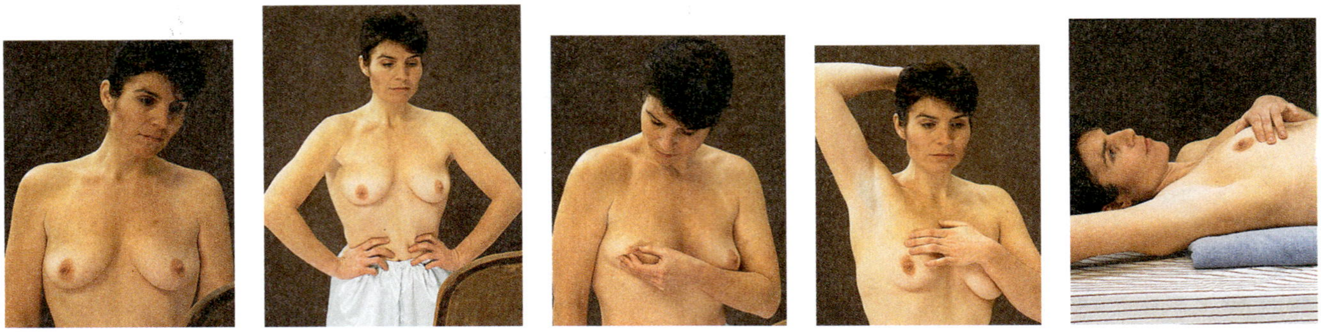

(A) (B) (C) (D) (E)

Figure 17-10 Breast self-examination

use three fingers of the right hand and firmly press a section at a time, in a circular motion. Continuing to press in the circular motion, she should move clockwise around the breast progressing toward the nipple of the breast with each round. The same process should be repeated with the right breast, palpating with the fingers of the left hand. See Figure 17-10D.

4. The process of checking the breasts for lumps in a clockwise pattern and checking the nipples for discharge, should now be performed while in the shower. The soap on the skin allows the fingers to glide more smoothly over the breasts. Check each breast in the careful manner as before.

5. Following the shower, or perhaps before the shower, the female should check both breasts while lying down. She should lie flat on her back with her left arm over her head and a small pillow or folded towel under her left shoulder. This will flatten the breast, making it easier to examine. Using the same clockwise pattern and the same circular motion, she should examine her left breast carefully with the flat part of the fingers of her right hand. This process should be repeated with the right breast. See Figure 17-10E.

---

colposcopy
(kol-**POSS**-koh-pee)
colp/o = vagina
-scopy = process of viewing

Visual examination of the vagina and cervix with a colposcope.

A colposcope is a lighted binocular microscope for direct examination of the surfaces of the vagina and cervix. The lenses of the microscope magnify the vaginal and cervical tissue for better viewing. See **Figure 17-11.** A colposcopy is advised for all women who have Pap smears showing dysplasia (abnormal cells).

After insertion of a speculum into the vagina and visualization of the cervix, the tissue is prepped by application of a 3% acetic acid (common household vinegar) solution. The solution is used to remove mucus and debris from the area and to slightly dehydrate the cells on the cervix, improving visibility of the cervical tissue. The physician observes the cervix and vagina with the colposcope, searching for any suspicious lesions. If a suspicious lesion or tissue is noted during the examination, a biopsy of the tissue will be obtained at that time.

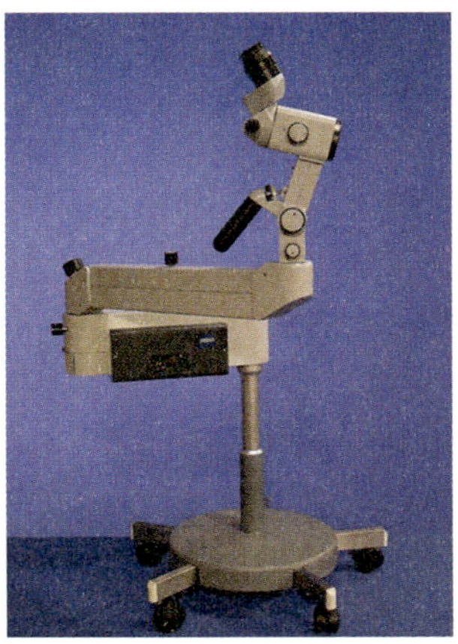

Figure 17-11 Colposcope 150 EC (Courtesy of Carl Zeiss Surgical, Inc.)

conization
(kon-ih-**ZAY**-shun)

Surgical removal of a cone-shaped segment of the cervix for diagnosis or treatment; also known as a cone biopsy.

When the lesion is in the inner lining of the cervical canal (endocervix) or when the Pap smear is suggestive of invasive carcinoma, a **conization** may be ordered. The lesion is removed from the endocervix, along with a margin of healthy tissue, in the cone-shaped segment that is removed. The patient should be observed for any unusual bleeding following a cone biopsy.

cryosurgery
(**cry**-oh **SER**-jer-ee)
cry/o = cold

The destruction of tissue by rapid freezing with substances such as liquid nitrogen.

The coolant is circulated through a metal probe, chilling it to subfreezing temperatures. When the cold metal probe touches the tissues, the moist tissues adhere to it and freeze. The tissues then become necrotic and slough off in a few days. Cryosurgery can be used for treatment of abnormal tissue of the cervix; it is frequently used to remove benign and/or malignant skin tumors and growths such as warts.

culdocentesis
(kull-doh-sen-**TEE**-sis)
culd/o = cul-de-sac
-centesis = surgical puncture

The surgical puncture through the posterior wall of the vagina into the cul-de-sac to withdraw intraperitoneal fluid for examination.

During a **culdocentesis** a culdoscope is inserted into the cul-de-sac to visualize the area for any evidence of inflammation, purulent drainage, bleeding, ovarian cysts, ectopic pregnancy, or ovarian malignancy. A needle is then inserted into the cul-de-sac through the scope and fluid is aspirated for examination.

dilatation and curettage
(dill-ah-**TAY**-shun and **koo**-reh-**TAHZ**)

Dilatation or widening of the cervical canal with a dilator, followed by scraping of the uterine lining with a curet; also termed D&C. See Figure 17-12A.

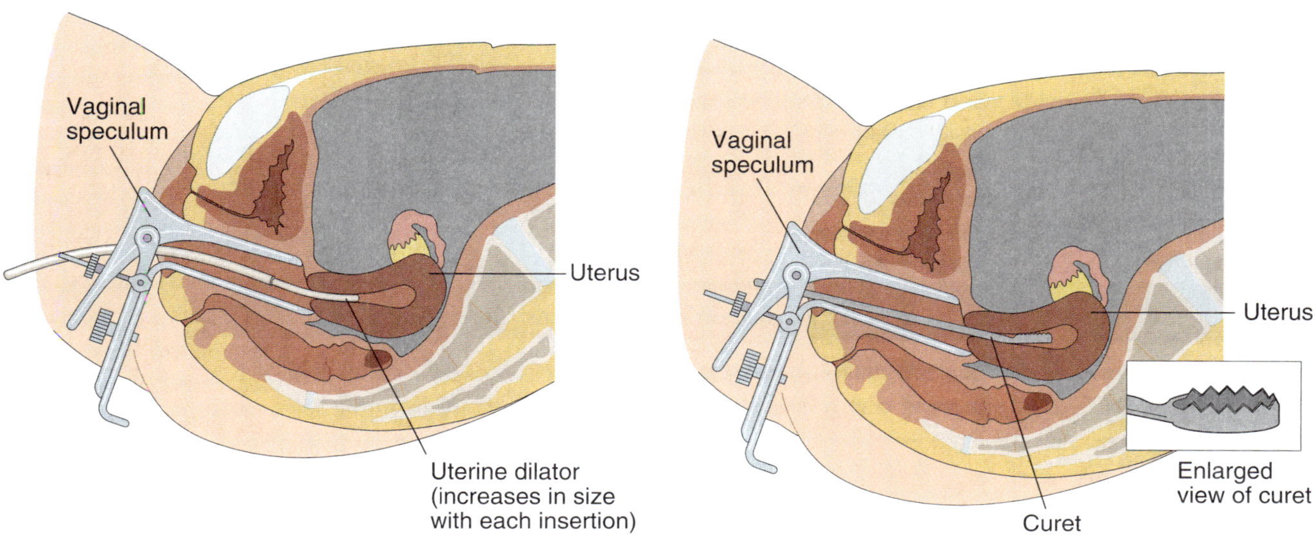

Figure 17-12 (A) Dilatation and curettage; (B) enlarged view of curet

During the dilatation, the cervix is expanded with a series of probes (increasing in diameter with each insertion); during the curettage, the lining of the uterine cavity is scraped with the cutting edge of a spoon-shaped metal loop (curet) See **Figure 17-12B**, for the purpose of diagnosing uterine disease, correcting heavy or prolonged uterine bleeding, or emptying the uterine contents. The patient should be observed for excessive bleeding within the first few hours after this procedure.

---

endometrial biopsy
(en-doh-**MEE**-tree-al **BYE**-op-see)
endo- = within
metri/o = uterus
-al = pertaining to

Endometrial biopsy is an invasive test for obtaining a sample of endometrial tissue with a small curet, for examination.

The endometrial tissue may be analyzed in cases of irregular bleeding, during infertility studies, and to examine tissue for possible endometrial cancer. During the procedure, the cervix is dilated and an instrument (uterine sound) is passed into the uterus to measure the depth of the uterine cavity (measures from the cervical os to the uterine fundus). A curet, or aspiration needle, is then inserted into the fundus of the uterus and a sample of endometrial tissue is extracted.

The patient will experience a "pinching" sensation during the procedure, followed by a short period of cramping after the procedure; this should be relieved by mild analgesics (pain relievers). The patient should experience only light bleeding following the procedure, but should be instructed to report any heavy bleeding.

---

hysterosalpingography
(**hiss**-ter-oh-**sal**-pin-**GOG**-rah-fee)
hyster/o = uterus
salping/o = eustachian tubes; also refers to fallopian tubes
-graphy = process of recording

X-ray of the uterus and the fallopian tubes, by injecting a contrast material into these structures.

The contrast medium is injected through a cannula inserted into the cervix. As the material is slowly injected, the filling of the uterus and fallopian tubes is observed with a fluoroscope. **Hysterosalpingography** is performed to evaluate the uterus for any abnormalities in structure, the presence of possible tumors, and to test for tubal obstructions. The patient may feel occasional menstrual-type cramping during the procedure and will have vaginal drainage for a couple of days after the procedure (from the drainage of the contrast material).

---

laparoscopy
(lap-ar-**OS**-koh-pee)
lapar/o = abdominal wall
-scopy = process of viewing

The process of viewing the abdominal cavity with a laparoscope (a thin-walled flexible tube with a telescopic lens and light).

A small incision is made into the abdominal wall near the umbilicus (navel) and the laparoscope is inserted. This procedure is used to visualize abdominal and pelvic organs. See **Figure 17-13.**

The reasons for performing a laparoscopy include, but are not limited to, diagnosing unexplained pelvic or abdominal pain, to confirm or rule out suspected cases of tubal pregnancy or endometriosis, to visualize and assess the female reproductive organs during various infertility studies, or for therapeutic procedures such as tubal ligations and other types of minor surgery.

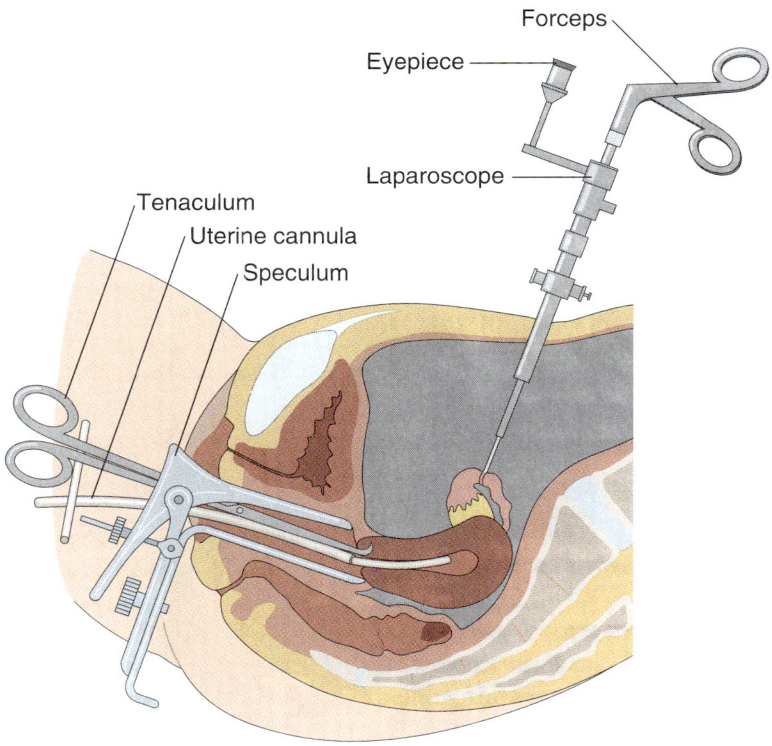

Figure 17-13 Laparoscopy

mammography
(mam-**OG**-rah-fee)
mamm/o = breasts
-graphy = process of recording

The process of examining with x-ray the soft tissue of the breast to detect various benign and/or malignant growths before they can be felt. See Figure 17-14.

The American College of Radiology recognizes the use of x-ray **mammography** as the approved method of screening for breast cancer. This procedure takes approximately 15 to 30 minutes to complete, and can be performed in an x-ray department of a hospital or in a private radiology facility. Each facility should have equipment that is designed and used exclusively for mammograms.

During the examination, the breast tissue is compressed between two clear disks for each x-ray view. The first view requires compressing the breast from top to bottom to take a top-to-bottom (craniocaudal) view. The second view requires compressing the breast from side to side to take a mediolateral view. The patient may experience fleeting discomfort as the breast tissue is compressed between the plates, but this is necessary to facilitate maximum visualization of the breast tissue.

The American Cancer Society recommends that women have their first mammogram between ages 35 and 39. This will provide a baseline for reference with future mammograms. Between ages 40 and 49, mammograms are usually recommended every 2 years, unless the woman is in a high-risk category. From age 50 and thereafter, mammograms are recommended annually.

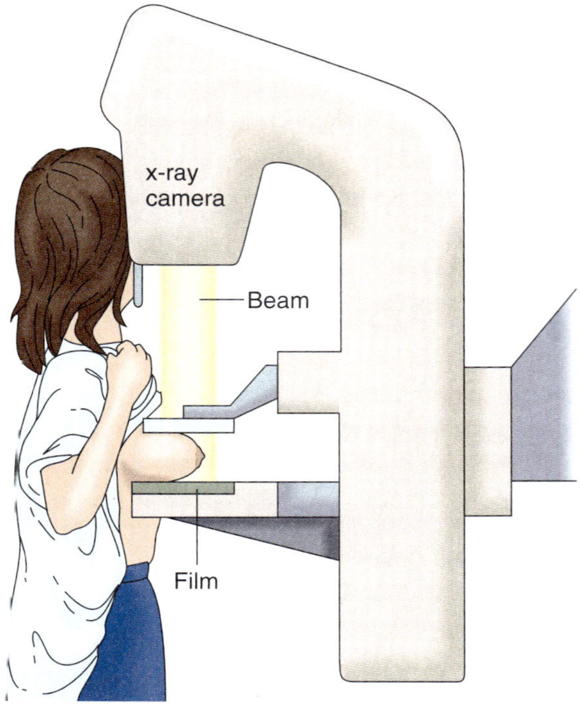

Figure 17-14 Mammography

Papanicolaou (Pap) smear
(pap-ah-**NIK**-oh-low smear)

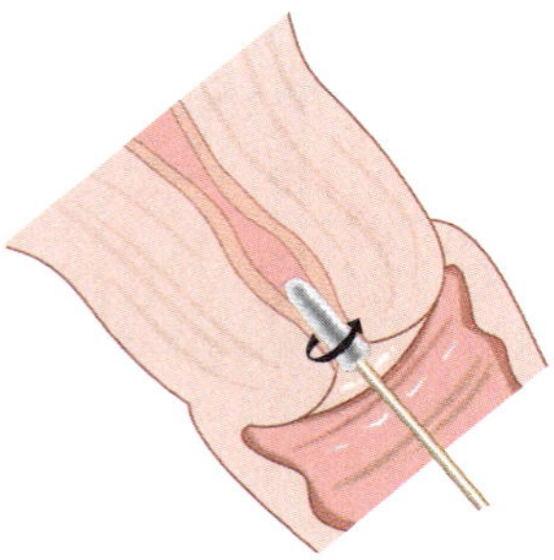

Figure 17-15
Endocervical smear

A diagnostic test for cervical cancer; that is, a microscopic examination of (Pap test) cells scraped from within the cervix (endocervix), from around the cervix (ectocervix), and from the posterior part of the vagina (near the cervix) to test for cervical cancer; also called Pap test.

As part of the annual gynecological examination, the Pap smear consists of obtaining a small amount of secretions taken from the endocervix (see **Figure 17-15**), and from the posterior vaginal area (nearest the cervix).

These secretions are smeared onto separate, clean microscope slides and are "set" with a spray fixative. The slides are marked for their source as either "C" for cervical or "V" for vaginal. The specimens obtained will be examined and interpreted by a pathologist.

Patients should be instructed not to douche or tub-bathe for at least 24 hours before a Pap smear, because this may cause cellular material to be washed away with the douching solution or the bath water. A lubricant is not used on the speculum for a Pap smear because this can interfere with the accurate reading of the slide. Furthermore, the Pap smear should be done during or close to the middle of the menstrual cycle because the presence of blood interferes with an accurate interpretation of the specimen and may camouflage atypical cells.

The Pap smear is up to 95% accurate in diagnosing early cervical cancer when the specimen sample is obtained correctly. When the Pap test is positive, additional tissue studies, that is, biopsy or even surgery, may be performed to confirm the diagnosis of cancer.

The traditional classification of Papanicolaou smears is as follows:

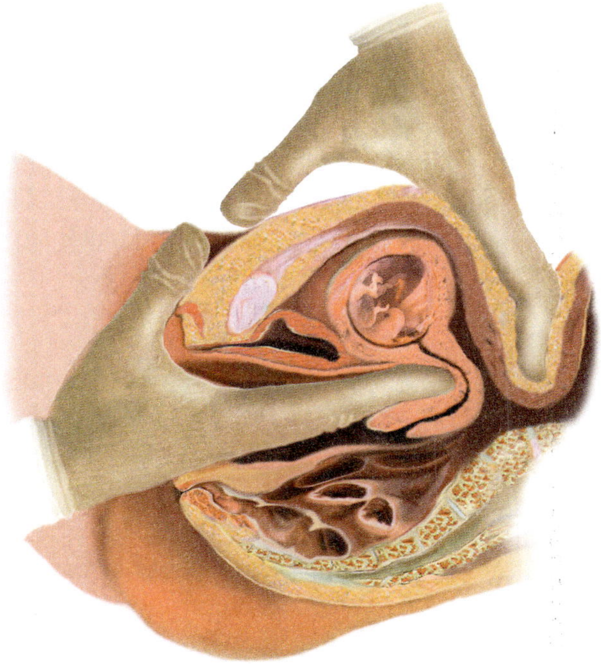

Figure 17-16 Bimanual examination

Class I—Absence of atypical or abnormal cells (negative)

Class II—Atypical cells present, but no evidence of malignancy (this is usually caused by cervical inflammation)

Class III—Cytology suggestive of, but not conclusive for, malignancy

Class IV—Cytology strongly suggestive of malignancy

Class V—Cytology conclusive for malignancy

Newer classifications for Pap smears are descriptive terms that omit the numbers for classifying; instead, they use terms descriptive of the cellular changes observed by the pathologist. The American Cancer Society recommends that women who are over 18 years of age or younger sexually active women should have yearly Pap smears and gynecological examinations. The annual exam will also include palpation of the female internal organs by bimanual examination (see **Figure 17-16**). When palpating the female pelvic organs by bimanual examination, the examiner places one hand on the abdomen and inserts one or two fingers of the other gloved hand into the vagina. This allows the examiner to feel the female organs between the two hands.

pelvic ultrasound
(**PELL**-vik **ULL**-trah-sound)
pelv/i = pelvis
-ic = pertaining to
ultra- = beyond

A noninvasive procedure that uses high-frequency sound waves to examine the abdomen and pelvis.

The sound waves pass through the abdominal wall from the transducer, which is moved back and forth across the abdomen. When the sound waves bounce off of the internal organs in the abdominopelvic region, these waves are converted to electrical impulses eventually recorded on an oscilloscope screen. The oscilloscope transforms the electrical impulses into visual images. A photograph of the images is then taken for further study.

Pelvic ultrasound can be used to locate a pelvic mass, an ectopic pregnancy, or an intrauterine device and to inspect and assess the uterus, ovaries, and fallopian tubes. Clearer ultrasonic pictures of the pelvic organs can be obtained by using **transvaginal ultrasonography.** This procedure produces the same type of picture as abdominal ultrasound, but involves the use of a vaginal probe inserted into the vagina while the patient is in **lithotomy position.** The probes are encased in a sterile sheath and placed in the transducer before it is inserted into the vagina. The sound waves function in the same way as those for the abdominopelvic ultrasound, but the transvaginal ultrasonic image is much clearer.

pelvimetry
(pell-**VIM**-eh-tree)
pelv/i = pelvis
-metry = the process of measuring

The process of measuring the female pelvis, manually or by x-ray, to determine its adequacy for childbearing.

Clinical pelvimetry is an estimate of the size of the birth canal by vaginal palpation of bony landmarks in the pelvis and a mathematical estimate of the distance between them. This is performed during the early part of the pregnancy and is recorded as "adequate," "borderline," or "inadequate."

X-ray pelvimetry is an actual x-ray of the pelvis to determine the dimensions of the bony pelvis of a pregnant woman; it is performed when there is doubt that the head of the fetus can safely pass through the pelvis during the labor process. Measurements are actually made on the x-ray, and the true dimensions of the birth canal and the head of the fetus can be calculated to determine if the proportions are suitable.

Sexually Transmitted Diseases (Male and Female)

Sexually transmitted diseases (STDs) in the female are the same as those in the male. These contagious diseases are spread from one person to another through contact with body fluids such as blood, semen, and vaginal secretions. STDs may be spread during vaginal, anal, or oral sex, or by direct contact with infected skin.

AIDS, which is a sexually transmitted disease, can also be transmitted through blood and blood products, sharing of needles (as in intravenous drug users), through the placenta of an infected mother to the baby (during the birth process), and through the breast milk of an infected mother to the baby (when nursing the baby).

The incidence of STDs is alarmingly high in the United States; it has greatly increased in recent years, especially among young people. Discussion of the more common STDs can be found in Chapter 16.

Common Abbreviations

ABBREVIATION	MEANING	ABBREVIATION	MEANING
AB	abortion	**LH**	luteinizing hormone
CIS	carcinoma in situ	**LMP**	last menstrual period
Cx	cervix	**LSO**	left salpingo-oophorectomy
D&C	dilatation and curettage	**Pap**	Papanicolaou smear
ECC	endocervical curettage	**Path**	pathology
EMB	endometrial biopsy	**PID**	pelvic inflammatory disease
ERT	estrogen replacement therapy	**PMS**	premenstrual syndrome
GYN	gynecology	**RSO**	right salpingo-oophorectomy
HSG	hysterosalpingography	**TAH**	total abdominal hysterectomy
IUD	intrauterine device; a particular type of contraceptive device	**TVH**	total vaginal hysterectomy

Written and Audio Terminology Review

Review each of the following terms from this chapter. Study the spelling of each term and write the definition in the space provided. If you have the Audio CD available, listen to each term, pronounce it, and check the box once you are comfortable saying the word. Check definitions by looking the term up in the glossary/index.

TERM	PRONUNCIATION	DEFINITION
abstinence	☐ **AB**-stih-nens	____________
adnexa	☐ add-**NEK**-sah	____________
amenorrhea	☐ ah-men-oh-**REE**-ah	____________
anteflexion	☐ an-tee-**FLEK**-shun	____________
areola	☐ ah-**REE**-oh-lah	____________
aspiration biopsy	☐ as-pih-**RAY**-shun **BYE**-op-see	____________
Bartholin's glands	☐ **BAR**-toh-linz glands	____________
carcinoma	☐ car-sin-**OH**-mah	____________
cervical	☐ **SER**-vih-kal	____________

Term		Pronunciation	
cervicitis	☐	ser-vih-**SIGH**-tis	________
cervix	☐	**SER**-viks	________
climacteric	☐	kly-**MAK**-ter-ik	________
clitoris	☐	**KLIT**-oh-ris	________
coitus	☐	**KOH**-ih-tus	________
colpodynia	☐	kol-poh-**DIN**-ee-ah	________
colposcopy	☐	kol-**POSS**-koh-pee	________
conization	☐	kon-ih-**ZAY**-shun	________
corpus luteum	☐	**KOR**-pus **LOO**-tee-um	________
cryosurgery	☐	**cry**-oh-**SER**-jer-ee	________
cul-de-sac	☐	**KULL**-dih-**SAK**	________
culdocentesis	☐	kull-doh-sen-**TEE**-sis	________
cystocele	☐	**SIS**-toh-seel	________
Depo-Provera injection	☐	**DEP**-oh proh-**VAIR**-ah injection	________
diaphragm	☐	**DYE**-ah-fram	________
dilatation and curettage	☐	dill-ah-**TAY**-shun and koo-reh-**TAHZ**	________
dysmenorrhea	☑	**dis**-men-oh-**REE**-ah	________
endometrial	☐	en-doh-**MEE**-tree-al	________
endometrial biopsy	☐	en-doh-**MEE**-tree-al **BYE**-op-see	________
endometriosis	☐	**en**-doh-**mee**-tree-**OH**-sis	________
endometrium	☐	en-doh-**MEE**-tree-um	________
estrogen	☐	**ESS**-troh-jen	________
fallopian tubes	☐	fah-**LOH**-pee-an **TOOBS**	________
fertilization	☐	fer-til-eye-**ZAY**-shun	________
fibrocystic	☐	figh-broh-**SIS**-tik	________
fibroid	☐	**FIGH**-broyd	________
fimbriae	☐	**FIM**-bree-**ay**	________
fourchette	☐	foor-**SHET**	________
fundus	☐	**FUN**-dus	________

Term	Pronunciation	
gamete	☐ **GAM**-eet	________
gonads	☐ **GOH**-nads	________
graafian follicles	☐ **GRAF**-ee-an **FALL**-ik-kls	________
gynecologist	☐ guy-neh-**KOL**-oh-jist	________
gynecology	☐ guy-neh-**KOL**-oh-jee	________
hymen	☐ **HIGH**-men	________
hysterectomy	☐ **hiss**-ter-**EK**-toh-mee	________
hysterosalpingography	☐ **hiss**-ter-oh-**sal**-pin-**GOG**-rah-fee	________
incompetent cervix	☐ in-**COMP**-eh-tent **SIR**-viks	________
intrauterine	☐ in-trah-**YOO**-ter-in	________
labia majora	☐ **LAY**-bee-ah mah-**JOR**-ah	________
labia minora	☐ **LAY**-bee-ah mih-**NOR**-ah	________
laparoscopy	☐ lap-ar-**OS**-koh-pee	________
leiomyoma	☐ **ligh**-oh-my-**OH**-mah	________
mammary	☐ **MAM**-ah-ree	________
mammography	☐ mam-**OG**-rah-fee	________
mastectomy	☐ mass-**TEK**-toh-mee	________
menarche	☐ men-**AR**-kee	________
menopause	☐ **MEN**-oh-pawz	________
menorrhagia	☐ **men**-oh-**RAY**-jee-ah	________
menorrhea	☐ men-oh-**REE**-ah	________
menstruation	☐ men-stroo-**AY**-shun	________
metrorrhagia	☐ **met**-roh-**RAY**-jee-ah	________
myometrium	☐ my-oh-**MEE**-tree-um	________
oligomenorrhea	☐ ol-ih-goh-**men**-oh-**REE**-ah	________
oogenesis	☐ oh-oh-**JEN**-eh-sis	________
oophoritis	☐ oh-off-oh-**RIGH**-tis	________
oral contraceptives	☐ **ORAL** con-trah-**SEP**-tivz	________
ovarian	☐ oh-**VAY**-ree-an	________
ovarian cysts	☐ oh-**VAY**-ree-an **SISTS**	________
ovariopexy	☐ oh-**vay**-ree-oh-**PEK**-see	________

ovary	☐	**OH**-vah-ree	______
ovulation	☐	ov-yoo-**LAY**-shun	______
ovum	☐	**OH**-vum	______
Pap smear	☐	**PAP** smear	______
Papanicolaou smear	☐	pap-ah-**NIK**-oh-low smear	______
pelvic	☐	**PELL**-vik	______
pelvic inflammatory disease	☐	**PELL**-vik in-**FLAM**-mah-toh-ree dih-**ZEEZ**	______
pelvic ultrasound	☐	**PELL**-vik **ULL**-trah-sound	______
pelvimetry	☐	pell-**VIM**-eh-tree	______
perineum	☐	pair-ih-**NEE**-um	______
pregnancy	☐	**PREG**-nan-see	______
premenstrual syndrome	☐	pre-**MEN**-stroo-al **SIN**-drom	______
progesterone	☐	proh-**JES**-ter-own	______
puberty	☐	**PEW**-ber-tee	______
retroversion	☐	ret-roh-**VER**-shun	______
salpingitis	☐	sal-pin-**JYE**-tis	______
tubal ligation	☐	**TOO**-bal lye-**GAY**-shun	______
uterus	☐	**YOO**-ter-us	______
vagina	☐	vah-**JEYE**-nah	______
vaginitis	☐	vaj-in-**EYE**-tis	______
vulva	☐	**VULL**-vah	______
vulvovaginitis	☐	**vull**-voh-**VAJ**-in-eye-tis	______

Chapter Review Exercises

The following exercises provide a more in-depth review of the chapter material. Your goal in these exercises is to complete each section at a minimum 80% level of accuracy. If you score below 80% in any area, return to the appropriate section in the chapter and read the material again. A place has been provided for your score at the end of each section.

A. Spelling

Circle the correctly spelled term in each pairing of words. Each correct answer is worth 10 points. Record your score in the space provided at the end of the exercise.

1.	ministration	menstruation
2.	meatus	meatis
3.	clitoris	clitorus
4.	menarkey	menarche
5.	mammogram	mammagram
6.	laproscope	laparoscope
7.	colposcopy	culposcopy
8.	coldocentesis	culdocentesis
9.	diaphram	diaphragm
10.	graffian follicles	graafian follicles

Number correct ______ × 10 points/correct answer: Your score _____%

B. Matching

Match the following terms on the left with the most appropriate definitions on the right. Each correct answer is worth 10 points. Record your score in the space provided at the end of the exercise.

_____	1. menstrual phase	a.	female reproductive organs are fully developed
_____	2. premenstrual phase	b.	absence of menstrual flow
_____	3. postmenstrual phase	c.	days 1 to 5; lasts for approximately 3 to 5 days
_____	4. ovulatory phase	d.	abnormally light or infrequent menstruation
_____	5. oligomenorrhea	e.	abnormally long or very heavy menstrual periods
_____	6. amenorrhea	f.	graafian follicle ruptures, releasing the mature ovum
_____	7. dysmenorrhea	g.	painful menstruation
_____	8. metrorrhagia	h.	interval between the menses and ovulation; days 6 to 12
_____	9. menorrhagia	i.	days 15 to 28; if pregnancy does not occur, hormone level drops causing irritability, fluid retention, and breast tenderness
_____	10. puberty		
		j.	uterine bleeding at times other than the menstrual period

Number correct ______ × 10 points/correct answer: Your score _____%

C. Crossword Puzzle

Read the clues carefully and complete the puzzle. Each crossword answer is worth 10 points. When you have completed the crossword puzzle, total your points and enter your score in the space provided.

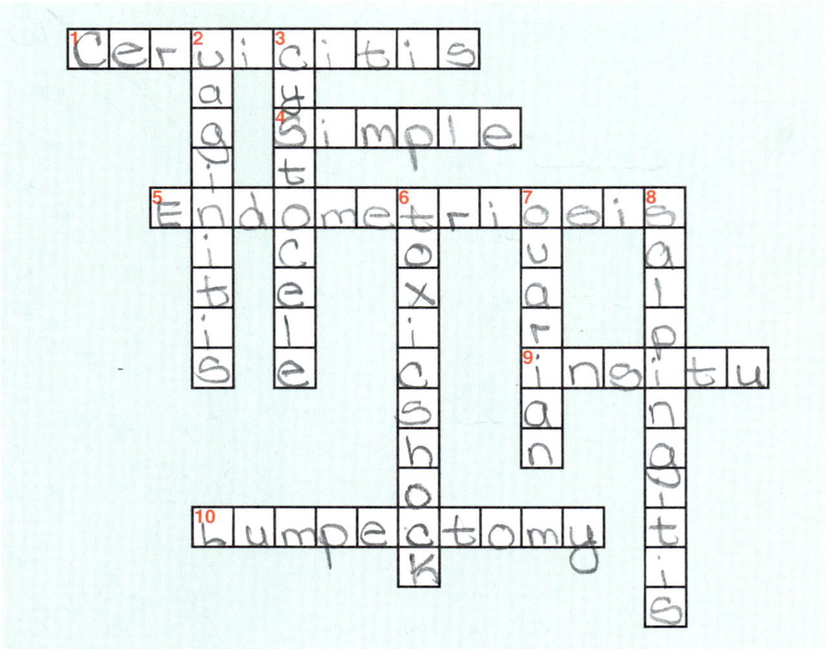

ACROSS

1 Inflammation of the uterine cervix
4 ___________ mastectomy; removal of only the breast
5 Uterine lining tissue out of place
9 Early-stage cancer: just sits there
10 Removal of tumor only and some breast tissue

DOWN

2 Inflammation of the vagina and vulva
3 Bladder protrudes into the vagina
6 Potentially fatal syndrome
7 Cancer, rarely detected early
8 Inflammation of the Fallopian tubes

***Number correct* ______ × *10 points/correct answer: Your score* _____%**

D. Proofreading Skills

Read the following excerpt from an operative report. For each boldface term, provide a brief definition in the space provided and indicate if the term is spelled correctly. If it is misspelled, provide the correct spelling. Each correct answer is worth 10 points. Record your score in the space provided at the end of the exercise.

Example:

fimbriated *Having fingerlike projections*

Spelled correctly? ☑ Yes ☐ No ______

1. **ectopic** Out of place

Spelled correctly? ☑ Yes ☐ No ______

2. **endometriosis** The presence and growth of tissue in areas outside the

Spelled correctly? ☑ Yes ☐ No endometrium (lining of the urterus

3. **ovarion** Ovarian

Spelled correctly? ☐ Yes ☑ No ______

NAME: Luna, Sophia

ROOM NO: 5261

HOSPITAL NO: 720431

SURGEON: Dr. I. Will Clampett

PREOPERATIVE DIAGNOSIS: Probable **ectopic** pregnancy

POSTOPERATIVE DIAGNOSIS:
1. Ectopic pregnancy, left tubule
2. Multiple cysts of both ovaries
3. Pelvic **endometriosis**

ANESTHESIA: General

OPERATION:
1. Left partial salpingectomy; removal of ectopic pregnancy
2. Lysis of pelvic adhesions
3. Coagulation of **ovarion** cysts

PROCEDURE: After successful general anesthesia, the patient was prepared for surgery. The pelvic cavity was entered without incident. Upon opening the abdomen, one could see some old dark blood and a modest amount of bright red blood. The **uteris** was held back and downwards, somewhat, by a mass filling the left side of the **col-de-sac** and extending over to the left lateral wall of the **pelvis.** This material was quite friable. The bowel seemed looped about it. Careful dissection freed the mass and brought it into view, revealing a tubal pregnancy in the outer portion of the left tube.

The left **ovary** was small but contained multiple tiny **cysks.** The right tube appeared normal with the **fimbriated** ends being open and intact. A partial **salpinjectomy** was carried out on the left side, removing the outer portion of the tube including the ectopic pregnancy.

After suctioning the blood from the cul-de-sac area, it was noted that there were massive adhesions of friable necrotic tissue on the posterior wall of the **fundus** of the uterus. The area was cleaned up as best as possible and tiny bleeders were coagulated. "......(material deleted)...."

The patient withstood the procedure well and was transferred to the recovery room in good condition.

SPONGE COUNT #1: One sponge missing

SPONGE COUNT #2: Reported correct

DATE OF DICTATION: 06-25-03

DICTATED BY: Dr. I Will Clampett

_________________________________ MD
Signature of surgeon

4. **uteris** uterus

Spelled correctly? ☐ Yes ☑ No ______

5. **col-de-sac** Cul-de-sac

Spelled correctly? ☐ Yes ☑ No ______

6. **pelvis** A lower part of the trunk of the body made up of

Spelled correctly? ☑ Yes ☐ No four bones

7. **ovary** A gamete-producing gland

Spelled correctly? ☑ Yes ☐ No ______

8. **cysks** Cysts

Spelled correctly? ☐ Yes ☑ No ______

9. **salpinjectomy** Salpingectomy

Spelled correctly? ☐ Yes ☑ No ______

10. **fundus** ______

Spelled correctly? ☑ Yes ☐ No ______

Number correct ______ × 10 points/correct answer: Your score _____%

E. Word Search

Using the definitions listed, identify the appropriate word and then find and circle it in the puzzle. The words may be read up, down, diagonally, across, or backward. Each correct answer is worth 10 points. Record your score in the space provided at the end of the exercise.

C O L P O S C O P Y A V E O L A R O S C O H
O R E E N D C M A N B R A D Y E V Y U S Q Y
N A Y C A R C I N O M E T F R I A B L U J S
I V Z O V A R I E N T E S I C P E L M I S T
Z I S I S E T N E C O D L U C I N V A S I E
A B C D E U S C O P I C A P E R Y A I P O R
T R I M E S R Y L T R A P S O U N D Y E A O
I A O M M A N G R U P H A C U L D H E L P S
O I N V A S I X E N T E R I E S P Y A V I A
N D I L A T I O X R S C O T Y A V E N I L L
C R Y O S U R G I N Y U S A R C O N I C U P
A S P I R A T U L V E M C G B I O L O U G I
S A L P Y I N G O S C E O R R H A P H L Y N
T Y P O G R A P I C U M P A R E O L U T E G
A D V E N T T U R E M S Y I N T M R M R L O
M E D I C A W E L A W O R D S W A T I A U G
R I G H E N D O M E T R I A L B I O P S Y R
Y O U R A N S W E I R I S C O R R U J O I A
T E R M I B O L O G V I N T R A U T E U R P
I N T R A V E N L P O L L A T E R O N N M H
C L A S S I F I C B R A E N D O S C O D U Y
P A P I N I R A E M S P A P A N I C O L A O

Example: A diagnostic test for cervical cancer

Pap smear

1. Visual examination of the vagina and cervix with a scope

____

2. Surgical removal of a cone-shaped segment of the cervix for diagnosis or treatment

____

3. The destruction of tissue by rapid freezing with substances such as liquid nitrogen

____

4. The surgical puncture through the posterior wall of the vagina into the cul-de-sac to withdraw intraperitoneal fluid for examination

____

5. An invasive test for obtaining a sample of endometrial tissue with a small curet for examination

____

6. The process of x-raying the uterus and the fallopian tubes

____

7. The process of viewing the abdominal cavity with a thin flexible tube with a telescopic lens and light

____

8. The process of x-raying the soft tissue of the breast

____

9. The process of measuring the female pelvis manually or by x-ray

____

10. A noninvasive procedure that uses high-frequency waves to examine the abdomen and pelvis

____

Number correct _______ × 10 points/correct answer: Your score ______%

F. Word Element Review

The following words relate to the female reproductive system. The word elements have been labeled (WR = word root, P = prefix, S = suffix, and V = combining vowel). Read the definition carefully and complete the word by filling in the blank, using the word elements provided in this chapter. If you have forgotten the word building rules, refer to Chapter 1. Each correct word is worth 10 points. Record your score in the space provided at the end of this exercise.

1. Surgical puncture of the amniotic sac:

amni / o / entesis

WR V S

2. Inflammation of the cervix:

cervic / itis

WR S

3. One who specializes in treating diseases/disorders of women:

gynec / o / logist

WR V S

4. Surgical removal of the uterus:

hyster / ectomy

WR S

5. Absence of menstrual flow:

a / men / o / rrhea

P WR V S

6. Condition of the inner lining of the uterus:

endo / metri / osis

P WR S

7. Surgical removal of the breast:

mast / ectomy

WR S

8. Inflammation of the fallopian tubes:

salping / itis

WR S

9. Beginning of menses; first menstrual period:

men / arche

WR S

10. Painful menstruation:

dys / men / o / rrhea

P WR V S

Number correct _______ × 10 points/correct answer: Your score _____%

G. Matching Abbreviations

Match the abbreviations on the left with the correct definition on the right. Each correct answer is worth 10 points. Record your score in the space provided at the end of the exercise.

e	1. D&C	a. last menstrual period
j	2. EMB	b. total abdominal hysterectomy
f	3. GYN	c. premenstrual syndrome
h	4. IUD	d. carcinoma in situ
g	5. Pap	e. dilatation and curettage
i	6. PID	f. gynecology
c	7. PMS	g. Papanicolaou smear
b	8. TAH	h. intrauterine device
d	9. CIS	i. pelvic inflammatory disease
a	10. LMP	j. endometrial biopsy

Number correct _______ × 10 points/correct answer: Your score _____%

H. Completion

The following is a discussion of secondary sex characteristic changes experienced by the female during puberty, and instructions for breast self-examination. Fill in the blanks with the most appropriate word(s). Each correct answer is worth 10 points. Record your score in the space provided at the end of the exercise.

> Puberty is the time during which the female experiences some secondary sex characteristic changes. These changes include the following: changes in the breast, which include (1) ______________ deposition of (2) ______________ in the buttocks and thighs, creating a more (3) ______________ appearance; widening of the (4) ______________ making it more appropriate for childbirth; growth of (5) ______________ and (6) ______________ hair. The most evident change during puberty is the onset of menstruation, with the first menstrual period being called the (7) ______________. By the time a young woman reaches the age of 20, she should perform the breast self-examination every month, about 7 to 10 days after the menstrual period. She should begin the process by standing (8) ______________ to observe the appearance of her breasts. As she palpates her breasts for the presence of any lumps, she should press firmly, moving in a circular motion, beginning at the armpit and progressing toward (9) ______________. Each breast should be checked in the same manner. After palpating the breasts for lumps, the female should then check her breast while in the (10a*) ______________ and while (10b*) ______________. **Note:* 10a and 10b count as one answer

Number correct ______ × 10 points/correct answer: Your score _____%

I. Matching

Match the terms on the left with the appropriate descriptions on the right. Each correct answer is worth 10 points. Record your score in the space provided at the end of the exercise.

_____ 1. lumpectomy
_____ 2. simple mastectomy
_____ 3. modified radical mastectomy
_____ 4. radical mastectomy
_____ 5. aspiration biopsy
_____ 6. Class I
_____ 7. Class II
_____ 8. Class III
_____ 9. Class IV
_____ 10. Class V

a. cytology conclusive for malignancy
b. tissue or fluid sample is withdrawn for microscopic examination and diagnosis
c. absence of atypical or abnormal cells
d. removal of only the tumor and a small margin of breast tissue
e. cytology suggestive of, but not conclusive for, malignancy
f. removal of the breast, chest muscles, and lymph nodes on the affected side
g. removal of the breast and lymph nodes on the affected side
h. this reading can be caused by cervical inflammation
i. cytology strongly suggestive of malignancy
j. only the breast is removed

Number correct ______ × 10 points/correct answer: Your score _____%

J. Label

Using the following figure, label the internal genitalia of the female reproductive system.

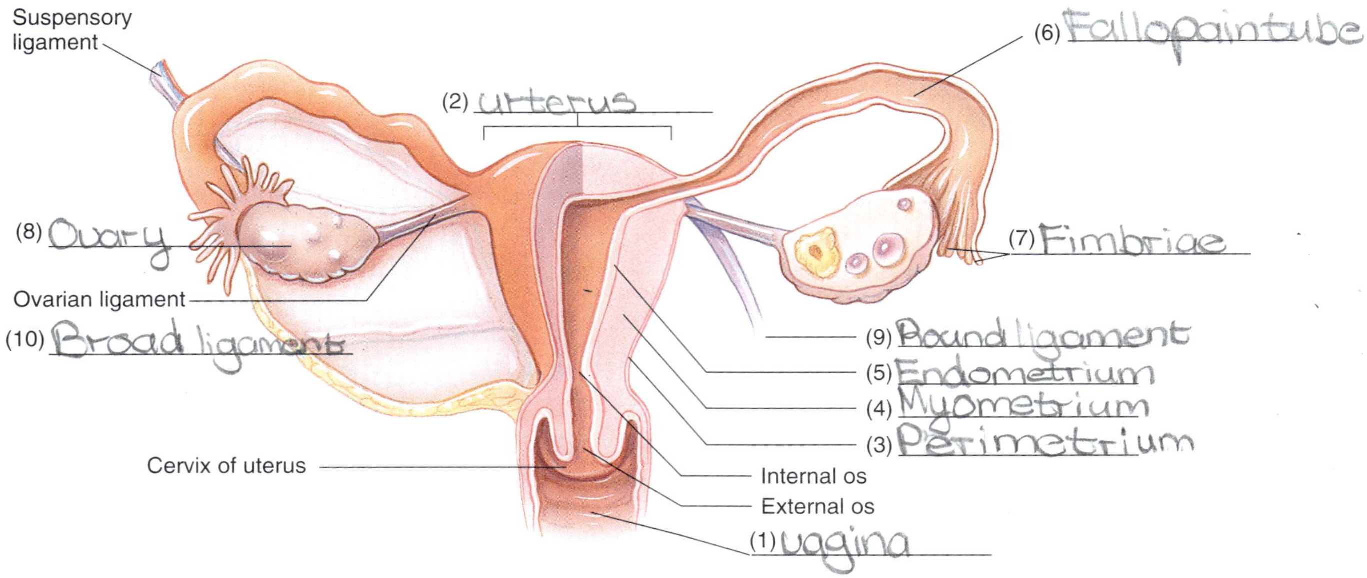

1. vagina	6. Fallopaintube
2. urterus	7. Fimbriae
3. Perimetrium	8. Ovary
4. Myometrium	9. Round ligament
5. Endometrium	10. Broad ligament

Number correct ______ × 10 points/correct answer: Your score _____%

Answers to Chapter Review Exercises

A. Spelling

1. menstruation	6. laparoscope
2. meatus	7. colposcopy
3. clitoris	8. culdocentesis
4. menarche	9. diaphragm
5. mammogram	10. graafian follicles

B. Matching

1. c	6. b
2. i	7. g
3. h	8. j
4. f	9. e
5. d	10. a

C. Crossword Puzzle

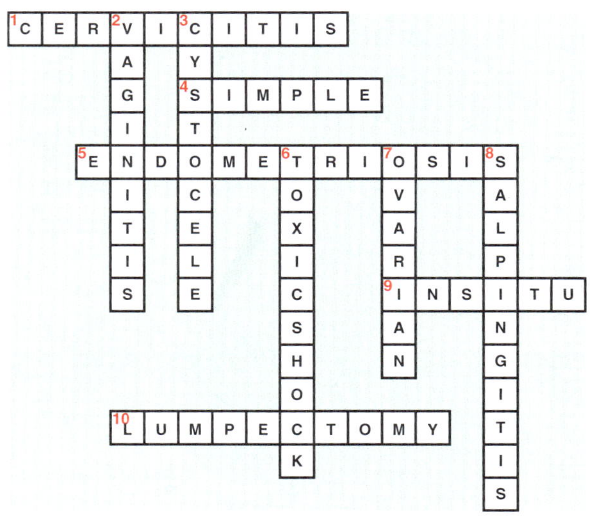

D. Proofreading Skills

1. Out of place.
   Spelled correctly? Yes
2. The presence and growth of tissue in areas outside the endometrium (lining of the uterus).
   Spelled correctly? Yes
3. Of or pertaining to the ovary.
   Spelled correctly? No **ovarian**
4. A pear-shaped, hollow, muscular organ that houses the fertilized, implanted ovum as it develops throughout pregnancy. It is also the source of the monthly menstrual flow if pregnancy does not occur.
   Spelled correctly? No **uterus**
5. A pouch that is located between the uterus and rectum within the peritoneal cavity.
   Spelled correctly? No **cul-de-sac**
6. The lower part of the trunk of the body made up of four bones.
   Spelled correctly? Yes
7. A gamete-producing gland.
   Spelled correctly? Yes
8. Closed sacs in or under the skin lined with epithelium and containing semisolid material or fluid.
   Spelled correctly? No **cysts**
9. Surgical removal of the fallopian tube(s).
   Spelled correctly? No **salpingectomy**
10. The small, dome-shaped portion of the uterus that rises above the area where the fallopian tubes enter.
    Spelled correctly? Yes

E. Word Search

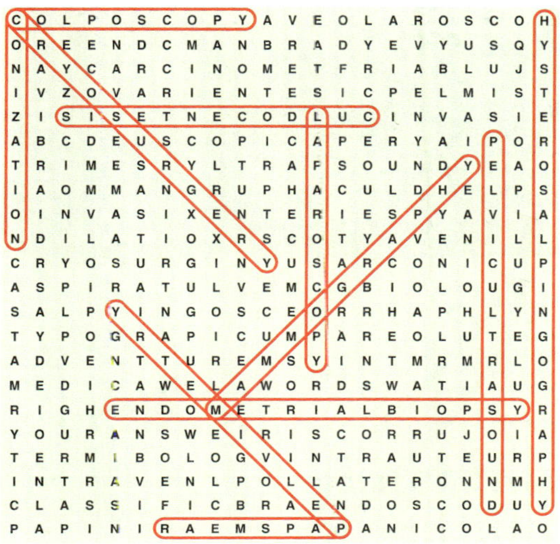

F. Word Element Review

1. amni /o/ entesis
   WR V S
2. cervic / itis
   WR S
3. gynec /o/ logist
   WR V S
4. hyster / ectomy
   WR S
5. a / men / o / rrhea
   P WR V S
6. endo /metri/ osis
   P WR S
7. mast / ectomy
   WR S
8. salping / itis
   WR S
9. men / arche
   WR S
10. dys / men / o / rrhea
    P WR V S

G. Matching Abbreviations

1. e.
2. j
3. f
4. h
5. g
6. i
7. c
8. b
9. d
10. a

H. Completion

1. development of glandular tissue
2. fat
3. rounded
4. pelvis
5. pubic
6. axillary
7. menarche
8. before a mirror
9. the nipple
10. a. shower b. lying down

I. Matching

1. d
2. j
3. g
4. f
5. b
6. c
7. h
8. e
9. i
10. a

J. Label

1. vagina
2. uterus
3. perimetrium
4. myometrium
5. endometrium
6. fallopian tube
7. fimbriae
8. ovary
9. round ligament
10. broad ligament

CHAPTER 18

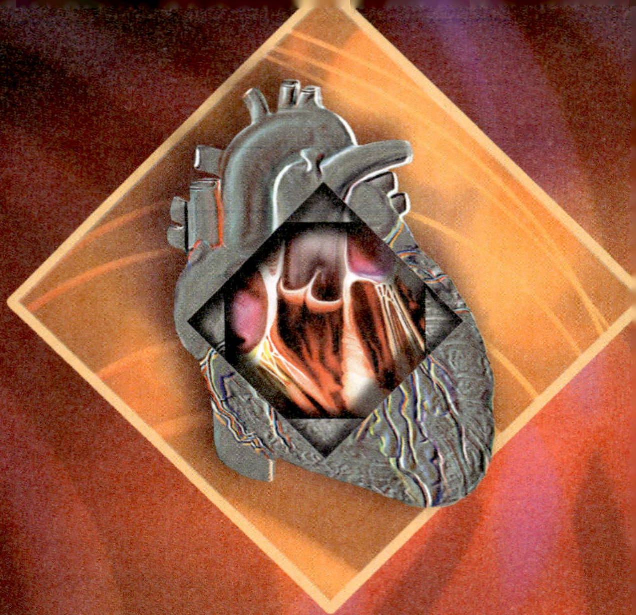

Obstetrics

CHAPTER CONTENT

KEY COMPETENCIES

Upon completing this chapter and the review exercises at the end of the chapter, the learner should be able to:

1. State the difference between presumptive and probable signs of pregnancy.
2. Correctly spell and pronounce each new term introduced in this chapter using the Activity CD-ROM and Audio CD, if available.
3. Define at least 20 abbreviations common to obstetrics.
4. Define 10 physiological changes that occur in the female during pregnancy.
5. List and define at least five diagnostic techniques used in treating obstetrical patients.
6. Demonstrate the ability to correctly construct words relating to the field of obstetrics by completing the word element review exercise at the end of the chapter.
7. List and define at least 10 complications of pregnancy.
8. Differentiate between the signs and symptoms of impending labor and those of false and/or true labor.

OVERVIEW

Obstetrics is the field of medicine that deals with pregnancy (prenatal), delivery of the baby, and the first 6 weeks after delivery (the **postpartum** period). The physician who specializes in the care of women during pregnancy, the delivery of the baby, and the first 6 weeks following the delivery is known as an **obstetrician**. Pregnancy signifies the fertilization of the ovum by the sperm: the creation of another human being. With this creation comes many changes, physiological as well as psychological. The physiological changes occur in a certain order as the fetus develops; many of the physiological changes will be discussed later in this chapter.

The psychological changes will vary with individuals. For some, pregnancy is desired and is perceived as one of the most exciting times of a woman's life. For others, pregnancy is not desired and may be the result of poor timing, ineffective birth control practices, or possibly rape. The psychological responses to pregnancy may vary from wonder and excitement to anxiety or despair.

Pregnancy is calculated to last 9 calendar months or 10 **lunar months,** 40 weeks or 280 days; for reference, it is divided into **trimesters**, or three intervals of 3 months each. Meeting the needs of the pregnant female is of utmost importance during this period between conception and labor, known as the **gestational period.** The health care professional in the obstetrician's office needs to be knowledgeable in all areas of obstetrical care to assist in providing the safest possible care during pregnancy.

Pregnancy

The female reproductive system provides an environment suitable for fertilization of the **ovum** (the female sex cell) and implantation of the fertilized ovum. This cyclic process repeats itself on a monthly basis throughout the female's reproductive years. The male reproductive system, on the other hand, functions to produce, store, and transmit the **sperm** (the male sex cell) that will fertilize the mature ovum. **Fertilization**, or **conception**, occurs when a sperm comes in contact with and penetrates a mature ovum. The time frame during which fertilization can occur is usually brief because of the short life span of the ovum; however, it may be as long as 5 days each month. After **ovulation**, a mature ovum survives for up to 24 hours. Sperm have been known to survive for 24 to 72 hours after **ejaculation** into the area of the female **cervix**.

Fertilization takes place in the outer third of the **fallopian tube** (that part closest to the ovary). The fertilized ovum, now called a zygote, continues to travel down the fallopian tube and burrows into the receptive uterine lining, where it will remain throughout the pregnancy as it continues to grow and develop. As development continues, the fertilized ovum, or product of conception, also changes; that is, it is called an **embryo** from the second through the eighth week of pregnancy, and a **fetus** beginning with the ninth week of pregnancy through the duration of the gestational period.

During pregnancy, two major accessory structures develop simultaneously with the baby's development. These two structures sustain the pregnancy and promote normal **prenatal** development. The first accessory structure is the **amniotic sac:** a strong, thin-walled membranous sac that envelops and protects the growing fetus. The amniotic sac

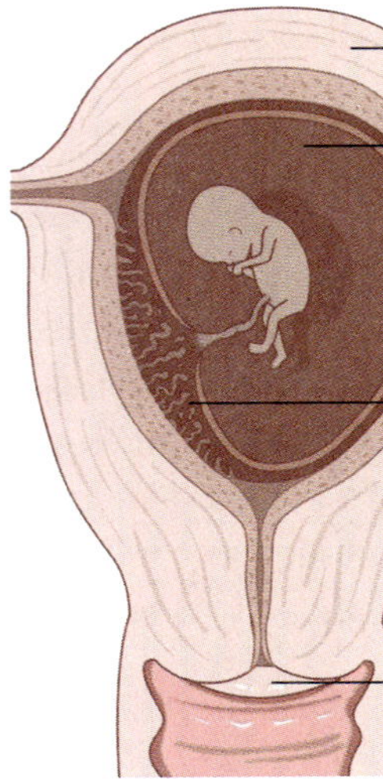

Figure 18-1 Amniotic sac

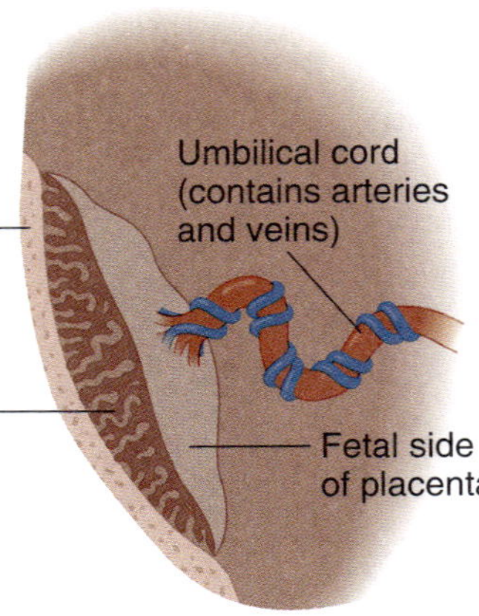

Figure 18-2 Placenta and umbilical cord

is also known as the fetal membrane. The outer layer of the sac is called the chorion and the inner layer is called the amnion. See **Figure 18-1.** Within the amniotic sac is a fluid that cushions and protects the fetus during pregnancy. This fluid is called the **amniotic fluid.**

The second accessory structure is the placenta: a temporary organ of pregnancy that provides for fetal respiration, nutrition, and excretion. It also functions as an endocrine gland in that it produces several hormones necessary for normal pregnancy (**human chorionic gonadotropin** [**HCG**], estrogen, progesterone) and human placental lactogen (HPL), also known as human chorionic somatomammotropin. The maternal side of the placenta is attached to the wall of the uterus and has a "beefy" red appearance. The fetal side of the placenta has a shiny, slightly grayish appearance; it contains the arteries and veins that intertwine to form the umbilical cord. See **Figure 18-2.**

The umbilical cord arises from the center of the placenta and attaches to the umbilicus of the fetus. It serves as the lifeline between the mother and the fetus, becoming the means of transport for the nutrients and waste products to and from the developing baby. The maternal blood and the fetal blood do not mix during pregnancy; however, they do pass very close to each other within the placenta. These two independent circulatory networks are separated by a very thin layer of tissues known as the placental membrane, or placental barrier. Oxygen and nutrients transfer across this membrane from the maternal circulation into the fetal circulation, and waste materials transfer across the membrane from the fetal circulation into the maternal circulation to be excreted.

The amniotic sac remains intact until uterine contractions begin with regularity and enough strength to indicate true labor. Sometimes the amniotic sac ruptures at the onset of labor, during the early stages of labor, or occasionally it is punctured by the physician at some point during the labor process. When this happens spontaneously, you may hear the woman describe it as "my membranes ruptured" or "my bag of water broke."

Barring any complications, the placenta remains intact and attached to the uterine lining until after the delivery of the baby. It then detaches from the uterus and is eliminated through the vaginal canal. Following childbirth, the placenta is known as the **afterbirth.**

Physiological Changes During Pregnancy

Pregnancy places increased demands on the expectant mother's body. Significant changes occur in her body that are necessary to support and nourish the fetus. These changes also prepare her body for childbirth and lactation (breastfeeding). The concept of being pregnant is oftentimes different from the reality of being pregnant. Some women find that they are psychologically unprepared for the physiological changes that occur during pregnancy. Each will need the support and guidance of a well-trained, perceptive staff within the obstetrician's office to better understand the changes her body is experiencing during this gestational period.

The health care professional must understand the physiological changes that occur during pregnancy and the effect they may have on the pregnant woman to provide the best care possible. The most obvious physiological changes that occur within the female reproductive system during pregnancy will be discussed in this segment.

Amenorrhea

Amenorrhea, or absence of menstruation, is usually one of the first things women consider being a sign of pregnancy. Although amenorrhea can occur for other reasons, it usually is a strong suggestion of pregnancy in women who have regular menstrual periods. The menstruation stops as a result of hormonal influence during pregnancy. Amenorrhea, alone, is not significant enough to confirm pregnancy. Other signs and tests will be necessary for confirmation; these will be discussed in the next section.

Changes in the Uterus

Before pregnancy, the uterus is a small, pear-shaped organ that weighs approximately 2 ounces. During pregnancy, the woman's uterus grows large enough to accommodate the growing fetus, placenta, amniotic sac, and amniotic fluid, increasing in size to over 2 pounds. As the uterus grows, and the fetus develops, it rises up and out of the pelvic cavity. By the end of the pregnancy, the top of the uterus (fundus) can be palpated (felt) just under the xiphoid process. See **Figure 18-3.**

Changes in the Cervix

The most obvious changes in the uterine cervix are those of color and consistency. After approximately the sixth week of pregnancy, the cervix and vagina take on a bluish-violet hue as a result of the local venous congestion. This is known as **Chadwick's sign,** and is an early sign of pregnancy. The changes in the cervix occur as a result of increased blood flow to the pregnant uterus. The increased fluid in this area also causes the cervix to soften in consistency, in preparation for childbirth. This softening of the cervix is a probable sign of pregnancy, and is known as **Goodell's sign.**

By the end of the pregnancy, the cervix has softened so significantly that it has a somewhat mushy feel to the examiner's touch. This marked softening of the cervix signifies that the cervix is ready for the dilatation and thinning that is necessary for the birth of the baby. At this time, the cervix is said to be "ripe" for birth.

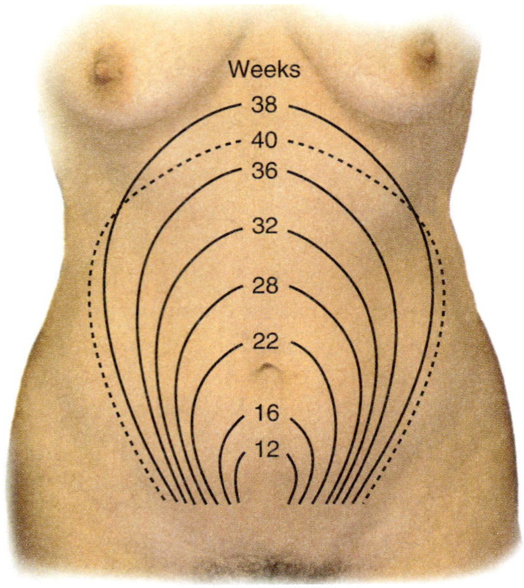

Figure 18-3 Changes in the uterus during pregnancy

Changes in the Vagina

The hormones secreted during pregnancy also prepare the vaginal canal for the great distention it will undergo during labor. As mentioned, the **vagina** takes on the same bluish-violet hue of the cervix during pregnancy. The hormonal influences during pregnancy generate increasing amounts of **glycogen** in the vaginal cells, which causes increased vaginal discharge and heavy shedding of vaginal cells; this in turn creates a thick, white vaginal discharge known as **leukorrhea**. It should be noted that the increase in glycogen in the cells favors the growth of *Candida albicans,* a causative organism in yeast infections of the vagina. Persistent yeast infections are not uncommon in pregnancy.

Changes in the Breasts

During pregnancy, the breasts undergo characteristic changes. Hormonal influences result in an increase in size and shape of the breasts, the nipples increase in size and become more erect, and the areola become larger and more darkly pigmented. The sebaceous glands within the areola (Montgomery's tubercles) become more active during pregnancy and secrete a substance that lubricates the nipples. The pregnant woman will also notice a thin, yellowish discharge from the nipples throughout the pregnancy. This is normal, and the discharge is called **colostrum**, a forerunner to breast milk. If the woman does not plan to breastfeed after delivery, natural suppression of lactation can be achieved by use of a snug-fitting support bra worn around the clock (except when bathing) and ice packs several times a day, to help reduce engorgement (swelling) of breasts. Pain medication may be necessary.

Changes in the Blood Pressure

The blood pressure of a pregnant woman should remain within fairly normal limits. It is important to monitor the woman's blood pressure carefully throughout the pregnancy, because a significant or continual increase in blood pressure may be indicative of complications of pregnancy, such as pregnancy-induced hypertension (which will be

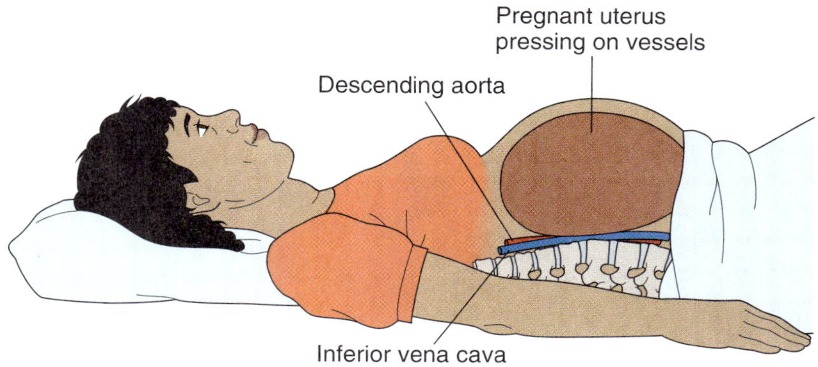

Figure 18-4 Example of supine hypotension

discussed in the next section). During the second and third trimesters (4 to 9 months), the expectant mother may experience **hypotension** when she is in the supine (lying on one's back) position. This happens because the weight of the pregnant uterus presses against the descending aorta and the inferior vena cava in the abdominal cavity when the woman is lying on her back. This pressure on these major blood vessels partially blocks the blood flow, therefore reducing the blood pressure. The pregnant female may complain of faintness, lightheadedness, and dizziness. It is important to advise these women to use the side-lying position when resting to relieve the pressure on the abdominal blood vessels. See **Figure 18-4.**

Changes in Urination

During the first 3 months of pregnancy (first trimester), the pregnant woman may experience urinary frequency due to the increasing size of the uterus, which creates pressure on the bladder. When the uterus rises up out of the pelvis during the second trimester, the pressure on the bladder is relieved. The urinary frequency will return during the last trimester due to the pressure of the baby's head on the bladder as it settles into the pelvis before delivery.

The increased demands placed on the urinary system during pregnancy can result in a minimal amount of spilling of glucose into the urine. Regular monitoring of the pregnant female's urine throughout the pregnancy is important, because a finding of more than a trace of glucose in a routine sample of urine may be indicative of problems, in particular **gestational diabetes**, which will be discussed in the next section.

Changes in Posture

As the pregnancy progresses, changes in the posture of the pregnant female are observable, beginning in the second trimester. The softening of the pelvic joints and relaxing of the pelvic ligaments may offset the pregnant woman's center of gravity, due to the pelvic instability. To compensate for this, the woman assumes a wider stance and a **waddling gait** as she walks.

The increasing size of the uterus places stress on the abdominal muscles particularly during the third trimester of pregnancy. During this time, one may observe that the pregnant female will stand straighter and taller with her shoulders back and her abdomen forward. This stance is in an effort to adjust her center of gravity to the changes that are

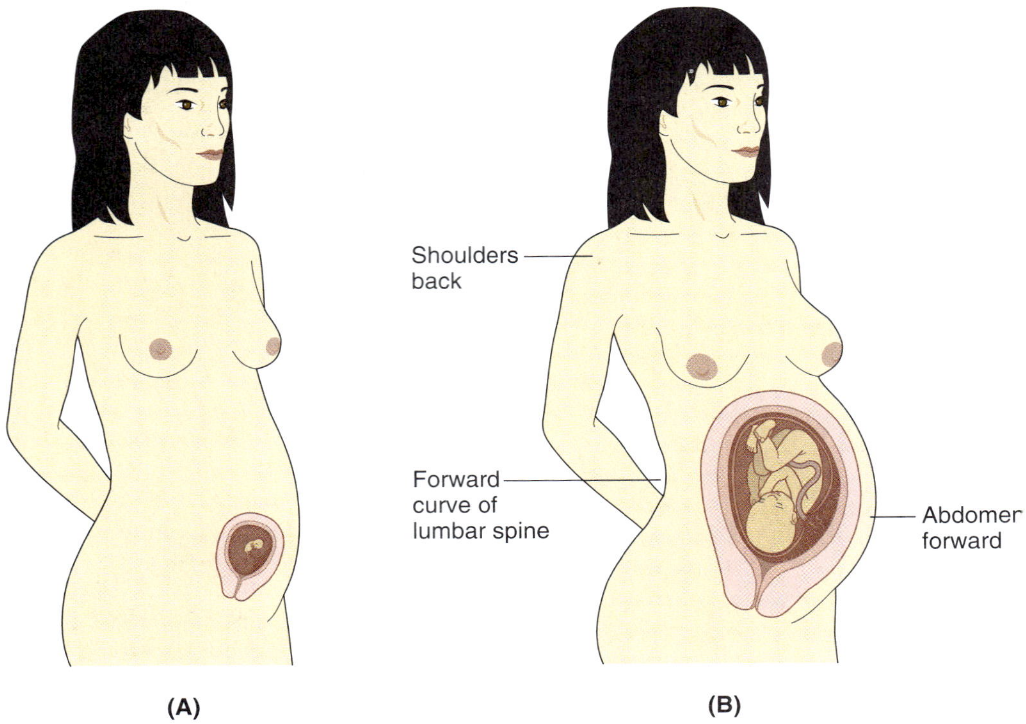

Figure 18-5 Changes in posture due to pregnancy: (A) 6 weeks; (B) 40 weeks

taking place within her body, and to make ambulation easier. Standing this way, however, creates a forward curve of the lumbar spine (**lordosis**), which may lead to complaints of backache. See **Figure 18-5.**

Changes in the Skin

During pregnancy some women may experience an increased feeling of warmth and sweating due to the increased activity of the sweat glands. They may also experience problems with facial blemishes due to the increased activity of the sebaceous glands during pregnancy. These, however, are not the most noticeable changes in the skin of the pregnant woman. What comes to mind as probably one of the most obvious skin changes during pregnancy is the increased pigmentation of the skin (**hyperpigmentation**).

The hyperpigmentation seen on the forehead, cheeks, and the bridge of the nose appears as brown patches called **chloasma,** or the "mask of pregnancy." Women who have brown hair or darker skin usually display more pigmentation than women who are fair skinned.

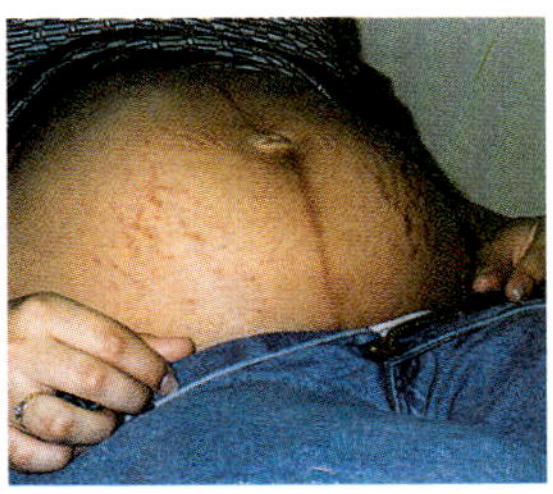

Figure 18-6 Linea nigra with striae gravidarum

The hyperpigmentation that appears on the abdomen of the pregnant female is seen as a darkened vertical midline between the fundus and the symphysis pubis, and is known as the **linea nigra**. See **Figure 18-6.** The **areola** of the breast (area surrounding the nipple) also becomes darker as pregnancy progresses.

During the second half of pregnancy, a woman may experience stretch marks on the abdomen, thighs, and breasts, known as **striae gravidarum**. These linear tears in the connective tissue usually occur in the areas of greatest stretch during pregnancy. The marks appear as slightly depressed, pinkish-purple streaks in these areas. See **Figure 18-6.** After pregnancy, the stretch marks fade to silvery lines, but they do not disappear completely. Some women may complain of an itching sensation when these stretch marks appear and may require relief for this.

Changes in Weight

Over the years there have been many theories concerning the acceptable amount of weight that could be gained during pregnancy. In the 1970s the recommended weight gain was 15 to 25 pounds, with some physicians even placing their patients on low sodium diets for the duration of the pregnancy. The belief then was that by restricting the weight gain during pregnancy, the patient was less likely to develop pregnancy-induced hypertension.

Today, the recommended weight gain during pregnancy ranges from 25 to 30 pounds for women who begin pregnancy at or near their normal weight. The weight gain during pregnancy, no matter what the mother's prepregnant weight, should be at least 15 pounds to ensure adequate nutrition to the developing fetus.

The pattern of weight gain during pregnancy is just as important as the amount of weight gained. In the early months of pregnancy, there is very little weight gain; only 3 to 4 pounds is recommended. During the remainder of the pregnancy (fourth to ninth month), the expected weight gain is about 1 pound per week. It is critical that the pregnant woman's weight be monitored during each prenatal visit. Significant, unexplained weight gains from one visit to the next may be indicative of fluid retention or problems such as pregnancy-induced hypertension.

Signs and Symptoms of Pregnancy

Traditionally, the confirmation of pregnancy has been based on **symptoms** experienced by the mother-to-be, as well as **signs** observed by the physician or health practitioner. These signs and symptoms are grouped into three categories, based on likelihood of accuracy. They are presumptive signs, probable signs, and positive signs of pregnancy.

Presumptive Signs

Presumptive signs of pregnancy are those experienced by the expectant mother, which suggest pregnancy but are not necessarily positive. These early symptoms experienced by the expectant mother include amenorrhea, nausea and vomiting, fatigue, urinary disturbances, and breast changes. A detailed discussion of these signs has been presented in the section on physiological changes of pregnancy. Another presumptive sign of pregnancy is **quickening**, or movement of the fetus felt by the mother. This usually occurs around 18 to 20 weeks' **gestation** and may be described as a faint abdominal fluttering.

Presumptive signs are slightly predictive of pregnancy as a group of symptoms, but taken individually they can be indicative of other conditions.

Probable Signs

Probable signs of pregnancy are those that are observable by the examiner. Even though they are much stronger indicators of pregnancy, they can be due to other pathological conditions and should not be used as the sole indicator of pregnancy. Probable signs that have already been discussed in the section on physiological changes of pregnancy include:

- Goodell's sign (softening of the cervix and vagina)
- Chadwick's sign (cervix and vagina take on a bluish-violet hue)
- Uterine enlargement
- Hyperpigmentation of the skin (mask of pregnancy)
- Abdominal stria (stretch marks)
- **Hegar's sign**, which is softening of the lower segment of the uterus
- **Braxton Hicks contractions,** which are irregular contractions of the uterus and may occur throughout the pregnancy and are relatively painless
- **Ballottement**, which is a technique of using the examiner's finger to tap against the uterus, through the vagina, to cause the fetus to "bounce" within the amniotic fluid and feeling it rebound quickly
- Fetal outline, which can be palpated by the examiner at approximately 24 weeks' gestation
- Pregnancy tests, which are commonly based on the presence of the hormone, human chorionic gonadotropin, secreted during pregnancy

To read the list of probable signs of pregnancy and then hear that they are not positive signs of pregnancy may sound a bit confusing to the individual just beginning in health care. It must be remembered that although the presumptive and probable signs of pregnancy are most often correct as indicators of pregnancy, they can be due to other causes. As you continue to read, we will discuss the positive signs of pregnancy.

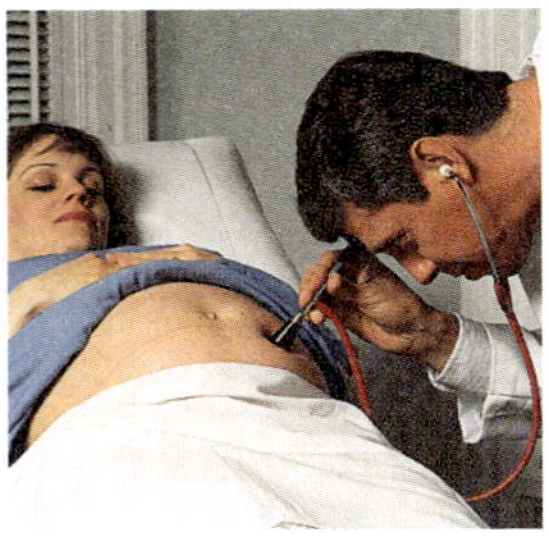

Figure 18-7
Fetoscope used to hear fetal heartbeat

Positive Signs

There are only three positive signs of pregnancy, which are the only absolute indicators of a developing fetus.

1. Fetal heartbeat, which can be detected by ultrasound at approximately 10 weeks' gestation, or by **fetoscope** at 18 to 20 weeks' gestation (a fetoscope is a special stethoscope for hearing the fetal heartbeat through the mother's abdomen). The fetal heart rate can vary from 120 to 180 beats per minute. See **Figure 18-7.**
2. Identification of an embryo or fetus by ultrasound, which can be detected as early as 5 to 6 weeks with 100% reliability, providing the earliest positive confirmation of a pregnancy.

   The **ultrasonography** is a noninvasive procedure that involves the use of reflected sound waves to detect the presence of the embryo or fetus. The waves that are reflected from the fetus are transmitted into a machine that converts them into an image produced on the screen.
3. Fetal movements felt by the examiner are palpable by the physician/examiner by the second trimester of the pregnancy. Fetal movements can also be observed by ultrasound earlier in the pregnancy.

For the learner's convenience, the presumptive, probable, and positive signs of pregnancy are presented in **Table 18-1.**

Table 18-1 Signs of Pregnancy

PRESUMPTIVE SIGNS	PROBABLE SIGNS	POSITIVE SIGNS
1. Amenorrhea 2. Nausea and vomiting 3. Fatigue 4. Urinary disturbances 5. Breast changes 6. Quickening	1. Goodell's sign 2. Chadwick's sign 3. Uterine enlargement 4. Hyperpigmentation of the skin 5. Abdominal stria 6. Hegar's sign 7. Braxton Hicks contractions 8. Ballottement 9. Fetal outline palpated 10. Pregnancy tests	1. Fetal heartbeat 2. Ultrasound identification of fetus 3. Palpated fetal movements

Calculation of Date of Birth

Everyone wants to know, "When will the baby be born?" It is not possible to predict the exact date of birth with a high degree of accuracy. The birth date, or due date, is determined based on the average length of a normal pregnancy, with a 2-week margin on either side of the date being considered within the normal limit.

The birth date for the baby is termed as the **expected date of confinement** (EDC), the **expected date of delivery** (EDD), or the **expected date of birth** (EDB). This date is determined using a formula that calculates from the date of the first day of the **last menstrual period** (LMP). The formula used to calculate the date of birth is known as **Nagele's rule**, named after the German obstetrician, Franz K. Nagele. *To calculate the estimated date of delivery, subtract 3 months from the beginning of the last normal menstrual period (LMP) and add 7 days to the date.*

Example: If the woman's last normal menstrual period began July 17, you would count back 3 months (which would be June . . . May . . . April . . . April 17) and add 7 days to the date (which would be April 24). The EDD, or expected date of delivery, would be April 24.

Vocabulary

The following vocabulary words are frequently used when discussing the field of obstetrics.

WORD	DEFINITION
afterbirth	The placenta, the amnion, the chorion, some amniotic fluid, blood, and blood clots expelled from the uterus after childbirth.
alpha-fetoprotein (**AL**-fah fee-toh-**PRO**-teen)	A protein found in the amniotic fluid. Measurements of the level of **alpha-fetoprotein** (AFP) in the amniotic sac are used for early diagnosis

	of fetal defects such as spina bifida (defective closure of the vertebrae of the spinal column) and anencephaly (congenital absence of the brain and spinal cord).
amenorrhea (ah-men-or-**REE**-ah) a- = without men/o = menstruation -rrhea = flow, drainage	Absence of menstrual flow.
amnion (**AM**-nee-on) amni/o = amnion	The inner of the two membrane layers that surround and contain the fetus and the amniotic fluid during pregnancy.
amniotic fluid (am-nee-**OT**-ik fluid) amni/o = amnion -tic = pertaining to	A liquid produced by and contained within the fetal membranes during pregnancy. This fluid protects the fetus from trauma and temperature variations, helps to maintain fetal oxygen supply, and allows for freedom of movement by the fetus during pregnancy.
amniotic sac (am-nee-**OT**-ik sack) amni/o = amnion -tic = pertaining to	The double layered sac that contains the fetus and the amniotic fluid during pregnancy.
areola (ah-**REE**-oh-lah)	The darker pigmented, circular area surrounding the nipple of each breast; also known as the areola mammae or the areola papillaris.
ballottement (bal-ot-**MON**)	A technique of using the examiner's finger to tap against the uterus, through the vagina, to cause the fetus to "bounce" within the amniotic fluid and feeling it rebound quickly.
Braxton Hicks contractions (**BRACKS**-ton **HICKS** con-**TRAK**-shuns)	Irregular, ineffective contractions of the uterus that occur throughout pregnancy.
cerclage (sair-**KLOGH**)	Suturing the cervix to keep it from dilating prematurely during the pregnancy. This procedure is sometimes referred to as a "purse string procedure." The sutures are removed near the end of the pregnancy.
cervix (**SER**-viks)	The part of the uterus that protrudes into the cavity of the vagina; the neck of the uterus.
cesarean section (see-**SAYR**-ee-an section)	A surgical procedure in which the abdomen and uterus are incised and a baby is delivered transabdominally.
Chadwick's sign	The bluish-violet hue of the cervix and vagina after approximately the sixth week of pregnancy.
chloasma (kloh-**AZ**-mah)	Patches of tan or brown pigmentation associated with pregnancy, occurring mostly on the forehead, cheeks, and nose; also called the "mask of pregnancy."
chorion (**KOH**-ree-on)	The outer of the two membrane layers that surround and contain the fetus and the amniotic fluid during pregnancy.
coitus (**KOH**-ih-tus)	Sexual intercourse; copulation.

colostrum (koh-**LOSS**-trum)	The thin, yellowish fluid secreted by the breasts during pregnancy and the first few days after birth, before lactation begins.
conception (con-**SEP**-shun)	The union of a male sperm and a female ovum; also termed fertilization.
copulation (**kop**-yoo-**LAY**-shun)	Sexual intercourse; **coitus**.
corpus luteum (**COR**-pus **LOO**-tee-um)	A mass of yellowish tissue that forms within the ruptured ovarian follicle after ovulation. It functions as a temporary endocrine gland for the purpose of secreting estrogen and large amounts of progesterone, which will sustain pregnancy, should it occur, until the placenta forms. If pregnancy does not occur, the **corpus luteum** will degenerate approximately 3 days before the beginning of menstruation.
culdocentesis (kull-doh-sen-**TEE**-sis) **culd/o** = cul-de-sac **-centesis** = surgical puncture	Needle aspiration, through the vagina, into the cul-de-sac area (area in the peritoneal cavity immediately behind the vagina) for the purpose of removing fluid from the area for examination or diagnosis. Aspiration of unclotted blood from the cul-de-sac area may indicate bleeding from a ruptured fallopian tube; the aspiration of clear fluid from the area would rule out a ruptured fallopian tube.
dilatation (of cervix) (dill-ah-**TAY**-shun)	The enlargement of the diameter of the cervix during labor. The calculation of the amount of **dilatation** is measured in centimeters (cm). When the cervix has dilated to 10 cm, it is said to be completely dilated.
Doppler 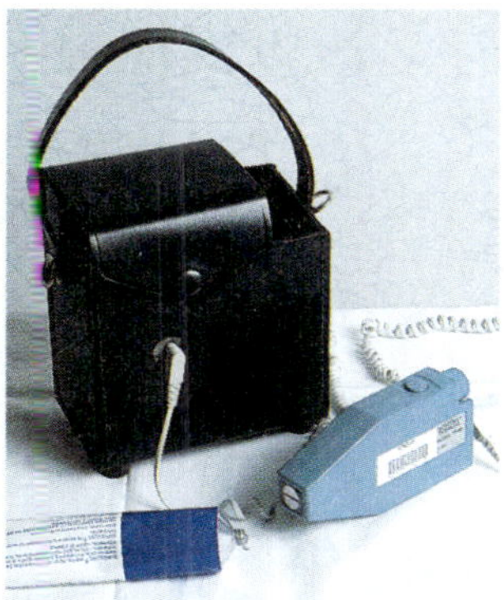	A technique used in **ultrasound** imaging to monitor the behavior of a moving structure, such as flowing blood or a beating heart. Fetal heart monitors operate on the Doppler sound wave principle to determine the fetal heart rate. See **Figure 18-8.** **Figure 18-8** Doppler
eclampsia (eh-**KLAMP**-see-ah)	The most severe form of hypertension during pregnancy, evidenced by seizures (convulsions).
edema (eh-**DEE**-mah)	Swelling, with water retention.
effacement (eh-**FACE**-ment)	Thinning of the cervix, which allows it to enlarge the diameter of its opening in preparation for childbirth; this occurs during the normal processes of labor.
ejaculation (eh-jak-yoo-**LAY**-shun)	The sudden emission of semen from the male urethra, usually occurring during sexual intercourse or masturbation.
embryo (**EM**-bree-oh)	The name given to the product of conception from the second through the eighth week of pregnancy (through the second month).

endometrium (en-doh-**MEE**-tree-um) endo- = within metri/o = uterine lining -um = noun ending	The inner lining of the uterus.
episiotomy (eh-**pis**-ee-**OT**-oh-mee) episi/o = vulva -tomy = incision into	A surgical procedure in which an incision is made into the woman's perineum to enlarge the vaginal opening for delivery of the baby. This incision is usually made shortly before the baby's birth (second stage of labor) to prevent tearing of the perineum.
estrogen (**ESS**-troh-jen)	One of the female hormones that promotes the development of the female secondary sex characteristics.
fallopian tubes (fah-**LOH**-pee-an tubes)	A pair of tubes opening at one end into the uterus and at the other end into the peritoneal cavity, over the ovary.
fertilization (fer-til-ih-**ZAY**-shun)	The union of a male sperm and a female ovum; also termed conception.
fetoscope (**FEET**-oh-scope) fet/o = fetus -scope = instrument for viewing	A special stethoscope for hearing the fetal heartbeat through the mother's abdomen.
fetus (**FEE**-tus) fet/o = fetus -us = noun ending	The name given to the developing baby from approximately the eighth week after conception until birth.
fimbriae (**FIM**-bree-ah)	The fringelike end of the fallopian tube.
fundus	Superior aspect of the uterus.
gamete (**GAM**-eet)	A mature sperm or ovum.
gastroesophageal reflux (**gas**-troh-eh-soff-ah-**JEE**-al) gastr/o = stomach esophag/o = esophagus -eal = pertaining to	A return, or reflux, of gastric juices into the esophagus, resulting in a burning sensation.
gestation (jess-**TAY**-shun)	The term of pregnancy, which equals approximately 280 days from the onset of the last menstrual period; the period of intrauterine development of the fetus from conception through birth; also termed the gestational period.
gestational hypertension (jess-**TAY**-shun-al **high**-per-**TEN**-shun)	A complication of pregnancy in which the expectant mother develops high blood pressure after 20 weeks' gestation, with no signs of proteinuria or edema.
glycogen (**GLYE**-koh-jen) glyc/o = sugar	The form of sugar that is stored in body cells, primarily the liver.

gonads (**GO**-nads)	A gamete-producing gland, such as an ovary or a testis.
Goodell's sign	The softening of the uterine cervix, a probable sign of pregnancy.
graafian follicles (**GRAF**-ee-an **FALL**-ih-kls)	A mature, fully developed ovarian cyst containing the ripe ovum.
gravida	A woman who is pregnant. She may be identified as **gravida I** if this is her first pregnancy, **gravida II** for a second pregnancy, and so on.
Hegar's sign (**HAY**-garz sign)	Softening of the lower segment of the uterus; a probable sign of pregnancy.
hyperpigmentation (**high**-per-**pig**-men-**TAY**-shun) hyper- = excessive	An increase in the pigmentation of the skin.
hypertension (high-per-**TEN**-shun) hyper- = excessive tens/o = strain, pressure -ion = state or condition	High blood pressure; a common, often asymptomatic disorder, in which the blood persistently exceeds 140/90 mmHg.
hypotension (**high**-poh-**TEN**-shun) hypo- = less than, low tens/o = strain -ion = state or condition	Low blood pressure; an abnormal condition in which the blood pressure is not adequate for normal passage through the blood vessels or for normal oxygenation of the body cells.
hypovolemic shock (**high**-poh-voh-**LEE**-mik) hypo- = under, below, beneath, less than normal	A state of extreme physical collapse and exhaustion due to massive blood loss; "less than normal" blood volume.
labor (**LAY**-bor)	The time and the processes that occur during birth, from the beginning of cervical dilatation to the delivery of the placenta.
lactation (lak-**TAY**-shun) lact/o = milk	The production and secretion of milk from the female breasts as nourishment for the infant. Lactation can be referred to as a process or as a period of time during which the female is breastfeeding.
lactiferous ducts (lak-**TIF**-er-us ducts) lact/o = milk	Channels or narrow tubular structures that carry milk from the lobes of each breast to the nipple.
laparoscopy (lap-ar-**OS**-koh-pee) lapar/o = abdominal wall -scopy = viewing	Visualization of the abdominal cavity with an instrument called a laparoscope through an incision into the abdominal wall.
leukorrhea (**loo**-koh-**REE**-ah) leuk/o = white -rrhea = discharge, flow	A white discharge from the vagina.

lightening	The settling of the fetal head into the pelvis, occurring a few weeks prior to the onset of labor.
linea nigra (**LIN**-ee-ah **NIG**-rah)	A darkened vertical midline appearing on the abdomen of a pregnant woman, extending from the fundus to the symphysis pubis.
lithotomy position (lith-**OT**-oh-mee position) 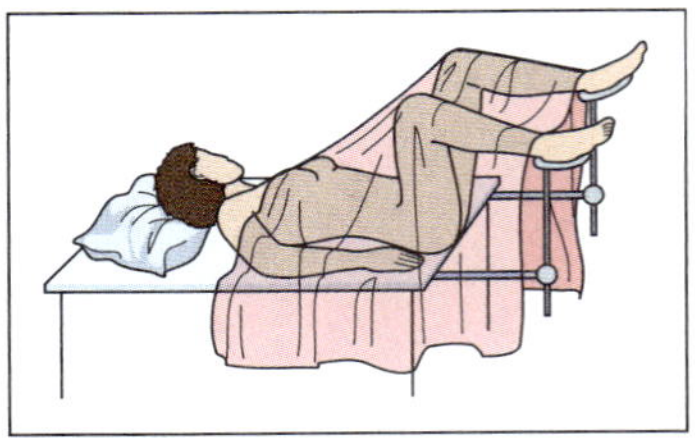	A position in which the patient lies on her back, buttocks even with the end of the table, with her knees bent back toward her abdomen and the heel of each foot resting in an elevated foot rest at the end of the examination table. See **Figure 18-9.** **Figure 18-9** Lithotomy position
lordosis (lor-**DOH**-sis) lord/o = bent -osis = condition 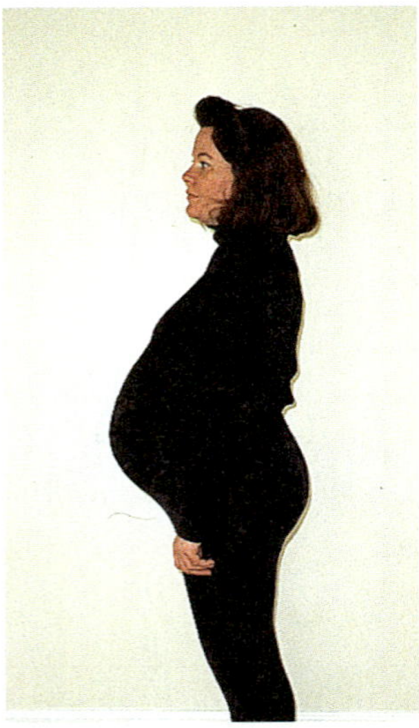	A forward curvature of the spine, noticeable if the person is observed from the side. See **Figure 18-10.** **Figure 18-10** Lordosis
lunar month (**LOON**-ar)	Four weeks or 28 days; approximately the amount of time it takes the moon to revolve around the earth.
mammary glands (**MAM**-ah-ree glands) mamm/o = breast -ary = pertaining to	The female breasts.
mask of pregnancy	Patches of tan or brown pigmentation associated with pregnancy, occurring mostly on the forehead, cheeks, and nose; also known as *chloasma.*
multigravida (**mull**-tih-**GRAV**-ih-dah) multi- = many -gravida = pregnancy	A woman who has been pregnant more than once.

multipara (**mull-TIP**-ah-rah) **multi-** = many **-para** = to bear	A woman who has given birth two or more times after 20 weeks' gestation.
Nagele's rule (**NAY**-geh-leez)	A formula that is used to calculate the date of birth: Subtract 3 months from the first day of the last normal menstrual period and add 7 days to that date to arrive at the estimated date of birth.
neonatology (nee-oh-nay-**TALL**-oh-jee) **ne/o** = new **nat/o** = birth **-logy** = the study of	The branch of medicine that specializes in the treatment and care of the diseases and disorders of the newborn through the first 4 weeks of life.
nullipara (null-**IP**-ah-rah) **nulli-** = none **-para** = to bear	A woman who has never completed a pregnancy beyond 20 weeks' gestation.
obstetrician (ob-steh-**TRISH**-an)	A physician who specializes in the care of women during pregnancy, the delivery of the baby, and the first 6 weeks following the delivery, known as the immediate postpartum period.
obstetrics (ob-**STET**-riks)	The field of medicine that deals with pregnancy, the delivery of the baby, and the first 6 weeks after delivery (the postpartum period).
ovary (**OH**-vah-ree) **ov/o** = ovum **-ary** = pertaining to	One of a pair of female gonads responsible for producing mature ova (eggs) and releasing them at monthly intervals (ovulation); also responsible for producing the female hormones, estrogen and progesterone.
ovulation (**ov**-yoo-**LAY**-shun)	The release of the mature ovum from the ovary; occurs approximately 14 days prior to the beginning of menses.
ovum (**OH**-vum) **ov/o** = egg **-um** = noun ending	The female reproductive cell; female sex cell or egg.
para	A woman who has produced an infant regardless of whether the infant was alive or stillborn. This term applies to any pregnancies carried to more than 20 weeks' gestation. The term may be written **para II, para III,** and so on, to indicate the number of pregnancies lasting more than 20 weeks' gestation, regardless of the number of offspring produced by the pregnancy. A woman who has had only one pregnancy resulting in multiple births is still a para I.
parturition (par-too-**RISH**-un)	The act of giving birth.
perineum (pair-ih-**NEE**-um)	The area between the vaginal orifice and the anus; it consists of muscular and fibrous tissue and serves as support for the pelvic structures.
placenta (plah-**SEN**-tah)	A highly vascular, disc-shaped organ that forms in the pregnant uterine wall for exchange of gases and nutrients between the mother and the fetus. The maternal side of the placenta attaches to the uterine

	wall, whereas the fetal side of the placenta gives rise to the umbilical cord, which connects directly to the baby. After the delivery of the baby, when the placenta is no longer needed, it separates from the uterine wall and passes to the outside of the body through the vagina, at which time it is called the afterbirth.
pre-eclampsia (**pre**-eh-**KLAMP**-see-ah)	A state during pregnancy in which the expectant mother develops high blood pressure, accompanied by proteinuria or edema, after 20 weeks' gestation.
pregnancy (**PREG**-nan-see)	The period of intrauterine development of the fetus from conception through birth. The average pregnancy lasts approximately 40 weeks; also known as the gestational period.
prenatal (pre-**NAY**-tl) **pre-** = before, in front **-natal** = pertaining to birth	Pertaining to the period of time, during pregnancy, that is before the birth of the baby.
primigravida (prigh-mih-**GRAV**-ih-dah) **primi-** = first **-gravida** = pregnancy	A woman who is pregnant for the first time.
primipara (prigh-**MIP**-ah-rah) **primi-** = first **-para** = to bear	A woman who has given birth for the first time, after a pregnancy of at least 20 weeks' gestation.
progesterone (proh-**JES**-ter-on)	A female hormone secreted by the corpus luteum and the placenta. It is primarily responsible for the changes that occur in the endometrium in anticipation of a fertilized ovum, and for development of the maternal placenta after implantation of a fertilized ovum.
proteinuria (**proh**-tee-in-**YOO**-ree-ah) **-uria** = urine condition	The presence of protein (albumin) in the urine; also called albuminuria. This can be a sign of pregnancy-induced **hypertension** (PIH).
puberty (**PEW**-ber-tee)	The period of life at which the ability to reproduce begins; that is, in the female, it is the period when the female reproductive organs become fully developed.
pyrosis (pye-**ROH**-sis) **pyr/o** = fire, heat **-osis** = condition	Heartburn; indigestion.
quickening (**KWIK**-en-ing)	The first feeling of movement of the fetus felt by the expectant mother; usually occurs around 18 to 20 weeks' gestation.
salpingectomy (**sal**-pin-**JEK**-toh-mee) **salping/o** = eustachian tubes; also refers to fallopian tubes **-ectomy** = surgical removal	Surgical removal of a fallopian tube.

sexual intercourse	The sexual union of two people of the opposite sex in which the penis is introduced into the vagina; also known as copulation or coitus.
signs	Objective findings as perceived by an examiner, such as the measurement of a fever on the thermometer, the observation of a rash on the skin, or the observation of a bluish-violet color of the cervix.
sperm	A mature male germ cell; spermatozoon.
striae gravidarum (**STRIGH**-ay grav-ih-**DAR**-um)	Stretch marks that occur during pregnancy due to the great amount of stretching that occurs. They appear as slightly depressed, pinkish-purple streaks in the areas of greatest stretch, which are the abdomen, the breasts, and the thighs.
symptoms (**SIM**-toms)	A subjective indication of a disease or a change in condition as perceived by the patient; something experienced or felt by the patient.
tachycardia (**tak**-eh-**CAR**-dee-ah) tachy- = rapid cardi/o = heart -a = noun ending	Rapid heartbeat, consistently over 100 beats per minute.
testes (**TESS**-teez)	The paired male gonads that produce sperm. They are suspended in the scrotal sac in the adult male.
transvaginal ultrasonography (trans-**VAJ**-in-al ull-trah-son-**OG**-rah-fee) trans- = across, through vagin/o = vagina -al = pertaining to ultra- = beyond son/o = sound -graphy = recording	An ultrasound image that is produced by inserting a transvaginal probe into the vagina. The probe is encased in a disposable cover and is coated with a gel for easy insertion. The gel also promotes conductivity. This procedure allows clear visualization of the uterus, gestational sac, and embryo in the early stages of pregnancy. It also allows the examiner to visualize deeper pelvic structures, such as the ovaries and fallopian tubes.
trimester (**TRY**-mes-ter)	One of the three periods of approximately 3 months into which pregnancy is divided. The first trimester consists of weeks 1 to 12, the second trimester consists of weeks 13 to 27, and the third trimester consists of weeks 28 to 40.
ultrasonography (ull-trah-son-**OG**-rah-fee) ultra- = beyond son/o = sound -graphy = recording	A noninvasive procedure that involves the use of reflected sound waves to detect the presence of the embryo or fetus.
umbilical cord (um-**BILL**-ih-kal cord)	A flexible structure connecting the umbilicus (navel) of the fetus with the placenta in the pregnant uterus. It serves as passage for the umbilical arteries and vein.
uterus (**YOO**-ter-us)	The hollow, pear-shaped organ of the female reproductive system that houses the fertilized, implanted ovum as it develops throughout pregnancy; also the source of the monthly menstrual flow from the nonpregnant uterus.

vagina (vah-**JIGH**-nah)	The muscular tube that connects the uterus with the vulva. It is approximately 3 inches in length, and rests between the bladder (anteriorly) and the rectum (posteriorly).
varicose veins (**VAIR**-ih-kohs veins)	Twisted, swollen veins that occur as a result of the blood pooling in the legs.
waddling gait (**WAH**-dl-ing gait)	A manner of walking in which the feet are wide apart and the walk resembles that of a duck.

Word Elements

The following word elements pertain to the field of obstetrics. As you review the list, pronounce each word element aloud twice and check the box after you "say it." Write the definition for the example word given for each word element. You may use your medical dictionary.

WORD ELEMENT	PRONUNCIATION	"SAY IT"	MEANING
amni/o **amni**ocentesis	**AM**-nee-oh am-nee-oh-sen-**TEE**-sis	☐	amnion
ante- **ante**flexion	**AN**-tee **an**-tee-**FLEK**-shun	☐	before; in front
culd/o **culd**ocentesis	**KULL**-doh **kull**-doh-sen-**TEE**-sis	☐	cul-de-sac
-cyesis pseudo**cyesis**	sigh-**EE**-sis **soo**-doh-sigh-**EE**-sis	☐	pregnancy
episi/o **episi**otomy	eh-**PIS**-ee-oh eh-pis-ee-**OT**-oh-mee	☐	vulva
fet/o **fet**oscope	**FEET**-oh **FEET**-oh-scope	☐	fetus
-gravida primi**gravida**	**GRAV**-ih-dah prigh-mih-**GRAV**-ih-dah	☐	pregnancy
hyper- **hyper**emesis	**HIGH**-per high-per-**EM**-eh-sis	☐	excessive, high
lact/o **lact**ation	**LAK**-toh lak-**TAY**-shun	☐	milk
multi- **multi**gravida	**MULL**-tih mull-tih-**GRAV**-ih-dah	☐	many
nat/o pre**nat**al	**NAY**-toh pre-**NAY**-tl	☐	birth

nulli- **nulli**para	**NULL**-ih null-ih-**PAIR**-ah	☐	none
-para multi**para**	**PAIR**-ah mull-tih-**PAIR**-ah	☐	to give birth
primi- **primi**gravida	**PRIGH**-mih prigh-mih-**GRAV**-ih-dah	☐	first
obstetr/o **obstetr**ics	ob-**STET**-roh ob-**STET**-riks	☐	midwife
pelv/i **pelv**imetry	**PELL**-vih pell-**VIM**-eh-tree	☐	pelvis
perine/o **perine**al	pair-ih-**NEE**-oh pair-ih-**NEE**-al	☐	perineum
salping/o **salping**ectomy	sal-**PIN**-go **sal**-pin-**JEK**-toh-mee	☐	eustachian tubes; also refers to fallopian tubes
-tocia dys**tocia**	**TOH**-see-ah dis-**TOH**-see-ah	☐	labor
vagin/o trans**vagin**al	**VAJ**-in-oh trans-**VAJ**-in-al	☐	vagina

Discomforts of Pregnancy

Throughout the pregnancy, the expectant mother will experience various discomforts. It is important that she realize these will be temporary discomforts and should subside after delivery. It is also important that the health care professional be aware of the difference between discomforts of pregnancy and signs of possible complications of pregnancy. The knowledgeable health care professional will have the responsibility of educating the patient regarding measures for relief of these temporary discomforts. The following list includes, but is not limited to, the more common discomforts of pregnancy.

backache

Backache is common during the second and third trimester of pregnancy and is due to the body's adaptation to the stresses placed upon the back as the pregnancy progresses.

Recommended treatment includes encouraging good posture, wearing comfortable shoes, getting adequate rest, and bending from the knees—not the waist.

edema

Edema, or swelling, of the lower extremities is not uncommon in pregnancy, particularly as the pregnancy progresses.

Recommended treatment includes elevating the feet and legs when sitting, lying down when resting, drinking plenty of water, and avoiding foods high in sodium. If the edema is present in the hands and face also, it should be reported immediately to the physician because this could be an indication of complications of pregnancy.

fatigue

Fatigue usually occurs during the first trimester of pregnancy, disappears during the second trimester, and returns toward the end of the pregnancy. This is due to the body's adjustment to the stresses of pregnancy.

Recommended treatment includes encouraging at least 8 to 10 hours of sleep per night and allowing for short naps during the day.

heartburn

Heartburn is also known as **pyrosis** (pyr/o = fever, fire + osis = condition). This discomfort occurs mainly in the last few weeks of pregnancy due to the pressure exerted on the esophagus by the enlarged pregnant uterus. This pressure may also cause a return, or reflux, of gastric juices into the esophagus, resulting in a burning sensation, a condition known as **gastroesophageal reflux**.

Recommended treatment includes avoiding spicy foods, drinking plenty of water, avoiding coffee, eating several small meals instead of three larger meals, and lying with head and shoulders elevated.

hemorrhoids

Hemorrhoids are swollen veins of the rectum and anus that develop as a result of the increasing pressure on the area due to the progressing pregnancy. They usually disappear after delivery, but can cause discomfort in the pregnant female.

Recommended treatment includes drinking plenty of fluids to avoid constipation, which causes hemmorrhoids to become more severe, soaking in warm water baths, and applying topical anesthetic ointments.

nausea

Nausea usually occurs during the first trimester of pregnancy and is known as "morning sickness," although it may occur during the morning, in the afternoon, or throughout the day.

Recommended treatment includes eating dry toast or crackers, eating small frequent meals, eating something before taking prenatal vitamins, or drinking fluids between meals instead of with meals.

Any prolonged nausea and vomiting should be reported to the physician immediately, that is, severe nausea that is preventing proper eating and hydration, or severe vomiting that persists.

varicose veins

Varicose veins are twisted, swollen veins that occur as a result of the blood pooling in the legs, due to the added weight (from the pregnancy) to the lower extremities of the body.

Recommended treatment includes the use of support hosiery, encouraging the pregnant woman to avoid crossing her legs, regular exercise of walking to increase the blood flow to the legs, and elevation of the feet and legs when sitting.

Complications of Pregnancy

For most women, pregnancy is a time of anticipation and excitement; most begin pregnancy in a state of seemingly good health. All women look forward to completing the pregnancy without any complications and to delivering a normal, healthy baby. For most women this will happen; for others it will not. Unfortunately, deviations from the normal course of pregnancy do occur in some women. Even though the reasons may be unclear as to why the complication occurs during the pregnancy, the warning signs may appear early enough to take preventative action.

Early and regular prenatal visits are essential to the well-being of the fetus and the mother. The regular monitoring of the fetus, the expectant mother, and her body's response to the pregnancy will provide the opportunity for skilled health professionals to anticipate some of the problems associated with pregnancy. Keen observation and listening skills are vital in an obstetrical office, because it may be *what the patient says* or *how the patient looks* that sets off the warning signal. Some complications of pregnancy can be made less severe if treated early enough; some may even be prevented.

Whether by phone or in person, the health care professional is often the first person to hear the complaints and concerns of the expectant mother. It is critical that this individual be knowledgeable of the signs and symptoms of complications of pregnancy, listening carefully as the patient describes her symptoms and immediately reporting deviations from the norm to the physician.

The following is a discussion of pregnancy-related complications, that is, those that occur during pregnancy and are not seen at other times in the female. These complications of pregnancy are listed in alphabetical order for easy reference; they are not listed in the order in which they might occur during pregnancy. Preexisting conditions that complicate pregnancy will not be discussed in this chapter.

abortion
(ah-**BOR**-shun)

Termination of a pregnancy before the fetus has reached a viable age, that is, an age at which the fetus could live outside of the uterine environment.

The medical consensus is that a fetus has not reached a viable age if it is under 20 weeks' gestation or under 500 g in weight.

The term **abortion** is a medical term used to denote any type of termination of pregnancy before the age of viability. Many lay people use the term *miscarriage* to describe a spontaneous abortion.

A spontaneous abortion is one that occurs on its own, as a result of abnormalities of the maternal environment or abnormalities of the embryo or fetus. Most spontaneous abortions occur within the first 3 months of pregnancy.

Symptoms include vaginal bleeding, rhythmic uterine cramping, continual backache, and a feeling of pressure in the pelvic area. Tissue may be passed through the vagina, depending on the type of abortion.

A spontaneous abortion may be a complete abortion in which all products of conception are expelled, an incomplete abortion in which some but not all products of conception are expelled, or a threatened abortion in which the symptoms of an impending abortion are present, but ultrasound indicates that a live fetus is present.

Under any circumstances, when vaginal bleeding is reported during pregnancy, the health care professional should obtain detailed information about the nature of the bleeding and the length of the pregnancy, and should report this to the physician immediately.

---

abruptio placenta
(ah-**BRUP**-she-oh pla-**SEN**-tah)

The premature separation of a normally implanted placenta from the uterine wall, after the pregnancy has passed 20 weeks' gestation or during labor (the birthing process).

Abruptio placenta is a dangerous and potentially life-threatening condition for both the mother and the fetus due to the potential for hemorrhage.

When bleeding occurs on the maternal side of the placenta (the side that attaches to the uterine lining), a clot (hematoma) forms in the area; this can lead to the premature separation of the placenta in the area. The severity of the complications from abruptio placenta depend on the amount of bleeding and the size of the clot that forms. The degree of separation may range from partial to complete, with bleeding being concealed or apparent.

Abruptio placenta does not usually occur alone, but may accompany other complications of pregnancy. Some of the conditions that may increase the risk of abruptio placenta are hypertension, use of cocaine by the expectant mother, trauma to the abdomen while pregnant (as in injury or abuse), and the presence of a short umbilical cord (creating tension on the placenta during the birth process).

A classic symptom of abruptio placenta is uterine tenderness with a board-like firmness to the abdomen. Additional symptoms include vaginal bleeding accompanied by abdominal or low back pain, or frequent cramplike contractions of the uterus (uterine irritability). If the bleeding is concealed, the patient may display other signs indicative of this, such as **tachycardia**, hypotension, and restlessness.

Treatment for abruptio placenta usually involves immediate delivery of the fetus by cesarean section if there are signs of fetal distress or if the expectant mother displays signs of hemorrhaging.

---

ectopic pregnancy
(ek-**TOP**-ic **PREG**-nan-see)
ecto- = out of place
-ic = pertaining to

Abnormal implantation of a fertilized ovum outside of the uterine cavity; also called a tubal pregnancy.

Approximately 90% of all **ectopic** pregnancies occur in the fallopian tubes; other sites for ectopic implantation are the ovaries and the abdomen. Rarely are abdominal pregnancies carried to full term.

Possible causes of ectopic pregnancy include scarring of the fallopian tubes due to infections, inflammation, or surgery; adhesions due to endometriosis; congenital defects causing deformity of the tubes; pregnancy occurring while an IUD (intrauterine device) is in place; and maternal age over 35 years.

Tubal pregnancies usually rupture between 6 and 12 weeks' gestation. Some women do not even realize that they are pregnant, because the more common signs of pregnancy may not be present during the early stage of gestation. Symptoms include vaginal spotting (usually dark) and sharp abdominal pain (usually described as colicky or cramping).

Diagnosis of an ectopic pregnancy is often confirmed with a positive pregnancy test, ruling out other conditions, and **transvaginal ultrasonography,** which will reveal the absence of a gestational sac within the uterus. The physician may perform a **culdocentesis** to rule out a ruptured ectopic pregnancy. The aspiration of unclotted blood from the cul-de-sac area may indicate bleeding from a ruptured fallopian tube. The aspiration of clear fluid from the area would rule out a ruptured fallopian tube.

If ultrasound and culdocentesis are inconclusive and symptoms indicate the possibility of an ectopic pregnancy, **laparoscopy** may be necessary to confirm the diagnosis.

For an unruptured ectopic pregnancy (tubal pregnancy), treatment includes surgery to remove the products of conception from the area. A ruptured ectopic pregnancy is much more serious, with the potential being present for hemorrhage and **hypovolemic shock** (diminished blood volume). The affected tube is surgically removed (**salpingectomy**) and the bleeding is brought under control by tying (ligating) the bleeding vessels.

Although the chances may decline, it is possible for a woman to have successful subsequent pregnancies with only one fallopian tube present.

---

gestational diabetes
(jess-**TAY**-shun-al dye-ah-**BEE**-teez)

A disorder in which women who are not diabetic before pregnancy develop diabetes during the pregnancy; that is, they develop an inability to metabolize carbohydrates (glucose intolerance), with resultant hyperglycemia.

This disorder develops during the latter part of pregnancy, with symptoms usually disappearing at the end of the pregnancy. Women who have gestational diabetes have a higher possibility of developing it with subsequent pregnancies; they are also at higher risk of developing diabetes later in life.

Factors that increase the risk of developing gestational diabetes include, but are not limited to, the following:

- Obesity
- Maternal age over 30 years
- History of birthing large babies (usually over 10 pounds)
- Family history of diabetes

- Previous, unexplained stillborn birth
- Previous birth with congenital anomalies (defects)

Symptoms vary from classic symptoms of diabetes, such as excessive thirst, hunger, and frequent urination, to being asymptomatic (no symptoms present). Because a high number of pregnant women have gestational diabetes without obvious symptoms, all pregnant women are routinely screened for diabetes with a blood test usually between weeks 24 and 28 of the pregnancy.

hydatidiform mole
(high-dah-**TID**-ih-form mohl)

An abnormal condition that begins as a pregnancy and deviates from normal development very early; the diseased ovum deteriorates (not producing a fetus), and the chorionic villi of the placenta (small vessels protruding from the outer layer) change to a mass of cysts resembling a bunch of grapes.

The growth of this mass progresses much more rapidly than uterine growth with a normal pregnancy. A **hydatidiform mole** is known as a molar pregnancy; also called a hydatid mole.

Symptoms include, but are not limited to, extreme nausea, uterine bleeding, anemia, an unusually large uterus for the duration of pregnancy (at 3 months the uterus may be the size expected at 5 or 6 months), absence of fetal heart sounds, edema, and hypertension.

Diagnosis is confirmed through the use of ultrasonography (no fetal skeleton will be visible), and laboratory findings (the HCG level will be extremely high).

Treatment options include evacuation of the uterus, followed by a dilatation and curettage when the uterine wall has regained its firmness (a few days later) or a hysterectomy, in which the uterus is removed. The age of the woman and the condition of the uterus will be factors determining the need for a hysterectomy. The tissue from the mass will be tested for presence of malignant (cancerous) cells.

Follow-up treatment involves close medical supervision for about 1 year following a molar pregnancy. This will include careful monitoring of the HCG levels (until they return to normal) and avoidance of another pregnancy for at least a year after all tests are negative. If no malignancy is detected and the HCG levels decrease, the prognosis (prediction of the outcome) is favorable.

hyperemesis gravidarum
(high-per-**EM**-eh-sis grav-ih-**DAR**-um)
hyper- = excessive
-emesis = to vomit
gravid/o = pregnancy

An abnormal condition of pregnancy characterized by severe vomiting that results in maternal dehydration and weight loss.

The nausea and vomiting associated with **hyperemesis gravidarum** persists beyond the first 3 months of pregnancy and persists throughout the day to the point that eventually nothing can be retained by mouth.

The exact cause of this condition is unknown, but the incidence seems to be greater in younger mothers, first-time mothers, and those with increased body weight. Psychological factors have been considered as being instrumental in the development of hyperemesis gravidarum (such as stress over the pregnancy, ambivalent feelings toward the pregnancy, and conflicting feelings over becoming a mother). Physical factors may include hyperthyroidism, elevated levels of estrogen, a multiple pregnancy, and the presence of a hydatidiform mole.

Treatment includes control of the vomiting, replacement of lost fluids and electrolytes, and emotional support for the woman. In most women, hyperemesis gravidarum is self-limiting and health is restored.

incompetent cervix
(in-**COMP**-eh-tent **SER**-viks)

A condition in which the cervical os (opening) dilates before the fetus reaches term, without labor or uterine contractions; usually occurring during the second trimester of pregnancy and resulting in a spontaneous abortion of the fetus.

Treatment for an **incompetent cervix** involves suturing the cervix to keep it from opening during the pregnancy; this is known as **cerclage**. If the woman is going to have a vaginal delivery, the sutures are removed near the end of the pregnancy. If she is to have a cesarean section delivery, the sutures may be left in place.

placenta previa
(plah-**SEN**-tah **PRE**-vee-ah)

A condition of pregnancy in which the placenta is implanted in the lower part of the uterus, and precedes the fetus during the birthing process.

The cause (etiology) is unknown.

The degree of **placenta previa** may range from marginal previa, where the placenta barely comes to the edge of the cervical os (opening), to partial previa, where the placenta partially covers the cervical os, to total previa, where the placenta completely covers the cervical os. See **Figure 18-11.**

The classic symptom of placenta previa is painless bleeding during the third trimester of pregnancy. The bleeding is usually abrupt and bright red, and very frightening to the expectant mother.

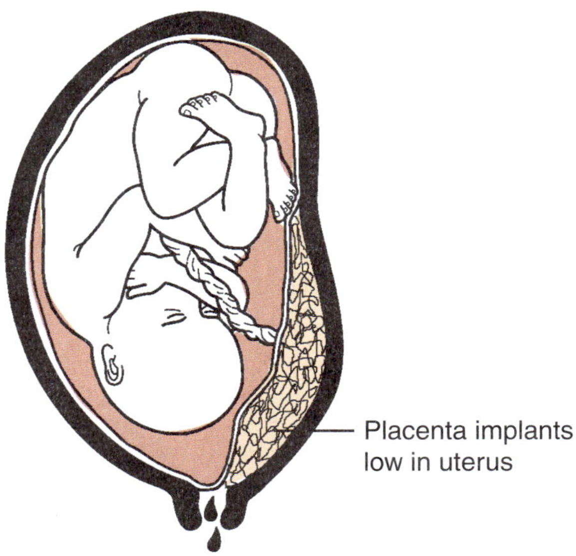

Figure 18-11 Example of placenta previa

Diagnosis of placenta previa is confirmed by ultrasonography; sometimes it is detected before symptoms occur, through routine use of ultrasonography.

Treatment ranges from conservative measures of bed rest to immediate delivery by cesarean section, depending on the condition of the expectant mother and the condition of the fetus, that is, maturity of fetus and whether fetal distress is detected.

pregnancy-induced hypertension

The development of hypertension (high blood pressure) during pregnancy, in women who had normal blood pressure readings (normotensive) prior to pregnancy.

For ease in understanding, pregnancy-induced hypertension (PIH) is divided into three categories based on degree of severity.

1. **Gestational hypertension** is the development of hypertension after 20 weeks' gestation with no signs of edema or proteinuria. A blood pressure reading of 140/90 mmHg or greater on more than one occasion, or a blood pressure reading of 30 mmHg systolic or 15 mmHg diastolic over the patient's normal baseline readings are indicative of gestational hypertension. The hypertension usually subsides after pregnancy.

2. **Pre-eclampsia** is the development of hypertension (as defined above) with proteinuria or edema after 20 weeks' gestation. The factor that distinguishes pre-eclampsia from gestational hypertension is the presence of proteinuria. The patient may also exhibit edema of the hands and face.

   Edema of the feet and legs is common during pregnancy; however, edema that occurs above the waist may be indicative of pregnancy-induced hypertension. One of the first signs of edema may be a sudden rapid weight gain of more than 4 pounds in a week. This may be followed by visible signs of edema, such as puffiness or swelling of the face and hands; the woman may remove the rings from her fingers as they seem increasingly tighter on the fingers.

   It is important that the health care professional carefully monitor the pregnant woman's weight and vital signs during each prenatal visit, and that any rise in blood pressure be taken seriously and be considered as a possible indication of impending complications. It is also important that early measures be taken to lower the blood pressure, reduce the edema, and correct the proteinuria.

   If the condition worsens, the patient with pre-eclampsia may experience blurred vision or see spots in front of the eyes, and complain of severe headaches. These symptoms are strong indicators of impending eclampsia and medical treatment will be necessary.

3. **Eclampsia** is the most severe form of hypertension during pregnancy and is evidenced by the presence of seizures. An eclamptic seizure may jeopardize the life of the expectant mother and her fetus.

   Delivery of the baby is the cure for pregnancy-induced hypertension. If it is determined that the fetus is mature enough for delivery, the pregnancy is ended by inducing labor or by performing a cesarean section. If the fetus is not mature enough for delivery, medical treatment will involve hospitalization of the expectant mother, bed rest, administration of medications to reduce her blood pressure, and administration of medications to prevent convulsions until the baby can be delivered.

Rh incompatibility

An incompatibility between an Rh negative mother's blood with her Rh positive baby's blood, causing the mother's body to develop antibodies that will destroy the Rh positive blood.

All blood types either have the Rh factor or they do not. Individuals who have the Rh factor present on their red blood cells are said to be Rh positive; those who do not have it are said to be Rh negative. Rh incompatibility can occur if the father of the baby is Rh positive and the mother of the baby is Rh negative; it does not occur when the expectant mother is Rh positive.

An Rh negative mother will give birth to either an Rh negative baby or an Rh positive baby. If her baby is Rh negative, the two are compatible. If her baby is Rh positive, the potential for incompatibility in subsequent births is present. During the birth process, if there is a mixing of Rh negative maternal and Rh positive fetal blood (as the placenta separates from the uterine wall), the mother's blood will recognize this as foreign to her body and will respond by producing antibodies to destroy the Rh positive blood.

The first Rh positive baby born to an Rh negative mother will not be affected by an Rh incompatibility; however, the antibodies that develop in response to the first pregnancy will be present during subsequent pregnancies. If a subsequent pregnancy produces an Rh positive fetus, the antibody production will increase. These antibodies are small enough to cross the placental barrier into the fetal circulation and destroy the red blood cells of the fetus, which have been recognized as "foreign" to the mother's body.

Treatment for prevention of Rh incompatibility is to administer an injection of Rh immune globulin (RhoGAM) to the Rh negative, pregnant woman during week 28 of pregnancy. If she gives birth to an Rh positive baby, she will be administered another injection of RhoGAM within 72 hours after the birth. The administration of this Rh immune globulin will prevent the formation of the antibodies in the Rh negative mother's blood.

It is important that an Rh negative woman realizes that if her first pregnancy ends in abortion, it is still counted as a pregnancy and she should receive the injection of RhoGAM after the abortion to prevent the formation of antibodies that will affect future pregnancies, should the fetus be Rh positive.

Signs and Symptoms of Labor

The material listed in this segment is an elementary discussion of the signs and symptoms of impending labor and comparison of true labor and false labor.

bloody show

A vaginal discharge that is a mixture of thick mucus and pink or dark brown blood.

It may begin a few weeks prior to the onset of labor and occurs as a result of the softening, dilation, and **effacement** (thinning) of the cervix in preparation for childbirth. The bloody show will continue and will increase during labor as the cervix continues to dilate and efface.

Braxton Hicks contractions	Mild, irregular contractions that occur throughout pregnancy. As full term approaches, these contractions intensify and are sometimes mistaken for true labor.
increased vaginal discharge	When the baby settles into the pelvis prior to the onset of labor, the pressure of the baby's head in the area creates congestion of the vaginal mucosa, which results in an increase in clear, nonirritating vaginal secretions.
lightening	The expectant mother will notice that she can breathe easier because the descent of the baby relieves some of the pressure from her diaphragm. When lightening occurs, most expectant mothers will refer to it by saying that the baby has "dropped." Lightening is more obvious in women who are having their first baby.
rupture of the amniotic sac	The rupture of the amniotic sac (membranes) may occur prior to the onset of labor, may occur during labor, or may not occur without assistance. Expectant mothers are usually advised to report to the hospital or birthing center for evaluation if the membranes rupture prior to the onset of labor. This is important because the amniotic sac serves as a barrier between the baby and the unsterile outside environment, and when broken, the chance for infection is increased. Women often refer to the rupture of the amniotic sac by saying their "water broke," because there may be a sudden gush of amniotic fluid as the membranes rupture.
sudden burst of energy	This occurs in some women shortly before the onset of labor. These women may suddenly have the energy to do major housecleaning duties—things they have not had the energy to do previously. They should be cautioned to save their energy during this time, so they will not be fatigued when labor actually begins.

The essential distinction between false labor and true labor is that true labor is characterized by progressive change in the cervix. For the baby to pass from the uterine cavity and descend through the vaginal canal to the outside of the body, the cervix must dilate (enlarge) and efface (thin) to allow passage. See **Figure 18-12.**

Preparations for childbirth should be discussed with the expectant mother regardless if she has attended prenatal classes. This will allow the health care professional the opportunity to review the signs and symptoms of impending labor, assist the expectant mother in distinguishing between false labor and true labor, and answer any questions that might follow the discussion. For the learner's convenience, the comparison of false labor to true labor is arranged in **Table 18-2.**

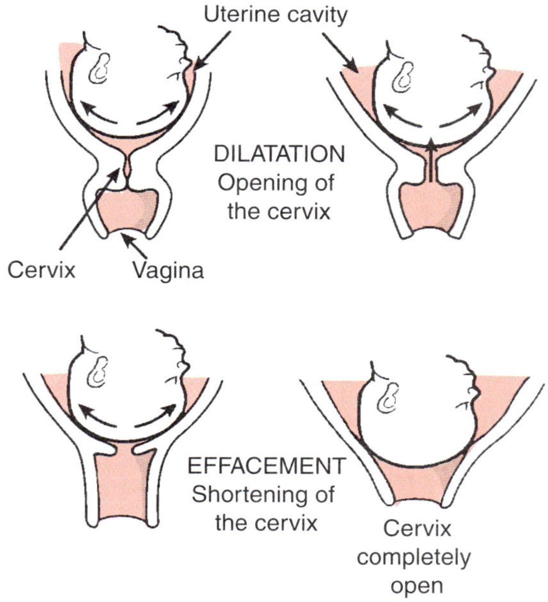

Figure 18-12 Dilatation and effacement of the cervix

Table 18-2 Comparison of False Labor and True Labor

FALSE LABOR	TRUE LABOR
1. Contractions Irregular Not too frequent Shorter duration Not too intense	1. Contractions Regular More frequent Longer duration More intense
2. Discomfort Felt in abdomen Felt in groin area	2. Discomfort Felt in lower back Radiates to lower abdomen Feels like menstrual cramps
3. Walking May relieve or decrease contractions	3. Walking May strengthen contraction
4. Effacement/Dilatation Dilatation and effacement of cervix does not change	4. Effacement/Dilatation Cervix progressively effaces (thins) and dilates (enlarges)

Diagnostic Techniques and Procedures

amniocentesis
(am-nee-oh-sen-**TEE**-sis)
amni/o = amnion
-centesis = surgical puncture

A surgical puncture of the amniotic sac for the purpose of removing amniotic fluid.

A needle is passed through the abdomen and uterus into the amniotic sac. Fluid is removed for laboratory analysis to detect fetal abnormalities and

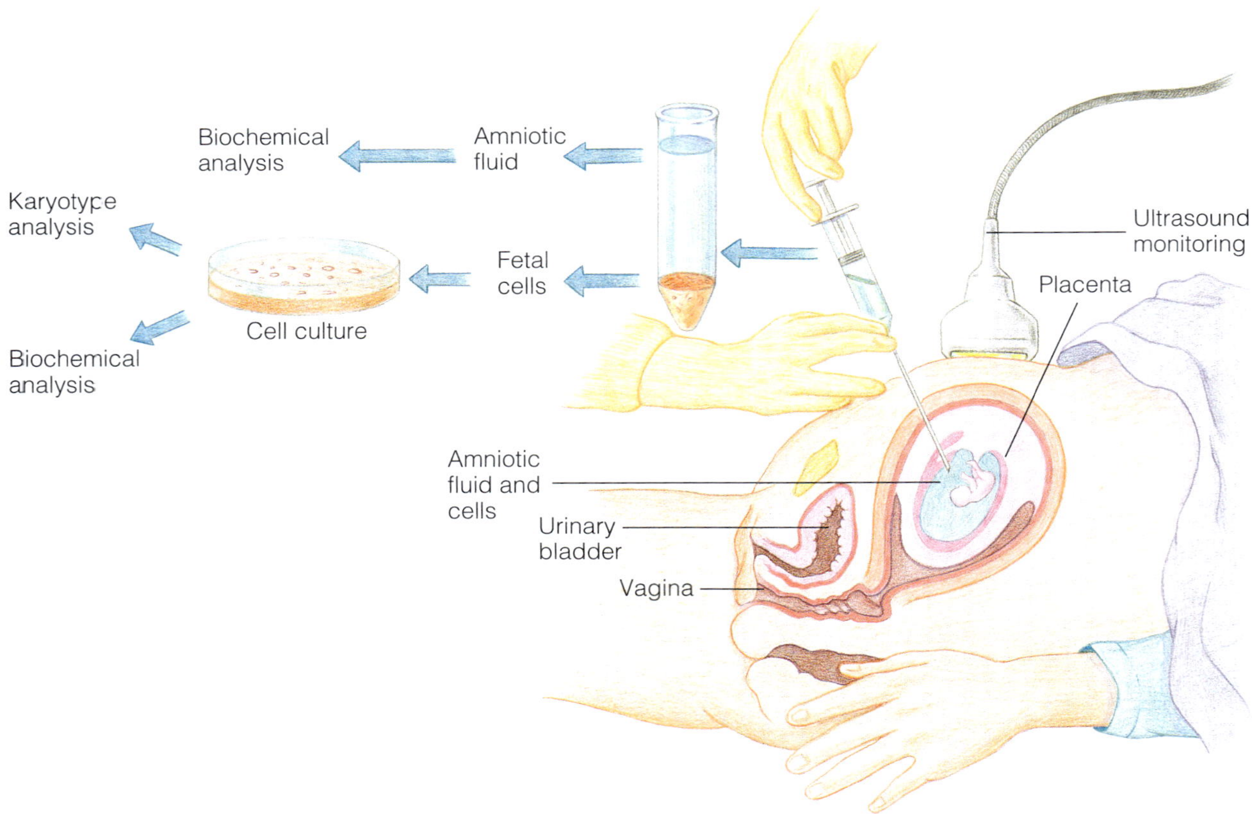

Figure 18-13 Amniocentesis

maternal-fetal blood incompatibilities, and to determine fetal maturity. If necessary, an amniocentesis is usually performed between 16 and 20 weeks' gestation. See **Figure 18-13.**

---

cesarean section
(see-**SAYR**-ee-an section)

A surgical procedure in which the abdomen and uterus are incised and a baby is delivered transabdominally.

It is performed when abnormal fetal or maternal conditions exist that are judged likely to make a vaginal delivery hazardous. See **Figure 18-14.**

---

contraction stress test

A stress test used to evaluate the ability of the fetus to tolerate the stress of labor and delivery (CST); also known as oxytocin challenge test.

The hormone, oxytocin, is diluted in an IV solution and is administered intravenously to the expectant mother to stimulate uterine contractions. The amount of oxytocin infused into the patient is monitored and is increased every 15 to 20 minutes until three uterine contractions, lasting approximately 30 to 40 seconds, are observed within a 10-minute period. The fetal heart rate (FHR) is then interpreted, and the infusion of oxytocin is discontinued.

The purpose of the oxytocin challenge test is to simulate labor for a measurable period of time to determine if the infant will tolerate labor well. During labor, uterine contractions decrease the oxygen supply to the fetus; if there is a significant decrease in the oxygen supply, then it may cause a decrease in the fetal heart rate.

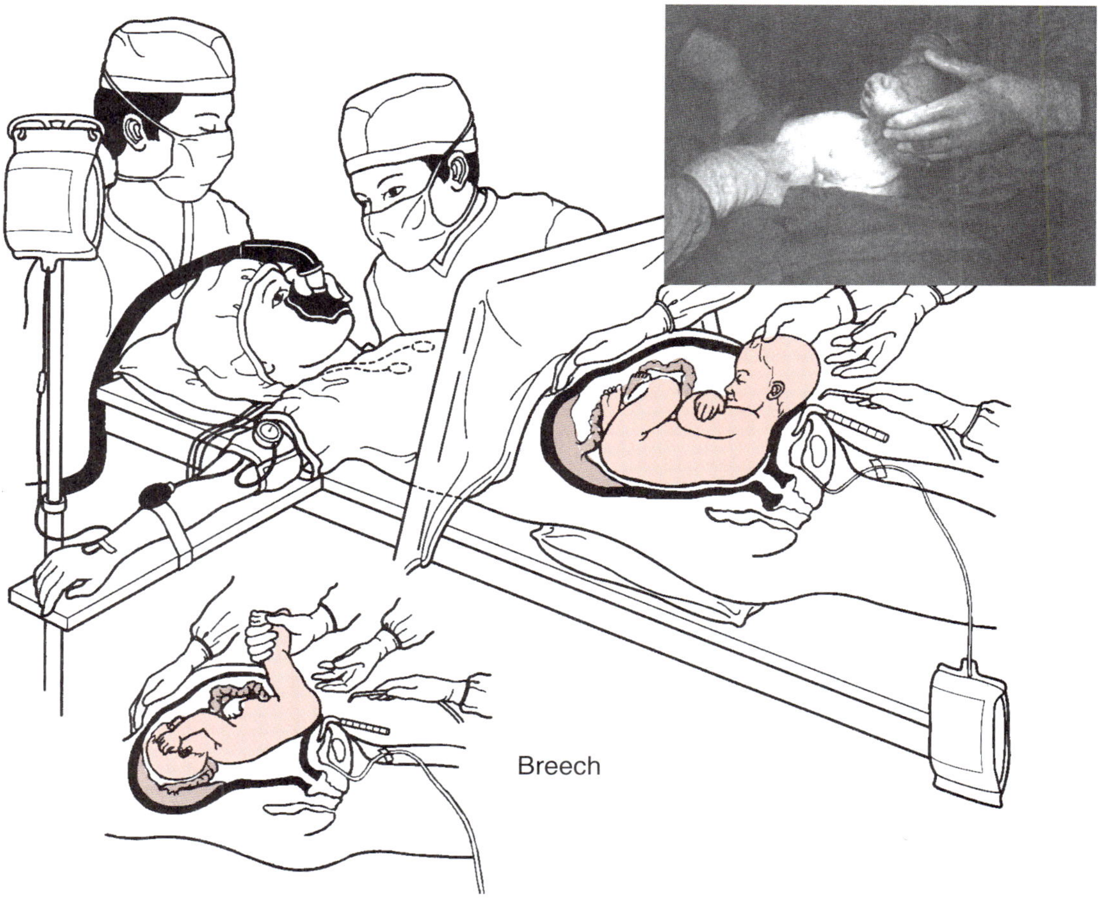

Figure 18-14 Cesarean section (Illustration adapted courtesy of Childbirth Graphics, Waco, Texas, ©1987; Photo by Marjorie Pyle, ©LIFECIRCLE)

The maternal uterine activity and the fetal heart rate are monitored closely during this stress test. If it appears that the contractions of the uterus will endanger the fetus as labor progresses, an emergency cesarean section may be indicated.

---

fetal monitoring (electronic)
(**FEE**-tal **MON**-ih-tor-ing)

The use of an electronic device to monitor the fetal heart rate and the maternal uterine contractions; this procedure can be done with external or internal devices.

This monitoring is valuable during labor to assess the quality of the uterine contractions and the effects of labor on the fetus. See **Figure 18-15.**

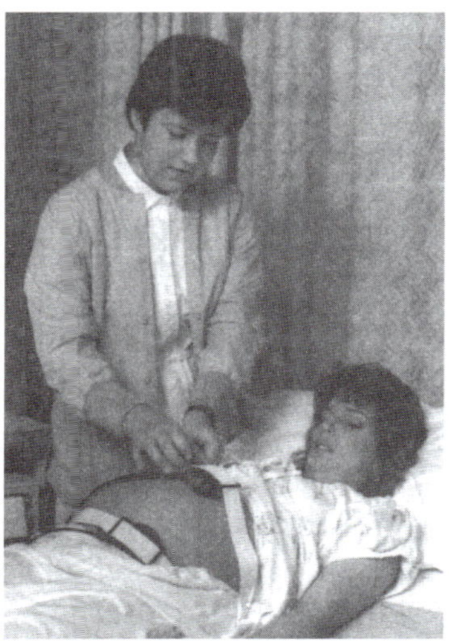

Figure 18-15 Fetal monitoring

nipple stimulation test

A noninvasive technique that produces basically the same results as the contraction stress test by having the pregnant woman stimulate the nipples of her breasts by rubbing them between her fingers.

This causes the natural release of oxytocin that causes contractions of the uterus. The nipple stimulation test is less stressing to the uterus.

pelvic ultrasound
(**PELL**-vik **ULL**-trah-sound)

A noninvasive procedure that uses high-frequency sound waves to examine the abdomen and pelvis.

The sound waves pass through the abdominal wall from the transducer, which is moved back and forth across the abdomen. When the sound waves bounce off of the internal organs in the abdominopelvic region, these waves are converted to electrical impulses eventually recorded on an oscilloscope screen. A photograph of the images is then taken for further study. See **Figure 18-16.**

Pelvic ultrasound can be used to locate a pelvic mass, an ectopic pregnancy, or an intrauterine device; and to inspect and assess the uterus, ovaries, and fallopian tubes. Clearer ultrasonic pictures of the pelvic organs can be obtained by using transvaginal ultrasonography. This procedure produces the same type of picture as abdominal ultrasound, but involves the use of a vaginal probe inserted into the vagina while the patient is in **lithotomy position.** The probes are encased in a sterile sheath and placed in the transducer before it is inserted into the vagina. The sound waves function in the same way as those for the abdominopelvic ultrasound, but the transvaginal ultrasonic image is much clearer.

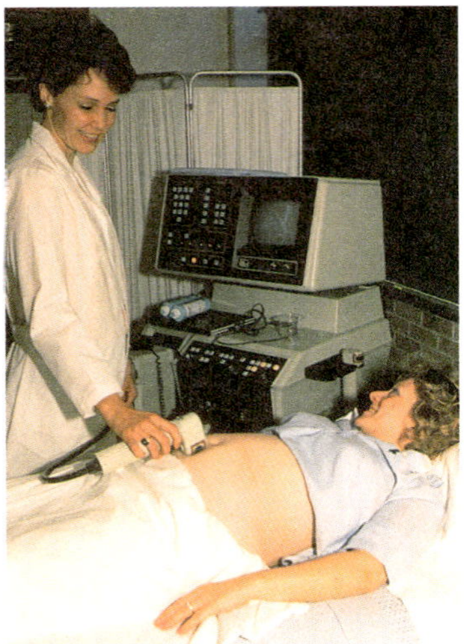

Figure 18-16 Pelvic ultrasound

pelvimetry
(pell-**VIM**-eh-tree)
pelv/i = pelvis
metr/o = measure
-y = noun ending

The process of measuring the female pelvis, manually or by x-ray, to determine its adequacy for childbearing.

Clinical **pelvimetry** is an estimate of the size of the birth canal by vaginal palpation of bony landmarks in the pelvis and a mathematical estimate of the distance between them. This is performed during the early part of the pregnancy and is recorded as "adequate," "borderline," or "inadequate."

X-ray pelvimetry is an actual x-ray of the pelvis to determine the dimensions of the bony pelvis of a pregnant woman; it is performed when there is doubt that the head of the fetus can safely pass through the pelvis during the labor process. Measurements are actually made on the x-ray, and the true dimensions of the birth canal and the head of the fetus can be calculated to determine if the proportions are suitable.

pregnancy testing

Tests performed on maternal urine and/or blood to determine the presence of the hormone, HCG (human chorionic gonadotropin); HCG is detected shortly after the first missed menstrual period.

Tests performed on blood are highly reliable and results are usually available in approximately 1 hour. Tests performed on urine are fairly accurate when done correctly, and are very popular in the form of home testing kits; results are available within minutes. Women using home testing kits should test the first voided urine specimen of the day, because the level of HCG is highest at that time.

Common Abbreviations

ABBREVIATION	MEANING	ABBREVIATION	MEANING
AFP	alpha-fetoprotein	**HCG**	human chorionic gonadotropin
C-section	cesarean section	**L & D**	labor and delivery
CS	cesarean section	**LMP**	last menstrual period
CST	contraction stress test	**LNMP**	last normal menstrual period
EDB	expected date of birth	**Multip**	multipara
EDC	expected date of confinement; estimated date of confinement (i.e., estimated date for birth of baby)	**NSD**	normal spontaneous delivery
		NST	non stress test
EDD	expected date of delivery	**OB**	obstetrics
EFM	electronic fetal monitoring	**Primip**	primipara
FHR	fetal heart rate	**SVD**	spontaneous vaginal delivery
FHS, FHT	fetal heart sound; fetal heart tone	**TPAL**	term, preterm, abortions, living (this is used on obstetrical history forms to obtain patient data)
FSH	follicle-stimulating hormone		
G	gravida (pregnant)	**UC**	uterine contractions
GPA	gravida, para, abortion		

Written and Audio Terminology Review

Review each of the following terms from this chapter. Study the spelling of each term and write the definition in the space provided. If you have the Audio CD available, listen to each term, pronounce it, and check the box once you are comfortable saying the word. Check definitions by looking the term up in the glossary/index.

TERM	PRONUNCIATION	DEFINITION
abortion	☐ ah-**BOR**-shun	______________
abruptio placenta	☐ ah-**BRUP**-she-oh plah-**SEN**-tah	______________

Term		Pronunciation	
alpha-fetoprotein	☐	**AL**-fah fee-toh-**PRO**-teen	________
amenorrhea	☐	ah-men-or-**REE**-ah	________
amnion	☐	**AM**-nee-on	________
amniotic	☐	am-nee-**OT**-ik	________
areola	☐	ah-**REE**-oh-lah	________
ballottement	☐	bal-ot-**MON**	________
cerclage	☐	sair-**KLOGH**	________
cervix	☐	**SER**-viks	________
chloasma	☐	kloh-**AZ**-mah	________
chorion	☐	**KOH**-ree-on	________
coitus	☐	**KOH**-ih-tus	________
colostrum	☐	koh-**LOSS**-trum	________
conception	☐	con-**SEP**-shun	________
copulation	☐	kop-you-**LAY**-shun	________
corpus luteum	☐	**COR**-pus **LOO**-tee-um	________
culdocentesis	☐	kull-doh-sen-**TEE**-sis	________
dilatation	☐	dill-ah-**TAY**-shun	________
eclampsia	☐	eh-**KLAMP**-see-ah	________
ectopic	☐	ek-**TOP**-ic	________
edema	☐	eh-**DEE**-mah	________
effacement	☐	eh-**FACE**-ment	________
ejaculation	☐	eh-jak-you-**LAY**-shun	________
embryo	☐	**EM**-bree-oh	________
endometrium	☐	en-doh-**MEE**-tree-um	________
episiotomy	☐	eh-peez-ee-**OT**-oh-mee	________
estrogen	☐	**ESS**-troh-jen	________
fallopian tubes	☐	fah-**LOH**-pee-an tubes	________
fertilization	☐	fer-til-ih-**ZAY**-shun	________
fetal	☐	**FEE**-tal	________
fetoscope	☐	**FEET**-oh-scope	________
fetus	☐	**FEE**-tus	________
fimbriae	☐	**FIM**-bree-ah	________

gamete	☐ **GAM**-eet	______
gastroesophageal reflux	☐ gas-troh-eh-soff-ah-**JEE**-al reflux	______
gestation	☐ jess-**TAY**-shun	______
gestational diabetes	☐ jess-**TAY**-shun-al dye-ah-**BEE**-teez	______
gestational hypertension	☐ jess-**TAY**-shun-al high-per-**TEN**-shun	______
glycogen	☐ **GLYE**-koh-jen	______
graafian follicles	☐ **GRAF**-ee-an **FALL**-ih-kls	______
Hegar's sign	☐ **HAY**-garz sign	______
hydatidiform mole	☐ high-dah-**TID**-ih-form mohl	______
hyperemesis gravidarum	☐ high-per-**EM**-eh-sis grav-ih-**DAR**-um	______
hyperpigmentation	☐ **high**-per-**pig**-men-**TAY**-shun	______
hypertension	☐ **high**-per-**TEN**-shun	______
hypotension	☐ **high**-poh-**TEN**-shun	______
hypovolemic shock	☐ **high**-poh-voh-**LEE**-mik shock	______
incompetent cervix	☐ in-**COMP**-eh-tent **SER**-viks	______
labor	☐ **LAY**-bor	______
lactation	☐ lak-**TAY**-shun	______
lactiferous ducts	☐ lak-**TIF**-er-us ducts	______
laparoscopy	☐ lap-ar-**OSS**-koh-pee	______
leukorrhea	☐ loo-koh-**REE**-ah	______
linea nigra	☐ **LIN**-ee-ah **NIG**-rah	______
lithotomy	☐ lith-**OT**-oh-mee	______
lordosis	☐ lor-**DOH**-sis	______
lunar	☐ **LOON**-ar	______
multigravida	☐ mull-tih-**GRAV**-ih-dah	______
multipara	☐ mull-**TIP**-ah-rah	______
Nagele's rule	☐ **NAY**-geh-leez rule	______
neonatology	☐ nee-oh-nay-**TALL**-oh-jee	______

Term		Pronunciation	
nullipara	☐	null-**IP**-ah-rah	________
obstetrician	☐	ob-steh-**TRISH**-an	________
obstetrics	☐	ob-**STET**-riks	________
ovary	☐	**OH**-vah-ree	________
ovulation	☐	ov-you-**LAY**-shun	________
ovum	☐	**OH**-vum	________
parturition	☐	par-too-**RISH**-un	________
pelvimetry	☐	pell-**VIM**-eh-tree	________
perineum	☐	pair-ih-**NEE**-um	________
placenta	☐	plah-**SEN**-tah	________
placenta previa	☐	plah-**SEN**-tah **PRE**-vee-ah	________
pre-eclampsia	☐	pre-eh-**KLAMP**-see-ah	________
prenatal	☐	pre-**NAY**-tl	________
primigravida	☐	prigh-mih-**GRAV**-ih-dah	________
progesterone	☐	proh-**JES**-ter-ohn	________
proteinuria	☐	proh-tee-in-**YOU**-ree-ah	________
puberty	☐	**PEW**-ber-tee	________
pyrosis	☐	pye-**ROH**-sis	________
quickening	☐	**KWIK**-en-ing	________
salpingectomy	☐	sal-pin-**JEK**-toh-mee	________
striae gravidarum	☐	**STRIGH**-ay grav-ih-**DAR**-um	________
symptoms	☐	**SIM**-toms	________
tachycardia	☐	tak-eh-**CAR**-dee-ah	________
testes	☐	**TESS**-teez	________
transvaginal	☐	trans-**VAJ**-in-al	________
trimester	☐	**TRY**-mes-ter	________
tubal ligation	☐	**TOO**-bal lye-**GAY**-shun	________
ultrasound	☐	**ULL**-tra-sound	________
ultrasonography	☐	ull-tra-son-**OG**-rah-fee	________
umbilical cord	☐	um-**BILL**-ih-kal cord	________
uterus	☐	**YOU**-ter-us	________

vagina	☐ vah-**JIGH**-nah	________________
waddling gait	☐ **WAH**-dl-ing gait	________________

Chapter Review Exercises

The following exercises provide a more in-depth review of the chapter material. Your goal in these exercises is to complete each section at a minimum 80% level of accuracy. If you score below 80% in any area, return to the appropriate section in the chapter and read the material again. A place has been provided for your score at the end of each section.

A. Spelling

Circle the correctly spelled term in each pairing of words. Each correct answer is worth 10 points. Record your score in the space provided at the end of the exercise.

1. areola	ariola
2. faloppian tubes	fallopian tubes
3. fimbrii	fimbria
4. graafian follicles	graffian follicles
5. partuition	parturition
6. preclampsia	pre-eclampsia
7. cesarean	ceserean
8. chloasthma	chloasma
9. effacement	efacement
10. obstetrics	obstetrix

Number correct _______ × 10 points/correct answer: Your score _______%

B. Is She or Isn't She?

The following exercise will review some of the presumptive and probable signs of pregnancy. Read each statement carefully, decide if the symptom is a presumptive or probable sign of pregnancy, and check your choice in the space provided. Each correct response is worth 20 points. Record your score in the space provided at the end of the exercise.

1. April Jones is a 21-year-old junior in college. She and her fiancé are sexually active and use condoms as a means of birth control. She is usually regular with her menstrual periods, but is 2 weeks late this month. At first she thought it might be due to the fact that she is preparing for end-of-semester exams, but now she is not sure.

   ☐ Presumptive sign ☐ Probable sign

2. Maria Quintana is a 35-year-old mother of three children, ages 2, 4, and 7. Lately she has experienced frequent fatigue and an increase in urination (urinary disturbances). Although Maria is using an IUD as a means of birth control, she is still concerned about the possibility of pregnancy, especially since she has had these symptoms with a previous pregnancy.

   ☐ Presumptive sign ☐ Probable sign

3. Chin Soo-Young is a 26-year-old female who has come to the office today to find out if she is pregnant. She has done a pregnancy test at home and it was positive, but she continues to have her menstrual periods even though they are irregular. Her last "normal" period was 4 months ago. She has had no nausea or vomiting. For the last week, however, she has felt a slight flutter in her abdomen, which concerns her.

   ☐ Presumptive sign ☐ Probable sign

4. Nicole Macormick is a 39-year-old mother of three children. She has come into the office today for her presurgery exam before having her tubal ligation next week. When the doctor performs the bimanual part of the pelvic examination, he notices that the lower segment of her uterus is soft and easy to palpate. He asks Nicole if she has missed a menstrual period; she confirms this, but states that it is not unusual for her to miss an occasional period.

   ☐ Presumptive sign ☐ Probable sign

5. Theresa Bustos is a 24-year-old female who has been coming to the office for the last year for infertility studies. Today she is being seen for her third artificial insemination treatment (using her husband's sperm). When the doctor performs the pelvic examination, prior to the procedure, he notices that Theresa's vagina has a bluish-violet color.

   ☐ Presumptive sign ☐ Probable sign

Number correct _______ × 20 points/correct answer: Your score _______%

C. Matching

Match the terms on the left with the appropriate definitions on the right. Each correct answer is worth 10 points. Record your score in the space provided at the end of the exercise.

_____ 1. Chadwick's sign
_____ 2. Goodell's sign
_____ 3. embryo
_____ 4. fetus
_____ 5. chloasma
_____ 6. linea nigra
_____ 7. striae gravidarum
_____ 8. quickening
_____ 9. Braxton Hicks
_____ 10. ballottement

a. A technique that causes the fetus to bounce within the amniotic fluid, with the examiner feeling it rebound quickly
b. Movement of the fetus felt by the mother
c. The name given to the product of conception from the second through the eighth week of pregnancy
d. A bluish-violet hue to the cervix and vagina
e. Absence of menstruation
f. Softening of the cervix, felt by the examiner
g. "Mask of pregnancy"
h. The name given to the product of conception from the ninth week through the duration of the gestational period
i. Stretch marks on the abdomen, thighs, and breasts during pregnancy
j. A dark line of pigmentation that may extend from the fundus to the symphysis pubis during pregnancy
k. Irregular contractions of the uterus that occur throughout pregnancy

Number correct _______ × 10 points/correct answer: Your score _______%

D. Word Element Review

The following words relate to the field of obstetrics. The prefixes and suffixes have been provided. Read the definition carefully and complete the word by filling in the blank, using the word elements provided in this chapter. If you have forgotten your word building rules, refer to Chapter 1. Each correct answer is worth 10 points. Record your score in the space provided at the end of this exercise.

1. Surgical puncture of the amniotic sac for the purpose of withdrawing amniotic fluid:
   ____________________ / centesis
2. Pertaining to before birth:
   pre / ____________________ / al
3. Surgical removal of a fallopian tube:
   ____________________ / ectomy
4. Pertaining to across the vagina:
   trans / ____________________ / al
5. A woman who is pregnant for the first time:
   primi / ____________________ / a
6. A woman who has borne no children:
   nulli / ____________________
7. Excessive vomiting:
   hyper / ____________________
8. Pertaining to the perineum:
   ____________________ / al
9. An instrument used to hear the fetal heartbeat through the mother's abdomen:
   ____________________ / _______ / scope
10. Difficult labor:
    dys / ____________________

Number correct _______ × 10 points/correct answer: Your score _______%

E. Completion

The following sentences provide a discussion of complications of pregnancy. Complete each sentence with the most appropriate word. Each correct answer is worth 10 points. Record your score in the space provided at the end of the exercise.

1. The premature separation of a normally implanted placenta from the uterine wall after the pregnancy has passed 20 weeks' gestation, or during labor, is known as:
   ____
2. The abnormal implantation of a fertilized ovum outside of the uterine cavity is known as:
   ____
3. Diabetes that develops during pregnancy is known as:
   ____
4. An abnormal condition of pregnancy characterized by severe vomiting that results in maternal dehydration and weight loss is known as:
   ____

5. A condition of pregnancy in which the placenta is implanted in the lower part of the uterus, and precedes the fetus during the birthing process, is known as:

____

6. A condition in which the cervical os dilates before the fetus reaches term, without uterine contractions, and results in a spontaneous abortion of the fetus is known as:

____

7. Hypertension that develops during pregnancy, after 20 weeks' gestation, with the presence of proteinuria or edema is known as:

____

8. The most severe form of hypertension during pregnancy that results in seizures is known as:

____

9. A miscarriage that occurs on its own as a result of abnormalities of the maternal environment or abnormalities of the embryo or fetus is known as:

____

10. An incompatibility between an Rh negative mother's blood with her Rh positive baby's blood, causing the mother's body to develop antibodies that will destroy the Rh positive blood is known as:

____

Number correct _______ × 10 points/correct answer: Your score _______%

F. Matching Abbreviations

Match the abbreviations on the left with the appropriate definitions on the right. Each correct answer is worth 10 points. Enter your score in the space provided at the end of the exercise.

_____	1. AFP	a. multipara
_____	2. EDC	b. fetal heart tone
_____	3. FHT	c. expected date of delivery
_____	4. HCG	d. alpha-fetoprotein
_____	5. LMP	e. cesarean section
_____	6. OB	f. fetal heart rate
_____	7. CS	g. last menstrual period
_____	8. EDD	h. expected date of confinement
_____	9. FHR	i. human chorionic gonadotropin
_____	10. Multip	j. obstetrics
		k. fetal heart reaction
		l. electronic fetal monitoring

Number correct _______ × 10 points/correct answer: Your score _______%

G. Multiple Choice

Read each statement carefully and select the correct answer from the choices provided. Each correct answer is worth 10 points. Record your score in the space provided at the end of the exercise.

1. The absence of menstruation is known as:
   a. amenorrhea
   b. oligomenorrhea
   c. metrorrhagia
   d. dysmenorrhea
2. The darker, pigmented, circular area surrounding the nipple of each breast is called the:
   a. chorion
   b. amnion
   c. areola
   d. alveoli
3. Patches of tan or brown pigmentation associated with pregnancy, occurring mostly on the forehead, cheeks, and nose, and also called the mask of pregnancy, is known as:
   a. corpus luteum
   b. cerclage
   c. effacement
   d. chloasma
4. Another name for sexual intercourse, other than coitus, is:
   a. copulation
   b. ballottement
   c. conception
   d. cerclage
5. The most severe form of hypertension during pregnancy, evidenced by seizures (convulsions) is known as:
   a. Goodell's sign
   b. Chadwick's sign
   c. eclampsia
   d. Hegar's sign
6. A probable sign of pregnancy is softening of the lower segment of the uterus, which is called:
   a. Goodell's sign
   b. Chadwick's sign
   c. eclampsia
   d. Hegar's sign
7. The bluish-violet hue of the cervix and vagina after approximately the sixth week of pregnancy is known as:
   a. Goodell's sign
   b. Chadwick's sign
   c. eclampsia
   d. Hegar's sign

8. The fringelike end of the fallopian tube is called:
   a. fimbriae
   b. gamete
   c. fundus
   d. striae
9. The first feeling of movement of the fetus felt by the expectant mother, usually occurring between 18 and 20 weeks' gestation, is termed:
   a. lightening
   b. Hegar's sign
   c. Chadwick's sign
   d. quickening
10. The settling of the fetal head into the pelvis, occurring a few weeks prior to the onset of labor, is known as:
    a. lightening
    b. Hegar's sign
    c. Chadwick's sign
    d. quickening

Number correct _______ × 10 points/correct answer: Your score _______%

H. True, False, or Nearing?

Read the following signs and symptoms and determine if they are signs and symptoms of false labor, true labor, or nearing labor. Enter your choice with a check mark (√) in the appropriate column. Each correct answer is worth 10 points. Record your score in the space provided at the end of the exercise.

	Signs/Symptoms	False	True	Nearing
1.	Irregular contractions, not too intense	☐	☐	☐
2.	Regular contractions, intense, longer duration	☐	☐	☐
3.	Lightening: the settling of the fetal head into the pelvis	☐	☐	☐
4.	Cervix does not change	☐	☐	☐
5.	Walking may relieve or decrease contractions	☐	☐	☐
6.	A sudden burst of energy, feels like doing major house cleaning duties	☐	☐	☐
7.	Discomfort felt in abdomen and groin area	☐	☐	☐
8.	Discomfort felt in lower back, radiates to abdomen; cramping	☐	☐	☐
9.	Walking strengthens contractions	☐	☐	☐
10.	Cervix progressively enlarges and thins	☐	☐	☐

Number correct _______ × 10 points/correct answer: Your score _______%

I. Crossword Puzzle

Read the clues carefully and complete the puzzle. Each crossword answer is worth 10 points. When you have completed the crossword puzzle, total your points and enter your score in the space provided at the end of the puzzle.

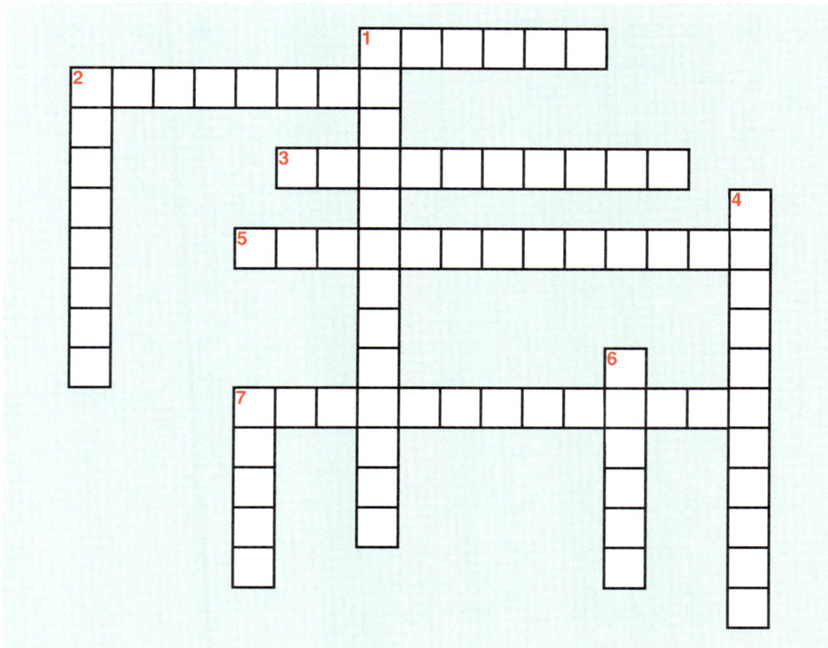

ACROSS

1 Inner layer of sac surrounding baby
2 Area between vaginal orifice and anus
3 Incision to enlarge vaginal opening
5 Union of sperm and ovum
7 Fertilization usually occurs here

DOWN

1 Fluid within the fetal membranes
2 Disc-shaped organ of pregnancy
4 Inner lining of the uterus
6 Houses the fertilized ovum
7 Name of baby from week 8 to birth

Number correct _______ × 10 points/correct answer: Your score _______%

J. Word Search

Using the definitions listed, identify the terms related to this chapter. After you have identified each term, find and circle it in the word search puzzle. The words may be read up, down, diagonally, across, or backward. Each correct answer is worth 10 points. Record your score in the space provided at the end of the exercise.

Example: Absence of menstruation.

amenorrhea

1. The inner of the two membrane layers that surround and contain the fetus and the amniotic fluid during pregnancy.

   ____

2. The darker pigmented, circular area surrounding the nipple of each breast.

   ____

3. Irregular, ineffective contractions of the uterus that occur throughout pregnancy.

   ____

4. Suturing the cervix to keep it from dilating prematurely during the pregnancy; sometimes referred to as the "purse string procedure."

   ____

F	L	O	A	M	N	I	O	N	O	L	E	M	I	C
A	C	Y	N	M	E	S	M	S	I	D	A	S	T	T
M	I	O	T	T	E	C	L	A	M	P	S	I	A	R
C	A	O	N	M	E	N	O	S	D	I	C	C	B	O
I	L	C	B	D	E	P	O	C	S	O	T	E	F	S
N	U	R	E	I	Y	T	T	R	T	E	L	N	L	T
C	Y	O	P	H	L	L	B	I	R	A	E	C	O	E
O	U	S	T	G	N	I	N	E	T	H	G	I	L	O
N	U	R	R	P	O	I	P	I	A	T	E	O	E	C
T	U	V	O	D	A	I	A	L	O	E	R	A	M	Y
E	A	L	C	G	R	S	P	I	N	E	C	S	E	E
B	R	A	X	T	O	N	H	I	C	K	S	A	I	G
E	S	P	A	D	R	U	Y	A	R	D	I	S	G	A
N	U	E	S	T	R	O	G	E	N	U	A	L	D	L
C	R	A	T	B	L	O	I	I	U	A	T	C	O	C
E	E	N	E	R	H	C	S	U	T	U	R	E	S	R
F	R	E	R	U	U	R	I	S	M	E	M	N	I	E
P	E	R	I	T	O	M	U	R	T	S	O	L	O	C

5. The thin, yellowish fluid secreted by the breasts during pregnancy and the first few days after birth, before lactation begins.

____

6. The most severe form of hypertension during pregnancy, evidenced by seizures (convulsions).

____

7. The name given to the product of conception from the second through the eighth week of pregnancy (through the second month).

____

8. A female hormone that promotes the development of the female secondary sex characteristics.

____

9. A special stethoscope for hearing the fetal heartbeat through the mother's abdomen.

____

10. The settling of the fetal head into the pelvis, occurring a few weeks prior to the onset of labor.

____

Number correct _______ × 10 points/correct answer: Your score _______%

Answers to Chapter Review Exercises

A. Spelling

1. areola
2. fallopian tubes
3. fimbria
4. graafian follicles
5. parturition
6. pre-eclampsia
7. cesarean
8. chloasma
9. effacement
10. obstetrics

B. Is She or Isn't She?

1. presumptive
2. presumptive
3. presumptive
4. probable
5. probable

C. Matching

1. d
2. f
3. c
4. h
5. g
6. j
7. i
8. b
9. k
10. a

D. Word Element Review

1. **amnio** / centesis
2. pre / **nat** / al
3. **salping** / ectomy
4. trans / **vagin** / al
5. primi / **gravid** / a
6. nulli / **para**
7. hyper / **emesis**
8. **perine** / al
9. **fet** / o / scope
10. dys / **tocia**

E. Completion

1. abruptio placenta
2. ectopic pregnancy
3. gestational diabetes
4. hyperemesis gravidarum
5. placenta previa
6. incompetent cervix
7. pre-eclampsia
8. eclampsia
9. spontaneous abortion
10. Rh incompatibility

F. Matching Abbreviations

1. d
2. h
3. b
4. i
5. g
6. j
7. e
8. c
9. f
10. a

G. Multiple Choice

1. a
2. c
3. d
4. a
5. c
6. d
7. b
8. a
9. d
10. a

H. True, False, or Nearing?

1. false
2. true
3. nearing
4. false
5. false
6. nearing
7. false
8. true
9. true
10. true

I. Crossword Puzzle

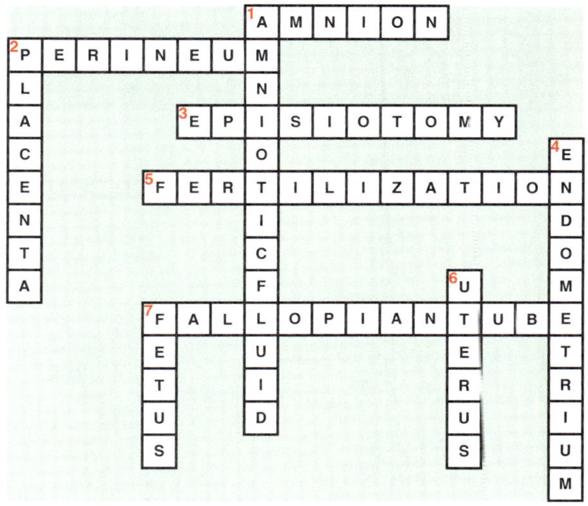

J. Word Search

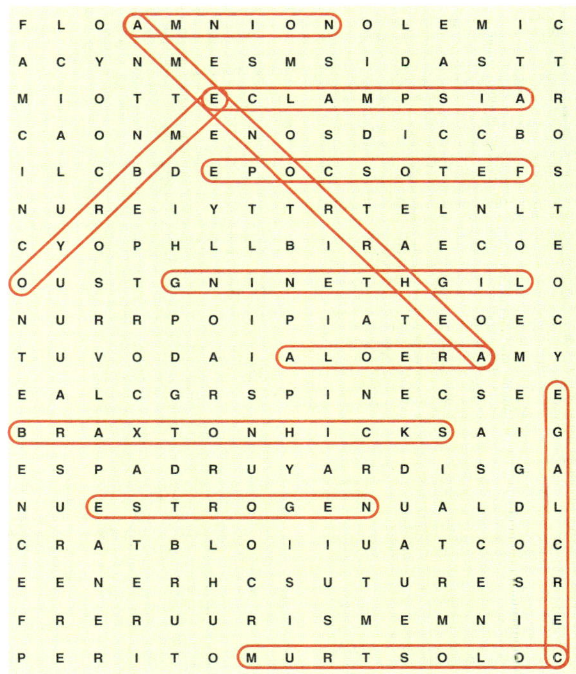

CHAPTER 19

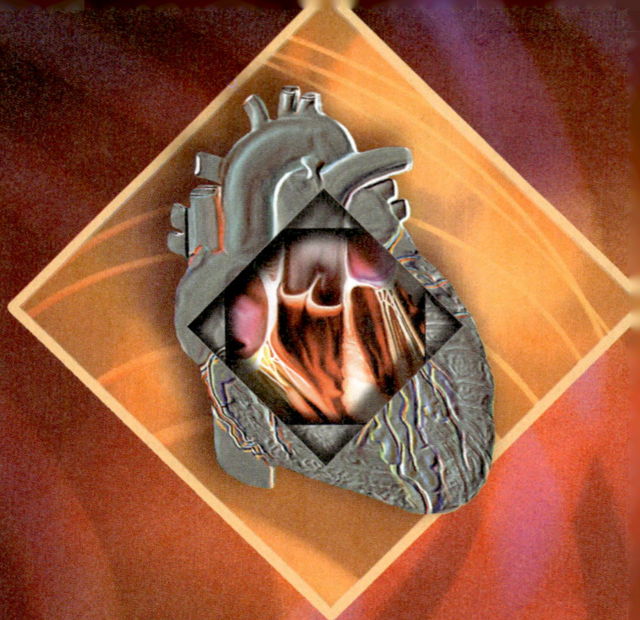

Child Health

CHAPTER CONTENT

KEY COMPETENCIES

Upon completing this chapter and the review exercises at the end of the chapter, the learner should be able to:

1. Identify and define at least 20 pathological conditions common to children.
2. List and define 10 communicable diseases seen in children.
3. Correctly spell and pronounce each new term introduced in this chapter using the Activity CD-ROM and Audio CD, if available.
4. Define at least 20 abbreviations common to the discussion of diseases and disorders of children.
5. State the recommended immunization schedule for infants and children.
6. Distinguish the differences between active and passive immunity.

OVERVIEW

Pediatrics is the field of medicine concerned with the development and care of children, specializing in the treatment and prevention of the diseases and disorders peculiar to children. In this chapter, the term "child health" will be synonymous with pediatrics. The physician who specializes in pediatrics is known as a **pediatrician**. Some pediatric offices employ a **pediatric nurse practitioner (PNP)**, who is a registered nurse practitioner with advanced study and clinical practice in pediatric nursing. The pediatric specialty concerned with the diseases and abnormalities of the newborn infant is known as **neonatology**. The physician who specializes in neonatology is known as a **neonatologist**.

There are many subspecialties that deal with the care of children, such as pediatric oncology, pediatric cardiology, and child psychology. No matter what the specialty, the health professional who cares for children must possess a broad base of knowledge in the growth and development of children as well as a clear understanding of the illnesses and diseases peculiar to children. This knowledge will be applied when assisting in the care of both the healthy and the sick child.

An instrumental part of the prevention of disease and early detection of deviations from the norm in children is the **well-child** visit. During this visit, health professionals will assess the current health status of the child, the progression of growth and development, and the need for **immunizations**. The well-child visit also provides the opportunity for teaching the parents what to expect in the various stages of their child's growth and development. The physical examination, the immunizations, and the health teachings are all designed to promote optimal health for the child.

The field of pediatrics encompasses a wide range of terms that will be used by the health professional. This chapter covers terms and concepts that deal with the normal growth and development of the child, the well-child visit, immunizations, and diseases and disorders common to children.

Growth and Development

Normal growth and development proceeds in a predictable and orderly sequence; however, the rate of growth and development in individuals will vary.

Growth is defined as the physical increase in the whole or any of its parts. Growth is the result of biological change and an increase in the size and number of cells. The parameters of a child's growth can be easily measured with accuracy through acquiring the child's weight, head circumference, length or height, and dentition.

Weight is an important indicator of the child's nutritional status and general growth. It is also used to calculate medication dosages for children. Weight should be measured at every well-visit for general indications about growth and at every sick-visit to determine the effects of illness on weight. See **Figure 19-1.**

Recording the weight of the infant or child is important to measure the child's progress. Weights should be plotted on a **growth chart** so that the growth pattern can be visualized.

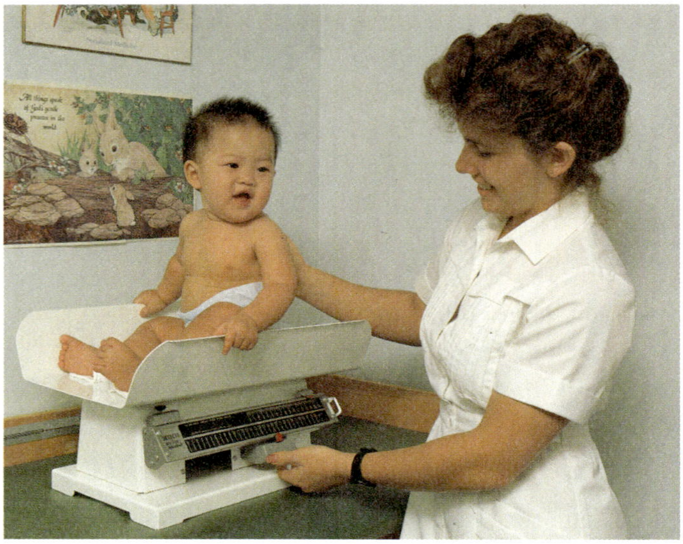

Figure 19-1 Measuring weight in the infant

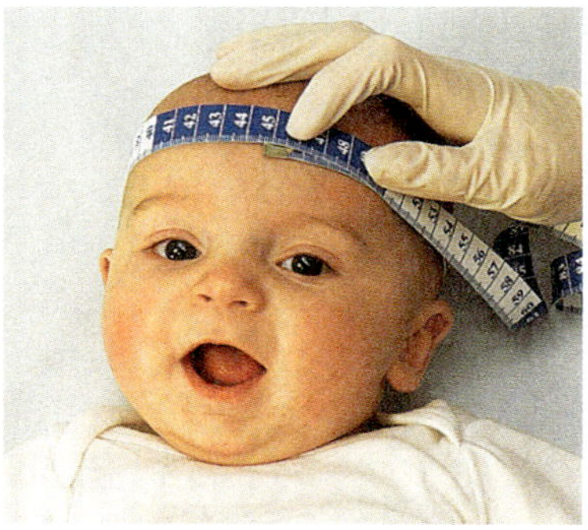

Figure 19-2 Measuring head circumference

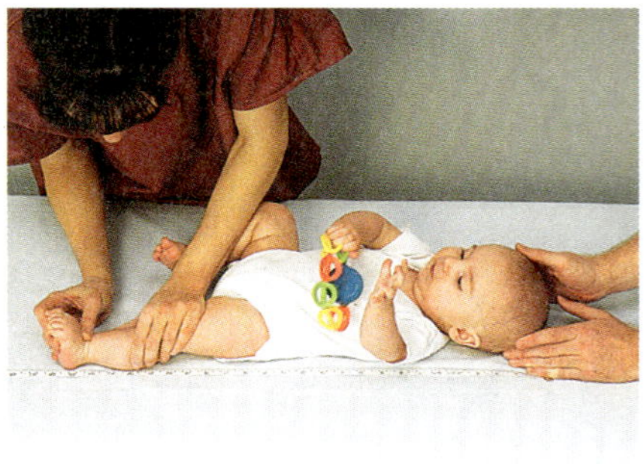

Figure 19-3 Recumbent length in infant

Head circumference is an important measurement because it is related to intracranial volume. Normal brain growth causes an increase in head circumference at an expected rate. Abnormal lags or surges in the increase of head circumference may indicate serious problems. Head circumference is measured during each well-child visit from birth to 2 to 3 years of age. See **Figure 19-2.**

An infant or child's head circumference is the measurement of the greatest circumference of the head. Head circumference is also plotted on a **nomogram** and is compared with weight and length for the particular age. Any inconsistencies in growth patterns will require further evaluation.

The **length** or **height** measurement is compared with the head circumference and weight measurement for an overall indicator of physical growth. Length or height is usually measured at every well-visit. The infant is measured from the crown of the head to the heel, with the child in a **recumbent** position. See **Figure 19-3.**

Standing height measurements are usually performed for children age 3 years or older. The child stands very still and straight, with his or her back against the measuring surface. Length or height is measured to the nearest 1/8 inch. This measurement is plotted on a growth chart for comparison with other measurements.

Dentition refers to the eruption of teeth and follows a sequential pattern. Twenty primary teeth erupt between 6 months and 30 months. Around the age of 6 years, the primary teeth are lost and permanent teeth begin to erupt. There are normally 32 permanent teeth. (See Figure 19-5 later in the chapter.)

Development refers to an increase in function and complexity that results through learning, maturation, and growth. Development is much more complicated to measure than growth. Observation of problem-solving skills, interaction patterns, the performance of daily activities (playing, dressing, eating, etc.) and the communication patterns used all provide useful data to evaluate the child's development. The child communicates through his or her universal language, "play."

Developmental screening can be achieved through standardized assessment tools. Examples are as follows:

- **Brazelton Neonatal Behavior Assessment (BNBA) Scale for newborns**—a scale developed for evaluating and assessing an infant's alertness, motor maturity, irritability, consolability, and interaction with people. Used as a tool for the evaluation of the neurological condition and the behavior of a newborn, the BNBA scale consists of a series of 27 reaction tests, including response to inanimate objects, pin prick, light, and the sound of a bell or rattle.
- **Dubowitz for newborns**—a system for estimating the gestational age of a newborn according to such factors as posture, ankle dorsiflexion, and arm and leg recoil.
- **Denver II Developmental Screening Test for infants and young children**—a test for evaluating development in children from 1 month to 6 years of age. Motor, social, and language development skills may be discovered by comparing the child's performance with the average performance of other children (in the same age group).

When working with children it is simple to refer to the child according to his or her age or stage of development. Following are stages of childhood growth and development.

- Newborn—birth to 1 month
- Infancy—1 month to 1 year
- Toddlerhood—1 to 3 years
- Preschool age—3 to 6 years
- School age—6 to 12 years
- Adolescents—12 to 18 years or 21 years

Growth and Development Principles

The patterns of growth and development are directional and predictable, including the following growth patterns.

cephalocaudal
cephal/o = head
caud/o = tail
-al = pertaining to

Growth and development proceeds from head to toe (cephalocaudal). See **Figure 19-4**. In the infant, muscular control follows the spine downward. For example, infants will hold up their head before they sit.

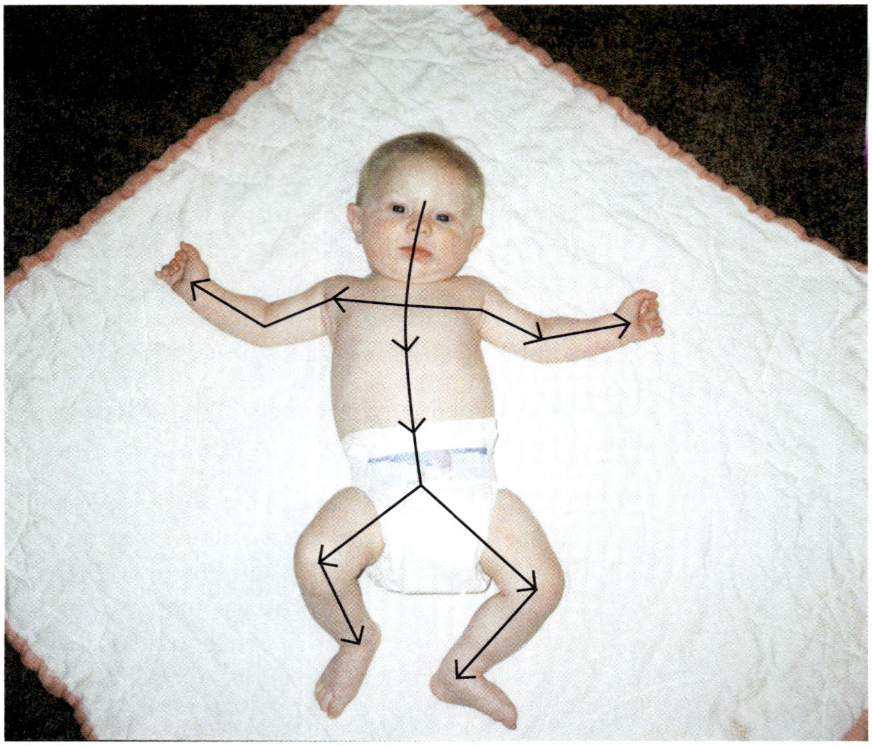

Figure 19-4 Cephalocaudal and proximodistal development (Courtesy of Vickie Rikard)

proximodistal proxim/o = near dist/o = away from -al = pertaining to	Growth and development proceeds from the center outward or from the midline to the periphery (proximodistal). See Figure 19-4. For example, the large muscles of the arms and legs are subject to voluntary control sooner than the fine muscles of the hands and feet.
general to specific	Activities move from being generalized toward being more focused (general to specific). For example, the child will use the whole hand before picking up a small object between the thumb and forefinger.
simple to complex	Language, for example, develops from simple to complex.
growth spurts	Occur throughout childhood alternating with periods of slow growth.

Children grow and learn and mature with the assistance of many factors. The factors can be an inspiration or stimulus or they can impede the process. Some of the factors that consistently have an influence on a child's growth and development, include, but are not necessarily limited to, genetics, environment and culture, nutrition and health status, play, family and parenteral attitudes, and child rearing philosophies.

Vocabulary

The following vocabulary words are frequently used when discussing child health.

WORD	DEFINITION
active acquired immunity (**AK**-tiv ih-**MEW**-nih-tee)	A form of long-term acquired immunity that protects the body against a new infection as the result of antibodies that develop naturally after an initial infection or artificially after a vaccination.
apical pulse (**AY**-pih-kal puhls)	The heart rate as heard with a stethoscope placed on the chest wall adjacent to the cardiac apex (top of the heart).
apnea (ap-**NEE**-ah) a- = without, not pne/o = breathing -a = noun ending	An absence of spontaneous respiration.
axillary temperature (**AK**-sih-lair-ee **TEMP**-per-ah-toor)	The body temperature as recorded by a thermometer placed in the armpit. The reading is generally 0.5 to 1.0 degree less than the oral temperature.
congenital	Present at birth.
crackles (**CRACK**-l'z)	A common abnormal respiratory sound heard on auscultation of the chest during inspiration, characterized by discontinuous bubbling noises.
cyanosis (sigh-ah-**NOH**-sis) cyan/o = blue -osis = condition	Bluish discoloration of the skin and mucous membranes caused by an excess of deoxygenated hemoglobin in the blood or a structural defect in the hemoglobin molecule.
deciduous teeth (dee-**SID**-yoo-us **TEETH**)	Baby teeth; the first set of teeth, also known as primary teeth.
dentition (den-**TIH**-shun)	The eruption of teeth; this occurs in a sequential pattern, with 20 primary teeth erupting between the ages of 6 to 30 months. See **Figure 19-5.**
development	An increase in function and complexity that results through learning, maturation, and growth.
febrile (**FEE**-brill)	Pertaining to or characterized by an elevated body temperature, such as a febrile reaction to an infectious agent.
friction rub (**FRICK**-shun rub)	A dry, grating sound heard with a stethoscope during auscultation.
growth	An increase in the whole or any of its parts physically.
grunting (**GRUNT**-ing)	Abnormal, short audible gruntlike breaks in exhalation that often accompany severe chest pain.

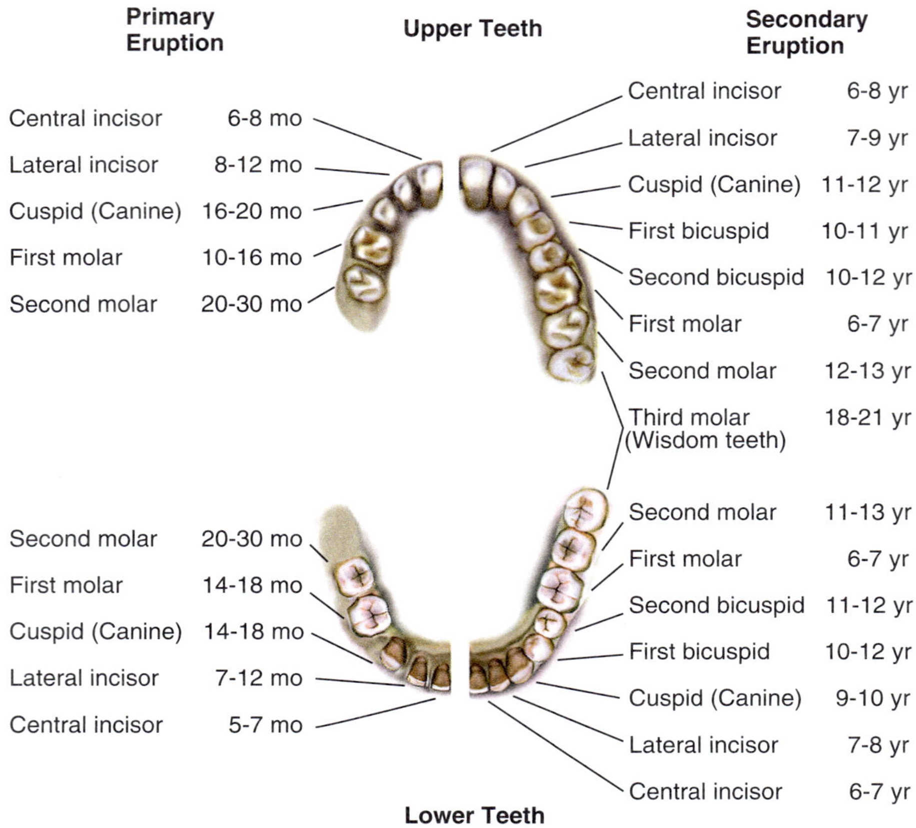

Figure 19-5 Deciduous and permanent teeth

head circumference (HEAD sir-**KUM**-fer-ens)	The measurement around the greatest circumference of the head of an infant. This measurement is plotted according to normal growth and development patterns for the infant's head; increased lags or surges in the increase of the head circumference may indicate serious problems.
hydrocephalus (high-droh-**SEFF**-ah-lus) hydr/o = water cephal/o = head -us = noun ending	A pathologic condition characterized by an abnormal accumulation of cerebrospinal fluid, usually under increased pressure, within the cranial vault and subsequent dilatation of the ventricles; also called **hydrocephaly**. See **Figure 19-6.**
immunity (ih-**MEW**-nih-tee)	The quality of being insusceptible to or unaffected by a particular disease or condition.
immunization (**im**-mew-nih-**ZAY**-shun)	A process by which resistance to an infectious disease is induced or augmented.
infant (**IN**-fant)	A child who is in the earliest stage of extrauterine life, a time extending from the first month after birth to approximately 12 months of age, when the baby is able to assume an erect posture; some extend the period to 24 months of age.
length (recumbent) (**LENGTH** [ree-**KUM**-bent])	The measurement of the distance from the crown of the infant's head to the infant's heel, while the infant is lying on the back with legs extended.

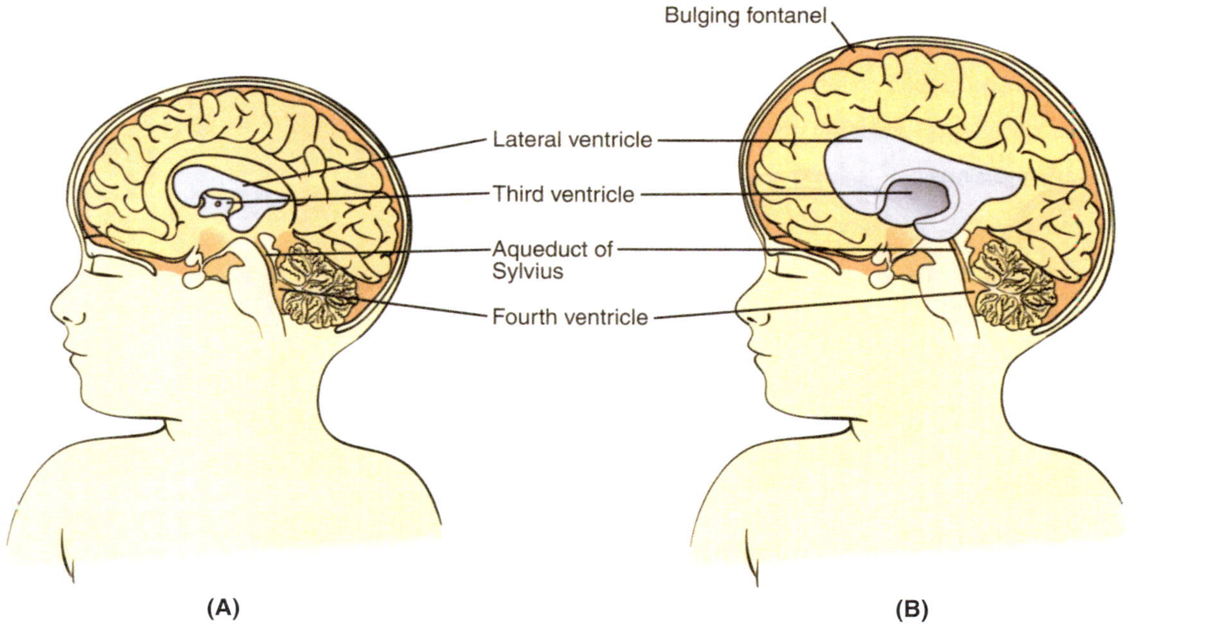

Figure 19-6 Comparison of (A) normal size ventricles and (B) enlarged ventricles associated with hydrocephalus

lumbar puncture (**LUM**-bar **PUNK**-choor)	The introduction of a hollow needle and stylet into the subarachnoid space of the lumbar portion of the spinal canal.
microcephalus (**my**-kroh-**SEFF**-ah-lus) micr/o = small cephal/o = head -us = noun ending	A congenital anomaly characterized by abnormal smallness of the head in relation to the rest of the body and by underdevelopment of the brain, resulting in some degree of mental retardation.
natural immunity (natural ih-**MEW**-nih-tee)	A usually innate and permanent form of immunity to a specific disease.
neonatologist (nee-oh-nay-**TALL**-oh-jist) ne/o = new nat/o = birth -logist = one who studies	A medical doctor who specializes in neonatology.
neonatology (**nee**-oh-nay-**TALL**-oh-jee) ne/o = new nat/o = birth -logy = the study of	The medical specialty concerned with the diseases and abnormalities of the newborn infant.
nomogram nom/o = of or relating to usage -gram = a record	A graphic representation, by any of various systems, of a numeric relationship.
omphalitis (om-fal-**EYE**-tis) omphal/o = navel -itis = inflammation of	An inflammation of the umbilical stump, marked by redness, swelling, and purulent exudate in severe cases.

omphalocele (om-**FAL**-oh-seel) **omphal/o** = navel **-cele** = swelling or herniation	Congenital herniation of intra-abdominal viscera through a defect in the abdominal wall around the umbilicus.
omphalorrhea (**om**-fal-oh-**REE**-ah) **omphal/o** = navel **-rrhea** = drainage	Drainage from the umbilicus (navel).
oral temperature **or/o** = mouth **-al** = pertaining to	The mean body temperature of a normal person as recorded by a clinical thermometer placed in the mouth.
passive acquired immunity (passive ih-**MEW**-nih-tee)	A form of acquired immunity resulting from antibodies that are transmitted naturally through the placenta to a fetus, through the colostrum to an infant, artificially by injection of antiserum for treatment or as a prophylaxis (protection against disease).
pediatrician (pee-dee-ah-**TRISH**-an) **pedi/a** = child **-iatrician** = one who treats; a physician	A physician who specializes in pediatrics.
pediatric nurse practitioner (pee-dee-**AT**-rik **NURSE** prac-**TIH**-shin-er) **pedi/a** = child **-iatric** = medicine, the medical profession, or physician	A registered nurse with advanced study and clinical practice in pediatric nursing.
pediatrics (pee-dee-**AT**-riks) **pedi/a** = child **-iatrics** = medicine, the medical profession, or physician	Pertaining to preventive and primary health care and treatment of children and the study of childhood diseases.
primary teeth (**PRYE**-mar-ee **TEETH**)	Baby teeth; the first set of teeth, also known as deciduous teeth.
pyrexia (pie-**REK**-see-ah) **pyr/o** = fire, heat	Fever.
rectal temperature **rect/o** = rectum **-al** = pertaining to	Temperature as measured in the rectum.
recumbent	Lying down.
retractions (rih-**TRAK**-shuns)	The displacement of tissues to expose a part or structure of the body.

stature (**STAT**-yoor)	Natural height of a person in an upright position.
stridor (**STRIGH**-dor)	An abnormal, high-pitched, musical sound caused by an obstruction in the trachea or larynx.
toxoid (**TOKS**-oyd) **tox/o** = poisons, toxins **-oid** = resembling	A toxin that has been treated with chemicals or with heat to decrease its toxic effect, but that retains its ability to cause the production of antibodies.
tympanic temperature (tim-**PAN**-ik **TEM**-per-ah-chur) **tympan/o** = eardrum **-ic** = pertaining to	The body temperature as measured electronically at the tympanic membrane.
vaccine (**VAK**-seen; vak-**SEEN**)	A suspension of attenuated or killed microorganisms administered intradermally, intramuscularly, orally, or subcutaneously to induce active immunity to infectious disease.
vertex (**VER**-teks)	The top of the head; crown.
well-child visit	Routine health visit in which health professionals assess the current health status of the child, the progression of growth and development, and the need for immunizations.
wheezing (**HWEEZ**-ing)	A breath sound, characterized by a high-pitched musical quality heard on both inspiration and expiration. Wheezes are associated with asthma and chronic bronchitis.

Word Elements

The following word elements pertain to the specialty of child health. As you review the list, pronounce each word element aloud twice and check the box after you "say it." Write the definition for the example word given for each word element. You may use your medical dictionary.

WORD ELEMENT	PRONUNCIATION	"SAY IT"	MEANING
blast/o erythro**blast**osis fetalis	**BLASS**-toh eh-rith-roh-blass-**TOH**-sis fee-**TAL**-is	☐	embryonic stage of development
cephal/o hydro**cephal**us	seff-**AH**-loh high-droh-**SEFF**-ah-lus	☐	head
crypt/o **crypt**orchidism	**KRIPT**-toh kript-**OR**-kid-izm	☐	hidden
epi- **epi**spadias	**EP**-ih ep-ih-**SPAY**-dee-ass	☐	upon, over

esophag/o **esophag**eal atresia	ee-**SOFF**-ah-goh ee-**soff**-ah-**JEE**-al ah-**TREE**-zee-ah	☐	esophagus
hydr/o **hydr**ocele	**HIGH**-droh **HIGH**-droh-seel	☐	water
hypo- **hypo**spadias	**HIGH**-poh **high**-poh-**SPAY**-dee-ass	☐	under, below, beneath, less than normal
-iatric ped**iatric**ian	ee-**AH**-trik pee-dee-ah-**TRISH**-an	☐	relating to medicine, physicians, or medical treatment
micr/o **micr**ocephalus	**MY**-kroh my-kroh-**SEFF**-ah-lus	☐	small
nat/o neo**nat**al	**NAY**-toh nee-oh-**NAY**-tal	☐	birth
ne/o **neo**natologist	**NEE**-oh **nee**-oh-nay-**TALL**-oh-jist	☐	new
omphal/o **omphal**orrhea	om-**FAL**-oh om-fal-oh-**REE**-ah	☐	navel
pedi/a **pedi**atrics	**PEE**-dee-ah pee-dee-**AT**-riks	☐	child
pyr/o **pyr**exia	**PIE**-roh pie-**REK**-see-ah	☐	fire, heat
rose/o **rose**ola infantum	**ROH**-zee-oh roh-zee-**OH**-lah in-**FAN**-tum	☐	rose colored
tetr/a **tetr**alogy of Fallot	**TEH**-trah teh-**TRALL**-oh-jee of fal-**OH**	☐	four
tympan/o **tympan**ic temperature	tim-**PAN**-oh tim-**PAN**-ik **TEM**-per-ah-chur	☐	eardrum

Immunizations

An important part of the normal growth, development, and health of a child is the prevention of disease. This is achieved partly through the administration of immunizations. Immunization is the process of creating immunity to a specific disease in an individual. Not only does immunization refer to a process, but also the word *immunization* is used to describe the medication that is administered to the child. The actual medication administered in the immunizing process is called a **vaccine**, a suspension of infectious agents, or some part of them, that is given for the purpose of establishing resistance to an infectious disease. The state of being immune to or protected from a disease, especially an infectious disease, is known as **immunity**.

The health professional will be involved in the administration of immunizations as well as the education of parents concerning the need for and importance of immunizations. The parents need to understand the risks involved in the administration of immunizations and the common side effects. They also need to know what to do to promote the comfort of their child after administration of the vaccine (side effects are usually mild). Additionally, parents should be taught to recognize severe side effects of immunizations and should be instructed in emergency follow-up, should serious reactions occur.

Immunizations are administered to the well child according to a specific schedule recommended by the American Academy of Pediatrics. Doctors who are responsible for the continuing health care of infants and children recommend a regular schedule of visits for both general physical checkups and immunizations throughout the childhood years. This general program of preventive care for infants is often referred to as "well-baby checkups." A typical schedule for well-baby care would include monthly visits for the first 6 months of life, followed by visits every 3 months from 6 months of age to approximately 2 years; then, general checkups every 6 months from 2 years of age to 6 years of age. After the child has reached 6 years of age, well-checkups usually occur annually.

The recommended vaccination schedule for infants and children is based on the fact that repeated doses of vaccine are necessary to ensure proper development of antibodies. The goal, with administration of immunizations, is to ensure complete vaccination of the child by the age of 15 to 18 months if no contraindications are present when immunizations are begun. **Table 19-1** illustrates the recommended immunization schedule for infants and children. This schedule is approved by the Advisory Committee on Immunization Practices (ACIP), the American Academy of Pediatrics (AAP), and the American Academy of Family Physicians (AAFP) (2002).

Communicable Diseases

This section concentrates on communicable diseases that are common to the child.

chickenpox (varicella)
(**CHICK**-en-pox)

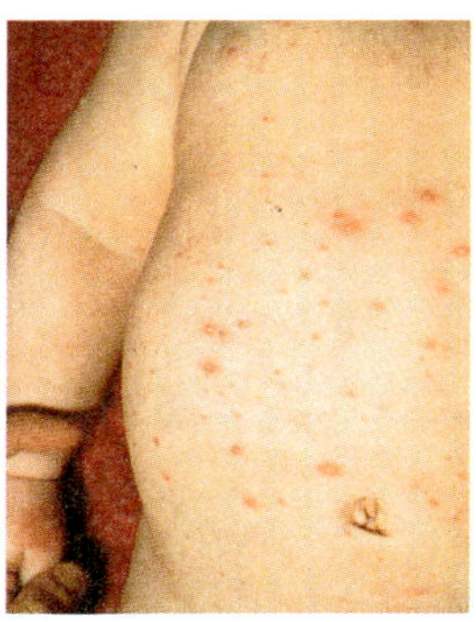

A viral disease of sudden onset with slight fever, successive eruptions of macules, papules, and vesicles on the skin, followed by crusting over of the lesions with a granular scab. Itching may be severe. (Macules are discolorations at normal skin level, papules are raised, pimplelike skin blemishes, and vesicles are blisterlike.) See Figure 19-7.

The infectious agent is the varicella-zoster virus, a member of the *Herpesvirus* group. Chickenpox is spread through direct contact, by droplet spread, or by contaminated objects. The incubation period is from 10 to 21 days. It is communicable from up to 5 days before skin eruptions occur until lesions are dry.

The immunization for chickenpox is called the varicella vaccine.

Figure 19-7 Varicella (chickenpox) (Courtesy of Robert A. Silverman, M.D., Pediatric Dermatology, Georgetown University)

Recommended Childhood Immunization Schedule
United States, 2002

range of recommended ages | catch-up vaccination | preadolescent assessment

Vaccine ▼ / Age ▶	Birth	1 mo	2 mos	4 mos	6 mos	12 mos	15 mos	18 mos	24 mos	4-6 yrs	11-12 yrs	13-18 yrs
Hepatitis B[1]	Hep B #1	only if mother HBsAg (-)										
			Hep B #2			Hep B #3					Hep B series	
Diphtheria, Tetanus, Pertussis[2]			DTaP	DTaP	DTaP		DTaP			DTaP	Td	
Haemophilus influenzae Type b[3]			Hib	Hib	Hib	Hib						
Inactivated Polio[4]			IPV	IPV		IPV				IPV		
Measles, Mumps, Rubella[5]						MMR #1				MMR #2	MMR #2	
Varicella[6]							Varicella				Varicella	
Pneumococcal[7]			PCV	PCV	PCV	PCV			PCV		PPV	
Vaccines below this line are for selected populations												
Hepatitis A[8]											Hepatitis A series	
Influenza[9]									Influenza (yearly)			

This schedule indicates the recommended ages for routine administration of currently licensed childhood vaccines, as of December 1, 2001, for children through age 18 years. Any dose not given at the recommended age should be given at any subsequent visit when indicated and feasible. ▨ Indicates age groups that warrant special effort to administer those vaccines not previously given. Additional vaccines may be licensed and recommended during the year. Licensed combination vaccines may be used whenever any components of the combination are indicated and the vaccine's other components are not contraindicated. Providers should consult the manufacturers' package inserts for detailed recommendations.

Approved by the Advisory Committee on Immunization Practices (www.cdc.gov/nip/acip) the American Academy of Pediatrics (www.aap.org), and the American Academy of Family Physicians (www.aafp.org).

Footnotes: Recommended Childhood Immunization Schedule United States, 2002

1. Hepatitis B vaccine (Hep B). All infants should receive the first dose of hepatitis B vaccine soon after birth and before hospital discharge; the first dose may also be given by age 2 months if the infant's mother is HBsAg-negative. Only monovalent hepatitis B vaccine can be used for the birth dose. Monovalent or combination vaccine containing Hep B may be used to complete the series; four doses of vaccine may be administered if combination vaccine is used. The second dose should be given at least 4 weeks after the first dose, except for Hib-containing vaccine which cannot be administered before age 6 weeks. The third dose should be given at least 16 weeks after the first dose and at least 8 weeks after the second dose. The last dose in the vaccination series (third or fourth dose) should not be administered before age 6 months.

Infants born to HBsAg-positive mothers should receive hepatitis B vaccine and 0.5 mL hepatitis B immune globulin (HBIG) within 12 hours of birth at separate sites. The second dose is recommended at age 1-2 months and the vaccination series should be completed (third or fourth dose) at age 6 months.

Infants born to mothers whose HBsAg status is unknown should receive the first dose of the hepatitis B vaccine series within 12 hours of birth. Maternal blood should be drawn at the time of delivery to determine the mother's HBsAg status; if the HBsAg test is positive, the infant should receive HBIG as soon as possible (no later than age 1 week).

2. Diphtheria and tetanus toxoids and acellular pertussis vaccine (DTaP). The fourth dose of DTaP may be administered as early as age 12 months, provided 6 months have elapsed since the third dose and the child is unlikely to return at age 15-18 months. **Tetanus and diphtheria toxoids (Td)** is recommended at age 11-12 years if at least 5 years have elapsed since the last dose of tetanus and diphtheria toxoid-containing vaccine. Subsequent routine Td boosters are recommended every 10 years.

3. *Haemophilus influenzae* type b (Hib) conjugate vaccine. Three Hib conjugate vaccines are licensed for infant use. If PRP-OMP (PedvaxHIB® or ComVax® [Merck]) is administered at ages 2 and 4 months, a dose at age 6 months is not required. DTaP/Hib combination products should not be used for primary immunization in infants at age 2, 4 or 6 months, but can be used as boosters following any Hib vaccine.

4. Inactivated poliovirus vaccine (IPV). An all-IPV schedule is recommended for routine childhood poliovirus vaccination in the United States. All children should receive four doses of IPV at age 2 months, 4 months, 6-18 months, and 4-6 years.

5. Measles, mumps, and rubella vaccine (MMR). The second dose of MMR is recommended routinely at age 4-6 years but may be administered during any visit, provided at least 4 weeks have elapsed since the first dose and that both doses are administered beginning at or after age 12 months. Those who have not previously received the second dose should complete the schedule by the visit at age 11-12 years.

6. Varicella vaccine. Varicella vaccine is recommended at any visit at or after age 12 months for susceptible children (i.e. those who lack a reliable history of chickenpox). Susceptible persons aged ≥ 13 years should receive two doses, given at least 4 weeks apart.

7. Pneumococcal vaccine. The heptavalent **pneumococcal conjugate vaccine (PCV)** is recommended for all children aged 2-23 months and for certain children aged 24-59 months. **Pneumococcal polysaccharide vaccine (PPV)** is recommended in addition to PCV for certain high-risk groups. See *MMWR* 2000;49(RR-9);1-37.

8. Hepatitis A vaccine. Hepatitis A vaccine is recommended for use in selected states and regions, and for certain high-risk groups; consult your local public health authority. See *MMWR* 1999;48(RR-12);1-37.

9. Influenza vaccine. Influenza vaccine is recommended annually for children age ≥ 6 months with certain risk factors (including but not limited to asthma, cardiac disease, sickle cell disease, HIV and diabetes; see *MMWR* 2001;50(RR-4);1-44), and can be administered to all others wishing to obtain immunity. Children aged ≤12 years should receive vaccine in a dosage appropriate for their age (0.25 mL if age 6-35 months or 0.5 mL if aged ≥ 3 years). Children aged ≤ 8 years who are receiving influenza vaccine for the first time should receive two doses separated by at least 4 weeks.

Additional information about vaccines, vaccine supply, and contraindications for immunization, is available at www.cdc.gov/nip or at the National Immunization Hotline, 800-232-2522 (English) or 800-232-0233 (Spanish).

diphtheria
(diff-**THEE**-ree-ah)

Serious infectious disease affecting the nose, pharynx, or larynx, usually resulting in sore throat, dysphonia (difficult speaking or hoarseness), and fever. The disease is caused by the bacterium *Corynebacterium diphtheriae,* which forms a white coating over the affected airways as it multiplies.

The bacterium releases a toxin into the bloodstream that can quickly damage the heart and nerves, resulting in heart failure, paralysis, and death. Diphtheria is uncommon in countries as the United States, where a vaccine against the disease is routinely given to children.

The immunization for diphtheria is one of the components of the DPT immunization.

erythema infectiosum (fifth disease)
(**air**-ih-**THEE**-mah in-**fek**-she-**OH**-sum)

A viral disease characterized by a face that appears as "slapped cheeks," a fiery red rash on the cheeks. See Figure 19-8.

In approximately 1 to 4 days after the appearance of the facial rash, a maculopapular rash appears on the trunk and extremities. There are usually only mild systemic responses during the course of this disease. This disease may last from 2 days up to 40 days.

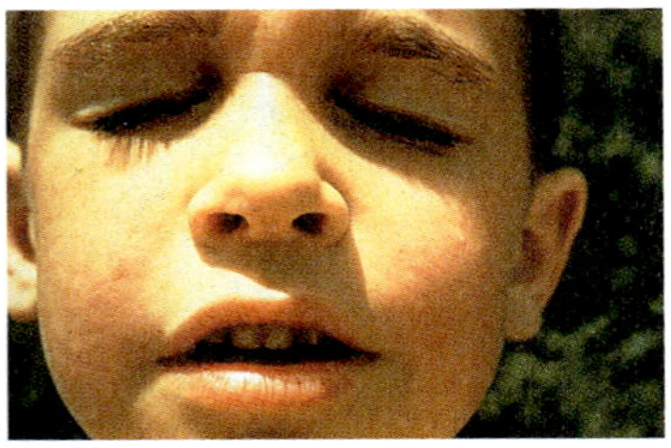

The infectious agent is the human parvovirus. The transmission of erythema infectiosum is through respiratory droplets, airborne particles, blood, and blood products. The incubation period is from 7 to 28 days. Its communicability is unknown, but believed to be up to 7 days before the initial rash on the face appears; therefore, isolation is not required.

Figure 19-8 Erythema infectiosum (Courtesy of the Centers for Disease Control and Prevention [CDC])

impetigo
(im-peh-**TYE**-goh)

Contagious superficial skin infection characterized by serous vesicles and pustules filled with millions of staphylococcus or streptococcus bacteria, usually forming on the face. See Figure 19-9.

Impetigo progresses to pruritic erosions and crusts with a honey-colored appearance. The discharge from the lesions allows the infection to be highly contagious.

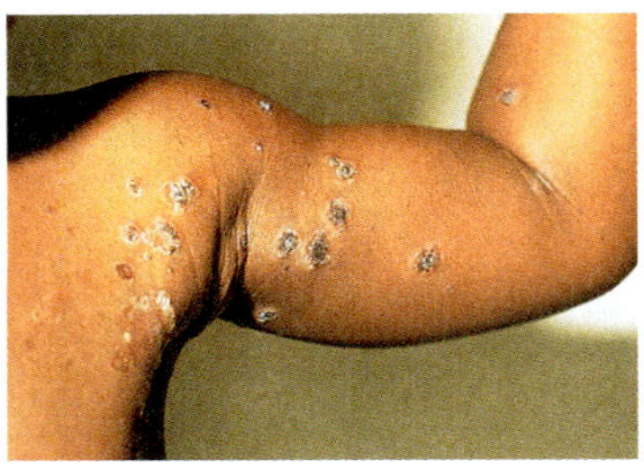

Treatment for impetigo includes the use of oral and topical antibiotics. It is important to instruct the individual to complete the entire regime of systemic antibiotics to prevent the possibility of complications due to secondary infections, such as acute glomerulonephritis (kidney infection, primarily in the glomeruli) and/or rheumatic fever.

Figure 19-9 Impetigo (Courtesy of Robert A. Silverman, M.D., Clinical Associate Professor, Department of Pediatrics, Georgetown University)

mumps (infectious parotitis)
(in-**FEK**-shus pah-roh-**TYE**-tis)

Acute viral disease characterized by fever, swelling, and tenderness of one or more salivary glands, usually the parotid glands (below and in front of the ears). See Figure 19-10.

The infectious agent is the mumps virus. It is transmitted by droplet spread or by direct contact with the saliva of an infected person.

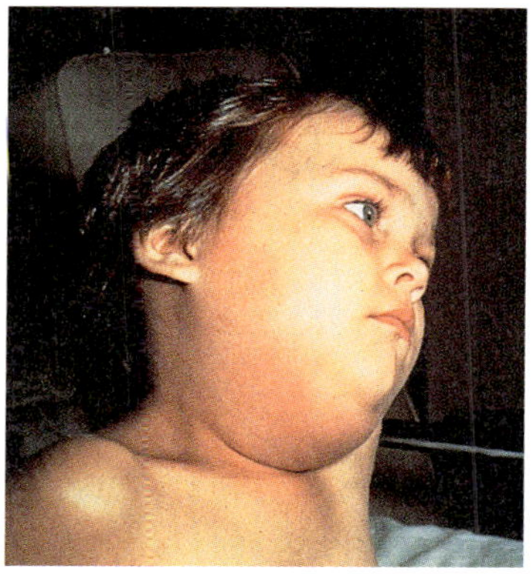

The incubation period is from 14 to 21 days. The period of maximum communicability is from immediately before to immediately after swelling begins.

The immunization for **mumps (infectious parotitis)** is a part of the MMR vaccine.

Figure 19-10 Mumps (parotitis) (Courtesy of the Centers for Disease Control and Prevention [CDC])

pertussis (whooping cough)
(per-**TUSS**-is)

An acute upper respiratory infectious disease caused by the bacterium *Bordetella pertussis*.

Pertussis (whooping cough) occurs mainly in children and infants. Early stages of pertussis are suggestive of the common cold with slight elevation of fever, sneezing, rhinitis, dry cough, irritability, and loss of appetite.

As the disease progresses (approximately 2 weeks later), the cough is more violent and consists of a series of several short coughs, followed by a long drawn inspiration during which the typical whoop is heard. The coughing episode may be severe enough to cause vomiting. If diagnosed early, pertussis can be treated with oral antibiotics. Otherwise, antibiotics are ineffective and treatment (when needed) consists of supportive care, such as the administration of sedatives to reduce coughing and oxygen to facilitate respiration. Pertussis may be prevented by immunization of infants beginning at 3 months of age.

The immunization for pertussis is one of the components of the DPT immunization.

roseola infantum
(roh-zee-**OH**-lah in-**FAN**-tum)
rose/o = rose colored

A viral disease with a sudden onset of a high fever for 3 to 4 days during which the child may experience mild coldlike symptoms and slight irritability.

When the fever falls rapidly on the third or fourth day, a macular or maculopapular rash appears on the trunk, expanding to the rest of the body, only to fade in 24 hours.

The infectious agent is the herpesvirus 6. The transmission of **roseola infantum** is unknown, as is the incubation period and the period of communicability.

rubella (German measles; 3-day measles)
(roo-**BELL**-lah)

A mild febrile (fever-causing) infectious disease resembling both scarlet fever and measles, but differing from these in its short course; characterized by a rash of both macules and papules that fades and disappears in 3 days. See Figure 19-11.

Koplik's spots and photophobia are not present with **rubella**. The infectious agent is the rubella virus, transmitted by direct contact or spread by infected persons (nasopharyngeal secretions), or by droplet spread.

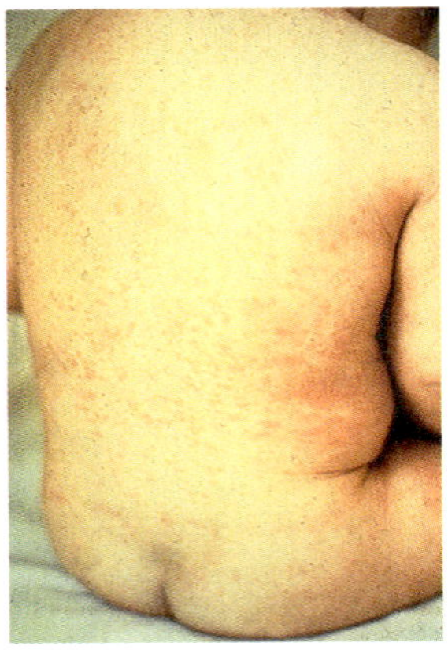

The incubation period for rubella is 14 to 21 days and the period of communicability is from 7 days before to about 5 days after rash appears. The immunization for rubella is a part of the MMR vaccine.

Figure 19-11 Rubella (Courtesy of the Centers for Disease Control and Prevention [CDC])

rubeola
("red measles," 7-day measles)
(roo-bee-**OH**-lah)

Acute, highly communicable viral disease that begins as an upper respiratory disorder with fever, sore throat, cough, runny nose, sensitivity to light, and possible conjunctivitis. Typical red, blotchy rash appears 4 to 5 days after onset of symptoms, beginning behind the ears, on the forehead, or cheeks, progressing to extremities and trunk and lasting about 5 days. See Figure 19-12.

Diagnosis is based on the presence of **Koplik's spots** in the mouth (spots with grayish centers and red, irregular outer rings). The measles virus is the infectious agent and is transmitted by droplet spread or by direct contact with secretions from an infected person.

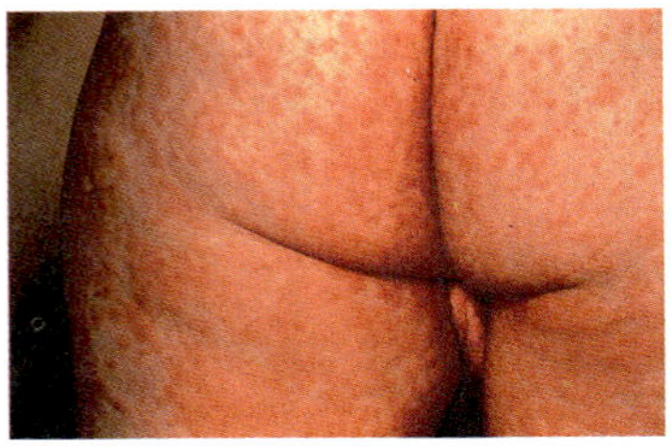

The incubation period is from 10 to 20 days. Rubeola is communicable from 4 days before to 5 days after the rash appears.

This immunization for measles is a part of the MMR vaccine.

Figure 19-12 Rubeola (Courtesy of the Centers for Disease Control and Prevention [CDC])

scarlet fever
(scarlatina)
(**SCAR**-let **FEE**-ver)
(**scar**-lah-**TEE**-nah)

An acute, contagious disease characterized by sore throat, abrupt high fever, increased pulse, strawberry tongue (red and swollen), and punctiform (pointlike) bright red rash on the body. See Figure 19-13.

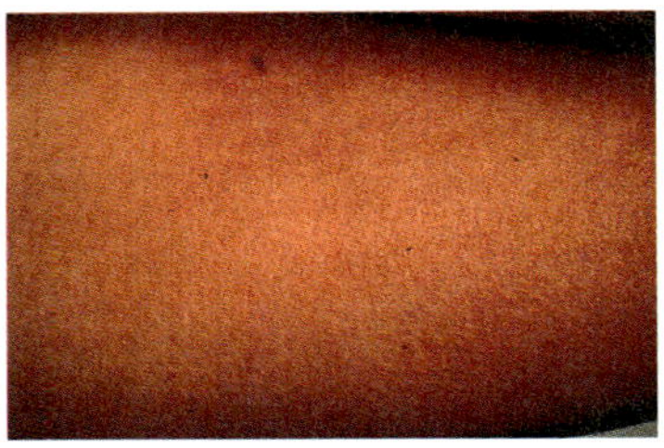

The infectious agent of scarlet fever (scarlatina) is group A, beta-hemolytic streptococci, transmitted by direct contact with an infected person or by droplet spread. Incubation period is 2 to 4 days and the period of communicability is from onset until approximately 10 days after onset.

Figure 19-13 Scarlet fever (Courtesy of the Centers for Disease Control and Prevention [CDC])

Pathological Conditions

As you study the pathological conditions seen in infants, toddlers, and children, note that the **basic definition** is in bold print, followed by a more detailed description in regular print. The phonetic pronunciation is directly beneath each term, and a breakdown of the component parts of the term when appropriate.

asthma
(**AZ**-mah)

Paroxysmal dyspnea (severe attack of difficult breathing), accompanied by wheezing caused by a spasm of the bronchial tubes or by swelling of their mucous membrane.

No age is exempt, but asthma occurs most frequently in childhood or early adulthood. Asthma differs from other obstructive lung diseases in that it is a reversible process. The attack may last from 30 minutes to several hours. In some circumstances the attack subsides spontaneously.

The asthmatic attack starts suddenly with coughing and a sensation of tightness in the chest; then slow, laborious, wheezy breathing begins. Expiration is much more strenuous and prolonged than inspiration and the patient may assume a "hunched forward" position in an attempt to get more air.

Recurrence and severity of attacks are greatly influenced by secondary factors, by mental or physical fatigue, by exposure to fumes or secondhand cigarette smoke, by endocrine changes at various periods in life, and by emotional situations. Acute attacks of asthma may be relieved by a number of drugs such as epinephrine.

Status asthmaticus is a severe asthma that is unresponsive to conventional therapy and lasts longer than 24 hours.

cleft lip and palate
(**CLEFT LIP** and **PAL**-at)

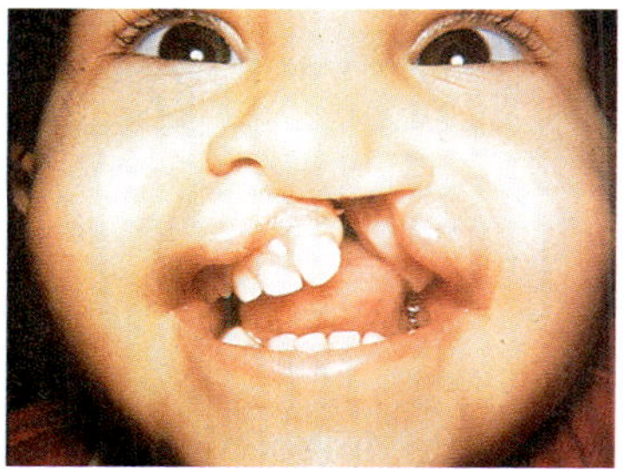
(A)

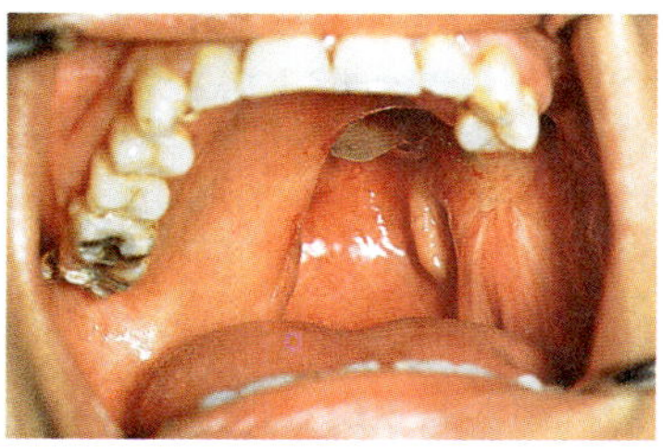
(B)

Cleft lip is a congenital defect in which there is an open space between the nasal cavity and the lip, due to failure of the soft tissue and bones in this area to fuse properly during embryologic development. See Figure 19-14A. With cleft palate there is failure of the hard palate to fuse, resulting in a fissure (cracklike sore) in the middle of the palate. See Figure 19-14B.

As a result of these abnormalities the newborn infant has difficulty with feeding and breathing. Dentition and speech can become problems as the child grows and develops.

The medical management of the child with a cleft lip and/or palate is based on the severity of the defect, but is focused on feeding techniques, which allow the newborn to have adequate intake and growth. Secondly, the surgical management will begin for the cleft lip as early as 2 to 4 days and will be completed by 4 weeks. Cosmetic modifications may be done around the age of 4 to 5 years. For the child with a cleft palate, the repair will begin between 6 months and 2 years.

Figure 19-14 (A) Cleft lip; (B) cleft palate (Photos courtesy of Dr. Joseph Konzelman, School of Dentistry, Medical College of Georgia)

coarctation of the aorta
(**koh**-ark-**TAY**-shun of the ay-**OR**-tah)

A congenital heart defect characterized by a localized narrowing of the aorta, which results in increased blood pressure in the upper extremities (area proximal to the defect) and decreased blood pressure in the lower extremities (area distal to the defect).

Refer to the cardiovascular system for a visual reference.

The classic sign of coarctation of the aorta is a contrast in pulsations and blood pressures in the arms and legs. The femoral, popliteal, and pedal pulses are weak or delayed in comparison with the strong, bounding pulses found in the arms and carotid arteries.

Surgical correction of the defect is curative if the disease is diagnosed early.

---

croup
(**CROOP**)

A childhood disease characterized by a barking cough, suffocative and difficult breathing, stridor (high-pitched musical sound when breathing in), and laryngeal spasm.

The symptoms of **croup** can be dramatic and anxiety producing to the parent and the child. It is important to approach the child and parents in a calm manner to reduce fears and anxiety.

Treatment includes providing a high humidity atmosphere with cool moisture (cool mist vaporizer) and rest to relieve the symptoms. Croup may result from an acute obstruction of the larynx caused by an allergen, foreign body, infection, or new growth.

---

cryptorchidism
(kript-**OR**-kid-izm)
crypt/o = hidden
orchid/o = testicle
-ism = condition

Condition of undescended testicle(s); the absence of one or both testicles from the scrotum.

The testicle may be located in the abdominal cavity or in the inguinal canal. If the testicle does not descend on its own, surgery will be necessary to correct the position.

The surgery for **cryptorchidism**, known as an **orchiopexy,** involves making an incision into the inguinal canal, locating the testicle, and bringing it back down into the scrotal sac. This surgery is usually done on an outpatient basis, with normal physical activity being restored within a few weeks to a month.

Down syndrome
(**DOWN SIN**-drohm)

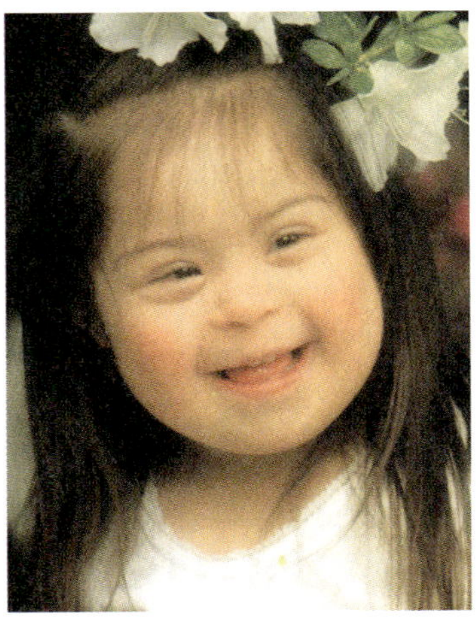

A congenital condition characterized by multiple defects and varying degrees of mental retardation. See Figure 19-15.

The cause of **Down syndrome** (DS) is unknown; however, maternal age over 35 years has consistently been noted as a risk factor. It is also called **trisomy 21**, indicating that there are three twenty-first chromosomes present instead of the normal two.

In addition to the mental retardation, specific clinical manifestations evident at birth include low set ears, a short broad appearance to the head (brachycephaly), protruding tongue, short thick neck, simian line (transverse crease on palm), broad short feet and hands, poor or diminished muscle tone, and hyperflexible joints. The diagnosis of Down syndrome can be made prenatally by testing the amniotic fluid.

Figure 19-15 Down syndrome (Marijane Scott, Marijane's Designer Portraits, Down Right Beautiful 1996 Calendar)

---

dwarfism
(**DWARF**-ism)

Generalized growth retardation of the body due to the deficiency of the human growth hormone; also known as congenital hypopituitarism or hypopituitarism. See Figure 19-16.

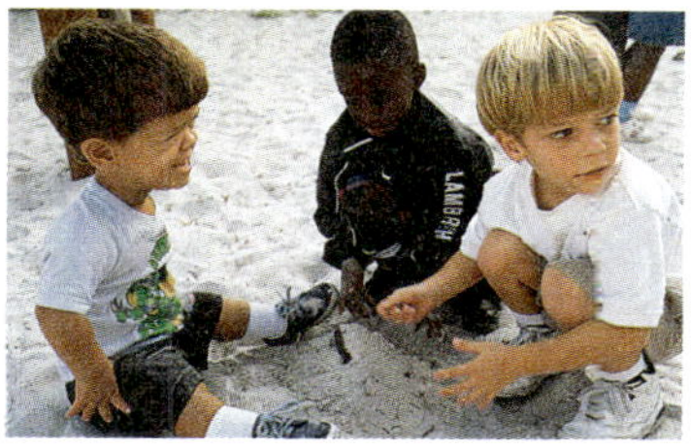

The abnormal underdevelopment leaves the child extremely short with a small body. There is an absence of secondary sex characteristics. The condition may have a connection with other defects or varying degrees of mental retardation.

Treatment may include administration of human growth hormone or somatotropin until a height of 5 feet is reached. These children may need replacement of other hormones, especially just before and during puberty.

Figure 19-16 Dwarfism

---

epispadias
(**ep**-ih-**SPAY**-dee-as)
epi- = upon, over

A congenital defect (birth defect) in which the urethra opens on the upper side of the penis at some point near the glans.

Refer to Chapter 16 for a visual reference.

Treatment for **epispadias** is surgical correction with redirection of the opening of the urethra to its normal position at the end of the penis.

---

erythroblastosis fetalis
(eh-**rith**-roh-blass-**TOH**-sis fee-**TAL**-iss)
erythr/o = red
blast/o = embryonic stage of development
-osis = condition

A form of hemolytic anemia that occurs in neonates due to a maternal-fetal blood group incompatibility, involving the ABO grouping or the Rh factors. This is also known as hemolytic disease of the newborn (HDN).

Erythroblastosis fetalis is caused by an antigen-antibody reaction. The incompatible antigens of fetal blood stimulates the mother to make antibodies against them. The hemolytic reaction typically occurs in subsequent pregnancies. This reaction can be prevented by giving the mother an injection of a high-titer anti-Rh gamma globulin after the delivery of an Rh positive fetus.

---

esophageal atresia
(ee-**soff**-ah-**JEE**-al ah-**TREE**-zee-ah)
esophag/o = esophagus
-eal = pertaining to

A congenital abnormality of the esophagus due to its ending before it reaches the stomach either as a blind pouch or as a fistula connected to the trachea.

Either type of **esophageal atresia** (EA) is a neonatal (newborn) surgical emergency. Death may result from aspiration pneumonia if prompt treatment is not instituted. The birth weight of infants with EA is significantly lower than average, and there is an unusually high incidence of prematurity in infants with this condition.

---

gigantism
(**JYE**-gan-tizm)

A proportional overgrowth of the body's tissue due to the hypersecretion of the human growth hormone before puberty.

The child experiences accelerated abnormal growth chiefly in the long bones.

The cause of oversecretion of the human growth hormone is most often due to an adenoma of the anterior pituitary. The treatment is aimed at reducing the size of the pituitary gland through surgery or radiation.

---

hyaline membrane disease
(**HIGH**-ah-lighn **MEM**-brayn dih-**ZEEZ**)

Also known as respiratory distress syndrome of the premature infant (RDS), hyaline membrane disease is severe impairment of

the function of respiration in the premature newborn. This condition is rarely present in a newborn of greater than 37 weeks' gestation or in one weighing at least 5 pounds.

Shortly after birth, the premature infant will have a low Apgar score and will develop signs of acute respiratory distress due to collapse of lung tissue; tachypnea (rapid breathing), tachycardia (rapid heartbeat), **retraction** of the rib cage during inspiration, **cyanosis**, and grunting during expiration will be present.

---

hydrocele
(**HIGH**-droh-seel)
hydro- = water
-cele = swelling or herniation

An accumulation of fluid in any saclike cavity or duct, particularly the scrotal sac or along the spermatic cord.

This condition is caused by inflammation of the epididymis or testis, or by obstruction of lymphatic or venous flow within the spermatic cord. Treatment for a **hydrocele** is surgery to remove the fluid pouch.

---

hydrocephalus
(high-droh-**SEFF**-ah-lus)
hydro- = water
cephal/o = head
-us = noun ending

An abnormal increase of cerebrospinal fluid (CSF) in the brain that causes the ventricles of the brain to dilate, resulting in an increased head circumference in the infant with open fontanel(s); congenital disorder. See Figure 19-17.

The increase in cerebrospinal fluid may be due to an increased production of CSF, a decreased absorption of CSF, or a blockage in the normal flow of CSF. The infant may also show frontal bossing (forehead protrudes out), which may cause the "setting sun" sign in which the upper scleras of the eyes show with the eyes directed downward. The infant will demonstrate other signs of increased pressure such as a high-pitched cry, a bulging fontanel, extreme irritability, and inability to sleep for long periods of time.

Hydrocephalus in the young infant may be detected by increased head circumferences resulting in an abnormal graphing curve. This may be detected when checking the head circumference of the infant on well-baby

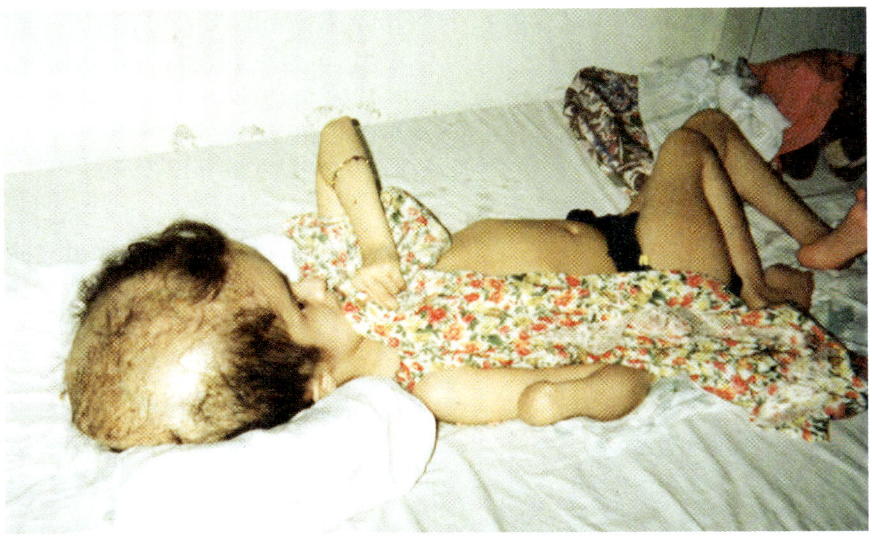

Figure 19-17 Untreated hydrocephalus (Courtesy of Dr. Russell Cox, Gastonia, NC)

checkups in the physician's office. Along with checking head circumference, the infant should be assessed for any signs and symptoms of increased intracranial pressure (IICP).

When the diagnosis of hydrocephalus is made, treatment to relieve or remove the obstruction is initiated. If there is no obstruction, a **shunt** is generally required to relieve the intracranial pressure by shunting the excess cerebrospinal fluid into another body space, thus preventing permanent damage to the brain tissue. As the child grows, the shunt will have to be replaced with a longer one.

Hydrocephalus is often a complication of another disease or disorder. The infant with spina bifida cystica may develop hydrocephalus. It can also occur as a result of an intrauterine infection such as rubella or syphilis.

---

hypospadias
(**high**-poh-**SPAY**-dee-as)
hypo- = under, below, beneath, less than normal

A congenital defect in which the urethra opens on the underside of the penis instead of at the end.

Refer to Chapter 16, for a visual reference.

Treatment for **hypospadias** involves surgery to redirect the opening of the urethra to its normal location at the end of the penis.

---

intussusception
(**in**-tuh-suh-**SEP**-shun)

Telescoping of a portion of proximal intestine into distal intestine usually in the ileocecal region causing an obstruction.

Refer to Chapter 12, for a visual reference.

Intussusception typically occurs in infants and young children. Clinical manifestations include intermittent, severe abdominal pain, vomiting, and a "currant jelly stool," which indicates the presence of bloody mucus.

Intussusception is diagnosed and medically treated with a barium enema. During examination, the telescoping is often reduced by the pressure created with a barium enema. When the obstruction is not reduced with the barium enema, immediate surgical intervention is necessary.

---

patent ductus arteriosus
(**PAY**-tent **DUK**-tus
ar-**tee**-ree-**OH**-suss)

An abnormal opening between the pulmonary artery and the aorta caused by failure of the fetal ductus arteriosus to close after birth. This defect is seen primarily in premature infants.

Refer to Chapter 10, for a visual reference.

During the prenatal period the ductus arteriosus serves as a normal pathway in the fetal circulatory system. It is a large channel between the pulmonary artery and the aorta that is open, allowing fetal blood to bypass the lungs, passing from the pulmonary artery to the descending aorta and ultimately to the placenta. This passageway is no longer needed after birth and usually closes during the first 24 to 72 hours of life, once the normal circulatory pattern of the cardiovascular system is established.

If the ductus arteriosus remains open after birth, blood under pressure from the aorta is shunted into the pulmonary artery, resulting in oxygenated blood *recirculating* through the pulmonary circulation. A strain is placed on the heart due to the pumping of blood, a second time, through the pulmonary circulation.

Treatment for **patent ductus arteriosus** is surgery to close the open channel.

---

phimosis
(fih-**MOH**-sis)

A tightness of the foreskin (prepuce) of the penis of the male infant that prevents it from being pulled back. The opening of the foreskin narrows due to the tightness and may cause some difficulty with urination.

The parents of the uncircumcised male infant may notice difficulty pulling the prepuce back for cleaning the area of the glans penis that the prepuce covers. If this occurs, it should be reported to the physician immediately.

Treatment for **phimosis** is circumcision (surgery to remove the foreskin).

Reye's syndrome
syn- = together, joined
drom/o = running
-e = noun ending

A syndrome marked by severe edema of the brain and increased intracranial pressure, hypoglycemia, and fatty infiltration and dysfunction of the liver. Symptoms may follow an acute viral infection, occurring in children below the age of 18, often with fatal results. There are confirmed studies linking the onset of Reye's syndrome to aspirin administration during a viral illness.

The symptoms of Reye's syndrome typically follow a pattern through stages:

1. Vomiting, confusion, and lethargy (sluggish and apathetic)
2. Irritability, hyperactive reflexes, delirium, and hyperventilation
3. Changes in level of consciousness progressing to coma, and sluggish pupillary response
4. Fixed dilated pupils, continued loss of cerebral function, periods of absent breathing
5. Seizures, loss of deep tendon reflexes, and respiratory arrest

The prognosis is directly related to the stage of Reye's syndrome at the time of diagnosis and treatment. Treatment includes decreasing intracranial pressure to prevent seizures, controlling cerebral edema, and closely monitoring the child for changes in level of consciousness. In some cases respiratory support and/or dialysis is necessary.

---

spina bifida occulta
(**SPY**-nah **BIH**-fih-dah oh-**KULL**-tah)

A congenital defect of the central nervous system in which the back portion of one or more vertebrae is not closed. A dimpling over the area may occur.

Other symptoms include hair growing out of this area, a port wine nevus (pigmented blemish) over the area, and/or a subcutaneous lipoma (fatty tumor) may occur in this area. **Spina bifida occulta** can occur anywhere along the vertebral column but usually occurs at the level of the fifth lumbar or first sacral vertebrae. There are usually very few neurological symptoms present. Without symptoms there is no treatment recommended.

sudden infant death syndrome (SIDS)

The completely unexpected and unexplained death of an apparently well, or virtually well, infant. SIDS, also known as "crib death," is the most common cause of death between the second week and first year of life.

In the United States, SIDS is responsible for the deaths of approximately 7,000 infants each year. This worldwide syndrome occurs more frequently in the third and fourth months of life, in premature infants, in males, and in infants living in poverty. The deaths usually occur during sleep and are more likely to happen in winter than in summer. These infants are monitored during their sleep and are sometimes placed on an **apnea** alarm mattress designed to sound an alarm when the infant lying on it ceases to breathe.

Tay-Sachs disease
(**TAY-SACKS** dih-**ZEEZ**)

A congenital disorder caused by altered lipid metabolism due to an enzyme deficiency.

An accumulation of a specific type of lipid occurs in the brain leading to progressive neurological deterioration with both physical and mental retardation. The symptoms of neurological deterioration begin around the age of 6 months. Deafness, blindness with a cherry red spot on each retina, convulsions, and paralysis all occur in the child with **Tay-Sachs disease** until death occurs around the age of 2 to 4 years. There is no specific therapy for this condition; therefore, supportive and symptomatic care are indicated.

Tay-Sachs disease occurs most frequently in families of Eastern European Jewish origin, precisely the Ashkenazic Jews. This disease can be diagnosed in utero through amniocentesis.

tetralogy of Fallot
(teh-**TRALL**-oh-jee of fal-**OH**)
tetr/a = four
-logy = the study of

A congenital heart anomaly that consists of four defects: pulmonary stenosis, interventricular septal defect, dextroposition (shifting to the right) of the aorta so that it receives blood from both ventricles, and hypertrophy of the right ventricle; named for the French physician, Etienne Fallot, who first described the condition.

Refer to Chapter 10, for a visual reference.

Further description of **tetralogy of Fallot** identifies the four defects in more detail.

1. The pulmonary stenosis restricts the flow of blood from the heart to the lungs.
2. The interventricular septal defect creates a right-to-left shunt between the ventricles, allowing deoxygenated blood from the right ventricle to communicate with the oxygenated blood in the left ventricle, which then exits the heart via the aorta.

3. The shifting of the aorta to the right causes it to override the right ventricle and thus communicate with the interventricular septal defect, thus allowing the oxygen-poor blood to pass more easily into the aorta.
4. The hypertrophy of the right ventricle occurs because of the increased work required to pump blood through the obstructed pulmonary artery.

Most infants born with tetralogy of Fallot display varying degrees of cyanosis, which may typically occur during activities that increase the need for oxygen, such as crying, feeding, or straining with a bowel movement. The cyanosis develops as a result of the decreased flow of blood to the lungs for oxygenation, and as a result of the mixing of oxygenated and deoxygenated blood released into the systemic circulation; these babies are termed "blue babies."

Treatment for tetralogy of Fallot involves surgery to correct the multiple defects.

---

transposition of the great vessels
(trans-poh-**SIH**-shun)

A condition in which the two major arteries of the heart are reversed in position, resulting in two noncommunicating circulatory systems.

The aorta arises from the right ventricle (instead of the left) and delivers unoxygenated blood to the systemic circulation. This blood is returned from the body tissues back to the right atrium and right ventricle without being oxygenated, because it does not pass through the lungs.

The pulmonary artery arises from the left ventricle (instead of the right) and delivers blood to the lungs for oxygenation. The oxygenated blood returns from the lungs, to the left atrium and the left ventricle, and back to the lungs, without sending the oxygenated blood throughout the systemic circulation.

This congenital **anomaly** creates an oxygen deficiency to the body tissues and an excessive workload on the right and left ventricles. The infant is usually severely cyanotic at birth.

Treatment involves surgical correction of the defect and repositioning of the vessels to reestablish a normal pattern of blood flow through the circulatory system. Surgical correction of the defect is an arterial switch that must be done as early as possible, usually within the first 2 weeks of life. When surgery must be delayed until the infant can better tolerate the procedure, an immediate **palliative** surgery, aimed at achieving adequate mixing of oxygenated and unoxygenated blood, enables the child to survive until the corrective surgery can be performed.

---

umbilical hernia
(um-**BILL**-ih-kahl **HER**-nee-ah)

An outward protrusion of the intestine through a weakness in the abdominal wall around the umbilicus (navel or "belly button").

An umbilical hernia usually closes spontaneously within the first 2 years of life. If it remains beyond that point, surgical closure of the weakened abdominal wall may be necessary. This defect is more likely to be seen in girls than boys, and in premature infants. See **Figure 19-18.**

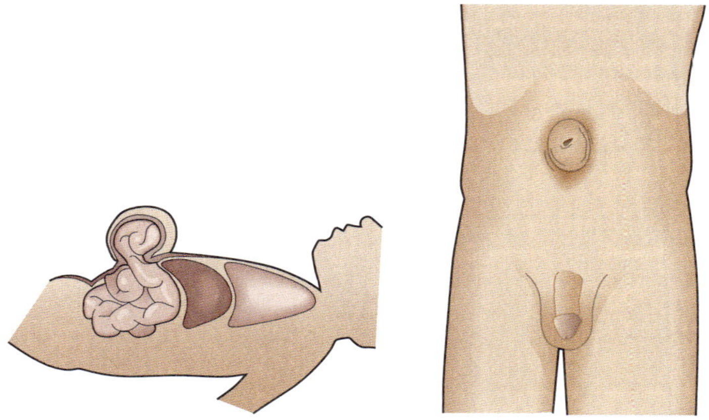

Figure 19-18 Umbilical hernia

Diagnostic Techniques and Procedures

heel puncture

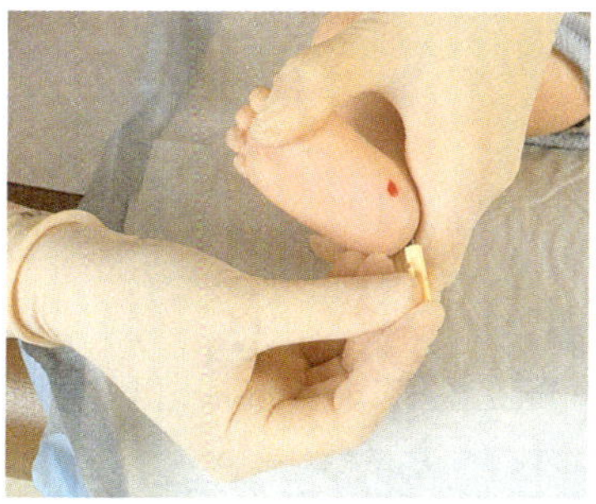

Heel puncture is a method of obtaining a blood sample from a newborn or premature infant by making a shallow puncture of the lateral or medial area of the plantar (sole of the foot) surface of the heel; also called a "heel stick." See Figure 19-19.

Figure 19-19 Capillary heel puncture

pediatric urine collection
(pee-dee-**AT**-rik)

A urine specimen may be requested as part of an infant's physical examination to determine the presence of a pathologic condition.

When a child is unable to produce a urine specimen upon request, a pediatric collection bag is used. Urine is collected as required for various diagnostic procedures. See **Figure 19-20.**

The disposable urine collection bag is applied to the perineal area of the infant so that urine can collect in the bag for a specimen. The skin must be completely dry for the bag to adhere to it. If the specimen is not needed immediately, the parent can attach the bag at home, place the diaper over the bag, and bring the infant to the office at a time when a specimen is available. The bag should be removed gently to avoid pulling or chafing the infant's skin.

The following should be recorded in the patient's chart: the date, time of collection, and purpose of the specimen, along with the results of any tests performed on the specimen. If the specimen is sent to a laboratory for testing, this should be noted in the chart.

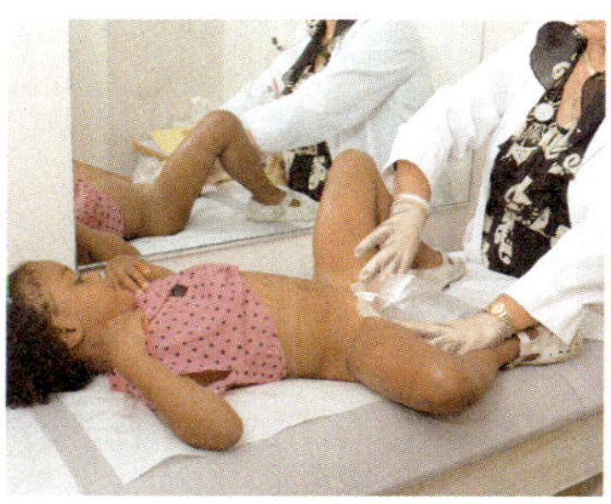

Figure 19-20 Application of a pediatric urine collector on a female

Common Abbreviations

ABBREVIATION	MEANING	ABBREVIATION	MEANING
BCG	bacille Calmette-Guérin [vaccine]	**HMD**	hyaline membrane disease
DDST	Denver II Developmental Screening Test	**MMR**	measles-mumps-rubella [vaccine]
DPT	diphtheria, pertussis, and tetanus [vaccine]	**PKU**	phenylketonuria
DS	Down syndrome	**PNP**	pediatric nurse practitioner
EA	esophageal atresia	**RDS**	respiratory distress syndrome
HDN	hemolytic disease of the newborn (erythroblastosis fetalis)	**SIDS**	sudden infant death syndrome
HIB	*Haemophilus influenzae* type B [vaccine]	**Tb**	tuberculosis
		Td	tetanus and diphtheria toxoid

Written and Audio Terminology Review

Review each of the following terms from this chapter. Study the spelling of each term and write the definition in the space provided. If you have the Audio CD available, listen to each term, pronounce it, and check the box once you are comfortable saying the word. Check definitions by looking the term up in the glossary/index.

TERM	PRONUNCIATION	DEFINITION
active immunity	☐ **AK**-tiv ih-**MEW**-nih-tee	____________
apical pulse	☐ **AY**-pih-kal pulhs	____________
apnea	☐ ap-**NEE**-ah	____________
asthma	☐ **AZ**-mah	____________
axillary temperature	☐ **AK**-sih-lair-ee **TEM**-per-ah-toor	____________
cleft	☐ **CLEFT**	____________
coarctation	☐ **koh**-ark-**TAY**-shun	____________
crackles	☐ **CRACK**-l's	____________
croup	☐ **CROOP**	____________

Term	Pronunciation	
cryptorchidism	☐ kript-**OR**-kid-izm	________
cyanosis	☐ sigh-ah-**NOH**-sis	________
dentition	☐ den-**TIH**-shun	________
diptheria	☐ diff-**THEE**-ree-ah	________
Down syndrome	☐ **DOWN SIN**-drom	________
epispadias	☐ **ep**-ih-**SPAY**-dee-as	________
erythema infectiosum	☐ air-ih-**THEE**-mah in-**fek**-she-**OH**-sum	________
erythroblastosis fetalis	☐ eh-**rith**-roh-blass-**TOH**-sis fee-**TAL**-iss	________
esophageal atresia	☐ ee-**soff**-ah-**JEE**-al ah-**TREE**-zee-ah	________
febrile	☐ **FEE**-brill *or* fee-**BRILL**	________
friction rub	☐ **FRICK**-shun rub	________
heel puncture	☐ heel **PUNK**-cher	________
hyaline membrane disease	☐ **HIGH**-ah-lighn **MEM**-brayn dih-**ZEEZ**	________
hydrocele	☐ **HIGH**-droh-seel	________
hydrocephalus	☐ high-droh-**SEFF**-ah-lus	________
hydrocephaly	☐ high-droh-**SEFF**-ah-lee	________
hypospadias	☐ **high**-poh-**SPAY**-dee-as	________
immunity	☐ ih-**MEW**-nih-tee	________
immunization	☐ **ih**-mew-nih-**ZAY**-shun	________
impetigo	☐ im-peh-**TYE**-goh	________
infectious parotitis	☐ in-**FEK**-shus pair-oh-**TYE**-tis	________
intussusception	☐ in-tus-suh-**SEP**-shun	________
microcephalus	☐ **my**-kroh-**SEFF**-ah-lus	________
mumps	☐ **MUMPS**	________
neonatal	☐ nee-oh-**NAY**-tal	________
neonatologist	☐ nee-oh-nay-**TALL**-oh-jist	________
neonatology	☐ nee-oh-nay-**TALL**-oh-jee	________
omphalitis	☐ om-fal-**EYE**-tis	________
omphalocele	☐ om-**FAL**-oh-seel	________

Term		Pronunciation	
omphalorrhea	☐	om-fal-oh-**REE**-ah	________
passive immunity	☐	passive ih-**MEW**-nih-tee	________
patent ductus arteriosus	☐	**PAY**-tent **DUK**-tus ar-**tee**-ree-**OH**-suss	________
pediatric	☐	pee-dee-**AT**-rik	________
pediatrician	☐	pee-dee-ah-**TRISH**-an	________
pertussis	☐	per-**TUSS**-is	________
phimosis	☐	fih-**MOH**-sis	________
pyrexia	☐	pie-**REK**-see-ah	________
retractions	☐	rih-**TRAK**-shuns	________
roseola infantum	☐	roh-zee-**OH**-lah in-**FAN**-tum	________
rubella	☐	roo-**BELL**-lah	________
rubeola	☐	roo-bee-**OH**-la	________
scarlatina, scarlet fever	☐	**scar**-lah-**TEE**-nah, **SCAR**-let **FEE**-ver	________
spina bifida occulta	☐	**SPY**-nah **BIH**-fih-dah oh-**KULL**-tah	________
stature	☐	**STAT**-yoor	________
stridor	☐	**STRIGH**-dor	________
Tay-Sachs disease	☐	**TAY**-sack dih-**ZEEZ**	________
tetralogy of Fallot	☐	teh-**TRALL**-oh-jee of fal-**OH**	________
toxoid	☐	**TOKS**-oyd	________
tympanic temperature	☐	tim-**PAN**-ik **TEM**-per-ah-chur	________
vaccine	☐	vak-**SEEN** *or* **VAK**-seen	________
vertex	☐	**VER**-teks	________
wheezing	☐	**HWEEZ**-ing	________

Chapter Review Exercises

The following exercises provide a more in-depth review of the chapter material. Your goal in these exercises is to complete each section at a minimum 80% level of accuracy. If you score below 80% in any area, return to the appropriate section in the chapter and read the material again. A place has been provided for your score at the end of each section.

A. Term to Definition

Define each diagnosis or procedure listed by writing the definition in the space provided. Check the box provided if you are able to complete this exercise correctly the first time (without referring to the answers). Each correct answer is worth 10 points. Record your score in the space provided at the end of the exercise.

☐ 1. transposition of the great vessels ________________

☐ 2. scarlet fever ________________

☐ 3. cleft lip ________________

☐ 4. intussusception ________________

☐ 5. cleft palate ________________

☐ 6. hyaline membrane disease ________________

☐ 7. phimosis ________________

☐ 8. erythema infectiosum ________________

☐ 9. impetigo ________________

☐ 10. sudden infant death syndrome ________________

Number correct ______ × 10 points/correct answer: Your score ______%

B. Matching Conditions

Match the descriptions of the pathological condition on the right with the appropriate pathological condition on the left. Each correct answer is worth 10 points. When you have completed the exercise, record your score in the space provided at the end of the exercise.

__c__ 1. spina bifida occulta

__j__ 2. Tay-Sachs disease

__e__ 3. roseola infantum disease

__f__ 4. rubella

__g__ 5. rubeola

__h__ 6. Down syndrome

__i__ 7. esophageal atresia

__a__ 8. tetralogy of Fallot

__d__ 9. erythroblastosis fetalis

__b__ 10. coarctation of the aorta

a. A congenital heart anomaly that consists of four defects: pulmonary stenosis; interventricular septal defect; dextroposition (shifting to the right) of the aorta so that it receives blood from both ventricles; and hypertrophy of the right ventricle

b. A congenital heart defect characterized by a localized narrowing of the aorta, which results in increased blood pressure in the upper extremities and decreased blood pressure in the lower extremities

c. A congenital defect of the central nervous system in which the back portion of one or more vertebrae is not closed

d. A form of hemolytic anemia, which occurs in neonates due to a maternal-fetal blood group incompatibility

e. A viral disease with sudden onset of a high fever for 3 to 4 days during which time the child may experience mild coldlike symptoms and slight irritability

f. A mild febrile infectious disease characterized by a rash of both macules and papules that fade and disappear in 3 days

g. acute, highly communicable viral disease with a red blotchy rash that begins as an upper respiratory disorder with fever, sore throat, cough, runny nose, and sensitivity to light

h. A congenital condition characterized by multiple defects and varying degrees of mental retardation

i. A congenital abnormality of the esophagus due to its ending before it reaches the stomach either as a blind pouch or as a fistula connected to the trachea

j. A congenital disorder caused by altered lipid metabolism due to an enzyme deficiency

Number correct ______ × 10 points/correct answer: Your score ______%

C. Crossword Puzzle

Each crossword answer is worth 10 points. When you have completed the crossword puzzle, total your points and enter your score in the space provided.

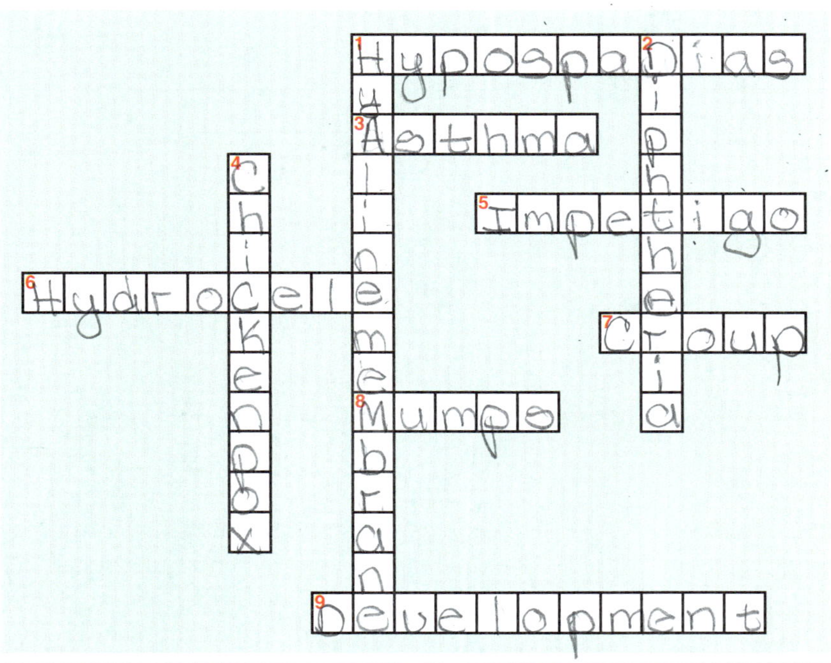

ACROSS

1 Urethra opens on underside of penis
3 Paroxysmal dyspnea with wheezing
5 Staphylococcal skin infection
6 Accumulation of fluid within a sac
7 Characterized by barking cough
8 Viral; swelling of parotid glands
9 Increase in function and complexity

DOWN

1 Respiratory distress syndrome
2 Forms false membrane on throat
4 Varicella

Number correct ______ × 10 points/correct answer: Your score ______%

D. Word Search

Using the definitions provided, identify the term relating to child health and then find and circle it in the puzzle. The words may be read up, down, diagonally, across, or backward. Each correct answer is worth 10 points. Record your score in the space provided at the end of the exercise.

Example: Also known as "German measles"

rubella

1. An increase in the whole or any of its parts physically

   ____

2. A congenital defect in which the urethra opens on the underside of the penis instead of at the end

   ____

3. A childhood disease characterized by a barking cough, suffocative and difficult breathing, stridor, and laryngeal spasm

   ____

4. Condition of undescended testicle(s); the absence of one or both testicles from the scrotum

   ____

C	L	E	X	R	U	B	E	L	L	A	S	I	S	L
R	O	I	R	E	T	S	O	P	O	R	E	T	N	A
Y	A	D	Y	A	H	U	T	E	M	A	G	R	Y	S
N	O	I	T	P	E	C	S	U	S	S	U	T	N	I
C	S	O	I	R	R	I	R	L	I	I	I	H	A	S
R	R	H	Y	O	O	T	H	O	T	S	H	P	D	Y
Y	T	O	D	E	U	H	I	M	N	E	I	A	I	L
P	I	S	U	M	S	I	F	R	A	W	D	R	O	A
T	V	O	A	P	T	N	G	N	G	N	P	G	P	S
O	N	M	C	I	I	N	I	I	I	E	N	O	A	I
R	N	E	E	R	D	A	A	R	G	C	A	I	Q	S
C	C	H	O	L	Y	A	A	J	I	O	V	D	U	S
H	Y	D	R	O	C	E	P	H	A	L	U	S	E	U
I	U	I	A	I	A	S	R	S	L	I	S	R	P	T
D	J	O	L	S	Y	H	S	H	O	M	S	Y	A	R
I	N	N	U	C	S	A	I	D	A	P	S	T	P	E
S	O	O	S	S	S	R	S	L	F	D	Y	P	X	P
M	C	A	I	M	I	G	A	I	U	B	H	H	Y	A
T	Q	S	D	A	G	R	O	W	T	H	K	L	T	R

5. Generalized growth retardation of the body due to the deficiency of the human growth hormone; also known as congenital hypopituitarism or hypopituitarism

____

6. A congenital defect (birth defect) in which the urethra opens on the upper side of the penis at some point near the glans

____

7. A proportional overgrowth of the body's tissue due to the hypersecretion of the human growth hormone before puberty

____

8. Telescoping of a portion of proximal intestine into distal intestine usually in the ileocecal region causing an obstruction

____

9. Also called "whooping cough"

____

10. An abnormal increase of cerebrospinal fluid (CSF) in the brain, which causes the ventricles of the brain to dilate, resulting in an increased head circumference in the infant with open fontanel(s)

____

Number correct _______ × 10 points/correct answer: Your score _______%

E. Matching Abbreviations

Match the abbreviation on the left with the appropriate definition on the right. Each correct response is worth 10 points. When you have completed the exercise, total your points and record your score in the space provided at the end of the exercise.

_____	1. PKU	a.	sudden infant death syndrome
_____	2. MMR	b.	tuberculosis
_____	3. DPT	c.	Denver Placement Test
_____	4. Td	d.	bacille Calmette-Guérin [vaccine]
_____	5. HMD	e.	measles, mumps, rubella [vaccine]
_____	6. DDST	f.	phenylketonuria
_____	7. HIB	g.	diphtheria, pertussis, tetanus [vaccine]
_____	8. BCG	h.	tetanus and diphtheria toxoid
_____	9. SIDS	i.	Standard Intelligence Developmental Screening
_____	10. Tb	j.	hyaline membrane disease
		k.	Denver Developmental Screening Test
		l.	*Haemophilus influenzae* type B [vaccine]
		m.	head circumference × months = dentition

Number correct _______ × 10 points/correct answer: Your score _______%

F. Spelling

Circle the correctly spelled term in each pairing of words. Each correct answer is worth 10 points. Record your score in the space provided at the end of the exercise.

1. dentition	dentishun
2. immunization	immanization
3. pediatrishun	pediatrician
4. omfalorrhea	omphalorrhea
5. stridor	strider
6. vacine	vaccine
7. pirexia	pyrexia
8. impetigo	infantigo
9. rubeyola	rubeola
10. hypospadias	hypospadius

Number correct ______ × 10 points/correct answer: Your score ______ %

G. Completion

The following sentences relate to the chapter on child health. Complete each sentence with the most appropriate word. Each correct answer is worth 10 points. Record your score in the space provided at the end of the exercise.

1. A communicable disease in children, caused by the varicella-zoster virus, that is characterized by eruptions of macules, papules, and vesicles on the skin followed by crusting over of the lesions with a granular scab, is known as Chickenpox.
2. A viral disease characterized by a face that appears as "slapped cheeks," with a fiery red rash on the cheeks, is called Fifth disease.
3. Another name for infectious parotitis is mumps.
4. The medical term for whooping cough is pertussis.
5. The medical term for the 3-day measles or German measles is rubella.
6. The medical term for the 7-day measles or "red measles" is rubeola.
7. A childhood disease characterized by a barking cough, suffocative and difficult breathing, stridor, and laryngeal spasms is called Croup.
8. An accumulation of fluid in any saclike cavity or duct, particularly the scrotal sac or along the spermatic cord, is known as hydrocele.
9. A congenital defect in which the urethra opens on the upper side of the penis at some point near the tip of the penis is known as epispadias.
10. A tightness of the foreskin (prepuce) of the penis of the male infant that prevents it from being pulled back, and causes difficulty with urination, is known as phimosis.

Number correct ______ × 10 points/correct answer: Your score ______ %

H. Word Element Review

The following words relate to the chapter on child health. The word elements have been labeled (WR = word root, P = prefix, S = suffix, and V = combining vowel). Read the definition carefully and complete the word by filling in the blank, using the word elements provided in this chapter. If you still have trouble with word building rules, refer to Chapter 1. Each correct word is worth 10 points. Record your score in the space provided at the end of this exercise.

1. A congenital anomaly characterized by abnormal smallness of the head in relation to the rest of the body and by underdevelopment of the brain:

   micr / o / cephal / us
   WR V WR S

2. The medical specialty concerned with the diseases and abnormalities of the newborn infant:

   neo / nat / o / ology
   P WR V S

3. A pathological condition characterized by an abnormal accumulation of cerebrospinal fluid, usually under increased pressure, within the cranium:

   hydro / cephal / us
   P WR S

4. Congenital herniation of intra-abdominal viscera through a defect in the abdominal wall around the umbilicus (umbilical hernia):

   Omphal / o / cele
   WR V S

5. A condition of undescended testicle(s); the absence of one or both testicles from the scrotum:

   Crypt / orchid / ism
   WR WR S

6. A condition of blueness; bluish discoloration of the skin and mucous membranes caused by an excess of deoxygenated hemoglobin in the blood or a structural defect in the hemoglobin molecule:

   Cyan / osis
   WR S

7. Pertaining to fever (other than pyrexia):

   Febr / ile
   WR S

8. Pertaining to the head and the tail, as in growth and development proceeding from the head to the toe:

   Cephal / o / caud / al
   WR V WR S

9. Pertaining to near and away from, as in growth and development proceeding from the center outward or from the midline to the periphery:

   Proxim / o / dist / al
   WR V WR S

10. Without breathing; an absence of spontaneous respiration:

    A / pne / a
    P WR S

Number correct ______ × 10 points/correct answer: Your score ______%

I. Definition to Term

Using the following definitions, identify and provide the word for the pathological condition to match the definition. (A clue has been provided for the number of words needed in your answer.) Each correct answer is worth 10 points. Record your score in the space provided at the end of the exercise.

1. The heart rate as heard with a stethoscope placed on the chest wall adjacent to the cardiac apex (top of the heart)
   Apical pulse ________
2. Abnormal, short, audible gruntlike breaks in exhalation that often accompany severe chest pain
   Grunting
3. The eruption of teeth; this occurs in a sequential pattern, with 20 primary teeth erupting between the ages of 6 months to 36 months
   Denition
4. A process by which resistance to an infectious disease is induced or augmented
   Immunization
5. A medical doctor who specializes in neonatology
   Neonatologist
6. Drainage from the umbilicus (navel)
   Omphalorrhea
7. A physician who specializes in pediatrics
   Pediatrician
8. Another name for fever, other than febrile
   Pyrexia
9. The body temperature as measured electronically at the eardrum
   Tympanic temperature
10. A breath sound, characterized by a high-pitched musical quality heard on both inspiration and expiration; associated with asthma and chronic bronchitis
    Wheezing

Number correct _______ × 10 points/correct answer: Your score _______%

J. Multiple Choice

Read each statement carefully and select the correct answer from the choices provided. Each correct answer is worth 10 points. Record your score in the space provided at the end of the exercise.

1. A process by which resistance to an infectious disease is induced or increased is called:
   a. immunization
   b. vaccine
   c. toxoid
   d. dentition

2. A graphic representation, by any of various systems, of a numeric relationship is called (a):
   a. stature
   b. nomogram
   c. head circumference
   d. growth spurt
3. A condition that is present at birth ("born with") is termed:
   a. grunting
   b. nomogram
   c. vertex
   d. congenital
4. The natural height of a person in an upright position is termed:
   a. stature
   b. nomogram
   c. vertex
   d. recumbent length
5. An acute, contagious disease characterized by sore throat, abrupt high fever, increased pulse, "strawberry" tongue, and a pointlike bright red rash on the body is:
   a. rubella (German measles)
   b. rubeola (red measles)
   c. scarlet fever (scarlatina)
   d. roseola infantum
6. A congenital defect in which there is an open space between the nasal cavity and the lip, due to failure of the soft tissue and bones in this area to fuse properly during embryological development is known as:
   a. coarctation of the aorta
   b. cleft lip
   c. croup
   d. tetralogy of Fallot
7. This condition is also known as respiratory distress syndrome of the premature infant:
   a. hyaline membrane disease
   b. esophageal atresia
   c. erythroblastosis fetalis
   d. epispadias
8. A congenital condition, also known as trisomy 21, and characterized by multiple defects and varying degrees of mental retardation, is called:
   a. dwarfism
   b. hyaline membrane disease
   c. Down syndrome
   d. patent ductus arteriosus
9. The telescoping of a portion of proximal intestine into distal intestine usually into the ileocecal region causing an obstruction is known as:
   a. phimosis
   b. intussusception
   c. Reye's syndrome
   d. Tay-Sachs disease

10. The completely unexpected and unexplained death of an apparently well, or virtually well, infant is known as SIDS or:
    a. crib death
    b. tetralogy of Fallot
    c. Reye's syndrome
    d. hyaline membrane disease

Number correct _______ × 10 points/correct answer: Your score _______%

Answers to Chapter Review Exercises

A. Term to Definition

1. a condition in which the two major arteries of the heart are reversed in position, which results in two noncommunicating circulatory systems
2. an acute, contagious disease characterized by sore throat, abrupt high fever, increased pulse, strawberry tongue (red and swollen), and punctiform (pointlike) bright red rash on the body
3. an abnormal opening in the lip that sometimes also is into the nose
4. telescoping of a portion of proximal intestine to distal intestine usually in the ileocecal region, causing an obstruction
5. failure of the palatal shelves to fuse resulting in a fissure in the middle of the palate
6. also known as respiratory distress syndrome (RDS) of the premature infant
7. a tightness of the foreskin (prepuce) of the penis of the male infant that prevents it from being pulled back
8. a viral disease characterized by a face that appears as "slapped cheeks," a fiery red rash on the cheeks
9. contagious superficial skin infection characterized by serous vesicles and pustules filled with millions of staphylococcus or streptococcus bacteria, usually forming on the face
10. the completely unexpected and unexplained death of an apparently well, or virtually well, infant

B. Matching Conditions

1. c	6. h
2. j	7. i
3. e	8. a
4. f	9. d
5. g	10. b

C. Crossword Puzzle

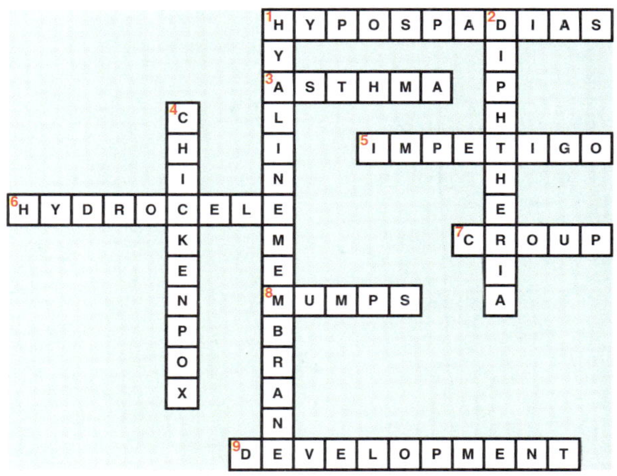

D. Word Search

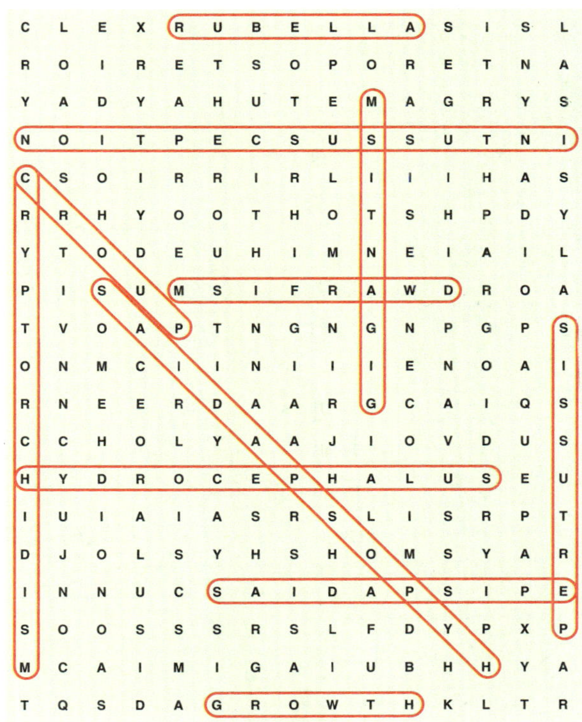

E. Matching Abbreviations

1. f
2. e
3. g
4. h
5. j
6. k
7. l
8. d
9. a
10. b

F. Spelling

1. dentition
2. immunization
3. pediatrician
4. omphalorrhea
5. stridor
6. vaccine
7. pyrexia
8. impetigo
9. rubeola
10. hypospadias

G. Completion

1. chickenpox, or varicella
2. erythema infectiosum, or fifth disease
3. mumps
4. pertussis
5. rubella
6. rubeola
7. croup
8. hydrocele
9. epispadias
10. phimosis

H. Word Element Review

1. micr / o/ cephal / us
   WR V WR S
2. neo / nat / o / logy
   P WR V S
3. hydro / cephal / us
   P WR S
4. omphal / o / cele
   WR V S
5. crypt / orchid / ism
   WR WR S
6. cyan / osis
   WR S
7. febr / ile
   WR S
8. cephal / o / caud / al
   WR V WR S
9. proxim / o / dist / al
   WR V WR S
10. a / pne / a
    P WR S

I. Definition to Term

1. apical pulse
2. grunting
3. dentition
4. immunization
5. neonatologist
6. omphalorrhea
7. pediatrician
8. pyrexia
9. tympanic
10. wheezing

J. Multiple Choice

1. a
2. b
3. d
4. a
5. c
6. b
7. a
8. c
9. b
10. a

CHAPTER 20

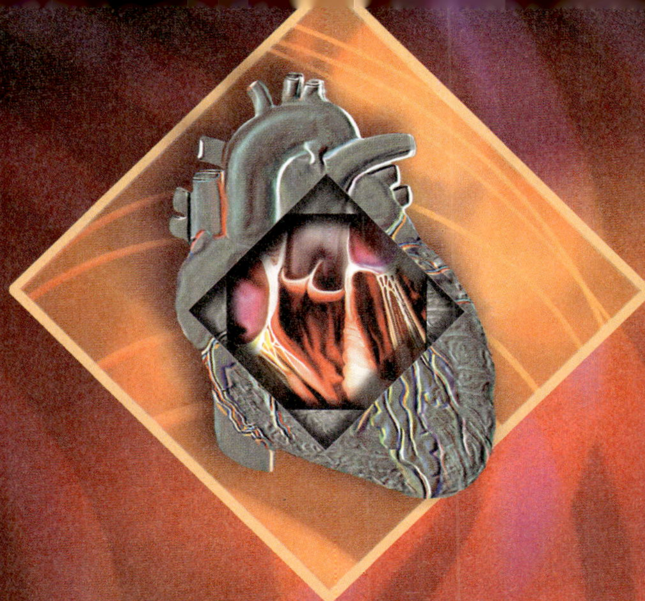

Radiology and Diagnostic Imaging

CHAPTER CONTENT

KEY COMPETENCIES

Upon completing this chapter and the review exercises at the end of the chapter, the learner should be able to:

1. Identify at least 20 diagnostic techniques/procedures relating to the specialty of radiology and diagnostic imaging.
2. Correctly spell and pronounce each new term introduced in this chapter using the Activity CD-ROM and Audio CD, if available.
3. Identify at least 10 radiological positions and/or movements based on their descriptions.
4. Demonstrate the ability to create at least 10 medical terms related to the specialty of radiology and diagnostic imaging by completing the "Definition to Term" exercise at the end of the chapter.
5. Identify at least 20 abbreviations common to the specialty of radiology and diagnostic imaging.

OVERVIEW

The specialty of radiology and diagnostic imaging evolved from an accidental discovery that occurred over 100 years ago. In 1895, Wilhelm Conrad Roentgen, a German physicist, was experimenting with electrical discharges in an evacuated glass tube called a Crookes' tube (cathode-ray tube). He accidentally discovered a new form of electromagnetic energy rays that could penetrate a person's hand, and cause the outline of bones to be seen on a chemically coated fluorescent screen behind the hand. Not knowing what the rays were, Roentgen coined the term x-ray (x represented the unknown). Roentgen developed a photographic film to replace the fluorescent screen to make lasting pictures of the image. The x-ray is also known as the roentgen ray, so named after its discoverer. Roentgen received the first Nobel prize for physics in 1901 for his discovery of the x-ray. From this simple beginning, a whole new world was opened to medicine.

X-rays are high-energy electromagnetic waves that travel in straight lines and have a shorter wavelength than visible light, enabling them to penetrate solid materials of varying densities. These invisible waves of radiant energy are capable of exposing a photographic plate (x-ray film) in much the same way as light rays expose the film in a camera. X-rays are used to visualize internal organs and structures of the body and provide a valuable means for verifying the presence of illness or disease. **Radiology** is the study of the diagnostic and therapeutic uses of x-rays. This branch of medicine is concerned with the use of x-rays, high-strength magnetic fields, high-frequency sound waves, and various radioactive compounds to diagnose and treat diseases. A **radiologist** is a medical doctor who specializes in radiology. A **radiologic technologist,** also known as a **radiographer**, is an allied health professional who is trained to use x-ray machines and other imaging equipment to produce images of the internal structures of the body. Most radiologic technologists are employed in hospital x-ray departments and work under the direction of a radiologist or other physicians.

Radiology and Diagnostic Imaging Procedures and Techniques

When the physician is confirming a diagnosis, he or she will sometimes find it necessary to view the internal structures of the body or observe them in action. Examples of procedures that aid in diagnosing include, but are not limited to, x-ray images of the body with or without a contrast medium, ultrasound images, body scans, and fluoroscopic procedures that allow the physician to observe the particular organ as it functions. This section provides a basic discussion of the most common radiologic and diagnostic imaging procedures and techniques used in medicine. The procedures and techniques are listed in alphabetical order.

angiocardiography (cardiac catheterization)
(**an**-jee-oh-kar-dee-**OG**-rah-fee **CAR**-dee-ak **kath**-eh-ter-ih-**ZAY**-shun)
angi/o = vessel
cardi/o = heart
-graphy = process of recording

A specialized diagnostic procedure in which a catheter (a hollow, flexible tube) is introduced into a large vein or artery, usually of an arm or a leg, and is then threaded through the circulatory system to the heart.

Cardiac catheterization is used to obtain detailed information about the structure and function of the heart chambers, valves, and the great vessels. Pressures within the chambers of the heart can be measured as can oxygen concentration, saturation, and tension. In the case of coronary artery disease, the patient may undergo a cardiac catheterization to determine the amount of occlusion of his or her coronary arteries for the physician to determine the most appropriate treatment; treatment may consist of coronary artery bypass surgery or percutaneous transluminal coronary angioplasty.

Immediately after the injection of the contrast medium, a series of x-ray films allowing visualization of the heart is taken. This sequence of films taken during a cardiac catheterization allows the radiologist to follow the circulation of blood through the great vessels, heart, and lungs.

The three major approaches used for the **angiocardiography** procedure for indicating the exact location of the contrast injection are right-sided angiocardiography, left-sided angiocardiography, and selective coronary artery angiocardiography.

This procedure is typically done in the special controlled environment of a cardiac catheterization lab under fluoroscopy and in the presence of a radiologist or a cardiologist. The person undergoing a cardiac catheterization is required to sign a consent form and is to have nothing by mouth (NPO) for 6 to 8 hours before the procedure. This procedure may be contraindicated for persons with allergies to shellfish, iodine, or other contrast media due to the possibility of experiencing an anaphylactic reaction.

angiography
(**an**-jee-**OG**-rah-fee)
angi/o = vessel
-graphy = process of recording

A series of x-ray films allowing visualization of internal structures after the introduction of a radiopaque substance. See Figure 20-1.

This recording is made possible by contrast medium, which promotes the imaging (makes them visible) of those structures that are otherwise difficult to see on x-ray film. This substance is injected into an artery or a vein.

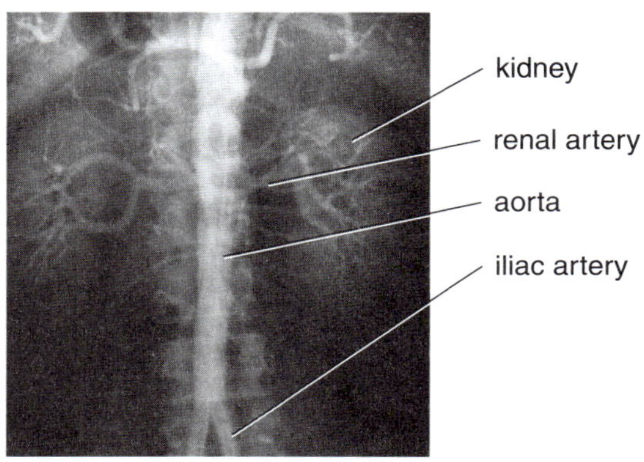

Figure 20-1 Angiogram of abdomen

Hypersensitivity tests are often performed before the radiographic material is used because the iodine in the contrast material has been known to cause severe allergic reactions in some persons. There are various types of **angiography** used to diagnose conditions such as myocardial infarction, occlusion of blood vessels, calcified atherosclerotic plaques, stroke (cerebrovascular accident), hypertension of the vessels leading to the liver (portal hypertension), and narrowing of the renal artery. The following are descriptions of some of the specific types of angiography.

---

cerebral angiography
(**SER**-eh-bral *or* seh-**REE**-bral **an**-jee-**OG**-rah-fee)
cerebr/o = cerebrum
-al = pertaining to
angi/o = vessel
-graphy = process of recording

The injection of a radiopaque contrast medium into an arterial blood vessel (carotid, femoral, or brachial) to make visualization of the cerebral vascular system via x-ray possible.

The arterial, capillary, and venous structures are outlined as the contrast medium flows through the brain.

Through the **cerebral angiography**, cerebral circulation abnormalities such as occlusions or aneurysms are visualized. Vascular and nonvascular tumors can be noted as well as hematomas and abscesses.

---

renal angiography
(**REE**-nal **an**-jee-**OG**-rah-fee)
ren/o = kidney
-al = pertaining to
angi/o = vessel
-graphy = process of recording

X-ray visualization of the internal anatomy of the renal blood vessels after injection of a contrast medium.

A radiopaque catheter is inserted into the femoral artery. Using fluoroscopy, the catheter is guided up the aorta to the level of the renal arteries. A contrast dye is then injected, and a series of x-rays are taken to visualize the renal vessels.

Renal angiography is used to detect narrowing of the renal vessels, vascular damage, renal vein thrombosis (clots), cysts, or tumors.

---

arteriography
(**ar**-tee-ree-**OG**-rah-fee)
arteri/o = artery
-graphy = process of recording

Arteriography is x-ray visualization of arteries following the introduction of a radiopaque contrast medium into the bloodstream through a specific vessel by way of a catheter.

---

arthrography
(ar-**THROG**-rah-fee)
arthr/o = joint
-graphy = process of recording

Arthrography is the process of taking x-rays of the inside of a joint, after a contrast medium (substance that makes the inside of the joint visible) has been injected into the joint.

---

barium enema (BE)
(**BAH**-ree-um **EN**-eh-mah)
(lower GI series)

Infusion of a radiopaque contrast medium, barium sulfate, into the rectum. The contrast medium is retained in the lower intestinal tract while x-ray films are obtained of the lower GI tract.

For the most definitive results, the colon should be empty of fecal material. Along with the use of a laxative and/or a cleansing enema, the person having a **barium enema (BE)** would be without food or drink from the midnight before the procedure. Abnormal findings include malignant tumors, colonic stenosis, colonic fistula, perforated colon, diverticula, and polyps. The barium will cause the stool (feces) to have a chalky appearance; patients are encouraged to drink plenty of fluids to help eliminate the barium.

barium swallow (upper GI series)
(**BAH**-ree-um **SWALL**-oh)

Oral administration of a radiopaque contrast medium, barium sulfate, which flows into the esophagus as the person swallows. See Figure 20-2.

During a **barium swallow**, x-ray films are obtained of the esophagus and borders of the heart in which esophageal varices (twisted veins) can be identified, and esophageal strictures, tumors or obstructions, achalasia, or abnormal motility of the esophagus can be identifiable.

As the barium sulfate continues to flow into the upper GI tract (lower esophagus, stomach, and duodenum), x-ray films are taken to reveal ulcerations, tumors, hiatal hernias, or obstructions.

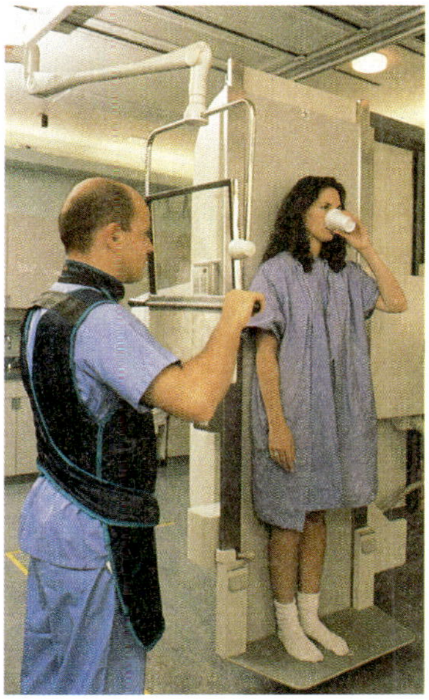

Figure 20-2 Barium swallow (upper GI series)

bronchography
(brong-**KOG**-rah-fee)
bronch/o = bronchus, airway
-graphy = process of recording

Bronchography is a bronchial examination via x-ray following the coating of the bronchi with a radiopaque substance.

cholangiography (intravenous)
(koh-**lan**-jee-**OG**-rah-fee)
(in-trah-**VEE**-nus)
chol/e = bile
angi/o = vessel
-graphy = process of recording

Visualizing and outlining of the major bile ducts following an intravenous injection of a contrast medium.

The bile duct structure can be observed for obstruction, strictures, anatomic variations, malignant tumors, and congenital cysts during an intravenous **cholangiography**.

cholangiography (percutaneous transhepatic) (PTC, PTHC)
(koh-**lan**-jee-**OG**-rah-fee)
(**per**-kyoo-**TAY**-nee-us
trans-heh-**PAT**-ik)
chol/e = bile
angi/o = vessel
-graphy = process of recording
per- = through
cutane/o = skin
-ous = pertaining to
trans- = across
hepat/o = liver
-ic = pertaining to

An examination of the bile duct structure using a needle to pass directly into an intrahepatic bile duct to inject a contrast medium. See Figure 20-3.

In bile duct structure, bile can be observed for obstruction, strictures, anatomic variations, malignant tumors, recording, and congenital cysts. If the cause is found to be extrahepatic in jaundiced persons, a catheter may be used for external drainage by leaving it in the bile duct.

There are special procedures and care required before, during, and after this procedure. It is an invasive procedure with significant morbidity due to the potential complications. Abnormal findings include:

- Tumors, gallstones, or strictures of the common bile or hepatic duct
- Biliary sclerosis
- Cysts of the common bile duct

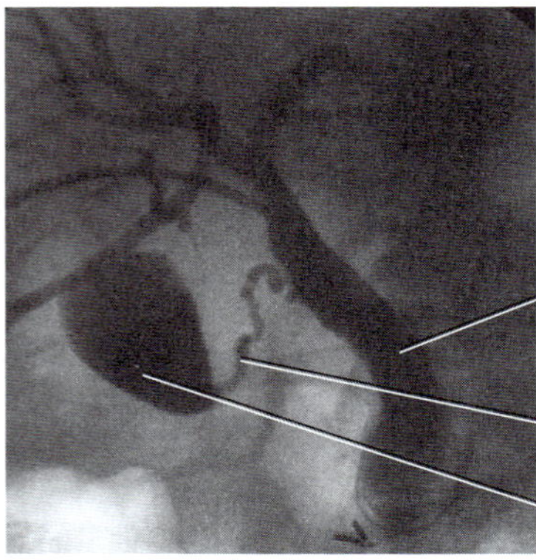

Figure 20-3 PTHC with common bile duct obstruction

- Tumors, inflammation, or pseudocysts of the pancreatic duct
- Anatomic biliary or pancreatic duct abnormalities

cholangiopancreatography (endoscopic retrograde) (ERCP)
(koh-**lan**-jee-oh-**pan**-kree-ah **TOG**-rah-fee)
(en-doh-**SKOP**-ic **RET**-roh-grayd)
chol/e = bile
angi/o = vessel
pancreat/o = pancreas
-graphy = process of recording
endo- = within
scop/o = to view
-ic = pertaining to
retr/o = behind

A procedure that examines the size of and the filling of the pancreatic and biliary ducts through direct radiographic visualization with a fiberoptic endoscope. See Figure 20-4.

During the ERCP procedure, a fiberoptic scope (flexible tube with a lens and a light source) passes through the patient's esophagus and stomach into the duodenum. Passage of the tube is observed on a fluoroscopic screen that makes it possible to view the procedure in action. The doctor locates the ampulla of Vater, a common passageway that connects the common bile duct and the pancreatic duct to the duodenum. Digestive enzymes can be removed from this area for analysis before a contrast medium is injected into the area for visualization upon x-ray.

This procedure requires the person to lie very still during the process. The patient is kept NPO (nothing by mouth) before the procedure and is mildly sedated during the procedure.

Abnormal findings include strictures (narrowing) of the common bile duct, tumors, gallstones, cysts, and anatomic variations of the biliary or pancreatic ducts.

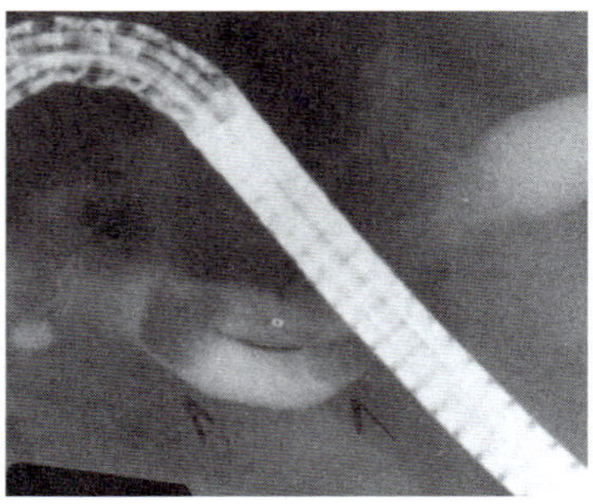

Figure 20-4 ERCP with stones

cholecystography (oral)
(koh-lee-sis-**TOG**-rah-fee)
chol/e = bile
cyst/o = bladder
-graphy = process of recording

Visualization of the gallbladder through x-ray following the oral ingestion of pills containing a radiopaque iodinated dye.

The oral **cholecystography** is not as accurate as the gallbladder ultrasound. Abnormal findings would include gallstones, gallbladder polyps, gallbladder cancer, or cystic duct obstruction.

cineradiography
(**sin**-eh-**ray**-dee-**OG**-rah-fee)
cine- = pertaining to movement
radi/o = radiation; also refers to radius
-graphy = process of recording

Cineradiography is a diagnostic technique combining the techniques of fluoroscopy, radiography, and cinematography by filming the images that develop on a fluorescent screen with a movie camera.

computed axial tomography (CT, CAT)
(kom-**PEW**-ted **AK**-see-al toh-**MOG**-rah-fee)
tom/o = to cut
-graphy = process of recording

A painless, noninvasive diagnostic x-ray procedure using ionizing radiation that produces a cross-sectional image of the body.

The image created by the computer represents a detailed cross section of the tissue structure being examined. See **Figure 20-5.**

Computed axial tomography (also called CAT or CT scan) is the analysis of a three-dimensional view of the tissue being evaluated as obtained from x-ray beams passing through successive horizontal layers of tissue. The computer detects the radiation absorption and the variation in tissue density in each layer. From this detection of radiation absorption and tissue density a series of anatomic pictures are produced in varying shades of gray.

When contrast is indicated for the CT scan, IV iodinated dye is injected via a peripheral IV site. If the procedure is ordered with contrast, the person needs to be NPO for 4 hours prior to the study because the contrast dye can cause nausea and vomiting.

This diagnostic procedure is used for various areas and systems of the body.

CAT scans are helpful in evaluating areas of the body that are difficult to assess using standard x-ray procedures. The CT scan provides information about the exact location, extent of involvement, and the direction needed for treatment.

As is true with magnetic resonance imaging, patients should be informed that the CAT is a very confining procedure because they are placed within a tubelike structure, and should be asked if they are claustrophobic (have fear of enclosed spaces). The following are descriptions of specific CT scans.

1. CT of the abdomen: The CT scan of the abdomen aids in the diagnosis of tumors, abscesses, cysts, inflammation, obstructions, perforation, bleeding, and aneurysms.
2. CT of the brain: The analysis of a three-dimensional view of brain tissue obtained as x-ray beams pass through successive horizontal layers of the brain. The images provided are as though you were looking down through the top of the head.

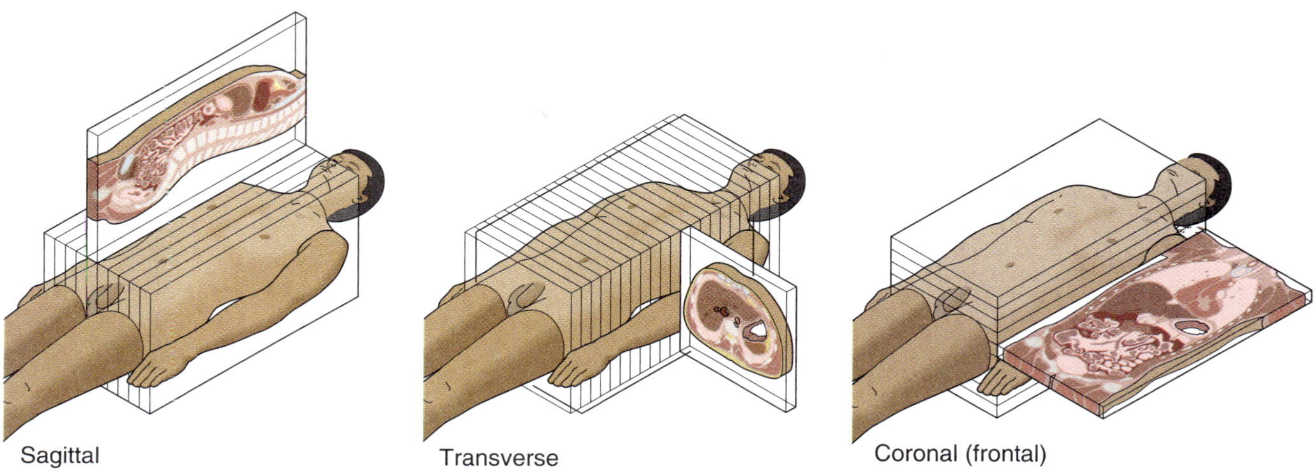

Figure 20-5 Computed tomography

CT scans of the brain are helpful in identifying intracranial tumors, areas of hemorrhage within the brain, cerebral aneurysm, multiple sclerosis, hydrocephalus, and brain abscess.

3. CT (CAT) of lymphoid tissue: Diagnosis of abnormalities in lymphoid organs are made in areas such as the spleen, thymus gland, and lymph nodes, with the collection of x-ray images taken from various angles following injection of a contrast medium.

---

voiding cystourethrography
(**VOYD**-ing **sis**-toh-yoo-ree-**THROG**-rah-fee)
cyst/o = bladder
urethr/o = urethra
-graphy = process of recording

X-ray visualization of the bladder and urethra during the voiding process, after the bladder has been filled with a contrast material; the record produced is known as a cystourethrogram.

A **radiopaque** dye is instilled into the bladder via a urethral catheter. The catheter is then removed and the patient is asked to void. X-ray pictures are taken as the patient is expelling the urine.

The **voiding cystourethrography** is helpful in diagnosing urethral lesions, bladder and urethral obstructions, and vesicoureteral reflux (abnormal backflow of urine from the bladder to the ureter).

---

digital subtraction angiography (DSA)
(**DIJ**-ih-tal sub-**TRAK**-shun an-jee-**OG**-rah-fee)
angi/o = vessel
-graphy = process of recording

X-ray images of blood vessels only, appearing without any background, due to the use of a computerized digital video subtraction process.

Through a central venous line a smaller than normal amount of contrast medium is injected. The raw data, in digital form, are stored and can be recovered at any time. The best images of the vessels are selected for electronic manipulation. The image is manipulated to provide specific detail.

A reaction to the contrast medium is the only potential complication of this procedure. The person undergoing a **digital subtraction angiography (DSA)** will need to be well hydrated and consume no solid food for 2 hours prior to the procedure. Persons with the following may be candidates for a DSA:

- Transient ischemic attacks (TIAs)
- Intracranial tumors
- Serial follow-up for individuals with known stenoses in the carotid artery
- Postoperative aneurysm

echocardiography
(**ek**-oh-**kar**-dee-**OG**-rah-fee)
echo- = sound
cardi/o = heart
-graphy = process of recording

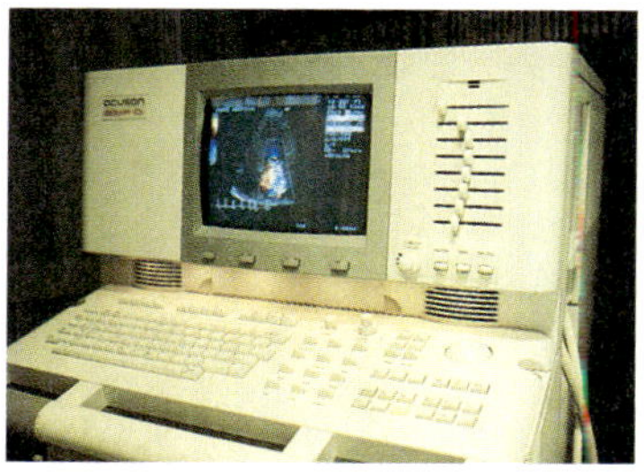

Echocardiography is a diagnostic procedure for studying the structure and motion of the heart. It is useful in evaluating structural and functional changes in a variety of heart disorders. See Figure 20-6.

Ultrasound waves pass through the heart, via a transducer, bounce off tissues of varying densities, and are reflected backward, or echoed, to the transducer, creating an image on the graph.

Figure 20-6 Echocardiography (Photo by Marcia Butterfield, Courtesy of W. A. Foote Memorial Hospital, Jackson, MI)

fluoroscopy
(**floor**-or-**OSS**-koh-pee)
fluor/o = luminous
-scopy = process of viewing

A radiological technique used to examine the function of an organ or a body part using a fluoroscope.

Fluoroscopy provides immediate serial images essential in many clinical procedures.

hysterosalpingography
(**his**-ter-oh-**sal**-pin-gog-rah-fee)
hyster/o = uterus
salping/o = fallopian tube
-graphy = process of recording

Hysterosalpingography is an x-ray of the uterus and the fallopian tubes by injecting a contrast material into these structures.

The contrast medium is injected through a cannula inserted into the cervix. As the material is slowly injected, the filling of the uterus and fallopian tubes is observed with a fluoroscope. This procedure is performed to evaluate abnormalities in structure, the presence of possible tumors, and to test for tubal obstructions. The patient may feel occasional menstrual-type cramping during the procedure and will have vaginal drainage for a couple of days after the procedure (from the drainage of the contrast material).

lymphangiography
(lim-**fan**-jee-**OG**-rah-fee)
lymph/o = lymph
angi/o = vessel
-graphy = process of recording

An x-ray assessment of the lymphatic system following injection of a contrast medium into the lymph vessels in the hand or foot.

The path of lymph flow is noted moving into the chest region. The assistance of a lymphangiography is helpful in diagnosing and staging lymphomas.

magnetic resonance imaging (MRI)
(mag-**NET**-ik **REZ**-oh-nans **IM**-ij-ing)

A noninvasive scanning procedure that provides visualization of fluid, soft tissue, and bony structures without the use of radiation. See Figure 20-7.

The person is placed inside a large electromagnetic, tubelike machine where specific radio frequency signals change the alignment of hydrogen atoms in the body. The absorbed radio frequency energy is analyzed by a computer and an image is projected on the screen.

A strong magnetic field is used and radio frequency waves produce the imaging valuable in providing images of the heart, large blood vessels, brain, and soft tissue. Magnetic resonance imaging (MRI) is also used to examine the aorta, to detect masses or possible tumors and pericardial

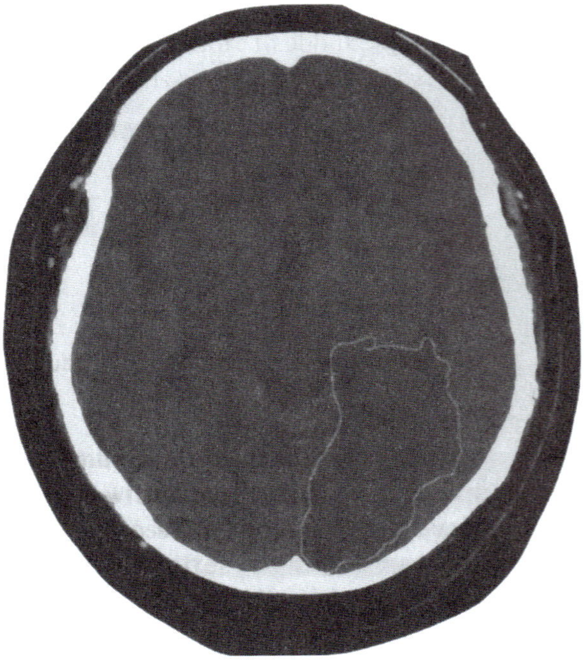

Figure 20-7 MRI of a brain with the area of a "bleed" visible in the lower right

disease; it can show the flowing of blood and the beating of the heart. The MRI provides far more preciseness and accuracy than most diagnostic tools.

Those persons with implanted metal devices cannot undergo an MRI due to the strong magnetic field and the possibility of dislodging a chip or rod. Thus, persons with pacemakers, any recently implanted wires or clips, or prosthetic valves are not eligible for MRI. Persons should be informed that MRI is a very confining procedure, because they are placed within a tube-like structure, and should be asked if they are claustrophobic (fear enclosed spaces).

---

mammography
(mam-**OG**-rah-fee)
mamm/o = breasts
-graphy = process of recording

The process of taking x-rays of the soft tissue of the breast to detect various benign and/or malignant growths before they can be felt.

The American College of Radiology recognizes the use of x-ray **mammography** as the approved method of screening for breast cancer. This procedure takes approximately 15 to 30 minutes to complete, and can be performed in an x-ray department of a hospital or in a private radiology facility. Each facility should have equipment designed and used exclusively for mammograms.

During the examination, the breast tissue is compressed between two clear disks for each x-ray view. The first view requires compressing the breast from top to bottom to take a top-to-bottom (craniocaudal) view. The second view requires compressing the breast from side to side to take a side-to-side (mediolateral) view.

Figures 20-8A and **B** illustrate the Cleopatra view for a mammogram. This view provides local compression of the lateral aspect of the breast close to the pectoral muscle.

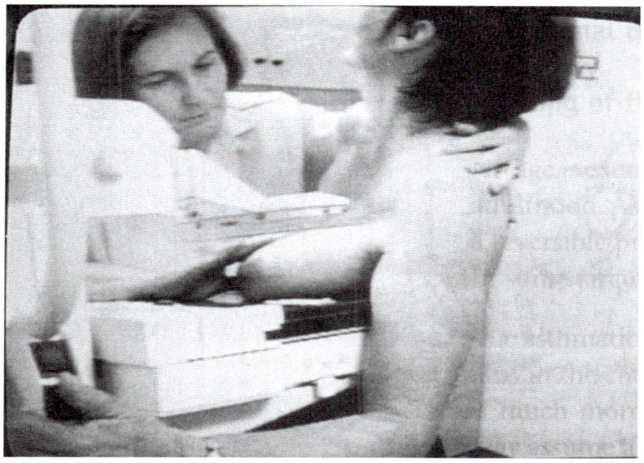

(A)

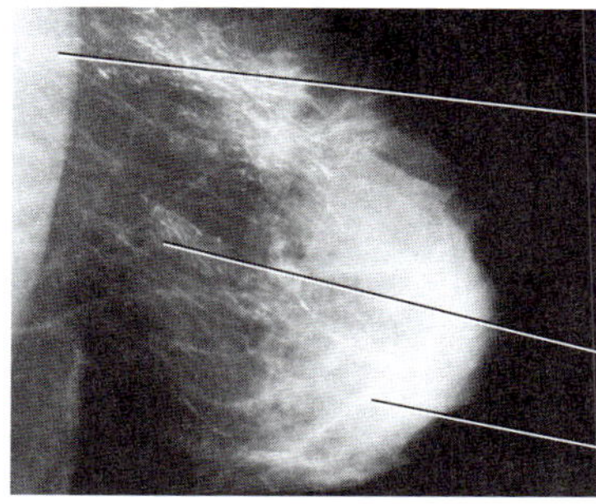

(B)

Figure 20-8 Mammography: (A) positioning for Cleopatra view; (B) Cleopatra view radiograph

The patient having a mammogram may experience fleeting discomfort as the breast tissue is compressed between the plates; but this is necessary to facilitate maximum visualization of the breast tissue.

The American Cancer Society and many personal physicians recommend that women have their first mammogram between ages 35 and 39. This will provide a baseline for reference with future mammograms. Between ages 40 and 49, mammograms are usually recommended every 2 years, unless the woman is in a high-risk category. From age 50 and thereafter, mammograms are recommended annually.

---

myelography
(my-eh-**LOG**-rah-fee)
myel/o = spinal cord or bone marrow
-graphy = process of recording

Introduction of contrast medium into the lumbar subarachnoid space through a lumbar puncture to visualize the spinal cord and vertebral canal through x-ray examination. See Figure 20-9.

Roughly 10 ml of CSF (cerebrospinal fluid) is removed and a radiopaque substance is injected slowly into the lumbar subarachnoid space.

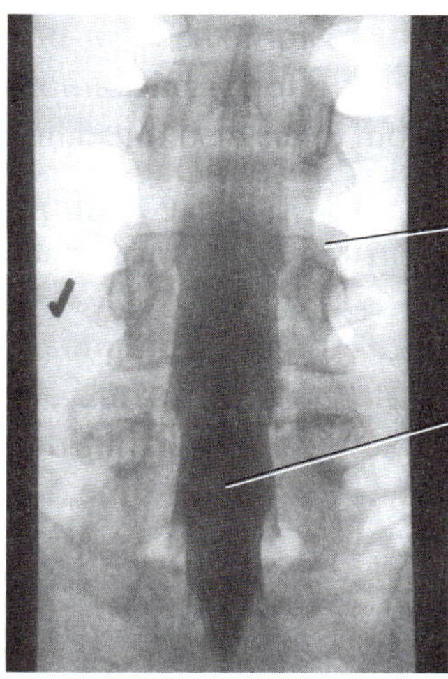

Figure 20-9 Posteroanterior (PA) lumbar myelogram

Myelography is accomplished on a tilt table in the radiology department to visualize the spinal canal in various positions. After a series of films are taken of the vertebral canal viewing various parts, the contrast medium is removed.

Myelography aids in the diagnosis of adhesions and tumors producing pressure on the spinal canal or intervertebral disc abnormalities.

---

positron emission tomography (PET) scan
(**POZ**-ih-tron ee-**MISH**-un toh-**MOG**-rah-fee)
tom/o = to cut
-graphy = process of recording

Computerized radiographic images of various body structures produced when radioactive substances are inhaled or injected. See Figure 20-10.

The metabolic activity of the brain and numerous other body structures are shown through computerized color-coded images that indicate the degree and intensity of the metabolic process. The positron emission tomography (PET) scan exposes persons to very little radiation because the radioactive substances used are short lived.

The PET scanner is helpful in detecting coronary artery disease, assessing the progression of narrowing of the coronary arteries (stenosis), and distinguishing between ischemic, infarcted, and normal cardiac tissue based on biochemical assessment of myocardial metabolism.

PET scans are used in assessing dementia, brain tumors, and cerebral vascular disease. In addition, there is a growing employment of the procedure to study biochemical activity of the brain as well as in the study and diagnosis of cancer.

One major disadvantage of the use of positron emission tomography is that it is very expensive. Due to the expense of a PET system, a modification called a single-photon emission computed tomography (SPECT) has been developed.

SPECT is an effective diagnostic tool, which is a variation of computed tomography using more stable but less precise measurements than the PET. The SPECT uses more readily accessible isotopes to measure, for example, cerebral blood flow rather than using metabolic activity like the PET scan. The SPECT also uses multiple detectors to reduce the imaging time.

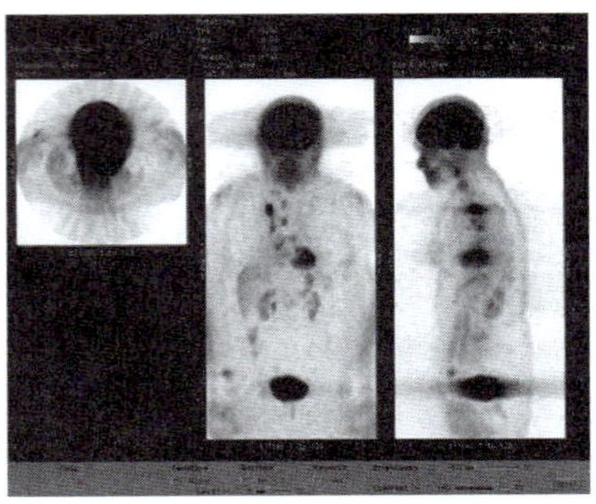

Figure 20-10 PET body scan demonstrates tumor in the right lung

---

pyelography (intravenous) (IVP)
(pye-eh-**LOG**-rah-fee)
(in-trah-**VEE**-nus)
pyel/o = renal pelvis
-graphy = process of
intra- = within
ven/o = vein
-ous = pertaining to

Also known as intravenous pyelogram or excretory urogram; this radiographic procedure provides visualization of the entire urinary tract, that is, the kidneys, ureters, bladder, and urethra. See Figure 20-11.

A contrast dye is injected intravenously and multiple x-ray films are taken as the medium is cleared from the blood by the glomerular filtration of the kidney.

The intravenous pyelography (IVP) is useful in diagnosing renal tumors, cysts, or stones, structural or functional abnormalities of the bladder, and ureteral obstruction.

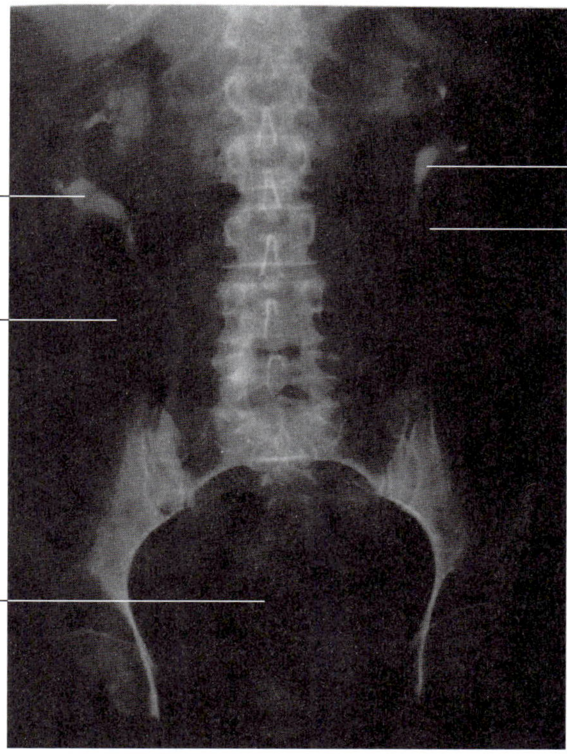

Figure 20-11 Intravenous pyelography (IVP) (Courtesy of Richard R. Carlton, Director of Radiography, Lima Technical College, Lima, OH)

radiation therapy
(ray-dee-**AY**-shun **THAIR**-ah-pee)

The delivery of ionizing radiation to accomplish one or more of the following:

1. **Destruction of tumor cells**
2. **Reduction of tumor size**
3. **Decrease in pain**
4. **Relief of obstruction**
5. **To slow or stop the spread of cancer cells**

The ionizing radiation of gamma and x-rays have proven to be lethal to the cell's DNA, especially rapidly dividing cells in faster growing tissues and tumors. **Radiation therapy** will destroy the rapidly multiplying cells regardless if they are cancerous. The cells of the skin and mucous membranes normally divide rapidly and may be affected by radiation therapy.

The goal of therapy with radiation is to reach maximum tumor control with no, or minimum, normal tissue damage. Radiation therapy may be delivered by **teletherapy** (external radiation) or **brachytherapy** (internal radiation) or a combination of both. A treatment method used to decrease the damage to normal tissue is fractionation, which involves giving radiation in repeated small doses at intervals.

The individual receiving external radiation (teletherapy) must lie still so that the radiation is delivered to the exact area that it is directed to prevent damage to other tissues. Side effects of external radiation include skin changes such as redness, blanching, scaling, sloughing, hyperpigmentation, pain or hemorrhage, ulcerations in the mucous membranes, and decreased secretions from the mucous membranes (thus posing the frequent ulcerations to become infected). Other common side effects are hair loss (hair cells multiply rapidly), tiredness, increased susceptibility to infection (bone marrow suppression), and GI symptoms including nausea, vomiting, anorexia, diarrhea, or bleeding. Radiation therapy affects the lungs through the development of an interstitial exudate that may lead to radiation pneumonia.

Internal radiation allows the radioactive material to be placed directly into the tumor site to dispense a high dose to the tumor itself and thus, the normal tissues receive a lower dose. The ingested or implanted radiation can be hazardous to those taking care of, living with, or treating the individual. Precautions are necessary for caregivers to protect themselves by using specific safety measures for handling secretions, maintaining a distance, and limiting the time of exposure. The side effects of internal radiation are the same as those of the external radiation.

radioactive iodine uptake
(**ray**-dee-oh-**AK**-tiv
EYE-oh-dine **UP**-tayk)

Radioactive iodine uptake is an examination that determines the position, size, shape, and physiological function of the thyroid gland through the use of radionuclear scanning.

An image of the thyroid is recorded and visualized after a radioactive substance is given. Nodules are readily noted with this scan and are classified as hot (functioning) or cold (nonfunctioning).

The thyroid scan is helpful in the diagnosis of the following cases:

1. Neck or substernal masses
2. Thyroid nodules (thyroid cancers are typically cold)
3. Cause of hyperthyroidism
4. Evaluating metastatic tumors with an unknown primary site

scanning

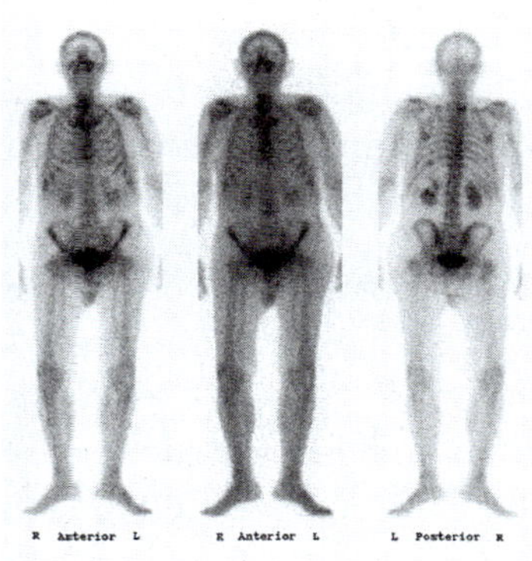

Figure 20-12 Complete bone scan

Scanning of the bones of the body with a gamma camera after an intravenous injection of a radionuclide material, which is absorbed by the bones.

The image of the area being studied is displayed by recording the concentration or collection of a radioactive substance specifically drawn to that area. There are a variety of scans used in diagnostic evaluations. The following are more distinct descriptions of some of the frequently used scans.

1. **Bone scan: A bone scan involves the intravenous injection of a radionuclide material absorbed by bone tissue. See Figure 20-12.**

   The degree of uptake of the radionuclide is directly related to the metabolism of the bone. After approximately 3 hours, the skeleton is scanned with a gamma camera (scanner), moving from one end of the body to the other. The scanner detects the areas of radioactive concentration (areas where the bone absorbs the isotope) and converts the radioactive image to a screen where the concentrations show up as pinpoint dots cast in the image of a skeleton. Areas of greater concentration of the radioisotope appear darker than other areas of distribution and are called "hot spots," which represent new bone growth around areas of pathology. These areas of pathology can be detected months earlier with a bone scan as compared to an x-ray film.

A bone scan is primarily used to detect spread of cancer to the bones (metastasis), osteomyelitis, and other destructive changes in the bone. It can be used to detect bone fractures when pathological fractures are suspected and multiple x-rays are not in the best interest of the patient. The "hot spots" on the scan will pinpoint the areas needing x-ray.

2. **Brain scan: Nuclear scanning of cranial contents 2 hours after an intravenous injection of radioisotopes.**

   Normally, blood does not cross the blood-brain barrier and come in contact with brain tissue; however, in localized pathological situations this barrier is disrupted allowing isotopes to gather. These isotopes concentrate in abnormal tissue of the brain indicating a pathological process. The scanner can localize any abnormal tissue where the isotopes have accumulated.

   The brain scan can assist in diagnosing abnormal findings such as an acute cerebral infarction, cerebral neoplasm, cerebral hemorrhage, brain abscess, aneurysms, cerebral thrombosis, hematomas, hydrocephalus, cancer metastasis to the brain, and bleeds.

3. **Liver scan: A noninvasive scanning technique that enables the visualization of the shape, size, and consistency of the liver after the IV injection of a radioactive compound.**

   This compound is readily taken up by the liver's Kupffer cells and later the distribution is recorded by a radiation detector. This scan can detect cysts, abscesses, tumors, granulomas, or diffuse infiltrative processes affecting the liver.

4. **Lung scan: The visual imaging of the distribution of ventilation or blood flow in the lungs by scanning the lungs after the patient has been injected with or has inhaled radioactive material.**

   The scanning device records the pattern of pulmonary **radioactivity** after the patient has received the medication.

5. **Spleen scan: A noninvasive scanning technique that enables the visualization of the shape, size, and consistency of the spleen after the IV injection of radioactive red blood cells.**

This scan can detect damage, tumors, or other problems.

---

small bowel follow-through

Oral administration of a radiopaque contrast medium, barium sulfate, which flows through the GI system. X-ray films are obtained at timed intervals to observe the progression of the barium through the small intestine. See Figure 20-13.

Notable delays in the time for transit may occur with both malignant and benign forms of obstruction or diminished intestinal motility. In hypermotility states, and malabsorption, the flow of barium is much quicker.

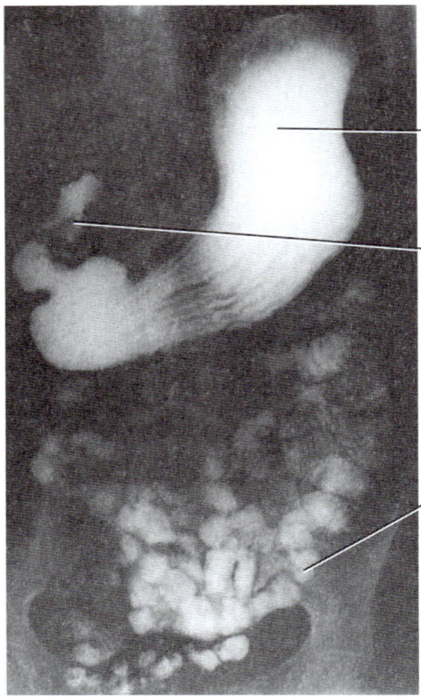

Figure 20-13 Fifteen-minute radiograph of small bowel study

Small bowel tumors, obstructions, inflammatory disease, malabsorption syndrome, congenital defects, or perforation may be identified with a small bowel follow-through study.

---

tomography
(toh-**MOG**-rah-fee)
tom/o = to cut; section
-graphy = process of recording

An x-ray technique used to construct a detailed cross section, at a predetermined depth, of a tissue structure.

Tomography is a useful diagnostic tool for finding and identifying space-occupying lesions in the liver, brain, pancreas, and gallbladder.

---

ultrasonography
(ull-trah-son-**OG**-rah-fee)
ultra- = beyond
son/o = sound
-graphy = process of recording

Also called ultrasound; this is a procedure in which sound waves are transmitted into the body structures as a small transducer is passed over the patient's skin. See Figure 20-14.

The area to be examined is lubricated before applying the transducer. As the sound waves are reflected back into the transducer, they are interpreted by a computer which, in turn, presents the composite in a picture form.

Frequently used types of ultrasonography are as follows:

1. **Abdominal ultrasound: Through the use of reflected sound waves abdominal ultrasound is able to provide reliable visualization of the liver, gallbladder, bile ducts, pancreas, kidneys, bladder, and ureters.**

   This noninvasive diagnostic procedure demonstrates normal or abnormal findings of the abdominal organs.

2. **Pelvic ultrasound: A noninvasive procedure that uses high-frequency sound waves to examine the abdomen and pelvis.**

   The sound waves pass through the abdominal wall from the transducer, which is moved back and forth across the abdomen. When the

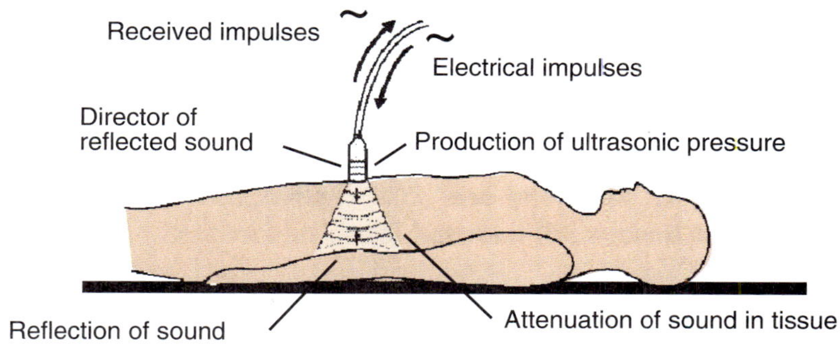

Figure 20-14 Ultrasonography

sound waves bounce off of the internal organs in the abdominopelvic region, these waves are converted to electrical impulses eventually recorded on an oscilloscope screen. A photograph of the images is then taken for further study.

Pelvic ultrasound can be used to locate a pelvic mass, an ectopic pregnancy, or an intrauterine device, and to inspect and assess the uterus, ovaries, and fallopian tubes. Clearer ultrasonic pictures of the pelvic organs can be obtained by using transvaginal ultrasonography. This procedure produces the same type of picture as abdominal ultrasound but involves the use of a vaginal probe, which is inserted into the vagina while the patient is in lithotomy position. The probes are encased in a sterile sheath and placed in the transducer before it is inserted into the vagina. The sound waves function in the same way as those for the abdominopelvic ultrasound, but the transvaginal ultrasonic image is much clearer.

3. **Renal ultrasound: An ultrasound of the kidneys is useful in distinguishing between fluid-filled cysts and solid masses, detecting renal calculi, identifying obstructions, and evaluating transplanted kidneys.**

   This noninvasive procedure requires no contrast medium.

4. **Thyroid echogram** (**ultrasound**)**: An ultrasound examiniation important in distinguishing solid thyroid nodules from cystic nodules.**

The type of nodule will provide information for treatment. In addition to differentiating the type of nodule, the thyroid echogram is used to evaluate the reaction to the medical therapy for a thyroid mass.

venography
(vee-**NOG**-rah-fee)
ven/o = vein
-graphy = process of recording

Also called phlebography, venography is a technique used to prepare an x-ray image of veins, which have been injected with a contrast medium that is radiopaque.

xeroradiography
(**zee**-roh-ray-dee-**OG**-rah-fee)
xer/o = dry
radi/o = radiation; also refers to radius
-graphy = process of recording

A diagnostic x-ray technique used to produce an electrical image rather than a chemical image.

Xeroradiography uses less radiation and decreased exposure time than ordinary x-rays. Similar to a powder toner used in a copy machine, the image is made visible when transferred to a sheet of paper. This technique

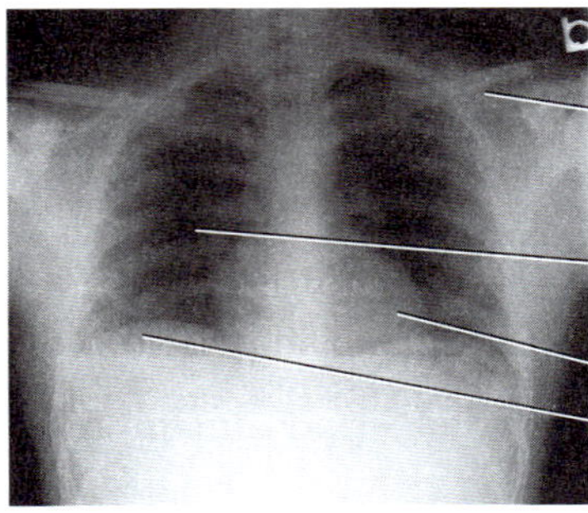

Figure 20-15 Anteroposterior (AP) view of the chest

is used primarily for mammography to identify very tiny calcifications in the breast.

---

x-rays

The use of high-energy electromagnetic waves, passing through the body onto a photographic film, to produce a picture of the internal structures of the body for diagnosis and therapy. A chest x-ray is a visualization of the interior of the chest; critical in the complete evaluation of the cardiac and pulmonary systems. See Figure 20-15.

Sites of abnormal density, such as collections of fluid or pus can be seen. In addition, the chest x-ray provides diagnostic information about the following:

1. Tumors—primary or metastatic lung, chest wall, heart, and bony thorax
2. Inflammation—pneumonia, pleuritis, and pericarditis
3. Accumulation of fluid—pleural effusion, pericardial effusion, pulmonary edema
4. Accumulation of air—chronic obstructive pulmonary disease (COPD), pneumothorax
5. Bone fractures—thorax, vertebrae
6. Diaphragmatic hernia
7. Size of the heart
8. Calcification—old lung granulomas, large vessel deterioration
9. Placement of centrally located intravenous access devices

Most chest x-rays are taken with the person standing at a distance of 6 feet. The **supine** or sitting position can be used but fluid levels cannot be visualized with chest x-rays taken in these positions. The chest x-ray can be viewed in the following ways:

1. **Posteroanterior (PA)**: The x-rays pass through the posterior (back) to the anterior (front).
2. **Lateral:** The x-rays pass through the person's side.
3. **Oblique:** The x-rays are taken from different angles.
4. **Decubitus:** The x-rays are taken with the person in recumbent lateral position, which aids in localizing fluid. Decubitus position also refers to the patient being on his or her back, or stomach.

A portable x-ray may be done at the bedside of a person who is in critical condition or who cannot be transported to an x-ray department.

Persons having a chest x-ray must remove clothing above the waist (wear an x-ray gown) and be able to take a deep breath and hold it while the x-ray is being taken. Precautions must be taken to be sure that the person has no metal objects on their body and that protection is provided for the testicles and ovaries to prevent radiation-induced abnormalities.

Vocabulary

The following vocabulary words are frequently used when discussing radiology and diagnostic imaging.

WORD	DEFINITION
abduction (ab-**DUCK**-shun) **ab-** = from, away from	Movement of a limb away from the body.
adduction (add-**DUCK**-shun) **ad-** = toward, increase	Movement of a limb toward the axis of the body.
anteroposterior (**an**-ter-oh-poss-**TEER**-ee-or) **anter/o** = front **poster/o** = back	From the front to the back of the body, commonly associated with the direction of the x-ray beam.
aortography (ay-or-**TOG**-rah-fee) **aort/o** = aorta **-graphy** = process of recording	A radiographic process in which the aorta and its branches are injected with any of various contrast media for visualization.
arthrography (ar-**THROG**-rah-fee) **arthr/o** = joint **-graphy** = process of recording	A method of radiographically visualizing the inside of a joint by injecting air or contrast medium.
axial (**AK**-see-al)	Pertaining to or situated on the axis of a structure or part of the body.
betatron (**BAY**-tah-tron)	A cyclic accelerator that produces high-energy electrons for radiotherapy treatments.
brachytherapy (**brak**-ee-**THAIR**-ah-pee)	The placement of radioactive sources in contact with or implanted into the tissues to be treated.
bronchography (brong-**KOG**-rah-fee) **bronch/o** = bronchus **-graphy** = process of recording	An x-ray examination of the bronchi after they have been coated with a radiopaque substance.
cineradiography (see-nee-ray-dee-**OG**-rah-fee)	The filming with a movie camera of the images that appear on a fluorescent screen, especially those images of body structures that have

cine- = pertaining to movement radi/o = radiation; also refers to radius -graphy = process of recording	been injected with a nontoxic, radiopaque medium for diagnostic purposes; also called cinefluorography.
computed tomography (CT) (computed toh-**MOG**-rah-fee) tom/o = to cut; section -graphy = process of recording	An x-ray technique that produces a film representing a detailed cross section of tissue structure.
digital radiography (di-gah-tull ray-dee-**OG**-rah-fee) radi/o = radiation; also refers to radius -graphy = process of recording	Any method of x-ray image formation that uses a computer to store and manipulate data.
Doppler effect (**DOP**-ler ee-fect)	The apparent change in frequency of sound or light waves emitted by a source as it moves away from or toward an observer.
eversion (ee-**VER**-zhun)	A turning outward or inside out, such as a turning of the foot outward at the ankle.
extension (eks-**TEN**-shun)	A movement allowed by certain joints of the skeleton that increases the angle between two adjoining bones, such as extending the leg, which increases the angle between the femur and the tibia.
flexion (**FLEK**-shun)	A movement allowed by certain joints of the skeleton that decreases the angle between two adjoining bones, such as bending the elbow, which decreases the angle between the humerus and the ulna.
fluorescence (floo-oh-**RES**-ens)	The emission of light of one wavelength (usually ultraviolet) when exposed to light of a different, usually shorter wavelength, a property possessed by certain substances.
fluoroscopy (**floo**-or-**OSS**-koh-pee) fluor/o = luminous -scopy = process of viewing	A technique in radiology for visually examining a part of the body or the function of an organ using a fluoroscope.
gamma camera (**GAM**-ah **CAM**-er-ah)	A device that uses the emission of light from a crystal struck by gamma rays to produce an image of the distribution of radioactive material in a body organ.
gamma rays (**GAM**-ah)	An electromagnetic radiation of short wavelength emitted by the nucleus of an atom during a nuclear reaction.
half-life	The time required for a radioactive substance to lose 50% of its activity through decay.
interstitial therapy (in-ter-**STISH**-al therapy)	Radiotherapy in which needles or wires that contain radioactive material are implanted directly into tumor areas.
inversion (in-**VER**-zhun)	An abnormal condition in which an organ is turned inside out, such as a uterine inversion; also refers to turning inward, as in inversion of the ankle.

ionization (eye-oh-nye-**ZAY**-shun)	The process in which a neutral atom or molecule gains or loses electrons and thus acquires a negative or positive electric charge.
irradiation (ih-ray-dee-**AY**-shun)	Exposure to any form of radiant energy such as heat, light, or x-ray.
lethal (**LEE**-thal)	Capable of causing death.
linear accelerator (**LIN**-ee-ar)	An apparatus for accelerating charged subatomic particles used in radiotherapy, physics research, and the production of **radionuclides**.
lymphangiography (lim-**fan**-jee-**OG**-rah-fee) **lymph/o** = lymph **angi/o** = vessel **-graphy** = process of recording	The x-ray examination of lymph glands and lymphatic vessels after an injection of contrast medium.
magnetic resonance imaging (mag-**NET**-ik **REZ**-oh-nans **IM**-ij-ing)	Medical imaging that uses radio frequency signals as its source of energy.
myelography (my-eh-**LOG**-rah-fee) **myel/o** = bone marrow or spinal cord **-graphy** = process of recording	A radiographic process by which the spinal cord and the spinal subarachnoid space are viewed and photographed after the introduction of a contrast medium.
nuclear medicine (**NOO**-klee-ar medicine)	A medical discipline that uses radioactive isotopes in the diagnosis and treatment of disease.
orthovoltage (**or**-thoh-**VOHL**-tij)	The voltage range of 100 to 350 KeV supplied by some x-ray generators used for radiation therapy.
palliative (**PAL**-ee-ah-tiv)	To soothe or relieve.
piezoelectric (pie-**EE**-zoh-eh-**lek**-trik)	The generation of a voltage across a solid when a mechanical stress is applied.
positron emission tomography (PET) (**POZ**-ih-tron ee-**MISH**-un toh-**MOG**-rah-fee) **tom/o** = to cut; section **-graphy** = process of recording	A computerized radiographic technique that employs radioactive substances to examine the metabolic activity of various body structures.
posteroanterior (**poss**-ter-oh-an-**TEER**-ee-or) **poster/o** = back **anter/o** = front	The direction from back to front.
prone (**PROHN**)	Being in horizontal position when lying face downward.

pyelography (pie-eh-**LOG**-rah-fee) pyel/o = renal pelvis -graphy = process of recording	A technique in radiology for examining the structures and evaluating the function of the urinary system.
rad (**RAD**)	Abbreviation for *radiation absorbed dose;* the basic unit of absorbed dose of ionizing radiation.
radiation therapy (ray-dee-**AY**-shun **THAIR**-ah-pee)	The treatment of neoplastic disease by using x-rays or gamma rays, usually from a cobalt source, to deter the growth of malignant cells by decreasing the rate of cell division or impairing DNA synthesis.
radioactivity (**ray**-dee-oh-**ak**-**TIV**-ih-tee)	The ability of a substance to emit rays or particles (alpha, beta, or gamma) from its nucleus.
radiographer (**ray**-dee-**OG**-rah-fer) radi/o = radiation; also refers to radius graph/o = to record -er = one who	An allied health professional trained to use x-ray machines and other imaging equipment to produce images of the internal structures of the body; also known as a radiologic technologist.
radioimmunoassay (**ray**-dee-oh-**im**-yoo-noh-**ASS**-ay) radi/o = radiation; also refers to radius immun/o = immune, protection -assay = to evaluate	A technique in radiology used to determine the concentration of an antigen, antibody, or other protein in the serum.
radioisotope (**ray**-dee-oh-**EYE**-soh-tohp)	A radioactive isotope of an element, used for therapeutic and diagnostic purposes.
radiologist (ray-dee-**ALL**-oh-jist) radi/o = radiation; also refers to radius -logist = one who specializes in the study of	A physician who specializes in radiology.
radiology (ray-dee-**ALL**-oh-jee) radi/o = radiation; also refers to radius -logy = the study of	The study of the diagnostic and therapeutic uses of x-rays; also known as **roentgenology**.
radiolucent (**ray**-dee-oh-**LOO**-sent)	Pertaining to materials that allow x-rays to penetrate with a minimum of absorption.
radionuclide (radioisotope) (ray-dee-oh-**NOO**-kleed) (**ray**-dee-oh-**EYE**-soh-tohp)	An isotope (or nuclide) that undergoes radioactive decay.
radiopaque (ray-dee-oh-**PAYK**)	Not permitting the passage of x-rays or other radiant energy.

radiopharmaceutical (**ray**-dee-oh-farm-ah-soo-tih-kal) radi/o = radiation; also refers to radius pharmac/o = drugs, medicine	A drug that contains radioactive atoms.
recumbent (rih-**KUM**-bent)	Lying down or leaning backward.
roentgenology (**rent**-jen-**ALL**-oh-jee)	See *radiology.*
scanning	A technique for carefully studying an area, organ, or system of the body by recording and displaying an image of the area.
single-photon emission computed tomography (single-**FOH**-ton ee-**MISH**-un kom-**PEW**-ted toh-**MOG**-rah-fee) **(SPECT)**	A variation of computerized tomography (CT) scanning in which gamma camera detectors rotate around the patient's body collecting data. The data are summarized into a three-dimensional representation.
supine (soo-**PIGHN**)	Lying horizontally on the back.
teletherapy (tell-eh-**THAIR**-ah-pee) tel/e = distance -therapy = treatment	Radiation therapy administered by a machine that is positioned at some distance from the patient.
tomography (toh-**MOG**-rah-fee) tom/o = to cut; section -graphy = process of recording	An x-ray technique that produces a film representing a detailed cross section of tissue structure at a predetermined depth.
transducer (trans-**DOO**-sir)	A handheld device that sends and receives a soundwave signal.
ultrasound (**ULL**-trah-sound) ultra- = beyond	Sound waves at the very high frequency of over 20,000 kHz (vibrations per second).
uptake (**UP**-tayk)	The drawing up or absorption of a substance.
xeroradiography (**zee**-roh-ray-dee-**OG**-rah-fee) xer/o = dry radi/o = radiation; also refers to radius -graphy = process of recording	A diagnostic x-ray technique in which an image is produced electrically rather than chemically, permitting lower exposure times and radiation of lower energy than that of ordinary x-rays.

Word Elements

The following word elements appear in terms used to describe radiology and diagnostic imaging treatments and procedures. As you review the list, pronounce each word element aloud twice and check the appropriate box after you "say it." Write the definition for the example word given for each word element. You may use your medical dictionary.

WORD ELEMENT	PRONUNCIATION	"SAY IT"	MEANING
angi/o **angi**ography	**AN**-jee-oh an-jee-**OG**-rah-fee	☐	vessel
anter/o **antero**posterior	**AN**-ter-oh **an**-ter-oh-poss-**TEER**-ee-or	☐	front
aort/o **aort**ogram	ay-**OR**-toh ay-**OR**-toh-gram	☐	aorta
arthr/o **arthr**ography	**AR**-throh ar-**THROG**-rah-fee	☐	joint
arteri/o **arteri**ogram	ar-**TEE**-ree-oh ar-**TEE**-ree-oh-gram	☐	artery
bronch/o **bronch**ography	**BRONG**-koh brong-**KOG**-rah-fee	☐	bronchus, airway
cardi/o **cardi**ocatheterization	**KAR**-dee-oh **kar**-dee-oh-**kath**-eh-ter-ih-**ZAY**-shun	☐	heart
chol/e **chol**ecystogram	**KOH**-lee **koh**-lee-**SIS**-toh-gram	☐	bile
cine- **cine**angiogram	**SIN**-ee **sin**-ee-**AN**-jee-oh-gram	☐	pertaining to movement
cyst/o **cyst**ourethrography	**SIS**-toh sis-toh-yoo-ree-**THROG**-rah-fee	☐	bladder, sac, or cyst
echo- **echo**cardiography	**EK**-oh **ek**-oh-**kar**-dee-**OG**-rah-fee	☐	sound
fluor/o **fluor**oscopy	**FLOO**-roh floo-or-**OSS**-koh-pee	☐	luminous
hyster/o **hyster**osalpingogram	**HIS**-ter-oh **his**-ter-oh-**sal**-**PING**-oh-gram	☐	uterus
immun/o radio**immun**oassay	im-**YOO**-noh **ray**-dee-oh-im-yoo-noh-**ASS**-ay	☐	immune, protection
lymph/o **lymph**angiogram	**LIM**-foh lim-**FAN**-jee-oh-gram	☐	lymph
mamm/o **mamm**ography	**MAM**-oh mam-**OG**-rah-fee	☐	breast
myel/o **myel**ography	**MY**-el-oh my-el-**OG**-rah-fee	☐	bone marrow, spinal cord

poster/o **poster**oanterior	**POSS**-ter-oh **poss**-ter-oh-an-**TEE**-ree-or	☐	back
pyel/o intravenous **pyel**ogram	**PYE**-eh-loh in-trah-**VEE**-nus **PYE**-eh-loh-gram	☐	renal pelvis
radi/o **radi**opaque	**RAY**-dee-oh ray-dee-oh-**PAYK**	☐	radiation; also refers to radius
ren/o **ren**al	**REE**-noh **REE**-nal	☐	kidney
son/o **son**ogram	**SOH**-noh **SOH**-noh-gram	☐	sound
tel/e **tel**etherapy	**TELL**-eh tell-eh-**THAIR**-oh-pee	☐	distance
tom/o **tom**ography	**TOH**-moh toh-**MOG**-rah-fee	☐	to cut; section
ultra- **ultra**sound	**ULL**-tra **ULL**-trah-sound	☐	beyond
ven/o **ven**ography	**VEE**-noh vee-**NOG**-rah-fee	☐	vein
xer/o **xer**oradiography	**ZEE**-roh **zee**-roh-ray-dee-**OG**-rah-fee	☐	dry

Common Abbreviations

ABBREVIATION	MEANING	ABBREVIATION	MEANING
AP	anteroposterior	**ERCP**	endoscopic retrograde cholangiopancreatography
Ba	barium	**Fx**	fracture
BE	barium enema	**IVC**	intravenous cholangiography
CAT	computed axial tomography	**IVP**	intravenous pyelogram
C-spine	cervical spine (film)	**IVU**	intravenous urography
CT	computed tomography	**KUB**	kidneys, ureters, bladder
CXR	chest x-ray	**LGI**	lower gastrointestinal (series)
DSA	digital subtraction angiography	**MRA**	magnetic resonance angiography
DSR	dynamic spatial reconstructor	**MRI**	magnetic resonance imaging
ECHO	echocardiogram		

NMR	nuclear magnetic resonance (imaging)
NPO	nothing by mouth
PA	posteroanterior
PET	positron emission tomography
PTC, PTHC	percutaneous transhepatic cholangiography
rad	radiation absorbed dose
RAI	radioactive iodine
RIA	radioimmunoassay
SBS	small bowel series
SPECT	single-photon emission computed tomography
UGI	upper gastrointestinal (series)
u/s	ultrasound

Written and Audio Terminology Review

Review each of the following terms from this chapter. Study the spelling of each term and write the definition in the space provided. If you have the Audio CD available, listen to each term, pronounce it, and check the box once you are comfortable saying the word. Check definitions by looking the term up in the glossary/index.

TERM	PRONUNCIATION	DEFINITION
angiocardiography	☐ an-jee-oh-kar-dee-**OG**-rah-fee	____________
angiography	☐ **an**-jee-**OG**-rah-fee	____________
anteroposterior	☐ **an**-ter-oh-poss-**TEER**-ee-or	____________
aortogram	☐ ay-**OR**-toh-gram	____________
aortography	☐ **ay**-or-**TOG**-rah-fee	____________
arteriogram	☐ ar-**TEE**-ree-oh-gram	____________
arteriography	☐ **ar**-tee-ree-**OG**-rah-fee	____________
arthrography	☐ ar-**THROG**-rah-fee	____________
axial	☐ **AK**-see-al	____________
barium enema (BE)	☐ **BAIR**-ree-um **EN**-eh-mah (BE)	____________
barium swallow	☐ **BAIR**-ree-um **SWALL**-oh	____________
betatron	☐ **BAY**-tah-tron	____________
brachytherapy	☐ **brak**-ee-**THAIR**-ah-pee	____________
bronchography	☐ brong-**KOG**-rah-fee	____________

cardiocatheterization	☐ kar-dee-o-**kath**-eh-ter-ih-**ZAY**-shun	________
cerebral angiography	☐ **SER**-eh-bral (seh-**REE**-bral) **an**-jee-**OG**-rah-fee	________
cholangiography	☐ koh-**lan**-jee-**OG**-rah-fee	________
cholecystogram	☐ koh-lee-**SIS**-toh-gram	________
cholecystography	☐ koh-lee-sis-**TOG**-rah-fee	________
cineangiogram	☐ sin-ee-**AN**-jee-oh-gram	________
cineradiography	☐ **sin**-eh-**ray**-dee-**OG**-rah-fee	________
computed axial tomography (CAT)	☐ kom-**PEW**-ted **AK**-see-al toh-**MOG**-rah-fee (CAT)	________
computed tomography	☐ kom-**PEW**-ted toh-**MOG**-rah-fee	________
cystourethrogram	☐ sis-toh-yoo-ree-**THROW**-gram	________
digital radiography	☐ **DIJ**-ih-tal ray-dee-**OG**-rah-fee	________
digital subtraction angiography (DSA)	☐ **DIJ**-ih-tal sub-**TRAK**-shun **an**-jee-**OG**-rah-fee (DSA)	________
Doppler	☐ **DOP**-ler	________
echocardiography	☐ **ek**-oh-kar-dee-**OG**-rah-fee	________
eversion	☐ ee-**VER**-shun	________
extension	☐ eks-**TEN**-shun	________
flexion	☐ **FLEK**-shun	________
fluorescence	☐ floo-oh-**RES**-ens	________
fluoroscopy	☐ floo-or-**OSS**-koh-pee	________
gamma	☐ **GAM**-ah	________
gamma rays	☐ **GAM**-ah rays	________
hysterosalpingogram	☐ **his**-ter-oh-**sal**-**PING**-oh-gram	________
hysterosalpingography	☐ **his**-ter-oh-**sal**-ping-**OG**-rah-fee	________
interstitial	☐ in-ter-**STISH**-al	________
intravenous pyelogram	☐ in-trah-**VEE**-nus **PYE**-eh-loh-gram	________

Term		Pronunciation	
inversion	☐	in-**VER**-zhun	______
ionization	☐	eye-oh-nye-**ZAY**-shun	______
irradiation	☐	ih-ray-dee-**AY**-shun	______
lethal	☐	**LEE**-thal	______
linear accelerator	☐	**LIN**-ee-ar ak-**SELL**-er-**ay**-tor	______
lymphangiogram	☐	lim-**FAN**-jee-oh-gram	______
lymphangiography	☐	lim-**fan**-jee-**OG**-rah-fee	______
magnetic resonance imaging (MRI)	☐	mag-**NET**-ik **REZ**-oh-nans **IM**-ij-ing (MRI)	______
mammography	☐	mam-**OG**-rah-fee	______
myelography	☐	my-eh-**LOG**-rah-fee	______
nuclear medicine	☐	**NOO**-klee-ar medicine	______
orthovoltage	☐	or-thoh-**VOHL**-tij	______
palliative	☐	**PAL**-ee-ah-tiv	______
piezoelectric	☐	pie-**EE**-zoh-eh-**lek**-trik	______
positron emission tomography (PET)	☐	**POZ**-ih-tron ee-**MISH**-un toh-**MOG**-rah-fee (PET)	______
posteroanterior	☐	poss-ter-oh-an-**TEER**-ee-or	______
prone	☐	**PROHN**	______
pyelography	☐	pie-eh-**LOG**-rah-fee	______
rad	☐	**RAD**	______
radiation therapy	☐	ray-dee-**AY**-shun **THAIR**-ah-pee	______
radioactive iodine uptake	☐	**ray**-dee-oh-**AK**-tiv **EYE**-oh-dine **UP**-tayk	______
radioactivity	☐	**ray**-dee-oh-ak-**TIV**-ih-tee	______
radiographer	☐	ray-dee-**OG**-rah-fer	______
radioimmunoassay	☐	**ray**-dee-oh-im-yoo-noh-**ASS**-ay	______
radioisotope	☐	**ray**-dee-oh-**EYE**-soh-tohp	______
radiologist	☐	ray-dee-**ALL**-oh-jist	______
radiology	☐	ray-dee-**ALL**-oh-jee	______
radiolucent	☐	ray-dee-oh-**LOO**-sent	______

Term		Pronunciation	
radionuclide	☐	ray-dee-oh-**NOO**-kleed	
radiopaque	☐	ray-dee-oh-**PAYK**	
radiopharmaceutical	☐	ray-dee-oh-farm-ah-**SOO**-tih-kal	
recumbent	☐	rih-**KUM**-bent	
renal angiography	☐	**REE**-nal an-jee-**OG**-rah-fee	
roentgenology	☐	rent-jen-**ALL**-oh-jee	
scanning	☐	**SCAN**-ing	
single-photon emission computed tomography (SPECT)	☐	single **FOH**-ton ee-**MISH**-un kom-**PEW**-ted toh-**MOG**-rah-fee (SPECT)	
sonogram	☐	**SOH**-noh-gram	
supine	☐	soo-**PIGHN**	
teletherapy	☐	tell-eh-**THAIR**-ah-pee	
tomography	☐	toh-**MOG**-rah-fee	
transducer	☐	trans-**DOO**-sir	
ultrasonography	☐	ull-trah-son-**OG**-rah-fee	
ultrasound	☐	**ULL**-trah-sound	
uptake	☐	**UP**-tayk	
venography	☐	vee-**NOG**-rah-fee	
voiding cystourethrography	☐	**VOYD**-ing sis-toh-yoo-ree-**THROG**-rah-fee	
x-rays	☐	**ECKS**-rays	
xeroradiography	☐	**zear**-roh-ray-dee-**OG**-rah-fee	

Chapter Review Exercises

The following exercises provide a more in-depth review of the chapter material. Your goal in these exercises is to complete each section at a minimum 80% level of accuracy. If you score below 80% in any area, return to the appropriate section in the chapter and read the material again. A place has been provided for your score at the end of each section.

A. Term to Definition

Define each term by writing the definition in the space provided. Check the box if you are able to complete this exercise correctly the first time (without referring to the answers). Each correct answer is worth 10 points. Record your score in the space provided at the end of the exercise.

☐ 1. mammography ______________________________

☐ 2. intravenous pyelogram ______________________________

☐ 3. hysterosalpingogram ______________________________

☐ 4. posteroanterior ______________________________

☐ 5. cystourethrogram ______________________________

☐ 6. fluoroscopy ______________________________

☐ 7. radiology ______________________________

☐ 8. radiation therapy ______________________________

☐ 9. lymphangiogram ______________________________

☐ 10. lethal ______________________________

Number correct ______ × 10 points/correct answer: Your score _____%

B. Matching Abbreviations

Match the abbreviations on the left with the correct definition on the right. Each correct response is worth 10 points. When you have completed the exercise, record your score in the space provided at the end of the exercise.

_____	1. AP	a. computed axial tomography
_____	2. BE	b. radioimmunoassay
_____	3. CXR	c. computed tomography
_____	4. IVP	d. retrograde pyelogram
_____	5. KUB	e. intravenous pyelogram
_____	6. MRI	f. anteroposterior
_____	7. PET	g. chest x-ray
_____	8. RIA	h. barium enema
_____	9. CAT	i. kidneys, ureters, bladder
_____	10. SPECT	j. magnetic resonance imaging
		k. positron emission tomography
		l. posteroanterior
		m. single-photon emission computed tomography

Number correct ______ × 10 points/correct answer: Your score _____%

C. Crossword Puzzle

Read the clues carefully and complete the puzzle. Each crossword puzzle answer is worth 10 points. When you have completed the puzzle, total your points and enter your score in the space provided at the end of the exercise.

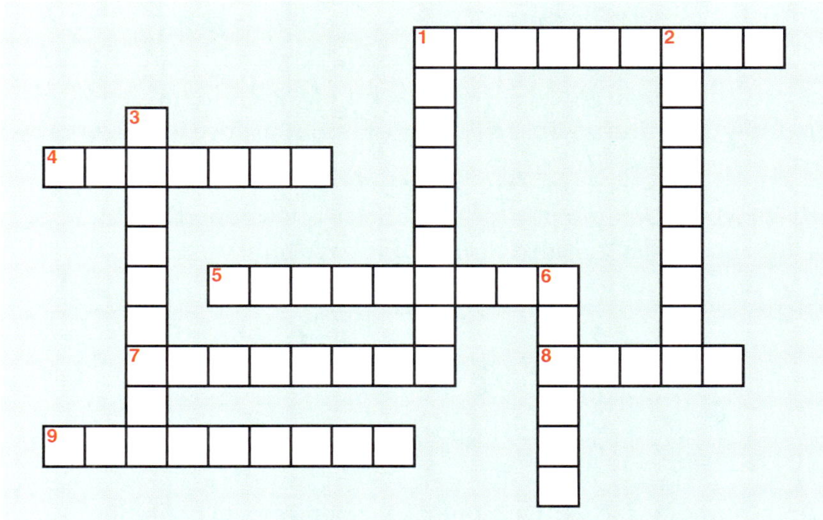

ACROSS
1 Movement toward the body
4 Bending (decreases the angle)
5 Recumbent lateral position for x-ray
7 Turning outward
8 Lying flat with face downward
9 Straightening (increases the angle)

DOWN
1 Movement away from the body
2 Turning inward
3 Lying down
6 Lying horizontally on the back

Number correct _______ × 10 points/correct answer: Your score ______%

D. Completion

Complete each sentence with the most appropriate answer. Each correct answer is worth 10 points. Record your score in the space provided at the end of the exercise.

1. X-ray of the uterus and the fallopian tubes, by injecting a contrast material into these structures is known as:

   ____

2. The introduction of contrast medium into the lumbar subarachnoid space through a lumbar puncture to visualize the spinal cord and vertebral canal through x-ray examination is known as:

   ____

3. The process of taking x-rays of the soft tissue of the breast, to detect various benign and/or malignant growths before they can be felt, is known as:

   ____

4. A procedure in which sound waves are transmitted into the body structures as a small transducer is passed over the patient's skin is called:

   ____

5. A diagnostic procedure for studying the structure and motion of the heart is known as:

   ____

6. A bronchial examination via x-ray following the coating of the bronchi with a radiopaque substance is termed:

   ____

7. The visualization of the gallbladder through x-ray following the oral ingestion of pills containing a radiopaque iodinated dye is known as an oral:

____

8. The visualization of the outline of the major bile ducts following an intravenous injection of a contrast medium is known as an intravenous:

____

9. A radiographic procedure that provides visualization of the entire urinary tract—the kidneys, ureters, bladder, and urethra—after intravenous injection of a contrast dye is known as an intravenous:

____

10. A specialized diagnostic procedure in which a catheter is introduced into a large vein or artery, usually of an arm or a leg, and is then threaded through the circulatory system to the heart is an:

____

Number correct ______ × 10 points/correct answer: Your score _____%

E. Matching Procedures

Match the diagnostic procedures on the left with one of the appropriate definitions on the right. Each correct answer is worth 10 points. When you have completed the exercise, record your score in the space provided at the end of the exercise.

_____ 1. ERCP

_____ 2. voiding cystourethrography

_____ 3. lung scan

_____ 4. MRI

_____ 5. cerebral angiography

_____ 6. xeroradiography

_____ 7. x-rays

_____ 8. small bowel follow-through

_____ 9. pelvic ultrasound

_____ 10. renal ultrasound

a. The visual imaging of the distribution of ventilation or blood flow in the lungs by scanning the lungs after the patient has been injected with, or has inhaled, radioactive material

b. Oral administration of a radiopaque contrast medium, barium sulfate, which flows through the GI system while x-ray films are obtained at timed intervals to observe the progression of the barium through the small intestines

c. A diagnostic x-ray technique used to produce an electrical image rather than a chemical image

d. A type of cholangiopancreatography that examines the filling of the pancreatic and biliary ducts through direct radiographic visualization with a fiberoptic endoscope

e. Visualization of the cerebrovascular system via x-ray made possible by the injection of a radiopaque contrast medium into an arterial blood vessel (carotid, femoral, or brachial)

f. The use of high-energy electromagnetic waves passing through the body onto a photographic film, to produce a picture of the internal structures of the body for diagnosis and therapy

g. A noninvasive procedure that uses high-frequency sound waves to examine the abdomen and pelvis

h. An ultrasound of the kidneys useful in distinguishing between fluid-filled cysts and solid masses, detecting renal calculi, identifying obstructions, and evaluating transplanted kidneys

i. A noninvasive scanning procedure that provides visualization of fluid, soft tissue, and bony structures without the use of radiation

j. X-ray visualization of the bladder and urethra during the voiding process, after the bladder has been filled with a contrast material

Number correct ______ × 10 points/correct answer: Your score _____%

F. Definition to Term

Using the following definitions, identify and provide the medical term(s) to match the definition. Each correct answer is worth 10 points. Record your score in the space provided at the end.

1. A series of x-ray films allowing visualization of internal structures after the IV introduction of a radiopaque substance

   ____

   (one word)

2. Infusion of a radiopaque contrast medium into the rectum and held in the lower intestinal tract while x-rays are made of the lower GI tract

   ____

   (two words)

3. A painless, noninvasive diagnostic x-ray using ionizing radiation and producing a cross-section image of the tissue structure being examined

   ____

   (two or three words)

4. Images of blood vessels only, appearing without any background

   ____

   (three words)

5. Visualization of the metabolic activity of body structures shown through computerized color-coded images, which indicate the degree and intensity of the metabolic process

   ____

   (three words)

6. Radiographic visualization of the entire urinary tract

   ____

   (one word)

7. Delivery of ionizing radiation to accomplish the destruction of rapidly multiplying tumor cells

   ____

   (two words)

8. Detection of the degree of uptake of a previous IV injection of a radionuclide material that has been absorbed by bone tissue

   ____

   (two words)

9. A noninvasive scanning technique that enables the visualization of the shape, size, and consistency of the spleen after the IV injection of radioactive red blood cells

   ____

   (two words)

10. An ultrasound examination important in distinguishing solid thyroid nodules from cystic nodules

    ____

    (two words)

Number correct ______ × 10 points/correct answer: Your score ______%

G. Word Search

Using the definitions listed, identify the radiological diagnostic imaging term, then find and circle it in the puzzle. The words may be read up, down, diagonally, across, or backward. Each correct answer is worth 10 points. Record your score in the space provided at the end of the exercise.

Example: Bending (decreases the angle)

flexion

1. A medical doctor who specializes in roentgenology is known as a:

2. A health professional who takes x-rays is known as a:

3. High-frequency sound waves are called:

4. Something that does not permit passage of x-rays is said to be:

5. Something that allows x-rays to penetrate is said to be:

F	L	E	X	I	O	N	O	A	T	T	S	I	S	L
R	O	I	R	E	T	S	O	P	O	R	E	T	N	A
L	A	B	Y	A	T	U	T	E	A	A	G	R	Y	C
T	A	D	S	A	I	H	S	D	I	N	E	E	R	I
I	S	D	I	R	G	I	I	L	E	S	I	H	A	T
P	I	S	Y	O	M	O	A	N	O	D	R	P	D	U
L	T	E	D	E	L	H	I	M	M	U	I	A	I	E
E	I	E	E	U	T	O	E	X	I	C	N	R	O	C
D	V	X	C	V	I	N	G	N	T	E	P	G	P	A
C	N	E	C	I	I	N	E	I	T	R	N	O	A	M
L	N	U	U	R	M	T	A	R	S	I	A	I	Q	R
T	C	H	O	L	Y	M	A	J	W	T	V	D	U	A
R	N	O	I	S	O	R	T	I	E	P	R	A	E	H
O	U	I	A	I	A	S	U	M	L	O	S	R	P	P
S	J	O	L	S	Y	R	S	H	C	L	S	Y	A	O
I	N	N	U	N	O	I	T	A	I	D	A	R	R	I
S	O	O	S	D	S	R	S	L	F	L	E	P	X	D
P	C	A	N	M	I	G	A	I	U	E	H	P	Y	A
T	Q	I	D	A	R	E	P	Y	M	C	K	L	T	R

6. The part of the sonograph that sends and receives sound wave signals is known as the:

____

7. A treatment or medication that soothes or relieves is said to be:

____

8. Exposure to radiant energy is called:

____

9. Direction of x-ray beam from front to back is termed:

____

10. A drug that contains radioactive atoms is called a:

____

Number correct ______ × 10 points/correct answer: Your score _____%

H. Spelling

Circle the correctly spelled term in each pairing of words. Each correct answer is worth 10 points. Record your score in the space provided at the end of the exercise.

1. flouroscopy	fluoroscopy
2. angography	angiography
3. cinoradiography	cineradiography
4. myelography	mylography
5. brachitherapy	brachytherapy
6. arterography	arteriography
7. rentgenology	roentgenology
8. cystourethrogram	cystourethergram
9. phlebography	phelbography
10. echogram	eckogram

Number correct ______ × 10 points/correct answer: Your score _____%

I. Word Element Review

Read the following definitions carefully and write the correct word element in the space provided. (Note: Each word element should be written as it appears in your textbook, using the combining vowel.) Each correct answer is worth 10 points. Record your score in the space provided at the end of the exercise.

Example: The word element for vessel is _angi/o_

1. The word element for *joint* is _______________
2. The word element for *bronchus* is _______________
3. The word element for *gall* or *bile* is _______________
4. The prefix that means "pertaining to movement" is _______________
5. The word element that means "luminous" is _______________
6. The word element that means "breast" is _______________
7. The word element that means "renal pelvis" is _______________
8. The word element that means "to cut or section" is _______________

9. The word element that means "dry" is ______________________

10. The prefix that means "beyond" is ______________________

Number correct ______ × 10 points/correct answer: Your score _______%

J. True or False

Read each statement carefully and circle the correct answer as true or false. HINT: Pay close attention to the word elements written in **bold** as you make your decision. If the statement is false, identify the meaning of that word element. Each correct answer is worth 10 points. Record your score in the space provided at the end of the exercise.

1. An angio**cardio**graphy is used to obtain detailed information about the structure and function of the heart chambers, valves, and the great vessels.

   True False

   If your answer is False, what does *cardi/o* mean? ______________________

2. An **arterio**graphy is the x-ray visualization of arteries following the introduction of a radiopaque contrast medium into the bloodstream through a specific vessel by way of a catheter.

   True False

   If your answer is False, what does *arteri/o* mean? ______________________

3. A **ren**al angiography is the x-ray visualization of the heart.

   True False

   If your answer is False, what does *ren/o* mean? ______________________

4. An **arthro**graphy is the process of taking x-rays inside of a joint, after a contrast medium has been injected into the joint.

   True False

   If your answer is False, what does *arthr/o* mean? ______________________

5. A **broncho**graphy is the x-ray examination of the stomach after coating it with a contrast medium.

   True False

   If your answer is False, what does *bronch/o* mean ______________________

6. An intravenous **chol**angiography is the process of visualizing and outlining the major bile ducts following an intravenous injection of a contrast medium.

   True False

   If your answer is False, what does *chol/e* mean? ______________________

7. A voiding **cysto**urethrography is the x-ray visualization of the bladder and urethra during the voiding process, after the bladder has been filled with a contrast material.

   True False

   If your answer is False, what does *cyst/o* mean? ______________________

8. A **lymph**angiography is an x-ray assessment of the urinary system.

   True False

   If your answer is False, what does *lymph/o* mean? ______________________

9. A hystero**salpingo**graphy is an x-ray of the uterus and the fallopian tubes by injecting a contrast material into these structures.

   True False

   If your answer is False, what does *salping/o* mean? ______________________

10. **Mammo**graphy is the process of taking x-rays of the soft tissue of the thigh.

True False

If your answer is False, what does *mamm/o* mean? ______________________

Number correct ______ × 10 points/correct answer: Your score ______%

Answers to Chapter Review Exercises

A. Term to Definition

1. the process of taking x-rays of breast tissue
2. the procedure in which a dye is introduced into a vein to visualize the renal pelvis
3. an x-ray of the uterus and fallopian tubes
4. an x-ray view that directs the beam from the back to the front
5. an x-ray of the urethra and bladder
6. the process of using x-ray and a fluorescent screen to view internal body organs as they function
7. the study of the diagnostic and therapeutic uses of x-rays
8. the treatment of neoplastic disease by using x-rays or gamma rays
9. the process of taking x-rays of the lymph glands and lymphatic vessels after injecting a contrast medium
10. something that is capable of causing death

B. Matching Abbreviations

1. f
2. h
3. g
4. e
5. i
6. j
7. k
8. b
9. a
10. m

C. Crossword Puzzle

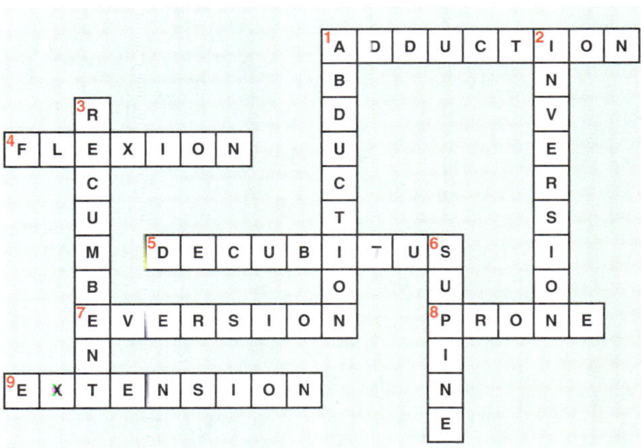

D. Completion

1. hysterosalpingography
2. myelography
3. mammography
4. ultrasonography
5. echocardiography
6. bronchography
7. cholecystography
8. cholangiography
9. pyelography
10. angiocardiography

E. Matching Procedures

1. d
2. j
3. a
4. i
5. e
6. c
7. f
8. b
9. g
10. h

Definition to Term

1. angiography
2. barium enema
3. computed tomography *or* computed axial tomography
4. digital subtraction angiography
5. positron emission tomography
6. pyelography
7. radiation therapy
8. bone scan
9. spleen scan
10. thyroid echogram

G. Word Search

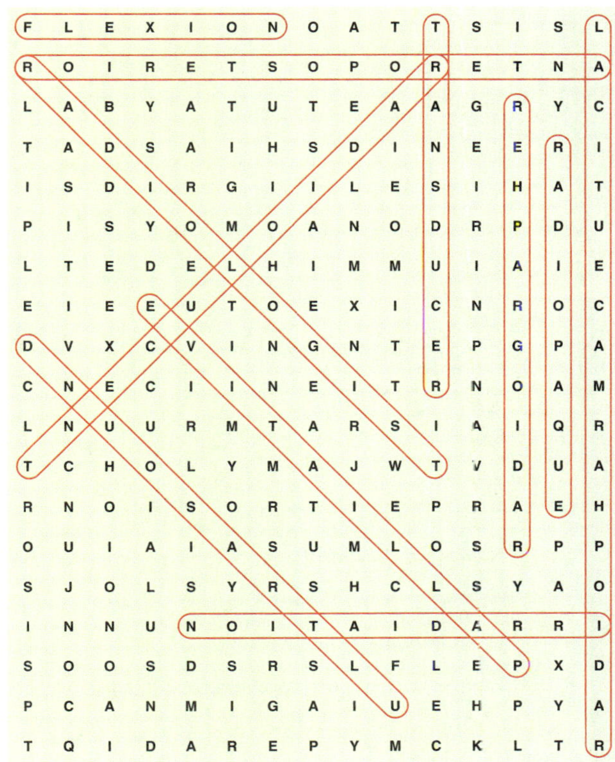

H. Spelling

1. fluoroscopy
2. angiography
3. cineradiography
4. myelography
5. brachytherapy
6. arteriography
7. roentgenology
8. cystourethrogram
9. phlebography
10. echogram

I. Word Element Review

1. arthr/o
2. bronch/o
3. chol/e
4. cine-
5. fluor/o
6. mamm/o
7. pyel/o
8. tom/o
9. xer/o
10. ultra-

J. True or False

1. True
2. True
3. False; ren/o = kidney
4. True
5. False; bronch/o = airway, bronchus
6. True
7. True
8. False; lymph/o = lymph
9. True
10. False; mamm/o = breast

CHAPTER 21

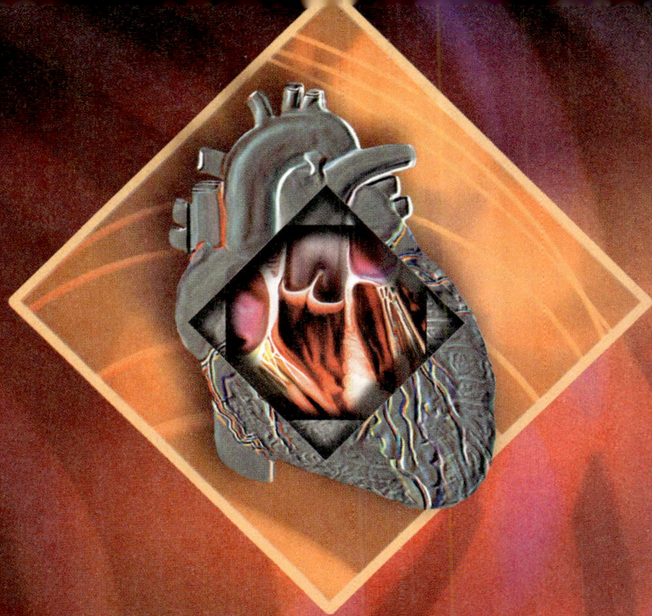

Oncology (Cancer Medicine)

CHAPTER CONTENT

KEY COMPETENCIES

Upon completing this chapter and the review exercises at the end of the chapter, the learner should be able to:

1. Identify and define 15 pathological conditions and five treatment methods associated with oncology.
2. Identify at least 10 diagnostic techniques used in diagnosis and treatment of oncological disorders.
3. Correctly spell and pronounce each new term introduced in this chapter using the Activity CD-ROM and Audio CD, if available.
4. Identify at least 10 abbreviations common to oncology.
5. List and define six surgical procedures used in the diagnosis or cure of malignant tumors.
6. List and define three tumor responses to radiation therapy.

OVERVIEW

When we hear that **cancer** causes more deaths in children between the ages of 3 and 15 than any other disease, it is a jolting reminder that cancer can strike at any age. It is estimated that one of every four Americans alive today will develop cancer during his or her lifetime. Cancer is now the second leading cause of death in the United States.

The term *cancer* does not refer to only one disease; it actually refers to a group of diseases, consisting of more than 100 different types. Although cancer can originate in almost any body organ, the most common site for cancer in women is the breast and the most common site for cancer in men is the prostate gland. The prognosis, or outlook, for a patient who is diagnosed with cancer will depend on many factors that include, but are not limited to, the type of cancer, the stage of the disease, the patient's age and general state of health, and the response to treatment.

This chapter concentrates on a discussion of many of the terms associated with the study of cancer, the characteristics of benign and malignant tumors, predisposing factors that influence one's susceptibility to developing cancer, some of the more common types of cancer, and the diagnostic techniques and procedures associated with the treatment of cancer. It is not designed to provide an in-depth study of cancer.

Many pathological conditions in this chapter have already been discussed in previous body system chapters. This should reinforce the concept that cancer can affect almost any body system.

Cancer Terms

Any discussion of cancer should begin with a review of some terms that provide a foundation for understanding this complex disease. The term **neoplasia** is used to define the development of an abnormal growth of new cells that is unresponsive to normal growth control mechanisms. This development may be **benign** or **malignant.** The term **neoplasm** refers to the growth itself; that is, any abnormal growth of new tissue that serves no useful purpose. It, too, may be benign or malignant. The term *neoplasm* is used synonymously with **tumor.** When the term *neoplasm* is used in the discussion of cancer, the word *malignant* must precede it, as in malignant neoplasm equals malignant tumor.

During the developmental stages, cells are under the control of **deoxyribonucleic acid (DNA)**—the carrier of genetic information. They undergo changes in their structural and functional properties as they form the different tissues of the body. In other words, the immature cell changes many times in its process of becoming a mature cell with clearly defined functions. This process of cells becoming specialized and differentiated both physically and functionally is known as **differentiation.** Cells that look and act like the parent cell, or tissue of origin, are said to be well differentiated.

Neoplasms that consist of cells that do not resemble the tissue of origin are said to be poorly differentiated or undifferentiated. The loss of cellular differentiation and reversion to a more primitive form is called **anaplasia.** Anaplastic cell division is not under the control of DNA. Anaplasia may occur as a response to overpowering destructive conditions in surrounding tissue or inside the cell. Anaplasia is not reversible and is considered a classic characteristic of malignant tumors.

Abnormal cells multiply to form nests of malignant tumors (malignant neoplasms). Malignant tumors contain cells that have the capability to detach from the tumor mass, overrun surrounding tissues, and spread to distant sites in the body via the lymph or blood. Cancers are inclined to grow rapidly, invade, crowd, and destroy normal tissues; they tend to recur when removed.

Malignant neoplasms that grow in the tissue of origin are called primary malignant tumors. Tumors that grow in tissues remote from the tissue of origin are called secondary or metastatic neoplasms. Malignant neoplasms that are untreated are usually fatal.

If the established growth is benign, it is noncancerous and the cells are well differentiated. If the established growth is malignant, it is cancerous and the cells are poorly differentiated. **Metastasis** is the term used to describe the process by which malignant cells spread to other parts of the body.

The medical specialty concerned with the study of malignancy is known as oncology. The physician who specializes in the study and treatment of neoplastic diseases, particularly cancer, is known as an oncologist.

Vocabulary

The following vocabulary words are frequently used when discussing cancer or oncology.

WORD	DEFINITION
adjuvant (**AD**-joo-vant)	A substance, especially a drug, added to a prescription to assist in the action of the main ingredient.
adjuvant therapy	Treatment of a disease with a substance, especially a drug, that enhances the main ingredient. For example, chemotherapy may be used as **adjuvant** therapy to radiation.
anaplasia (**an**-ah-**PLAY**-zee-ah) ana- = not, without plas/o = formation, development -ia = condition	A change in the structure and orientation of cells characterized by a loss of specialization and reversion to a more primitive form.
antimetabolite (**an**-tih-meh-**TAB**-oh-light)	A class of **antineoplastic** drugs used to treat cancer; these drugs are most effective against rapidly growing tumors.
antineoplastic (**an**-tih-**nee**-oh-**PLASS**-tik) anti- = against ne/o = new plas/o = formation, development -tic = pertaining to	Of or pertaining to a substance, procedure, or measure that prevents the proliferation of malignant cells.
benign (bee-**NINE**)	Noncancerous and therefore not an immediate threat, even though treatment eventually may be required for health or cosmetic reasons; not life threatening.

cancer	A neoplasm characterized by the uncontrolled growth of anaplastic cells that tend to invade surrounding tissue and to metastasize to distant body sites.
carcinogen (kar-**SIN**-oh-jen) **carcin/o** = cancer **-gen** = that which generates	A substance or agent that causes the development or increases the incidence of cancer.
carcinoma (kar-sin-**NOH**-mah) **carcin/o** = cancer **-oma** = tumor	A malignant neoplasm.
carcinoma in situ (CIS) **carcin/o** = cancer **-oma** = tumor	A premalignant neoplasm that has not invaded the basement membrane but shows cytologic characteristics of cancer.
chemotherapy (**kee**-moh-**THAIR**-ah-pee) **chem/o** = chemical reaction **-therapy** = treatment	The use of chemical agents to destroy cancer cells on a selective basis.
dedifferentiation (dee-diff-er-en-she-**AY**-shun)	See *anaplasia*.
deoxyribonucleic acid (DNA) (dee-ock-see-rye-boh-noo-**KLEE**-ic **ASS**-id)	A large nucleic acid molecule found principally in the chromosomes of the nucleus of a cell that is the carrier of genetic information.
differentiation (diff-er-en-she-**AY**-shun)	A process in development in which unspecialized cells or tissues are systemically modified and altered to achieve specific and characteristic physical forms, physiologic functions, and chemical properties.
encapsulated (en-**CAP**-soo-**LAY**-ted)	Enclosed in fibrous or membranous sheaths.
fractionation (frak-shun-**AY**-shun)	In radiology, the division of the total dose of **radiation** into small doses administered at intervals in an effort to minimize tissue damage.
infiltrative (in-fill-**TRAY**-tiv)	Possessing the ability to invade or penetrate adjacent tissue.
invasive (in-**VAY**-siv)	Characterized by a tendency to spread, infiltrate, and intrude.
ionizing radiation (**EYE**-oh-nigh-zing ray-dee-**AY**-shun)	High-energy x-rays that possess the ability to kill cells or retard their growth.
linear accelerator (**LIN**-ee-ar ak-**SELL**-er-**ay**-tor)	An apparatus for accelerating charged subatomic particles used in **radiotherapy**, physics research, and the production of radionuclides.
lumpectomy (lum-**PEK**-toh mee)	Surgical removal of only the tumor and the immediate adjacent breast tissue; a method of treatment for breast cancer when detected in the early stage of the disease.
malignant (mah-**LIG**-nant)	Tending to become worse and cause death.

metastasis (meh-**TASS**-tah-sis) **meta-** = beyond, after **-stasis** = stopping; controlling	The process by which tumor cells spread to distant parts of the body.
mitosis (my-**TOH**-sis)	A type of cell division that results in the formation of two genetically identical daughter cells.
mixed-tissue tumor (mixed-tissue **TOO**-mor)	A growth of more than one kind of neoplastic tissue.
modality (moh-**DAL**-ih-tee)	A method of application; i.e., a treatment method.
morbidity (mor-**BID**-ih-tee)	An illness or an abnormal condition or quality.
mutation (mew-**TAY**-shun)	A change or transformation.
neoplasm (**NEE**-oh-plazm) **ne/o** = new **-plasm** = growth, formation	Any abnormal growth of new tissue, benign or malignant.
oncogene (**ONG**-koh-jeen) **onc/o** = swelling, mass, or tumor **-gene** = that which generates	A gene in a virus that has the ability to cause a cell to become malignant.
oncogenesis (**ong**-koh-**JEN**-eh-sis) **onc/o** = swelling, mass, or tumor **-genesis** = production of, formation of	The formation of a tumor.
papillary (**PAP**-ih-lar-ee)	Of or pertaining to a papilla, or nipplelike projections.
papilloma (pap-ih-**LOH**-mah) **papill/o** = resembling a nipple **-oma** = tumor	A benign epithelial neoplasm characterized by a branching or lobular tumor.
pedunculated (peh-**DUN**-kyoo-**LAY**-ted)	Pertaining to a structure with a stalk.
protocol (**PROH**-toh-kall)	A written plan or description of the steps to be taken in an experiment.

radiation (ray-dee-**AY**-shun)	The emission of energy, rays, or waves.
radiocurable tumor (**ray**-dee-oh-**KYOOR**-oh-b'l **TOO**-mor)	Pertaining to the susceptibility of tumor cells to destruction by **ionizing radiation.**
radioresistant tumor (**ray**-dee-oh-ree-**SIS**-tant **TOO**-mor)	A tumor that resists the effects of radiation.
radioresponsive tumor (**ray**-dee-oh-ree-**SPON**-siv **TOO**-mor)	A tumor that reacts favorably to radiation.
radiosensitive tumor (**ray**-dee-oh-**SEN**-sih-tiv **TOO**-mor)	A tumor that is capable of being changed by or reacting to radioactive emissions such as x-rays, alpha particles, or gamma rays.
radiotherapy (ray-dee-oh-**THAIR**-ah-pee)	The treatment of disease by using x-rays or gamma rays.
relapse (ree-**LAPS**)	To exhibit again the symptoms of a disease from which a patient appears to have recovered.
remission (rih-**MISH**-un)	The partial or complete disappearance of the symptoms of a chronic or malignant disease.
ribonucleic acid (RNA) (**rye**-boh-**new**-**KLEE**-ik **ASS**-id)	A nucleic acid found in both the nucleus and cytoplasm of cells that transmits genetic instructions from the nucleus to the cytoplasm.
sarcoma (sar-**KOM**-ah) **sarc/o** = flesh **-oma** = tumor	A malignant neoplasm of the connective and supportive tissues of the body, usually first presenting as a painless swelling.
scirrhous (**SKIR**-us) **scirrh/o** = hard **-ous** = pertaining to	Pertaining to a carcinoma with a hard structure.
sessile (**SESS'l**)	Attached by a base rather than by a stalk or a peduncle.
staging (**STAJ**-ing)	The determination of distinct phases or periods in the course of a disease.
stem cell (**STEM SELL**)	A formative cell; a cell whose daughter cells may give rise to other cell types.
tumor (**TOO**-mor)	A new growth of tissue characterized by progressive, uncontrolled proliferation (growth) of cells. The tumor may be localized or invasive, benign or malignant.
verrucous (ver-**ROO**-kus)	Rough; warty.

Word Elements

The following word elements pertain to the medical specialty of oncology. As you review the list, pronounce each word element aloud twice and check the box after you "say it." Write the definition for the example word given for each word element. You may use your medical dictionary.

WORD ELEMENT	PRONUNCIATION	"SAY IT"	MEANING
ana- **ana**plasia	**AN**-ah an-ah-**PLAY**-zee-ah	☐	not, without
-blast melano**blast**	**BLAST** **MELL**-an-oh-**blast**	☐	embryonic stage of development
carcin/o **carcin**oma	kar-**SIH**-noh kar-sih-**NOH**-mah	☐	cancer
chem/o **chem**otherapy	**KEE**-moh kee-moh-**THAIR**-ah-pee	☐	pertaining to a chemical
cry/o **cry**osurgery	**KRIGH**-oh krigh-oh-**SIR**-jer-ee	☐	cold
cyst/o **cyst**ic carcinoma	**SIS**-toh **SIS**-tik kar-sih-**NOH**-mah	☐	bladder, sac, or cyst
epi- **epi**dermoid carcinoma	**EP**-ih ep-ih-**DER**-moyd kar-sih-**NOH**-mah	☐	on, upon
fibr/o **fibr**osarcoma	**FY**-broh fy-broh-sar-**KOH**-mah	☐	pertaining to fiber
meta- **meta**stasis	**MEH**-tah meh-**TASS**-tah-sis	☐	beyond, after
-oma melan**oma**	**OH**-mah mell-ah-**NOH**-mah	☐	tumor
onc/o **onc**ogenic	**ONG**-koh ong-koh-**JEN**-ik	☐	swelling, mass, or tumor
papill/o **papill**ocarcinoma	pap-**ILL**-oh **pap**-ill-oh-kar-sih-**NOH**-mah	☐	resembling a nipple
-plasia hyper**plasia**	**PLAY**-zee-ah **high**-per-**PLAY**-zee-ah	☐	formation or development
-plasm neo**plasm**	**PLAZM** **NEE**-oh-plazm	☐	living substance

radi/o **radi**ocurable	**RAY**-dee-oh **ray**-dee-oh-**KYOOR**-oh-bl	☐	radiation; also refers to radius
sarc/o **sarc**oma	**SAR**-koh sar-**KOM**-ah	☐	of or related to the flesh
scirrh/o **scirrh**ous carcinoma	**SKIR**-oh **SKIR**-us kar-sih-**NOH**-mah	☐	hard

Benign Versus Malignant Tumors

A benign tumor is a neoplasm that does not invade other tissues or metastasize to other sites. Characteristics of a benign tumor include the following:

- Usually **encapsulated** (tumor cells usually remain within a connective tissue capsule)
- Cells similar in structure to cells from which they originate (well differentiated)
- Well-defined borders
- Slow growing and limited to one area
- Possible growth displacement (but not invasion) to adjacent tissue

A malignant tumor is a neoplasm that can invade surrounding tissue and can metastasize to distant sites. Characteristics of a malignant tumor include the following:

- Not encapsulated; not cohesive, and irregular pattern of growth
- No resemblance to cell of origin
- No well-defined borders; distinct separation from surrounding tissue difficult
- Growth into adjacent cells rather than displacing or pushing them aside
- Able to metastasize or spread to distant sites through the blood or lymph systems
- Rapid growth through rapid cell division and multiplication

Classification of Neoplasms

There is a system for naming, or classifying, neoplasms that uses a root word to indicate the type of body tissue that gives rise to the neoplasm, and a suffix to indicate whether the tumor is benign or malignant. If the tumor is benign, the root word is usually followed by the suffix *-oma*. If the tumor is malignant, the root word will be followed by the suffix *carcinoma* or *sarcoma*. For example, a benign tumor of the epithelium is termed a **papilloma,** whereas a malignant tumor of the epithelium is termed a *carcinoma;* a benign tumor of the adipose tissue is called a *lipoma,* whereas a malignant tumor of the adipose tissue is called a *liposarcoma*. Exceptions to this rule include neoplastic disorders that have distinct names of their own such as leukemia, Hodgkin's disease, Wilms' tumor, and lymphomas.

Two main categories of neoplasms are carcinomas and sarcomas:

1. **Carcinomas** make up the largest group of neoplasms. They are solid tumors that originate from epithelial tissue which covers the external and internal body surfaces, the lining of vessels, body cavities, glands, and organs. An example of a name of a carcinoma of the stomach follows:

   gastric adenocarcinoma

   gastr/o = stomach

   aden/o = gland

   carcin/o = cancer

   -oma = tumor

2. **Sarcomas** are less common than carcinomas. These tumors originate from supportive and connective tissue such as bone, fat, muscle, and cartilage. An example of a name of a sarcoma arising from bone tissue follows:

   osteosarcoma

   oste/o = bone

   sarc/o = connective tissue

   -oma = tumor

Grading of Neoplasms

Grading measures the extent to which tumor cells differ from their parent tissue. Well-differentiated cells function most like the parent tissue and thus are graded as the least malignant, or grade 1. Those cells that are the least differentiated (not like the parent tissue) and most rapidly increasing in number are grade 4. There may be some variation in the grading criteria with tumors of different type locations.

Staging of Neoplasms

Staging refers to the extent of disease and relative size of the tumor. All of the following are used in the staging of neoplasms.

- The "TNM staging classification system" is an internationally recognized system used for staging neoplasms. Every metastatic disease will have specific criteria that will differ regarding the following categories.

  T: (0–4) = tumor size (primary)

  N: (0–3) = degree of regional lymph node involvement

  M: (0–3) = presence or absence of distant metastases. In all of the above, zero equals no evidence and the scale moves toward increased involvement as each number increases.

- Cytologic examination of biopsied tissues, tumors, body fluids, and/or body secretions further evaluates the extent of the disease.

- Tumor markers are biochemical indicators that a malignancy is present in the body when these molecules (tumor markers) are detectable in any body fluids, particularly blood. If high levels are detected, a diagnostic follow-up is necessary.

- Oncologic imaging includes CT scans, MRIs, x-ray imaging, radioisotope scans, ultrasonography, use of tagged antibodies, angiography, and use of direct visualization (endoscopy, sigmoidoscopy, etc.).

Risk Factors

Many factors have been identified by cancer researchers as those that predispose, or influence, one's susceptibility to developing cancer. Research indicates that a large majority of cancers are related to lifestyle and environmental factors such as tobacco, alcohol, diet, sunlight, radiation, industrial agents and chemicals, and hormones. These factors can be controlled to some degree. An uncontrollable factor that influences one's susceptibility to developing cancer is heredity.

Who is at risk of developing cancer? Anyone. Cancer researchers define two different risk categories for developing cancer.

1. Lifetime risk refers to the probability that an individual, over the course of his or her lifetime, will develop cancer or will die from cancer. Men have a 1 in 2 lifetime risk of developing cancer; women have a 1 in 3 lifetime risk of developing cancer.
2. Relative risk measures the strength of the relationship between risk factors and particular types of cancer. For example, smokers have a 10 times greater chance of developing cancer than do nonsmokers; and women who have a mother, sister, or daughter with a history of breast cancer are twice as likely to develop breast cancer as women who do not have a family history of breast cancer.

Some of the preventive measures recommended by the American Cancer Society in relation to risks of developing cancer include the following:

- Avoid smoking and heavy intake of alcohol. All cancers caused by cigarette smoking and heavy use of alcohol could be prevented completely.
- Avoid excessive exposure to the sun's rays.
- Participate in health screening examinations on a regular basis: Screening examinations conducted regularly by a health care professional are important in early detection of cancers, with treatment being more likely to be successful.
- Know how to and perform self-examinations. For possible cancer of the breast, testicle, and skin, these may result in early detection with more successful treatment results.

Warning Signs of Cancer

It is essential that all individuals know the warning signals of possible cancer to promote early detection, because any delay in the diagnosis and treatment of cancer can influence the prognosis significantly. The American Cancer Society lists several warning signs of cancer that would indicate the need for immediate medical follow-up. These warning signs are listed in a particular order to make them easier to remember; by using the first letter of each statement and putting them together, one forms the acronym **CAUTION.** The individual is "cautioned" to report the following:

C = **C**hange in bowel or bladder habits

A = **A** sore that does not heal

Cancer Cases by Site and Sex*		Cancer Deaths by Site and Sex*	
Male	**Female**	**Male**	**Female**
Prostate 189,000 (30%)	Breast 203,500 (31%)	Lung & bronchus 89,200 (31%)	Lung & bronchus 65,700 (25%)
Lung & bronchus 90,200 (14%)	Lung & bronchus 79,200 (12%)	Prostate 30,200 (11%)	Breast 39,600 (15%)
Colon & rectum 72,600 (11%)	Colon & rectum 75,700 (12%)	Colon & rectum 27,800 (10%)	Colon & rectum 28,800 (11%)
Urinary bladder 41,500 (7%)	Uterine corpus 39,300 (6%)	Pancreas 14,500 (5%)	Pancreas 15,200 (6%)
Melanoma of the skin 30,100 (5%)	Non-Hodgkin's lymphoma 25,700 (4%)	Non-Hodgkin's lymphoma 12,700 (5%)	Ovary 13,900 (5%)
Non-Hodgkin's lymphoma 28,200 (4%)	Melanoma of the skin 23,500 (4%)	Leukemia 12,100 (4%)	Non-Hodgkin's lymphoma 11,700 (4%)
Kidney 19,100 (3%)	Ovary 23,300 (4%)	Esophagus 9,600 (3%)	Leukemia 9,600 (4%)
Oral cavity 18,900 (3%)	Thyroid 15,800 (2%)	Liver 8,900 (3%)	Uterine corpus 6,600 (2%)
Leukemia 17,600 (3%)	Pancreas 15,600 (2%)	Urinary bladder 8,600 (3%)	Brain 5,900 (2%)
Pancreas 14,700 (2%)	Urinary bladder 15,000 (2%)	Kidney 7,200 (3%)	Multiple myeloma 5,300 (2%)
All Sites 637,500 (100%)	All Sites 647,400 (100%)	All Sites 288,200 (100%)	All Sites 267,300 (100%)

* Excludes basal and squamous cell skin cancers and insitu carcinoma except urinary bladder. Percentages may not total 100% due to rounding.

Figure 21-1 Leading sites of new cancer cases and deaths—2002 estimates (Reprinted by the permission of the American Cancer Society, Inc.)

U = **U**nusual bleeding or discharge

T = **T**hickening or lump in breast or elsewhere

I = **I**ndigestion or difficulty in swallowing

O = **O**bvious change in a wart or mole

N = **N**agging cough or hoarseness

When suspicious symptoms are present, further testing is indicated to rule out or confirm the possibility of cancer. A Pap test or a biopsy may be performed to establish a diagnosis. These procedures will be discussed later in this chapter.

Specific Types of Cancers

For a general grouping of the leading sites of new cancer cases and deaths as estimated by a 2002 American Cancer Society Surveillance Research report, refer to **Figure 21-1.**

The following is a discussion of some of the more commonly known types of cancers.

basal cell carcinoma
(**BAY**-sal-sell **kar**-sih-**NOH**-mah)
carcin/o = cancer
-oma = tumor

The most common malignant tumor of the epithelial tissue that occurs most often on areas of the skin exposed to the sun. See Figure 21-2.

Basal cell carcinoma presents as a nodule slightly elevated with a depression or ulceration in the center that becomes more obvious as the tumor grows.

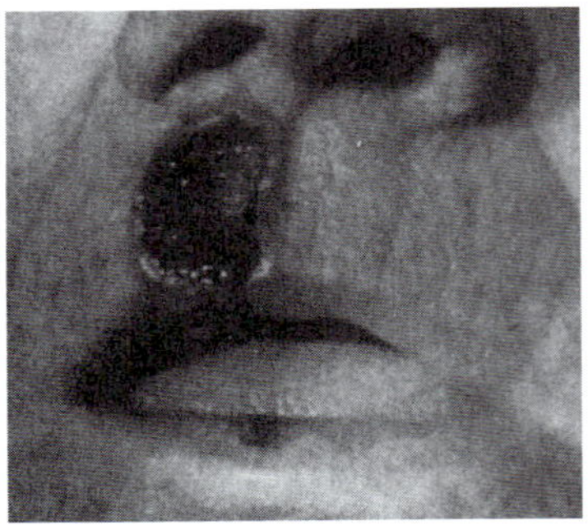

If not treated, the basal cell carcinomas will invade surrounding tissue, which can lead to destruction of body parts (such as a nose). Treatment includes surgical excision, curettage and electrodesiccation, **cryosurgery**, or **radiation therapy.**

Basal cell carcinomas rarely metastasize but they tend to recur, especially those larger than 2 cm in diameter.

Figure 21-2 Basal cell carcinoma (Courtesy of Delmar Learning)

breast cancer (carcinoma of the breast)
(**kar**-sih-**NOH**-mah of the breast)
carcin/o = cancer
-oma = tumor

A malignant tumor of the breast tissue; the most common type, ductal carcinoma, originates in the mammary ducts.

In advanced cases, symptoms such as dimpling of the breast, peau d'orange appearance of the breast (breast skin will have the appearance of an orange peel), and retraction of the breast nipple may occur. See **Figure 21-3.**

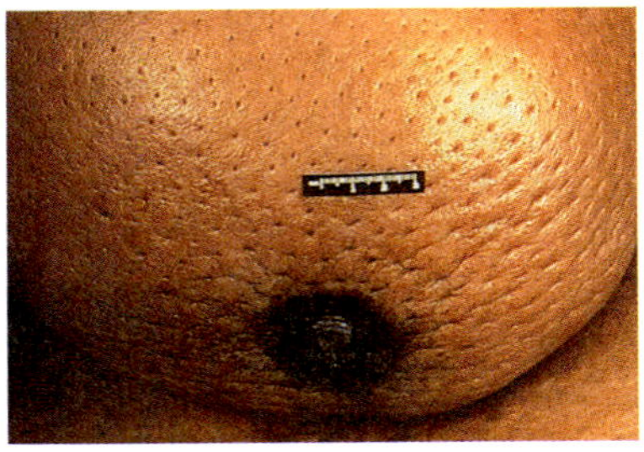

Figure 21-3 Peau d'orange (Courtesy of Dr. S. Eva Singletary, University of Texas, Anderson Cancer Center, Houston, TX)

Carcinoma of the breast has the ability to invade surrounding tissue if not detected early enough. Once the cancer cells penetrate the duct, they will metastasize (spread) through the surrounding breast tissue, eventually reaching the axillary lymph nodes. Through the lymph vessels, the cancer cells can spread to distant parts of the body.

The symptoms of breast cancer have a gradual onset. A nontender lump, which may be movable, develops in the breast. This is usually noticed in the upper outer quadrant. Most breast lumps are discovered by either the woman or her sexual partner. Many women, however, fail to follow through with seeking medical attention when they discover a lump in their breast. Any lump, no matter how small, should be reported to a physician immediately! Some women have no noticeable symptoms or palpable lump, but will have an abnormal mammogram.

Once a lump has been discovered in the female breast, and has been palpated (felt) by the physician, a mammogram is ordered to confirm the presence of a suspicious mass. This is usually followed with a biopsy of the lump, to confirm the diagnosis.

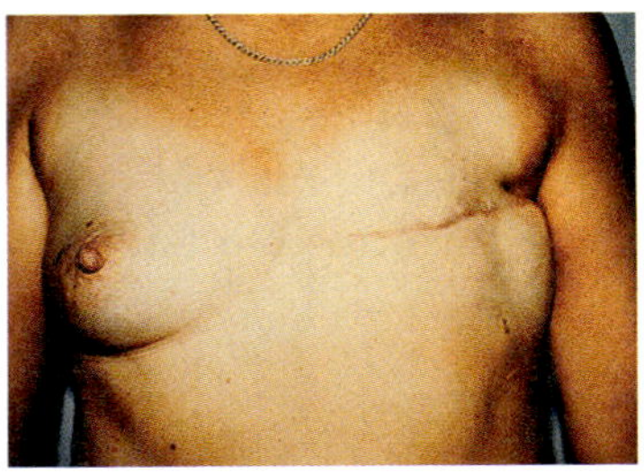

Figure 21-4 Modified radical mastectomy (*Courtesy of Dr. Steven M. Lynch*)

Most women with early-stage breast cancer are successfully treated. Treatment involves surgical removal of the lump and any diseased tissue surrounding it. If the lump is detected in the early stage of the disease, a lumpectomy may be the only surgery necessary. This involves removal of only the tumor and the immediate adjacent breast tissue. Other treatment options include a simple mastectomy in which only the breast is removed, a modified radical mastectomy (see **Figure 21-4**) in which the breast is removed, along with the lymph nodes in the axilla (armpit), and a radical mastectomy in which the breast, the chest muscles on the affected side, and the lymph nodes in the axilla are removed. Surgery is usually followed by a series of radiation treatments (radiation therapy), chemotherapy, or sometimes both.

Some women opt to have reconstructive breast surgery after having had a mastectomy. The type of material used to reconstruct the breast includes silicone implants and transplanting tissue from one part of the patient's body (such as the hips or thighs) to the breast. Patients considering breast reconstruction should discuss this thoroughly with the physician to ensure their understanding of breast reconstruction.

Cancer of the breast is estimated to be the second major cause of cancer deaths in 2002 (American Cancer Society, *Cancer Facts & Figures,* 2002). It is estimated that one in eight women in the United States will develop breast cancer during her lifetime, based on a 100-year life expectancy.

Factors that place some women in a higher risk category than others include a family history of breast cancer, nulliparity (having borne no children), early menarche, late menopause, hypertension, obesity, diabetes, chronic cystic breast disease, exposure to radiation, and possibly postmenopausal estrogen therapy.

Early detection and treatment is of the utmost importance when the diagnosis is cancer. Women should be encouraged to perform breast self-examinations monthly, have yearly physical examinations by their physicians, have a baseline mammogram done at age 35, or have mammograms as recommended by their physician. The procedure for breast self-examination is described in the section on diagnostic techniques.

---

bronchogenic carcinoma
(brong-koh-**JEN**-ik kar-sih-**NOH**-mah)
- **bronch/o** = bronchus
- **-genic** = producing
- **carcin/o** = cancer
- **-oma** = tumor

A malignant lung tumor that originates in the bronchi; lung cancer.

Bronchogenic carcinoma is usually associated with a history of cigarette smoking. It is increasing at a greater rate in women than in men. Since 1987, more women have died each year of lung cancer than breast cancer, which, for over 40 years, was the major cause of cancer death in women (American Cancer Society, *Cancer Facts & Figures,* 2002). The survival rate for lung cancer is low due to usually significant metastasis at the time of diagnosis. More than one-half of the tumors are advanced and inoperable when diagnosed.

---

cervical carcinoma
(**SER**-vih-kal kar-sih-**NOH**-mah)
- **cervic/o** = cervix
- **-al** = pertaining to
- **carcin/o** = cancer
- **-oma** = tumor

A malignant tumor of the cervix.

Cervical cancer is one of the most common malignancies of the female reproductive tract. Symptoms include bleeding between menstrual periods, after sexual intercourse, or after menopause; and an abnormal Pap smear.

Cervical cancer appears to be most frequent in women from ages 30 to 50. Factors that increase the risk of developing cervical cancer at a later age are as follows:

- First sexual intercourse before the age of 20
- Having many sex partners
- Having certain sexually transmitted diseases
- History of smoking
- Presence of condylomata (genital warts)

In the earliest stage of cervical cancer, the cancer remains in place without spreading. This early stage is known as **carcinoma in situ (CIS)** (it just sits there). The progression into a more advanced stage that can metastasize to other parts of the body is usually slow. This particular quality of cervical cancer makes the prognosis excellent if the disease is detected in its earliest stage.

The Papanicolaou (Pap) smear is used to detect early changes in the cervical tissue that may indicate cervical cancer. The Pap test consists of obtaining scrapings from the cervix and examining them under a microscope to detect any abnormalities in cervical tissue. Approximately 90% of the early changes in the cervical tissue are detected by this test. The diagnosis of cervical cancer is confirmed with a tissue biopsy.

Treatment for cervical cancer includes surgery to remove the diseased tissue and a margin of healthy tissue. This may involve removing the cervix or may be more extensive, involving removal of the uterus, fallopian tubes, and ovaries as well. Surgery may be followed with radiation therapy.

---

colorectal cancer
(koh-lon-**REK**-tal **CAN**-ser)
col/o = colon
rect/o = rectum
-al = pertaining to

The presence of a malignant neoplasm in the large intestine.

Most neoplasms in the large intestine are adenocarcinomas and at least 50% originate in the rectum, causing bleeding and pain.

A personal or family history of **colorectal cancer** or polpys and inflammatory bowel disease have been associated with increased colorectal cancer risk. Other possible risk factors include physical inactivity, high-fat and/or low-fiber diet, as well as inadequate intake of fruits and vegetables (American Cancer Society, *Cancer Facts & Figures*, 2002).

Diagnostic procedures include a rectal examination, barium enema, sigmoidoscopy and/or colonoscopy, and examination of a stool specimen for occult blood.

---

endometrial carcinoma
(**en**-doh-**MEE**-tree-al kar-sih-**NOH**-mah)
endo- = within
metri/o = uterus
-al = pertaining to
carcin/o = cancer
-oma = tumor

Malignant tumor of the inner lining of the uterus; also known as adenocarcinoma of the uterus.

This is the most common cancer of the female reproductive tract, occurring in women during or after menopause (peak incidence between the ages 50 and 60).

The classic symptom of **endometrial carcinoma** is inappropriate uterine bleeding. This includes any postmenopausal bleeding or recurrent metrorrhagia in the premenopausal patient. An abnormal discharge (mucoid or watery discharge) may precede the bleeding by weeks or months.

Diagnosis is usually confirmed with an endometrial biopsy or dilatation and curettage, with microscopic examination of the tissue sample. Dilatation involves enlarging the cervical opening, and curettage involves scraping tissue cells from the uterine lining for sampling.

Treatment involves a total abdominal hysterectomy (removal of the uterus, fallopian tubes, and ovaries) followed by radiation.

Kaposi's sarcoma
(**KAP**-oh-seez sar-**KOH**-mah)
sarc/o = flesh
-oma = tumor

Rare malignant lesions that begin as soft purple-brown nodules or plaques on the feet and gradually spread throughout the skin. See Figure 21-5.

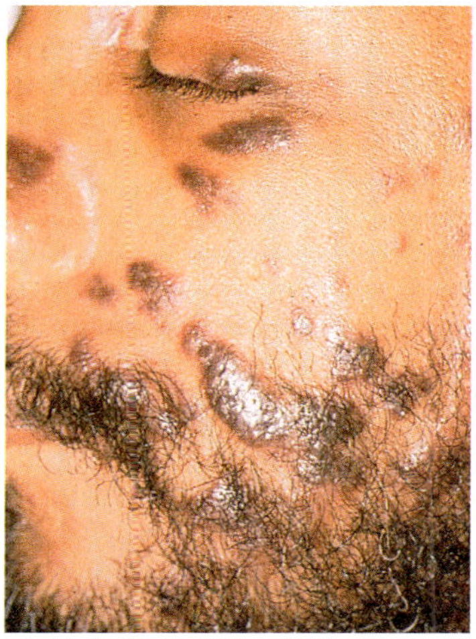

This is a systemic disease also involving the GI tract and lungs. Kaposi's sarcoma occurs most often in men and there is an increased incidence in individuals infected with AIDS; it is also associated with diabetes and malignant lymphoma (tumor of lymphatic tissue).

Radiotherapy and **chemotherapy** are usually recommended as methods of treatment. Kaposi's sarcoma may also be treated with cryosurgery or laser surgery.

Figure 21-5 Kaposi's sarcoma (Courtesy of Robert A. Silverman, M.D., Pediatric Dermatology, Georgetown University)

---

malignant melanoma
(mah-**LIG**-nant **mell**-ah-**NOH**-mah)
melan/o = black, dark
-oma = tumor

Malignant skin tumor originating from melanocytes in preexisting nevi (moles), freckles, or skin with pigment; darkly pigmented cancerous tumor. See Figure 21-6.

These tumors have irregular surfaces and borders, variable colors, and are generally located on the trunk in men and on the legs in women. The diameter of most malignant **melanomas** measures more than 6 mm. Around the primary lesion, small satellite lesions 1 to 2 cm in diameter are often noted.

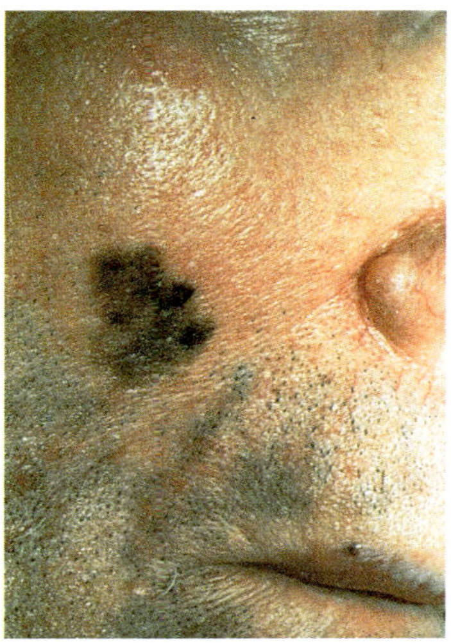

Figure 21-6 Malignant melanoma (Courtesy of Robert A. Silverman, M.D., Pediatric Dermatology, Georgetown University)

Persons at risk for malignant melanomas include those with a family history of melanoma and those with fair complexions. There is also an increased risk with excessive sun exposure to develop particular forms of malignant melanomas. Generally, most melanomas are extremely **invasive** and spread first to the lymphatic system and then metastasize throughout the body to any organ with fatal results.

All nevi and skin should be inspected and self-examined regularly, remembering the ABCDs of malignant melanoma:

> Asymmetry—Any pigmented lesion that has flat and elevated parts should be considered potentially malignant.
>
> Borders—Any leakage across the borders of brown pigment or irregular shaped margins are suspicious.
>
> Color—Variations whether red, black, dark brown, or pale are suspicious.
>
> Diameter—Any lesions with the above characteristics measuring more than 6 mm in diameter should be removed.

Treatment is surgical removal and for distant metastases, chemotherapy and radiation therapy. The depth of surgical dissection and the prognosis depends on the staging classification of the tumor. The 5-year survival rate is approximately 60% for all forms of malignant melanomas.

neuroblastoma
(**noo**-roh-blass-**TOH**-mah)
neur/o = nerve
blast/o = embryonic stage of development
-oma = tumo

A highly malignant tumor of the sympathetic nervous system.

Neuroblastoma most commonly occurs in the adrenal medulla with early metastasis spreading widely to the liver, lungs, lymph nodes, and bone.

oral leukoplakia
(**OR**-al **loo**-koh-**PLAY**-kee-ah)
or/o = mouth
-al = pertaining to
leuk/o = white

Oral leukoplakia is a precancerous lesion occurring anywhere in the mouth.

These elevated gray-white or yellow-white leathery surfaced lesions have clearly defined borders. Causative factors include chronic oral mucosal irritation, which occurs with the use of tobacco and alcohol. For a visual reference, refer to Chapter 12.

ovarian carcinoma
(oh-**VAY**-ree-an kar-sih-**NOH**-mah)
ovari/o = ovary
-an = characteristic of
carcin/o = cancer
-oma = tumor

A malignant tumor of the ovaries, most commonly occurring in women in their 50s.

It is rarely detected in the early stage and is usually far advanced when diagnosed. Ovarian carcinoma causes more deaths than any other cancer in the female reproductive system (American Cancer Society, *Cancer Facts & Figures,* 2002).

Symptoms usually do not appear with ovarian cancer until the disease is well advanced. The earliest symptoms of ovarian cancer are swelling, bloating or discomfort in the lower abdomen, and mild digestive complaints (loss of appetite, feeling of fullness, indigestion, nausea, and weight loss). As the tumor increases in size it may create pressure on adjacent organs, such as the urinary bladder or the rectum, causing frequent urination and dysuria or constipation. Later developments in the course of the disease include an accumulation of fluid within the abdominal cavity (ascites), resulting in swelling and discomfort.

Diagnosis is confirmed with examination of a sample of the tumor tissue under a microscope. This is achieved through surgical removal of the affected ovary. If the ovary is diseased with cancer, the surgeon will then remove the other ovary, the uterus, and the fallopian tubes. A process called staging is important to determine the amount of metastasis, if any. This process involves taking samples (biopsy) of nearby lymph nodes, the diaphragm, and sampling the fluid from the abdomen.

Treatment involves the use of surgery, chemotherapy, or radiation therapy. It may involve one or a combination of the treatment choices, depending on the extent of the disease.

pancreatic cancer
(**pan**-kree-**AT**-ik **CAN**-ser)
pancreat/o = pancreas
-ic = pertaining to

A life-threatening primary malignant neoplasm typically found in the head of the pancreas.

Of those diagnosed with pancreatic cancer, 95% lose their lives 1 to 3 years after diagnosis. The occurrence of pancreatic cancer for smokers is twice the number that it is for nonsmokers. Other related risk factors include a diet high in fat, pancreatitis, exposure to chemicals and toxins, and diabetes mellitus.

With a slow onset, pancreatic cancer causes very nonspecific symptoms such as nausea, anorexia, dull epigastric pain, weight loss, and flatulence. As the tumor grows, the pain worsens. If there is an early diagnosis, surgical removal of the tumor may be possible.

---

prostatic cancer (carcinoma of the prostate)
(kar-sih-**NOH**-mah of the **PROSS**-tayt
carcin/o = cancer
-oma = tumor

Malignant growth within the prostate gland, creating pressure on the upper part of the urethra.

Cancer of the prostate is estimated to be the second leading cause of cancer death in men (American Cancer Society, *Cancer Facts & Figures*, 2002). Unfortunately, symptoms are not usually present in the early stages of cancer of the prostate. By the time symptoms are evident, the cancer may have already metastasized (spread) to other areas of the body.

When symptoms of prostate cancer do occur, they may include any of the following:

1. A need to urinate frequently (i.e., urinary frequency), especially at night
2. Difficulty starting or stopping urine flow
3. Inability to urinate
4. Weak or interrupted flow of urine when urinating (patient may complain of "dribbling," instead of having a steady stream of urine)
5. Pain or burning when urinating
6. Pain or stiffness in the lower back, hips, or thighs
7. Painful ejaculation

Because the presence of symptoms usually mean that the disease is more advanced, early detection of cancer of the prostate is essential to successful treatment. All men over the age of 40 should have a yearly physical examination that includes a digital rectal examination of the prostate gland. The rectal examination can reveal a cancerous growth before symptoms appear. A **PSA blood test** may be performed during the examination to detect increased growth of the prostate (the growth could be benign or malignant). The PSA test measures a substance called prostate-specific antigen. The level of PSA in the blood may rise in men who have prostate cancer or benign prostatic hypertrophy. If the level is elevated, the physician will order additional tests to confirm a diagnosis of cancer of the prostate.

The most common procedure used to treat or relieve the urinary obstruction resulting from cancer of the prostate is surgery to remove the prostate tissue that is pressing against the upper part of the urethra. This procedure also is used to treat benign prostatic hypertrophy. This surgery, called transurethral resection of the prostate (TUR or TURP), will be discussed in the diagnostic procedures section of the chapter.

Other methods of treatment include a radical prostatectomy (removal of the prostate gland), radiation therapy, hormone therapy, or chemotherapy. The treatment of choice is dependent on the patient's age, medical history, risks and benefits of treatment, and the stage of the disease.

renal cell carcinoma
(**REE**-nal **SELL** kar-sih-**NOH**-mah)
ren/o = kidney
-al = pertaining to
carcin/o = cancer
-oma = tumor

A malignant tumor of the kidney, occurring in adulthood.

The patient is asymptomatic (symptom-free) until the latter stages of the disease. The most common symptom of **renal cell carcinoma** is painless hematuria, with later development of flank pain and intermittent fever. Once the diagnosis is confirmed, the treatment of choice is surgery to remove the tumor before it can metastasize. Chemotherapy and radiation treatment may also follow surgery.

squamous cell carcinoma
(**SKWAY**-mus **SELL** kar-sih-**NOH**-mah)
carcin/o = cancer
-oma = tumor

A malignancy of the squamous cells of epithelial tissue, which is a much faster growing cancer than basal cell carcinoma and has a greater potential for metastasis if not treated. See Figure 21-7.

Squamous cell lesions are seen most frequently on sun-exposed areas such as the following:

1. Top of the nose
2. Forehead
3. Margin of the external ear
4. Back of the hands
5. Lower lip

The squamous cell lesion begins as a firm, flesh-colored or red, firm papule sometimes with a crusted appearance. As the lesion grows it may bleed or ulcerate and become painful. When squamous cell carcinoma recurs, it can be highly invasive and present an increased risk of metastasis.

Treatment is surgical excision with the goal to remove the tumor completely along with a margin of healthy surrounding tissue. Cryosurgery for low-risk squamous cell carcinomas is also common.

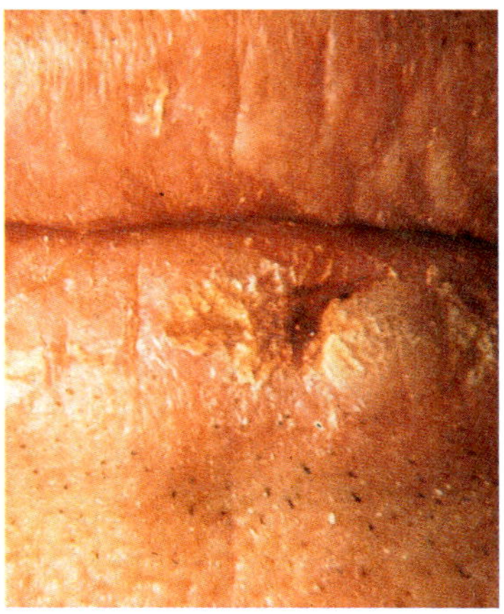

Figure 21-7 Squamous cell carcinoma (Courtesy of Dr. Joseph Konzelman, School of Dentistry, Medical College of Georgia)

testicular cancer (carcinoma of the testes)
(kar-sih-**NOH**-mah of the **TESS**-teez)
carcin/o = tumor
-oma = tumor

A malignant tumor of the testicle that appears as a painless lump in the testicle.

This type of tumor is rare and usually occurs in men under the age of 40. The cause is basically unknown.

The diagnosis of testicular cancer is usually confirmed by biopsy, after the physician has palpated the lump in the testicle. Treatment of choice is surgery to remove the diseased testicle, followed by radiation therapy and chemotherapy. The healthy testicle is not removed, thus fertility and potency should not be altered in the male. Chances for complete recovery are excellent if the malignancy is detected in the early stages.

Testicular cancer can spread throughout the body via the lymphatic system if not treated in the early stages. Early treatment is essential to complete recovery. Therefore, it is recommended that all men perform monthly testicular self-examinations. If a lump is discovered, it should be reported immediately to a physician.

thyroid cancer (cancer of the thyroid gland)
(**CAN**-ser, **THIGH**-royd gland)

Malignant tumor of the thyroid gland that leads to dysfunction of the gland and thus inadequate or excessive secretion of the thyroid hormone.

The presence of a palpable nodule or lump may be the first indication of thyroid cancer.

A needle aspiration biopsy is used to confirm the diagnosis. A malignant tumor of the thyroid is classified and staged according to the site of origin, size of tumor, amount of lymph node involvement, and the presence of metastasis.

Treatment typically consists of partial or complete removal of the thyroid gland. Lifelong thyroid hormone replacement is then required.

tumors, intracranial
(**TOO**-mors in-trah-**KRAY**-nee-al)
intra- = within
crani/o = cranium, skull
-al = pertaining to

Intracranial tumors occur in any structural region of the brain and they may be malignant or benign, classified as primary or secondary, and are named according to the tissue from which they originate.

An intracranial tumor causes the normal brain tissue to be displaced and compressed, leading to progressive neurological dysfunctions. The symptoms of intracranial tumors include headaches, dizziness, vomiting, problems with coordination and muscle strength, personality changes, altered mental function, seizures, paralysis, and sensory disturbances.

Surgical removal is the desired treatment when possible. Radiation and/or chemotherapy are used according to location, classification, and type of tumor.

tumors, metastatic intracranial
(**TOO**-mors, **met**-ah-**STAT**-ik in-trah-**KRAY**-nee-al)
intra- = within
crani/o = cranium, skull
-al = pertaining to

Tumors occurring as a result of metastasis from a primary site such as the lung or (secondary) breast.

A **metastatic intracranial tumor** is a common occurrence, comprising approximately 15% of intracranial tumors. The tissue in the brain reacts intensely to the presence of a metastatic tumor and usually progresses rapidly. Surgical removal of a single metastasis to the brain can be achieved if the tumor is located in an operable region. The removal may provide the individual with several months or years of life.

tumors, primary intracranial
(**TOO**-mors, primary in-trah-**KRAY**-nee-al)
intra- = within
crani/o = cranium, skull
-al = pertaining to

Tumors that arise from gliomas (malignant glial cells which are a support for nerve tissue), and tumors arising from the meninges are known as primary intracranial tumors.

Gliomas are classified according to the principal cell type, shape, and size. The following are classified as gliomas.

1. *Glioblastoma multiforme* comprises approximately 20% of all intracranial tumors. They arise in the cerebral hemisphere and are the most rapidly growing of the gliomas.
2. *Astrocytoma* comprises approximately 10% of all intracranial tumors and is a slow-growing primary tumor of astrocytes. Astrocytomas tend to invade surrounding structures and over time become more anaplastic. A highly malignant glioblastoma may develop within the tumor mass.

3. *Ependymomas* comprise approximately 6% of all intracranial tumors. They commonly arise from the ependymomal cells that line the fourth ventricle wall and often extend into the spinal cord. An ependymoma occurs more commonly in children and adolescents and is usually encapsulated and benign.
4. *Oligodendrogliomas* comprise approximately 5% of all intracranial tumors and are usually slow growing. At times, the oligodendrogliomas imitate the glioblastomas with rapid growth. Oligodendrogliomas occur most often in the frontal lobe.
5. *Medulloblastoma* comprises approximately 4% of all intracranial tumors. Medulloblastoma occurs most frequently in children between 5 and 9 years of age. It affects more boys than girls and typically arises in the cerebellum growing rapidly. The prognosis is poor.

Meningiomas comprise approximately 15% of all intracranial tumors. They originate from the meninges, grow slowly, and are largely vascular. Meningiomas largely occur in adults.

Wilms' tumor
(**VILMZ TOO**-mor)

A malignant tumor of the kidney occurring predominately in childhood.

The most frequent finding is a palpable mass in the abdomen. The child may also be experiencing abdominal pain, fever, anorexia, nausea, vomiting, and hematuria. Secondary hypertension may also occur.

Once diagnosis is confirmed the treatment of choice is surgery to remove the tumor, followed by chemotherapy and radiation. With treatment and no evidence of metastasis, the cure rate is high for patients with **Wilms' tumors.**

Treatment Techniques and Procedures

The treatment of cancer may be used in conjunction with some other course of treatment, may only provide symptomatic relief (palliative treatment), or may cure the cancer. Techniques used to treat cancer may be used alone or in combination. Following are three major treatment procedures used and one treatment procedure occasionally used against cancer.

chemotherapy
(**kee**-moh-**THAIR**-ah-pee)
chem/o = chemical reaction
-therapy = treatment

The use of cytotoxic drugs and chemicals to achieve a cure, decrease tumor size, provide relief of pain, or slow metastasis.

Chemotherapy is often used in conjunction with surgery, radiation therapy, or immunotherapy.

Chemotherapy destroys cells by disrupting the cell cycle in various phases of metabolism and reproduction. Chemotherapy also interferes with the malignant cell's ability to synthesize needed chemicals and enzymes. Chemotherapy drugs are phase specific (only work during a specific phase of the cell cycle) or nonphase specific (works throughout the cell cycle). The following describes the classes or categories of chemotherapeutic drugs.

Alkylating agents are nonphase specific and work by altering DNA synthesis and the cell's ability to replicate. The toxic effects include delayed, prolonged, or permanent bone marrow failure, a treatment-resistant form of acute myelogenous leukemia, irreversible infertility, hemorrhagic cystitis, and nephrotoxicity.

Antimetabolites are a group of chemotherapy drugs that are phase specific and alter the cell's ability to replicate or copy the DNA, consequently preventing cell replication. The toxic effects relate to cells that rapidly proliferate (GI, hair, skin, and WBCs) and include nausea and vomiting, stomatitis, decreased WBC count, diarrhea, and alopecia (baldness).

Cytotoxic antibiotics are nonphase specific and act in several ways to damage the cell membrane and kill cells. The main toxic effect occurs as damage to the cardiac muscle, which restricts the duration and amount of treatment.

Plant alkaloids include two groups: vinca alkaloids and etoposide. The vinca alkaloids are phase specific. The toxicity is seen as depression of deep-tendon reflexes, motor weakness, pain and altered sensation, paralytic ileus, and cranial nerve disruptions. Etoposide affects all phases of the cell cycle. The most common toxic effect is hypotension, which results from the IV administration being too rapid. Other toxic effects are nausea, vomiting, and bone marrow suppression.

Hormones and hormone antagonists: Corticosteroids and prednisone, the main hormones used in cancer therapy, are phase specific and alter cell function and growth. Side effects include hyperglycemia, hypertension, impaired healing, osteoporosis, fluid retention, and hirsutism. Hormone antagonists are used with hormone-binding tumors (prostate, breast, and endometrium) to deprive them of their hormones. The goal of these drugs is to cause regression of the tumor, not to cure it. Toxic effects include change in the secondary sex characteristics.

---

immunotherapy
(**im**-yoo-noh-**THAIR**-ah-pee)
immun/o = immune, protection
-therapy = treatment

Agents that are capable of changing the relationship between a tumor and the host are known as biologic response modifiers (BRMs). These agents are used to strengthen the individual's immune responses.

Because the role of various immune cells against different malignancies is not clear, **immunotherapy** is only used to halt disease that is advanced and/or metastasizing.

---

radiation therapy
(ray-dee-AY-shun **THAIR**-ah-pee)

The use of ionizing radiation to interrupt cellular growth. The goal of radiation therapy is to reach maximum tumor control with minimum normal tissue damage.

The delivery of ionizing radiation is used to accomplish one or more of the following:

1. Destruction of tumor cells
2. Reduction of tumor size
3. Decrease in pain

4. Relief of obstruction
5. To slow or stop metastasis

Low-energy beams called electron beams are used for the treatment of surface and skin tumors. High-energy x-ray beams are delivered by a large electronic device called a linear accelerator, and are required for the treatment of deep-seated tumors.

Radiation therapy may be delivered by teletherapy (external radiation) or brachytherapy (internal radiation) or a combination of both. A treatment method used to decrease damage to normal tissue is **fractionation.** With fractionation, the radiation is given in repeated small doses at intervals.

Radiocurable tumors are very sensitive to radiation and can be totally eradicated by radiation therapy (Hodgkin's disease and lymphomas). Drugs that increase the sensitivity of tumors to radiation are called radiosensitizers.

In radiosensitive tumors, irradiation is able to cause cell death without seriously damaging normal surrounding tissue. Hematopoietic and lymphatic origin tumors are radiosensitive.

Radioresistant tumors require large doses of radiation to produce death of the tumor cells. Connective tissue tumors are highly radioresistant.

---

surgery
(**SIR**-jer-ee)

In more than 90% of all cancers, surgery is used for diagnosing and staging. In more than 60% of all cancers, surgery is the primary treatment. When feasible, the primary tumor is excised in its entirety.

Tumor removal may necessitate the reconstruction of tissues or organs affected by the surgery. An example is the creation of a colostomy when a portion of the colon is removed.

Common surgical procedures used for diagnosis or cure of malignant tumors are as follows:

1. **Incisional biopsies** are used to remove a piece of a tumor for examination and diagnosing.
2. **Excisional biopsies** are used to remove the tumor and a portion of normal tissue, which provide a specimen for examination and diagnosis. Sometimes this excisional biopsy results in a cure when the neoplasm is small.
3. An **en bloc** resection includes the removal of a tumor and a large area of surrounding tissue that contains lymph nodes. An example is a modified radical mastectomy.
4. **Fulguration** is the destruction of tissue with electric sparks and **electrocauterization** is destruction of tissue by burning.
5. Cryosurgery is often used to treat bladder or brain tumors by freezing the malignant tissue, which results in its destruction.
6. **Exenteration** is a wide resection that removes the organ of origin and surrounding tissue.

Common Abbreviations

ABBREVIATION	MEANING	ABBREVIATION	MEANING
Bx, bx	biopsy	**MTX**	an anticancer drug combination of methotrexate, mercaptopurine, and cyclophosphamide
Ca	cancer	**NHL**	non-Hodgkin's lymphoma
CEA	carcinoembryonic antigen	**Pap smear**	a simple smear method of examining stained exfoliative cells; the Papanicolaou test
CMF	an anticancer drug combination of cyclophosphamide, methotrexate, and fluorouracil	**POMP**	an abbreviation for a combination drug regimen used in the treatment of cancer, containing three antineoplastics: Purinethos (mercaptopurine), Oncovin (vincristine sulfate), methotrexate, and prednisone (a glucocorticoid)
DES	diethylstilbestrol	**PSA**	prostate-specific antigen
DNA	deoxyribonucleic acid	**RNA**	ribonucleic acid
mets	metastasis	**TNM**	tumor, nodes and metastasis (a system for staging malignant neoplastic disease)
MOPP	an abbreviation for a combination drug regimen used in the treatment of cancer, containing three antineoplastics, Mustargen (mechlorethamine), Oncovin (vincristine sulfate), and Matulane (procarbazine hydrochloride), and prednisone (a glucocorticoid). MOPP is prescribed in the treatment of Hodgkin's disease.		

Written and Audio Terminology Review

Review each of the following terms from this chapter. Study the spelling of each term and write the definition in the space provided. If you have the Audio CD available, listen to each term, pronounce it, and check the box once you are comfortable saying the word. Check definitions by looking the term up in the glossary/index.

TERM	PRONUNCIATION	DEFINITION
adjuvant	☐ **AD**-joo-vant	______
anaplasia	☐ **an**-ah-**PLAY**-zee-ah	______
antimetabolite	☐ **an**-tih-meh-**TAB**-oh-lite	______
antineoplastic	☐ **an**-tih-**nee**-oh-**PLASS**-tik	______
benign	☐ bee-**NINE**	______
bronchogenic carcinoma	☐ brong-koh-**JEN**-ik kar-sih-**NOH**-mah	______

Term		Pronunciation	
cancer	☐	**CAN**-ser	______
carcinogen	☐	kar-**SIN**-oh-jen	______
carcinoma	☐	kar-sih-**NOH**-mah	______
carcinoma in situ (CIS)	☐	kar-sih-**NOH**-mah in **SIT**-oo (CIS)	______
chemotherapy	☐	kee-moh-**THAIR**-ah-pee	______
colorectal cancer	☐	koh-loh-**REK**-tal **CAN**-ser	______
cryosurgery	☐	krigh-oh-**SIR**-jer-ee	______
cystic carcinoma	☐	**SIS**-tik kar-sih-**NOH**-mah	______
dedifferentiation	☐	dee-diff-er-en-she-**AY**-shun	______
deoxyribonucleic acid (DNA)	☐	dee-ock-see-rye-boh-noo-**KLEE**-ic **ASS**-id (DNA)	______
differentiation	☐	diff-er-en-she-**AY**-shun	______
encapsulated	☐	en-**CAP**-soo-lay-ted	______
endometrial carcinoma	☐	**en**-doh-**MEE**-tree-al **kar**-sih-**NOH**-mah)	______
epidermoid carcinoma	☐	ep-ih-**DER**-moyd kar-sih-**NOH**-mah	______
fibrosarcoma	☐	fy-broh-sar-**KOH**-mah	______
fractionation	☐	frak-shun-**AY**-shun	______
hyperplasia	☐	high-per-**PLAY**-zee-ah	______
immunotherapy	☐	im-yoo-noh-**THAIR**-ah-pee	______
infiltrative	☐	in-fill-**TRAY**-tiv	______
intracranial tumors	☐	in-trah-**KRAY**-nee-al **TOO**-mors	______
invasive	☐	in-**VAY**-siv	______
ionizing radiation	☐	**EYE**-oh-nigh-zing ray-dee-**AY**-shun	______
linear accelerator	☐	**LIN**-ee-ar ak-**SELL**-er-ay-tor	______
malignant	☐	mah-**LIG**-nant	______
melanoblast	☐	**MELL**-an-oh-blast	______
melanoma	☐	mell-ah-**NOH**-mah	______
metastasis	☐	meh-**TASS**-tah-sis	______

Term	Pronunciation	
metastatic intracranial tumors	☐ **met**-ah-**STAT**-ik in-trah-**KRAY**-nee-al **TOO**-mors	___
mitosis	☐ my-**TOH**-sis	___
mixed-tissue tumor	☐ mixed-tissue **TOO**-mor	___
modality	☐ moh-**DAL**-ih-tee	___
morbidity	☐ mor-**BID**-ih-tee	___
mutation	☐ mew-**TAY**-shun	___
neoplasm	☐ **NEE**-oh-plazm	___
neuroblastoma	☐ **noo**-roh-blass-**TOH**-mah	___
oncogene	☐ **ONG**-koh-jeen	___
oncogenesis	☐ **ong**-koh-**JEN**-eh-sis	___
oncogenic	☐ ong-koh-**JEN**-ik	___
oral leukoplakia	☐ **OR**-al **loo**-koh-**PLAY**-kee-ah	___
ovarian carcinoma	☐ oh-**VAY**-ree-an kar-sih-**NOH**-mah	___
pancreatic cancer	☐ pan-kree-**AT**-ik **CAN**-ser	___
papillary	☐ **PAP**-ih-lar-ee	___
papilloma	☐ pap-ih-**LOH**-mah	___
papillocarcinoma	☐ pap-ill-oh-kar-sih-**NOH**-mah	___
pedunculated	☐ peh-**DUN**-kyoo-lay-ted	___
primary intracranial tumors	☐ primary in-trah-**KRAY**-nee-al **TOO**-mors	___
protocol	☐ **PROH**-toh-kall	___
radiation	☐ ray-dee-**AY**-shun	___
radiation therapy	☐ ray-dee-**AY**-shun **THAIR**-ah-pee	___
radiocurable tumor	☐ **ray**-dee-oh-**KYOOR**-ah-b'l **TOO**-mor	___
radioresistant tumor	☐ **ray**-dee-oh-ree-**SIS**-tant **TOO**-mor	___
radioresponsive tumor	☐ **ray**-dee-oh-ree-**SPON**-siv **TOO**-mor	___
radiotherapy	☐ ray-dee-oh-**THAIR**-ah-pee	___
relapse	☐ ree-**LAPS**	___

remission	☐	rih-**MISH**-un	______
renal cell carcinoma	☐	**REE**-nal sell kar-sih-**NOH**-mah	______
ribonucleic acid (RNA)	☐	rye-boh-new-**KLEE**-ik **ASS**-id (RNA)	______
sarcoma	☐	sar-**KOM**-ah	______
scirrhous	☐	**SKIR**-us	______
sessile	☐	**SESS**'l	______
staging	☐	**STAJ**-ing	______
stem cell	☐	**STEM SELL**	______
surgery	☐	**SIR**-jer-ee	______
verrucous	☐	ver-**ROO**-kus	______
Wilms' tumor	☐	**VILMZ TOO**-mor	______

Chapter Review Exercises

The following exercises provide a more in-depth review of the chapter material. Your goal in these exercises is to complete each section at a minimum 80% level of accuracy. If you score below 80% in any area, return to the appropriate section in the chapter and read the material again. A place has been provided for your score at the end of each section.

A. Term to Definition

Define each diagnosis or procedure by writing the definition in the space provided. Check the box if you are able to complete this exercise correctly the first time (without referring to the answers). Each correct answer is worth 10 points. Record your score in the space provided at the end.

☐ 1. simple mastectomy ______

☐ 2. modified radical mastectomy ______

☐ 3. radical mastectomy ______

☐ 4. Papanicolaou smear ______

☐ 5. endometrial carcinoma ______

☐ 6. Kaposi's sarcoma ______

☐ 7. transurethral resection ______

☐ 8. intracranial tumors ______

☐ 9. Wilm's tumor ______

☐ 10. oral leukoplakia ______

Number correct ______ × 10 points/correct answer: Your score _____%

B. Matching

Match the descriptions of the tumor on the right with the appropriate tumor name on the left. Each correct answer is worth 10 points. When you have completed the exercise, record your score in the space provided at the end of the exercise.

_____ 1. astrocytoma
_____ 2. glioblastoma
_____ 3. meningioma
_____ 4. medulloblastoma
_____ 5. ependymoma
_____ 6. oligodendroglioma
_____ 7. bronchogenic carcinoma
_____ 8. cervical cancer
_____ 9. colorectal cancer
_____ 10. malignant melanoma

a. A malignant tumor of the cervix
b. The presence of a malignant multiform neoplasm in the large intestine
c. Malignant skin tumor originating from melanocytes in preexisting nevi, freckles, or skin with pigment
d. Arises in the cerebral hemisphere and is the most rapidly growing of the gliomas
e. Typically arises in the cerebellum and grows rapidly, occurs most frequently in children between 5 and 9 years of age
f. Originates from the meninges, grows slowly, and is largely vascular
g. Comprises approximately 10% of all intracranial tumors; is a slow-growing primary tumor of star-shaped cells
h. Commonly arises from the ependymomal cells that line the fourth ventricle wall and often extends into the spinal cord
i. Occurs most often in the frontal lobe of the brain, usually grows slowly, and comprises approximately 5% of all intracranial tumors
j. A malignant lung tumor that originates in the bronchi; lung cancer usually associated with a history of cigarette smoking

Number correct ______ × 10 points/correct answer: Your score _____%

C. Crossword Puzzle

Read the clues carefully and complete the puzzle. Each crossword answer is worth 10 points. When you have completed the crossword puzzle, total your points and enter your score in the space provided.

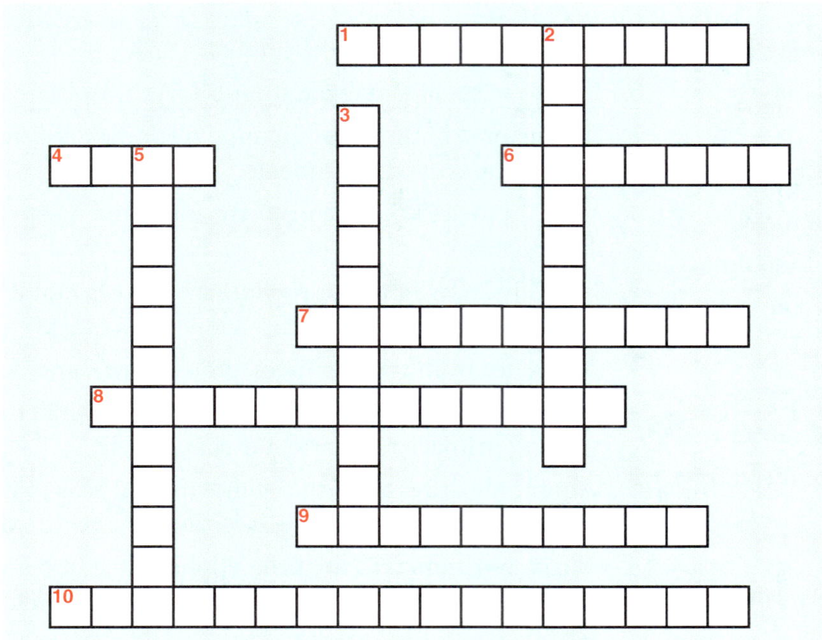

ACROSS

1 Spread of cancer
4 Formative cell is a ________ cell
6 Recurrence of symptoms
7 Freezes malignant tissues to destroy
8 Internal radiation
9 ____biopsy removes piece of tumor
10 Apparatus for accelerating charged subatomic particles used in radiotherapy

DOWN

2 External radiation
3 Destruction with electric sparks
5 Remove organ and surrounding tissue

Number correct ______ × 10 points/correct answer: Your score _____%

D. Definition to Term

Using the following definitions, identify and provide the medical term(s) to match the definition. Each correct answer is worth 10 points. Record your score in the space provided at the end.

1. A substance, especially a drug, added to a prescription to assist in the action of the main ingredient

   ____

   (one word)

2. Noncancerous and therefore not an immediate threat

   ____

   (one word)

3. A substance or agent that causes the development or increases the incidence of cancer

   ____

   (one word)

4. A premalignant neoplasm that has not invaded the basement membrane but shows cytologic characteristics of cancer

 ____

 (three words)

5. In radiology, the division of the total dose of radiation into small doses administered at intervals, in an effort to minimize tissue damage

 ____

 (one word)

6. Characterized by a tendency to spread, infiltrate, and intrude

 ____

 (one word)

7. The process by which tumor cells spread to distant parts of the body

 ____

 (one word)

8. A method of application; that is, a treatment method

 ____

 (one word)

9. A written plan or description of the steps to be taken in an experiment

 ____

 (one word)

10. To exhibit again the symptoms of a disease from which a patient appears to have recovered

 ____

 (one word)

Number correct ______ × 10 points/correct answer: Your score _____%

E. Word Search

Using the definitions listed, identify the medical term, then find and circle it in the puzzle. The words may be read up, down, diagonally, across, or backward. Each correct answer is worth 10 points. Record your score in the space provided at the end of the exercise.

Example: Bending (decreases the angle)

 flexion

1. Use of biologic response modifiers (BRMs)

 ____

2. Destroys cells by disrupting the cell cycle in various phases through interruption of cell metabolism and replication

 ____

3. Irradiation is able to cause cell death without damaging normal surrounding tissue

 ____

4. Drugs that increase the sensitivity of tumors to radiation

 ____

5. A highly malignant tumor of the sympathetic nervous system

____

6. The type of tumor very sensitive to radiation and can be totally eradicated by radiation

____

7. The main hormones used in cancer therapy

____

8. The main toxic effect of this chemotherapy drug occurs as damage to the cardiac muscle; this drug is known as a ____________________ antibiotic.

9. ____________________ cell carcinoma is the most common malignant tumor of the epithelial tissue and occurs most often on areas of the skin exposed to the sun.

10. This carcinoma most commonly occurs in women in their 50s and is rarely detected in the early stage

____

F	L	E	X	I	O	N	O	A	T	T	S	I	S	L
R	S	I	R	M	T	S	O	P	O	R	Y	T	N	A
A	R	B	Y	M	T	U	T	E	A	P	R	Y	C	L
D	E	D	S	U	I	H	S	D	I	N	A	E	R	I
I	Z	D	I	N	G	I	I	L	E	R	H	A	S	S
O	I	S	Y	O	M	O	A	N	O	D	E	P	D	U
S	T	E	D	T	V	H	I	M	B	U	H	I	I	E
E	I	E	E	H	T	A	E	X	I	C	O	R	O	L
N	S	X	C	E	I	N	R	N	T	R	O	G	P	B
S	N	E	C	R	I	N	E	I	E	R	M	O	A	A
I	E	U	B	A	S	A	L	T	A	I	E	I	Q	R
T	S	H	O	P	Y	M	S	J	W	N	H	D	U	U
I	O	O	C	Y	T	O	T	O	X	I	C	A	E	C
V	I	I	A	I	C	S	U	M	L	O	S	R	P	O
E	D	O	L	I	Y	R	S	H	C	L	S	Y	A	I
I	A	N	T	N	O	I	T	A	I	D	A	R	R	D
S	R	R	S	D	S	R	S	L	F	L	E	P	X	A
C	O	C	H	E	M	O	T	H	E	R	A	P	Y	R
C	Q	A	M	O	T	S	A	L	B	O	R	U	E	N

Number correct ______ × *10 points/correct answer: Your score* _____%

F. Matching Abbreviations

Match the abbreviations on the left with the correct definition on the right. Each correct answer is worth 10 points. When you have completed the exercise, record your score in the space provided at the end of the exercise.

_____	1. bx	a. metastasis
_____	2. Ca	b. deoxyribonucleic acid
_____	3. mets	c. a system for staging malignant neoplastic disease
_____	4. NHL	d. a simple smear method of examining stained exfoliative cells
_____	5. PSA	e. cancer
_____	6. RNA	f. biopsy
_____	7. TNM	g. carcinoembryonic antigen
_____	8. DES	h. ribonucleic acid
_____	9. DNA	i. non- Hodgkin's lymphoma
_____	10. Pap smear	j. prostate- specific antigen
		k. diethylstilbestrol

Number correct _______ × 10 points/correct answer: Your score _____%

G. Spelling

Circle the correctly spelled term in each pairing of words. Each correct answer is worth 10 points. Record your score in the space provided at the end of the exercise.

1. melanoma	melenoma
2. scirrous	scirrhous
3. neaplasm	neoplasm
4. metastasis	metastisis
5. papillary	papilarry
6. incapsulated	encapsulated
7. mytosis	mitosis
8. benign	bening
9. adjuvant	ajudvant
10. antimetabolyte	antimetabolite

Number correct _______ × 10 points/correct answer: Your score _____%

H. True or False

Read each statement carefully and circle the correct answer as true or false. HINT: Pay close attention to the word elements written in **bold** as you make your decision. If the statement is false, identify the meaning of the word element written in bold. Each correct answer is worth 10 points. Record your score in the space provided at the end of the exercise.

1. A **carcin**oma is a benign tumor.

   True False

   If your answer is False, what does *carcin/o* mean? ______________________

2. **Meta**stasis is the process by which tumor cells spread beyond or to distant parts of the body.

   True False

   If your answer is False, what does *meta-* mean? ______________________

3. The term ***scirrh**ous* pertains to a carcinoma with a hard structure.

   True False

   If your answer is False, what does *scirrh/o* mean? ______________________

4. The medical term **ana**plasia means complete formation.

   True False

   If your answer is False, what does *ana-* mean? ______________________

5. **Cryo**surgery is the use of heat to treat tissues.

   True False

   If your answer is False, what does *cry/o* mean? ______________________

6. The term *hyper**plasia*** refers to excessive formation or development.

   True False

   If your answer is False, what does *-plasia* mean? ______________________

7. A melan**oma** is a dark spot on the nailbed.

   True False

   If your answer is False, what does *-oma* mean? ______________________

8. **Chemo**therapy is treatment with a drug or chemical.

   True False

   If your answer is False, what does *chem/o* mean? ______________________

9. The term ***anti**neoplastic* means "of or pertaining to a substance, procedure, or measure that prevents (works against) the proliferation (increase) of malignant cells."

   True False

   If your answer is False, what does *anti-*mean? ______________________

10. The medical term *onco**genesis*** means "destruction of a tumor."

    True False

    If your answer is False, what does *-genesis* mean? ______________________

Number correct _____ × 10 points/correct answer: Your score _____%

I. Multiple Choice

Read each statement carefully and select the correct answer from the choices provided. Each correct answer is worth 10 points. Record your score in the space provided at the end of the exercise.

1. The medical term for rough or warty is:
   a. verrucous
   b. papillary
   c. neoplasm
   d. pedunculated
2. A substance, especially a drug, added to a prescription to assist in the action of the main ingredient is a(n):
   a. antimetabolite
   b. carcinogen
   c. adjuvant
   d. protocol
3. High-energy x-rays that possess the ability to kill cells or retard their growth are known as:
   a. ionizing radiation
   b. linear accelerator
   c. fractionation
   d. protocol
4. A tumor or growth that is enclosed in a fibrous or membranous sheath is:
   a. infiltrative
   b. anaplastic
   c. sessile
   d. encapsulated
5. A tumor that possesses the ability to invade or penetrate adjacent tissue is:
   a. infiltrative
   b. anaplastic
   c. sessile
   d. encapsulated
6. The medical term that means "pertaining to a structure with a stalk" is:
   a. sessile
   b. pedunculated
   c. verrucous
   d. papillary
7. The medical term that means "pertaining to nipplelike projections" is:
   a. sessile
   b. pedunculated
   c. verrucous
   d. papillary
8. A written plan or description of the steps to be taken in an experiment is known as:
   a. protocol
   b. staging
   c. grading
   d. differentiation

9. The medical term that means to exhibit again the symptoms of a disease from which a patient appears to have recovered is:
   a. remission
   b. mutation
   c. relapse
   d. protocol
10. The medical term that means the partial or complete disappearance of the symptoms of a chronic or malignant disease is:
    a. remission
    b. mutation
    c. relapse
    d. protocol

Number correct _____ × 10 points/correct answer: Your score _____%

J. Completion

Complete each statement with the most appropriate prefix. (Note: Because you are just beginning your study of medical terminology, the meaning of the prefix has been italicized for you.) Each correct answer is worth 10 points. Record your score in the space provided at the end of the exercises.

1. High-energy x-rays that possess the ability to kill cells or retard their growth are known as ____________________ radiation.
2. A gene in a virus that has the ability to cause a cell to become malignant is known as an ____________________.
3. To exhibit again the symptoms of a disease form which a patient appears to have recovered is known as ____________________.
4. The partial or complete disappearance of the symptoms of a chronic or malignant disease is known as ____________________.
5. The probability that an individual, over the course of his or her lifetime, will develop cancer or will die from cancer is known as ____________________ risk.
6. The measure of the strength of the relationship between risk factors and particular types of cancer is known as ____________________ risk.
7. The most common malignant tumor of the epithelial tissue that occurs most often on areas of the skin exposed to the sun is ____________________ ____________________ carcinoma.
8. The classic symptom of endometrial cancer is inappropriate ____________________ bleeding.
9. A malignant skin tumor originating from melanocytes in the preexisting nevi, freckles, or skin with pigment is known as malignant ____________________.
10. A precancerous lesion occurring anywhere in the mouth, that has elevated gray-white or yellow-white leathery surfaces with clearly defined borders is known as oral ____________________.

Number correct _____ × 10 points/correct answer: Your score _____%

Answers to Chapter Review Exercises

A. Term to Definition

1. only the breast is removed
2. the breast is removed, along with the lymph nodes in the axilla (armpit)
3. the breast, chest muscles on the affected side, and lymph nodes in the axilla are removed
4. used to detect early changes in the cervical tissue that may indicate cervical cancer. The Pap test consists of obtaining scrapings from the cervix and examining them under a microscope to detect any abnormalities in cervical tissue
5. malignant tumor of the inner lining of the uterus; also known as adenocarcinoma
6. rare malignant lesions that begin as soft purple-brown nodules or plaques on the feet and gradually spread throughout the skin. This is a systemic disease also involving the GI tract and lungs.
7. surgery to remove the prostate tissue that is pressing against the upper part of the urethra causing urinary obstruction
8. occur in any structural region of the brain and they may be malignant or benign, classified as primary or secondary, and are named according to the tissue from which they originate
9. a malignant tumor of the kidney occurring predominantly during childhood
10. a precancerous lesion occurring anywhere in the mouth

B. Matching

1. g	6. i
2. d	7. j
3. f	8. a
4. e	9. b
5. h	10. c

C. Crossword Puzzle

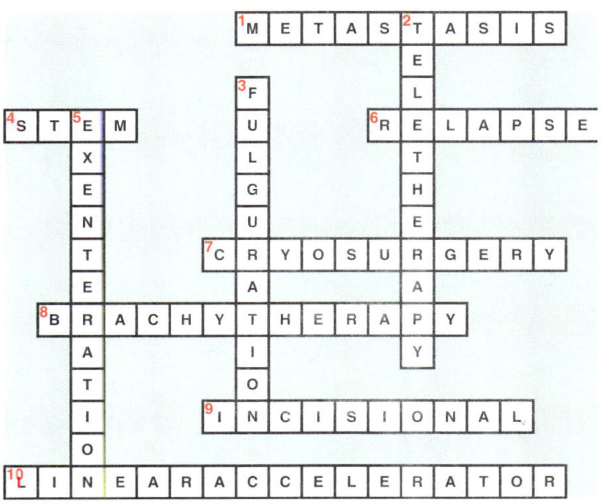

D. Definition to Term

1. adjuvant	6. invasive
2. benign	7. metastasis
3. carcinogen	8. modality
4. carcinoma in situ	9. protocol
5. fractionation	10. relapse

E. Word Search

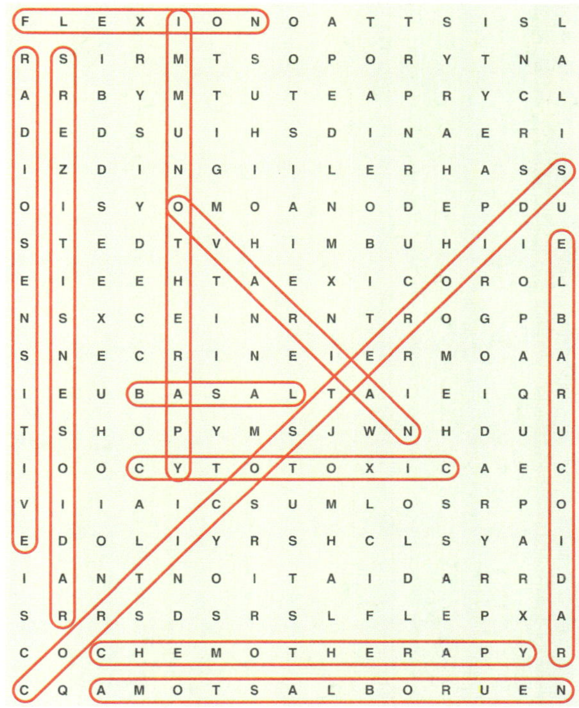

F. Matching Abbreviations

1. f	6. h
2. e	7. c
3. a	8. k
4. i	9. b
5. j	10. d

G. Spelling

1. melanoma	6. encapsulated
2. scirrhous	7. mitosis
3. neoplasm	8. benign
4. metastasis	9. adjuvant
5. papillary	10. antimetabolite

H. True or False

1. False; carcin/o = cancer
2. True
3. True
4. False; ana- = not, without
5. False; cry/o = cold
6. True
7. False; -oma = tumor
8. True
9. True
10. False; -genesis = production of, formation of

I. Multiple Choice

1. a
2. c
3. a
4. d
5. a
6. b
7. d
8. a
9. c
10. a

J. Completion

1. ionizing
2. oncogene
3. relapse
4. remission
5. lifetime
6. relative
7. basal cell
8. uterine
9. melanoma
10. leukoplakia

CHAPTER 22

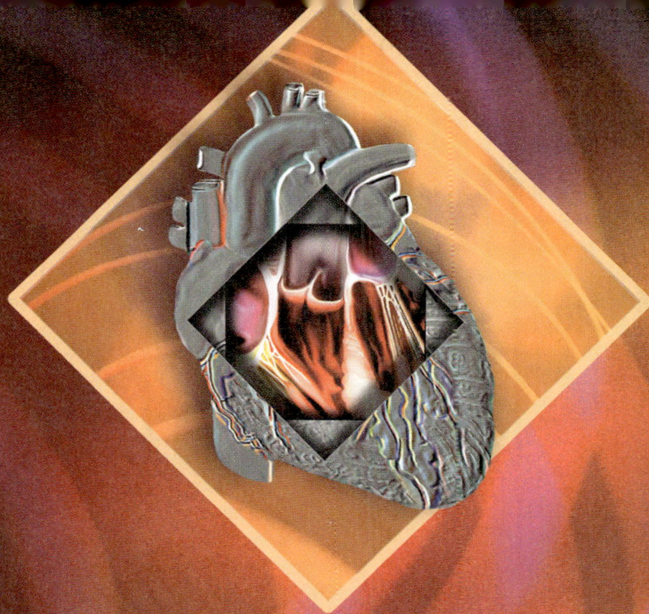

Pharmacology

CHAPTER CONTENT

KEY COMPETENCIES

Upon completing this chapter and the review exercises at the end of the chapter, the learner should be able to:

1. Identify the laws and governing agencies that enforce the safe manufacture, distribution, and use of foods, drugs, and cosmetics.
2. List five drug schedules used for categorizing controlled substances as identified in this chapter.
3. List four drug references identified in this chapter.
4. Identify four sources of drugs, giving examples for each source, as identified in this chapter.
5. Identify five different names given to drugs to identify either their chemical formula, their manufacturer's original name, or the name under which they are sold.
6. Identify at least 10 drug actions/interactions that occur within the body.
7. Identify 10 different forms of administration of medications.
8. Identify at least 14 classifications of drugs identified in this chapter.
9. Correctly spell and pronounce each new term introduced in this chapter using the Activity CD-ROM and Audio CD, if available.
10. Identify at least 30 abbreviations related to pharmacology.

OVERVIEW

Health care professionals must know the basics of pharmacology and understand the interactions of drugs within the body. A knowledge of the sources, forms, routes of administration, classifications, indications, range of dosages, desired effects, and side effects of drugs is essential. Additionally, health care professionals must know the laws regulating the distribution and use of medications. A concentrated study of pharmacology will provide the background necessary for understanding the need for safe administration of medications as prescribed by the physician, and for acquiring a strong sense of responsibility concerning administering medications.

Pharmacology is the field of medicine that specializes in the study of drugs, their sources, appearance, chemistry, actions, and uses. A **drug** is any substance that, when taken into the body, may modify one or more of its functions. **Pharmacodynamics** is the study of how drugs interact in the human body. A **pharmacist** is one who is licensed to prepare and dispense drugs. A **pharmacy** is a drugstore. **Chemotherapy** is the study of drugs that have a specific and deadly effect on disease-causing microorganisms. These drugs are used in the treatment of certain infectious diseases and cancer. **Toxicology** is the study of poisons, their detection, their effects, and establishing antidotes (substances that oppose the action of poisons) and methods of treatment for conditions they produce.

There are many terms related to pharmacology. Health care professionals may use these terms on a day-to-day basis when involved in administering medications, instructing patients in the use of medications, charting the administration of medications, or transcribing information regarding medications in the patient's chart. This chapter is devoted to the study of terms that relate to the field of pharmacology. Where appropriate throughout the chapter, word elements will be identified and defined.

Drug Laws

To ensure the safe manufacture, distribution, and use of medications, drugs are subject to numerous state and federal laws. The **Food, Drug, and Cosmetic Act (FDCA)** was passed in 1938. This law regulates the quality, purity, potency, effectiveness, safety, labeling, and packaging of food, drug, and cosmetic products. The government agency responsible for administering and enforcing the FDCA within the United States is the **Food and Drug Administration (FDA).** The federal law concerned with the manufacture, distribution, and dispensing of controlled substances, those drugs that have the potential of being abused and of causing physical or psychological dependence, administering, and enforcing the Controlled Substances Act is the **Drug Enforcement Administration (DEA).** Physicians who administer controlled substances must enter their DEA number on the prescription. Drugs that fall under the Controlled Substances Act are known as **controlled substances** or **schedule drugs.** These drugs are identified by a classification system that categorizes them by their potential for abuse. The schedule is divided into five categories: Schedules I to V. The five schedules for controlled substances are listed in **Table 22-1** with examples of specific medicines appearing in each schedule.

Table 22-1 Schedule of Controlled Substances

DRUG SCHEDULE	DESCRIPTION	EXAMPLE DRUGS
I	Schedule I drugs are not considered to be legitimate for medical use in the United States. They are used for research only and they cannot be prescribed, having a high risk for abuse.	LSD, heroin, marijuana*
II	Schedule II drugs have accepted medical use but have a high potential for abuse or addiction. These drugs must be ordered by written prescription and cannot be refilled without a new, written prescription.	Morphine, cocaine, codeine, demerol, dilaudid
III	Schedule III drugs have moderate potential for abuse or addiction, low potential for physical dependence. These drugs may be ordered by written prescription or by telephone order. Prescription expires in 6 months. They may not be refilled more than five times in a 6-month period .	Tylenol with codeine, butisol, hycodan
IV	Schedule IV drugs have less potential for abuse or addiction than those of Schedule III, with limited physical dependence. These drugs may be ordered by written prescription or by telephone order. They may be refilled up to five times over a 6-month period. Prescription expires in 6 months.	Librium, valium, darvon, equanil
V	Schedule V drugs have a small potential for abuse or addiction. These drugs may be ordered by written prescription or by telephone order and there is no limit on prescription refills. Some of these drugs may not need a prescription.	Robitussin A-C, donnagel-PG, lomotil

**Limited special permission has been obtained in some states for MDs to prescribe marijuana for treatment of side effects, such as nausea and vomiting, in patients receiving chemotherapy.*

Drug Standards

The law requires that all preparations called by the same drug name must be of a uniform strength, quality, and purity. This assures the patient of getting the same quality, purity, and strength of medication from the pharmacy each time it is prescribed and anywhere in the United States that it is prescribed. These rules, or **standards,** have been established to control the strength, quality, and purity of medications prepared by various manufacturers. The **United States Pharmacopeia/National Formulary (USP/NF)** is an authorized publication of the United States Pharmacopeial Convention, Inc. It contains formulas and information that provide the standard for preparation and dispensation of drugs. The USP/NF is recognized by the U.S. government as the official listing of standardized drugs in the United States. The FDCA specifies that a drug is official when it is listed in the USP/NF. This publication is updated every 5 years.

Drug References

There are several reference books available to physicians, nurses, and other health care professionals who are responsible for the safe administration of medications. These references normally provide the following information about drugs listed within them: composition, action, indications for use, contraindications for use, precautions, side effects, adverse reactions, route of administration, dosage range, and what forms are available.

The **Hospital Formulary** is a reference listing of all the drugs commonly stocked in the hospital pharmacy. This reference provides information about the characteristics of drugs and their clinical usage. This information is continuously revised to provide the most up-to-date information available.

The **Physicians' Desk Reference (PDR)** is published yearly by Medical Economics Company. See **Figure 22-1.**

Manufacturers pay to list information about their products in the PDR. The information provided by the manufacturers is the same basic information that is found in **package inserts** that accompany each container of medication. The FDA requires that the

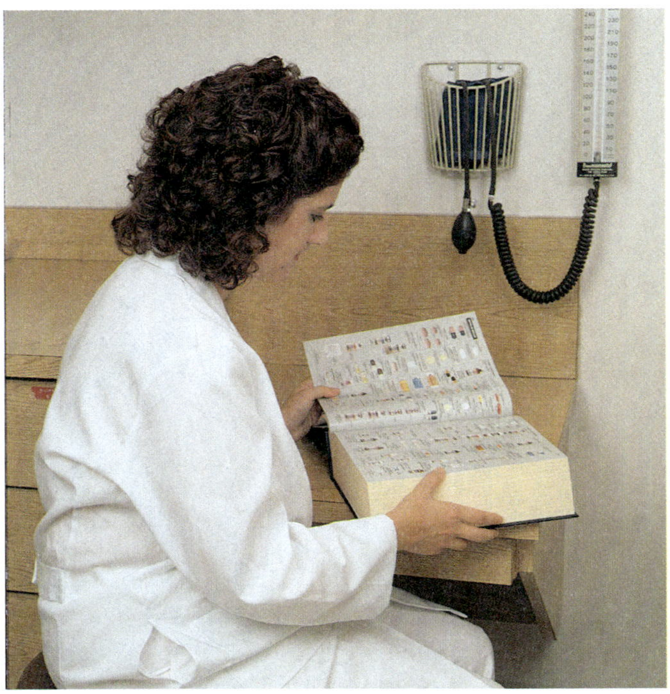

Figure 22-1 Physicians' Desk Reference (PDR)

drug's **generic** name, indications, contraindications, adverse effects, dosage, and route of administration be described in package inserts. Four additional references published by the Medical Economics Company are as follows:

1. Physicians' Desk Reference for Nonprescription Drugs
2. Physicians' Desk Reference for Ophthalmology
3. Drug Interactions and Side Effects Index
4. Indications Index

The **Drug Facts and Comparisons** is a reference for health care professionals. It is issued yearly and is updated monthly. This loose-leaf binder reference provides information on drugs according to their **therapeutic** classifications. It contains the same basic facts as the other drug references listed and is particularly helpful in comparing the various drugs within each category to other products in reference to effectiveness, content, and cost.

Vocabulary

The following vocabulary words are frequently used when discussing pharmacology.

WORD	DEFINITION
adverse reaction	The body's reaction to a drug in an unexpected way that may endanger a patient's health and safety.
anaphylactic shock (**an**-ah-fih-**LAK**-tic **SHOCK**)	A life-threatening, hypersensitive reaction to food or drugs. The patient experiences acute respiratory distress, **hypotension**, edema, tachycardia, cool pale skin, **cyanosis**, and possibly convulsions shortly after administration of the medication.
bacteriostatic **bacteri/o** = bacteria	Stopping or controlling the growth of bacteria.
brand name	The name under which the drug is sold by a specific manufacturer. This name is owned by the manufacturer and no other company may use that name. Each brand name carries a registered trademark symbol.
buccal medication (**BUCK**-al med-ih-**KAY**-shun) **bucc/o** = cheek **-al** = pertaining to	Medication that is placed in the mouth next to the cheek, where it is absorbed into the mucous membrane lining of the mouth.
chemical name	The **chemical name** for a drug is the description of the chemical structure of the drug. It is listed in the *Hospital Formulary* along with the chemical formula diagram.
chemotherapy (**kee**-moh-**THAIR**-ah-pee) **chem/o** = chemical reaction **-therapy** = treatment	The treatment of diseases using drugs that have a specific deadly effect on disease-causing microorganisms. These drugs are used in the treatment of certain infections and cancer.

contraindication (**kon**-trah-**in**-dih-**KAY**-shun)	Any special symptom or circumstance that indicates that the use of a particular drug or procedure is dangerous, not advised, or has not been proven safe for administration.
controlled substances	Drugs that have a potential for abuse. These drugs are placed into five categories ranging from Schedule I drugs, which are the most dangerous and most likely to be abused, to Schedule V drugs, which are the least dangerous and least likely to be abused; also known as schedule drugs.
Controlled Substances Act	The federal law concerned with the manufacture, distribution, and dispensing of controlled substances. These drugs have the potential of being abused and of causing physical or psychological dependence.
cumulation (**KYOO**-mew-**lay**-shun)	**Cumulation** means that a drug level begins to accumulate in the body with repeated doses because the drug is not completely excreted from the body before another dose is administered.
desired effect	The effect that was intended; that is, if the drug lowered the blood pressure as was intended, the desired effect was achieved.
drug	Any substance that, when taken into the body, may modify one or more of its functions.
drug action	Drug action describes how a drug produces changes within the body.
drug effect	Drug effect describes the change that takes place in the body as a result of the drug action.
Drug Enforcement Administration	The government agency responsible for administering and enforcing the Controlled Substances Act.
Drug Facts and Comparisons	A reference book for health care professionals that provides information on drugs according to their therapeutic classifications. This reference compares the various drugs within each category with other products.
druggist	Pharmacist.
first dose	Initial dose.
first-dose effect	An undesired effect of a medication that occurs within 30 to 90 minutes after administration of the first dose.
Food and Drug Administration	The government agency responsible for administering and enforcing the Food, Drug, and Cosmetic Act within the United States.
Food, Drug, and Cosmetic Act	A law that regulates the quality, purity, **potency**, effectiveness, safety, labeling, and packaging of food, drug, and cosmetic products.
generic name (jeh-**NAIR**-ik)	The name that is established when the drug is first manufactured. This name is protected for use only by the original manufacturer for a period of 17 years; after that time, the name of the drug becomes public property and can be used by any manufacturer.
Hospital Formulary (**FORM**-yoo-lair-ee)	A reference book that lists all of the drugs commonly stocked in the hospital pharmacy. This book provides information about the characteristics of drugs and their clinical usage.

hypotension (high-poh-**TEN**-shun) hypo- = under, below, beneath, less than normal	Low blood pressure; less than normal blood pressure.
idiosyncrasy (id-ee-oh-**SIN**-krah-see)	An unusual, inappropriate response to a drug or to the usual effective dose of a drug. This reaction can be life threatening.
inhalation medication (**in**-hah-**LAY**-shun)	Medication is sprayed or breathed into the nose, throat, and lungs. It is absorbed into the mucous membrane lining of the nose and throat and by the alveoli of the lungs.
initial dose	The first dose of a medication.
intradermal medication (**in**-trah-**DER**-mal) intra- = within derm/o = skin -al = pertaining to	Medication that is inserted just beneath the epidermis using a syringe and needle.
intramuscular medication (**in**-trah-**MUSS**-kyoo-lar) intra- = within muscul/o = muscle -ar = pertaining to	Medication that is injected directly into the muscle.
intravenous medication (in-trah-**VEE**-nus) intra- = within ven/o = vein -ous = pertaining to	Medication that is injected directly into the vein, entering the blood stream immediately.
local effect	A response to a medication that is confined to a specific part of the body.
maintenance dose	The dose of a medication that will keep the concentration of the medication in the bloodstream at the desired level.
official name	Generic name.
package insert	An information leaflet placed inside the container or package of prescription drugs. The FDA requires that the drug generic name, indications, contraindications, adverse effects, dosage, and route of administration be described in the leaflet.
parenteral medication (par-**EN**-ter-al)	Medication that is injected into the body using a needle and syringe.
pharmacist (**FAR**-mah-sist) pharmac/o = drugs, medicine -ist = specialist	One who is licensed to prepare and dispense drugs; also known as a druggist.
pharmacodynamics (**far**-mah-koh-dye-**NAM**-iks)	The study of how drugs interact in the human body.

pharmacology (**far**-mah-**KALL**-oh-jee) pharmac/o = drugs, medicine -logy = the study of	The field of medicine that specializes in the study of their sources, appearance, chemistry, actions, and uses.
pharmacy (**FAR**-mah-see)	Drugstore.
Physicians' Desk Reference	A reference book that provides the same information that is found in package inserts that accompany each container of medication: description of the drug, actions, indications and usage (why medication is prescribed), contraindications, warnings, precautions, adverse reactions, overdosage, and dosage and administration.
potency (**POH**-ten-see)	Strength.
potentiation (poh-**ten**-she-**AY**-shun)	The effect that occurs when two drugs administered together produce a more powerful response than the sum of their individual effects.
rectal medication (**REK**-tal) rect/o = rectum -al = pertaining to	Medication that is inserted into the rectum and is slowly absorbed into the mucous membrane lining of the rectum. It is in the form of a suppository, which melts as the body temperature warms it.
route of administration	The method of introducing a medication into the body.
side effect	An additional effect on the body by a drug that was not part of the goal for that medication. Nausea is a common side effect of many drugs.
standards	Rules that have been established to control the strength, quality, and purity of medications prepared by various manufacturers.
subcutaneous medication (**sub**-kyoo-**TAY**-nee-us) sub- = under, below cutane/o = skin -ous = pertaining to	Medication that is injected into the subcutaneous layer, or fatty tissue, of the skin.
sublingual medication (sub-**LING**-gwal) sub- = under lingu/o = tongue -al = pertaining to	Medication that is placed under the tongue, where it dissolves in the patient's saliva and is quickly absorbed through the mucous membrane lining of the mouth.
systemic effect (sis-**TEM**-ik effect)	A generalized response to a drug by the body. The drug has a widespread influence on the body because it is absorbed into the bloodstream.
tachycardia (**tak**-ee-**KAR**-dee-ah) tachy- = rapid cardi/o = heart -ia = noun ending	Rapid heartbeat, over 100 beats per minute.

therapeutic dose (thair-ah-**PEW**-tik)	The dose of a medication that achieves the desired effect.
tolerance (**TALL**-er-ans)	The body's resistance to the effect of a drug.
topical medication (**TOP**-ih-kal)	Medication that is applied directly to the skin or mucous membrane for a local effect to the area.
toxicology (**tocks**-ih-**KALL**-oh-jee) toxic/o = poisons, toxins -logy = the study of	The study of poisons, their detection, their effects, and establishing antidotes and methods of treatment for conditions they produce.
trade name	Brand name.
United States Pharmacopeia (**far**-mah-koh-**PEE**-ah)	An authorized publication of the United States Pharmacopeial Convention, Inc. that contains formulas and information that provide a standard for preparation and dispensation of drugs. Recognized by the U.S. government as the official listing of standardized drugs.
vaginal medication (**VAJ**-in-al) vagin/o = vagina -al = pertaining to	Medication that is inserted into the vagina; may be in the form of a suppository, cream, foam, or tablet.

Word Elements

The following word elements pertain to pharmacology. As you review the list, pronounce each word element aloud twice and check the box after you "say it." Write the definition for the example word given for each word element. You may use your medical dictionary.

WORD ELEMENT	PRONUNCIATION	"SAY IT"	MEANING
alges/o an**alges**ic	al-**JEE**-soh **an**-al-**JEE**-sik	☐	sensitivity to pain
anti- **anti**depressant	**AN**-tih **an**-tih-dee-**PRESS**-ant	☐	against
arrhythm/o anti**arrhythm**ic	ah-**RITH**-moh **an**-tee-ah-**RITH**-mik	☐	rhythm
bi/o anti**bi**otic	**BYE**-oh an-tih-**BYE**-ot-ik	☐	life
bronch/o **bronch**odilator	**BRONG**-koh **brong**-koh-**DYE**-lay-tor	☐	airway
bucc/o **bucc**al	**BUCK**-oh **BUCK**-al	☐	cheek

chem/o **chemo**therapy	**KEE**-moh kee-moh-**THAIR**-ah-pee	☐	drug
coagul/o anti**coagul**ant	koh-**AG**-yoo-loh an-tih-koh-**AG**-yoo-lant	☐	clotting
cutane/o sub**cutane**ous	kyoo-**TAY**-nee-oh sub-kyoo-**TAY**-nee-us	☐	skin
cyan/o **cyan**osis	sigh-**AN**-oh sigh-ah-**NOH**-sis	☐	blue
esthesi/o an**esthesi**a	ess-**THEEZ**-ee-oh an-ess-**THEEZ**-ee-ah	☐	feeling, sensation
fung/o anti**fung**al	**FUNG**-oh **an**-tih-**FUNG**-al	☐	fungus
gloss/o hypo**gloss**al	**GLOSS**-oh high-poh-**GLOSS**-al	☐	tongue
hyper- anti**hyper**tensive	**HIGH**-per an-tih-high-per-**TEN**-siv	☐	excessive, high
hypno- **hypno**tic	**HIP**-noh hip-**NOT**-ik	☐	sleep
-ia analges**ia**	**EE**-ah an-al-**JEE**-see-ah	☐	condition; noun ending
immun/o **immun**osuppressant	**IM**-yoo-noh **im**-yoo-noh-suh-**PRESS**-ant	☐	immune, protection
intra- **intra**dermal	**IN**-trah **in**-trah-**der**-mal	☐	within
-ist pharmac**ist**	**IST** **FAR**-mah-sist	☐	a specialist in a field of study
lingu/o sub**lingu**al	**LING**-yoo-oh sub-**LING**-gwal	☐	tongue
lip/o **lip**id	**LIP**-oh **LIP**-id	☐	fat
-logy pharmaco**logy**	**LOH**-jee **far**-mah-**KALL**-oh-jee	☐	the study of
muscul/o intra**muscul**ar medication	**MUSS**-kyoo-loh **in**-trah-**MUSS**-kyoo-lar	☐	muscle
ne/o anti**ne**oplastic	**NEE**-oh **an**-tih-**nee**-oh-**PLASS**-tic	☐	new

or/o **or**al medication	**OR**-oh **OR**-al	☐	mouth
pharmac/o **pharmac**y	**FAR**-mah-koh **FAR**-mah-see	☐	drugs, medicine
rect/o **rect**al medication	**REK**-toh **REK**-tal	☐	rectum
skelet/o **skelet**al muscle relaxant	**SKELL**-eh-toh **SKELL**-eh-tal muscle rih-**LAK**-sant	☐	skeleton
sub- **sub**ungual	**SUB** sub-**UNG**-gwal	☐	under, below
toxic/o **toxic**ology	**TOCKS**-ih-koh **tocks**-ih-**KALL**-oh-jee	☐	poison
vagin/o **vagin**al medication	**VAJ**-in-oh **VAJ**-in-al	☐	vagina
ven/o intra**ven**ous	**VEE**-noh in-trah-**VEE**-nus	☐	vein

Drug Sources

The origin of many of the drugs used today can be traced to ancient civilizations. Many drugs were prepared from plants, leaves, herbs, roots, and barks, with plants being a primary source of medicinal substances. Examples of plant sources of medications are the purple fox glove, which is a source for digitalis, a medication used to treat heart arrhythmias and congestive heart failure, and the poppy plant, which is a source of opium, and is used in **antidiarrheal** medications and **analgesics**. Leaves and herbs were sources of medicinal-type teas in the earlier generations.

As time evolved, animals and minerals became additional sources of drugs. An example of an animal source for drugs commonly used today is insulin, which is extracted from the pancreas of animals (hogs and cows). An example of a mineral source of drugs is sulphur, which is used in many bacteriostatic medications.

A more recent source of drugs has been pharmaceutical laboratories that produce synthetic drugs. Medications such as Demerol, a narcotic analgesic, and Lomotil, an antidiarrheal, are examples of synthetic forms of medications. Insulin and sulphur drugs are also produced synthetically in pharmaceutical laboratories. See **Figure 22-2.**

Drug Names

The chemical name of a drug describes the chemical structure of the drug. It is the formula that indicates the composition of the drug.

The **generic** name or official name of a drug is the name that was established when the drug was first manufactured. The spelling of the generic name is written in lowercase

Source	Example	Drug name	Classification
Plants 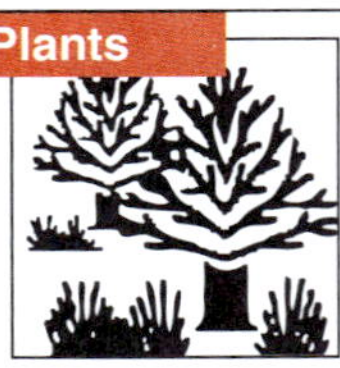	cinchona bark purple foxglove	quinidine digitalis	antiarrhythmic cardiotonic
Minerals 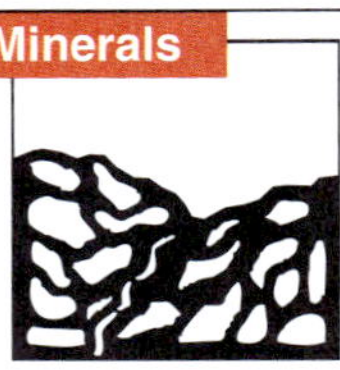	magnesium gold	Milk of Magnesia Solganal; auranofin	antacid, laxative anti-inflammatory used to treat rheumatoid arthritis
Animals 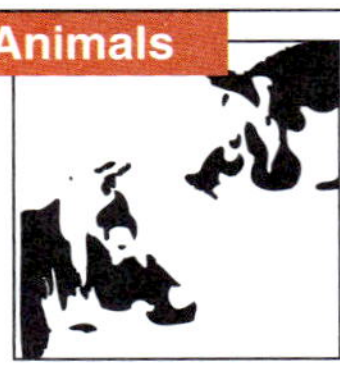	pancreas of cow, hog thyroid gland of animals	insulin thyroid, USP	antidiabetic hormone hormone
Synthetic 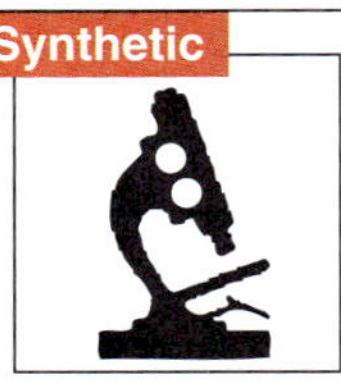	meperidine diphenoxylate	Demerol Lomotil	analgesic antidiarrheal

Figure 22-2 Drug sources

letters. The original manufacturer of the drug is the only company that can use the generic name for the drug for the first 17 years of its use; then the name of the drug becomes public property and can be used by any manufacturer. Each drug has only one generic name. The official (generic) name for each drug is listed in the USP/NF.

The brand name or trade name of a drug is the name under which the drug is sold by a specific manufacturer. The name is owned by the drug company and no other company may use that name. Each brand name drug carries a registered trademark symbol (®) after its name, showing that it is restricted to the particular manufacturer. A drug may be known by several different brand names. The spelling of the brand name or trade name always begins with a capital letter.

Drug Actions/Interactions

When drugs are ingested or administered into the body, they are absorbed into the bloodstream or into the body tissues. The drugs then combine with, or alter, the molecules in the body cells, changing the way the cells work. How the drugs produce these changes within the body is known as drug action. The changes that take place in the body as a result of the drug action is known as the drug effect. Some drugs act in the body by either slowing down or speeding up the ordinary processes that the cells carry out. Other drugs destroy certain cells or parts of cells, such as drugs that destroy disease-producing microorganisms and cancer cells. Yet other drugs act by replacing substances that the body lacks or fails to produce, such as **vitamins**.

The effect of the drug in the body may be a desired effect, achieving the response by the body that is intended; that is, the desired effect was to lower the blood sugar, and the patient's blood sugar level did drop. A drug is usually prescribed for its desired effect. A side effect, is an additional effect on the body by the drug that was not part of the goal for that medication; nausea is a common side effect of many drugs. Even though side effects are bothersome, they are not usually severe enough to warrant discontinuing the medication. An **adverse reaction** is one in which the body reacts to a drug in an unexpected way that may endanger a patient's health and safety. A **contraindication** is any special symptom or circumstance that indicates that the use of a particular drug or procedure is dangerous, not advised, or has not been proven safe for administration.

Drugs may affect only a specific part of the body, having a local effect, or they may affect the body as a whole, having a systemic effect. A local effect of a drug is one that is confined to a specific part of the body; for example, the dentist may administer a medication to numb only one tooth, thus, the medication has a local effect on that particular area of the body.

A systemic effect of a drug is one that has a widespread influence on the body because it is absorbed into the bloodstream. The remaining terms in this section describe the action and interaction of drugs in the body after they have been absorbed into the bloodstream; that is, those having a systemic effect on the body.

---

cumulation
(**KYOO**-mew-lay-shun)

Cumulation occurs when a drug is not completely excreted from the body before another dose is given.

When repeated doses of the drug are given, the drug starts to accumulate in the body tissues and **toxic** effects may occur.

---

idiosyncrasy
(**id**-ee-oh-**SIN**-krah-see)

An idiosyncrasy is an unusual, inappropriate response to a drug or to the usual effective dose of a drug.

This reaction may be life threatening. An example of a severe idiosyncratic reaction to a drug or its dosage is anaphylactic shock in which the patient experiences acute respiratory distress, hypotension, edema, tachycardia, cool pale skin, cyanosis, and possibly convulsions shortly after administration of the medication; penicillin is a medicine that is known to cause anaphylactic reactions in some individuals.

---

potentiation
(poh-**ten**-**she**-**AY**-shun)

Potentiation occurs when two drugs administered together produce a more powerful response than the sum of their individual effects.

Patients who are taking blood thinners are advised to avoid taking aspirin, which will potentiate the thinning effect on the blood.

---

tolerance
(**TALL**-er-ans)

Tolerance is resistance to the effect of a drug.

The individual develops a decreased sensitivity to subsequent doses of the drug and requires increasingly larger doses to get the full effect of the drug. Tolerance is also a characteristic of drug addiction.

When a drug is given for the first time by whatever method, it is called the initial dose. The initial dose is also known as the first dose. Sometimes patients will have an undesired effect after the initial or first dose of a medication, particularly with some medications given for treatment of hypertension; that is, a sharp drop in blood pressure and fainting within 30 to 90 minutes after the first dose of the medication. This response to the initial dose of a medication is known as first-dose effect.

The dose of a medication that achieves the desired effect is known as the **therapeutic** dose. Some medications have to be given in increasing doses until the desired level of concentration in the bloodstream is achieved. A maintenance dose will keep the concentration of the medication in the bloodstream at the desired level. Medications given to slow and strengthen the heartbeat are often given in increments until the maintenance dose level is achieved.

Routes of Administration for Medications

Medications can be introduced into the body using several different methods, referred to as the route of administration. The route of administration determines how rapidly a drug is absorbed into the bloodstream, how well the drug is absorbed, and how long the drug acts within the body. The route of administration is usually based on the type of medication given, the dosage form, and the desired effect. The following is a list of the major routes of administration for medications. The list is not alphabetized, but is presented in the order in which routes of administration of medications are usually discussed in pharmacology textbooks.

oral
(**OR**-al)
or/o = mouth
-al = pertaining to

An oral medication is one that is given by mouth and swallowed.

This drug is then slowly absorbed into the bloodstream through the lining of the stomach and intestines. See **Figure 22-3.**

Advantage: easiest and safest method, most economical method.

Disadvantage: slow method of absorption, possibility of being destroyed by the gastric juices.

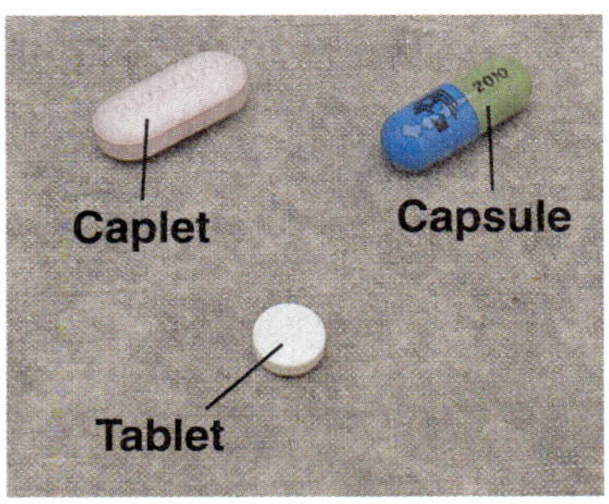

Figure 22-3 Oral medications

sublingual
(sub-**LING**-gwal)
sub- = under, below
lingu/o = tongue
-al = pertaining to

A sublingual medication is one that is placed under the tongue.

It dissolves in the patient's saliva and is quickly absorbed through the mucous membrane lining of the mouth; also known as **hypoglossal**.

Advantage: more rapid absorption rate than oral, higher concentration of medication reaches the bloodstream by not passing through the stomach.

Disadvantage: not a convenient route of administration for bad-tasting medications or those that might irritate the mucous membrane.

buccal
(**BUCK**-a.)
bucc/o = cheek
-al = pertaining to

A buccal medication is one that is placed in the mouth next to the cheek; it is in tablet form.

The medication is absorbed into the mucous membrane lining of the mouth.

Advantage: more rapid absorption rate than oral, higher concentration of medication reaches the bloodstream by not passing through the stomach, effects of the medication stop if the tablet is removed.

Disadvantage: possibility of swallowing the pill.

inhalation
(**in**-hah-**LAY**-shun)

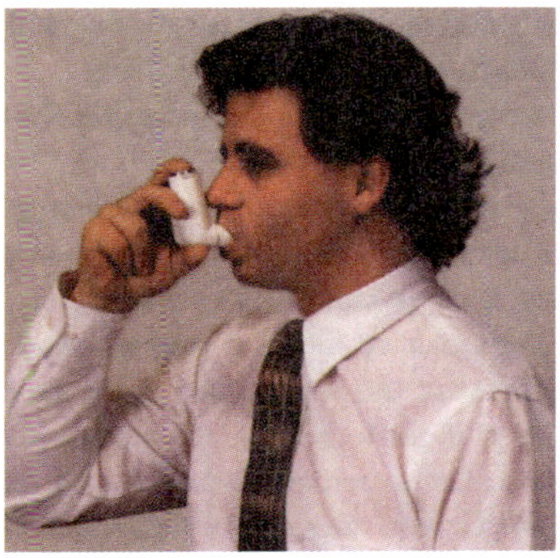

Medications administered by inhalation are those that are sprayed or inhaled into the nose, throat, and lungs. See Figure 22-4.

The medication is absorbed into the mucous membrane lining of the nose and throat and by the alveoli of the lungs. These drugs are in the form of inhalers, sprays, mists, and sometimes steam vapor.

Advantage: good absorption due to large surface contact area, provides rapid treatment.

Disadvantage: sometimes difficult to regulate the dosage, not suitable for medications that might irritate the mucous membrane lining, sometimes considered to be an awkward method of administering medication.

Figure 22-4 Medications by inhalation

rectal
(**REK**-tal)
rect/o = rectum
-al = pertaining to

Rectal medications are those that are inserted into the rectum and are slowly absorbed into the mucous membrane lining of the rectum.

This medication is in the form of a suppository, which dissolves as the body temperature warms and melts it. See **Figure 22-5A.**

Advantage: one method of choice when the patient is nauseated or cannot take medications orally.

Disadvantage: absorption is slow and irregular.

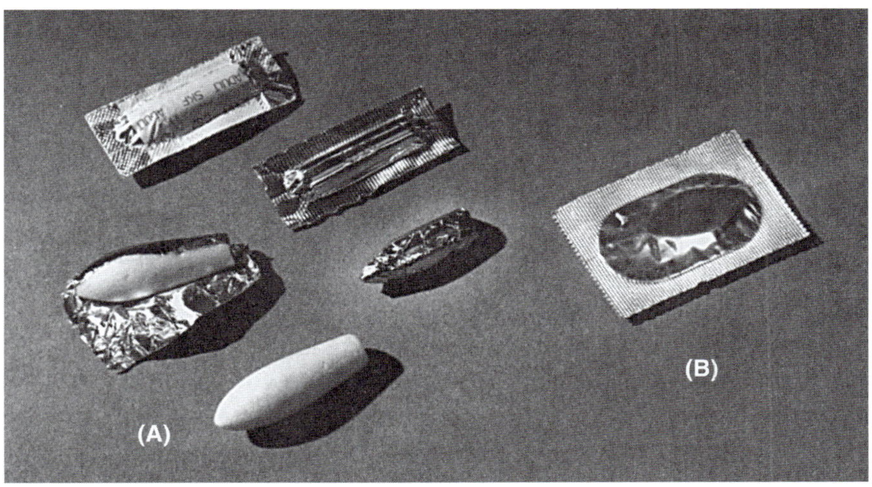

Figure 22-5 (A) Rectal medications; (B) vaginal medications

vaginal
(**VAJ**-in-al)
vagin/o = vagina
-al = pertaining to

Vaginal medications are those that are inserted into the vagina.

This medication may be in the form of a suppository, cream, foam, or tablet. The medication dissolves as the body temperature warms and melts it. See **Figure 22-5B.** Vaginal medications are usually given for their local effect on the mucous membrane lining the vagina.

Advantage: easiest method for treating the specific area.

Disadvantage: no particular disadvantage, other than the fact that medications sometimes stain underwear.

topical
(**TOP**-ih-kal)

A topical medication is one that is applied directly to the skin or mucous membrane for a local effect to the area.

These medications are in the form of creams, ointments, sprays, lotions, liniments, liquids, and powders.

Advantage: easy method, convenient.

Disadvantage: slow absorption through the skin.

transdermal
trans- = across
derm/o = skin
-al = pertaining to

A method of applying a drug to unbroken skin. The drug is absorbed continuously and produces a systemic effect.

Medications administered by the transdermal infusion system are packaged in an adhesive-backed disk. The disk contains a premeasured amount of medication. When the disk is applied, the medication is released through the skin into the bloodstream at a controlled rate, producing a systemic effect. Examples of transdermal medications include vasodilators such as nitroglycerin, hormones such as estrogen, and medications used to help stop smoking.

Advantage: good method for administering medications that need to be released slowly into the bloodstream over a period of time.

Disadvantage: units can be dangerous if they come in contact with the skin of children or pets. There are a very limited number of drugs available at this time that can be administered by the transdermal patch. Removal of the patch does not guarantee immediate stoppage of absorption of the medication, should an adverse reaction occur. See **Figure 22-6.**

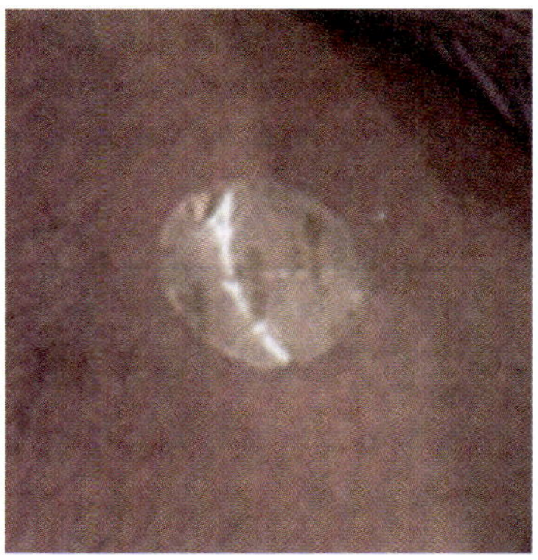

Figure 22-6 Transdermal delivery system

parenteral
(par-**EN**-ter-al)
par- = apart from
enter/o = intestine
-al = pertaining to

Parenteral medications are those administered by injecting the medication into the body using a needle and syringe. See Figure 22-7.

Parenteral medication must be in a liquid form and is administered by one of the following four methods.

intradermal
(**in**-trah-**der**-mal)
intra- = within
derm/o = skin
-al = pertaining to

A small amount of medication is injected just beneath the epidermis.

Intradermal injections are used for allergy testing, tuberculin skin testing, and some vaccinations.

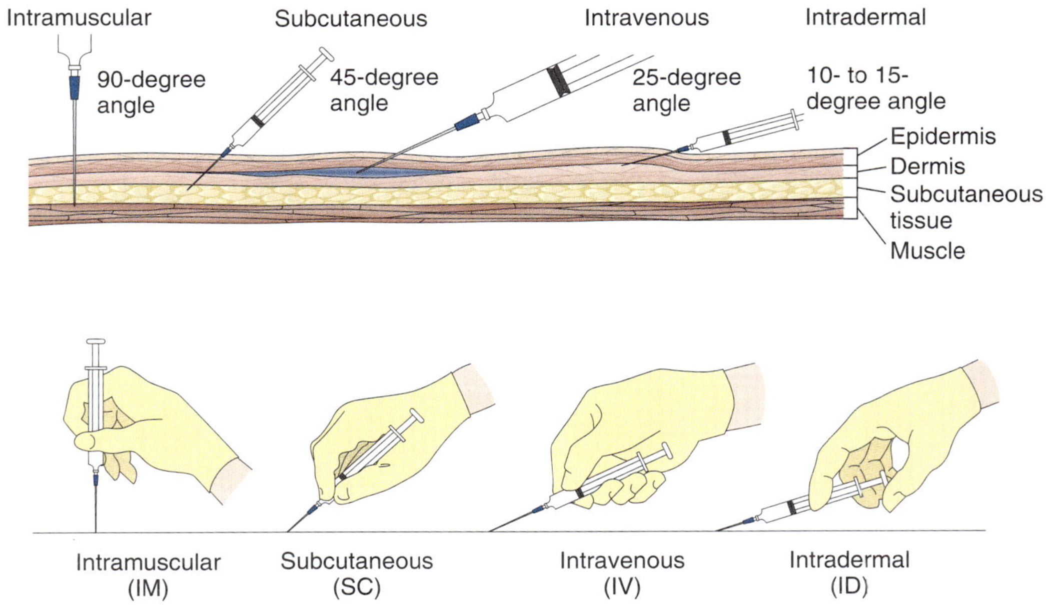

Figure 22-7 Parenteral medications

---

intramuscular
(in-trah-**MUSS**-kyoo-lar)
intra- = within
muscul/o = muscle
-ar = pertaining to

The medication is injected directly into the muscle.

Intramuscular injections are used for administering antibiotics, medications that might be irritating to the layers of the skin, and medications that require dosages larger than the amount allowed for a subcutaneous injection.

---

intravenous
(in-trah-**VEE**-nus)
intra- = within
ven/o = vein
-ous = pertaining to

The medication is injected directly into the vein, entering the bloodstream immediately.

Intravenous injections are used when medication is needed quickly, and for administering medication over a period of time, by adding the medication to a bag of intravenous fluids (a process known as infusion).

---

subcutaneous
(**sub**-kyoo-**TAY**-nee-us)
sub- = under, below
cutane/o = skin
-ous = pertaining to

The medication is injected into the subcutaneous layer, or fatty tissue, of the skin.

Subcutaneous injections are used for administering insulin, hormones, and local **anesthetics**.

Drug Classification

Drugs are classified, or categorized, according to their primary or main effect(s) in the body. **Table 22-2** lists most of the major classifications of drugs, along with a basic description of each category and a common example of a medicine from each classification. The generic name is written in lowercase letters and the brand name begins with a capital letter.

Table 22-2 Major Drug Classifications

DRUG CLASSIFICATION	GENERAL-PURPOSE DEFINITION	COMMON EXAMPLE
analgesic (**an**-al-**JEE**-sik) an- = without alges/o = pain -ic = pertaining to	Relieves pain	acetylsalicylic acid (aspirin, Bayer Children's Aspirin) acetaminophen (Tylenol)
anesthetic (**an**-ess-**THET**-ik) an- = without esthet/o = feeling nervous sensation or sense of perception -ic = pertaining to	Partially or completely numbs or eliminates sensitivity with or without loss of consciousness	lidocaine (Xylocaine)
antiarrhythmic (**an**-tee-ah-**RITH**-mik) anti- = against arrhythm/o = rhythm -ic = pertaining to	Corrects cardiac arrhythmias (irregular beats)	digoxin (Lanoxin) propranolol hydrochloride (Inderal)
antibiotic **(anti-infective)** (**an**-tih-**BYE**-ot-ik) anti- = against bi/o = life -tic = pertaining to	Stops or controls the growth of infection-causing microorganisms	phenoxymethyl-penicillin sodium (Pen-Vee-K, Penicillin VK, Veetids, V-Cillin K) trimethoprim and sulfameth-oxazole (Bactrim, Bactrim DS)
anticoagulant (**an**-tih-koh-**AG**-yoo-lant) anti- = against coagul/o = clotting	Prevents clot continuation and formation	heparin calcium (Calcilean) warfarin sodium (Coumadin)
anticonvulsant (**an**-tih-kon-**VULL**-sant)	Prevents or relieves convulsions (seizures)	phenobarbital sodium (Luminal Sodium) diazepam (Valium)
antidepressant (**an**-tih-dee-**PRESS**-ant)	Prevents, cures, or alleviates mental depression	amitriptyline hydrochloride (Elavil, Amitril) imipramine hydrochloride (Tofranil)
antidiabetic (**an**-tih-**dye**-ah-**BET**-ik)	Helps control the blood sugar level	chlorpropamide (Diabenese) tolazamide (Tolinase) insulin
antidiarrheal (**an**-tih-dye-ah-**REE**-ul)	Prevents or treats diarrhea	diphenoxylate-atropine sulfate (Lomotil) loperamide hydrochloride (Imodium)

antidiuretic (an-tih-dye-yoo-**REH**-tic)	Suppresses the formation of urine	vasopressin (Pitressin)
antiemetic (**an**-tih-ee-**MET**-ik)	Prevents or relieves nausea and vomiting	chlorpromazine (Thorazine) meclizine hydrochloride (Bonine, Dramamine II, Antivert)
antifungal (**an**-tih-**FUNG**-gal) **anti-** = against **fung/o** = fungus **-al** = pertaining to	Destroys or inhibits the growth of fungi	miconazole (Monistat) nystatin (Mycostatin) clotrimazole (Gyne-Lotrimin)
antihistamine (an-tih-**HISS**-tah-meen)	Opposes the action of histamine, which is released in allergic reactions	diphenhydramine hydrochloride (Benadryl) brompheniramine maleate (Dimetane)
antihypertensive (**an**-tih-**high**-per-**TEN**-siv) **anti-** = against **hyper-** = excessive	Prevents or controls high blood pressure	nadolol (Corgard) furosemide (Lasix) diltiazem hydrochloride (Cardizem, Cardizem CD)
anti-infective (antibiotic) (an-tih-in-**FEK**-tiv)	Stops or controls the growth of infection-causing microorganisms	amoxycillin (Amoxil, Polymox) doxycycline hyclate (Vibramycin)
anti-inflammatory (an-tih-in-**FLAM**-ah-toh-ree)	Counteracts inflammation in the body	nabumetone (Relafen) naproxen sodium (Anaprox, Aleve)
antineoplastic (**an**-tih-**nee**-oh-**PLASS**-tik) **anti-** = against **ne/o** = new **plas/o** = formation **-tic** = pertaining to	Prevents the development, growth, or reproduction of cancerous cells	fluorouracil (Adrucil) methotrexate (Rheumatrex Dose Pack)
antitussive (an-tih-**TUSS**-iv)	Relieves cough due to various causes	dextromethorphan hydrobromide (Benylin DM, Robitussin Pediatric, Vick's Formula 44, Vick's Formula 44 Pediatric Formula) pseudoephedrine hydrochloride and guaifenesin (Novahistex Expectorant with Decongestant, Robitussin PE, Sudafed Expectorant)
antiulcer agent (an-tih-**ULL**-ser)	Treats and prevents peptic ulcer and gastric hypersecretion	ranitidine hydrochloride (Zantac) nizatidine (Axid)
antiviral agent (an-tih-**VYE**-ral)	Treats various viral conditions such as serious herpes virus infection, chicken-pox, and influenza A	acyclovir (Zovirax) vidarabine (Vira-A)

beta blocker (**BAY**-tah block-er)	Treats hypertension, angina, and various abnormal heart rhythms	metoprolol tartrate (Lopressor) carteolol hydrochloride (Ocupress, Cartrol)
bronchodilator (**brong**-koh-**DYE**-lay-tor) **bronch/o** = bronchus; airway	Expands the bronchial tubes by relaxing the bronchial muscles	theophylline (Bronkodyl, Quibron-T/SR, Theobid Duracaps) aminophylline (Aminophylline, Truphyllin)
calcium channel blocker (**KAL**-see-um **CHAN**-ell **BLOCK**-er)	Treats hypertension, angina, and various abnormal heart rhythms	nicardipine hydrochloride (Cardene) bepridil hydrochloride (Vascor)
diuretic (**dye**-yoor-**RET**-ik)	Increases urine secretion	furosemide (Lasix) hydrochlorothiazide (Hydro-Diuril)
hormone (**HOR**-mohn)	Treats deficiency states where specific hormone level is abnormally low	estrogen, conjugated (Premarin) glucagon (Glucagon)
hypnotic (hip-**NOT**-ik) **hypno-** = sleep **-tic** = pertaining to	Induces sleep or dulls the senses	pentobarbital (Nembutal) secobarbital sodium (Seconal Sodium)
immunosuppressant (**im**-yoo-noh-suh-**PRESS**-ant) **immun/o** = immunity	Suppresses the body's natural immune response to an antigen, as in treatment for transplant patients	cyclosporine (Sandimmune) azathioprine (Imuran)
laxative (**LACK**-sah-tiv)	Prevents constipation or promotes the emptying of the bowel contents with ease	docusate calcium (Surfak) bisacodyl (Dulcolax) psyllium hydrophilic muciloid (Metamucil)
lipid-lowering agent (**LIP**-id) **lip/o** = fat	Reduces blood lipid (fat) levels	niacin (Nicobid) lovastatin (Mevacor)
sedative (**SED**-ah-tiv)	Exerts a soothing or tranquilizing effect on the body	phenobarbital (Nembutal) diazepam (Valium) flurazepam hydrochloride (Dalmane)
skeletal muscle relaxant (**SKELL**-eh-tal muscle rih-**LAK**-sant) **skelet/o** = skeleton **-al** = pertaining to **muscul/o** = muscle **-e** = noun ending	Relieves muscle tension	dantrolene sodium (Dantrium) carisoprodol (Soma) cyclobenzaprine- hydrochloride (Flexiril)
vitamin (**VIGH**-tah-min)	Prevents and treats vitamin deficiencies and used as dietary supplement	Vitamins A, D, E, etc. ascorbic acid (vitamin C) cyanocobalamin (vitamin B_{12})

Common Charting Abbreviations

Medical abbreviations are a form of shorthand that serve as a universal language for medical professionals to provide specific information and/or orders in an abbreviated format. These abbreviations may be used on a daily basis by those involved in all aspects of health care. It is essential that health care professionals commit these abbreviations to memory to transmit and receive clear and concise meanings. Some of the more commonly used abbreviations that relate to pharmacology and are used for charting are listed below. As you continue your studies in pharmacology and other aspects of the medical field, your list of abbreviations will expand.

ABBREVIATION	MEANING
$\overline{aa}$	of each
a.c.	before meals
ad lib.	as desired
AM	morning
AQ, aq	water
b.i.d.	twice a day
C	Celsius (Centigrade)
$\bar{c}$	with
cap(s)	capsule, capsules
cc	cubic centimeter
cm	centimeter
dc, D/C	discontinue
DEA	Drug Enforcement Administration
disp	dispense
dr	dram
DS	double strength
elix	elixir
F	Fahrenheit
FDA	Food and Drug Administration
FDCA	Food, Drug, and Cosmetic Act
gal	gallon
Gm., g, gm	gram
gr	grain
gtt	drops
h, hr	hour
h.s.	hour of sleep
H_2O	water
ID	intradermal
IM	intramuscular
inj.	injection
I.U.	International Units
IV	intravenous
kg	kilogram
L or l	liter
lb	pound
mg	milligram
mEq	milliequivalent
mL or ml	milliliter
♏	minim
n.p.o., NPO	nothing by mouth
O_2	oxygen
O.D.	right eye
oint., ung	ointment
O.S.	left eye
OTC	over the counter (drugs)
O.U.	both eyes
oz	ounce
$\bar{p}$	after

p.c.	after meals
PDR	Physicians' Desk Reference
PM	afternoon
p.o.	by mouth (per os)
p.r.n.	as needed
pt	pint
q.	every
q. a.m.	every morning
q.d.	every day
q.h.	every hour
q.2 h., q.3 h.,. . . .	every 2 hours, every 3 hours . . . .
q. h.s.	at bedtime (every hour of sleep)
q.i.d.	four times a day
q.o.d.	every other day
q.s.	quantity sufficient
qt	quart
R	rectal
R_x	take; treatment; prescription
$\bar{s}$	without
SC, subq, sub-Q	subcutaneous
sig	write on label (let it be labeled)
sol	solution
sos	if necessary
$\overline{ss}$	one-half
stat.	immediately
supp.	suppository
T, Tbsp.	tablespoon
t, tsp.	teaspoon
tab.	tablet
t.i.d.	three times a day
tinct.	tincture
TO	telephone order
U	unit
ung, oint.	ointment
USP/NF	United States Pharmacopeia/ National Formulary
VO	verbal order
x	times, multiplied by

Written and Audio Terminology Review

Review each of the following terms from this chapter. Study the spelling of each term and write the definition in the space provided. If you have the Audio CD available, listen to each term, pronounce it, and check the box once you are comfortable saying the word. Check definitions by looking the term up in the glossary/index.

TERM	PRONUNCIATION	DEFINITION
adverse reaction	☐ **AD**-vers reaction	______________
analgesic	☐ an-al-**JEE**-sik	______________
anaphylactic shock	☐ an-ah-fih-**LAK**-tic **SHOCK**	______________
anesthesia	☐ an-ess-**THEEZ**-ee-ah	______________
anesthetic	☐ an-ess-**THET**-ik	______________

Term	Pronunciation	
antiarrhythmic	☐ **an**-tee-ah-**RITH**-mik	______
antibiotic	☐ **an**-tye-**BYE**-ot-ik	______
anticoagulant	☐ **an**-tih-koh-**AG**-yoo-lant	______
anticonvulsant	☐ **an**-tih-kon-**VULL**-sant	______
antidepressant	☐ **an**-tih-dee-**PRESS**-ant	______
antidiabetic	☐ **an**-tih-**dye**-ah-**BET**-ik	______
antidiarrheal	☐ **an**-tih-dye-ah-**REE**-al	______
antiemetic	☐ **an**-tih-ee-**MET**-ik	______
antifungal	☐ **an**-tih-**FUNG**-gal	______
antihistamine	☐ **an**-tih-**HISS**-tah-meen	______
antihypertensive	☐ **an**-tih-**high**-per-**TEN**-siv	______
anti-infective	☐ **an**-tih-in-**FEK**-tiv	______
anti-inflammatory	☐ **an**-tih-in-**FLAM**-ah-toh-ree	______
antineoplastic	☐ **an**-tih-nee-oh-**PLASS**-tik	______
antitussive	☐ **an**-tih-**TUSS**-iv	______
antiulcer	☐ **an**-tih-**ULL**-ser	______
antiviral	☐ **an**-tih-**VYE**-ral	______
beta blocker	☐ **BAY**-tah blocker	______
bronchodilator	☐ **brong**-koh-**DYE**-lay-tor	______
buccal medication	☐ **BUCK**-al med-ih-**KAY**-shun	______
calcium channel blocker	☐ **KAL**-see-um **CHAN**-ell **BLOCK**-er	______
chemical name	☐ **KEM**-ih-cal name	______
chemotherapy	☐ kee-moh-**THAIR**-ah-pee	______
contraindication	☐ **kon**-trah-**in**-dih-**KAY**-shun	______
cumulation	☐ **KYOO**-mew-lay-shun	______
cyanosis	☐ sigh-ah-**NOH**-sis	______
diuretic	☐ **dye**-yoor-**RET**-ik	______
generic	☐ jeh-**NAIR**-ik	______
hormone	☐ **HOR**-mohn	______
Hospital Formulary	☐ hospital **FORM**-you-lair-ee	______
hypnotic	☐ hip-**NOT**-ik	______

Term		Pronunciation	
hypoglossal	☐	high-poh-**GLOSS**-al	______
hypotension	☐	high-poh-**TEN**-shun	______
idiosyncrasy	☐	**id**-ee-oh-**SIN**-krah-see	______
immunosuppressant	☐	**im**-yoo-noh-suh-**PRESS**-ant	______
inhalation	☐	**in**-hah-**LAY**-shun	______
intradermal	☐	**in**-trah-**der**-mal	______
intramuscular	☐	**in**-trah-**MUSS**-kyoo-lar	______
intravenous	☐	in-trah-**VEE**-nus	______
laxative	☐	**LACK**-sah-tiv	______
lipid-lowering agent	☐	**LIP**-id lowering agent	______
oral	☐	**OR**-al	______
parenteral	☐	par-**EN**-ter-al	______
pharmacist	☐	**FAR**-mah-sist	______
pharmacodynamics	☐	**far**-mah-koh-dye-**NAM**-iks	______
pharmacology	☐	**far**-mah-**KALL**-oh-jee	______
pharmacopeia	☐	**far**-mah-koh-**PEE**-ah	______
pharmacy	☐	**FAR**-mah-see	______
potency	☐	**POH**-ten-see	______
potentiation	☐	poh-**ten**-she-**AY**-shun	______
rectal	☐	**REK**-tal	______
sedative	☐	**SED**-ah-tiv	______
skeletal muscle relaxant	☐	**SKELL**-eh-tal muscle rih-**LAK**-sant	______
subcutaneous	☐	**sub**-kyoo-**TAY**-nee-us	______
sublingual	☐	sub-**LING**-gwal	______
subungual	☐	sub-**UNG**-gwal	______
systemic	☐	sis-**TEM**-ik	______
therapeutic	☐	thair-ah-**PEW**-tik	______
tolerance	☐	**TAHL**-er-ans	______
topical	☐	**TOP**-ih-kal	______
toxicology	☐	**tocks**-ih-**KAHL**-oh-jee	______
vaginal	☐	**VAJ**-in-al	______
vitamin	☐	**VIGH**-tah-min	______

Chapter Review Exercises

The following exercises provide a more in-depth review of the chapter material. Your goal in these exercises is to complete each section at a minimum 80% level of accuracy. If you score below 80% in any area, return to the appropriate section in the chapter and read the material again. A space has been provided for your score at the end of each section.

A. Matching

Match the terms on the left with the most appropriate definition on the right. Each correct answer is worth 10 points. Record your score in the space provided at the end of the exercise.

_____	1. pharmacology	a.	pharmacist
_____	2. drug	b.	rules that have been established to control the strength, quality, and purity of medications
_____	3. pharmacodynamics	c.	the field of medicine that specializes in the study of drugs
_____	4. pharmacist	d.	an information leaflet placed inside the container of a package of prescription drugs
_____	5. pharmacy	e.	any substance that, when taken into the body, may modify one or more of its functions
_____	6. chemotherapy	f.	treatment using drugs that have a specific and deadly effect on disease-causing microorganisms
_____	7. toxicology	g.	one who is licensed to prepare and dispense drugs
_____	8. standards	h.	the study of poisons, their detection, their effects, and establishing antidotes and methods of treatment
_____	9. package insert	i.	drugstore
_____	10. druggist	j.	the study of how drugs interact in the human body

Number correct _______ × 10 points/correct answer: Your score _______%

B. Multiple Choice

Read each question carefully and circle the most appropriate response for each statement. Each correct answer is worth 10 points. When you have completed this exercise, record your score in the space provided at the end of the exercise.

1. The Food, Drug, and Cosmetic Act is a law that regulates:
   a. the quality, purity, potency, effectiveness, safety, labeling, and packaging of food, drugs, and cosmetics
   b. the quality, purity, potency, effectiveness, safety, labeling, and packaging of drugs only
   c. the quality, purity, potency, effectiveness, safety, labeling, and packaging of prescription cosmetics
   d. the quality, purity, labeling, and packaging of food only
2. The government agency responsible for administering and enforcing the Food, Drug, and Cosmetic Act within the United States is the:
   a. FDA
   b. FNA
   c. DEA
   d. CSA

3. The federal law that is concerned with the manufacture, distribution, and dispensing of drugs that have the potential of being abused and of causing physical or psychological dependence is the:
   a. Food, Drug, and Cosmetic Act
   b. Controlled Substance Act
   c. Drug Enforcement Act
   d. Schedule Drug Control Act
4. The government agency responsible for administering and enforcing the Controlled Substance Act within the United States is the:
   a. FDA
   b. FNA
   c. DEA
   d. CSA
5. The drug schedule that includes drugs that are not acceptable for medical use and are used for research only is the:
   a. Schedule I
   b. Schedule II
   c. Schedule III
   d. Schedule IV
6. The drug schedule that includes drugs that are considered to have a strong potential for abuse or addiction, and cannot be refilled without a new, written prescription is:
   a. Schedule I
   b. Schedule II
   c. Schedule III
   d. Schedule IV
7. The drug schedule that includes drugs that have a small potential for abuse or addiction is:
   a. Schedule I
   b. Schedule II
   c. Schedule IV
   d. Schedule V
8. The official publication that contains formulas and information that provide a standard for preparation and dispensation of drugs is the:
   a. Physicians' Desk Reference
   b. United States Pharmacopeia/National Formulary
   c. Drug Facts and Comparisons
   d. Compendium of New Drugs/New Standards
9. The drug reference published annually by Medical Economics Company is:
   a. Physicians' Desk Reference
   b. United States Pharmacopeia
   c. Drug Facts and Comparisons
   d. Compendium of New Drugs/New Standards

10. The drug reference that lists all of the drugs commonly stocked by the hospital pharmacy is:
    a. Physician's Hospital Reference
    b. Hospital Drug Facts and Comparisons
    c. Compendium of New Drugs/New Standards
    d. Hospital Formulary

Number correct _______ × 10 points/correct answer: Your score _______%

C. Completion

Complete each sentence with the most appropriate answer. Each correct answer is worth 10 points. Record your score in the space provided at the end of the exercise.

1. The name that describes the chemical structure of a drug is the ____________________ name.
2. The name of a drug that is established when the drug is first manufactured is known as the ______________ name.
3. The name by which a drug is sold by a specific manufacturer is known as the ______________ name.
4. The name that is the same as the official name of a drug is the ____________________ name.
5. The name that is the same as the trade name of a drug is the ____________________ name.
6. How the drug produces changes within the body is known as drug ____________________.
7. The change that takes place in the body as a result of the drug action is known as drug ______________.
8. An additional effect on the body by a drug that was not part of the goal for that medication is known as a ____________________.
9. When the body reacts to a drug in an unexpected way that may endanger a patient's health and safety, the patient is said to have had the following type of reaction to the medication: ____________________.
10. Any special symptom or circumstance that indicates that the use of a particular drug or procedure is dangerous, not advised, or has not been proven safe for administration is known as a ____________________.

Number correct _______ × 10 points/correct answer: Your score _______%

D. Crossword Puzzle

Identify the various routes of administration of medications based on the clues provided. Each correct answer is worth 10 points. When you have completed this exercise, record your score in the space provided at the end.

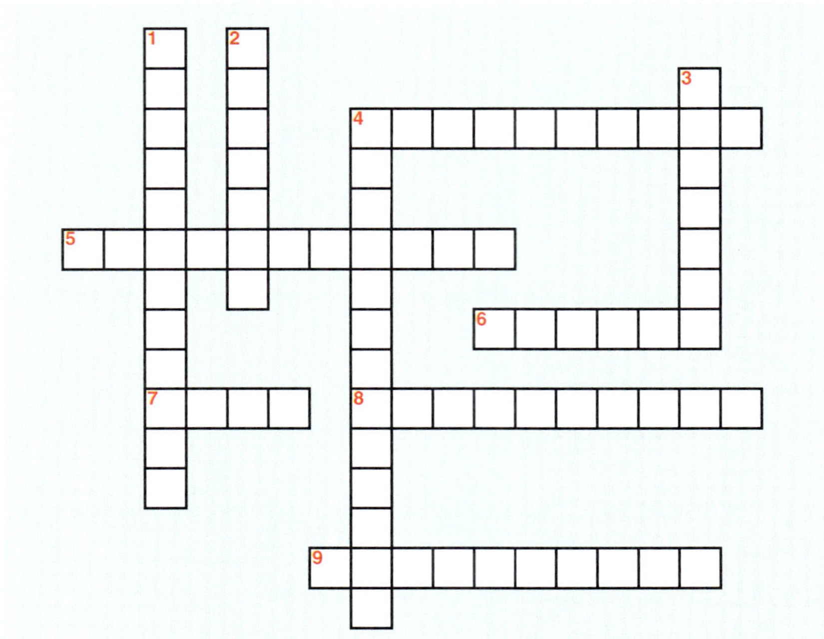

ACROSS

4 Medicine breathed in through nose
5 Medicine injected within the dermis
6 Medication placed next to cheek
7 Medication swallowed by mouth
8 Medication placed under the tongue
9 Medication injected into the body

DOWN

1 Medicine injected into fatty layer
2 Medication inserted into vagina
3 Medication applied directly to skin
4 Medication injected into the muscle

Number correct _______ × 10 points/correct answer: Your score _______%

E. Drug Classification Selection

Using the following drug classifications, enter the most appropriate response in the space provided. Each correct answer is worth 10 points. When you have completed the exercise, record your score in the space provided. If you can answer all of the questions without assistance from your text or notes, give yourself 10 extra bonus points!

antiulcer agent	antitussive	anticonvulsant
diuretic	antihistamine	anesthetic
antihypertensive	antiemetic	anticoagulant
antidepressant	antibiotic	antidiabetic
analgesic	bronchodilator	antifungal

1. Juan Miguel is complaining of a headache. His doctor told him to take Tylenol (acetaminophen) to relieve the pain. You know that acetaminophen is classified as a(n):

   ____

2. Judy Silverstein's mother recently died shortly after Judy lost her job. For the last 2 months Judy has been having difficulty coping with her situation. She has been extremely depressed and cries excessively. The

doctor has placed Judy on Elavil (amitriptyline hydrochloride), a medication used to alleviate mental depression. You know that amitriptyline hydrochloride is classified as a(n):

____

3. Latasha Smith has had a cold for 3 days. She has developed a scratchy cough that keeps her awake at night. Her doctor recommended that she purchase Robitussin PE (pseudoephedrine hydrochloride and guaifenesin) at her local pharmacy. You know that pseudoephedrine hydrochloride and guaifenesin is a medication given to relieve coughing, and is classified as a(n):

____

4. Pearl Henderson suffers from high blood pressure. The doctor has placed her on Corgard (nadolol), a medication used to control hypertension. You know that nadolol is classified as a(n):

____

5. Bette Daves was stung by a wasp while working in her garden. Shortly after the sting, her finger was throbbing and she noticed some swelling. She immediately took one of her Benadryl capsules (diphenhydramine hydrochloride) to relieve the allergic response to the sting. You know that diphenhydramine hydrochloride is classified as a(n):

____

6. Mark Jones has an ear infection. His pediatrician has prescribed Bactrim (trimethoprim and sulfamethoxazole) to stop the infection. You know that trimethoprim and sulfamethoxazole is classified as a(n):

____

7. Alicia Montoya suffers from asthma. Her physician has prescribed Bronkodyl (theophylline), a medication given to expand the bronchial tubes, to relieve her symptoms. You know that theophylline is classified as a(n):

____

8. Helen Bell has experienced a good bit of swelling in her legs lately. Her physician has prescribed Lasix (furosemide), a medication used to increase urine secretion, in hopes of relieving the edema in her legs. You know that furosemide is classified as a(n):

____

9. Jennifer Allran is 4 months pregnant and is still complaining of nausea. Her physician has prescribed Bonine (meclizine hydrochloride) to relieve the nausea. You know that meclizine hydrochloride is classified as a(n):

____

10. Matt King went to the dentist today to have a filling replaced. His dentist used Xylocaine (lidocaine) to completely numb the tooth before replacing the filling. You know that lidocaine is classified as a(n):

____

Number correct _______ × 10 points/correct answer: Your score _______%

Bonus points for answering all questions without assistance: _______

Your score + bonus points: Grand total _______%

F. Definition to Term

Using the word definitions in each statement, identify and provide the appropriate medical term to match the definition. Each correct response is worth 10 points. When you complete the exercise, record your score in the space provided at the end of the exercise.

1. Without sensitivity to pain (adjective):

   ____

2. Treatment with drugs:

   ____

3. Within the skin (adjective):

   ____

4. Without sensation or feeling:

   ____

5. Pertaining to the rectum (adjective):

   ____

6. The study of drugs:

   ____

7. Under the tongue (adjective):

   ____

8. The study of poisons:

   ____

9. Within the vein (adjective):

   ____

10. One who is licensed to dispense drugs:

   ____

Number correct _______ × 10 points/correct answer: Your score _______%

G. Matching

Match the abbreviations on the left with the appropriate definition on the right. Each correct answer is worth 5 points. Record your score in the space provided at the end of the exercise.

_____	1. a.c.	a. ounce
_____	2. b.i.d.	b. rectal
_____	3. $\bar{c}$	c. three times a day
_____	4. Gm, g	d. one-half
_____	5. gr	e. quantity sufficient
_____	6. gtt	f. after meals
_____	7. ID	g. ointment
_____	8. IM	h. milliequivalent
_____	9. cc	i. intradermal
_____	10. mEq	j. drops

_____	11. NPO	k.	gram
_____	12. ung	l.	twice a day
_____	13. $\overline{p}$	m.	before meals
_____	14. p.c.	n.	with
_____	15. p.r.n.	o.	grain
_____	16. q.s.	p.	intramuscular
_____	17. R_x	q.	cubic centimeter
_____	18. $\overline{ss}$	r.	nothing by mouth
_____	19. stat.	s.	after
_____	20. t.i.d.	t.	as needed
		u.	take
		v.	immediately
		w.	tablet
		x.	every night

Number correct _______ × 5 points/correct answer: Your score _______%

H. Word Search

Using the following definitions, identify the appropriate word and then find and circle it in the puzzle. The words may be read up, down, diagonally, across, or backward. Each correct word is worth 10 points. Record your score in the space provided at the end of the exercise.

Example: A drug effect confined to a specific part of the body is known as a *local* effect.

1. Drug _____________________ is defined as how the drugs produce changes within the body.
2. The _____________________ effect is when a drug achieves the response in the body that is intended.
3. A _____________________ effect is when a medication has a widespread influence on the body because it is absorbed into the bloodstream.
4. An _____________________ reaction is one in which the body reacts to a drug in an unexpected way that may endanger a patient's health and safety.
5. A _____________________ is a special symptom or circumstance that indicates that the use of a particular drug is dangerous.
6. A _____________________ effect is an additional effect on the body by the drug that was not part of the goal for that medication.
7. _____________________ occurs when a drug is not completely excreted from the body before another dose is given and the drug starts to accumulate within the body tissues with each successive dose.
8. _____________________ is an unusual inappropriate response to a drug or to the usual effective dose of a drug.
9. _____________________ occurs when two drugs administered together produce a more powerful response than the sum of their individual effects.
10. _____________________ is the resistance to the effect of a drug; the individual requires increasingly higher doses to achieve the full effect of the drug.

B	R	P	O	N	C	H	S	Y	S	T	E	M	I	C	B	R	E	A	T	H	I
A	N	A	O	G	E	S	I	C	A	N	E	S	T	H	E	T	I	C	R	A	D
M	I	C	K	T	M	N	M	E	T	L	O	C	A	L	N	O	T	O	M	E	I
C	A	R	V	E	E	O	O	S	D	I	A	C	B	A	C	R	F	E	S	R	O
I	L	E	T	Y	T	N	L	I	E	O	Y	N	T	I	C	H	A	I	Y	I	S
M	U	C	O	I	O	T	T	O	T	E	B	R	L	N	E	E	R	R	O	N	Y
L	R	O	T	H	L	O	E	I	U	A	S	C	O	A	S	E	I	D	R	T	N
P	U	D	L	M	E	I	D	N	A	U	L	I	R	R	D	I	B	I	C	R	C
L	E	U	V	D	R	N	I	A	C	T	Y	U	E	N	O	M	L	U	P	H	R
S	A	C	U	D	A	D	S	O	D	E	I	V	M	A	C	T	I	O	N	B	A
L	A	C	I	G	N	L	E	R	U	E	D	O	R	U	Q	W	E	A	R	Y	C
N	O	I	T	A	C	I	D	N	I	A	R	T	N	O	C	V	E	N	O	U	Y
B	U	T	T	E	E	R	U	M	A	I	D	I	S	G	O	O	D	Y	E	S	E

Number correct ______ × 10 points/correct answer: Your score ______%

I. Terms to Definition

Define the following drug classification terms. Where possible, break the word down into its word elements in the space provided. Each correct definition is worth 10 points and each correct "breakdown" of the word is worth 10 points. When you have completed the exercise, record your score in the space provided at the end of the exercise.

Term: analgesic

1. Definition: ____
2. Breakdown: ____________ / ____________ / ____________
   (prefix) (word root) (suffix)

Term: antiarrhythmic

3. Definition: ____
4. Breakdown: ____________ / ____________ / ____________
   (prefix) (word root) (suffix)

Term: anticonvulsant

5. Definition ____

Term: antidepressant

6. Definition: ____

Term: antifungal

7. Definition: ____
8. Breakdown: ____________ / ____________ / ____________
   (prefix) (word root) (suffix)

Term: antineoplastic

9. Definition: ____
10. Breakdown: ____________ / ____________ / ____________ / ____________
    (prefix) (combining form) (word root) (suffix)

Number correct ______ × 10 points/correct answer: Your score ______%

J. Interpret the Doctor's Orders

The following is an example of some written orders that may be seen on a prescription or may have to be called into the hospital for the physician. Read each order carefully in its abbreviated form, then write the definition for each abbreviation in the space provided. Each correct response is worth 10 points. Record your score in the space provided when you have completed the exercise.

1. Physician's order: Give Tylenol, gr. X for T. above 101 degrees F. prn.
   a. gr. X ______
   b. T ______
   c. F ______
   d. prn ______
2. Physician's order: Seconal gr. $\overline{\text{iss}}$ h.s. for sleep.
   a. gr. $\overline{\text{iss}}$ ______
   b. h.s. ______
3. Physician's order: Normal Saline Solution 0.5% IV × 8 hr, D/C when absorbed.
   a. IV ______
   b. x ______
   c. hr ______
   d. D/C ______

Number correct ______ × 10 points/correct answer: Your score ______%

Answers to Chapter Review Exercises

A. Matching

1. c
2. e
3. j
4. g
5. i
6. f
7. h
8. b
9. d
10. a

B. Multiple Choice

1. a
2. a
3. b
4. c
5. a
6. b
7. d
8. b
9. a
10. d

C. Completion

1. chemical
2. generic or official
3. trade or brand
4. generic
5. brand
6. action
7. effect
8. side effect
9. adverse
10. contraindication

D. Crossword Puzzle

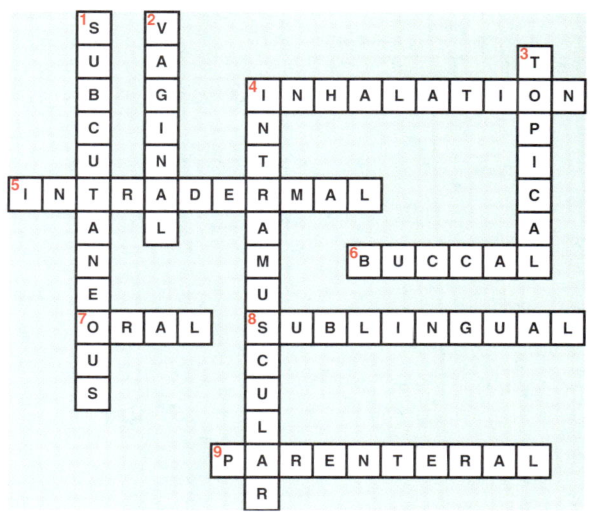

E. Drug Classification Selection

1. analgesic
2. antidepressant
3. antitussive
4. antihypertensive
5. antihistamine
6. antibiotic
7. bronchodilator
8. diuretic
9. antiemetic
10. anesthetic

F. Definition to Term

1. analgesic
2. chemotherapy
3. intradermal
4. anesthesia
5. rectal
6. pharmacology
7. sublingual, hypoglossal
8. toxicology
9. intravenous
10. pharmacist

G. Matching

1. m
2. l
3. n
4. k
5. o
6. j
7. i
8. p
9. q
10. h
11. r
12. g
13. s
14. f
15. t
16. e
17. u
18. d
19. v
20. c

H. Word Search

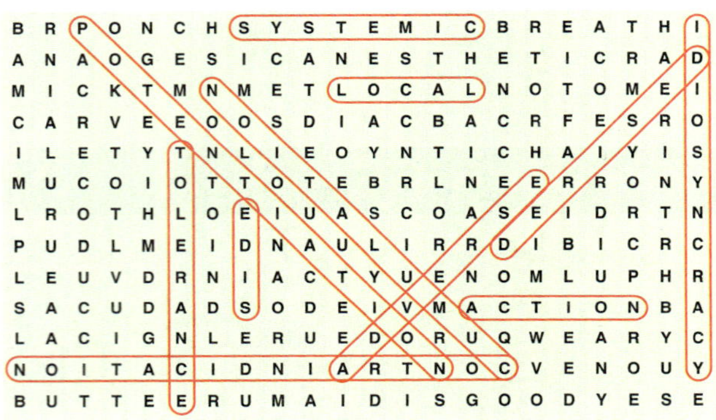

I. Terms to Definition

1. an agent that relieves pain without causing loss of consciousness
2. an / alges / ic
   prefix word root suffix
3. an agent that controls cardiac arrhythmias
4. anti / arrhythm / ic
   prefix word root suffix
5. an agent that prevents or relieves convulsions
6. an agent that prevents or relieves the symptoms of depression
7. an agent that destroys or inhibits the growth of fungi
8. anti / fung / al
   prefix word root suffix
9. an agent that prevents the replication of neoplastic cells
10. anti / ne/o / plas / tic
    prefix combining form word root suffix

J. Interpret the Doctor's Orders

1. a. grains 10
   b. temperature
   c. Fahrenheit
   d. as needed
2. a. grains one and one-half
   b. hour of sleep; at bedtime
3. a. intravenously
   b. times
   c. hour
   b. discontinue

CHAPTER 23

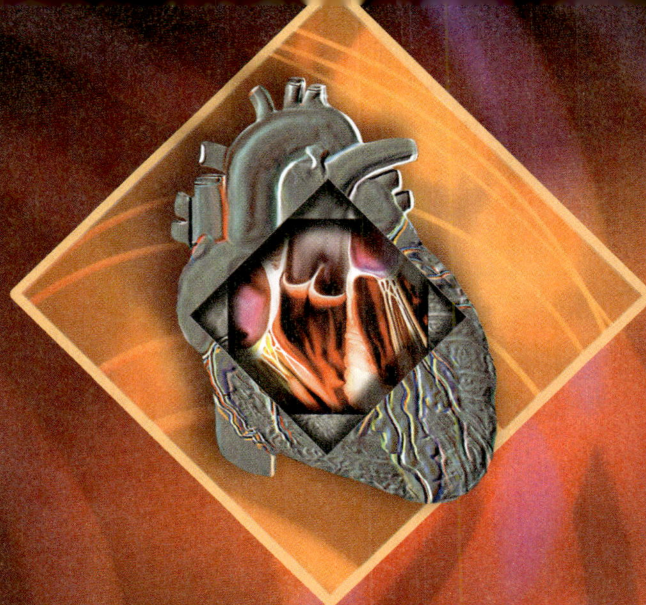

Mental Health

CHAPTER CONTENT

KEY COMPETENCIES

Upon completing this chapter and the review exercises at the end of the chapter, the learner should be able to:

1. Correctly spell and pronounce each new term introduced in this chapter using the Activity CD-ROM and Audio CD, if available.
2. List and define 10 defense mechanisms studied in this chapter.
3. List and define at least five phobias studied in this chapter.
4. List and define at least 20 mental disorders discussed in this chapter.
5. Identify at least 10 abbreviations common to mental health.
6. Identify 10 treatments, therapies, and tests used in the practice of mental health.

OVERVIEW

Physical symptoms have been first and foremost in the previous chapters of this textbook as we have discussed the various pathological conditions of each body system. We now turn from the physical to the study of psychological symptoms that often impact the physical condition of the patient. A general discussion of defense mechanisms, phobias, mental disorders, and therapeutic treatments is included in this chapter. The topics of discussion are alphabetized under each category heading.

Mental health is a relative state of mind in which the person who is healthy is able to cope with and adjust to the recurrent stresses of everyday living in an acceptable way. **Mental disorders** are disturbances of emotional stability, as manifested in maladaptive behavior and impaired functioning. This may be caused by genetic, physical, chemical, biologic, psychologic, or social and cultural factors. A mental disorder may be referred to as mental illness, emotional illness, or psychiatric disorder.

Many of us use **defense mechanisms** on a normal day-to-day basis when dealing with areas of conflict in our lives. It is when the defense mechanisms become a way of dealing with life that they may be indicative of the need for psychological or psychiatric help.

Psychology is the study of behavior and the processes of the mind, especially as it relates to the individual's social and physical environment. A **psychologist** is a professional who specializes in the study of the structure and function of the brain and related mental processes. A psychologist is not a physician, but one who earns either a master's or doctoral degree in some area of psychology. A **clinical psychologist** provides testing and counseling services to patients with mental and emotional disorders. **Psychiatry** is the branch of medicine that deals with the causes, treatment, and prevention of mental, emotional, and behavioral disorders. A **psychiatrist** is a medical doctor who specializes in diagnosing, preventing, and treating mental disorders—an educational process that involves several additional years beyond medical school. Psychiatrists may specialize in various areas of practice in the field of psychiatry. If a psychiatrist chooses to specialize in **psychoanalysis**, he or she would be known as a **psychoanalyst** and would complete additional special training in psychotherapeutic techniques. Psychoanalysis involves the use of free association, dream interpretation, and the analysis of defense mechanisms. The psychoanalyst applies the techniques of psychoanalytic theory to help the patient become aware of repressed emotional conflicts and seeks ways to help the individual to bring the conflicts to a conscious level so they can be resolved.

Defense Mechanisms

The body's unconscious reaction used to protect itself from conflicts or anxieties is known as a defense mechanism. There is, however, one conscious defense mechanism, **sublimation**, which is included in this section. Some defense mechanisms are designed to lessen or deal with anxiety or conflict, allowing normal function to continue. Others are designed to conceal the anxiety or conflict.

The following is an alphabetical listing and a general discussion of some of the more commonly used defense mechanisms, with an example of each. Keep in mind that each of these defense mechanisms operates on an unconscious level.

compensation
(kom-pen-**SAY**-shun)

Compensation is an effort to overcome, or make up for, real or imagined inadequacies.

An individual may compensate for a deficiency in physical size by excelling in academics.

denial
(dee-**NYE**-al)

Denial is a refusal to admit or acknowledge the reality of something, thus avoiding emotional conflict or anxiety.

A child may deny that he or she is being abused by a parent.

displacement
(dis-**PLACE**-ment)

Displacement is the process of transferring a feeling or emotion from the original idea or object to a substitute idea or object.

An individual is angry at the "boss," and cannot express that anger; the feelings are displaced by criticizing everyone else.

introjection
(in-troh-**JEK**-shun)

An ego defense mechanism whereby an individual unconsciously identifies with another person or with some object. The individual assumes the supposed feelings and/or characteristics of the other personality or object.

A child develops his or her conscience by internalizing what the parents believe is right and wrong. The child may say to a friend while playing, "Don't hit people. Nice people don't do that."

projection
(proh-**JEK**-shun)

Projection is the act of transferring one's own unacceptable thoughts or feelings on to someone else.

A worker who dislikes his or her boss accuses the boss of disliking him or her.

rationalization
(rash-un-al-ih-**ZAY**-shun)

Rationalization is attempting to make excuses or invent logical reasons to justify unacceptable feelings or behaviors.

A student may rationalize that he or she failed a test because the questions were too confusing.

regression
(rih-**GRESH**-un)

Regression is a response to stress in which the individual reverts to an earlier level of development and the comfort measures associated with that level of functioning.

A child may regress to an earlier stage of development, such as bedwetting, when confronted with a stress in his or her life, such as a new baby in the family.

repression
(ree-**PRESH**-un)

Repression is an involuntary blocking of unpleasant feelings and experiences from one's conscious mind.

An individual involved in a tragic automobile accident may have no memory of the sequence of events.

sublimation
(sub-lih-**MAY**-shun)

Rechanneling or redirecting one's unacceptable impulses and drives into constructive activities.

Sublimation is a conscious defense mechanism. The positive aspect of sublimation is that the individual participates in constructive activities. Parents of children who were victimized by violence may redirect their expected anger and outrage into working with other victims of violent crimes.

suppression
(suh-**PRESH**-un)

Suppression is the voluntary blocking of unpleasant feelings and experiences from one's mind.

An individual faced with a frustrating or painful situation may consciously choose not to confront the situation.

Vocabulary

The following vocabulary words are frequently used when discussing mental health.

WORD	DEFINITION
affect (**AFF**-fekt)	Observable evidence of a person's feelings or emotions.
amnesia (am-**NEE**-zee-ah)	Loss of memory caused by severe emotional trauma, brain injury, substance abuse, or reaction to medications or toxins.
amphetamines (am-**FET**-ah-meenz)	A group of nervous system stimulants that produce alertness and a feeling of well-being (**euphoria**).
anorexia (an-oh-**REK**-see-ah)	Lack of appetite, resulting in the inability to eat.
anorexia nervosa (an-oh-**REK**-see-ah ner-**VOH**-suh)	A disorder seen primarily in adolescent girls, characterized by an emotional disturbance concerning body image, prolonged refusal to eat followed by extreme weight loss, amenorrhea, and a lingering, abnormal fear of becoming obese.
anxiety (**ang-ZY**-eh-tee)	A state of mind in which the individual feels increased tension, apprehension, a painfully increased sense of helplessness, a feeling of uncertainty, fear, jitteriness, and worry. Observable signs of **anxiety** include, but are not limited to, restlessness, poor eye contact, glancing about, facial tension, dilated pupils, increased perspiration, and a constant focus on self.
anxiety disorders	Disorders characterized by chronic worry.
apathy (**AP**-ah-thee)	Absence or suppression of observable emotion, feeling, concern, or passion.
autism (**AW**-tizm)	A mental disorder characterized by the individual being extremely withdrawn and absorbed with fantasy. The individual suffers from impaired communication/social interaction skills; and activities and interests are very limited.

behavior therapy	A form of **psychotherapy** that seeks to modify observable, maladjusted patterns of behavior by substituting new responses to given stimuli.
bulimia nervosa (boo-**LIM**-ee-ah)	An uncontrolled craving for food, often resulting in eating binges, followed by vomiting to eliminate the food from the stomach. The individual may then feel depressed, go through a period of self-deprivation, followed by another eating binge, and the cycle continues.
cannabis (**CAN**-ah-bis)	A mind-altering drug derived from the flowering top of hemp plants; also called **marijuana**. This drug is classified as a controlled substance, Schedule I drug.
cataplexy (**CAT**-ah-pleks-ee)	A sudden loss of muscle tone in which the individual's head may drop, the jaw may sag, the knees become weakened, and the individual may collapse or fall to the ground; may accompany a **narcolepsy** attack (sudden, uncontrollable attack of sleep).
compensation (kom-pen-**SAY**-shun)	An effort to overcome, or make up for, real or imagined inadequacies.
compulsions (kom-**PUHL**-shuns)	Irresistible, repetitive, irrational impulses to perform an act; these behavior patterns are intended to reduce anxiety, not provide pleasure or gratification.
conversion disorder (kon-**VER**-zhun)	A disorder in which the individual represses anxiety experienced by emotional conflicts by converting the anxious feelings into physical symptoms that have no organic basis, but are perceived to be real by the individual; the individual may experience symptoms such as paralysis, pain, loss of sensation, or some other form of dysfunction of the nervous system; also called conversion hysteria.
cyclothymic disorder (sigh-cloh-**THIGH**-mic)	A chronic (of long duration) mood disorder characterized by numerous periods of mood swings from **depression** to happiness; the period of mood disturbance is at least 2 years duration.
defense mechanism	An unconscious, intrapsychic (within one's mind) reaction that offers protection to the self from a stressful situation.
delirium (dee-**LIR**-ee-um)	A state of frenzied excitement or wild enthusiasm.
delirium tremens (DTs) (dee-**LIR**-ee-um **TREE**-menz)	An acute and sometimes fatal psychotic reaction caused by cessation of excessive intake of alcoholic beverages over a long period of time.
delusion (dee-**LOO**-zhun)	A persistent abnormal belief or perception is firmly held by a person despite evidence to the contrary. Two forms of **delusions** are delusions of persecution in which the person thinks others are following him, spying on him, or trying to torment him, and delusions of grandeur in which the person has a false sense of possessing wealth or power.
dementia (dee-**MEN**-shee-ah)	A progressive, organic mental disorder characterized by chronic personality disintegration, confusion, disorientation, stupor, deterioration of intellectual capacity and function, and impairment of control of memory, judgment, and impulses.

denial	A refusal to admit or acknowledge the reality of something, thus avoiding emotional conflict or anxiety.
depression	A mood disturbance characterized by exaggerated feelings of sadness, discouragement, and hopelessness that are inappropriate and out of proportion with reality; may be relative to some personal loss or tragedy.
displacement (dis-**PLACE**-ment)	The process of transferring a feeling or emotion from the original idea or object to a substitute idea or object.
dissociation (dis-**soh**-shee-**AY**-shun)	An unconscious defense mechanism by which an idea, thought, emotion, or other mental process is separated from the consciousness and thereby loses emotional significance.
drug therapy	The use of psychotherapeutic drugs to treat mental disorders.
dysphoria (dis-**FOH**-ree-ah) dys- = bad, difficult, painful, disordered phor/o = bearing -ia = condition	A disorder of affect (mood) characterized by depression and anguish.
electroconvulsive therapy (ECT)	The process of passing an electrical current through the brain to create a brief seizure in the brain.
euphoria (yoo-**FOR**-ee-ah) eu- = well, easily, good, normal phor/o = bearing -ia = condition	A sense of well-being or elation.
exhibitionism	A sexual disorder involving the exposure of one's genitals to a stranger.
factitious disorders	Disorders that are characterized by physical or psychological symptoms that are intentionally produced or feigned to assume the sick role.
family therapy	A form of psychotherapy that focuses the treatment on the process between family members that supports and sustains symptoms.
fetishism, transvestic	A sexual disorder in which the focus of the fetish involves cross-dressing.
free association	The spontaneous, consciously unrestricted association of ideas, feelings, or mental images.
frotteurism	A sexual disorder in which the person gains sexual stimulation or excitement by rubbing against a nonconsenting person.
group therapy	The application of psychotherapeutic techniques within a small group of people who experience similar difficulties.
hallucination (hah-loo-sih-**NAY**-shun)	A subjective (existing in the mind) perception of something that does not exist in the external environment. Hallucinations may be visual, olfactory (smell), gustatory, (taste), tactile (touch), or auditory (hear).

hallucinogens (hah-**LOO**-sih-non-jens)	Substances that cause excitation of the central nervous system, characterized by symptoms such as hallucinations, mood changes, anxiety, increased pulse and blood pressure, and dilation of the pupils.
hypnosis	A passive, trancelike state of existence that resembles normal sleep during which perception and memory are altered, resulting in increased responsiveness to suggestion.
hypochondriasis (high-poh-kon-**DRY**-ah-sis)	A chronic, abnormal concern about the health of the body, characterized by extreme anxiety, depression, and an unrealistic interpretation of real or imagined physical symptoms as indications of a serious illness or disease despite rational medical evidence that no disorder is present. A person affected by **hypochondriasis** is referred to as a hypochondriac.
hypomania (high-poh-**MAY**-nee-ah) hypo- = under, below, beneath, less than normal -mania = madness	A mild degree of **mania** characterized by optimism, excitability, energetic and productive behavior, marked hyperactivity and talkativeness, heightened sexual interest, quick to anger, irritability, and a decreased need for sleep.
intoxication (in-**toks**-ih-**KAY**-shun)	A state of being characterized by impaired judgment, slurred speech, loss of coordination, irritability, and mood changes; may be due to drugs, including alcohol.
introjection	An ego defense mechanism whereby an individual unconsciously identifies with another person or with some object, assuming the supposed feelings and/or characteristics of the other personality or object.
lithium (**LITH**-ee-um)	A drug that is particularly useful in treating the manic phase of **bipolar disorders** (manic-depressive disorders).
major depressive disorder	A disorder characterized by one or more episodes of depressed mood that lasts at least 2 weeks and is accompanied by at least four additional symptoms of depression.
malingering (mah-**LING**-er-ing)	A willful and deliberate faking of symptoms of a disease or injury to gain some consciously desired end.
mania (**MAY**-nee-ah)	Madness; an emotional state characterized by symptoms such as extreme excitement, hyperactivity, overtalkativeness, agitation, flight of ideas, fleeting attention, and sometimes violent, destructive, and self-destructive behavior.
marijuana	See *cannabis.*
mood disorders	An affective state characterized by any of a variety of periods of depression or depression elation.
mutism (**mew**-tizm)	The inability to speak because of a physical defect or emotional problem.
neurosis (noo-**ROH**-sis) neur/o = nerve -osis = condition	A psychological or behavioral disorder in which anxiety is the primary characteristic, thought to be related to unresolved conflicts.

obsession (ob-**SESS**-shun)	A persistent thought or idea with which the mind is continually and involuntarily preoccupied.
panic attack	An episode of acute anxiety during which the individual may experience intense feelings of uneasiness or fright accompanied by dyspnea, dizziness, sweating, trembling, and palpitations of the heart. Panic attacks, which occur unexpectedly, may last a few minutes and may return.
panic disorder	A disorder characterized by recurrent panic attacks that come on unexpectedly.
paranoia (pair-ah-**NOY**-ah)	A mental disorder characterized by an elaborate overly suspicious system of thinking, with delusions of persecution and grandeur usually centered on one major theme, such as a financial matter, a job situation, an unfaithful spouse, or other problem.
paraphilia (pair-ah-**FILL**-ee-ah) para- = near, beside, beyond, two like parts phil/o = attraction to -ia = condition	Sexual perversion or deviation; a condition in which the sexual instinct is expressed in ways that are socially prohibited, unacceptable, or biologically undesirable.
pedophilia	A sexual disorder in which the individual is sexually aroused and engages in sexual activity with children (generally age 13 or younger).
personality disorders	Any of a large group of mental disorders characterized by rigid, inflexible, and maladaptive behavior patterns that impair a person's ability to function in society by severely limiting adaptive potential.
phobia (**FOH**-bee-ah)	An anxiety disorder characterized by an obsessive, irrational, and intense fear of a specific object, of an activity, or of a physical situation. **Phobias** are usually characterized by symptoms such as faintness, fatigue, palpitations, perspiration, nausea, tremor, and panic.
play therapy	A form of psychotherapy in which a child plays in a protected and structured environment with games and toys provided by a therapist.
projection (proh-**JEK**-shun)	The act of transferring one's own unacceptable thoughts or feelings on to someone else.
psychiatrist (sigh-**KIGH**-ah-trist) psych/o = mind, soul -iatrist = one who treats; a physician	A physician who specializes in the diagnosis, prevention, and treatment of mental disorders.
psychiatry (sigh-**KIGH**-ah-tree) psych/o = mind, soul -iatry = medical treatment, medical profession	The branch of medicine that deals with the causes, treatment, and prevention of mental, emotional, and behavioral disorders.
psychoanalysis (**sigh**-koh-an-**NAL**-ih-sis)	A form of psychotherapy that uses free association, dream interpretation, and analysis of defense mechanisms to help the patient become aware of repressed emotional conflicts.

psychoanalyst (**sigh**-koh-**AN**-ah-list)	A psychotherapist, usually a psychiatrist, who has had special training in psychoanalysis and who applies the techniques of psychoanalytic theory.
psychodrama (sigh-koh-**DRAM**-ah)	A form of group psychotherapy in which people act out their emotional problems through unrehearsed dramatizations; also called role-playing therapy.
psychologist (sigh-**KALL**-oh-jist) psych/o = mind, soul -logist = one who specializes	A person who specializes in the study of the structure and function of the brain and related mental process of animals and humans. A clinical psychologist has a graduate degree with specialized training in providing testing and counseling to patients with mental and emotional disorders.
psychology (sigh-**KALL**-oh-jee) psych/o = mind, soul -logy = the study of	The study of behavior and the processes of the mind, especially as it relates to the individual's social and physical environment.
psychosis (sigh-**KOH**-sis) psych/o = mind, soul -osis = condition	Any major mental disorder of organic or emotional origin characterized by a loss of contact with reality.
psychosomatic (**sigh**-koh-soh-**MAT**-ik) psych/o = mind, soul somat/o = body -ic = pertaining to	Pertaining to the expression of an emotional conflict through physical symptoms.
psychotherapy (sigh-koh-**THAIR**-ah-pee) psych/o = mind, soul -therapy = treatment	Any of a large number of related methods of treating mental and emotional disorders using psychological techniques instead of physical means of treatment.
purging (**PERJ**-ing)	The means of ridding the body of what has been consumed; that is, the individual may induce vomiting or use laxatives to rid the body of food that has just been eaten.
rationalization (**rash**-un-al-ih-**ZAY**-shun)	Attempting to make excuses or invent logical reasons to justify unacceptable feelings or behaviors.
regression (rih-**GRESH**-un)	A response to stress in which the individual reverts to an earlier level of development and the comfort measures associated with that level of functioning.
repression (ree-**PRESH**-un)	An involuntary blocking of unpleasant feelings and experiences from one's conscious mind.
schizophrenia (skiz-oh-**FREN**-ee-ah) schiz/o = split phren/o = mind; also refers to the diaphragm -ia = condition	Any of a large group of psychotic disorders characterized by gross distortion of reality, disturbances of language and communication, withdrawal from social interaction, and the disorganization and fragmentation of thought, perception, and emotional reaction.

sedative	An agent that decreases functional activity and has a calming effect on the body.
senile dementia (**SEE**-nyl dee-**MEN**-shee-ah)	An organic mental disorder of the aged resulting from the generalized atrophy (wasting) of the brain with no evidence of cerebrovascular disease. This condition is characterized by loss of memory, impaired judgment, decreased moral and ethical values, inability to think abstractly, and periods of confusion and irritability; these symptoms may range from mild to severe.
sexual sadism/sexual masochism	A sexual disorder that involves the act (real, not simulated) of being humiliated, beaten, bound, or otherwise made to suffer; or, the act of inflicting psychological or physical suffering on the victim.
somatoform disorders (soh-**MAT**-oh-form)	Any group of neurotic disorders characterized by symptoms suggesting physical illness or disease, for which there are no demonstrable organic causes or physiologic dysfunctions.
sublimation (sub-lih-**MAY**-shun)	Rechanneling or redirecting one's unacceptable impulses and drives into constructive activities.
suppression (suh-**PRESH**-un)	The voluntary blocking of unpleasant feelings and experiences from one's mind.
tolerance	The ability to endure unusually large doses of a drug without apparent adverse effects, and with continued use of the drug, to require increased dosages to produce the same effect.

Word Elements

The following word elements pertain to the specialty of mental health. As you review the list, pronounce each word element aloud twice and check the box after you "say it." Write the definition for the example word given for each word element. You may use your medical dictionary.

WORD ELEMENT	PRONUNCIATION	"SAY IT"	MEANING
cata- **cata**tonia	**KAT**-ah kat-ah-**TOH**-nee-ah	☐	down, under, against, lower
hypn/o **hypn**otize	**HIP**-noh **HIP**-noh-tize	☐	sleep
-iatrist psych**iatrist**	eye-**AH**-trist sigh-**KIGH**-ah-trist	☐	one who treats; a physician
-mania klepto**mania**	**MAY**-nee-ah klep-toh-**MAY**-nee-ah	☐	a mental disorder; a "madness"
ment/o **ment**al	**MEN**-toh **MEN**-tal	☐	mind

neur/o psycho**neur**osis	**NOO**-roh sigh-koh-noo-**ROH**-sis	☐	nerves
phil/o necro**phil**ia	**FILL**-oh nek-roh-**FILL**-ee-ah	☐	attraction to
-phobia claustro**phobia**	**FOH**-bee-ah klaws-troh-**FOH**-bee-ah	☐	abnormal fear
-phoria eu**phoria**	**FOR**-ee-ah yoo-**FOR**-ee-ah	☐	emotional state
psych/o **psych**osis	**SIGH**-koh sigh-**KOH**-sis	☐	mind
schiz/o **schizo**phrenia	**SKIZ**-oh skiz-oh-**FREN**-ee-ah	☐	split, divided
somat/o psycho**somat**ic disorder	soh-**MAT**-oh **sigh**-koh-soh-**MAT**-ik dis-**OR**-der	☐	body
-thymia cyclo**thymia**	**THIGH**-mee-ah **sigh**-kloh-**THIGH**-mee-ah	☐	condition of the mind or will

Mental Disorders

In the United States, the initial motivation for developing a classification of mental disorders was the need to collect statistical data. Through the years, this system of classification has been refined. The *Diagnostic and Statistical Manual of Mental Disorders (DSM-IV-TR) (2000)* is the principal guide for mental health professionals today. The DSM-IV-TR uses the term *mental disorder* to mean "a mental disturbance."

> The DSM-IV-TR conceptualizes mental disorders as, "a clinically significant behavioral or psychological syndrome or pattern that occurs in an individual and that is associated with present distress (e.g., a painful symptom) or disability (i.e., impairment in one or more important areas of functioning) or with a significantly increased risk of suffering death, pain, disability, or an important loss of freedom.
>
> In addition, this syndrome or pattern must not be merely an expectable and culturally sanctioned response to a particular event, for example, the death of a loved one.
>
> Whatever its original cause, it must currently be considered a manifestation of a behavioral, psychological, or biological dysfunction in the individual." (*DSM-IV-TR*, p. xxxi)

The DSM-IV-TR disorders are grouped into 16 major diagnostic classes (e.g., substance-related disorders, mood disorders, anxiety disorders) and one additional section on other conditions that may be a focus of clinical attention. (*DSM-IV-TR:* p. 10). Within each major diagnostic classification

Table 23-1 DSM-IV-TR Multiaxial Classification System

AXIS I
Clinical Disorders
Other Conditions that May Be a Focus of Clinical Attention
AXIS II
Personality Disorders
Mental Retardation
AXIS III
General Medical Conditions
AXIS IV
Psychosocial and Environmental Problems
AXIS V
Global Assessment of Functioning

are several mental disorders. The organizing principle for most of the classification sections is to group disorders based on their shared features to facilitate differential diagnosis.

The DSM-IV-TR includes a multiaxial classification system that involves an assessment of information from several domains, or axes. The information from each axis is designed to help the mental health professional plan treatment and predict outcome for clients. This format is convenient for organizing and communicating clinical information, for capturing the complexity of clinical situations, and for describing the differences among individuals presenting with the same diagnosis. The five axes included in the DSM-IV-TR multiaxial classification are presented in **Table 23-1.**

In this chapter, the categories for discussion of mental disorders are:

- Cognitive disorders
- Substance-related disorders
- Schizophrenia
- Mood disorders
- Anxiety disorders
- Somatoform, sleep, and factitious disorders
- Dissociative identify disorders
- Sexual and gender identity disorders
- Eating disorders
- Personality disorders

They are alphabetized within each category. These disorders fall within the first two axes of the multiaxial classification system. A quick reference of the categories of mental disorders discussed in this chapter can be found in **Table 23-2.** Note that the appropriate DSM-IV-TR axis has been identified for each category within the table.

Table 23-2 Categories of Mental Disorders

COGNITIVE DISORDERS (AXIS I)	SUBSTANCE-RELATED DISORDERS (AXIS I)	SCHIZOPHRENIA (AXIS I)	MOOD DISORDERS (AXIS I)	ANXIETY DISORDERS (AXIS I)	SOMATOFORM DISORDERS*, SLEEP DISORDERS**, & FACTITIOUS DISORDERS*** (AXIS I)	DISSOCIATIVE IDENTITY DISORDERS (AXIS I)	SEXUAL AND GENDER IDENTITY DISORDERS (AXIS I)	EATING DISORDERS (AXIS I)	PERSONALITY DISORDERS (AXIS II)
Amnesia	Substance Abuse	Paranoid Schizophrenia	Major Depressive Disorder	Panic Disorder	Conversion Disorder*	Dissociative Identity Disorder (formerly Multiple Personality Disorder)	Gender Identity Disorder	Anorexia Nervosa	Antisocial Personality Disorder
Delirium	Substance Dependence		Cyclothymic Disorder	Phobic Disorder	Pain Disorder*	Dissociative Amnesia (formerly Psychogenic Amnesia)	Transvestic Fetishism	Bulimia	Borderline Personality Disorder
Dementia	Substance Intoxication		Bipolar Disorders	Obsessive-Compulsive Disorder	Hypochondriasis*	Dissociative Fugue (formerly Psychogenic Fugue)	Sexual Sadism		Narcissistic Personality Disorder
				Posttraumatic Stress Disorder	Narcolepsy**		Sexual Masochism		Paranoid Personality Disorder
					Munchausen Syndrome***		Exhibitionism		Schizoid Personality Disorder
					Malingering***		Frotteurism		
							Pedophilia		

Cognitive Disorders

Cognitive disorders are those that affect the individual's ability to perceive, think, reason, and remember. The following cognitive disorders deal with a deficiency in memory. They may also be termed as **organic mental disorders**. The incidence of these disorders, which may be related to the aging of the brain or to the body's reaction to the ingestion of a substance, is increasing and is expected to continue increasing in this century.

amnesia disorders
(am-**NEE**-zee-ah)

Amnesia disorders, or amnestic disorders, are characterized by short-term and long-term memory deficits.

These individuals have normal attention but are unable to learn new information (short-term memory) and are unable to recall previously learned information (long-term memory). Individuals with amnesia are able to remember things from the distant past easier than things from the recent past. These individuals have no personality change, no impairment in judgment, and no impairment in abstract thinking.

Causes of amnestic disorders include, but are not limited to, medical conditions such as head injury, cerebrovascular disease, poorly controlled insulin-dependent diabetes mellitus, substance abuse, reaction to medications, and exposure to toxins. Treatment is directed at the underlying cause.

delirium
(dee-**LEER**-ee-um)

A delirium is a state of frenzied excitement. It occurs rapidly and is characterized by difficulty maintaining and shifting attention.

The individual is easily distracted and must be constantly reminded to focus attention. Thinking is disorganized and speech is irrelevant, rambling, and sometimes incoherent. The individual is disoriented to time and place and has lost the ability to reason.

Causes of delirium include, but are not limited to, medical conditions such as systemic infections, severe hypoglycemia, injury to the head, substance abuse, or withdrawal from certain substances.

One particular type of delirium is **delirium tremens (DTs)**, an acute and sometimes fatal psychotic reaction caused by cessation of excessive intake of alcoholic beverages over a long period of time.

The duration of delirium is usually short term and subsides completely after treating the underlying cause.

dementia
(dee-**MEN**-she-ah)

Dementia is a progressive, organic mental disorder characterized by chronic personality disintegration, confusion, disorientation, stupor, deterioration of intellectual capacity and function, and impairment of control of memory, judgment, and impulses.

Dementia of the Alzheimer's type is the most common form of dementia. The onset of symptoms is slow and not easily detected at first, with the course of the disorder becoming progressive and deteriorating. If the onset is early, the symptoms will appear before the age of 65; if the onset is late, the symptoms will appear after the age of 65. A definitive diagnosis of Alzheimer's disease is not possible until death, because biopsy or autopsy examination of the brain tissue is required for a diagnosis.

However, the symptoms of dementia of the Alzheimer's type may begin as forgetfulness, followed by the individual becoming suspicious of others as his or her memory deteriorates. The individual may become apathetic and socially withdrawn, or may become more untidy in appearance. Irritability, moodiness, and sudden outbursts over trivial issues may become apparent. These individuals may wander away from home, forgetting where they are and where they live. As the condition progresses, the ability to work or care for personal needs independently is no longer possible and the individual requires supervised care.

Substance-Related Disorders

Substance-related disorders are those associated with the use of drugs. Characteristics include psychological dependence on the substance, daily use, frequent intoxication by the ingestion of the substance, and an inability to control use of the substance. Physical dependence on the substance involves serious withdrawal problems if use of the substance is stopped.

The following drugs are involved in most of the substance-related disorders.

- Central nervous system depressants: substances that slow the activity of the central nervous system, causing impaired motor activity, judgment, and concentration. Examples of central nervous system depressants are alcohol, barbiturates, and opium derivatives.
- Central nervous system stimulants: substances that increase the activity of the central nervous system, causing an increase in heart rate and blood pressure, heightened behavioral activity, and increased alertness. Examples of central nervous system stimulants are cocaine and amphetamines.
- **Hallucinogens**: substances that create perceptual distortions of the mind. Examples of hallucinogens are LSD and **cannabis** (marijuana).

The misuse of drugs may lead to a state of **intoxication**, characterized by impaired judgment, slurred speech, loss of coordination, irritability, and mood changes. Continued use of drugs will lead to a pattern of maladaptive behavior and dependence on the drug. The individual develops a pattern of substance abuse in which the drug is used excessively on a regular basis, allowing it to become a major part of his or her life. The drug is used for a nontherapeutic effect. Drug abuse may begin to affect the individual's relationships with family members, friends, and employers.

The continued abuse of the drug will create a physical dependence in which serious withdrawal symptoms would occur if the use of the drug were stopped. Withdrawal symptoms include a physical craving for the drug characterized by muscle aches, cramps, anxiety, sweating, and nausea. In addition to the physical dependence, the individual develops a **tolerance** to the drug and requires increasing strengths of the drug with each use to achieve the desired effect. Physical dependence and tolerance are classic symptoms of drug addiction.

Individuals who become physically dependent on drugs or alcohol may need to enroll in a detoxification program. This medically supervised treatment program is designed to counteract or destroy toxic properties within the patient. Withdrawal may take several days and may require a week or more of treatment in a medical center. After detoxification, the patient should attend drug therapy sessions to learn the steps necessary to remain free of drugs or alcohol.

Schizophrenia

A **psychosis** is described as a condition characterized by loss of contact with reality. The individual's ability to comprehend and react to environmental stimuli becomes impaired and distorted. The impairment can become so severe that the individual may be reduced to limited functioning and may withdraw into a private world. Most commonly, psychosis appears in the form of **schizophrenia**.

schizophrenia
(skiz-oh-**FREN**-ee-ah)
schiz/o = split
phren/o = mind; also refers to the diaphragm
-ia = condition

Any of a large group of psychotic disorders characterized by gross distortion of reality, disturbances of language and communication, withdrawal from social interaction, and the disorganization and fragmentation of thought, perception, and emotional reaction. See Figure 23-1.

This complex disorder is diagnosed most frequently in the early 20s for men and the late 20s for women.

The diagnosis of schizophrenia requires not only the presence of distinct symptoms but the persistence of those symptoms over a period of time;

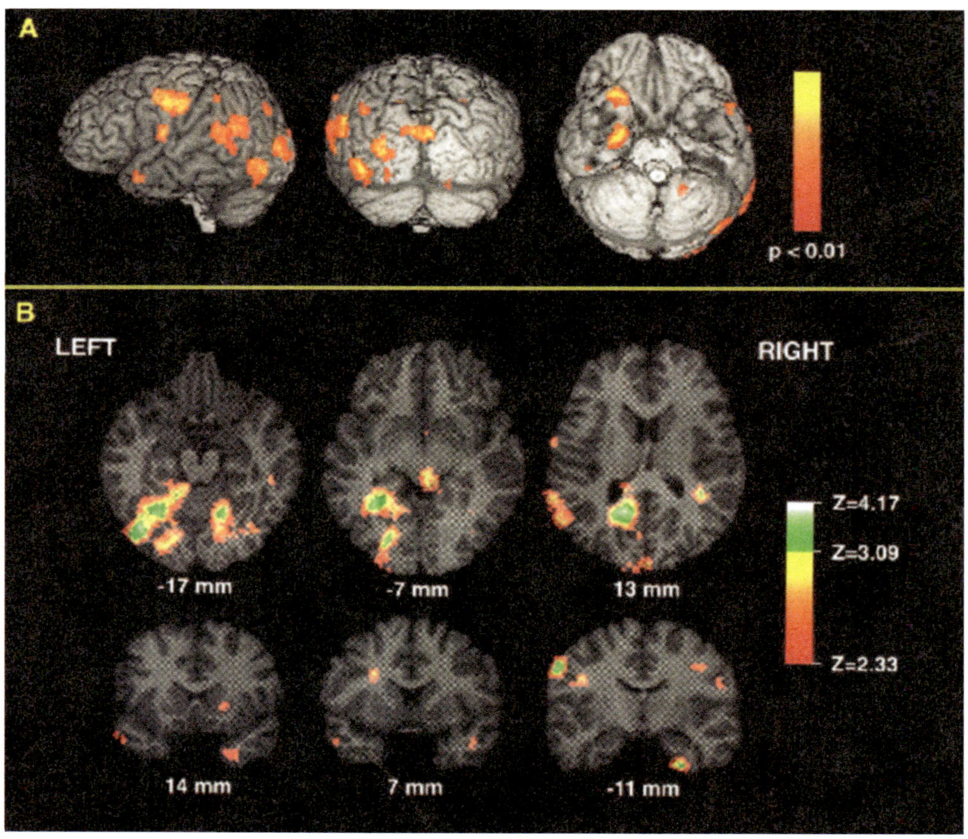

Figure 23-1 Surface and slice images of the brain of a patient with schizophrenia (Courtesy of D. Silbersweig, M.D., and E. Stern, M.D., Functional Neuroimaging Laboratory, The New York Hospital–Cornell Medical Center)

that is, the symptoms must be present for at least 6 months with two or more of the characteristic symptoms being present for at least a 1-month period during that time frame.

Characteristic symptoms of schizophrenia include the following:

1. Hallucinations—in which the person perceives something that does not exist in the external environment. The hallucination may be visual, olfactory (smell), gustatory (taste), tactile (touch), or auditory (hear). The most common form of hallucination in schizophrenia is hearing voices that are distinct from the person's own thoughts. The voices may be friendly or hostile.
2. Delusions—in which the person firmly holds to a persistent abnormal belief or perception despite evidence to the contrary. Two forms of delusions are delusions of persecution in which the person believes others are following him, spying on him, or trying to torment him and delusions of grandeur in which the person believes that newspaper articles and/or radio-television stories are about him or her.
3. Disorganized speech—in which the person may move rapidly from one topic to another, making little sense.
4. Disorganized or catatonic (unresponsive) behavior—in which the person may alternate between agitation and nonpurposeful or random body movements to little or no behavioral response to the environment.
5. Flattened affect—in which the individual shows little or no emotional response to the environment.

paranoid schizophrenia
(**PAIR**-ah-noyd skiz-oh-**FREN**-ee-ah)
schiz/o = split
phren/o = mind; also refers to the diaphragm
-ia = condition

Paranoid schizophrenia is a condition characterized by the individual being overly suspicious of others and having hallucinations and delusions.

Delusions of persecution or delusions of grandeur, accompanied by auditory hallucinations, are usually centered on one major theme, such as a financial matter, a job situation, an unfaithful spouse, or some other problem. The individual is often distrustful, suspicious, and may be argumentative, hostile, and aggressive.

Mood Disorders

Mood disorders are a group of psychiatric disorders characterized by disturbances in physical, emotional, and behavioral response patterns. These patterns range from extreme elation and agitation to extreme depression with suicidal potential. A listing of the more common mood disorders follows.

bipolar disorders (manic-depressive)
(by-**POHL**-ar)

A psychological disorder characterized by episodes of mania, depression, alternating between the two, or a mixture of the two moods simultaneously.

The mania is characterized by extreme excitement, hyperactivity, agitation, overly talkative, flight of ideas, fleeting attention, and sometimes violent, destructive, and self-destructive behavior; the individual may have a decreased need for sleep, and seemingly limitless energy.

The depression is characterized by exaggerated feelings of sadness, discouragement, and hopelessness that are inappropriate and out of proportion with reality.

cyclothymic disorder (sigh-cloh-**THIGH**-mic)

A chronic mood disorder characterized by numerous periods of mood swings from depression to happiness; the period of mood disturbance is at least 2 years duration.

The symptoms of the **cyclothymic disorder** are similar to, but less severe, than those of major depressive disorder.

major depressive disorder

A disorder characterized by one or more episodes of depressed mood that lasts at least 2 weeks and is accompanied by at least four additional symptoms of depression.

These symptoms of depression must exist for most of the day and must exist for at least 2 consecutive weeks to be categorized as a major depressive episode.

Major depressive disorder is characterized by exaggerated feelings of sadness, discouragement, hopelessness, worthlessness, or guilt that are inappropriate and out of proportion with reality; the individual may experience changes in appetite, weight, or sleep, have decreased energy, have difficulty concentrating or making decisions, and have recurrent thoughts of death or suicide. The depressive episode may be relative to some personal loss or tragedy; however, it is different from the normal sadness and grief that follow a personal loss or tragedy.

Symptoms of a major depressive episode usually develop over a period of time. If a full major depressive episode is left untreated, the depression may last 6 months or more.

Anxiety Disorders

Anxiety is state of mind in which the individual feels increased tension, apprehension, a painfully increased sense of helplessness, a feeling of uncertainty, fear, jitteriness, and worry. Observable signs of anxiety include, but are not limited to, restlessness, poor eye contact, glancing about, facial tension, dilated pupils, increased perspiration, and a constant focus on self. Anxiety is usually considered a normal reaction to a realistic danger or threat to the body or self-concept. Normal anxiety disappears when the danger or threat is no longer present. The discussion that follows will deal with disorders that precipitate unrealistic feelings of anxiety in individuals.

generalized anxiety disorder

A disorder characterized by chronic, unrealistic, and excessive anxiety and worry. The symptoms have usually existed for at least 6 months or more and have no relation to any specific causes.

Symptoms of **generalized anxiety disorder** include excessive worry about numerous events, restlessness, feeling keyed up, being easily fatigued, irritability, difficulty concentrating, muscle tension, and sleep disturbance.

Generalized anxiety tends to be chronic with recurrence being associated with stress-related situations.

panic disorder

Panic disorder is characterized by recurrent panic attacks that come on unexpectedly, followed by at least one month of persistent concern about having another panic attack.

The individual experiences intense apprehension, fear, or terror, often associated with feelings of impending doom. The person may experience dyspnea, dizziness, sweating, trembling, and chest pain or palpitations of the heart. The attack may last a few seconds, to several minutes, to an hour or longer and may repeat itself in certain situations.

phobic disorder
(**FOH**-bik)

An anxiety disorder characterized by an obsessive, irrational, and intense fear of a specific object, of an activity, or of a physical situation; also called phobia disorder.

Phobias are usually characterized by symptoms such as faintness, fatigue, palpitations, perspiration, nausea, tremor, and panic. The individual recognizes that the fear is excessive or unreasonable in proportion to the actual danger of the object, activity, or situation even though the feelings are still present.

Phobias are normal, common experiences in childhood with fear of animals, darkness, strangers, etc.; however, phobias in adulthood can become a debilitating experience. Several classifications of phobias are listed, with a brief definition of each.

1. Acrophobia: fear of high places that results in extreme anxiety
2. Aerophobia: morbid fear of fresh air or drafts
3. Agoraphobia: fear of being in an open, crowded, or public place, such as a field, congested street, or busy department store, where escape may be difficult
4. Arachnophobia: fear of spiders
5. Claustrophobia: fear of being in or becoming trapped in enclosed or narrow places; fear of closed spaces
6. Nyctophobia: an obsessive, irrational fear of darkness
7. Zoophobia: a persistent, irrational fear of animals, particularly dogs, snakes, insects, and mice

obsessive-compulsive disorder
(ob-**SESS**-iv kom-**PUHL**-siv)

A disorder characterized by recurrent obsessions or compulsions that are severe enough to be time consuming, (they take more than one hour a day), or to cause obvious distress or a notable handicap.

Obsessions are repeated, persistent thoughts or impulses that are irrational and with which the mind is continually and involuntarily preoccupied. Examples of obsessions are repetitive doubts that something is not right, that a tragic event may occur, thoughts of contamination, or thoughts of violence. Compulsions are irresistible, repetitive, irrational impulses to perform an act; these behavior patterns are intended to reduce anxiety, not to provide pleasure or gratification. Examples of compulsions are touching repeatedly, often combined with counting, washing the hands repeatedly when they have come in contact with contaminants, or checking repeatedly to make sure that no disaster has occurred.

The individual affected with **obsessive-compulsive disorder** recognizes that his or her behavior is excessive or unreasonable. The disorder also causes obvious distress, is time consuming, and interferes with the individual's normal daily routine.

---

posttraumatic stress disorder
(post-trah-**MAT**-ik)

A disorder in which the individual experiences characteristic symptoms following exposure to an extremely traumatic event. The individual reacts with horror, extreme fright, or helplessness to the event.

Experiences that may produce this type of response include, but are not limited to, military combat, being kidnapped, being raped, being tortured, natural or manmade disasters, or automobile accidents.

Symptoms may include reexperiencing the traumatic event, flashbacks, feeling emotionally detached, startling easily, having trouble sleeping, and having difficulty concentrating when awake. **Posttraumatic stress disorder** may last from a few months to several years, depending on the severity of the trauma; it is often more severe or long lasting when the trauma was due to an act of human violence, such as rape. Complete recovery can occur within a few months in approximately half of the individuals; relapse can also occur.

Somatoform, Sleep, and Factitious Disorders

Somatoform disorders are described as any group of neurotic disorders characterized by symptoms suggesting physical illness or disease, for which there are no demonstrable organic causes or physiologic dysfunctions. Sleep disorders are a problem for many individuals, be they temporary or long standing. The causes of sleep disorders may be related to stress, anxiety, or physiological problems. Factitious disorders are characterized by physical or psychological symptoms that are intentionally produced or feigned to assume the sick role. **Malingering** is a term used to describe a willful and deliberate faking of symptoms of a disease or injury to gain some consciously desired end. It differs from somatoform disorders in that it is of the conscious mind instead of being unconsciously motivated, and it usually results in secondary gain as opposed to the somatoform disorders resulting in reduction of anxiety.

---

conversion disorder

A disorder in which the individual represses anxiety experienced by emotional conflicts by converting the anxious feelings into physical symptoms that have no organic basis, but are perceived to be real by the individual.

The individual may experience symptoms such as paralysis, pain, loss of sensation, or some other form of dysfunction of the nervous system; also called conversion hysteria.

The symptoms that occur with **conversion disorder** usually occur after a situation that produces extreme psychological stress. The conversion symptoms, which usually appear suddenly, prevent the individual from experiencing the internal conflict and pain associated with the incident. The individual's lack of concern, over the problem, however, is not in keeping with the severity of the symptoms. This relative lack of concern for the severity of the symptoms displayed is often a clue to the physician that the problem may be psychological rather than physiological.

---

hypochondriasis
(high-poh-kon-**DRY**-ah-sis)

A chronic, abnormal concern about the health of the body, characterized by extreme anxiety, depression, and an unrealistic interpretation of real or imagined physical symptoms as indications of a serious illness or disease despite rational medical evidence that no disorder is present.

The individual is preoccupied with fear of having a serious illness. This fear becomes disabling despite reassurance that no organic disease exists.

Individuals with **hypochondriasis** complain of minor physical problems, worry unrealistically about having or developing a serious illness, constantly seek professional care, and consume multiple over-the-counter remedies. They are so consumed with their fears of illness that it impairs their social and/or occupational functioning. These individuals are so convinced that their symptoms are related to organic disease that they firmly reject any implication that their problems may be due to stress and/or psychosocial problems instead of true medical conditions. Their fear of serious illness may persist for a period of 6 months or more despite medical reassurance. They may become irritated with their physician's suggestion of something other than medical problems. Individuals with hypochondriasis often have a long history of "doctor shopping" and are convinced that they are not receiving the proper care.

Munchausen syndrome (by proxy)
(mun-**CHOW**-zen **SIN**-drom)

A somewhat rare form of child abuse in which a parent of a child falsifies an illness in a child by fabricating or creating the symptoms, and then seeks medical care for the child.

The children usually range in age from infancy to around 6 years. The parent will take the child to the doctor for repeated treatment and possible hospitalization for acute illnesses. Frequently, the mother is the one who actually triggers the symptoms in the child by giving insulin to induce hypoglycemia, laxatives to induce diarrhea, or syrup of ipecac to induce vomiting. When the child is admitted to the hospital for testing and treatment, the mother rarely leaves the child's bedside and appears genuinely concerned about her child's illness.

The most common symptoms that the child will be presented with are bleeding, vomiting, diarrhea, fever, seizures, and apnea. **Munchausen syndrome by proxy** may be suspected when the following criteria become evident.

1. The child is presented for recurrent illnesses for which a cause cannot be identified.

2. The symptoms presented by the parent are unusual and they do not make sense or come together as a particular illness/condition.

3. The symptoms are only observed by the parent.

4. The child's history and the physical findings by the physician do not match.

5. The child has frequent hospital visits (particularly emergency room visits) resulting in normal physical findings.

6. The child has had numerous hospital admissions at several different hospitals (if this can be determined).

Munchausen syndrome in adults is characterized by the adult making habitual pleas for treatment and hospitalization for a symptomatic but imaginary illness. The affected person may logically and convincingly present the symptoms and history of a real illness or disease. Oftentimes, the individual has enough health-related background to make the information appear believable. The symptoms may disappear after treatment, but the individual may seek further treatment for another imaginary illness or condition.

Adults with Munchausen syndrome are mentally ill and need treatment. When they do not get the necessary help, they frequently turn their "perceived illnesses and symptoms" toward their child in the form of Munchausen syndrome by proxy.

---

narcolepsy
(**NAR**-coh-**lep**-see)
narc/o = sleep
-lepsy = seizure, attack

A sleep disorder that is characterized by a repeated, uncontrollable desire to sleep, often several times a day. The sleep attacks must occur daily over a period of at least 3 months to establish the diagnosis of narcolepsy.

The individual cannot prevent falling asleep. He or she may be in the middle of a task or a conversation when the attack occurs. **Cataplexy** may accompany the sleep attack; this is characterized by a sudden loss of muscle tone in which the individual's head may drop, the jaw may sag, the knees may become weakened, and the individual may collapse and fall to the ground. The individual will regain full muscle strength after the sleep episode.

The attacks of sleep usually last 10 to 20 minutes, but can last for as long as an hour. They can occur at any time, are unpredictable, and therefore can be dangerous if the individual is driving or operating heavy equipment or machinery. The condition is treated effectively with amphetamines and other stimulant drugs.

---

pain disorder

A psychological disorder in which the patient experiences pain in the absence of physiologic findings.

Pain disorder is essentially the same as conversion disorder except that the symptom is limited to physical pain. As a result of the pain, the individual often experiences unemployment, disability, and/or family problems. The pain not only limits the individual's ability to function, but also becomes the central focus of the individual's life. He or she may spend much time and money trying to find the right doctor to "cure" the pain.

Dissociative Identity Disorders

Dissociative identity disorders are those in which the individual has emotional conflicts that are so repressed into the subconscious mind that a separation or split in personality occurs. This results in an altered state of consciousness or a confusion in identity. Examples of dissociative disorder include amnesia, fugue, and multiple personality; these disorders will be discussed individually.

dissociative amnesia
(formerly: psychogenic amnesia)
(diss-**SOH**-see-ah-tiv am-**NEE**-zee-ah)

Dissociative amnesia is a disorder in which the individual is unable to recall important personal information, usually of a traumatic or stressful nature; the loss of memory is more than simple forgetting.

This disorder, although rare, is more common in adolescents and young adult women.

dissociative fugue
(formerly: psychogenic fugue)
(diss-**SOH**-see-ah-tiv **FYOOG**)

Dissociative fugue is a disorder in which the individual separates from a past life and associations, wanders away for a period of time, and returns with no recollection of the disappearance.

This disorder appears to be due to the individual's inability to cope with a severe emotional conflict. He or she usually wanders far away from home, staying for several days at a time to weeks. The individual may assume a new identity during the time of absence and may enter a new occupation, appearing and acting consciously aware of his or her behavior and activities. After the episode, however, the individual does not remember the period of absence or actions.

dissociative identity disorder
(formerly: multiple personality disorder)

A disorder in which there is the presence of two or more distinct personalities within one individual. At some point in time, each personality takes complete control of the person's behavior.

Sexual and Gender Identity Disorders

Sexual and gender identity disorders include sexual dysfunctions, paraphilias, and gender identity disorders. **Sexual dysfunctions** are characterized by disturbance in sexual desire and sexual response, and cause marked distress and interpersonal difficulty. **Paraphilias** are characterized by recurrent, intense sexual urges, fantasies, or behaviors that involve unusual objects, activities, or situations. These sexual perversions or deviations are expressed in ways that are socially prohibited or unacceptable, or are biologically undesirable. **Gender identity disorders** are characterized by strong and persistent cross-gender identification accompanied by persistent discomfort with one's assigned sex. The discussion in this section is limited to paraphilias.

exhibitionism
(egs-hih-**BIH**-shun-izm)

Exhibitionism is a sexual disorder involving the exposure of one's genitals to a stranger.

The episode may or may not be accompanied by masturbation. In some cases, the individual is aware of a desire to surprise or shock the observer.

In other cases, the individual has the sexually arousing fantasy that the observer will become sexually aroused.

---

fetishism, transvestic
(**FEH**-tish-izm)

Transvestic fetishism is a sexual disorder in which the focus of the fetish involves cross-dressing. The male usually keeps a collection of female clothing that he intermittently uses to cross-dress.

While cross-dressed, the individual with the fetish may masturbate while holding, smelling, or rubbing the object; or, the individual may have his sexual partner wear the object during sexual activity to achieve sexual excitement.

---

frotteurism
(**FROH**-chur-izm)

Frotteurism is a sexual disorder in which the person gains sexual stimulation or excitement by rubbing against a nonconsenting person. The sexual arousal is achieved through the act of rubbing and/or touching, which includes fondling.

The incident usually occurs in crowded places such as buses and subway transportation, and involves the rubbing of the individual's genitalia against the victim's thighs or buttocks, or fondling the victim. During this brief encounter, the individual fantasizes a relationship with the victim. Escape is usually easy after the episode due to the victim's initial shock and disbelief that something of this nature could occur in such a public place.

---

pedophilia
(**pee**-doh-**FILL**-ee-ah)
ped/o = child; foot
phil/o = attraction to
-ia = condition

Pedophilia is a sexual disorder in which the individual is sexually aroused and engages in sexual activity with children (generally age 13 or younger); this individual is known as a pedophile.

The child usually knows the pedophile, who may be a family member, neighbor, or older friend; the pedophile is at least 16 years of age and is at least 5 years older than the child. The molestation by pedophiles may involve exposing genitalia to the child, genital touching and fondling of the child, masturbating in the presence of a child, or undressing and looking at the child.

---

sexual sadism/sexual masochism

A sexual disorder that involves the act (real, not simulated) of being humiliated, beaten, bound, or otherwise made to suffer; or, the act of inflicting psychological or physical suffering on the victim.

Examples of sexual sadism or masochism include, but are not limited to, restraining by holding down or tying down, slapping, spanking, blindfolding, beating, burning, rape, cutting, and torturing. If the sadistic urges are intense enough, there is danger of serious harm or even death to the victim.

Eating Disorders

The eating disorders discussed in this section are characterized by severe disturbances in eating behavior; the individuals have a morbid fear of gaining weight. Anorexia nervosa is characterized by a refusal to maintain a minimally normal body weight. Bulimia nervosa is characterized by

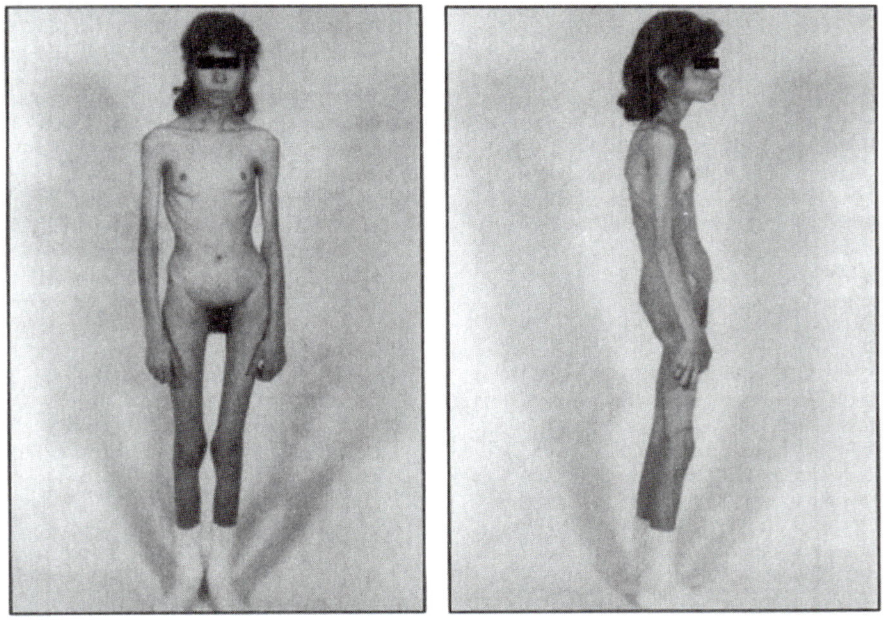

Figure 23-2 Physical manifestations of extreme wasting in an adolescent with anorexia nervosa (From *Mental Health—Psychiatric Nursing,* 3rd ed., by R. P. Rawlings, S. R. Williams, and C. K. Beck, 1992, St. Louis, MO: Mosby-Year Book)

repeated episodes of binge eating followed by inappropriate behaviors such as self-induced vomiting, excessive exercise, misuse of laxatives, or fasting. A disturbance in perception of body shape and weight is an essential feature of both anorexia nervosa and bulimia nervosa. A discussion of each disorder follows.

anorexia nervosa
(an-oh-**REK**-see-ah ner-**VOH**-suh)

A disorder seen primarily in adolescent girls, characterized by an emotional disturbance concerning body image, prolonged refusal to eat followed by extreme weight loss, amenorrhea, and a lingering, abnormal fear of becoming obese. See Figure 23-2.

This potentially life-threatening disorder is most common in young women, beginning sometimes as early as the age of 12. Weight loss is usually achieved by reduction in food intake (may be as little as 300 calories per day) and considerable exercise; the individual may also abuse the use of laxatives and diuretics and induce vomiting after meals to ensure the weight loss.

bulimia nervosa
(boo-**LIM**-ee-ah ner-**VOH**-suh)

An uncontrolled craving for food, often resulting in eating binges, followed by vomiting to eliminate the food from the stomach. The individual may then feel depressed, go through a period of self-deprivation, followed by another eating binge, and the cycle continues.

The individual may consume as many as 5,000 or more calories in one eating binge episode, with several episodes occurring within one day. Immediately after the episode the individual feels depressed, guilty, and ashamed of the binge episode. This may be followed by purging, a means of ridding the body of what has been consumed; that is, the individual may induce vomiting, use laxatives or diuretics to rid the body of the food. Vomiting is the most common method used for purging following an eating binge. Individuals with **bulimia** often avoid social eating events, disappear after meals, and express overly concern about their body weight. They may experience some weight fluctuations due to the alternating food binges and food fasting, although the weight of the bulimic individual usually stays close to the normal ranges.

Personality Disorders

Personality disorders are rigid, inflexible, and maladaptive patterns of behavior that impair a person's ability to function well in society due to a limited ability to adapt. Following are some of the more common personality disorders.

---

antisocial personality disorder
(**an**-tih-**SOH**-shal)

Antisocial personality disorder is characterized by repetitive behavioral patterns that lack moral and ethical standards, keeping the individual in continuous conflict with society.

The individual demonstrates socially irresponsible, guiltless behavior. He or she manipulates others for personal gain, deceives others, and fails to establish stable relationships.

---

borderline personality disorder

Borderline personality disorder is characterized by an extensive pattern of instability of interpersonal relationships, self-image, and marked impulsivity that begins by early adulthood and is present in a variety of contexts.

Characteristics of this disorder include the following:

1. Frantic efforts to avoid real or imagined abandonment. These individuals experience intense abandonment fears and inappropriate anger even when faced with a realistic time-limited separation or when there are unavoidable changes in plans (e.g., panic or fury when someone important to them arrives late or cancels an appointment).
2. A pattern of unstable and intense interpersonal relationships characterized by alternating between extremes of idealization and devaluation.
3. An unstable self-image or sense of self. There may be sudden changes in opinions and plans about career, sexual identity, values, and types of friends.
4. Impulsivity in at least two areas that are potentially self-damaging (e.g., they may gamble, spend money irresponsibly, binge eat, abuse substances, engage in unsafe sex, or drive recklessly).
5. May express inappropriate, intense anger or have difficulty controlling anger, as evidenced by frequent displays of temper, constant anger, or verbal outbursts.

Because of the similarity of characteristics, borderline personality disorder must be distinguished from personality changes due to a general medical condition. It should also be distinguished from symptoms that may develop in association with chronic substance abuse.

narcissistic personality disorder
(nar-sis-**SIST**-ik)

Narcissistic personality disorder is characterized by an abnormal interest in oneself, especially in one's own body and sexual characteristics.

This individual has an exaggerated sense of self-worth, lacks empathy, appears to lack humility, and tends to exploit others to fulfill his or her own needs and desires. The narcissistic individual is usually jealous of others and feels that others are jealous of him or her. Due to his or her fragile self-esteem, the narcissistic individual is hypersensitive to the evaluation of others and may quickly shift from an optimistic, cheerful mood to a mood of shame, humiliation, or rage. Following this feeling of disapproval, the narcissistic individual may withdraw from others and fantasize or rationalize about his or her continued superiority over others.

paranoid personality disorder
(**PAIR**-ah-noyd)

Paranoid personality disorder is characterized by a generalized distrust and suspiciousness of others, so much so that the individual blames them for his or her own mistakes and failures.

These individuals are constantly "on guard" for any real or imagined threat, they appear tense and irritable, and they feel that others are trying to take advantage of them. The paranoid personality trusts no one and anticipates humiliation and betrayal by others. As a result of this distrust and suspicion, the paranoid individual is quick to react angrily or to counterattack when perceiving that someone has attacked his or her character or reputation.

schizoid personality disorder
(**SKIZ**-oyd)

Schizoid personality disorder is characterized by the inability to form social relationships. The individual may appear as emotionally cold or indifferent.

These individuals almost always choose solitary activities, are quiet and rarely speak to coworkers or neighbors, and have no close friends.

Treatments and Therapies

Psychotherapy is defined as any of a large number of related methods of treating mental and emotional disorders using psychological techniques instead of physical means of treatment; it may involve talking, interpreting, listening, rewarding, and role play. Many people seek **therapy** at some point in their lives. We often think of therapy for the obvious needs, such as receiving help in overcoming the trauma of physical or emotional abuse, or seeking help in overcoming fears and depressions. Therapy can also be used to improve the quality of one's life. In any case, the therapies are designed to help the individual learn ways of dealing with emotional conflict and helping them to find positive ways to heal and move forward with their lives. These treatment methods may be conducted by a psychiatrist or by a clinical psychologist.

Following are some of the more commonly practiced treatments and therapies in the field of psychiatry or psychology, with a brief definition of each.

behavior therapy

A form of psychotherapy that seeks to modify observable, maladjusted patterns of behavior by substituting new responses to given stimuli; also called behavior modification.

Behavior therapy is used to treat conditions such as anxieties, phobias, panic disorders, and stuttering. The therapist strives to change the individual's feelings of fear and panic to a belief that he or she is able to master the situation.

drug therapy

The use of psychotherapeutic drugs to treat mental disorders. Psychotherapeutic drugs are those prescribed for their effects in relieving symptoms of anxiety, depression, or other mental disorders, such as schizophrenia.

This section will be devoted to the discussion of three main types of psychotherapeutic drugs: antianxiety agents, antidepressants, and antipsychotic agents.

1. **Antianxiety agents,** commonly known as tranquilizers, are used to calm anxious or agitated people without decreasing their consciousness. Popular antianxiety drugs used are Xanax, Valium, and Ativan.
2. Antidepressants regulate mood and reduce the symptoms of depression. Some common agents used to relieve or reduce the symptoms of depression are Elavil, Prozac, and Nardil.
3. Antipsychotic agents are strong drugs that work to block the receptors in the brain responsible for psychotic behavior, including hallucinations, delusions, and paranoia. These agents lessen agitated behavior, reduce tension, decrease hallucinations and delusions, improve the individual's social behavior, and produce better sleep patterns of the disturbed individual. Some of the most effective drugs used to treat schizophrenia are Clozaril, Zyprexa, and Resperdol.

electroconvulsive therapy (ECT)
(ee-**lek**-troh-kon-**VULL**-siv)

The process of passing an electrical current through the brain to create a brief seizure in the brain, much like a spontaneous seizure from some forms of epilepsy; also called shock therapy.

Electroconvulsive therapy is used mainly to treat severe depression that has not responded to drug treatment. The patient is given anesthesia and muscle relaxants before the current is applied, and usually sleeps through the procedure. A small electric current lasting no longer than a second passes through two electrodes that have been placed on the individual's head. The current excites the nerve tissue and stimulates a brain seizure that lasts from 60 to 90 seconds. Upon awakening after the procedure, the individual usually has no conscious memory of the treatment. Positive results are usually seen after several treatments, as evidenced by the reduction of depression.

family therapy

A form of psychotherapy that focuses the treatment on the process between family members that supports and sustains symptoms. It is a group therapy with family members composing the group.

The therapist may focus on validating the importance of each member in the family, concentrating on the fact that the problem is a "family" problem—not an individual's problem, and leading the family members toward focusing on ways to solve the central conflict within the family.

group therapy

The application of psychotherapeutic techniques within a small group of people who experience similar difficulties; also known as encounter groups.

Although **group therapy** is not as popular today as 20 years ago, the sessions are designed to promote self-understanding through candid group interactions. These encounter groups are not necessarily positive experiences nor are they helpful to all participants.

hypnosis
(hip-**NOH**-sis)

A passive, trancelike state of existence that resembles normal sleep during which perception and memory are altered, resulting in increased responsiveness to suggestion.

Hypnosis is used in psychotherapy, medicine, and in some criminal investigations. While the individual is in the trancelike state of existence, the hypnotist may direct the individual to stop certain behaviors (such as smoking or overeating), may question the individual about forgotten events (as in a criminal investigation), or may suggest the absence of pain upon awakening (as in use with dentistry or medicine).

play therapy

A form of psychotherapy in which a child plays in a protected and structured environment with games and toys provided by a therapist, who observes the behavior, effect, and conversation of the child to gain insight into thoughts, feelings, and fantasies.

The therapist will help the child work through any conflicts that are discovered during the sessions.

psychoanalysis
(**sigh**-koh-ah-**NAL**-ih-sis)

A form of psychotherapy that analyzes the individual's unconscious thought, using free association, questioning, probing, and analyzing.

The therapist uses a technique known as **free association**, which allows the individual to say aloud anything that comes to mind no matter how minor or embarrassing. The therapist interprets the statements to understand what is truly causing the individual's conflict. This form of psychotherapy is designed to bring the unconscious thoughts, often repressed since childhood, to a conscious level so the individual can deal with the emotional conflict.

Personality Tests

Psychologists use a variety of scientifically developed tests and methods to evaluate personality. The reasons for evaluating personality are also varied; for example, a clinical or school psychologist may assess personality to

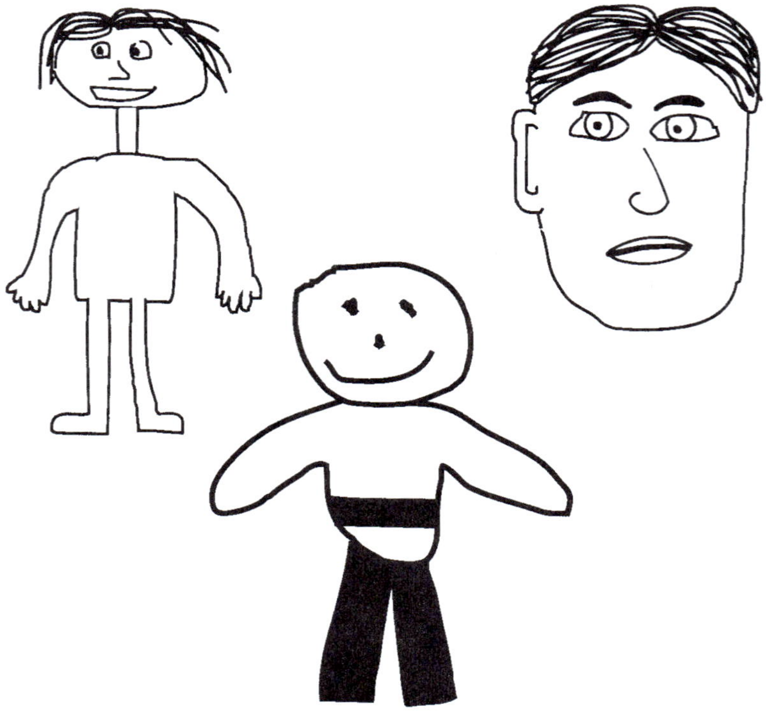

Figure 23-3 Draw-a-person (DAP) test

gain a better understanding of an individual's psychological problems, an industrial psychologist may evaluate personality to help an individual trying to select a career, and a research psychologist may assess personality to investigate theories of personality. The following list is a sample of some of the more commonly used personality tests today in the field of psychiatry or psychology.

draw-a-person (DAP) test

A personality test that is based on the interpretation of drawings of human figures of both sexes. See Figure 23-3.

The individual is asked to draw human figures and talk about them. Evaluations of the drawings are based on the quality and shape of the drawings, the location of the drawing on the paper, how solid the pencil stroke lines appear, the features of the figures drawn, and whether the individual used any background in the drawing.

It is believed that the individual's interpretations of the drawings will reveal valuable information about his or her personality.

Minnesota multiphasic personality inventory (MMPI)
(mull-tih-**FAYZ**-ic)

A self-report personality inventory test that consists of 567 items that can be answered "true," "false," or "cannot say." The items vary widely in content and are sometimes repeated in various ways throughout the test.

The individual's answers are grouped according to 10 clinical categories that detect various disorders such as depression, schizophrenia, and social introversion.

Rorschach inkblot test
(**ROR**-shak)

Rorschach inkblot test is a personality test that involves the use of 10 inkblot cards, half black and white and half in color. The cards are shown to the individual, one at a time. The person is shown a card, and asked to describe what he or she sees in the card.

The examiner records the responses and notes the individual's mannerisms, gestures, and attitude during the responses. After the 10 cards have been shown and described, the examiner presents each inkblot again and this time, asks the individual questions about the previous responses that were made; that is, "how" and "what" questions to determine characteristics about the individual's true personality.

thematic apperception test (TAT)
(thee-**MAT**-ik **ap**-er-**SEP**-shun)

Thematic apperception test is designed to elicit stories that reveal something about an individual's personality. This test consists of a series of 30 black-and-white pictures, each on an individual card.

When the cards are shown, the individual being tested is asked to tell a story about each picture, providing all of the background information and all of the details of the story. The assumption in this test is that the individual will project his or her own unconscious feelings and thoughts into the story he or she tells.

Common Abbreviations

ABBREVIATION	MEANING	ABBREVIATION	MEANING
AD	attention deficit	**M.A.**	mental age
ADHD	attention deficit hyperactivity disorder	**MMPI**	Minnesota multiphasic personality inventory
C.A.	chronological age	**OCD**	obsessive-compulsive disease
CNS	central nervous system	**PCP**	phencyclidine (a psychoactive drug)
DAP	draw-a-picture personality test	**SAD**	seasonal affective disorder
DSM	diagnostic and statistical manual of mental disorders	**TAT**	thematic apperception test (personality test)
DT	delirium tremens	**WAIS**	Wechsler Adult Intelligence Scale
ECT	electroconvulsive therapy	**WISC**	Weschler Intelligence Scale for Children
I.Q.	intelligence quotient		
LSD	lysergic acid diethylamide (an hallucinogenic drug)		

Written and Audio Terminology Review

Review each of the following terms from this chapter. Study the spelling of each term and write the definition in the space provided. If you have the Audio CD available, listen to each term, pronounce it, and check the box once you are comfortable saying the word. Check definitions by looking the term up in the glossary/index.

TERM	PRONUNCIATION	DEFINITION
affect	☐ **AFF**-fekt	____________________
amnesia	☐ am-**NEE**-zee-ah	____________________
amphetamine	☐ am-**FET**-ah-meen	____________________
anorexia nervosa	☐ an-oh-**REK**-see-ah ner-**VOH**-suh	____________________
antisocial personality disorder	☐ an-tih-**SOH**-shal per-son-**AL**-ih-tee dis-**OR**-der	____________________
anxiety	☐ **ang**-**ZY**-eh-tee	____________________
apathy	☐ **AP**-ah-thee	____________________
autism	☐ **AW**-tizm	____________________
behavior therapy	☐ bee-**HAY**-vyhor **THAIR**-ah-pee	____________________
bipolar disorder	☐ by-**POHL**-ar dis-**OR**-der	____________________
borderline personality disorder	☐ **BOR**-der-line per-son-**AL**-ih-tee dis-**OR**-der	____________________
bulimia	☐ boo-**LIM**-ee-ah	____________________
bulimia nervosa	☐ boo-**LIM**-ee-ah ner-**VOH**-suh	____________________
cannabis	☐ **CAN**-ah-bis	____________________
cataplexy	☐ **CAT**-ah-pleks-ee	____________________
catatonia	☐ kat-ah-**TOH**-nee-ah	____________________
claustrophobia	☐ kloss-troh-**FOH**-bee-ah	____________________
compensation	☐ kom-pen-**SAY**-shun	____________________
compulsions	☐ kom-**PUHL**-shuns	____________________

Term		Pronunciation	
conversion disorder	☐	kon-**VER**-zhun dis-**OR**-der	______
cyclothymia	☐	**sigh**-kloh-**THIGH**-mee-ah	______
cyclothymic disorder	☐	sigh-cloh-**THIGH**-mic dis-**OR**-der	______
defense mechanism	☐	dee-**FENCE MEH**-kan-izm	______
delirium	☐	dee-**LEER**-ee-um	______
delirium tremens (DTs)	☐	dee-**LEER**-ee-um **TREE**-menz (DTs)	______
delusion	☐	dee-**LOO**-zhun	______
dementia	☐	dee-**MEN**-she-ah	______
denial	☐	dee-**NYE**-al	______
depression	☐	dee-**PRESH**-un	______
displacement	☐	dis-**PLACE**-ment	______
dissociation	☐	dis-soh-shee-**AY**-shun	______
dissociative amnesia	☐	diss-**OH**-see-ah-tiv am-**NEE**-zee-ah	______
dissociative fugue	☐	diss-**OH**-see-ah-tiv **FYOOG**	______
dysphoria	☐	dis-**FOH**-ree-ah	______
electroconvulsive therapy (ECT)	☐	ee-**lek**-troh-kon-**VULL**-siv **THAIR**-ah-pee (ECT)	______
euphoria	☐	yoo-**FOR**-ee-ah	______
exhibitionism	☐	egs-hih-**BIH**-shun-izm	______
fetishism	☐	**FEH**-tish-izm	______
free association	☐	free ah-soh-shee-**AY**-shun	______
frotteurism	☐	**FROH**-chur-izm	______
generalized anxiety disorder	☐	generalized ang-**ZY**-eh-tee dis-**OR**-der	______
group therapy	☐	groop **THAIR**-ah-pee	______
hallucination	☐	hah-loo-sih-**NAY**-shun	______
hallucinogens	☐	hah-**LOO**-sih-noh-jens	______
hypnosis	☐	hip-**NOH**-sis	______
hypnotize	☐	**HIP**-noh-tize	______
hypochondriasis	☐	high-poh-kon-**DRY**-ah-sis	______

Term		Pronunciation	
hypomania	☐	high-poh-**MAY**-nee-ah	________
intoxication	☐	in-toks-ih-**KAY**-shun	________
kleptomania	☐	klep-toh-**MAY**-nee-ah	________
lithium	☐	**LITH**-ee-um	________
major depressive disorder	☐	**MAY**-jer dee-**PRESS**-iv dis-**OR**-der	________
malingering	☐	mah-**LING**-er-ing	________
mania	☐	**MAY**-nee-ah	________
marijuana	☐	mar-ih-**WAH**-nah	________
mental	☐	**MEN**-tal	________
Minnesota multiphasic personality inventory (MMPI)	☐	min-eh-**SOH**-tah mull-tih-**FAYZ**-ic per-son-**AL**-ih-tee **IN**-ven-toh-ree	________
mood disorders	☐	mood dis-**OR**-ders	________
Munchausen syndrome (by proxy)	☐	mun-**CHOW**-zen **SIN**-drom by **PROCKS**-ee	________
mutism	☐	**MEW**-tism	________
narcissistic personality disorder	☐	nar-sis-**SIST**-ik per-son-**AL**-ih-tee dis-**OR**-der	________
narcolepsy	☐	**NAR**-coh-**lep**-see	________
necrophilia	☐	nek-roh-**FILL**-ee-ah	________
neurosis	☐	noo-**ROH**-sis	________
obsession	☐	ob-**SESS**-shun	________
obsessive-compulsive disorder	☐	ob-**SESS**-siv kom-**PUHL**-siv dis-**OR**-der	________
organic mental disorder	☐	or-**GAN**-ik **MEN**-tal dis-**OR**-der	________
pain disorder	☐	pain dis-**OR**-der	________
panic disorder	☐	**PAN**-ik dis-**OR**-der	________
paranoia	☐	pair-ah-**NOY**-ah	________
paranoid personality disorder	☐	**PAIR**-ah-noyd per-son-**AL**-ih-tee dis-**OR**-der	________

Term	Pronunciation	
paranoid schizophrenia	☐ **PAIR**-ah-noyd skiz-oh-**FREN**-ee-ah	______
paraphilia	☐ pair-ah-**FILL**-ee-ah	______
pedophilia	☐ **pee**-doh-**FILL**-ee-ah	______
phobia	☐ **FOH**-bee-ah	______
phobia disorder	☐ **FOH**-bee-ah dis-**OR**-der	______
posttraumatic stress disorder	☐ post-trah-**MAT**-ik stress dis-**OR**-der	______
projection	☐ proh-**JEK**-shun	______
psychiatrist	☐ sigh-**KIGH**-ah-trist	______
psychiatry	☐ sigh-**KIGH**-ah-tree	______
psychoanalysis	☐ **sigh**-koh-ah-**NAL**-ih-sis	______
psychoanalyst	☐ sigh-koh-**AN**-ah-list	______
psychodrama	☐ sigh-koh-**DRAM**-ah	______
psychologist	☐ sigh-**KALL**-oh-jist	______
psychology	☐ sigh-**KALL**-oh-jee	______
psychoneurosis	☐ sigh-koh-noo-**ROH**-sis	______
psychosis	☐ sigh-**KOH**-sis	______
psychosomatic	☐ sigh-koh-soh-**MAT**-ik	______
psychotherapy	☐ sigh-koh-**THAIR**-ah-pee	______
purging	☐ **PERJ**-ing	______
rationalization	☐ rash-un-al-ih-**ZAY**-shun	______
regression	☐ rih-**GRESH**-un	______
repression	☐ ree-**PRESH**-un	______
Rorschach inkblot test	☐ **ROR**-shak **INK**-blot test	______
schizoid personality disorder	☐ **SKIZ**-oyd per-son-**AL**-ih-tee dis-**OR**-der	______
schizophrenia	☐ skiz-oh-**FREN**-ee-ah	______
sedative	☐ **SED**-ah-tiv	______
senile dementia	☐ **SEE**-nile dee-**MEN**-she-ah	______
sexual masochism	☐ **SEKS**-yoo-al **MASS**-oh-kism	______
sexual sadism	☐ **SEKS**-yoo-al **SAY**-dizm	______

somatoform disorders	☐ soh-**MAT**-oh-form dis-**OR**-ders	______________
sublimation	☐ sub-lih-**MAY**-shun	______________
suppression	☐ suh-**PRESH**-un	______________
thematic apperception test	☐ thee-**MAT**-ik ap-er-**SEP**-shun test	______________
therapy	☐ **THAIR**-ah-pee	______________
tolerance	☐ **TAHL**-er-ans	______________

Chapter Review Exercises

The following exercises provide a more in-depth review of the chapter material. Your goal in these exercises is to complete each section at a minimum 80% level of accuracy. If you score below 80% in any area, return to the appropriate section in the chapter and read the material again. A place has been provided for your score at the end of each section.

A. Spelling

Circle the correctly spelled term in each pairing of words. Each correct answer is worth 10 points. Record your score in the space provided at the end of the exercise.

1.	bulemia	bulimia
2.	hypochondriasis	hypocondriasis
3.	schizophrenia	skitzophrenia
4.	bipoler	bipolar
5.	claustrophobia	claustraphobia
6.	malingering	melingering
7.	Munchousen	Munchausen
8.	frotteurism	frotturism
9.	narcalepsy	narcolepsy
10.	hallucination	halucination

Number correct ______ × 10 points/correct answer: Your score ______%

B. Crossword Puzzle

Read the clues carefully and complete the puzzle. Each crossword answer is worth 10 points. When you have completed the crossword puzzle, total your points and enter your score in the space provided.

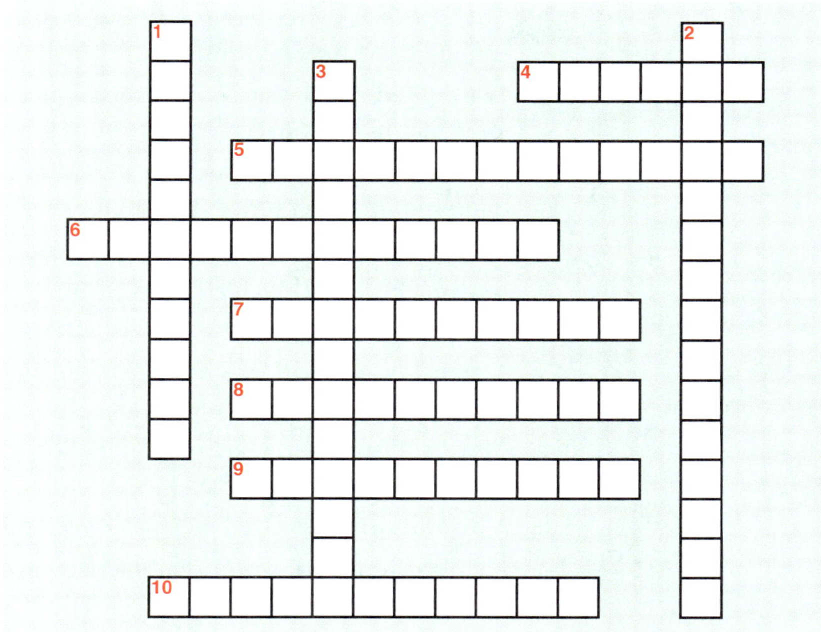

ACROSS
4 Refusal to acknowledge problem
5 Abnormal fear of spiders
6 Emphasizing a stronger trait
7 Abnormal fear of heights
8 Blocking unpleasant thoughts
9 To assign one's feelings to another
10 Abnormal fear of open spaces

DOWN
1 Rechanneling unacceptable impulses
2 Making excuses for behavior
3 Fear of closed space

Number correct _______ × 10 points/correct answer: Your score _______%

C. Term to Definition

Define each term listed by writing the definition in the space provided. Check the box if you are able to complete this exercise correctly the first time (without referring to the answers). Each correct answer is worth 10 points. Record your score in the space provided at the end of the exercise.

☐ 1. affect ______________________________

☐ 2. amnesia ______________________________

☐ 3. apathy ______________________________

☐ 4. delirium ______________________________

☐ 5. euphoria ______________________________

☐ 6. malingering ______________________________

☐ 7. phobia ______________________________

☐ 8. tolerance ______________________________

☐ 9. sedative ______________________________

☐ 10. compulsion ______________________________

Number correct _______ × 10 points/correct answer: Your score _______%

D. Matching Mental Disorders

Match the mental disorders on the left with the appropriate description on the right. Each correct answer is worth 10 points. Record your score in the space provided at the end of the exercise.

_____ 1. anorexia nervosa
_____ 2. bipolar disorder
_____ 3. paranoid schizophrenia
_____ 4. cyclothymic disorder
_____ 5. obsessive-compulsive disorder
_____ 6. conversion disorder
_____ 7. Munchausen syndrome (by proxy)
_____ 8. narcolepsy
_____ 9. exhibitionism
_____ 10. pedophilia

a. Characterized by recurrent obsessions or compulsions severe enough to be time consuming
b. The individual converts anxious feelings into physical symptoms that have no organic basis
c. A parent makes up an illness in a child by creating the symptoms and then seeks medical care for the child
d. A sleep disorder characterized by an uncontrollable desire to sleep
e. A sexual disorder in which an individual repeatedly exposes himself to unsuspecting women or girls
f. A sexual disorder in which the person becomes sexually aroused by inanimate objects
g. A sexual disorder in which the individual engages in sexual activity with children
h. A disorder characterized by a prolonged refusal to eat
i. A chronic mood disorder characterized by mood swings; lasts approximately 2 years
j. A psychological disorder alternating between mania and depression
k. A condition characterized by the individual being overly suspicious of others and having hallucinations and delusions

Number correct _______ × 10 points/correct answer: Your score _______%

E. Matching Abbreviations

Match the abbreviations on the left with the correct definition on the right. Each correct answer is worth 10 points. Record your score in the space provided at the end of the exercise.

_____ 1. SAD
_____ 2. TAT
_____ 3. DSM
_____ 4. ECT
_____ 5. IQ
_____ 6. MMPI
_____ 7. WAIS
_____ 8. OCD
_____ 9. DTs
_____ 10. AD

a. Minnesota Math Placement Test
b. intelligence quotient
c. obsessive-compulsive disorder
d. mental age
e. Weschler Adult Intelligence Scale
f. seasonal affective disorder
g. thematic apperception test
h. Diagnostic and Statistical Manual of Mental Disorders
i. Minnesota multiphasic personality inventory
j. electroconvulsive therapy
k. delirium tremens
l. attention deficit

Number correct _______ × 10 points/correct answer: Your score _______%

F. Word Search

Using the following definitions, identify the mental disorder and then find and circle it in the puzzle. The words may be read up, down, diagonally, across, or backward. Each correct answer is worth 10 points. Record your score in the space provided at the end of the exercise.

Example: A sexual disorder involving the exposure of one's genitals to strangers. In some cases, the individual is aware of a desire to shock the observer.

exhibitionism

1. A sexual disorder in which the individual is sexually aroused and engages in sexual activity with children (generally age 13 or younger)

   ____

2. A personality disorder characterized by an abnormal interest in oneself especially in one's own body and sexual characteristics is known as a ______________________ personality disorder.
3. An uncontrollable craving for food, often resulting in eating binges, followed by vomiting to eliminate the food from the stomach

   ____

4. A disorder characterized by an emotional disturbance concerning body image, prolonged refusal to eat followed by extreme weight loss, amenorrhea, and a lingering, abnormal fear of becoming obese is known as _______ nervosa.
5. A sexual disorder in which the individual derives sexual excitement or gratification from inflicting pain and suffering on another person, either a consenting or nonconsenting partner

   ____

6. A sexual disorder in which the person gains sexual stimulation or excitement by rubbing against a non-consenting person

   ____

7. A sexual disorder in which the focus of the fetish involves cross-dressing. This is known as ___________ fetishism.
8. A sleep disorder that is characterized by a repeated, uncontrollable desire to sleep, often several times a day

   ____

9. A somewhat rare form of child abuse in which a parent of a child falsifies an illness in a child by fabricating or creating the symptoms, and then seeks medical care for the child is known as ________________ syndrome by proxy.
10. A chronic, abnormal concern about the health of the body, characterized by extreme anxiety, depression, and unrealistic worry over the possibility of having a serious illness or disease despite rational medical evidence that no disorder is present

    ____

Number correct _______ × 10 points/correct answer: Your score _______%

B	R	H	O	N	C	H	S	Y	S	T	N	M	I	C
A	N	Y	O	G	E	S	M	S	I	D	A	S	T	T
M	I	P	K	T	M	N	M	E	T	T	R	N	V	R
C	A	O	V	E	E	O	O	S	D	I	C	C	B	A
I	L	C	T	Y	T	N	L	I	E	O	O	N	T	N
M	U	H	O	I	O	T	T	O	T	E	L	R	L	S
L	R	O	T	H	L	O	B	I	U	A	E	C	O	V
P	U	N	L	M	E	I	U	N	A	R	P	I	R	E
P	E	D	O	P	H	I	L	I	A	T	S	U	E	S
S	A	R	U	D	A	D	I	N	D	E	Y	V	M	T
L	A	I	I	G	R	L	M	R	U	E	D	O	R	I
N	I	A	N	A	R	C	I	S	S	I	S	T	I	C
B	S	S	N	E	R	U	A	A	I	D	I	S	G	O
P	U	I	A	I	X	E	R	O	N	A	L	I	R	R
L	R	S	T	H	L	O	E	I	U	A	S	C	O	A
N	E	S	U	A	H	C	N	U	M	I	A	C	B	A
F	R	O	T	T	E	U	R	I	S	M	E	M	I	C
E	X	H	I	B	I	T	I	O	N	I	S	M	N	T

G. Completion

The following statements describe various treatments and therapies used in the field of psychiatry and psychology. Read each statement carefully and complete the sentences with the most appropriate answer. Each correct answer is worth 10 points. Record your score in the space provided at the end of the exercise.

1. A form of psychotherapy that analyzes the individual's unconscious thought, using free association, questioning, probing, and analyzing is known as:

   ____

2. The application of psychotherapeutic techniques with a small number of people who experience similar difficulties is known as:

   ____

3. A form of psychotherapy that seeks to modify observable, maladjusted patterns of behavior by substituting new responses to given stimuli is known as:

   ____

4. A passive, trancelike state of existence that resembles normal sleep during which perception and memory are altered, resulting in increased responsiveness to suggestion is known as:

   ____

5. The process of passing an electrical current through the brain to create a brief seizure in the brain, much like a spontaneous seizure from some forms of epilepsy is known as:

____

6. A form of psychotherapy in which a child plays in a protected and structured environment with games and toys provided by a therapist, who observes the behavior, affect, and conversation of the child to gain insight into thoughts, feelings, and fantasies is known as:

____

7. A personality test in which 10 inkblot cards are shown to the individual, one at a time, and the person is asked to describe what he or she sees in the card is known as the:

____

8. A form of psychotherapy that focuses the treatment on the process between family members, that supports and sustains symptoms is known as:

____

9. A personality test that is based on the interpretation of drawings of human figures of both sexes is known as the:

____

10. A personality test in which the person is shown 30 black-and-white picture cards and is asked to tell an elaborate story about each picture, filling in all of the details, is known as:

____

Number correct _______ × 10 points/correct answer: Your score _______%

H. Multiple Choice

Read the definition of each commonly used defense mechanism and select the correct answer from the choices provided. Each correct answer is worth 10 points. Record your score in the space provided at the end of the exercise.

1. An effort to overcome, or make up for, real or imagined inadequacies is known as:
   a. repression
   b. regression
   c. compensation
   d. projection
2. The voluntary blocking of unpleasant feelings and experiences from one's mind is known as:
   a. repression
   b. regression
   c. suppression
   d. sublimation
3. A refusal to admit or acknowledge the reality of something, thus avoiding emotional conflict or anxiety is known as:
   a. displacement
   b. denial
   c. rationalization
   d. suppression

4. The process of transferring a feeling or emotion from the original idea or object to a substitute idea or object is known as:
   a. displacement
   b. introjection
   c. projection
   d. rationalization
5. Rechanneling or redirecting one's unacceptable impulses and drives into constructive activities is known as:
   a. projection
   b. sublimation
   c. compensation
   d. displacement
6. An involuntary blocking of unpleasant feelings and experiences from one's conscious mind is known as:
   a. denial
   b. regression
   c. repression
   d. suppression
7. An ego defense mechanism whereby an individual unconsciously identifies with another person or with some object and assumes the supposed feelings and/or characteristics of the other personality or object is known as:
   a. introjection
   b. rationalization
   c. compensation
   d. sublimation
8. A response to stress in which the individual reverts to an earlier level of development and the comfort measures associated with that level of functioning is known as:
   a. repression
   b. regression
   c. rationalization
   d. projection
9. The act of transferring one's own unacceptable thoughts or feelings on to someone else is known as:
   a. compensation
   b. displacement
   c. projection
   d. sublimation
10. Attempting to make excuses or invent logical reasons to justify unacceptable feelings or behaviors is known as:
    a. rationalization
    b. projection
    c. denial
    d. introjection

Number correct _______ × 10 points/correct answer: Your score _______%

I. Definition to Term

Using the following definitions, identify and provide the word for the pathological condition to match the definition. Each correct answer is worth 10 points. Record your score in the space provided at the end of the exercise.

1. Observable evidence of a person's feelings or emotions

   ____

2. Loss of memory caused by severe emotional trauma, brain injury, substance abuse, or reaction to medications or toxins

   ____

3. A mental disorder characterized by the individual being extremely withdrawn and absorbed with fantasy

   ____

4. Absence or suppression of observable emotion, feeling, concern, or passion

   ____

5. A state of frenzied excitement or wild enthusiasm

   ____

6. A passive, trancelike state of existence that resembles normal sleep during which perception and memory are altered, resulting in increased responsiveness to suggestion

   ____

7. A persistent thought or idea with which the mind is continually and involuntarily preoccupied

   ____

8. The inability to speak because of a physical defect or emotional problem

   ____

9. A willful and deliberate faking of symptoms of a disease or injury to gain some consciously desired end

   ____

10. Any major mental disorder of organic or emotional origin characterized by a loss of contact with reality

   ____

Number correct _______ × points/correct answer: Your score _______%

J. True or False

Read each statement carefully and circle the correct answer as true or false. HINT: Pay close attention to the word elements written in **bold** as you make your decision. If the statement is false, identify the meaning of the word element written in bold. Each correct answer is worth 10 points. Record your score in the space provided at the end of the exercise.

1. The term ***hypn****osis* means "condition of sleep" or "a passive, trancelike state of existence."

   True False

   If the answer is False, what does *hypn/o* mean? ______________________________

2. The term ***psych****iatry* refers to the branch of medicine that deals with physical therapy.

   True False

   If your answer is False, what does *psych/o* mean? ______________________________

3. **Dys**phoria is a disorder of affect (mood) characterized by difficult or bad feelings such as depression and anguish.

   True False

   If your answer is False, what does *dys*-mean? ____________________

4. The term ***euphoria*** is used to express a sense of well-being or elation.

   True False

   If you answer is False, what does *eu*-mean? ____________________

5. Psycho**somat**ic means "pertaining to the expression of an emotional conflict by making excuses."

   True False

   If your answer is False, what does *somat/o* mean? ____________________

6. **Schiz**ophrenia literally means "split mind."

   True False

   If your answer is False, what does *schiz/o* mean? ____________________

7. A person suffering from kleptomania has a love for shopping.

   True False

   If your answer is False, what does *-mania* mean? ____________________

8. Someone with claustro**phobia** has an abnormal fear of enclosed spaces.

   True False

   If your answer is False, which does *-phobia* mean? ____________________

9. Someone suffering from necro**philia** has an abnormal fear of dead bodies.

   True False

   If your answer is False, what does *-philia* mean? ____________________

10. The term *psycho**neur**osis* literally means "a condition of the mind and nerves."

    True False

    If your answer is False, what does *neur/o* mean? ____________________

Number correct _______ × 10 points/correct answer: Your score _______%

Answers to Chapter Review Exercises

A. Spelling

1 bulimia
2. hypochondriasis
3. schizophrenia
4. bipolar
5. claustrophobia
6. malingering
7. Munchausen
8. frotteurism
9. narcolepsy
10. hallucination

B. Crossword Puzzle

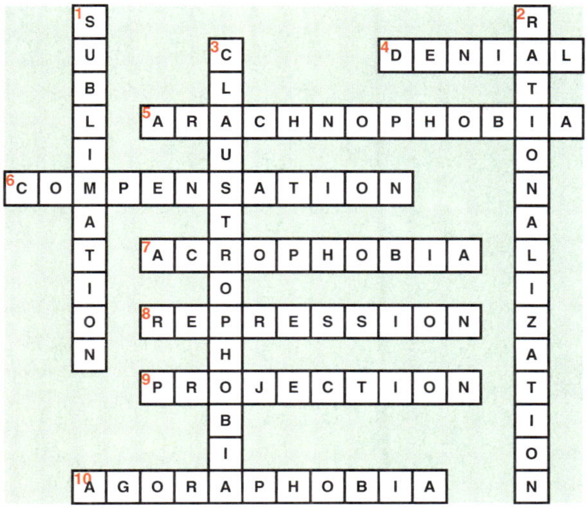

C. Term to Definition

1. observable evidence of a person's feelings or emotions
2. loss of memory
3. absence or suppression of observable emotion, feeling, concern, or passion
4. a state of frenzied excitement or wild enthusiasm
5. a sense of well-being or elation
6. deliberately faking symptoms of a disease or injury to gain some consciously desired end
7. an abnormal fear
8. the ability to endure unusually large doses of a drug without apparent adverse effects, requiring increased doses each time to achieve the same effect
9. an agent that has a calming effect on the body
10. irresistible, repetitive, irrational impulses to perform an act

D. Matching Mental Disorders

1. h
2. j
3. k
4. i
5. a
6. b
7. c
8. d
9. e
10. g

E. Matching Abbreviations

1. f
2. g
3. h
4. j
5. b
6. i
7. e
8. c
9. k
10. l

F. Word Search

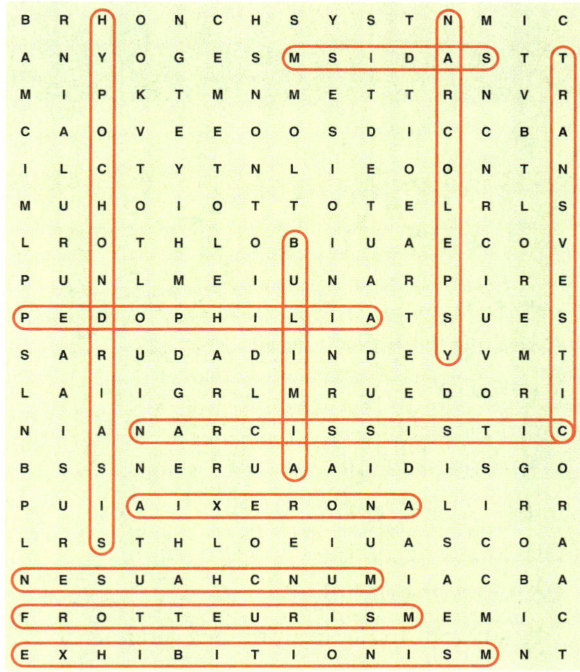

G. Completion

1 psychoanalysis
2. group therapy
3. behavior therapy
4. hypnosis
5. electroconvulsive therapy
6. play therapy
7. Rorschach test
8. family therapy
9. draw-a-person test
10. thematic apperception test

H. Multiple Choice

1. c
2. c
3. b
4. a
5. b
6. c
7. a
8. b
9. c
10. a

I. Definition to Term

1. affect
2. amnesia
3. autism
4. apathy
5. delirium
6. hypnosis
7. obsession
8. mutism
9. malingering
10. psychosis

J. True or False

1. True
2. False; psych/o = mind, soul
3. True
4. True
5. False; somat/o = body
6. True
7. False; -mania = madness
8. True
9. False; -philia = attracted to
10. True

CHAPTER 24

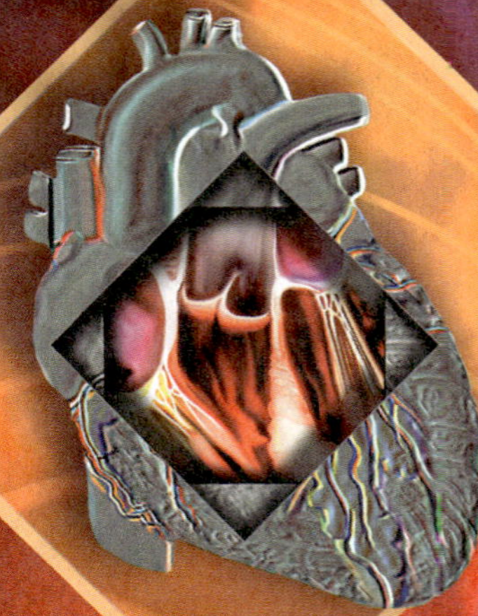

Gerontology

CHAPTER CONTENT

KEY COMPETENCIES

Upon completing this chapter and the review exercises at the end of the chapter, the learner should be able to:

1. Identify and define 10 pathological conditions related to gerontology.
2. Identify at least five diagnostic techniques and procedures used in diagnosis and treatment of disorders of the elderly.
3. Correctly spell at least 20 medical terms that relate to gerontology.
4. Identify at least 10 medical terms related to gerontology based on their descriptions.
5. Create at least 10 medical terms related to gerontology and identify the appropriate combining form(s) for each term.
6. Identify at least 10 abbreviations related to gerontology.
7. Identify and define 10 word elements related to gerontology.

OVERVIEW

"Come grow old with me, the best is yet to be." Is it? "Life begins at 40." Does it? The poetic statements regarding aging are sometimes quite different from reality. Abraham Lincoln once said, "And in the end, it's not the years in your life that count. It's the life in your years." People age in different ways and at different rates. For those who enjoy good health and a clear mind, the years beyond the age of 60 can be most productive and rewarding. For others, who do not enjoy good health, the scenario is quite different. Longevity (living a long life) can be influenced by many factors such as heredity, improved medical treatments, and lifestyle. In the United States, the fastest growing age group is individuals over the age of 85. The health care professional must have an understanding of the normal changes that occur with aging versus changes or signs that indicate a disease process, to provide the best care possible for the patient.

Aging, or **senescence**, is the process of growing old. This process can be positive in that the individual possesses desirable traits such as increased wisdom and experience. On the other hand, the aging process can have negative traits such as decreased capacity to remember things, poorer vision, and a less steady gait (way of walking). The study of all aspects of the aging process, including the clinical, psychological, economical, and sociological issues encountered by older persons and the consequences for both the individual and society, is known as **gerontology**. The branch of medicine that deals with the physiological characteristics of aging and the diagnosis and treatment of diseases affecting the aged is known as **geriatrics**. A **geriatrician** is a physician who has specialized postgraduate education and experience in the medical care of the older person. A **geriatric nurse practitioner** is a registered nurse with additional education obtained through a master's degree program that prepares the nurse to deliver primary health care to elderly adults. **Gerontic nursing** is the nursing care of the elderly, a compromise between caring for the elderly who are ill (geriatric nursing) and a more holistic view of the nursing care of the elderly (gerontological nursing). A **gerontologist** is one who specializes in the study of gerontology.

This chapter will be devoted to the discussion of some of the changes and conditions that occur in the elderly adult. Many of the pathological conditions in this chapter have already been discussed in previous body system chapters. They are presented again in this chapter as they relate to the elderly, and are presented by body systems.

Assessing the Elderly Adult

When conducting a physical assessment on an elderly adult, some of the following observations may be noted. There will be a decrease in adipose tissue. The skin becomes drier and the individual experiences a decrease in skin **turgor**. The individual also may notice some flaking of the skin on the extremities due to the dryness. Additionally, the skin in the elderly person may be thin, almost transparent. There may be an increase in skin tags as well as age spots.

There will be evidence of graying of the hair (**hypopigmentation**), as well as a decrease in the amount of hair on the head. Male pattern baldness may be evident. Men may develop thicker eyebrow hair, coarse nasal hair, and hair in the ear canal. The nailbeds may become more brittle and there is usually a thickening of the toenails. The toenails may also become malformed and yellowish.

Observation of the face will reveal wrinkles and sagging of the skin. The lips may wrinkle due to the degeneration of elastin. The individual may have a pursed-lip appearance. Further observation of the mouth may reveal receding gum lines, some exposure of the root of the tooth, and some yellowing of the teeth. The eyes may appear sunken and the lids may droop due to loss of fatty tissue in the area. Visual acuity for far vision (hyperopia) will increase with aging and visual acuity for near vision (**myopia**) will decrease. The change that occurs in the near vision due to the aging process is known as **presbyopia** (poor vision due to the natural aging process).

The stature (height) of the elderly female may be several inches shorter than in earlier years, as a result of estrogen depletion. The abdomen of both the male and female may have a rounder appearance due to the redistribution of subcutaneous (fatty) tissue. The female breasts become more elongated and appear flatter with advanced age.

Accurate observations by the health care professional will assist the physician in proper diagnosis of the patient's condition. Not all deviations from the norm, in the elderly patient, are due to pathological conditions. Some are simply the normal process of aging. Every body system undergoes change with aging.

As you read through the chapter section on pathological conditions, you will find observations concerning the normal changes that occur in the particular body system as it ages (at the beginning of each body system discussed), followed by a discussion of the various pathological conditions related to that particular body system.

Vocabulary

The following vocabulary words are frequently used when discussing the diseases and disorders of the elderly.

WORD	DEFINITION
acrochordon (ak-roh-**KOR**-don)	Skin tag; a benign growth that hangs from a short stalk, commonly occurring on the neck, eyelids, axilla, or groin.
aging	The process of growing old.
alopecia (al-oh-**PEE**-she-ah)	Partial or complete loss of hair. **Alopecia** may result from normal aging, a reaction to a medication such as anticancer medications, an endocrine disorder, or a skin disease.
anastomosis (ah-**nas**-toh-**MOH**-sis)	A surgical joining of two ducts, blood vessels, or bowel segments to allow flow from one to the other; **anastomosis** of blood vessels may be performed to bypass an occluded area and restore normal blood flow to the area.
anorexia (an-oh-**REK**-see-ah)	Lack or loss of appetite, resulting in the inability to eat. **Anorexia** is seen in individuals who are depressed, with the onset of fever and illness, with stomach disorders, or as a result of excessive intake of alcohol or drugs.

ascites (ah-**SIGH**-teez)	An abnormal intraperitoneal (within the peritoneal cavity) accumulation of a fluid containing large amounts of protein and electrolytes.
atherosclerosis (**ath**-er-**oh**-scleh-**ROH**-sis) ather/o = fatty scler/o = hard -osis = condition	A form of **arteriosclerosis** (hardening of the arteries) characterized by fatty deposit buildup within the inner layers of the walls of larger arteries.
atrophic (aye-**TROH**-fik) a- = without troph/o = development -ic = pertaining to	Characterized by a wasting of tissues, usually associated with general malnutrition or a specific disease state.
atrophy (**AT**-roh-fee) a- = without troph/o = development -y = noun ending	Wasting away; literally "without development."
bruit (brew-**EE**)	An abnormal sound or murmur heard when listening to a carotid artery, organ, or gland with a stethoscope (e.g., during auscultation).
bunionectomy (bun-yun-**ECK**-toh-mee) -ectomy = surgical removal	Surgical removal of a bunion; removing the bony overgrowth and the bursa.
claudication (klaw-dih-**KAY**-shun)	Cramplike pains in the calves of the legs caused by poor circulation to the muscles of the legs; commonly associated with **atherosclerosis**.
crepitation (crep-ih-**TAY**-shun)	Clicking or crackling sounds heard upon joint movement.
cryosurgery (cry-oh-**SER**-jer-ee) cry/o = cold	A noninvasive treatment for nonmelanoma skin cancer using liquid nitrogen, which freezes the tissue. It is also used to remove benign skin tumors and growths such as warts.
curettage (koo-**REH**-tazh)	The process of scraping material from the wall of a cavity or other surface for the purpose of removing abnormal tissue or unwanted material.
dyskinesia (dis-kih-**NEE**-see-ah) dys- = bad, difficult, painful, disordered -kinesia = movement	An impairment of the ability to execute voluntary movements.
ectropion (ek-**TROH**-pee-on)	Eversion (turning outward) of the edge of the eyelid.
edema (eh-**DEE**-ma)	The abnormal accumulation of fluid in interstitial spaces of tissues.
electrodesiccation (ee-**lek**-troh-**des**-ih-**KAY**-shun) electr/o = electricity	A technique using an electrical spark to burn and destroy tissue; used primarily for the removal of surface lesions.

entropion (en-**TROH**-pee-on)	Inversion (turning inward) of the edge of the eyelid.
geriatrician (**jer**-ee-ah-**TRIH**-shun)	A physician who has specialized postgraduate education and experience in the medical care of the older person.
geriatric nurse practitioner (jer-ee-**AT**-rik)	A registered nurse with additional education obtained through a master's degree program that prepares the nurse to deliver primary health care to elderly adults.
geriatrics (jer-ee-**AT**-riks)	The branch of medicine that deals with the physiological characteristics of aging and the diagnosis and treatment of diseases affecting the aged.
gerontics	Pertaining to old age.
gerontologist	One who specializes in the study of gerontology.
gerontology (**jer**-on-**TAHL**-oh-jee)	The study of all aspects of the aging process, including the clinical, psychological, economic, and sociologic issues encountered by older persons and their consequences for both the individual and society.
gerontophobia	An abnormal fear of growing old; fear of aging.
geropsychiatry	The study and treatment of psychiatric aspects of aging and mental disorders of elderly people.
glucagon (**GLOO**-kah-gon)	A hormone produced by the alpha cells of the pancreas that stimulates the liver to convert **glycogen** into glucose when the blood sugar level is dangerously low.
glycosuria (glye-kohs-**YOO**-ree-ah) glyc/o = sugar -uria = urine condition	The presence of sugar in the urine.
hyperglycemia (high-per-glye-**SEE**-mee-ah) hyper- = excessive glyc/o = sugar -emia = blood condition	Elevated blood sugar level.
hypopigmentation (**high**-poh-pig-min-**TAY**-shun) hypo- = less than normal	Unusual lack of skin color.
ischemia (iss-**KEY**-mee-ah) -emia = blood condition	Decreased supply of oxygenated blood to a body part or organ.
ketones (**KEE**-tohnz)	Substances that increase in the blood as a result of improper carbohydrate metabolism; fats are broken down for energy when the body is unable to utilize carbohydrates for energy and the result is a buildup of ketone bodies in the blood and the urine.
kyphosis (ki-**FOH**-sis)	An abnormal outward curvature of a portion of the spine, commonly known as humpback or hunchback.

lichenification (lye-**ken**-ih-fih-**KAY**-shun)	Thickening and hardening of the skin.
malabsorption (**mal**-ab-**SORP**-shun)	Impaired absorption of nutrients into the bloodstream from the gastrointestinal tract.
middle-old	A term used to describe an individual between the ages of 75 and 84 years.
myopia (my-**OH**-pee-ah) my/o = muscle -opia = visual condition	A refractive error in which the lens of the eye cannot focus on an image accurately, resulting in impaired distant vision that is blurred due to the light rays being focused in front of the retina because the eyeball is longer than normal; nearsightedness.
nocturia (nok-**TOO**-ree-ah) noct/o = night -uria = urine condition	Urination at night.
old-old	A term used to describe an individual 85 years of age and older. The fastest number of older adults is in the old-old age group.
pitting edema (pitting ee-**DEE**-mah)	Swelling, usually of the skin of the extremities, that when pressed firmly with a finger will maintain the dent produced by the finger.
presbycusis (prez-bee-**KOO**-sis) presby/o = old age	Loss of hearing due to the natural aging process.
presbyopia (prez-bee-**OH**-pee-ah) presby/o = old, elderly -opia = vision	Loss of accommodation for near vision; poor vision due to the natural aging process.
senescence (seh-**NESS**-ens)	The process of growing old.
senile lentigines (**SEE**-nyle lin-**TIH**-jeh-nez)	Age spots; brown macules found on areas of the skin that are frequently exposed to the sun, such as the face, neck, or back of the hands of many older people; the singular version of the word is lentigo.
stent	A rod or threadlike device (mesh tube) for supporting tubular structures during surgical anastomosis or for holding arteries open during angioplasty.
turgor (**TURH**-gor)	A reflection of the skin's elasticity. Turgor can be checked by lightly pinching the skin of the forearm between the examiner's thumb and forefinger and releasing it. The time it takes for the skin to return to its normal position is the measure of skin turgor, with the normal return time being approximately 3 seconds.
urinary incontinence (**YOO**-rih-**nair**-ee in-**CON**-tin-ens) urin/o = urine -ary = pertaining to	Inability to control urination; the inability to retain urine in the bladder.
young-old	A term used to describe an individual between the ages of 65 and 74 years.

Word Elements

The following word elements pertain to gerontology and diseases and disorders of the elderly. As you review the list, pronounce each word element aloud twice and check the box after you "say it." Write the definition for the example word given for each word element. You may use your medical dictionary.

WORD ELEMENT	PRONUNCIATION	"SAY IT"	MEANING
ankyl/o **ankyl**osis	**ANG**-kih-loh ang-kih-**LOH**-sis	☐	stiff
arter/o, arteri/o **arteri**osclerosis	ar-**TEE**-roh, ar-**TEE**-ree-oh ar-tee-ree-oh-skleh-**ROH**-sis	☐	artery
arthr/o **arthr**itis	**AR**-throh ar-**THRY**-tis	☐	joint
carcin/o **carcin**oma	kar-**SIN**-noh kar-sih-**NOH**-mah	☐	cancer
corne/o **corne**itis	**COR**-nee-oh cor-nee-**EYE**-tis	☐	cornea
coron/o **coron**ary arteries	cor-**OH**-no **KOR**-oh-nah-ree **AR**-ter-eez	☐	heart
cry/o **cry**osurgery	**KRY**-oh kry-oh-**SIR**-jeer-ee	☐	cold
glauc/o **glauc**oma	**GLAW**-koh glaw-**KOH**-mah	☐	gray, silver
glyc/o **glyc**ogen	**GLIGH**-koh **GLIGH**-koh-jen	☐	sugar
hyper- **hyper**glycemia	**HIGH**-per high-per-glye-**SEE**-mee-ah	☐	excessive
hypo- **hypo**glycemia	**HIGH**-poh high-poh-glye-**SEE**-mee-ah	☐	less than normal
-itis prostat**itis**	**EYE**-tiss pross-tah-**TYE**-tis	☐	inflammation
kerat/o **kerat**osis	kair-**AH**-toh kair-ah-**TOH**-sis	☐	hard, horny; also refers to the cornea of the eye
-malacia osteo**malacia**	mah-**LAY**-she-ah **oss**-tee-oh-mah-**LAY**-she-**ah**	☐	softening

Word part / Term	Pronunciation		Meaning
myx/o **myx**edema	**MIKS**-oh miks-eh-**DEE**-mah	☐	relating to mucus
neur/o **neur**opathy	**NOO**-roh noo-**ROP**-ah-thee	☐	nerve
-opia my**opia**	**OH**-pee-ah my-**OH**-pee-ah	☐	visual condition
-osis thromb**osis**	**OH**-sis throm-**BOH**-sis	☐	condition
oste/o **oste**oarthritis	**OSS**-tee-oh oss-tee-oh-ar-**THRY**-tis	☐	bone
ovari/o **ovari**an carcinoma	oh-**VAY**-ree-oh oh-**VAY**-ree-an car-sin-**OH**-ma	☐	ovary
-porosis osteo**porosis**	por-**ROW**-sis **oss**-tee-oh-por-**ROW**-sis	☐	passage or pore
presby/o **presby**opia	**PREZ**-bee-oh prez-bee-**OH**-pee-ah	☐	old, elderly
prostat/o **prostat**itis	pross-**TAH**-toh pross-tah-**TYE**-tis	☐	prostate gland
pulmon/o **pulmon**ary	pull-**MON**-oh **PULL**-mon-air-ee	☐	lung
retin/o **retin**itis	**RET**-in-oh ret-in-**EYE**-tis	☐	retina
scler/o **scler**osis	**SKLAIR**-oh sklair-**OH**-sis	☐	hard
spondyl/o **spondyl**osis	**SPON**-dih-loh spon-dih-**LOH**-sis	☐	spine
troph/o hyper**trophy**	**TROH**-foh high-**PER**-troh-fee	☐	development, growth
ur/o **ur**inary incontinence	**YOO**-roh **YOO**-rih-nair-ee in-**CON**-tin-ens	☐	urine
urethr/o **urethr**itis	yoo-**REE**-throh yoo-ree-**THRIGH**-tis	☐	urethra
-uria poly**uria**	**YOO**-ree-ah pall-ee-**YOO**-ree-ah	☐	urine condition

Pathological Conditions and Changes in the Elderly Person

The following is a discussion of some of the more commonly occurring pathological conditions and changes in the elderly than in other age groups. These conditions and changes are presented by body systems.

Integumentary System

When observing the elderly person and considering the integumentary system, the obvious changes due to the aging process are the graying of hair and the wrinkling of skin. Wrinkling of the skin is caused by the loss of subcutaneous fat and water in the epidermal layers of the skin and exposure to the sun over the course of a lifetime. The elderly person will also have reduced skin turgor, possible dry scaly skin, and thinning epidermis (paper-thin skin). Sometimes the skin seems almost transparent over the underlying blood vessels. See **Figure 24-1.**

The nails of the elderly person may become thick and prone to splitting. Additionally, the elderly person will develop brown, pigmented areas on the back of the hands, arms, and face. These spots are known as age spots. The elderly person may also be prone to the development of precancerous and cancerous skin growths due to the lifetime exposure to the sun.

The pathological conditions related to aging skin include, but are not limited to the following:

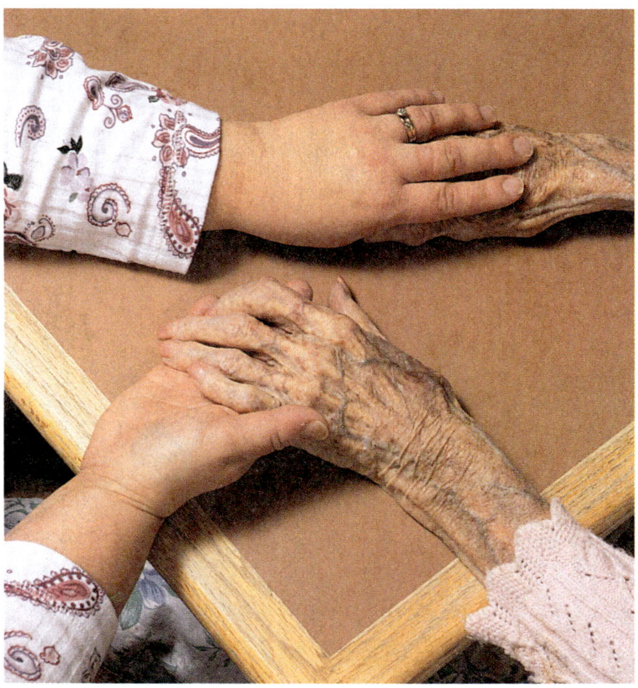

Figure 24-1 Transparent appearance of aging skin

acrochordon
(ak-roh-**KOR**-don)

A benign growth that hangs from a short stalk, commonly occurring on the neck, eyelids, axilla, or groin of an older person.

Acrochordon is also known as cutaneous papilloma or skin tag.

actinic keratosis
ak-**TIN**-ic kair-ah-**TOH**-sis
kerat/o = hard
-osis = condition

Actinic keratosis is identified by raised areas that appear scaly and may bleed at the edges. An area of inflammation around the border of the lesion may be noted.

This premalignant warty lesion, occurring on the sun-exposed skin of the face or hands in aged light-skinned persons, should be checked by a physician if any change in its status occurs. Also known as senile lentigines.

carcinoma, basal cell
car-sih-**NOH**-mah,
BAY-sal sell
carcin/o = cancer
-oma = tumor

The most common malignant tumor of the epithelial tissue which occurs most often on areas of the skin that are exposed to the sun. See Figure 24-2.

Older adults exposed to the sun or other irritants for long intervals are susceptible to the development of skin cancer on the exposed surfaces of the skin. Basal cell **carcinoma** presents as a nodule slightly elevated with a depression or ulceration in the center that becomes more obvious as the tumor grows.

If not treated, the basal cell carcinomas will invade surrounding tissue, which can lead to destruction of body parts (such as a nose). Treatment includes surgical excision, **curettage** and **electrodesiccation, cryosurgery,** or radiation therapy (see the section on diagnostic tests and procedures for description).

Basal cell carcinomas rarely metastasize, but they tend to recur, especially those larger than 2 cm in diameter.

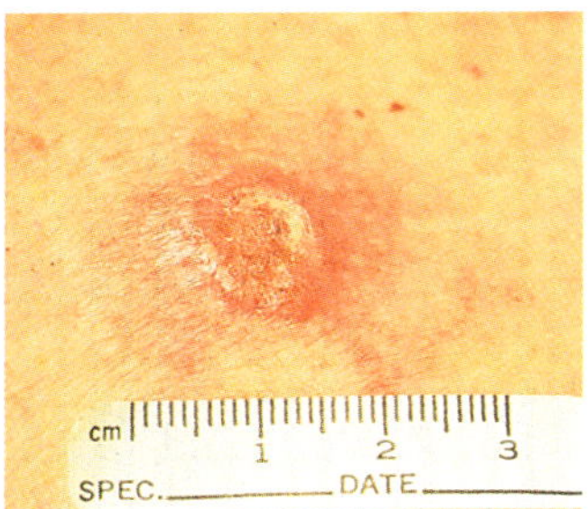

Figure 24-2 Basal cell carcinoma (Courtesy of Robert A. Silverman, M.D., Pediatric Dermatology, Georgetown University)

carcinoma, squamous cell
car-sih-**NOH**-mah,
SKWAY-mus sell
carcin/o = cancer
-oma = tumor

A malignancy of the squamous, or scalelike, cells of the epithelial tissue. Squamous cell carcinoma is a much faster growing cancer than basal cell carcinoma and has a greater potential for metastasis if not treated. See Figure 24-3.

These squamous cell lesions are seen most frequently on these sun-exposed areas:

1. Top of the nose
2. Forehead
3. Margin of the external ear
4. Back of the hands
5. Lower lip

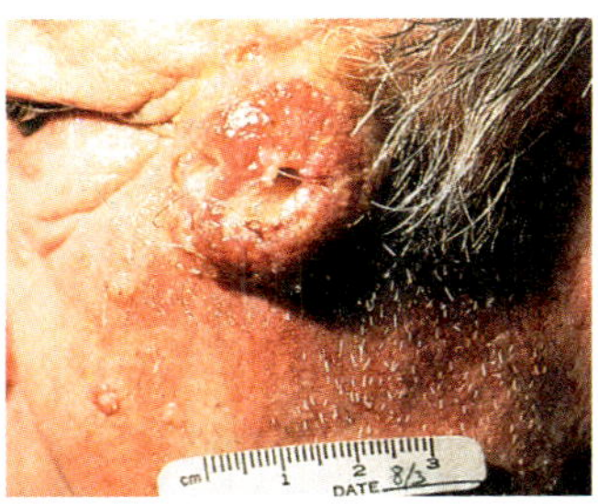

Figure 24-3 Squamous cell carcinoma (Courtesy of Robert A. Silverman, M.D., Pediatric Dermatology, Georgetown University)

The squamous cell lesion begins as a firm flesh-colored or red papule sometimes with a crusted appearance. As the lesion grows it may bleed or ulcerate and become painful. When squamous cell carcinoma recurs, it can be highly invasive and have an increased risk of metastasis.

Treatment is surgical excision with the goal to remove the tumor completely along with a margin of healthy surrounding tissue. Cryosurgery for low-risk squamous cell carcinomas is also common.

eczema

Eczema is an acute or chronic inflammatory skin condition characterized by erythema, papules, vesicles, pustules, scales, crusts, or scabs; accompanied by intense itching.

These lesions may occur alone or in any combination. They may be dry or may produce a watery discharge with resultant itching. Although eczema is not limited to the elderly, it is discussed in this section due to the fact that it also affects the aging skin.

Long-term effects of eczema may result in thickening and hardening of the skin, known as **lichenification**, which is due to irritation caused from repeated scratching of the itchy area; redness and scaling of the skin may also accompany the condition. Severe itching predisposes the areas to secondary infections and possible invasion by viruses.

An estimated 9% to 12% of the population is affected by eczema occurring most commonly during infancy and childhood. The incidence decreases in adolescence and adulthood. There is no exact cause known; however, statistics support a convincing genetic component in that when both mother and father are affected, the child has an 80% chance of developing eczema. This inflammatory response is believed to be initiated by histamine release with lesions usually occurring on the flexor surfaces of the arms and legs, hands, feet, and upper trunk of the body.

There is no specific treatment to cure eczema; however, local and systemic medications may be prescribed to prevent itching. It is important to stress daily skin care and avoidance of known irritants. Chronic eczema is often frustrating to control and may have to be dealt with throughout most of the individual's life as it is prone to recur.

psoriasis

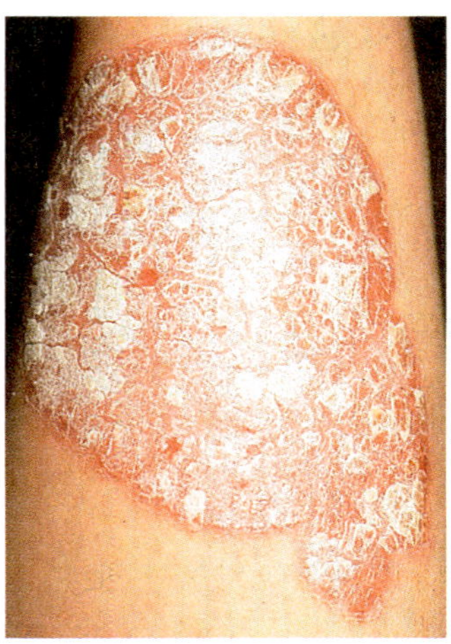

Psoriasis is a common noninfectious chronic disorder of the skin manifested by silvery white scales over round raised reddened plaques producing pruritus.

The process of hyperkeratosis produces various size lesions occurring largely on the scalp, ears, extensor surfaces of the extremities, bony prominences, and perianal and genital areas. See **Figure 24-4** for a visual reference.

Onset of psoriasis is usually between the ages of 10 and 40, but no age is exempt. Treatment includes topical application of various medications, phototherapy, and ultraviolet light therapy in an attempt to slow the hyperkeratosis.

Figure 24-4 Psoriasis (Courtesy of Robert A. Silverman, M.D., Pediatric Dermatology, Georgetown University)

seborrheic keratosis
(seb-oh-**REE**-ik kair-ah-**TOH**-sis)
kerat/o = hard
-osis = condition

Seborrheic keratosis appears as a brown or waxy yellow wartlike lesion(s), 5 to 20 mm in diameter, loosely attached to the skin surface.

Seborrheic keratosis is also known as seborrheic warts.

Skeletal System

The normal age-related changes of the musculoskeletal system generally affect mobility. After about the age of 50, the process of bone formation and resorption becomes unstable, causing the musculoskeletal system to gradually lose bone mass. When discussing the skeletal system of the elderly person, one must consider the decrease in total body mass, bone mass, and bone density. The elderly person will also experience an increase in bone fragility and a decrease in bone strength. These factors influence the types of skeletal system diseases and disorders experienced by the elderly.

The pathological conditions related to the aging skeletal system include, but are not limited to, the following:

fracture of the hip

A break in the continuity of the bone involving the upper third of the femur.

A hip fracture is classified as either intracapsular (within the joint capsule) or extracapsular (outside of the joint capsule). See **Figure 24-5.**

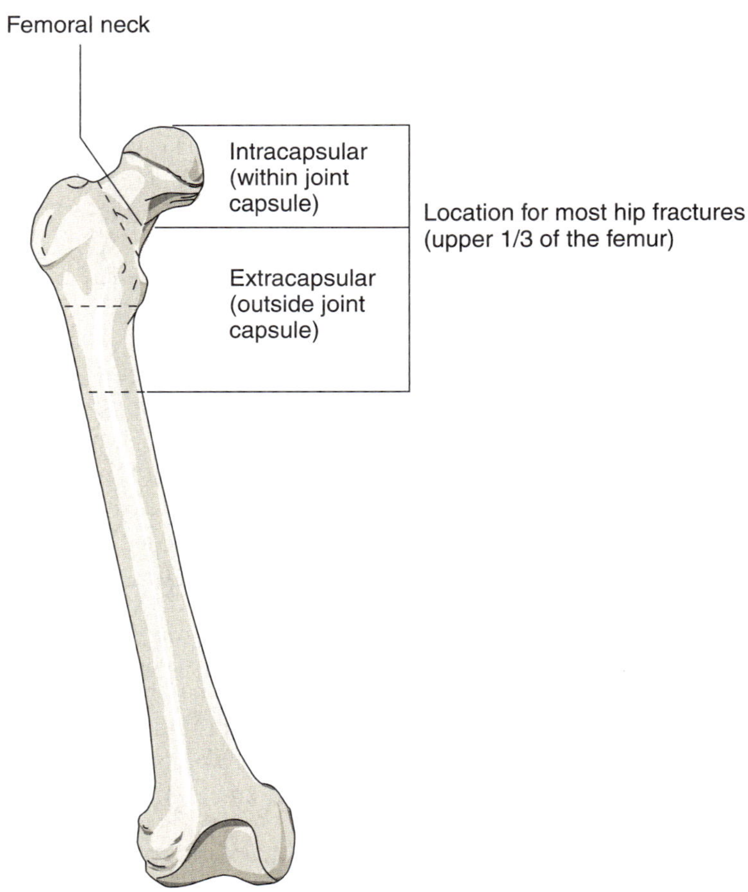

Figure 24-5 Location of hip fractures

Hip fractures occur most often in elderly adults. This may be partly due to the fact that the senses that help maintain equilibrium, coordination, and body position are diminished in the elderly adult, resulting in a general unsteadiness and a lack of coordination in movements.

Women who have osteoporosis are more susceptible to fractures of the hip. Most hip fractures, impactions (the adjacent fragmented ends of the fractured bone are wedged together), or dislocations (femoral head is out of the hip joint) are caused by falls.

Repair of hip fractures has rapidly become one of the most common surgeries among the elderly. Many of the elderly patients who sustain a hip fracture do not experience a rapid or full recovery. Some may die within a year of injury due to medical complications or immobility as a result of the fracture.

The treatment of choice for a fractured hip is surgery, which may involve open reduction and internal fixation. (Figure 24-16 later in the chapter provides a visual reference for internal fixation of a fracture.)

---

osteomalacia
(oss-tee-oh-mah-**LAY**-she-ah)
oste/o = bone
malac/o = softening
-ia = condition

Osteomalacia is a disease in which the bones become abnormally soft, due to a deficiency of calcium and phosphorus in the blood (which is necessary for bone mineralization). This disease results in fractures and noticeable deformities of the weight-bearing bones. This disease is the adult equivalent of rickets.

The deficiency of these minerals is due to a lack of vitamin D, which is necessary for the absorption of calcium and phosphorus by the body. The vitamin D deficiency may be caused by a diet lacking in vitamin D, a lack of exposure to sunlight, or by a metabolic disorder causing malabsorption.

Treatment includes daily administration of vitamin D in addition to a diet sufficient in calcium, phosphorus, and protein. Supplemental calcium may also be prescribed. The elderly adult should be encouraged to be as active as possible, because active exercise and a nutritionally adequate diet are now thought to decrease the speed at which muscle mass and bone density decrease.

---

osteoporosis
(oss-tee-oh-poh-**ROW**-sis)
oste/o = bone
por/o = cavity, passage
-osis = condition

Osteoporosis literally means porous bones; that is, bones that were once strong become fragile due to loss of bone density.

Osteoporosis is a common manifestation of bone abnormality in older adults and occurs more frequently and at an earlier age in women than in men. The patient is more susceptible to fractures, especially in the wrist, hip, and vertebral column.

Osteoporosis occurs most frequently in postmenopausal women, in sedentary or immobilized individuals, and in patients on long-term steroid treatment.

A major factor in osteoporosis is hormonal: Postmenopausal women are at a high risk for osteoporosis, because estrogen production and bone calcium storage decrease with menopause. Other risk factors tend to be hereditary.

Classic characteristics of osteoporosis are fractures that occur in response to normal activity or minimal trauma, a loss of standing height of greater than 2 inches, and the development of the typical kyphosis (dowager's hump). See **Figure 24-6.**

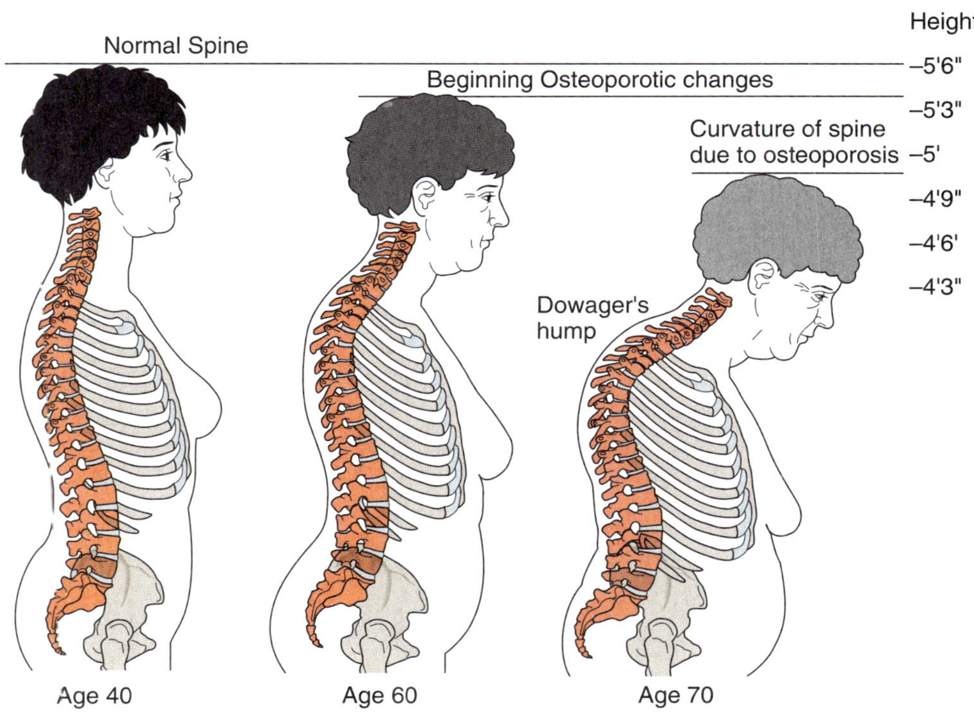

Figure 24-6 Structural changes due to osteoporosis

Treatment includes, but is not limited to, prescribing drug therapy such as estrogen replacement and calcium supplements, promoting calcium intake, and promoting active weight-bearing exercises. Studies indicate that women age 65 years and older should consume dairy products to provide 1500 mg calcium daily or take calcium fortified with vitamin D.

Paget's disease
(Osteitis deformans)

A chronic disease of bone, affecting middle-age and elderly people, characterized by thickening and hypertrophy of the long bones and deformity of the flat bones, due to excessive bone destruction (by the osteoclasts) and unorganized, abnormal bone formation (by the osteoblasts). The new bone is not replaced at the lines of stress, resulting in large malformed bones with poor mineralization.

Most individuals with Paget's disease are asymptomatic. Those with symptoms usually experience bone pain at first. The pain may be described as aching, deep, and worsened by pressure and weight bearing. The mild to moderate pain is most noticeable at night or when resting. Additional manifestations of Paget's disease are bowing of the tibias, kyphosis, frequent fractures (due to the weakened bones), and enlargement of the cranium. The patient may also experience low back and sciatic nerve pain due to loss of normal spinal curvature.

The exact cause of Paget's disease is unknown. One theory is that it may be the result of a virus that remains dormant in the body for many years and activates itself later in life. Paget's disease is more common in males than females.

Treatment is directed at relieving the pain and decreasing bone resorption.

Muscles and Joints

Loss of muscle mass due to a decline in the number of muscle fibers is significant in the aging individual. This process occurs more slowly in men than in women, because men have more muscle mass than women. Many elderly adults also experience a decline in muscle strength, depending on the muscle group. By the time a person is 80 years old, he or she may lose 30% or more skeletal muscle mass.

Cartilage in the joints eventually erodes in the elderly individual, increasing stress on the underlying bone. This leads to changes secondary to inflammation, which decreases flexibility. Joint mobility in the elderly adult is also hampered by the elastic synovial tissue being replaced with collagen fibers and the synovial fluid within the joint increasing in viscosity.

The ability to move around independently is one of the most important issues to elderly individuals. Many of the diseases and disorders of the musculoskeletal system limit mobility. The pathological conditions related to the aging muscles and joints include, but are not limited to, the following:

---

ankylosing spondylitis
ankyl/o = stiff
spondyl/o = spine
-itis = inflammation

Ankylosing spondylitis is a type of arthritis that affects the vertebral column and causes deformities of the spine; also known as Marie-Strümpell disease and as rheumatoid spondylitis.

Patient symptoms include other joint involvement, **arthralgia** (pain in the joints), weight loss, and generalized **malaise** (weakness). As the disease progresses, the spine becomes increasingly stiff, with fusion of the spine into a position of **kyphosis** (humpback).

Treatment includes prescribing medications to reduce inflammation and relieve pain, as well as physical therapy to keep the spine as straight as possible and to promote mobility.

---

bunion
(hallux valgus)

An abnormal enlargement of the joint at the base of the great toe. See Figure 24-7.

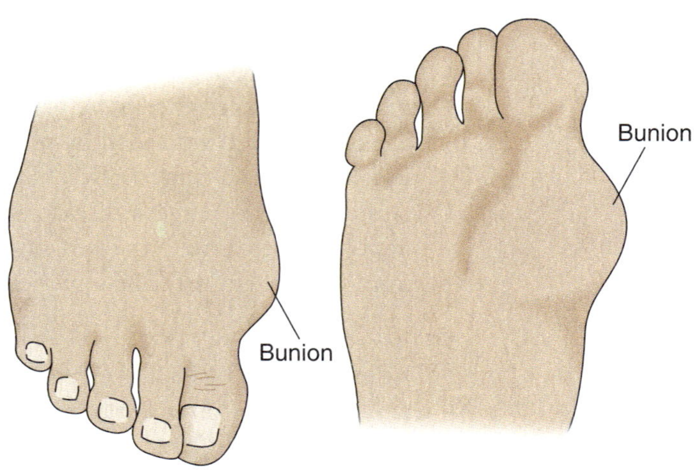

Figure 24-7 Bunion

The great toe deviates laterally, causing it to either override or undercut the second toe. As the condition worsens, the bony prominence enlarges at the base of the great toe, causing pain and swelling of the joint.

A bunion often occurs as a result of arthritis or as a result of chronic irritation and pressure from wearing poorly fitting shoes, although it can be congenital. Treatment for a bunion may include application of padding between the toes or around the bunion to relieve pressure when wearing shoes, medications to relieve the pain and inflammation, or a **bunionectomy**, which involves removal of the bony overgrowth and the bursa.

---

gout
(GOWT)

Gout is a form of acute arthritis that is characterized by inflammation of the first metatarsal joint of the great toe. Although the great toe is the most common site for gout, it can occur in other parts of the foot and body. Men between the ages of 40 and 60 are more commonly affected by gout than women. Gout usually appears in women in the postmenopausal period.

Gout, also known as gouty arthritis, is a hereditary disease in which the individual does not metabolize uric acid properly. Large amounts of uric acid accumulate in the blood and in the synovial fluid of the joints. (The body produces uric acid from metabolism of ingested purines in the diet, especially from eating red meats.) The uric acid crystals are responsible for the inflammatory reaction that develops in the joint, causing intense pain. The pain reaches a peak after several hours and then gradually declines; the attack may be accompanied by a slight fever and chills.

Treatment for gout may include bed rest, immobilizing the affected part, and application of a cold pack (if the area is not too painful to touch). Anti-inflammatory medications may be given to lessen the inflammation of the area; analgesics may be given to relieve the pain; and medications such as allopurinol may be prescribed to lower the uric acid level in the blood. The individual will be instructed to avoid eating foods high in purine (i.e., decrease the red meats) and increase fluid intake.

---

osteoarthritis
(**oss**-tee-oh-ar-**THRY**-tis)
oste/o = bone
arthr/o = joint
-itis = inflammation

Osteoarthritis is also known as degenerative joint disease. It is the most common form of arthritis, having universal prevalence in those age 80 and over. It results from wear and tear on the joints, especially weight-bearing joints such as the hips and knees.

As this chronic disease progresses, the repeated stress to the joints results in degeneration of the joint cartilage. The joint space becomes narrower, taking on a flattened appearance. See **Figure 24-8.**

Symptoms include joint soreness and pain; stiffness, especially in the mornings; and aching, particularly with changes in the weather. Joint movement may elicit clicking or crackling sounds, known as **crepitation**. The individual may also experience a decrease in the range of motion of a joint and increased pain with use of the joint.

The objectives of treatment for osteoarthritis are to reduce inflammation, lessen the pain, and maintain the function of the affected joints. Osteoarthritis cannot be cured. Medications may be prescribed to reduce

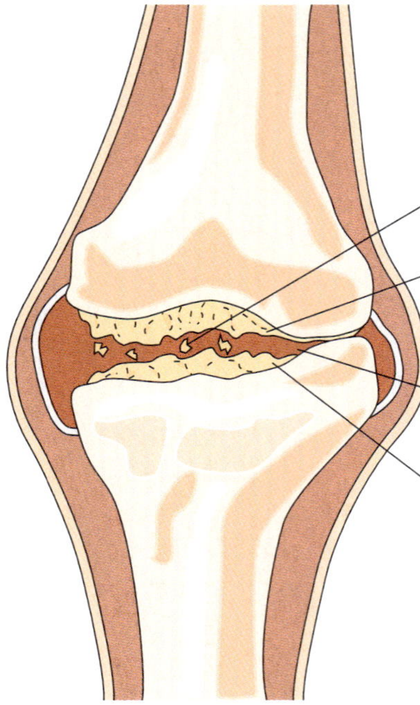

Figure 24-8 Osteoarthritis (knee joint)

the inflammation and to relieve the pain. Physical therapy may be prescribed to promote the function of the joint. If the condition becomes severe, joint replacement surgery may become necessary.

restless legs syndrome (RLS)

A condition of the legs involving annoying sensations of uneasiness, tiredness, itching, or tingling of the leg muscles while resting. The individual feels an overwhelming desire to get up and move around, due to the jerking sensation and painful twitching of the muscles. It is sometimes referred to as Ekbom's syndrome, after the doctor who first recognized it.

Elderly persons often experience restless legs syndrome, although it is not limited to this age group. RLS tends to run in families and is most common in middle-age women, the elderly, pregnancy, people who drink large quantities of caffeine-containing drinks, and people who smoke heavily. Individuals who have RLS experience repeated awakenings during the night and experience daytime sleepiness.

Treatment involves the use of skeletal muscle relaxants to decrease the movements and awakenings.

Nervous System

The rate at which neurological changes occur in the elderly adult vary among individuals. In very old people there is a decrease in the size and weight of the brain, with some decrease in the number of functioning neurons, although there is no real correlation between the size of the brain and functioning. Changes in the brain can include decreased cerebral blood flow, cerebral atrophy, and ventricular dilation, and alterations in the production and metabolism of various neurotransmitters. Generally, nerve transmission is slower in the elderly; and around age 70, the individual may be noted to have somewhat slower voluntary movement, may be slower in decision-making processes, and have a slowed startle response.

Noticeable nervous system changes that are common in the elderly adult may include, but are not limited to, slower voluntary movement, stooped forward-flexed posture, slowed gait (way of walking), dry eyes, impaired ability to hear high-pitched sounds, and decreased ability to maintain balance and correct imbalance.

The pathological conditions related to the aging nervous system include, but are not limited to, the following:

Alzheimer's disease
(**ALTS**-high-merz dih-**ZEEZ**)

A progressive, degenerative disease that affects the cortex of the brain and results in deterioration of a person's intellectual functioning. Alzheimer's disease (AD) is progressive and extremely debilitating. It begins with minor memory loss and progresses to complete loss of mental, emotional, and physical functioning frequently occurring in persons over 65 years of age.

Approximately 10% of individuals over the age of 65, and almost 50% of those over the age of 85, will develop Alzheimer's disease, although it can strike in those aged 40 to 50.This process occurs through three identified stages over a number of years.

Stage 1 lasts for approximately 1 to 3 years and includes loss of short-term memory; decreased ability to pay attention or learn new information; gradual personality changes such as increased irritability, denial, and depression; and difficulties in depth perception. The person with AD in stage 1 will often recognize and attempt to adjust or cover up mental errors.

Stage 2 lasts approximately 2 to 10 years during which time the person loses the ability to write, to identify objects by touch, to accomplish purposeful movements, and to perform simple tasks such as getting dressed. During this progressive deterioration, safety is a major concern. Also during the second stage, the person with AD loses the ability to socially communicate with others; he or she uses the wrong words in conversation, tends to repeat phrases, and may eventually develop total loss of language function, called aphasia.

Stage 3 lasts for 8 to 10 years during which time the person with AD has very little, if any, communication skills due to disorientation to time, place, and person. There is bowel and bladder incontinence, posture flexion, and limb rigidity noted during this stage as well. This increasing deterioration tends to render the person with AD dependent on others to provide for basic needs. This individual may be cared for by family members or need placement in a long-term care facility. The person with AD is prone to additional complications such as malnutrition, dehydration, and pneumonia.

There is no single clinical test to identify Alzheimer's disease. Before a diagnosis is made, other conditions that mimic the symptoms must be excluded. A clinical diagnosis of Alzheimer's is then based upon tests such as physical, psychological, neurological, and psychiatric examinations plus various laboratory tests. With today's new diagnostic tools and criteria, it is possible for physicians to make a positive clinical diagnosis of Alzheimer's with approximately 90% accuracy. A confirmation of the diagnosis of Alzheimer's disease is not possible until death, because biopsy or autopsy examination of the brain tissue is required for diagnosis.

Treatment for Alzheimer's disease includes the use of tacrine hydrochloride (Cognex), which is approved for use in mild to moderate cases due to its ability to improve memory in approximately 40% of persons with AD. Antidepressants and tranquilizers are also frequently used to treat the symptoms of AD.

The persons and families experiencing AD need a great deal of education and support to endure this difficult disease.

---

cerebrovascular accident (CVA)

Neurological deficit(s) resulting from a decrease in blood (ischemia) to a specific localized area in the brain; also called "stroke."

The deficits will differ widely according to the degree of involvement, the amount of time the blood flow is decreased or stopped, and the region of the brain involved. If only a small area of the brain is involved for a short period of time, the deficit may be small or even go unnoticed; however, if there is significant loss of blood supply to a large area, the deficit may be a severe disability or death. Due to the crossing of the sensory-motor pathways at the junction of the medulla and spinal cord, neurological deficits from the **cerebrovascular accident** (CVA) on one side of the brain will show manifestations on the opposite side of the body.

Cellular death and altered level of consciousness occurs if the ischemia is severe and prolonged. Vasospasm and increased blood viscosity may also occur with a CVA and cause decreased circulation to the specific area(s) of the brain causing even more complex deficits. Other typical clinical manifestations of the person experiencing a CVA are motor deficits (frequently hemiplegia), language disorders, visual alterations, headache, dizziness, and various sensory deficits. The elderly have a higher mortality rate than younger individuals; however, those who do survive a stroke have an excellent chance of recovery with proper care.

The onset of a CVA may be gradual or rapid. A number of factors that cause the alteration in cerebral blood flow leading to neurological deficits include transient ischemic attacks, cerebral thrombosis, cerebral embolism, and cerebral hemorrhage. These will be described below.

Transient ischemic attacks (TIAs) are very brief periods of ischemia in the brain lasting from minutes to hours, which can cause a variety of symptoms. TIAs or "mini strokes" often precede a full-blown thrombolytic CVA. The neurological symptoms range according to the amount of ischemia and the location of the vessels involved. The person experiencing a TIA may complain of numbness or weakness in the extremities or corner of the mouth, difficulty communicating, or maybe a visual disturbance. Sometimes the symptoms are vague and difficult to describe. The person may simply complain of a "funny feeling."

Cerebral thrombosis (clot), also called thrombolytic CVA, makes up 50% of all CVAs and occurs largely in individuals older than 50, and often during rest or sleep. The cerebral clot is typically caused by atherosclerosis, which is a thickened, fibrotic vessel wall, causing the diameter of the vessel to be decreased or completely closed off from the buildup of plaque. The thrombolytic CVA is often preceded by one or many TIAs. The occurrence of the CVA caused by a cerebral thrombosis is rapid but the progression is slow. It is often called a "stroke-in-evolution," sometimes taking 3 days to become a "completed stroke" when the maximum neurological deficit has been accomplished and the affected area of the brain is swollen and necrotic.

Cerebral embolism occurs when an embolus or fragments of a blood clot, fat, bacteria, or tumor lodge in a cerebral vessel and cause an occlusion. This occlusion renders the area supplied by this vessel ischemic. A heart problem may lead to the occurrence of a cerebral embolus such as endocarditis, atrial fibrillation, and valvular conditions. A piece of a thrombosis may break off in the carotid artery and move into the circulation causing a cerebral embolism. A fat emboli can occur from the fracture of a long bone. The cerebral emboli will cause immediate neurological deficits. If the emboli breaks up and is consumed by the body, the deficits will disappear; if not, the deficits will remain. Even when the emboli breaks up, the vessel wall is often left weakened, thus increasing the possibility of a cerebral hemorrhage at this site.

Cerebral hemorrhage occurs when a cerebral vessel ruptures allowing bleeding into the CSF, brain tissue, or the subarachnoid space. High blood pressure is the most common cause of a cerebral hemorrhage. The symptoms occur rapidly and generally include a severe headache along with other neurological deficits (related to the area involved).

Parkinson's disease

A degenerative, slowly progressive deterioration of nerves in the brain stem's motor system, characterized by a gradual onset of symptoms, such as a stooped posture with the body flexed forward, a bowed head, a shuffling gait, pill-rolling gestures, an expressionless masklike facial appearance, muffled speech, and swallowing difficulty.

The cause of **Parkinson's disease** is not known, although a neurotransmitter deficiency (dopamine) has been clinically noted in persons with Parkinson's disease. Parkinson's disease is seen more often in males with the onset of symptoms beginning during the ages of 50 to 60 years.

The clinical symptoms can be divided into three groups.

1. **Motor dysfunction** demonstrated by the nonintentional tremors (pill-rolling), slowed movements, inability to start voluntary movements, speech problems, muscle rigidity, gait and posture disturbances.
2. **Autonomic system dysfunction** demonstrated by mottled skin, problems from seborrhea and excess sweating on the upper neck and face, absence of sweating on the lower body, abnormally low blood pressure when standing, heat intolerance, and constipation.
3. **Mental and emotional dysfunction** demonstrated by loss of memory, declining mental processes, lack of problem-solving skill, uneasiness, and depression.

Treatment for Parkinson's disease, in addition to drug therapy, consists of control of symptoms and supportive measures with physical therapy playing a very important role in keeping the person's mobility maximized.

A recent surgical technique utilized for the person with Parkinson's disease is a **pallidotomy.** This procedure involves the destruction of the involved tissue in the brain to reduce tremors and severe dyskinesia. The goal of this procedure, to restore a more normal ambulatory function to the individual, is not always successful.

shingles (herpes zoster)

An acute viral infection seen mainly in adults, characterized by inflammation of the underlying spinal or cranial nerve pathway producing painful, vesicular eruptions on the skin following along these nerve pathways.

This acute eruption is caused by reactivation of latent varicella virus (the same virus that causes chickenpox).

Ten to 20% of the population is affected by **herpes zoster**, with the highest incidence in adults over 50.

Symptoms include severe pain before and during eruption, fever, itching, GI disturbances, headache, general tiredness, and increased sensitivity of the skin around the area. The lesions usually take 3 to 5 days to erupt, then progress to crusting and drying with recovery in approximately 3 weeks. Treatment with antiviral medications, analgesics, and sometimes corticosteroids aids in decreasing the severity of symptoms.

Blood and Lymphatic Systems

The effect of the aging process on the blood results mainly from the reduced capacity to make new blood cells quickly when disease has occurred. After about the age of 70, the percentage of bone marrow space occupied by tissue that produces blood cells declines progressively. This decreased ability to produce new blood cells when disease has occurred can be a problem for the elderly.

Age-related changes in the lymphatic system affect the immune responses. The aging process impairs specific antibody responses to foreign antigens. Due to the decreased immunity, the elderly individual may be more susceptible to infections and malignancy. Infections are a leading cause of morbidity and mortality in the elderly.

The pathological conditions related to the aging blood and lymphatic systems include, but are not limited to, the following:

influenza

A highly contagious viral infection of the respiratory tract, transmitted by airborne droplet infection; also known as the flu. Influenza can occur in isolated cases or can be epidemic. The incubation period is usually 1 to 3 days after exposure. The elderly may be more prone to developing bacterial influenza, as are those individuals who have chronic pulmonary disease.

Symptoms of the flu include sore throat, cough, fever, muscular pains, and generalized weakness. The onset is usually sudden, with the individual experiencing fever, chills, respiratory symptoms, headache, muscle pain, and extreme tiredness.

Treatment for influenza is symptomatic and involves bed rest, plenty of fluids, and medications for pain. Recovery usually occurs within 3 to 10 days.

Yearly vaccination with current prevailing strain of influenza virus is recommended for elderly or debilitated individuals.

---

pneumonia

An acute inflammation of the lungs caused mainly by inhaled pneumococci of the species *Streptococcus pneumoniae.* It may also be caused by other bacteria, as well as viruses.

Pneumonia is a common infection in the elderly and one of the leading causes of death. Aging tends to predispose the elderly adult to pneumonia as a result of the lowered immune status and less efficient ventilation. Some of the predisposing factors to the elderly developing pneumonia are chronic obstructive pulmonary disease (COPD), nutritional deficiencies, or changes in mental status.

Treatment for pneumonia includes medication for the causative organism or virus, proper diet, increased fluid intake, analgesics for pain and or nonsteroidal anti-inflammatory drugs (NSAIDS) for inflammation, plenty of rest, and proper clearing of mucus from the respiratory passages. Depending on the age of the individual and the general health status, the individual may be treated at home. The recovery period for the elderly person varies. It may take weeks to feel normal again.

Prevention is important in the elderly patient. This can be achieved through administration of the pneumonia vaccine. The general rule of thumb is to administer the pneumonia vaccine once before the age of 80 and to repeat it every 5 to 7 years thereafter.

---

purpura
(**PER**-pew-rah)

Collection of blood beneath the skin in the form of pinpoint hemorrhages appearing as red-purple skin discolorations.

Purpura are small hemorrhages caused from a decreased number of circulating platelets (thrombocytopenia). The body may produce an antiplatelet factor that will damage its own platelets.

Idiopathic thrombocytopenic purpura is a disorder in which the individual produces antibodies that destroy his or her own platelets. The cause of the prolonged bleeding time is unknown. Corticosteroids are administered and many times the individuals require the removal of the spleen to stop platelet destruction.

Purpura is also seen in persons with low platelet counts for other associated reasons such as drug reactions and leukemia.

Cardiovascular System

As one ages, the workload and efficiency of the heart may be compromised due to accumulation of excess fat surrounding the heart. This may be brought about by poor dietary and exercise habits. Studies have shown that cardiovascular disease is nearly twice as likely to develop in sedentary people than in those who continue to be active. Cardiovascular disease can be quite severe in the elderly, with approximately 85% of all cardiovascular deaths occurring in those over the age of 65. The risk for cardiovascular disease increases significantly in women after menopause. After the age of 65, the incidence of coronary heart disease in women is about one in three.

The pathological conditions related to the aging cardiovascular system include, but are not limited to, the following:

arteriosclerosis
(ar-tee-ree-oh-skleh-**ROH**-sis)
arteri/o = artery
scler/o = hard
-osis = condition

An arterial condition in which there is thickening, hardening, and loss of elasticity of the walls of the arteries, resulting in decreased blood supply, especially to the lower extremities and cerebrum; also called hardening of the arteries.

Symptoms include intermittent **claudication,** changes in skin temperature and color, altered peripheral pulses, **bruits** over the involved artery, headache, dizziness, and memory defects (depending on the organ system involved).

Risk factors for arteriosclerosis include hypertension, increased blood **lipids** (particularly cholesterol and triglycerides), obesity, diabetes, cigarette smoking, inability to cope with stress, and family history of early-onset atherosclerosis.

Treatment options may include a diet low in saturated fatty acids, medications to lower the blood lipid levels (in conjunction with the low-fat diet), proper rest and regular exercise, avoidance of stress, discontinuing cigarette smoking, and additional treatment specific to the condition for factors such as hypertension, diabetes, and obesity.

congestive heart failure (CHF)

Condition characterized by weakness, breathlessness, abdominal discomfort; edema in the lower portions of the body results from the flow of the blood through the vessels being slowed (venous stasis) and the outflow of blood from the left side of the heart is reduced; the pumping ability of the heart is progressively impaired to the point that it no longer meets bodily needs; also known as cardiac failure. Congestive heart failure is the single most frequent cause of hospitalization for those individuals 65 years of age and older.

The principal feature in congestive heart failure is increased intravascular volume. Congestion of the tissues results from increased arterial and venous pressure due to decreased cardiac output in the failing heart.

Left-sided cardiac failure is more common in the elderly. It occurs when the left ventricle is unable to sufficiently pump the blood that enters it from the lungs. This causes increased pressure in the pulmonary circulation, which results in the forcing of fluid into the pulmonary tissues, creating pulmonary edema ("congestion"). The patient experiences dyspnea, cough (mostly moist sounding), fatigue, tachycardia, restlessness, and anxiety.

Right-sided cardiac failure occurs when the right side of the heart is unable to sufficiently empty its blood volume and cannot accommodate all of the blood that it receives from the venous circulation. This results in congestion of the viscera and the peripheral tissues. The patient experiences edema of the lower extremities (**pitting edema**), weight gain, enlargement of the liver (hepatomegaly), distended neck veins, **ascites,** anorexia, nocturia, and weakness.

Treatment involves promoting rest to reduce the workload on the heart, medications to increase the strength and efficiency of the heartbeat, and medications to eliminate the accumulation of fluids within the body. Dietary sodium may also be restricted. The elderly adult with moderate to severe symptoms may require hospital admission for proper treatment.

coronary artery disease (CAD)

coron/o = heart
-ary = pertaining to
arter/o = artery
-y = noun ending

Narrowing of the coronary arteries to the extent that adequate blood supply to the myocardium is prevented.

Coronary artery disease is usually caused by atherosclerosis; it may progress to the point where the heart muscle is damaged due to lack of blood supply (ischemia), as the lumen of the coronary artery narrows. When the lumen of the artery is narrowed and the wall is rough, there is a great tendency for clots to form, creating the possibility for **thrombotic occlusion** of the vessel.

As a result of the ischemia of the myocardial muscle, the individual experiences a burning, squeezing, or tightness in the chest that may radiate to the neck, shoulder blade, and left arm; nausea, vomiting, sweating, and anxiety may also accompany the pain.

Accepted treatments for occluded coronary arteries (that reduce or prevent sufficient flow of blood to the myocardium) include medications that may be used alone or in conjunction with other types of therapy, and diagnostic and treatment procedures such as percutaneous transluminal coronary angioplasty (PTCA), directional coronary atherectomy (DCA), and coronary bypass graft (CABG). The PTCA, DCA, and CABG procedures will be discussed later in the chapter.

Respiratory System

When considering the respiratory system of the elderly adult, it is important to remember some of the changes that occur in the aging lungs; most notably, the elderly adult experiences decreased volume during inspiration and expiration. Aging also affects the mechanical aspects of ventilation. Pulmonary tissue in the elderly adult has an altered level of function because of loss of elasticity, which leads to some degree of hyperinflation of the lung. The cilia within the respiratory tract show decreased action as the lung ages and the respiratory muscle strength and endurance also decreases. With these changes there is a corresponding decrease in strength for breathing and/or coughing. The respiratory system generally is able to meet the needs of a normal elderly adult; however, when illness or stress triggers a need for increased respiratory function, the reserve capacity may be inadequate to meet the need.

The pathological conditions related to the aging respiratory system include, but are not limited to, the following:

emphysema

A chronic pulmonary disease characterized by increase beyond the normal in the size of air spaces distal to the terminal bronchiole, either from dilatation of the alveoli or from destruction of their walls. See Figure 24-9.

This nonuniform pattern of abnormal permanent distention of the air spaces appears to be the end stage of a process that has progressed slowly for many years. By the time the patient develops the symptoms of **emphysema,** pulmonary function is often so impaired that it is irreversible.

The major cause of emphysema is cigarette smoking. The person with emphysema has a chronic obstruction (increase in airway resistance) to the inflow and outflow of air from the lungs. The lungs lose their elasticity and are in a chronic state of hyperexpansion, making expiration of air more difficult. The act of expiration then becomes one of active muscular movement in order to force the air out. The patient takes on a "barrel chest" appearance due to the loss of elasticity of lung tissue, becoming increasingly short of breath.

Treatment for emphysema is directed at improving the quality of life for the patient and to slow the progression of the disease. This may involve measures to improve the patient's ventilation (with the use of bronchodilators and medicine to thin the mucous secretions), as well as administration of medications to treat any infection present, and the administration of oxygen to treat the hypoxia that may be present.

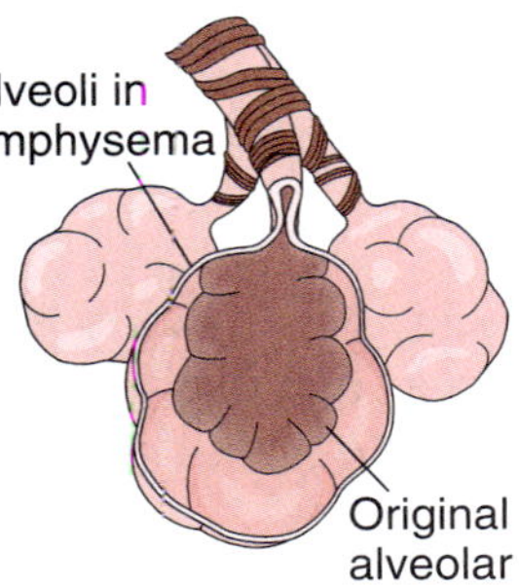

Figure 24-9 Emphysema

pulmonary edema
(**PULL**-mon-air-ree eh-**DEE**-mah)
pulmon/o = lung
-ary = pertaining to

Swelling of the lungs caused by an abnormal accumulation of fluid in the lungs, either in the alveoli or the interstitial spaces.

The most common cause of pulmonary edema is cardiac disease. The pulmonary congestion occurs when the pulmonary vessels receive more blood from the right ventricle of the heart than the left ventricle can accommodate and remove. This congestion (or backup of fluid) causes the fluid to leak through the capillary walls and permeate into the airways, creating a sudden onset of breathlessness and a sense of suffocation. The patient's nailbeds become cyanotic and the skin becomes gray. As the condition progresses, breathing is noisy and moist. The patient needs immediate medical attention.

pulmonary heart disease (cor pulmonale)
(**PULL**-mon-air-ree heart dih-**ZEEZ**)
(**COR**-pull-mon-**ALL**-ee)
pulmon/o = lung
-ary = pertaining to

Hypertrophy of the right ventricle of the heart (with or without failure) resulting from disorders of the lungs, pulmonary vessels, or chest wall; heart failure resulting from disorders of the lungs; pulmonary disease.

Pulmonary heart disease reduces proper ventilation to the lungs resulting in increased resistance in the pulmonary circulation. This, in turn, raises the pulmonary blood pressure. **Cor pulmonale** develops because of the pulmonary hypertension, which causes the right side of the heart to work harder to pump the blood against the resistance of the pulmonary vascular circulation, thus creating hypertrophy of the right ventricle of the heart.

Chronic obstructive pulmonary disease (COPD), the most frequent cause of cor pulmonale, produces shortness of breath and cough. The patient develops edema of the feet and legs, distended neck veins, an enlarged liver, pleural effusion, ascites, and a heart murmur.

Treatment is related to treating the underlying cause of cor pulmonale and is often a long-term process. In the case of COPD, treatment involves improving the patient's ventilation (airways must be dilated to improve gas exchange within the lungs). The improved transport of oxygen to the blood and body tissues will reduce the strain on the pulmonary circulation, thus relieving the pulmonary hypertension that leads to cor pulmonale.

Digestive System

As the digestive system ages, many elderly adults experience significant changes in the gastrointestinal system that not only affect the nutritional status but also cause pain and discomfort. For the most part, however, gastrointestinal function remains intact even when some changes are present. Some of the notable changes include loss of teeth related to dental or periodontal problems, decrease in the quality and quantity of saliva, some decrease in normal peristalsis in the esophagus, a weakness in the musculature of the large intestine that results in decreased forcefulness of contractions and a slowing of peristaltic activity, and a tendency toward formation of diverticula or herniations of the mucosa into the weakened intestinal musculature. The elderly adult may also experience some difficulty metabolizing some medications, making it necessary to adjust medication dosages to prevent cumulative effects and to ensure proper excretion of drugs.

The pathological conditions related to the aging digestive system include, but are not limited to, the following:

achalasia
(**ack**-al-**LAY**-zee-ah)

Decreased mobility of the lower two thirds of the esophagus along with constriction of the lower esophageal sphincter (LES); making it difficult for food and liquids to move down the esophagus.

Due to the lack of nerve impulses and the absence of sympathetic receptors, the relaxation of the lower LES fails to happen with swallowing.

Food and fluid accumulate in the lower esophagus due to the decreased mobility there and the constriction of the LES. **Achalasia** is a progressive disease, and generally gets worse not better.

The individual may complain of difficulty in swallowing fluids and food, retrosternal chest pain or discomfort (a sensation of great fullness in the lower chest), and regurgitation of undigested food.

Among the diagnostic tests used to diagnose achalasia are barium swallow and endoscopy studies. Medical intervention may be more suitable for the elderly adult, although achalasia can also be treated surgically.

colorectal cancer
(**koh**-lo-**REK**-tal **CAN**-sir)

The presence of a malignant neoplasm in the large intestine.

Most neoplasms in the large intestine are adenocarcinomas and at least 50% originate in the rectum causing bleeding and pain. Next to cancer of the lung, colon cancer is the most commonly occurring cause of death. The incidence of **colorectal cancer** increases in individuals over 70 years of age with a death rate of almost 50% of those affected.

Symptoms of colorectal cancer vary according to tumor location. Two-thirds of all colorectal cancers occur in the lower sigmoid colon and the rectum. The most common symptoms include rectal bleeding, followed by bowel changes, abdominal pain or cramping, unexplained weight loss, and anemia.

Although the cause of colorectal cancer is unknown, it has been suggested that a diet high in beef and refined carbohydrates and low in roughage leads to the formation of bacteria boosting the amount of fatty acids and bile which behave as carcinogens. Other factors which predispose one to colorectal cancer are history of Crohn's disease, ulcerative colitis, irritable bowel syndrome, or familial polyposis.

Along with the rectal exam, a barium enema, sigmoidoscopy and/or colonoscopy, and stool exam for occult blood will be used for diagnosis. Prognosis is dependent on the extent of the disease and surgery is usually the treatment of choice.

constipation

A state in which the individual's pattern of bowel elimination is characterized by a decrease in the frequency of bowel movements and the passage of hard, dry stools. The individual experiences difficult defecation.

Constipation is a common complaint among older patients. Contributing factors include decreased peristalsis in the intestinal tract, decreased appetite, inadequate fluid intake, and lack of exercise. Repeated overuse or abuse of laxatives over the years worsens the problem.

Dietary concerns are important in preventing constipation in the elderly adult. The individual should be encouraged to eat small frequent meals, increase dietary fiber, and drink plenty of fluids daily.

diverticular disease

An expression used to characterize both diverticulosis and diverticulitis. Diverticulosis describes the noninflamed outpouchings or herniations through the muscular layer of the intestine, typically the sigmoid colon. Inflammation of the outpouchings called diverticulum is referred to as diverticulitis.

Diverticular disease is an increasingly common occurrence in persons over 45 years of age. Persons eating diets low in fiber predispose themselves to the formation of diverticulum.

Symptoms of diverticulosis may include mild cramps, bloating, and constipation. The most common symptom of diverticulitis is abdominal pain; more severe symptoms include cramping, fever, increased flatus, and elevated WBC count (leukocytosis). The severity of symptoms depend on the extent of the infection and/or complications.

Proctoscopy and barium enemas are used in the diagnostic process.

Endocrine System

When considering the aging endocrine system, there is a noted overall decline in hormone secretion and diminished tissue sensitivity to secreted hormones. The most notable decrease in hormones is that of estrogen and testosterone. The elderly adult also experiences a change in glucose tolerance, which results in a prolonged elevated blood sugar level in response to a meal. As a result of the physiological changes that occur in the endocrine system, endocrine diseases are most common in later years.

The pathological conditions related to the aging endocrine system include, but are not limited to, the following:

diabetes mellitus
(dye-ah-**BEE**-teez **MELL**-ih-tus)

A disorder of the pancreas in which the beta cells of the islets of Langerhans of the pancreas fail to produce an adequate amount of insulin, resulting in the body's inability to appropriately metabolize carbohydrates, fats, and proteins.

Diabetes mellitus affects approximately 10% of individuals over 65 years of age and approximately 20% of individuals over 80 years of age.

Two classic characteristics of the disease are **hyperglycemia** and ketosis. First, the individual will experience abnormally elevated blood glucose levels, known as hyperglycemia, due to the body's inability to utilize glucose for energy. Insulin is necessary for the body cells to utilize glucose for energy. Second, when the body cannot utilize glucose for energy, the cells begin to break down fats and proteins for energy. This breakdown of fats and proteins releases waste products known as ketones into the bloodstream, which spill over into the urine due to abnormal accumulations. These two conditions, hyperglycemia and ketosis (the presence of ketone bodies in the bloodstream) are at the root of the major symptoms of diabetes mellitus.

The classic symptoms of diabetes mellitus are **glycosuria, polydipsia,** and **polyuria.** Other symptoms include increased eating (**polyphagia**) and weight loss, presence of ketones in the urine, itching (pruritus), muscle weakness, and fatigue.

Diabetes mellitus is classified as either insulin-dependent diabetes (Type I) or non-insulin-dependent diabetes (Type II). All diabetics are encouraged to wear emergency alert bracelets. This discussion will be limited to Type II, or non-insulin-dependent diabetes, which usually occurs later in life.

Non-insulin-dependent diabetes mellitus (NIDDM), also known as Type II diabetes, usually appears in adults after the age of 40 having a gradual onset; the majority of these individuals are obese. Individuals with NIDDM usually have some pancreatic activity making it possible to control the disease with diet and exercise. These individuals usually do not rely on insulin to control the disease and they are not prone to developing ketosis. Approximately 80% of all diabetics have NIDDM, which is also known as adult-onset diabetes.

Despite the name, non-insulin-dependent diabetes, a few Type II diabetics *are* insulin dependent. This often makes it difficult for the individual to understand how he or she can be a Type II diabetic (non insulin dependent) and still require insulin injections. These individuals are usually able to control their diabetes with diet and exercise in the beginning, but eventually have to convert to the administration of insulin injections for proper control, when the pancreatic activity becomes insignificant or it ceases completely. The individual with adult-onset diabetes (Type II) who requires insulin injections to control the disease, experiences all of the symptoms and problems that accompany Type I diabetes or IDDM.

Diagnosis of diabetes mellitus is confirmed with a glucose tolerance test, which is described later in the chapter.

Individuals with NIDDM usually control their diabetes with diet and exercise, occasionally requiring the use of oral **hypoglycemia** agents to stimulate the production of insulin by the pancreas.

Complications of long-term diabetes vary according to the individual and the type of diabetes. These complications include poor circulation in the extremities, especially the lower legs and feet; infections that heal poorly, due to the decreased circulation; kidney disease and renal failure; diabetic retinopathy, which is a leading cause of blindness; and involvement of the nervous system (diabetic neuropathy), characterized by numbness (decreased sensitivity of the fingers to touch and grasp), and intermittent but severe episodes of pain in the extremities.

Diabetics who maintain near normal blood glucose levels can reasonably expect to live for many years without major complications.

Special Senses (Eye and Ear)

Impairment of vision is one of the three most common medical problems among the elderly. Of elderly individuals over the age of 85, at least 25% have significant visual difficulties to cause trouble reading or difficulty conducting daily activities independently. The size of the pupil decreases with aging, which necessitates a brighter light for vision. Sensitivity to glare also increases with age because of changes in the opacity of the lens. Color discrimination decreases with aging and depth perception is altered.

Hearing impairment is the second most common health problem affecting the elderly population. The ability to discriminate among high frequencies is often impaired by the age of 50 and shows a marked decline after the age of 65. The elderly adult who is described as "hard of hearing" may actually have more of a high-frequency loss than a generalized decline in hearing perception. It is, therefore, easier for an elderly adult to hear voices, telephones, doorbells, and horns that have lower tones and high intensity.

The pathological conditions related to the aging eye and ear include, but are not limited to, the following:

cataract
(**KAT**-ah-rakt)

The lens in the eye becomes progressively cloudy losing its normal transparency and thus altering the perception of images due to the interference of light transmission to the retina.

The occurrence of cataracts can be classified as senile or secondary on the basis of etiology. See **Figure 24-10.**

Senile cataracts typically begin after the age of 50 years, at which time degenerative changes occur resulting in the gradual clouding of the crystalline lens due to wear and tear and the change in fibers and protein as it ages. Senile cataracts are common and can be found in an estimated 95% of persons over 65 years.

Secondary cataracts result from trauma, radiation injury, inflammation, taking certain medications such as corticosteroids, or due to metabolic diseases such as diabetes mellitus.

Immature cataracts, those in which only a portion of the lens is affected, are diagnosed through ophthalmoscopy and the person's history. Mature cataracts, those in which the entire lens is clouded, can be visualized with the naked eye and appear as a gray-white area behind the pupil. A loss of the red reflex is noted as the cataract matures.

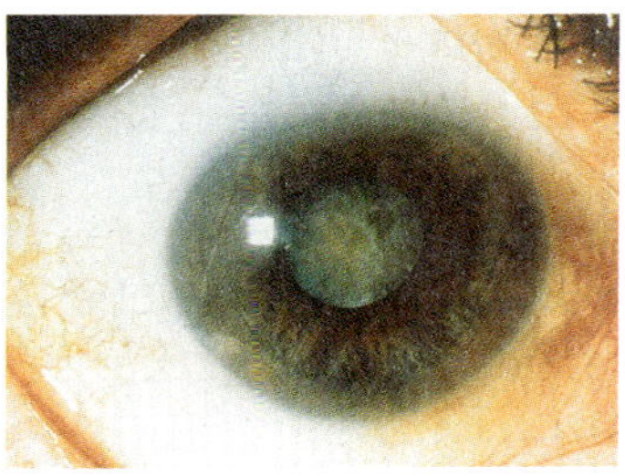

Treatment includes surgical intervention to remove the cataract. Surgery is indicated when the vision loss handicaps the person in the accomplishment of daily activities or when glaucoma or another secondary condition occurs. Surgical intervention for cataract removal is typically completed on an outpatient basis. There is no medical treatment available for cataracts at present.

Figure 24-10 Cataract (Courtesy of the National Eye Institute, NIH)

deafness, sensorineural
(sen-soh-ree-**NOO**-ral)
neur/o = nerve
-al = pertaining to

Hearing loss caused by the inability of nerve stimuli to be delivered to the brain from the inner ear due to damage to the auditory nerve or the cochlea.

The results vary from a mild hearing loss to a profound hearing loss. This sensorineural hearing loss can occur due to the aging process or damaged hair cells of the organ of Corti, which may occur in relation to loud machinery noise, loud music, or medication side effects. Other causes of sensorineural hearing loss include tumors, infections (such as bacterial meningitis), trauma altering the central auditory pathways, vascular disorders, and degenerative or demyelinating diseases. Sensorineural deafness makes speech discrimination difficult, primarily in noisy surroundings.

Diagnosis is based on the person's history and the results of the audiometry test. The best treatment is prevention when possible, accomplished by avoiding exposure to loud noises and being aware of medication with ototoxic effects both of which may cause this damage. If the person cannot totally avoid the loud noises, wearing earplugs will be helpful to prevent or escape further damage. Hearing aids are helpful in some cases; however, the person with sensorineural hearing loss may require a cochlear implant to have sound perception restored.

diabetic retinopathy
(dye-ah-**BET**-ik reh-tin-**OP**-ah-thee)
retin/o = retina
-pathy = disease

Occurs as a consequence of an 8- to 10-year duration of diabetes mellitus in which the capillaries of the retina experience scarring due to the following:

1. Abnormal dilatation and constriction of vessels
2. Hemorrhages
3. Microaneurysm
4. Abnormal formation of new vessels causing leakage of blood into the vitreous humor

The scarring and leakage of blood causes a permanent decline in the sharpness of vision. The inability to get the oxygen and nutrients needed for good vision to the retina eventually will lead to permanent loss of vision. In the United States, **diabetic retinopathy** is the leading cause of blindness.

Diagnosis is made from the person's history and a thorough examination of the internal eye via ophthalmoscopy during which the changes in the retinal vasculature can be seen. The person with diabetes mellitus should be followed regularly with ophthalmoscopic exams to identify the changes taking place due to the available treatment with vitrectomy (removal of vitreous hemorrhages) and laser photocoagulation, which are normally useful in managing diabetic retinopathy.

ectropion
(ek-**TROH**-pee-on)

"Turning out" or eversion of the eyelash margins (especially the lower eyelid) from the eyeball leading to exposure of the eyelid and eyeball surface and lining. See Figure 24-11.

When an individual is affected by **ectropion**, tears are unable to flow into the tear ducts to keep the eyes moist and therefore flow down the face. This exposure and lack of moisture leads to dryness and irritation of the eye.

Ectropion frequently affects the older population as a result of aging. This occurs with the development of a weakened muscle in the lower eyelid resulting in eversion of the eyelid causing the outward turning of the eyelid. Facial nerve paralysis and eyelid tissue atrophy are also causes of ectropion as well as scarring of the cheek or eyelid that pull down on the eyelid.

Ectropion is diagnosed through a visual exam. Treatment with a minor surgical process to correct ectropion is usually required because the condition rarely resolves on its own. The dryness and irritation remain a constant threat to the cornea and the development of permanent damage and/or corneal ulcers.

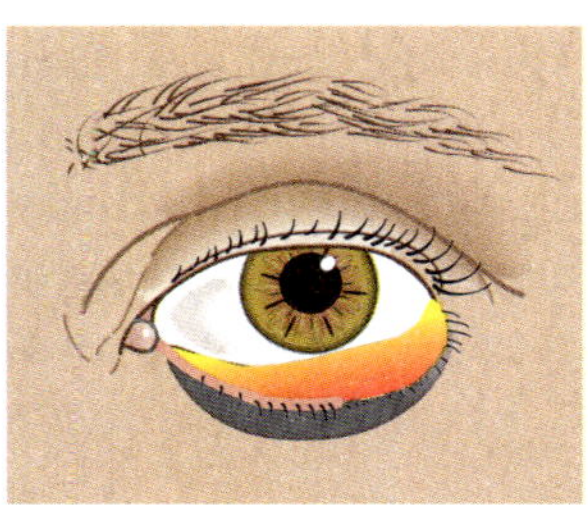

Figure 24-11 Ectropion

entropion
(en-TROH-pee-on)

"Turning in" of the eyelash margins (especially the lower margins) resulting in the sensation similar to that of a foreign body in the eye (redness, tearing, burning, and itching). See Figure 24-12.

Entropion may result in damage to the cornea in the form of corneal ulcers due to the constant irritation of the conjunctiva from the rubbing of the lashes.

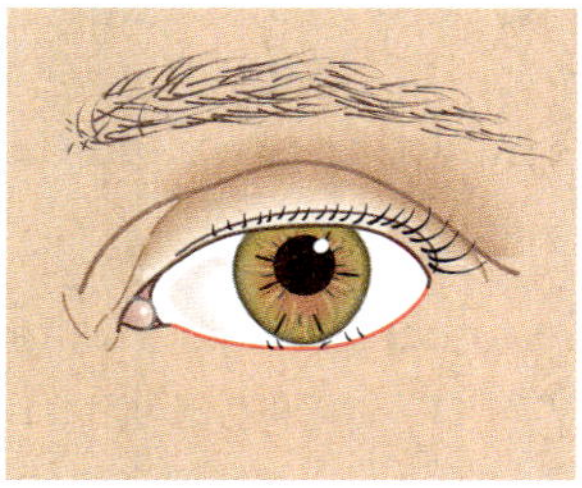

Entropion frequently affects the older population as a result of aging. This occurs with the development of loose fibrous tissue in the lower eyelid resulting in extreme tightening of the eyelid muscle causing the inward turning of the eyelid. This is diagnosed through a visual exam. Treatment with a minor surgical process to correct entropion is required if the condition does not resolve and remains a constant irritant to the conjunctiva and cornea.

Figure 24-12 Entropion

glaucoma
(glau-**KOH**-mah)

Ocular disorders identified as a group due to the increase in intraocular pressure. This increase in intraocular pressure may be primary or secondary, acute or chronic, and described as open or closed angle.

These disorders occur due to a barrier in the normal outflow of aqueous humor or an increased production of aqueous humor. Increased intraocular pressure leads to an inhibited blood supply of the optic neurons, which will lead to degeneration and atrophy of the optic nerve and finally total loss of vision. Glaucoma is the second leading cause of blindness in the United States. The incidence of glaucoma increases rapidly after 40 years of age. Chronic open-angle glaucoma, acute closed-angle glaucoma, and secondary glaucoma will be discussed.

Chronic open-angle glaucoma occurs as a primary disorder with a breakdown in the drainage system of the circulation of aqueous humor. A gradual elevation of internal pressure leads to a decreased blood supply to the optic nerve and the retina. The most common type of glaucoma, chronic open angle, is so gradual that the presence in most individuals is longstanding before any symptoms are recognized.

When chronic open-angle glaucoma is untreated, peripheral vision is gradually lost. The central vision will eventually be lost as well, rendering the individual completely blind. Routine ophthalmic examinations, which include optic nerve evaluation and readings of intraocular pressure, are important to pick up as well as evaluate the development and presence of chronic open-angle glaucoma.

Along with the person's history and the identified symptoms, the diagnosis of open-angle glaucoma can be confirmed through an ophthalmic exam with tonometry (measurement of intraocular pressure). When diagnosis is made and early treatment is started with medication to open the drainage system or reduce the production of aqueous humor, the intraocular pressure is controlled to a certain extent. When medication does not adequately control the intraocular pressure, surgery may be required to bypass the faulty drainage system.

Acute angle-closure glaucoma is a rapid primary occurrence of increased intraocular pressure in a short period of time. It is due to the mouth of the drainage system being narrow and closing completely, allowing no flow of aqueous humor. This rapid occurrence is characterized by severe pain, blurred vision, photophobia, redness, and seeing " halos" around light. Within several days the person with untreated acute angle-closure glaucoma can lose his or her sight.

Treatment is aimed at quickly reducing the pressure inside the eye to avoid vision loss. The creation of a small hole between the posterior and anterior chambers through a procedure called laser iridotomy has been effective in opening the filtering angle, allowing the aqueous humor to flow, and thus decreasing the intraocular pressure.

Secondary glaucoma occurs as a complication of another disorder, trauma, or surgery. Swelling of eye tissue from the trauma of surgery, injury, or inflammation causes the flow pattern or system to be affected. This leads to impeded drainage of aqueous humor and increased intraocular pressure.

---

macular degeneration

Progressive deterioration of the retinal cells in the macula due to aging. Known as senile or age-related macular degeneration (ARMD), this condition is a common and progressive cause of visual deficiency and permanent reading impairment in the adult over 65 years of age.

The macular area is the area of central vision. During the aging process, the macula may undergo a degenerative process that results in the loss of central vision. The peripheral or side vision remains in tact. The elderly individual with age-related macular degeneration rarely experiences complete blindness. Because only the macula is affected, these individuals maintain their peripheral vision and can walk without assistance and carry out many activities by using side vision.

There are two types of macular degeneration. The dry form causes a slow, gradual deterioration of the function of the macula. Individuals affected by this form of macular degeneration may note distortion or blind spots in their vision. They experience slow, progressive, and painless decrease in vision. The second type is the wet form, which is more serious and is responsible for the majority of the cases of severe visual loss due to macular degeneration. Individuals affected by the wet form of macular degeneration experience a leakage of fluid from abnormal vessels under the retina.

There is no known treatment for the dry type of ARMD. The wet type of macular degeneration is often treatable with laser therapy in the early stages; however, the laser is not used in the center of the macula if abnormal vessels already occupy it because the laser destroys the area treated.

---

presbyopia
(prez-bee-**OH**-pee-ah)
presby/o = old, elderly
-opia = visual condition

A refractive error occurring after the age of 40, when the lens of the eye(s) cannot focus on an image accurately due to its decreasing loss of elasticity resulting in a firmer and more opaque lens; poor vision due to the natural aging process.

This results in decreased color vision and a decline in refraction and accommodation for close vision. There is diminished ability to focus clearly on close objects and fine print. Presbyopia is also called farsightedness due to better clarity of distant objects.

In addition to blurred vision of close objects, the individual may also complain of headaches and frequent squinting. The diagnosis presbyopia is verified through an ophthalmoscopic exam and is corrected through the use of contact lenses or eyeglasses.

The Urinary System

During the aging process, there are both structural and functional changes in the kidneys. The aging kidney is more susceptible to trauma or disease. The number of nephron units of the kidney decreases during the aging process and there is a gradual degenerative change in the remaining number of nephrons. By the time the elderly adult reaches the age of 70 to 80 years, the glomerular filtration rate is approximately 50% of what it was when the individual was 30 years of age. With this decreased glomerular filtration, drugs may not be excreted as rapidly as possible and they may remain in the bloodstream, producing toxic levels.

The aging kidney is inefficient in its ability to regain normal fluid and electrolyte balance after a rapid loss of fluids, thus requiring a longer time to correct fluid and electrolyte imbalances. The ureters and bladder tend to lose muscle tone and the bladder loses enough tone to result in incomplete emptying that leads to accumulation of residual urine, increasing the risk of retention and cystitis.

The pathological conditions related to the aging urinary system include, but are not limited to, the following:

---

urinary incontinence
urin/o = urine
-ary = pertaining to

The inability to retain urine in the bladder; the loss of urine from the bladder due to loss of sphincter control. This involuntary loss of urine is severe enough to cause social or hygienic problems.

Urinary incontinence affects mostly older adults; however, it is not a normal consequence of aging. Bladder incontinence may be due to abnormalities of bladder contraction, abnormalities of urethral relaxation, or in some of the elderly patients, dementia.

Many older women suffer from **stress incontinence,** which is the inability to hold urine when the bladder is stressed by sneezing, coughing, laughing, or lifting.

A common method of treating stress incontinence is through the use of isometric exercises known as **Kegel exercises.** The woman executes a series of voluntary contractions or squeezing of the muscles required to stop the urinary stream while voiding (a tightening and relaxation of the pelvic muscles). Repetition of this tightening and relaxation exercise, 20 to 40 times, several times a day, has proven successful in controlling some types of stress incontinence.

The older adult may also suffer other types of urinary incontinence, such as the following:

1. *Functional incontinence.* The individual experiences an involuntary, unpredictable passage of urine. This is characterized by the urge to void, or bladder contractions that are strong enough to result in loss of urine before reaching an appropriate receptacle.
2. *Urge incontinence.* The urge to empty the bladder is sudden and uncontrollable, and the individual experiences involuntary passage of urine soon after the strong sense of urgency to void. The individual may not be able to reach a toilet in time when suffering from urge incontinence.

3. *Overflow incontinence.* The involuntary loss of urine is associated with overdistention of the bladder, when the bladder's capacity has reached its maximum. The individual may experience a constant dribbling of urine. This type of incontinence may be the result of complications of long-term diabetes (diabetic neuropathy) or the side effect of medication.

It is estimated that up to 30% of older adults over the age of 60, not living in nursing homes, are affected by urinary incontinence and that over 50% of those residing in nursing homes are affected by urinary incontinence. In many cases, once the underlying cause of the urinary incontinence is determined, it can be treated and often times cured.

The Male Reproductive System

As men age, they experience a decrease in testosterone level, sperm production, muscle tone of the scrotum, and the size and firmness of the testicles. The prostate gland enlarges considerably with age. Sexual activity is normal and possible in the older age group if there are no major health problems.

The pathological conditions related to the aging male reproductive system include, but are not limited to, the following:

benign prostatic hypertrophy
(bee-**NYEN**-pross-**TAT**-ik high-**PER**-troh-fee)
prostat/o = prostate gland
-ic = pertaining to
hyper- = excessive
troph/o = development, growth
-y = noun ending

A benign (noncancerous) enlargement of the prostate gland, creating pressure on the upper part of the urethra or neck of the bladder, causing obstruction of the flow of urine.

This is a common condition occurring in men over the age of 50. Approximately 25% of males older than 80 years will require prostatic surgery due to the obstructive symptoms caused by the enlarged prostate gland.

Men with **benign prostatic hypertrophy** (**BPH**) may complain of symptoms such as difficulty in starting urination, a weak stream of urine (not being able to maintain a constant stream), the inability to empty the bladder completely, or "dribbling" at the end of voiding.

Diagnosis is usually confirmed by thorough patient history and a rectal examination by the physician to confirm prostatic enlargement. The physician may order a urinalysis and culture of the urine to check for urinary tract infection or any abnormalities in the urine, such as blood. Other diagnostic tests may be a **cystourethroscopy** to visualize the interior of the bladder and the urethra; a **KUB** x-ray (kidneys, ureters, bladder) to visualize the urinary tract; or a **residual urine test** to check for incomplete emptying of the bladder. If a malignancy (cancer) is suspected, a biopsy of the prostatic tissue may be ordered.

Treatment for BPH is dependent upon the degree of urinary obstruction noted. For patients with mild cases of prostatic enlargement (which is normal as the male ages), the condition may simply be monitored. For patients with recurrent and obstructive problems due to hyperplasia of the prostate gland, surgery is usually indicated to remove the prostate gland. Two types of surgery used are **transurethral resection of the prostate**

(**TURP**) and **suprapubic prostatectomy**, each of which will be discussed in the diagnostic procedures section of this chapter.

---

carcinoma of the prostate
(car-sin-**OH**-mah of the **PROSS**-tayt)
carcin/o = cancer
-oma = tumor

Malignant growth within the prostate gland, creating pressure on the upper part of the urethra.

Cancer of the prostate is the most common cause of cancer among men, and the most common cause of cancer death due to cancer in men over the age of 55. Unfortunately, symptoms are not usually present in the early stages of cancer of the prostate. By the time symptoms are evident, the cancer may have already metastasized (spread) to other areas of the body.

When symptoms of prostate cancer occur, they may include any of the following:

1. A need to urinate frequently (i.e., urinary frequency), especially at night
2. Difficulty starting or stopping urine flow
3. Inability to urinate
4. Weak or interrupted flow of urine when urinating (patient may complain of "dribbling" instead of having a steady stream of urine)
5. Pain or burning when urinating
6. Pain or stiffness in the lower back, hips, or thighs
7. Painful ejaculation

Since the presence of symptoms usually means that the disease is more advanced, early detection of cancer of the prostate is essential to successful treatment. All men over the age of 40 should have a yearly physical exam which includes a digital rectal examination of the prostate gland.

The rectal exam can reveal a cancerous growth before symptoms appear. A prostate-specific antigen (PSA) blood test may be performed during the exam to detect increased growth of the prostate (the growth could be benign or malignant). The level of PSA in the blood may rise in men who have prostate cancer, or benign prostatic hypertrophy. If the level is elevated, the physician will order additional tests to confirm a diagnosis of cancer of the prostate.

The most common procedure used to treat or relieve the urinary obstruction resulting from cancer of the prostate is surgery (TURP) to remove the prostate tissue that is pressing against the upper part of the urethra. TURP is also used to treat benign prostatic hypertrophy.

Other methods of treatment include a radical prostatectomy (removal of the prostate gland), radiation therapy, hormone therapy, or chemotherapy. The treatment of choice is dependent upon the patient's age, medical history, risks and benefits of treatment, and the stage of the disease.

The Female Reproductive System

Physical changes occur in women after menopause. The ovaries cease to produce ova (eggs) and have less estrogen hormone that may cause physiological symptoms. As women age, they experience a general atrophy of the genitalia related to the hormonal changes. These changes in the genitalia include less fat, external hair loss, and flattening of the labia. The uterus of the elderly female is approximately one-half the size of the uterus of the young adult female. The vagina becomes drier and narrower. As a result of less vaginal lubrication, postmenopausal women may experience dyspareunia (pain during sexual intercourse).

After menopause and the decrease in estrogen levels, women experience changes in breast tissue that result in less glandular tissue, reduced elasticity, and more connective tissue and fat. These changes can cause sagging breasts, although the size of the breasts may not change.

The pathological conditions related to the aging female reproductive system include, but are not limited to, the following:

atrophic vaginitis

Degeneration of the vaginal mucous membrane after menopause. Also known as senile vaginitis, this condition is common in estrogen-deprived older women. The tissues of the vagina become drier and thinner.

Symptoms of atrophic vaginitis include pruritus (itching), burning, dyspareunia (pain during sexual intercourse), and bleeding. Treatment includes estrogen replacement therapy, vaginal hormone creams, and lubricants.

ovarian carcinoma
(oh-**VAY**-ree-an car-sin-**OH**-mah)
ovari/o = ovary
-an = characteristic of
carcin/o = cancer
-oma = tumor

A malignant tumor of the ovaries, most commonly occurring in women in their 50s. It is rarely detected in the early stage and is usually far advanced when diagnosed.

Symptoms usually do not appear with **ovarian cancer** until disease is well advanced. The earliest symptoms of ovarian cancer are swelling, bloating, or discomfort in the lower abdomen, and mild digestive complaints (loss of appetite, feeling of fullness, indigestion, nausea, and weight loss). As the tumor increases in size it may create pressure on adjacent organs, such as the urinary bladder or the rectum, causing frequent urination and dysuria or constipation. Later developments in the course of the disease include an accumulation of fluid within the abdominal cavity (ascites), resulting in swelling and discomfort.

Diagnosis is confirmed with examination of a sample of the tumor tissue under a microscope. This is achieved through surgical removal of the affected ovary. If the ovary is diseased with cancer, the surgeon will then remove the other ovary, the uterus, and the fallopian tubes. A process called staging is important to determine the amount of metastasis, if any. This process involves taking samples (biopsy) of nearby lymph nodes, the diaphragm, and sampling the fluid from the abdomen.

Treatment involves the use of surgery, chemotherapy, or radiation therapy. It may involve one or a combination of the treatment choices, depending on the extent of the disease.

Mental Health

Oliver Wendell Homes, U.S. physician, poet, and humorist, once commented, "To be 70 years young is sometimes far more cheerful and hopeful than to be 40 years old." How true! Can you think of an elderly friend or relative who seems young, although this person is over 65? What is it that allows this individual to age successfully and to enjoy a mentally healthy attitude about aging?

Many factors contribute to successful aging and a continued sense of self-worth. Factors such as maintaining positive social relationships, continuing to be independent, having adequate personal income, and maintaining the best possible level of health contribute to successful aging. It is important that aging adults become acquainted with the normal changes that occur with aging and understand that some adjustments may be required to meet these changes. Normal physiological changes do occur with aging, but at an individualized pace and in a unique manner for each individual. Some approach these changes in a positive way; others find aging to be a negative event.

Although normal aging does not imply disease, the incidence of chronic diseases increases with age. This has been clearly depicted in the previous pages of this chapter. Mental health is defined as a relative state of mind in which a person is able to cope with and adjust to the repeated stresses of everyday living in an acceptable way. The majority of elderly adults have successfully coped with life crises and the aging process. A small percentage find difficulty in coping with life changes as they age. For those individuals, a common mental health problem is depression, which often goes undiagnosed. Furthermore, many elderly adults experience a co-occurrence of depression with heart disease.

This segment of the chapter will be devoted to the discussion of dementia and depression as related to the elderly.

dementia
(dee-**MEN**-she-ah)

A progressive, organic mental disorder characterized by chronic personality disintegration, confusion, disorientation, stupor, deterioration of intellectual capacity and function, and impairment of control of memory, judgment, and impulses.

Dementia of the Alzheimer's type is the most common form. The onset of symptoms is slow and not easily detected at first, with the course of the disorder becoming progressive and deteriorating. If the onset is early, the symptoms will appear before the age of 65; if the onset is late, the symptoms will appear after the age of 65. It has been projected that approximately 10% of individuals over the age of 65 and 50% of those over the age of 85 will develop Alzheimer's disease.

The symptoms of dementia of the Alzheimer's type may begin as forgetfulness, followed by the individual becoming suspicious of others as the memory deteriorates. The individual may become apathetic and socially withdrawn or untidier in appearance. Irritability, moodiness, and sudden outbursts over trivial issues may become apparent. These individuals may wander away from home, forgetting where they are and where they live. As the condition progresses, the ability to work or care for personal needs independently is no longer possible and the individual requires supervised care.

depression

A mood disturbance characterized by exaggerated feelings of sadness, discouragement, and hopelessness that are inappropriate and

out of proportion to reality; may be relative to some personal loss or tragedy.

Depression is one of the most common, and most treatable, of all mental disorders in older adults—if it is recognized. There are many factors in the lives of the elderly that place them at high risk, for the development or recurrence of depression, such as biological, psychological, and social changes. The lack of treatment, however, for depression in the elderly adult may be attributed to the reluctance of the elderly adult to seek psychiatric care, the tendency of the elderly to insist that physical illness rather than an emotional problem is at the root of their concern, and the failure of many health care professionals to recognize that depressive symptoms are not a natural part of growing old.

Depression can affect every aspect of an elderly adult's life. It may be characterized by some of the following behavioral signs: sadness, discouragement, crying, irritability, withdrawing from usual activities, being critical of self and others, becoming passive, decreased or increased appetite, fatigue, weight loss or sometimes weight gain, and thoughts of death. Some of these symptoms can be easily overlooked by the health care professional, as physical illness can mask the symptoms of depression.

Several types of therapies have been found to be beneficial in treating depression in the elderly adult. The goals of treatment are designed to improve the quality of life and functional ability of these individuals, as well as reducing morbidity and mortality.

Diagnostic Techniques and Procedures

barium enema (lower GI series)
(**BEAR**-ee-um **EN**-eh-mah)

Infusion of a radiopaque contrast medium, barium sulfate, into the rectum and held in place in the lower intestinal tract while x-ray films are obtained of the lower GI tract.

For the most definitive results, the colon should be empty of fecal material. Along with the use of a laxative and/or a cleansing enema, the person having a barium enema should be without food or drink from midnight before the procedure. Abnormal findings include malignant tumors, colonic stenosis, colonic fistula, perforated colon, diverticula, and polyps.

barium swallow (upper GI series)
(**BEAR**-ee-um swallow)

Oral administration of a radiopaque contrast medium, barium sulfate, which flows into the esophagus as the person swallows.

X-ray films are obtained of the esophagus and borders of the heart in which varices can be identified, as well as strictures, tumors, obstructions, achalasia, or abnormal motility of the esophagus. As the barium sulfate continues to flow into the upper GI tract (lower esophagus, stomach, and duodenum), x-ray films are taken to reveal ulcerations, tumors, hiatial hernias, or obstruction.

colonoscopy
(**koh**-lon-**OSS**-koh-pee)
colon/o = colon
-scopy = the process of viewing

The direct visualization of the lining of the large intestine using a fiberoptic colonoscope.

A colonoscopy is indicated for individuals with a history of undiagnosed constipation and diarrhea, loss of appetite (anorexia), persistent rectal bleeding, or lower abdominal pain. The procedure is also used to check for colonic polyps or possible malignant tumors.

corneal transplant
(**COR**-nee-al)
corne/o = cornea
-al = pertaining to

Surgical transplantation of a donor cornea (cadaver's) into the eye of a recipient usually under local anesthesia.

Young donor corneas are preferred for **corneal transplant,** because the endothelial layer of the cornea has a direct relationship to age and health.

coronary artery bypass graft (CABG) surgery

A surgical procedure designed to increase the blood flow to the myocardial muscle and involves bypass grafts to the coronary arteries that reroute the blood flow around the occluded area of the coronary artery. See Figure 24-13.

Grafts are made from veins taken from other parts of the body (usually the saphenous vein from the leg), and are connected to the coronary artery above and below the occlusion. This anastomosis (plural: anastomoses) joins the two vessels, restoring the normal flow of oxygenated blood to the myocardium.

directional coronary atherectomy

A procedure that uses a catheter (AtheroCath) which has a small mechanically driven cutter that shaves the plaque and stores it in a collection chamber. See Figure 24-14.

The plaque is then removed from the artery when the device is withdrawn. This procedure usually lasts from 1 to 3 hours and requires overnight hospitalization.

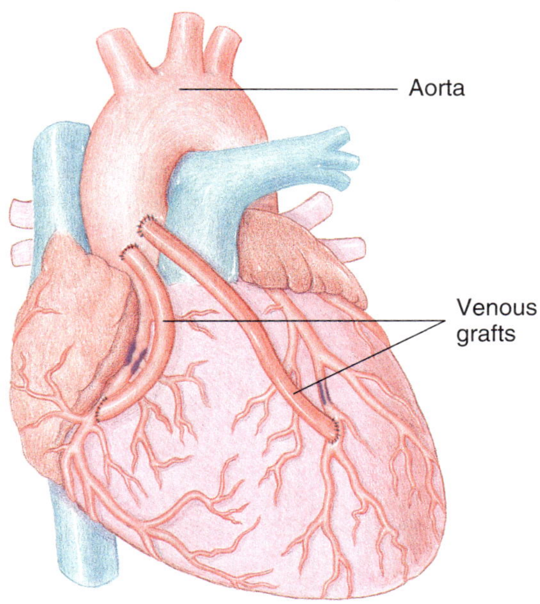

Figure 24-13 Coronary artery bypass surgery

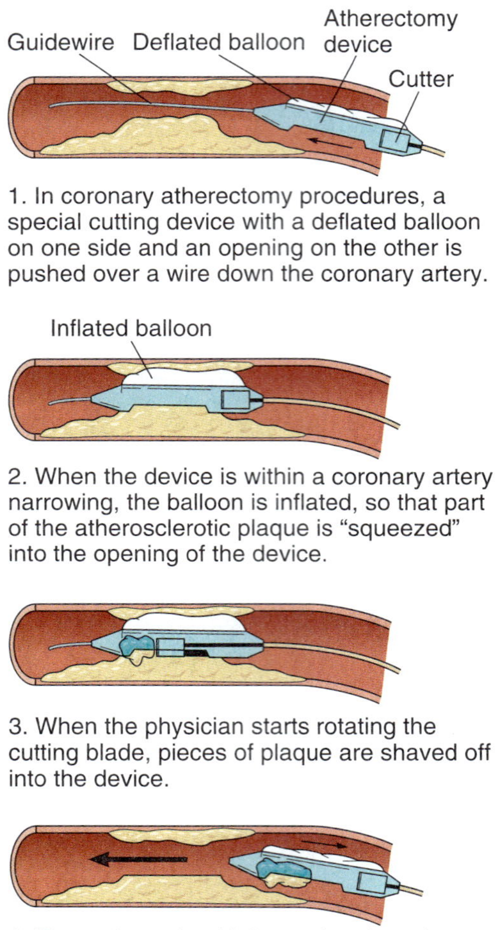

1. In coronary atherectomy procedures, a special cutting device with a deflated balloon on one side and an opening on the other is pushed over a wire down the coronary artery.

2. When the device is within a coronary artery narrowing, the balloon is inflated, so that part of the atherosclerotic plaque is "squeezed" into the opening of the device.

3. When the physician starts rotating the cutting blade, pieces of plaque are shaved off into the device.

4. The catheter is withdrawn, leaving a larger opening for blood flow.

Figure 24-14 Directional coronary atherectomy

During the atherectomy procedure, the patient remains awake, but sedated. The catheter is inserted into the femoral artery and is advanced into position using x-ray visualization as a guide. Once in place, the catheter balloon is inflated, pressing the cutting device against the plaque on the opposite wall of the artery. This causes the plaque to protrude into the window of the cutting device. As this happens, the rotating blade of the cutting device then shaves off the plaque, storing it in the tip of the catheter until removal from the body. The process is repeated several times to widen the opening of the artery at the blockage site.

If the medications, angioplasty, and atherectomy are not successful methods of treatment, or the coronary artery disease is severe, then coronary bypass surgery will be the treatment of choice.

dual photon absorptiometry
(dual **FOH**-ton ab-sorp-she-**AHM**-eh-tree)

Dual photon absorptiometry is a noninvasive procedure for evaluating bone density. This procedure involves beaming a minimal amount of radiation (from a radioactive isotope) through the bones. A computer then evaluates the amount of radiation

absorbed by the bones and summarizes the findings, which are then interpreted by the physician.

This procedure measures the bone density within 2% to 3% accuracy of the bone's actual density.

---

dual energy x-ray absorptiometry (DEXA)

This newer technique is also a noninvasive procedure that measures bone density. In the dual energy x-ray absorptiometry (DEXA) procedure, an x-ray machine generates the energy photons that pass through the bones. A computer evaluates the amount of radiation absorbed by the bones, and the findings are interpreted by a physician.

This procedure measures the bone density more accurately than the dual photon absorptiometry, taking less time and emitting less radiation to the patient.

---

extracapsular cataract extraction (ECCE)
(eks-trah-**KAP**-syoo-lar **KAT**-ah-rakt eks-**TRAK**-shun)

Extracapsular cataract extraction is the surgical removal of the anterior segment of the lens capsule and the lens, allowing for the insertion of an intraocular lens implant.

The insertion of a posterior chamber intraocular lens has proven to result in less complications.

---

hearing aids

Devices that amplify sound to provide more precise perception and interpretation of words communicated to the individual with a hearing deficit.

This improved interpretation and perception is made possible by the amplification of sound above the individual's hearing threshold as it is introduced to the ear's hearing apparatus.

Hearing aids are accessible in an assortment of styles.

1. The " in-canal style" hearing aid is the newest and least conspicuous of the devices, fitting completely into the ear canal and allowing for exercise and talking on the telephone without being obtrusive. The disadvantages of using this style of hearing aid occur for those individuals who do not have good dexterity with their hands. Due to the size of the hearing aid, the handling, cleaning, and changing of batteries require good manual dexterity, which can be difficult for many older individuals. Cleaning is important because of the possible accumulation of earwax, which will plug the small portals and disrupt sound transmission.
2. The "in-ear style" hearing aid is worn in the external ear and is larger and more noticeable than the in-canal style. The care of the in-ear style also requires manual dexterity, which is often a concern for the older individual. Advantages of the in-ear style include a greater degree of amplification and toggle switches that allow for usage of the telephone. Cleaning is important because of the possible accumulation of earwax, which will plug the small portals and disrupt sound transmission. See **Figure 24-15A.**

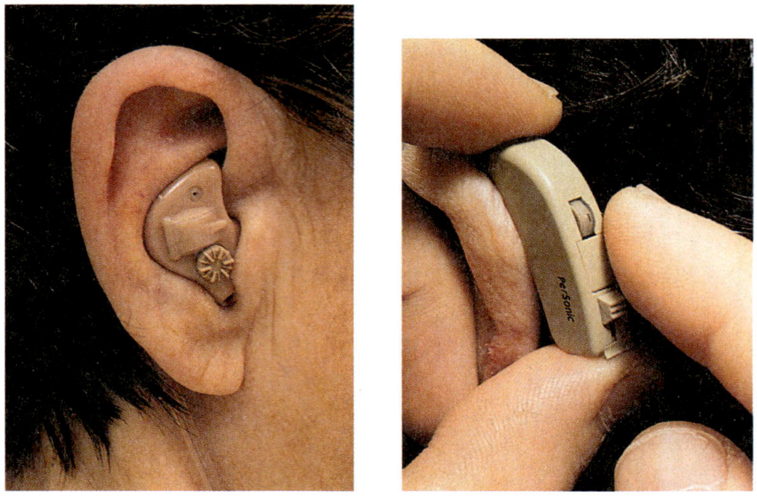

Figure 24-15 Hearing aids: (A) in-ear style; (B) behind-ear style

3. The "behind-ear style" hearing aid allows for even greater amplification of sound than the in-ear style and is much easier to manipulate manually for care and control. If the user wears glasses, components are available that fit into the earpiece of the eyeglasses for convenience and comfort. See **Figure 24-15B.**

4. A "body hearing aid" is used by individuals who have a profound hearing loss. Sound is delivered to the ear canal by way of a microphone and amplifier clipped on the clothing in a pocket-sized container that is connected to a receiver, which is clipped onto the ear mold.

---

internal fixation devices

The treatment of choice for a fractured hip is usually surgery. Devices such as screws, pins, wires, and nails may be used to internally maintain the bone alignment while healing takes place. These internal fixation devices are more commonly used with fractures of the femur and fractures of joints. See Figure 24-16.

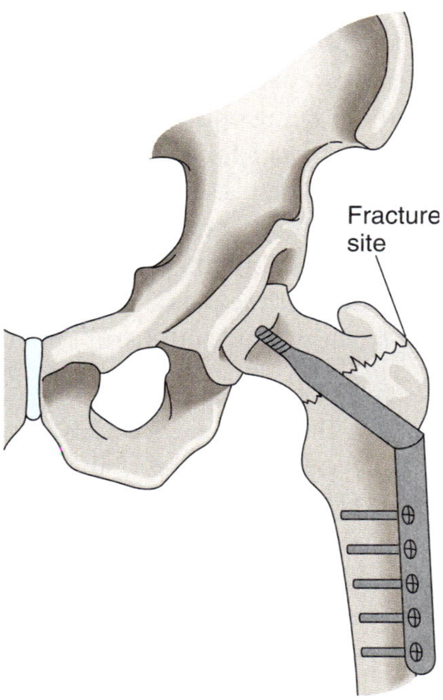

Figure 24-16 Internal fixation device

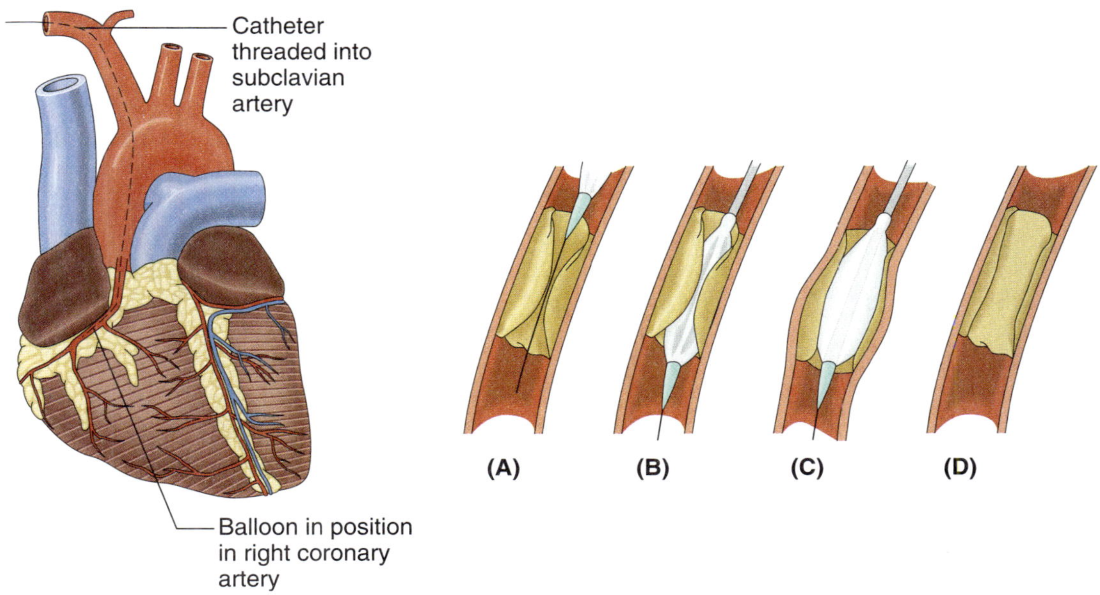

Figure 24-17 Balloon angioplasty

intraocular lens implant
(in-trah-**OCK**-yoo-lar **LENZ IM**-plant)
intra- = within
ocul/o = eye
-ar = pertaining to

Intraocular lens implant is the surgical process of cataract extraction, which restores visual acuity and provides depth perception, light refraction, and binocular vision.

The lens can be implanted in the anterior chamber or the posterior chamber.

percutaneous transluminal coronary angioplasty (PTCA)

A nonsurgical procedure in which a catheter, equipped with a small inflatable balloon on the end, is inserted into the femoral artery and is threaded up the aorta (under x-ray visualization) into the narrowed coronary artery.

When properly positioned, the balloon is carefully inflated, compressing the fatty deposits against the side of the walls of the artery, thus enlarging the opening of the artery to increase blood flow through the artery.

Once the plaque is compressed against the walls of the artery, the balloon-tipped catheter is then removed or replaced with a **stent** (a mesh tube used to hold the artery open). Typically, the stent remains in place permanently unless reocclusion occurs. This procedure is also called a balloon catheter dilatation or a balloon angioplasty. See **Figure 24-17.**

retinal photocoagulation
(**RET**-in-al **foh**-toh-coh-**ag**-yoo-**LAY**-shun)
retin/o = retina
-al = pertaining to
phot/o = light

Retinal photocoagulation is a surgical procedure that uses an argon laser to treat conditions such as glaucoma, retinal detachment, and diabetic retinopathy.

Following are different treatment methods.

1. In glaucoma, the argon laser destroys portions of the ciliary body to allow flow of aqueous humor.
2. In retinal detachment, the argon laser is used to create an area of inflammation, which will develop adhesions, causing a "welding" of the layers.

3. In diabetic retinopathy, the argon laser is used to seal microaneurysms and to reduce the risk of hemorrhage.

serum glucose tests

Measures the amount of glucose in the blood at the time the sample was drawn.

True serum glucose elevations are indicative of diabetes mellitus; however, the value must be evaluated according to the time of day and the last time the person has eaten. A glucose level can be collected in a tube or evaluated with a finger stick.

suprapubic prostatectomy
(**soo**-prah-**PEW**-bik pross-tah-**TEK**-toh-mee)
supra- = above
pub/o = pubis
-ic = pertaining to
prostat/o = prostate gland
-ectomy = surgical removal of

The surgical removal of the prostate gland by making an incision into the abdominal wall, just above the pubis.

A small incision is then made into the bladder which has been distended with fluid. The prostate gland is removed through the bladder cavity.

The removal of the prostate gland by the suprapubic approach is done when the surgeon believes that the prostate gland is too enlarged to be removed through the urethra, or more likely, for malignancies.

transurethral resection of the prostate (TURP)
(trans-you-**REE**-thral **REE**-sek-shun of the **PROSS**-tayt)
trans- = across
urethr/o = urethra
-al = pertaining to

The surgical removal of the prostate gland by inserting a resectoscope (an instrument used to remove tissue from the body) through the urethra and into the bladder to remove small pieces of tissue from the prostate gland.

Common Abbreviations

ABBREVIATION	MEANING	ABBREVIATION	MEANING
AAA	Area Agency on Aging	**DEXA**	dual energy x-ray absorptiometry
AD	Alzheimer's disease	**ECG**	electrocardiogram
ADL	activities of daily living	**ECHO**	echocardiogram
BPH	benign prostatic hypertrophy	**GCNS**	gerontological clinical nurse specialist
CABG	coronary artery bypass graft	**GNP**	gerontological nurse practitioner
CAD	coronary artery disease	**IDDM**	insulin-dependent diabetes mellitus
Cath	catheterization	**KUB**	kidneys, ureters, bladder (an x-ray)
CHF	congestive heart failure	**NIDDM**	non-insulin-dependent diabetes mellitus
CVA	cerebrovascular accident; stroke		
CVD	cardiovascular disease		

PTCA	percutaneous transluminal coronary angioplasty
RSVP	retired seniors volunteer program
SOB	shortness of breath
TIA	transient ischemic attack
TURP	transurethral resection of the prostate
URI	upper respiratory infection

Written and Audio Terminology Review

Review each of the following terms from this chapter. Study the spelling of each term and write the definition in the space provided. If you have the Audio CD available, listen to each term, pronounce it, and check the box once you are comfortable saying the word. Check definitions by looking the term up in the glossary/index.

TERM	PRONUNCIATION	DEFINITION
acrochordon	☐ ak-roh-**KOR**-don	______________
alopecia	☐ **al**-oh-**PEE**-shee-ah	______________
Alzheimer's disease	☐ **ALTS**-high-merz dih-**ZEEZ**	______________
ankylosing spondylitis	☐ **ang**-kih-**LOH**-sing spon-dil-**EYE**-tis	______________
arteriosclerosis	☐ ar-tee-ree-oh-skleh-**ROH**-sis	______________
arthralgia	☐ ar-**THRAL**-jee-ah	______________
arthritis	☐ ar-**THRY**-tis	______________
atherosclerosis	☐ ath-er-**oh**-scleh-**ROH**-sis	______________
benign prostatic hypertrophy	☐ bee-**NYEN** pross-**TAT**-ik high-**PER**-troh-fee	______________
bunionectomy	☐ bun-yun-**ECK**-toh-mee	______________
cataract	☐ **KAT**-ah-rakt	______________
cerebrovascular accident	☐ seh-**ree**-broh-**VASS**-kyoo-lar **AK**-sih-dent	______________
claudication	☐ klaw-dih-**KAY**-shun	______________
constipation	☐ **kon**-stih-**PAY**-shun	______________
coronary artery disease	☐ **KOR**-ah-nair-ree **AR**-ter-ee dih-**ZEEZ**	______________
crepitation	☐ crep-ih-**TAY**-shun	______________

Term		Pronunciation	
cystourethroscopy	☐	**siss**-toh-yoo-ree-**THROSS**-koh-pee	___
deafness, sensorineural	☐	**DEFF**-ness, sen-soh-ree-**NOO**-ral	___
dementia	☐	dee-**MEN**-shee-ah	___
diabetes mellitus	☐	dye-ah-**BEE**-teez **MELL**-ih-tus	___
diabetic retinopathy	☐	dye-ah-**BET**-ik ret-in-**OP**-ah-thee	___
ectropion	☐	ek-**TROH**-pee-on	___
eczema	☐	**EK**-zeh-mah	___
entropion	☐	en-**TROH**-pee-on	___
geriatrician	☐	**jer**-ee-ah-**TRIH**-shun	___
geriatrics	☐	jer-ee-**AT**-riks	___
gerontology	☐	**jer**-on-**TAHL**-oh-jee	___
glaucoma	☐	glah-**KOH**-mah	___
herpes zoster	☐	**HER**-peez **ZOS**-ter	___
intraocular lens implant	☐	in-trah-**OCK**-yoo-lar **LENZ IM**-plant	___
ketones	☐	**KEY**-tonz	___
kyphosis	☐	ki-**FOH**-sis	___
lichenification	☐	lye-**ken**-ih-fih-**KAY**-shun	___
nocturia	☐	nok-**TOO**-ree-ah	___
osteoarthritis	☐	**oss**-tee-oh-ar-**THRY**-tis	___
osteoporosis	☐	oss-tee-oh-poh-**ROW**-sis	___
Parkinson's disease	☐	**PARK**-in-sons dih-**ZEEZ**	___
presbyopia	☐	prez-bee-**OH**-pee-ah	___
purpura	☐	**PER**-pew-rah	___
retinal photocoagulation	☐	**RET**-in-al **foh**-toh-coh-**ag**-yoo-**LAY**-shun	___
seborrheic keratosis	☐	seb-or-**REE**-ik kair-ah-**TOH**-sis	___
senescence	☐	seh-**NESS**-ens	___

Term		Pronunciation	
senile lentigines	☐	**SEE**-nyle lin-**TIH**-jeh-nez	______
suprapubic prostatectomy	☐	**soo**-prah-**PEW**-bik pross-tah-**TEK**-toh-mee	______
thrombosis	☐	throm-**BOH**-sis	______
transurethral resection of the prostate	☐	trans-yoo-**REE**-thral **REE**-sek-shun of the **PROSS**-tayt	______
turgor	☐	**TURH**-gor	______
urinary incontinence	☐	**YOO**-rih-nair-ee in-**CON**-tin-ens	______

Chapter Review Exercises

The following exercises provide a more in-depth review of the chapter material. Your goal in these exercises is to complete each section at a minimum 80% level of accuracy. A space has been provided for your score at the end of each section.

A. Define the Abbreviation

Define each abbreviation by writing the definition in the space provided. Confirm your answers with the text. Place a check in the space provided if you were able to complete this exercise correctly the first time (without referring to the text). Each correct answer is worth 10 points. Record your score in the space provided at the end of the exercise.

( ) 1. CVA ______

( ) 2. CAD ______

( ) 3. CABG ______

( ) 4. CHF ______

( ) 5. BPH ______

( ) 6. TURP ______

( ) 7. SOB ______

( ) 8. PTCA ______

( ) 9. ECG ______

( ) 10. KUB ______

Number correct ______ × 10 points/correct answer: Your score ______%

B. Name the Pathological Condition

Read the descriptions of the pathological conditions on the right and match them with the appropriate pathological condition on the left. Each correct answer is worth 10 points. When you have completed the exercise, record your score in the space provided at the end of the exercise.

_____ 1. eczema
_____ 2. seborrheic keratosis
_____ 3. psoriasis
_____ 4. achalasia
_____ 5. osteoporosis
_____ 6. osteomalacia
_____ 7. Paget's disease
_____ 8. osteoarthritis
_____ 9. gout
_____ 10. bunion

a. A common noninfectious chronic disorder of the skin manifested by silvery white scales over round, raised, reddened plaques producing pruritus
b. Bones that were once strong become fragile due to loss of bone density
c. An abnormal enlargement of the joint at the base of the great toe
d. An acute or chronic inflammatory skin condition characterized by erythema, papules, vesicles, pustules, scales, crusts, or scabs; accompanied by intense itching
e. Osteitis deformans
f. Also known as degenerative joint disease, results from wear and tear on the joints, especially weight-bearing joints such as the hips and knees
g. Abnormal softening of the bones due to a deficiency of calcium and phosphorus in the blood (which is necessary for bone mineralization)
h. Brown or yellow wartlike lesions loosely attached to the skin surface; also known as senile warts
i. Decreased mobility of the lower two thirds of the esophagus along with constriction of the lower esophageal sphincter
j. A form of acute arthritis that is characterized by inflammation of the first metatarsal joint of the great toe

Number correct _______ × 10 points/correct answer: Your score _______%

C. Word Element Review

The following words relate to the chapter on gerontology. The word elements have been labeled (WR = word root, P = prefix, S = suffix, and V = combining vowel). Read the definition carefully and complete the word by filling in the blank, using the word elements provided in this chapter. If you have forgotten the word building rules, refer to Chapter 1. Each correct answer is worth 10 points. Record your score in the space provided at the end of this exercise.

1. A refractive error in which the lens of the eye cannot focus on an image accurately, resulting in impaired distant vision that is blurred, due to the image being focused in front of the retina; nearsightedness.

   ____________________/____________________
   WR S

2. A form of arteriosclerosis (hardening of the arteries) characterized by fatty deposits building up within the inner layers of the walls of larger arteries.

   ____________________/____________________/____________________/____________________
   WR V WR S

3. Urination at night.

   ____________________/____________________
   WR S

4. Elevated blood sugar level.

_______________/_______________/_______________

P WR S

5. Poor vision due to the natural aging process.

_______________/_______________

WR S

6. Pertaining to the heart.

_______________/_______________

WR S

7. An arterial condition in which there is thickening, hardening, and loss of elasticity of the walls of the arteries; hardening of the arteries.

_______________/_______________/_______________/_______________

WR V WR S

8. Any disease of the retina.

_______________/_______________/_______________

WR V S

9. A cancerous tumor.

_______________/_______________

WR S

10. A condition of hardness.

_______________/_______________

WR S

Number correct _______ × 10 points/correct answer: Your score _______%

D. Spelling

Circle the correctly spelled term in each pairing of words. Each correct answer is worth 10 points. Record your score in the space provided at the end of the exercise.

1. geriatrics — geriatricks
2. turger — turgor
3. ekzema — eczema
4. soriasis — psoriasis
5. osteomalacia — osteomalasha
6. purpera — purpura
7. Alzhimer's — Alzheimer's
8. arteriosclerosis — arteriosclerosus
9. emphyzema — emphysema
10. cateract — cataract

Number correct _______ × 10 points/correct answer: Your score _______%

E. Word Search

Using the definitions, write the appropriate answer in the space provided. After you have written each answer, find it in the word search puzzle and circle the word. The words may be read up, down, diagonally, across, or backward. Each correct answer is worth 10 points. Record your score in the space provided at the end of the exercise.

Example: The process of growing old.

aging

1. The study of all aspects of the aging process.

____

2. Partial or complete loss of hair.

____

3. A reflection of the skin's elasticity.

____

4. An abnormal sound or murmur heard when listening to a carotid artery, organ, or gland with a stethoscope.

____

5. Another name for nearsightedness.

____

6. Another name for humpback.

____

7. Clicking or crackling sounds heard upon joint movement.

____

8. Another name for swelling.

____

9. Lack or loss of appetite.

____

G	E	R	O	N	T	O	L	O	G	Y	N	M	I	A
P	L	E	U	R	U	I	D	A	G	I	N	G	M	L
E	I	O	K	T	R	N	M	E	T	T	R	N	V	O
X	A	O	N	E	G	L	O	S	D	I	C	C	B	P
I	L	C	T	D	O	P	A	R	A	G	M	D	N	E
M	U	H	O	B	R	U	I	T	E	L	R	O	T	C
C	R	O	T	H	L	Y	P	U	A	S	C	P	E	I
R	U	R	R	E	P	N	O	M	A	T	O	F	E	A
E	U	D	O	S	I	X	Y	T	U	I	P	E	E	E
P	D	R	C	D	A	D	M	R	D	E	Y	S	M	N
I	R	E	I	N	O	R	I	H	E	A	D	S	R	P
T	I	A	M	A	R	A	H	S	S	S	S	A	I	Y
A	S	S	N	A	T	U	Y	A	I	D	I	S	G	D
T	U	I	T	C	E	S	P	I	N	A	E	N	P	A
I	R	S	O	H	L	O	S	I	S	O	H	P	Y	K
O	A	N	O	R	E	X	I	A	T	U	R	E	S	B
N	R	O	T	T	E	U	R	I	S	M	E	M	I	C
E	X	H	I	B	I	T	D	I	O	M	A	S	E	S

10. Urination at night.

____

Number correct _______ × 10 points/correct answer: Your score _______%

F. True or False

Read each statement carefully and circle the correct answer as true or false. HINT: Pay close attention to the word elements written in **bold** as you make your decision. If the statement is false, identify the meaning of that word element. Each correct answer is worth 10 points. Record your score in the space provided at the end of the exercise.

1. Urination at night is known as **noct**uria.

   True False

   If your answer is False, what does *noct/o* mean? ______________________
2. **Hyper**glycemia means a low blood sugar level.

   True False

   If your answer is False, what does *hyper* mean? ______________________
3. Diabetic **retin**opathy is a disease of the retina of the eye in which the capillaries of the retina experience scarring.

   True False

   If your answer is False, what does *retin/o* mean? ______________________
4. Loss of vision due to the aging process is known as **presby**opia.

   True False

   If your answer is False, what does *presby/o* mean? ______________________
5. Benign **prostat**ic hypertrophy is enlargement of the epididymis.

   True False

   If your answer is False, what does *prostat/o* mean? ______________________
6. **Endo**metrial carcinoma refers to a malignant tumor of the outside of the uterus.

   True False

   If your answer is False, what does *endo-* mean? ______________________
7. Osteo**porosis** refers to softening of the bones.

   True False

   If your answer is False, what does *-porosis* mean? ______________________
8. Osteo**malacia** is a disease in which the bones become porous.

   True False

   If your answer is False, what does *-malacia* mean? ______________________
9. **Kyph**osis is another name for humpback.

   True False

   If your answer is False, what does *kyph/o* mean? ______________________
10. Osteo**arthr**itis is inflammation of the bones and the cartilage.

    True False

    If your answer is False, what does *arthr/o* mean? ______________________

Number correct _______ × 10 points/correct answer: Your score _______%

G. Completion

The following sentences relate to the chapter on gerontology. Complete each sentence with the most appropriate word. Each correct answer is worth 10 points. Record your score in the space provided at the end of the exercise.

1. A condition of the legs involving annoying sensations of uneasiness, tiredness, itching, or tingling of the leg muscles while resting is known as ____________________.
2. An abnormal enlargement of the joint at the base of the great toe is known as a ____________________.
3. A form of acute arthritis that is characterized by inflammation of the first metatarsal joint of the great toe is known as ____________________.
4. A disease in which the bones become abnormally soft, due to a deficiency of calcium and phosphorus in the blood, resulting in fractures and noticeable deformities of the weight-bearing bones is known as ____________________.
5. A type of arthritis, also known as Marie-Strümpell disease, that affects the vertebral column and causes deformities of the spine is known as ____________________.
6. Cramplike pains in the calves of the legs caused by poor circulation to the muscles of the legs, and commonly associated with atherosclerosis, is known as ____________________.
7. A progressive and extremely debilitating disease that results in deterioration of a person's intellectual functioning is ____________________.
8. A degenerative, slowly progressive deterioration of nerves in the brain stem's motor system, characterized by stooped posture, bowed head, shuffling gait, pill-rolling gestures, and an expressionless masklike facial appearance is known as ____________________.
9. ____________________ is an acute viral infection seen mainly in adults, characterized by inflammation of the underlying spinal or cranial nerve pathway producing painful, vesicular eruptions on the skin following along these nerve pathways.
10. Another name for a cerebrovascular accident is a ____________________.

Number correct _______ × 10 points/correct answer: Your score _______%

H. Crossword Puzzle

Each crossword answer is worth 10 points. When you have completed the crossword puzzle, total your points and enter your score in the space provided.

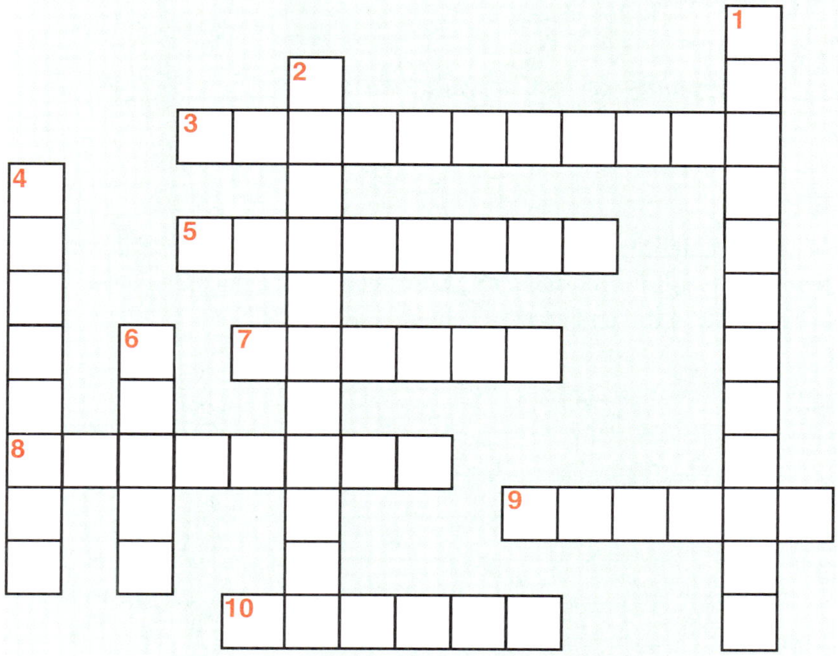

ACROSS

3 Clicking or crakling sounds heard upon joint movement
5 Partial or complete loss of hair
7 Cerebrovascular accident
8 Herpes zoster
9 Reflection of the skin's elasticity
10 Nearsightedness

DOWN

1 Surgical removal of a bunion
2 Study of all aspects of the aging process
4 Humpback
6 The process of growing old

Number correct* _______ × *10 points/correct answer: Your score* _______*%

I. Matching Abbreviations

Match the abbreviations on the left with the most appropriate definition on the right. Each correct response is worth 10 points. When you have completed the exercise, record your score in the space provided at the end of the exercise.

_____	1. ECG	a. benign prostatic hypertrophy
_____	2. KUB	b. electroencephalogram
_____	3. TURP	c. coronary artery bypass graft
_____	4. CVD	d. electrocardiogram
_____	5. CVA	e. coronary artery disease
_____	6. TIA	f. kidneys, ureters, bladder
_____	7. DEXA	g. transient urinary retrograde pyelogram
_____	8. CAD	h. cardiovascular disease

_____ 9. CABG

_____ 10. BPH

i. transient ischemic attack

j. dual energy x-ray absorptiometry

k. cerebrovascular accident; stroke

l. transurethral resection of the prostate

Number correct _______ × 10 points/correct answer: Your score _______%

J. Term to Definition

Define each term by writing the definition in the space provided. Check the box if you are able to complete this exercise correctly the first time (without referring to the answers). Each correct answer is worth 10 points. Record your score in the space provided at the end of the exercise.

☐ 1. kyphosis ______________________________

☐ 2. crepitation ______________________________

☐ 3. edema ______________________________

☐ 4. ascites ______________________________

☐ 5. lichenification ______________________________

☐ 6. myopia ______________________________

☐ 7. alopecia ______________________________

☐ 8. acrochordon ______________________________

☐ 9. senile lentigines ______________________________

☐ 10. senescence ______________________________

Number correct _______ × 10 points/correct answer: Your score _______%

Answers to Chapter Review Exercises

A. Define the Abbreviation

1. CVA = cerebrovascular accident; stroke
2. CAD = coronary artery disease
3. CABG = coronary artery bypass graft
4. CHF = congestive heart failure
5. BPH = benign prostatic hypertrophy
6. TURP = transurethral resection of the prostate
7. SOB = shortness of breath
8. PTCA = percutaneous transluminal coronary angioplasty
9. ECG = electrocardiogram
10. KUB = kidneys, ureters, bladder (x-ray)

B. Name the Pathological Condition

1. d
2. h
3. a
4. i
5. b
6. g
7. e
8. f
9. j
10. c

C. Word Element Review

1. my / opia
   WR S
2. ather / o / scler / osis
   WR V WR S
3. noct / uria
   WR S
4. hyper / glyc / emia
   P WR S
5. presby / opia
   WR S
6. coron / ary
   WR S
7. arteri / o / scler / osis
   WR V WR S
8. retin / o / pathy
   WR V S
9. carcin / oma
   WR S
10. kerat / osis
    WR S

D. Spelling

1. geriatrics
2. turgor
3. eczema
4. psoriasis
5. osteomalacia
6. purpura
7. Alzheimer's
8. arteriosclerosis
9. emphysema
10. cataract

E. Word Search

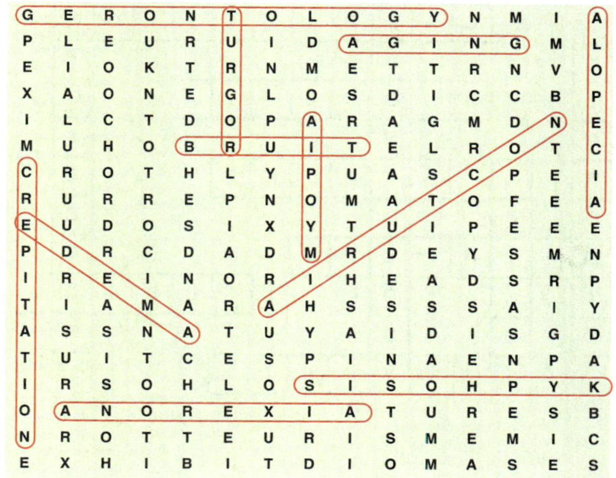

F. True or False

1. True
2. False; hyper = excessive
3. True
4. True
5. False; prostat/o = prostate gland
6. False; endo- = within
7. False; -porosis = passage or pore
8. False; -malacia = softening
9. True
10. False; arthr/o = joint

G. Completion

1. restless legs syndrome
2. bunion
3. gout
4. osteomalacia
5. ankylosing spondylitis
6. claudication
7. Alzheimer's disease
8. Parkinson's disease
9. shingles or herpes zoster
10. stroke

H. Crossword Puzzle

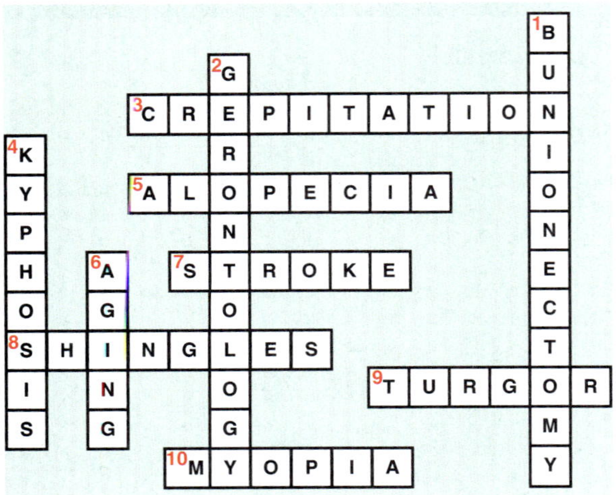

I. Matching Abbreviations

1. d
2. f
3. l
4. h
5. k
6. i
7. j
8. e
9. c
10. a

J. Term to Definition

1. humpback or hunchback (an abnormal outward curvature of a portion of the spine)
2. clicking or crackling sounds heard upon joint movement
3. the abnormal accumulation of fluid in interstitial spaces of tissues
4. an abnormal intraperitoneal accumulation of a fluid (containing large amounts of protein and electrolytes)
5. thickening and hardening of the skin
6. nearsightedness
7. partial or complete loss of hair
8. skin tag(s)
9. age spots
10. the process of growing old

Glossary/Index

A

C

foreign body, contact lenses, or a scratch from a fingernail, 532
Corneal transplant (COR-nee-al), **surgical transplantation of a donor cornea into the eye of a recipient, 540, 979**
Corneitis (cor-nee-EYE-tis), 527
Coron/o, 347, 946
Coronary artery (KOR-oh nair-ree AR-ter-ee), **one of a pair of arteries that branch from the artery, 338, 343**
Coronary artery disease (KOR-oh-nair-ree AR-ter-ee dih-ZEEZ), **narrowing of the coronary arteries to the extent that adequate blood supply to the myocardium is prevented, 349–352, 963**
Coronary bypass surgery, 350, 352, 979
Corpus luteum (KOR-pus LOO-tee-um), **a yellowish mass that forms within the ruptured ovarian follicle after ovulation containing high levels of progesterone and some estrogen, 660, 661, 713**
Corpuscle, 289
Cortex (COR-tex), **pertaining to the outer region of an organ or structure, 482, 574, 580**
Cortic/o, 488
Corticosteroid, 502
Cortisol (cor-tih-sal), **a steroid hormone occurring naturally in the body, 478, 482**
Coryza (kor-RYE-zuh), **inflammation of the respiratory mucous membranes, known as the common cold, which is an upper respiratory tract infection, 395**
Cost/o, 152
Costal cartilage, 143
Costochondral, pertaining to a rib and its cartilage, 152
Cough, a forceful and sometimes violent expiratory effort preceded by a preliminary inspiration. The glottis is partially closed, the accessory muscles of expiration are brought into action, and the air is noisily expelled, 392
Cowper's gland (KOW-perz). *See* Bulbourethral glands, 619, 621
Crackles (CRACK-l'z), **a common abnormal respiratory sound heard on auscultation of the chest during inspiration, characterized by discontinuous bubbling noises, 753**
Crani/o, 70, 152, 238
Cranial (KRAY-nee-al)
cavity, contains the brain
pertaining to the head, 63, 65
Craniotomy, a surgical incision into the cranium or skull, 231, 256, 260
Creatinine clearance test (kree-AT-in-in), **a diagnostic test for kidney function that measures the filtration rate of creatinine, a waste product (of muscle metabolism), which is normally removed by the kidney, 599**
Crepitation (crep-ih-TAY-shun), **clicking or crackling sounds heard upon joint movement, 197, 203, 943, 955**
Crest, a distinct border or ridge; an upper, elevated edge as in the upper part of the hip bone (the iliac crest); generally a site for muscle attachment, 136, 149
Cretinism (KREE-tin-izm), **a congenital condition (one that occurs at birth) caused by a lack of thyroid secretion. This condition is characterized by dwarfism, slowed mental development, puffy facial features, dry skin, and large tongue, 483, 492**
Crin/o, 488
-crine, 489
Crohn's disease (KROHNZ), **digestive tract inflammation of a chronic nature causing fever, cramping, diarrhea, weight loss, and anorexia, 442**
Cross-matching, 287
Croup (KROOP), **a childhood disease characterized by a barking cough, suffocative and difficult breathing, stridor, and laryngeal spasm, 396, 766**
Crown, the part of the tooth that is visible above the gum line, 428, 430
Cry/o, 624, 831, 946
Cryosurgery (cry-oh-SER-jer-ee), **a noninvasive treatment that uses subfreezing temperature to freeze and destroy the tissue. Coolants such as liquid nitrogen are used in the metal probe, 91, 106, 115, 621, 633, 675, 683, 836, 846, 943, 949**
Crypt/o, 624, 757
Cryptorchidism (kript-OR-kid-izm), **condition of undescended testicle(s); the absence of one or both testicles from the scrotum, 627, 766**
CT scan, a collection of x-ray images taken from various angles following injection of a contrast medium, 156, 318, 366, 793–794, 806
abdomen (AB-doh-men), **computerized tomography a painless, noninvasive x-ray procedure that produces an image created by the computer representing a detailed cross section of the tissue structure within the abdomen, 450**
of the brain, computerized tomography is the analysis of a three-dimensional view of brain tissue obtained as x-ray beams pass through successive horizontal layers of the brain, 260
Culd/o, 720
Cul-de-sac (kull-dih-SAK), **a pouch that is located between the uterus and rectum within the peritoneal cavity, 661**
Culdocentesis (kull-doh-sen-TEE-sis), **needle aspiration, through the vagina, into the cul-de-sac area for the purpose of removing fluid from the area for examination or diagnosis, 683, 713, 725**
Cumulation (KYOO-mew-lay-shun), **means that a drug level begins to accumulate in the body with repeated doses because the drug is not completely excreted from the body before another dose is administered, 866, 873**
Curettage and electrodesiccation (koo-REH-tahz and ee-lek-troh-des-ih-KAY-shun), **this procedure is a combination of curettage, which involves scraping away abnormal tissue, followed by electrodesiccation, which involves destroying the tumor base with a low-voltage electrode, 91, 115**
Curettage (koo-REH-tazh), **the process of scraping material from the wall of a cavity or other surface for the purpose of removing abnormal tissue or unwanted material, 91, 106, 115, 943, 949**
Cushing's syndrome (CUSH-ings SIN-drom), **a condition of the adrenal gland in which there is a cluster of symptoms occurring as a result of an excessive amount of cortisol or ACTH circulating in the blood, 495–496**
Cusp, any one of the small flaps on the valves of the heart, 343
Cuspid tooth (CUSS-pid). *See* Canine tooth, 428, 430
Cutane/o, 99, 870
Cutaneous membrane (kew-TAY-nee-us), **the skin.** *See also* Integument, 85, 91
Cuticle (KEW-tikl), **a fold of skin that covers the root of the fingernail or toenail, 88, 91**
Cyan/o, 24, 26, 870
Cyanosis (sigh-ah-NO-sis), **slightly bluish, grayish, slatelike, or dark discoloration of the skin due to the presence of abnormal amounts of reduced hemoglobin in the blood, 91, 348, 392–393, 753, 768, 865**
Cycloplegia (sigh-kloh-PLEE-jee-ah), **paralysis of the ciliary muscle of the eye, 523**
Cyclothymia, 927

D

the terminal bronchiole, either from dilatation of the alveoli or from destruction of their walls, 398–399, 964

Empyema (em-pye-**EE**-mah), **pus in a body cavity, especially in the pleural cavity (pyothorax); usually the result of a primary infection in the lungs, 399**

Emulsify (eh-**MULL**-sih-figh), **to disperse a liquid into another liquid, making a colloidal suspension, 426, 431**

En bloc resection, 846

Enamel (en-**AM**-el), **a hard, white substance that covers the dentin of the crown of a tooth; enamel is the hardest substance in the body, 428, 431**

Encapsulated (en-**CAP**-soo-**LAY**-ted), **enclosed in fibrous or membranous sheats, 828, 832**

Encephal/o, 238

Encephalitis (en-**seff**-ah-**LYE**-tis), **inflammation of the brain or spinal cord tissue largely caused by viruses, 245**

Encephalography, 267

Endo-, 23, 27, 347, 664

Endocarditis (**en**-doh-car-**DYE**-tis), **inflammation of the membrane lining the valves and chambers of the heart caused by direct invasion of bacteria or other organisms and leading to deformity of the valve cusps. Abnormal growth called vegetations are formed on or within the membrane, 343, 354**

Endocardium (en-doh-**CAR**-dee-um), **within the heart, the lining of the heart, 7, 335**

Endocrine gland (**EN**-doh-krin), **a ductless gland that produces a hormone, which is secreted directly into the bloodstream via the capillaries instead of being transported through the body through ducts, 427, 431, 483**

Endocrine system, 473
 anatomy/physiology of, 473–481
 diagnostic techniques, 500–501
 pathological conditions, 490–499

Endocrinologist (en-doh-krin-**ALL**-oh-jist), **a physician who specializes in the medical practice of treating the diseases and disorders of the endocrine system, 483**

Endocrinology (en-doh-krin-**ALL**-oh-jee), **the field of medicine that deals with the study of the endocrine system and of the treatment of the diseases and disorders of the endocrine system, 483**

Endolymph, 545

Endometrial biopsy (en-doh-**MEE**-tree-al **BYE**-op-see), **an invasive test for obtaining a sample of endometrial tissue with a small curet, for examination, 684**

Endometrial carcinoma, malignant tumor of the inner lining of the uterus, 675–676, 838

Endometriosis (**en**-doh-**mee**-tree-**OH**-sis), **the presence and growth of endometrial tissue in the areas outside the endometrium, 676–677**

Endometrium (en-doh-**MEE**-tree-um), **the inner lining of the uterus, 656, 661, 714**

Endoscopic retrograde cholangiopancreatography (ERCP) (en-doh-**SKOP**-ic **RET**-roh-grayd koh-**lan**-jee-oh-**pan**-kree-ah-**TOG**-rah-fee), **a procedure that examines the size of and the filling of the pancreatic and biliary ducts through direct radiographic visualization with a fiberoptic endoscope, 450–451, 792**

Enter/o, 436

Enteritis, 458

Entropion (en-**TROH**-pee-on), **"turning in" of the eyelash margins resulting in the sensation similar to that of a foreign body in the eye, 523, 533, 944, 970–971**

Enuresis (in-yoo-**REE**-sis), **a condition of urinary incontinence, especially in bed at night; bedwetting, 588**

Enzyme (**EN**-zime), **an organic substance that initiates and accelerates a chemical reaction, 289, 422–423, 431**

Eosin/o, 24, 27, 293

Eosinophil (**ee**-oh-**SIN**-oh-fill), **a granulocytic, bilobed leukocyte somewhat larger than a neutrophil characterized by large numbers of coarse, refractile, cytoplasmic granules that stain with the acid dye, eosin, 285, 289**

Ependymomas, 251, 844

Epi-, 23, 27, 70, 527, 757, 831

Epicardium (**ep**-ih-**CARD**-ee-um), **the inner layer of the pericardium, which is the double-faced membrane that encloses the heart, 335, 343**

Epidermis, anatomy/physiology, 85–86

Epidermis (ep-ih-**DER**-mis), **the outermost layer of the skin, 92**

Epidermoid carcinoma, 848

Epidermoid cyst (ep-ih-**DER**-moid). *See* sebaceous cyst

Epididym/o, 624

Epididymectomy (**ep**-ih-**DID**-ih-**MEK**-toh-mee), **surgical removal of the epididymis, 621**

Epididymis (**ep**-ih-**DID**-ih-mis), **a tightly coiled tubule that resembles a comma, 619, 620**

Epididymitis (**ep**-ih-**did**-ih-**MY**-tis), **inflammation of the epididymis, 621**

Epidural space (**ep**-ih-**DOO**-ral space), **the space immediately outside of the dura mater that contains a supporting cushion of fat and other connective tissues, 225, 232**

Epigastric, 57, 66

Epigastric region (**ep**-ih-**GAS**-trik **REE**-jun), **the region of the abdomen located between the right and left hypochondriac regions in the upper section of the abdomen, beneath the cartilage or the ribs, 57, 66**

Epiglott/o, 390

Epiglottis (**ep**-ih-**GLOT**-iss), **a thin, leaf-shaped structure located immediately posterior to the root of the tongue; covers the entrance of the larynx when the individual swallows, 384, 388**

Epilepsy (**EP**-ih-**lep**-see), **a syndrome of recurring episodes of excessive irregular electrical activity of the central nervous system called seizures, 232, 245**

Epinephrine (ep-ih-**NEF**-rin), **a hormone produced by the adrenal medulla, 478–479, 483**

Epiphyseal, 133

Epiphyseal line (**ep**-ih-**FIZZ**-e-al), **a layer of cartilage that separates the diaphysis from the epiphysis of a bone, 133, 149**

Epiphysis, the end of a bone, 132–133, 149

Episcleritis (ep-ih-skleh-**RYE**-tis), **inflammation of the outermost layers of the sclera, 523**

Episi/o, 720

Episiotomy (eh-**peez**-ee-**OT**-oh-mee), **a surgical procedure in which an incision is made into the woman's perineum to enlarge the vaginal opening for delivery of the baby, 714**

Epispadias (**ep**-ih-**SPAY**-dee-as), **a congenital defect in which the urethra opens on the upper side of the penis at some point near the glans, 628, 767**

Epistaxis (ep-ih-**STAKS**-is), **hemorrhage from the nose; nosebleed, 393**

Epithelial tissue (**ep**-ih-**THEE**-lee-al **TISH**-oo), **the tissue that covers the internal and external organs of the body; it also lines the vessels, body cavities, glands, and body organs, 54, 66**

Epithelium (ep-ih-**THEE**-lee-um), **the tissue that covers the internal and external surfaces of the body, 93, 97**

G

H

I

J

K

M

Microcephalus (**my**-kroh-**SEFF**-ah-lus), **a congenital anomaly characterized by abnormal smallness of the head in relation to the rest of the body and by underdevelopment of the brain, resulting in some degree of mental retardation, 755**
Microglia (my-**KROG**-lee-ah), **small, neuroglial cells found in the interstitial tissue of the nervous system that engulf cellular debris, waste products, and pathogens within the nerve tissue, 224–225, 233**
Micturition, the act of eliminating urine from the bladder, 578, 581
Midbrain, the uppermost part of the brain stem, 228, 233
Middle ear, 545
Middle-old, a term used to describe an individual between the ages of 75 and 84 years, 945
Midline of the body, the imaginary "line" that is created when the body is divided into equal right and left halves, 67
Midsagittal plane (mid-**SAJ**-ih-al), **the plane that divides the body or a structure into right and left equal portions, 55, 67**
Midstream specimen, 603
Migraine headache (**MY**-grain headache), **a recurring, pulsating, vascular headache usually developing on one side of the head; characterized by a slow onset that may be preceded by an "aura" during which a sensory disturbance occurs, such as confusion or some visual interference, 247**
Milli-, one-thousandth, 21, 28
Mineralocorticoids, 478
Minnesota multiphasic personality inventory (MMPI) (mull-tih-**FAYZ**-ic), **a self-report personality inventory test that consists of 567 items that can be answered "true", "false", or "cannot say." The items vary widely in content and are sometimes repeated in various ways throughout the test, 924**
Miosis (my-**OH**-sis), **abnormal constriction of the pupil of the eye, 525**
Miotic (my-**OT**-ik), **an agent that causes the pupil of the eye to constrict, 525**
Mitochondria (my-toh-**KOH**-dree-ah), **cell organs, or organelles, which provide the energy needed by the cell to carry on its essential functions, 52, 67**
Mitosis (my-**TOH**-sis), **a type of cell division that results in the formation of two genetically identical daughter cells, 829**
Mitral valve, 338
Mitral valve prolapse (**my**-tral valve proh-**LAPS**), **drooping of one or both cusps of the mitral valve back into the left atrium during ventricular systole, resulting in complete closure of the valve and mitral insufficiency, 356**
Mitrochondria, 52, 67
Mixed cerebral palsy, 243
Mixed-tissue tumor (mixed-tissue **TOO**-mor), **a growth composed of more than one kind of neoplastic tissue, 829**
Modality (moh-**DAL**-ih-tee), **a method of application i.e., a treatment method, 829**
Moist gangrene, 108
Molar tooth (**MOH**-lar), **any one of 12 molar teeth, 6 in each dental arch, located posterior to the premolar teeth; the molar teeth have a flat surface with multiple projections (cusps) for crushing and grinding food, 433**
Mole (**MOHL**). *See* Nevus
Mon/o, 311
Mono-, 21, 28, 294
Monochromatism, 530
Monocyte (**MON**-oh-sight), **a large mononuclear leukocyte, 286, 291**
Monocytopenia, 322
Mononucleosis (mon-oh-**noo**-klee-**OH**-sis), **usually caused by the Epstein-Barr virus (EBV); typically a benign, self-limiting acute infection of the B lymphocytes, 316–317**
Mons pubis, 654
Montgomery's glands, 657
Montgomery's tubercles, 657
Mood disorders, an affective state characterized by any of a variety of periods of depression or depression and elation, 901, 911–912
Morbidity (mor-**BID**-ih-tee), **an illness or an abnormal condition or quality, 829**
Morph/o, 294
Morphology, 322
Motility (moh-**TILL**-ih-tee), **the ability to move spontaneously, 620, 622**
Motor dysfunction, 254, 959
Motor nerves (**MOH**-tor nerves). *See* Efferent nerves
Movements of joints, 194–196
MRI. *See* Magnetic resonance imaging
MRI of the brain, 262
MSH (melanocyte-stimulating hormone), 475
Mucoid, 392
Mucopurulent (mew-koh-**PEWR**-yoo-lent), **characteristic of a combination of mucus and pus, 392, 622, 632**
Multi-, 22, 28, 720
Multigravida (**mull**-tih-**GRAV**-ih-dah), **a woman who has been pregnant more than once, 716**
Multipara (**mull**-**TIP**-ah-rah), **a woman who has been pregnant more than one time, 717**
Multiple myeloma (plasma cell myeloma) (**MULL**-tih-pl my-eh-**LOH**-mah), **a malignant plasma cell neoplasm causing an increase in the number of both mature and immature plasma cells, which often entirely replace the bone marrow and destroy the skeletal structure, 298**
Multiple sclerosis (MS) (**MULL**-tih-pl **SKLEH**-roh-sis), **a degenerative inflammatory disease of the central nervous system attacking the myelin sheath in the spinal cord and brain, leaving it sclerosed (hardened) or scarred, 252–253**
Mumps, acute viral disease characterized by fever and by swelling and tenderness of one or more salivary glands, usually the parotid glands, 762–763
Munchausen syndrome (by proxy) (mun-**CHOW**-zen **SIN**-drom), **a somewhat rare form of child abuse in which a parent of a child falsifies an illness in a child by fabricating or creating the symptoms, and then seeks medical care for the child, 915–916**
Munro's point (mun-**ROHZ**), **a point on the left side of the abdomen, about halfway between the umbilicus and the anterior bony prominence of the hip, 58, 68**
Murmur, a low-pitched humming or fluttering sound, as in a "heart murmur," heard on auscultation, 344
Muscle, tissue composed of fibers or cells that are able to contract, causing movement of body parts and organs, 180
Muscle biopsy (muscle **BYE**-op-see), **extraction of a specimen of muscle tissue, through either a biopsy needle or an incisional biopsy, for the purpose of examining it under a microscope, 189, 191**
Muscle fibers, the name given to the individual muscle cell, 181, 187
Muscle tissue, the tissue that is capable of producing movement of the parts and organs of the body by contracting and relaxing its fibers, 54, 68

N

O

Psychosis (sigh-**KOH**-sis), **any major mental disorder of organic or emotional origin characterized by a loss of contact with reality, 903**
Psychosomatic (**sigh**-koh-soh-**MAT**-ik), **pertaining to the expression of an emotional conflict through physical symptoms, 903**
Psychotherapy (sigh-koh-**THAIR**-ah-pee), **any of a large number of related methods of treating mental and emotional disorders using psychological techniques instead of physical means of treatment, 903**
Pterygium (ter-**IJ**-ee-um), **an irregular growth developing as a fold in the bulbar conjunctiva on the nasal side of the cornea that can disrupt vision if it extends over the pupil, 538**
-ptosis, 45, 529
Pub/o, 153
Puberty (**PEW**-ber-tee), **the period of life at which the ability to reproduce begins; that is, in the female, it is the period when the female reproductive organs are fully developed, 654, 659–661, 664, 718**
Pubic, pertaining to the region of the symphysis pubis of the pelvis, 146
Pudendum, 654
Pulmon/o, 391, 947
Pulmonary arteries (**PULL**-mon-air-ree artery), **one of a pair of arteries that transports deoxygenated blood from the right ventricle of the heart to the lungs for oxygenation, 337, 345**
Pulmonary circulation (**PULL**-mon-air-ree), **the circulation of deoxygenated blood from the right ventricle of the heart to the lungs for oxygenation, 337, 345**
Pulmonary edema (**PULL**-mon-air-ree eh-**DEE**-mah), **swelling of the lungs caused by an abnormal accumulation of fluid in the lungs, either in the alveoli or the interstitial spaces, 401, 964**
Pulmonary embolism (**PULL**-mon-air-ree **EM**-boh-lizm), **the obstruction of one or more pulmonary arteries by a thrombus (clot) that dislodges from another location, and is carried through the venous system to the vessels of the lung, 401**
Pulmonary function tests, a variety of tests to assess respiratory function, 405
Pulmonary heart disease (cor pulmonale) (**PULL**-mon-air-ree heart dih-**ZEEZ, COR** pull-mon-**ALL**-ee), **hypertrophy of the right ventricle of the heart (with or without failure) resulting from disorders of the lungs, pulmonary vessels, or chest wall; heart failure resulting from pulmonary disease, 401, 964–965**
Pulmonary parenchyma (**PULL**-mon-air-ee par-**EN**-kih-mah), **the functional units of the lungs; for example, the alveoli, which have very thin walls that allow for the exchange of gases between the lungs and the blood, 385, 390**
Pulmonary valve, 337
Pulmonary vein (**PULL**-mon-air-ree vein), **one of four large veins that return oxygenated blood from the lungs back to the left atrium of the heart, 337, 345**
Pulp, any soft, spongy tissue, such as that contained within the spleen, the pulp chamber of the tooth, or the distal phalanges of the fingers and the toes, 433
Punch biopsy, 117
Pupil, 518, 520
Pupill/o, 529
Pupillary (**PEW**-pih-lair-ee), **pertaining to the pupil of the eye, 526**
Purging (**PERJ**-ing), **the means of ridding the body of what has been consumed by inducing vomiting or using laxatives, 903, 919**
Purkinje fibers, 340
Purpur/o, 25, 28
Purpura (**PER**-pew-rah), **a group of bleeding disorders characterized by bleeding into the skin and mucous membranes; small, pinpoint hemorrhages are known as petechia and larger hemorrhagic areas are known as ecchymoses or bruises, 97, 299, 961**
Purulent (**PEWR**-yoo-lent), **containing pus, 156, 392, 548, 622, 634**
Pustule (**PUS**-tool), **a small elevation of the skin filled with pus; a small abscess, 97, 103**
Py/o, 585
Pyel/o, 584, 811
Pyelitis (pye-eh-**LYE**-tis), **inflammation of the renal pelvis, 582**
Pyelography (pie-eh-**LOG**-rah-fee), **a technique in radiology for examining the structures and evaluating the function of the urinary system, 798, 808**
Pyelonephritis (acute) (pye-eh-loh-neh-**FRYT**-tis), **a bacterial infection of the renal pelvis of the kidney, 592**
Pyloric sphincter (pigh-**LOR**-ik **SFINGK**-ter), **a thickened muscular ring in the stomach that regulates the passage of food from the pylorus of the stomach into the duodenum, 433**
Pylorus, 423
Pyr/o, 758
Pyrexia (pie-**REK**-see-ah), **fever, 756**
Pyrosis (pye-**ROH**-sis), **heartburn; indigestion, 718, 722**
during pregnancy, 722
Pyuria (pye-**YOO**-ree-ah), **the presence of pus in the urine, usually a sign of an infection of the urinary tract, 585, 589**

Q

Quadri-, 22, 28
Quadriceps femoris muscle (**KWAHD**-rih-seps **FEM**-or-iss), 186
Quadriplegia (**KWOD**-rih-**PLEE**-jee-ah), **follows severe trauma to the spinal cord between the fifth and eighth cervical vertebrae, generally resulting in loss of motor and sensory function below the level of the injury, 236, 257–258**
Quickening (**KWIK**-en-ing), **the first feeling of movement of the fetus felt by the expectant mother, 709, 718**

R

Rach/i, 153
Rachitis, inflammation of the spine; also known as rickets, 153
Rad, abbreviation for radiation absorbed dose; the basic unit of absorbed dose of ionizing radiation, 808
Radi/o, 154, 811, 832
Radial, pertaining to the radius, 153
Radiation (ray-dee-**AY**-shun), **the emission of energy, rays, or waves, 156, 828, 830**
Radiation therapy (ray-dee-**AY**-shun **THAIR**-ah-pee), **the delivery of ionizing radiation to accomplish one or more of the following: destruction of tumor cells; reduction of tumor size; decrease in pain; relief of obstruction; slowing or stopping the spread of cancer cells, 799–800, 808, 836, 845–846**
Radiculotomy (rah-dick-you-**LOT**-oh-mee). *See* Rhizotomy
Radioactive iodine uptake (RAIU) test (ray-dee-o-**AK**-tiv **EYE**-oh-dine **UP**-tayk), **a thyroid function test that evaluates the function of the**

thyroid gland by administering a known amount of radioactive iodine and later placing a gamma ray detector over the thyroid gland to determine the percentage or quantity of radioactive iodine absorbed by the gland over specific time periods, 493, 500, 800

Radioactivity (ray-dee-oh-ak-TIV-ih-tee), **the ability of a substance to emit rays or particles (alpha, beta, or gamma) from its nucleus, 808**

Radiocurable tumor (ray-dee-oh-KYOOR-oh-bl TOO-mur), **pertaining to the susceptibility of tumor cells to destruction by ionizing radiation, 830, 846**

Radiographer (ray-dee-OG-rah-fer), **an allied health professional trained to use x-ray machines and other imaging equipment to produce images of the internal structures of the body; also known as a radiologic technologist, 788, 808**

Radioimmunoassay (ray-dee-oh-im-yoo-noh-ASS-ay), **a technique in radiology used to determine the concentration of an antigen, antibody, or other protein in the serum, 808**

Radioisotope (ray-dee-oh-EYE-soh-tohp), **a radioactive isotope of an element, used for therapeutic and diagnostic purposes, 808**

Radiologic technologist, 788

Radiologist (ray-dee-ALL-oh-jist), **a physician who specializes in radiology, 788, 808**

Radiology (ray-dee-ALL-oh-jee), **the study of the diagnostic and therapeutic uses of x-rays; also known as roentgenology, 788, 808**

Radiolucent (ray-dee-oh-LOO-sent), **pertaining to materials that allow x-rays to penetrate with a minimum of absorption, 808**

Radionuclide (radioisotope) (ray-dee-oh-NOO-kleed) (ray-dee-oh-EYE-soh-tohp), **an isotope (or nuclide) that undergoes radioactive decay, 808**

Radiopaque (ray-dee-oh-PAYK), **not permitting the passage of x-rays or other radiant energy; appears white on an exposed x-ray film, 582, 600, 794, 808**

Radiopharmaceutical (ray-dee-oh-farm-ah-soo-tih-kal), **a drug that contains radioactive atoms, 808**

Radioresistant tumor (ray-dee-oh-ree-SIS-tant TOO-mur), **a tumor that resists the effects of radiation, 830, 846**

Radioresponsive tumor (ray-dee-oh-ree-SPON-siv TOO-mor), **a tumor that reacts favorably to radiation, 830**

Radiosensitive tumor (ray-dee-oh-SEN-sih-tiv TOO-mur), **a tumor that reacts favorably to radiation, 830**

Radiotherapy (ray-dee-oh-THAIR-ah-pee), **the treatment of disease by using x-rays or gamma rays, 828, 830**

Radius (RAY-dee-us), **one of the two lower arm bones that joins the humerus to the wrist bones, 145**

Rales (ralz), **an abnormal sound heard on auscultation of the chest, produced by passage of air through bronchi that contain secretion or exudate or that are constricted by spasm or a thickening of their walls, 394**

Random specimen, 603

Rationalization (rash-un-al-ih-ZAY-shun), **attempting to make excuses or invent logical reasons to justify unacceptable feelings or behavior, 897, 903**

Raynaud's phenomenon (ray-NOZ), **intermittent attacks of vasoconstriction of the arterioles, causing pallor of the fingers or toes, followed by cyanosis, then redness, before returning to normal color, 360**

RBC count, 301, 303

RBC indices, 301

Receptor (ree-SEP-tor), **a sensory nerve ending, 236**

Recipient, 287

Rect/o, 437, 871

Rectal medication (REK-tal), **medication that is inserted into the rectum and is slowly absorbed into the mucous membrane lining of the rectum. It is in the form of a suppository, which melts as the body temperature warms it, 868**

Rectal temperature, temperature as measured in the rectum, 756

Rectocele, 437

Rectoscope (REK-toh-skohp), **an instrument used to view the rectum that has a cutting and cauterizing loop, 623**

Rectum (REK-tum), **the portion of the large intestine, about 12 cm long, continuous with the descending sigmoid colon, just proximal to the anal canal, 425, 434**

Recumbent (rih-KUM-bent), **lying down or leaning backward, 750, 756, 809**

Red blood cell count (RBC), the measurement of the circulating number of RBCs in one cubic millimeter of peripheral blood, 301, 303

Red blood cell morphology (mor-FALL-oh-jee), **an examination of the RBC on a stained blood smear that enables the examiner to identify the form and shape of the RBCs, 303**

Red bone marrow, soft, semifluid substance located in the small spaces of cancellous bone that is the source of blood cell production, 134, 150

Red measles, acute, highly communicable viral disease that begins as an upper respiratory disorder with fever, sore throat, cough, runny nose, sensitivity to light, and possible conjunctivitis, 764

Refraction, 521

Regression (rih-GRESH-un), **a response to stress in which the individual reverts to an earlier level of development and the comfort measure associated with that level of functioning, 897, 903**

Relapse (ree-LAPS), **to exhibit again the symptoms of a disease from which a patient appears to have recovered, 830**

Remission (rih-MISH-un), **the partial or complete disappearance of the symptoms of a chronic or malignant disease, 830**

Ren/o, 585, 811

Renal angiography (REE-nal an-jee-OG-rah-fee), **x-ray visualization of the internal anatomy of the renal blood vessels after injection of a contrast medium, 600–601, 790**

Renal artery (REE-nal AR-ter-ree), **one of a pair of large arteries branching from the abdominal aorta that supplies blood to the kidneys, adrenal glands, and the ureters, 577, 582**

Renal calculi, stone formations in the kidney, 582, 592

Renal calculus, a stone formation in the kidney (plural: renal calculi); also called a nephrolith, 582, 592

Renal capsule, 574

Renal cell carcinoma (REE-nal SELL car-sin-OH-mah), **a malignant tumor of the kidney occurring in adulthood, 592, 842**

Renal failure, chronic (REE-nal FAIL-yoor KRON-ik) **(uremia), progressively slow development of kidney failure occurring over a period of years. The late stages of chronic renal failure are known as end-stage renal disease (ESRD), 592–593**

Renal pelvis (REE-nal PELL-vis), **the central collecting part of the kidney that narrows into the large upper end of the ureter; it receives urine**

T

U

V

W

X

Y

Z

Getting Started with Comprehensive Medical Terminology, Second Edition Activity CD-ROM

Setup Instructions

1. Double click my Computer.
2. Double click the Control panel icon.
3. Double click Add/Remove Programs.
4. Click the Install button and follow the on-screen prompts from there.

System Requirements

- Microsoft® Windows® 95 or better
- Pentium or faster processor
- 24 MB or more of RAM
- Double-spin CD-ROM drive
- 10 MB or more free hard drive space